Orthopaedic Surgery
The Essentials

Orthopaedic Surgery
The Essentials

Edited by

Mark E. Baratz, MD
Vice Chairman of Research and Academic Affairs
Department of Orthopaedic Surgery
Allegheny University of the Health Sciences
Allegheny General Hospital
Pittsburgh, Pennsylvania

Anthony D. Watson, MD
Director of Clinical Research
Clinical Instructor
Department of Orthopaedic Surgery
Allegheny University of the Health Sciences
Allegheny General Hospital
Pittsburgh, Pennsylvania

Joseph E. Imbriglia, MD
Director, Division of Hand and Upper Extremity Surgery
Department of Orthopaedic Surgery
Allegheny University of the Health Sciences
Allegheny General Hospital
Pittsburgh, Pennsylvania

Assistant Editor

Jodi Lyn Fowler, MS
Clinical Research Associate
Department of Orthopaedic Surgery
Allegheny University of the Health Sciences
Allegheny General Hospital
Pittsburgh, Pennsylvania

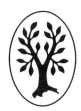

1999
Thieme
New York • Stuttgart

Thieme New York
333 Seventh Avenue
New York, NY 10001

Executive Editor: Jane E. Pennington, Ph. D.
Editorial Director: Avé McCracken
Assistant Editor: Jinnie Kim
Developmental Editor: Regina C. Paleski
Director, Production & Manufacturing: Maxine Langweil
Production Editor: Janice G. Stangel
Marketing Director: Phyllis Gold
Sales Manager: David Bertelsen
Chief Financial Officer: Seth S. Fishman
President: Brian D. Scanlan
Medical Illustrator: Anthony Pazos
Cover Designer: Jeanette Jacobs
Designer: Jose Fonfrias
Compositor: Prepare
Printer: Maple-Vail Book Manufacturing Group

Library of Congress Cataloging-in-Publication Data

Orthopaedic surgery: the essentials / editors, Mark E. Baratz,
    Anthony D. Watson, Joseph E. Imbriglia; assistant editor, Jodi Lyn
    Fowler.
        p.   cm.
    Includes bibliographical references and index.
    ISBN 0-86577-779-9 (TMP). -- ISBN 3-13-116291-0 (GTV)
    1. Orthopedic surgery.   I. Baratz, Mark.   II. Watson, Anthony D.
III. Imbriglia, Joseph E.
    [DNLM: 1. Orthopedics.   2. Orthopedic Procedures. WE 168 076274
1999]
    RD731.O775   1999
    617.4'7--dc21
    DNLM/DLC
    for Library of Congress   98-45052
                                                                    CIP

Important note: Medical knowledge is ever-changing. As new research and clinical experience broaden our knowledge, changes
in treatment and drug therapy may be required. The authors and editors of the material herein have consulted sources believed
to be reliable in their efforts to provide information that is complete and in accord with the standards accepted at the time of publication. However, in view of the possibility of human error by the authors, editors, or publisher of the work herein, or changes
in medical knowledge, neither the authors, editors, publisher, nor any other party who has been involved in the preparation of
this work, warrants that the information contained herein is in every respect accurate or complete, and they are not responsible
for any errors or omissions or for the results obtained from use of such information. Readers are encouraged to confirm the information contained herein with other sources. For example, readers are advised to check the product information sheet included in
the package of each drug they plan to administer to be certain that the information contained in this publication is accurate and
that changes have not been made in the recommended dose or in the contraindications for administration. This recommendation
is of particular importance in connection with new or infrequently used drugs.

Some of the product names, patents, and registered designs referred to in this book are in fact registered trademarks or
proprietary names even though specific reference to this fact is not always made in the text. Therefore, the appearance of a name
without designation as proprietary is not to be construed as a representation by the publisher that it is in the public domain.

Printed in the United States of America
Compositor: Prepare   Printer: Maple-Vail Book Manufacturing Group

5   4   3   2   1

TNY ISBN 0-86577-779-9

GTV ISBN 3-13-116291-0

To Arlene.
In Memory of Morton S. Baratz, PhD (1924-1998).

Contents

Section I. Basic Science

Section II. Diagnostic Studies

Section III. Trauma

Section IV. Soft Tissue Coverage

Section V. Spine

Section VI. Shoulder

Section VII. Elbow

Section VIII. Wrist/Hand

Section IX. Pelvis, Hip, and Femur

Section X. Knee and Leg

Section XVIII. Ethics

Section XIX. Economic, Legal, and Political Issues in Orthopaedics

Contributors

Donald D. Anderson, BSE, MS, PhD
Director
Biomechanics Laboratory
Minneapolis Sports Medicine Center
Minneapolis, Minnesota

Rey Aponte, PA-C
Divisions of Plastic and Orthopaedic Surgery
Duke University Medical Center
Durham, North Carolina

Julian S. Arroyo, MD
Lakewood Orthopaedic Surgeons, PS
Tacoma, Washington

Mark E. Baratz, MD
Vice Chairman of Research and
  Academic Affairs
Department of Orthopaedic Surgery
Allegheny University of the Health Sciences
Allegheny General Hospital
Pittsburgh, Pennsylvania

John M. Bednar, MD
Assistant Professor
Department of Orthopaedic Surgery
Thomas Jefferson University School of Medicine
The Philadelphia Hand Center
Philadelphia, Pennsylvania

Don C. Beringer, MD
Department of Orthopaedic Surgery
University of Florida
Gainesville, Florida

Louis U. Bigliani, MD
Chairman
Chief, The Shoulder Service
Department of Orthopaedic Surgery
New York Orthopaedic Hospital
Professor of Orthopaedic Surgery
College of Physicians and Surgeons
Columbia-Presbyterian Medical Center
New York, New York

Betsy W. Blazek-O'Neill, MD
Department of Occupational Medicine
Allegheny University of the Health Sciences
Allegheny General Hospital
Pittsburgh, Pennsylvania

Fredrick W. Bode, III, JD
Shareholder/Director
Dickie, McCamey & Chilcote
Pittsburgh, Pennsylvania

Heather Brien, MD, FRCSC
Clinical Fellow
Department of Orthopaedic Surgery
Hand and Upper Limb Centre
University of Western Ontario
London, Ontario
CANADA

Joseph A. Buckwalter, MS, MD
Professor
Department of Orthopaedic Surgery
University of Iowa Hospitals
Iowa City, Iowa

John T. Campbell, MD
Instructor
Department of Surgery
Uniformed Services University of the Health Sciences
Bethesda, Maryland

Paul S. Cederna, MD
Section of Plastic Surgery
University of Michigan Medical Center
Ann Arbor, Michigan

Hugh P. Chandler, MD
Department of Orthopaedic Surgery
Massachusetts General Hospital
Harvard Medical School
Boston, Massachusetts

John Clifford, MD
Department of Orthopaedics
Kaiser Santa Theresa
San Jose, California

Brian J. Cole, MD, MBA
Assistant Professor
Section of Sports Medicine
Rush Presbyterian-St. Luke's Medical Center
Chicago, Illinois

Richard H. Daffner, MD, FACR
Professor of Radiologic Sciences
Chief of the Division of Musculoskeletal and
*   Emergency Radiology*
Department of Diagnostic Radiology
Allegheny University of the Health Sciences
Allegheny General Hospital
Pittsburgh, Pennsylvania

Gregory G. Degnan, MD
Assistant Professor
Department of Orthopedic Surgery
University of Virginia Health Sciences Center
Charlottesville, Virginia

Thomas T. Dovan, MD
Department of Orthopaedic Surgery
Vanderbilt University
Nashville, Tennessee

Michael T. Dye, MD
Department of Orthopaedic Surgery
Allegheny University of the Health Sciences
Allegheny General Hospital
Pittsburgh, Pennsylvania

Neal S. ElAttrache, MD
Associate and Fellowship Instructor
Department of Sports Medicine
Kerlan-Jobe Orthopaedic Clinic
Los Angeles, California

Lucio S. Ernlund, MD
Department of Orthopaedic Surgery
Curtiba, Paranam
BRAZIL

Christopher H. Evans, PhD, DSc
Henry J. Mankin Professor of Orthopaedic Surgery
Department of Orthopaedic Surgery and
*   Molecular Genetics and Biochemistry;*
Director
Ferguson Laboratory
University of Pittsburgh Medical Center
Pittsburgh, Pennsylvania

Joseph M. Failla, MD
William Clay Ford Center for Athletic Medicine
Detroit, Michigan

Evan L. Flatow, MD
Associate Chief
The Shoulder Service
New York Orthopaedic Hospital;
Professor of Orthopaedic Surgery
College of Physicians and Surgeons
Columbia-Presbyterian Medical Center
New York, New York

Guy Foucher MD
Department of Hand Surgery
Chiurgie de la Main et Microchirugie
Strasbourg
FRANCE

Freddie H. Fu, MD
Professor of Orthopaedics
Chairman
Department of Orthopaedic Surgery
Center for Sports Medicine
University of Pittsburgh
Pittsburgh, Pennsylvania

Mark A. Fye, MD
Clinical Instructor
Department of Orthopaedic Surgery
Allegheny University of the Health Sciences
Allegheny General Hospital
Pittsburgh, Pennsylvania

Lars Gilbertson, PhD
Assistant Professor
Department of Orthopedic Surgery
University of Pittsburgh School of Medicine
Pittsburgh, Pennsylvania

Samuel Goldblatt, JD
Buffalo, New York

Joseph E. Hale, PhD
Research Engineer
Biomechanics Laboratory
Minneapolis Sports Medicine Center
Minneapolis, Minnesota

Suzanne E. Hall, MD
Fellow in Shoulder Service
Department of Orthopaedic Surgery
Hospital for Joint Diseases New York University
New York, New York

B. David Horn, MD
Assistant Professor
Department of Orthopaedic Surgery
St. Christopher's Hospital for Children
Philadelphia, Pennsylvania

Robert Hube, MD
Martin Luther University
Halle Wittenberg
GERMANY

David Hungerford, MD
Department of Orthopaedic Surgery
Johns Hopkins University
Baltimore, Maryland

Joseph P. Iannotti, MD, PhD
Professor of Orthopaedic Surgery
Department of Orthopaedic Surgery
Penn Musculoskeletal Institute
Hospital University of Pennsylvania
Philadelphia, Pennsylvania

Joseph E. Imbriglia, MD
Director, Division of Hand and Upper
  Extremity Surgery
Department of Orthopaedic Surgery
Allegheny University of the Health Sciences
Allegheny General Hospital
Pittsburgh, Pennsylvania

Bruce Jacobs, OT
Allegheny University of the Health Sciences
Allegheny General Hospital
Pittsburgh, Pennsylvania

Matthew L. Jimenez, MD
Illinois Bone & Joint Institute
Lutheran General Hospital;
Clinical Instructor
Department of Orthopaedic Surgery
University of Chicago;
Clinical Associate Professor
Finch University of Health Sciences
The Chicago School of Medicine
Chicago, Illinois

James D. Kang, MD
Assistant Professor
Department of Orthopedic Surgery
University of Pittsburgh School of Medicine
Pittsburgh, Pennsylvania

Morton L. Kasdan, MD
Clinical Professor
Department of Preventive Medicine and
  Environmental Health
University of Kentucky
Clinical Professor
Department of Plastic Surgery
University of Louisville
Louisville, Kentucky

Douglas K. Kehl, MD
Associate Clinical Professor
Department of Orthopaedic Surgery
Emory University School of Medicine
Scottish Rite Children's Medical Center
Atlanta, Georgia

Ario B. Keyarash, MD
Department of Orthopaedic Surgery
Allegheny University of the Health Sciences
Allegheny General Hospital
Pittsburgh, Pennsylvania

Graham J.W. King, MD, MSc, FRCSC
Associate Professor
Department of Orthopaedic Surgery
Hand and Upper Limb Centre
University of Western Ontario
London, Ontario
CANADA

Scott H. Kozin, MD
Assistant Professor
Department of Orthopaedic Surgery
Temple University School of Medicine;
Attending Hand Surgeon
Shriner's Hospital for Children
Philadelphia, Pennsylvania

Richard Lackman, MD
Department of Orthopaedic Surgery
Allegheny University of the Health Sciences
Hahnemann School of Medicine
Philadelphia, Pennsylvania

Joseph M. Lane, MD
Professor and Assistant Dean
Department of Orthopaedic Surgery
Cornell University Medical College
Hospital for Special Surgery
New York, New York

Jon P. Leimkuehler, CPO
Union Orthotics and Prosthetics
Pittsburgh, Pennsylvania

L. Scott Levin, MD
Chief
Division of Plastic, Reconstructive,
  & Maxillofacial Surgery
Associate Professor
Orthopaedic & Plastic Surgery
Duke University Medical Center
Durham, North Carolina

Norbert J. Lindner, MD
Klinikym Und Polikinik
Fur Allgemeine Orthopadie
Albert-Schweitzer, Munster

Mark R. LoDico, MD
Allegheny University of the Health Sciences
Allegheny General Hospital
Pittsburgh, Pennsylvania

Dean S. Louis, MD
Chairman
Chief of Hand Surgery
Department of Orthopaedic Surgery
University of Michigan
Ann Arbor, Michigan

Susan E. Mackinnon, MD
Shoenberg Professor and Chief
Division of Plastic and Reconstructive Surgery
Department of Surgery
Washington University School of Medicine
St. Louis, Missouri

Peter G. Mangone, MD
Foot and Ankle Surgery
Center for Orthopaedic Care
The Christ Hospital
Cincinnati, Ohio

Stanley Marczyk, MD
Atlantic Shore Orthopaedics Assoc.
Northfield, New Jersey

Gregory A. Mencio, MD
Associate Professor
Department of Orthopaedics and Rehabilitation
Vanderbilt University Medical Center
Nashville, Tennessee

Mark S. Meyer, MD
Department of Orthopaedic Surgery
University of Florida
Gainesville, Florida

Michael A. Miranda, MD
Assistant Clinical Professor of Medicine
Department of Orthopedics
University of Connecticut
Hartford Hospital
Hartford, Connecticut

Richard S. Moore, Jr., MD
Hand & Microvascular Surgery
Division of Orthopaedic Surgery
Duke University Medical Center
Durham, North Carolina

Thomas Mutschler, MD, MS
Department of Orthopaedic Surgery
Allegheny University of the Health Sciences
Allegheny General Hospital
Pittsburgh, Pennsylvania

David C. Napoli, MD
State College, Pennsylvania

Clayton A. Peimer, MD
Chief of Hand Surgery
Professor of Orthopaedic Surgery
Department of Orthopaedic Surgery
State University at Buffalo School of Medicine
Buffalo, New York

Dennis B. Phelps, MD, FACS
Department of Orthopedics
Santa Barbara Cottage Hospital
Santa Barbara, California

Reed E. Pyeritz, MD, PhD
Professor of Human Genetics, Medicine, and Pediatrics
Chair
Department of Human Genetics
Allegheny University of the Health Sciences
Allegheny General Hospital
Pittsburgh, Pennsylvania

Richard L. Ray, MD
Associate Professor
Department of Orthopedic Surgery
Allegheny University of the Health Sciences
Allegheny General Hospital
Pittsburgh, Pennsylvania

David C. Rehak, MD
The Hughston Clinic, P.C.
Columbus, Georgia

Robin R. Richards, MD, FRCS (C)
Professor of Surgery
Division of Orthopaedic Surgery
Department of Surgery
University of Toronto
St. Michael's Hospital
Toronto, Ontario
CANADA

Jory D. Richman, MD
Chief
Department of Orthopaedic Surgery
Mercy Hospital of Pittsburgh
Pittsburgh, Pennsylvania

Barry Riemer, MD
Department of Orthopaedics
Henry Ford Clay Hospital
Detroit, Michigan

Enrico B. Robotti, MD
Acting Chief
Department of Plastic Surgery
Ospedali Riuniti di Bergamo
Paladina,
ITALY

Mark W. Rodosky, MD
Chief, Division of Shoulder Surgery
Assistant Professor
Department of Orthopaedic Surgery
University of Pittsburgh Medical Center
Pittsburgh, Pennsylvania

Mark J. Sangimino, MD
Department of Orthopaedic Surgery
Children's Hospital of Pittsburgh
Pittsburgh, Pennsylvania

Mark T. Scarborough, MD
Associate Professor
Department of Orthopaedic Surgery
University of Florida
Gainesville, Florida

Michael Scarpone, DO
Trinity Sports Medicine
Steubenville, Ohio

Stephanie L. Schneck-Jacob, MD
Instructor
Department of Orthopaedic Surgery
Allegheny University of the Health Sciences
Allegheny General Hospital
Pittsburgh, Pennsylvania

Lew C. Schon, MD
Assistant Director
Foot and Ankle Services
Department of Orthopaedic Surgery
The Union Memorial Hospital
Baltimore, Maryland

John G. Seiler, III, MD
Clinical Associate Professor
Department of Orthopaedic Surgery
Emory University School of Medicine
Atlanta, Georgia

Abraham Shurland, MD
Department of Orthopaedic Surgery
Temple University
Philadelphia, Pennsylvania

David J. Smith, MD, Jr.
Section of Plastic Surgery
University of Michigan Medical Center
Ann Arbor, Michigan

Edward Snell, MD
Department of Orthopaedic Surgery
Allegheny University of the Health Sciences
Allegheny General Hospital
Pittsburgh, Pennsylvania

Trevor Soergel, BA
University of Louisville
Louisville, Kentucky

Nicholas G. Sotereanos, MD
Department of Orthopaedic Surgery
Allegheny University of the Health Sciences
Allegheny General Hospital
Pittsburgh, Pennsylvania

Anthony A. Stans, MD
Senior Associate Consultant
Department of Orthopedic Surgery
Mayo Clinic
Rochester, Minnesota

George N. Stewart, JD
Partner
Zimmer Kunz, PC
Pittsburgh, Pennsylvania

James D. Strader, JD
Dickie, McCamey & Chilcote, PC
Pittsburgh, Pennsylvania

William M. Swartz, MD
Clinical Associate Professor of Surgery
Division of Plastic Surgery
University of Pittsburgh School of Medicine
Pittsburgh, Pennsylvania

Vishwas R. Talwalkar, MD
Department of Orthopaedics and Rehabilitation
Vanderbilt University Medical Center
Nashville, Tennessee

Joseph J. Thoder, MD
Assistant Professor
Department of Orthopaedic Surgery
Temple University School of Medicine
Attending Hand Surgeon
Shriner's Hospital for Children
Philadelphia, Pennsylvania

Joeseph E. Tomaro, MS, PT
Senior Director of Clinical Development
Department of Human Motion Rehabilitation
Allegheny General Hospital
Pittsburgh, Pennsylvania

Adrienne J. Towsen, MD
Department of Orthopaedic Surgery
Allegheny University of the Health Sciences
Allegheny General Hospital
Pittsburgh, Pennsylvania

Jon B. Tucker, MD
Clinical Instructor
Department of Orthopaedic Surgery
University of Pittsburgh
Pittsburgh, Pennsylvania

Arthur L. Valadie, III, M.D.
Private practice, Sports Medicine
Bradenton Orthopaedic Clinic
Bradenton, Florida

Vincent J. Vigorita, MD
Professor of Pathology and Orthopedic Surgery
State University Health Sciences Center at Brooklyn
Medical Director
Lutheran Medical Center
Brooklyn, New York

Keith L. Wapner, MD
Professor
Department of Orthopaedic Surgery
Allegheny University of the Health Sciences
Allegheny General Hospital
Pittsburgh, Pennsylvania;
Director
Foot and Ankle Division
Department of Orthopaedic Surgery
Hahneman School of Medicine
Philadelphia, Pennsylvania

Raymond C. Wasielewski, MD
Department of Orthopaedics
Ohio State University Medical Center
Columbus, Ohio

Greg P. Watchmaker, MD
St. Mary's Hospital
Mequon, Wisconsin

Anthony D. Watson, MD
Director of Clinical Research
Clinical Instructor
Department of Orthopaedic Surgery
Allegheny University of the Health Sciences
Allegheny General Hospital
Pittsburgh, Pennsylvania

Kelly L. Welsh, RN
Hartford Hospital
Hartford, Connecticut

John J. Williams, MD
Pediatric Orthopaedic Surgeon
Central Texas Pediatric Orthopaedics and
    Scoliosis Surgery
Austin, Texas

Scott C. Wilson, MD
Assistant Professor
Department of Orthopaedics
Louisiana State University Medical Center at New Orleans
New Orleans, Louisiana

Thomas W. Wright, MD
Associate Professor
Department of Orthopaedics
University of Florida
Gainesville, Florida

Joseph D. Zuckerman, MD
Professor and Chairman
New York University-Hospital for Joint Diseases
Department of Orthopaedic Surgery
New York University School of Medicine
New York, New York

Preface

Next week a new group of residents will begin their careers in orthopaedic surgery. Most were born in the early seventies: a period of renaissance in the field of orthopaedics. Total joint arthroplasty, arthroscopy, and microsurgery were techniques that were changing the complexion of orthopaedic practice. Medical resources seemed infinite. Resident education took place in the operating room and in the hospital wards. Basic science education emphasized growth and development, fracture healing, and bone metabolism. Over the last 27 years, the rules have changed. Residents in the new millenium will be expected to understand gene therapy, outpatient orthopaedics, a host of orthopaedic procedures, resource management, and both the legal and ethical issues in orthopaedic care. This text has been designed to help educate the next generation of orthopaedic surgeons.

This book is divided into three parts: Basic Science, Clinical Orthopaedics, and Ethical, Legal and Economic issues relevant to orthopaedic surgeons. Each clinical chapter follows a consistent format including relevant basic science, anatomy and surgical approaches, evaluation, and treatment with anticipated outcome. Special highlights include musculoskeletal soft tissues, the scientific method, musculoskeletal imaging, a comprehensive review of adult and pediatric orthopaedics, economics of orthopaedic practice, critical pathways, and medical malpractice.

Our goal was to create a single volume text that could be used as the core reference for orthopaedic residents. An exceptional group of international physicians and scientists were recruited in preparation of this text, including Christopher Evans, Ph D, Joseph Buckwalter, MD, Guy Foucher, MD, Joseph Iannotti, MD, Barry Riemer, MD, Evan Flatow, MD, Louis Bigliani, MD, Robin Richards, MD, Freddie Fu, MD, Keith Wapner, MD, Mark Scarborough, MD, Richard Lackman, MD, Susan Mackinnon, MD, and Clayton Peimer, MD. The authors were asked to provide the essence of their topic in a concise, readable fashion. The information is presented in a way that will hopefully be as useful to a first-year resident as to a chief resident.

Mark E. Baratz, MD

Foreword

As Benjamin Disraeli pointed out in the 19th century, change is inevitable, and in a progressive society, change is constant. The maturation of scientific research and improved communication have accelerated the rate of change throughout the 20th century. This last decade prior to the 21st century has experienced an explosion in scientific knowledge, and developments in electronic communication have vastly accelerated information exchange. This has led to profound advances in the science of the musculoskeletal system, medical and surgical treatment of related disorders, and unexpected changes in the cultural, political, and economic environment in which musculoskeletal medicine and surgery must be practiced. Mark Baratz and his contributors in this text on the essentials of orthopaedic surgery provide students of orthopaedic surgery, from the medical school undergraduate to the mature surgeon, a succinct text that addresses these issues.

This text approximating a thousand pages provides nearly comprehensive coverage. In the basic science section the prestigious group of contributors provides the most up-to-date knowledge about the science of the musculoskeletal system, including an important chapter on the scientific method. When read and applied this will permit readers to evaluate more accurately scientific literature in the future. The section on diagnostic studies includes a section on imaging that features many of the advances that have been made in magnetic resonance imaging. Fourteen sections containing 41 chapters provide a comprehensive review of the medical and surgical aspects of the musculoskeletal system. An improvement in society's habits, nutrition, and exercise, combined with advances in modern health care, is leading to a rapid expansion in our geriatric population. The chapter on orthopaedic issues in aging is therefore very timely and important for practitioners just entering orthopaedic surgery or related fields. In this age of shifting public ethics, managed health care, and increasing medical-legal complexity, the ten chapters on ethics and economic, legal, and political issues in orthopaedics are essential for residents, registrars and fellows leaving training who wish to provide optimal care for their patients, ensure that their practices survive economically, and avoid unnecessary pitfalls.

"Essentials" is user-friendly, providing excellent illustrations, pearls, a very selective bibliography for each chapter, and sample questions with answers that allow readers to assess their understanding of the material. Although this text is written primarily for the use of residents and registrars in training, I commend it to medical students, other practitioners involved in the care of patients with musculoskeletal system problems, and to those seeking readily available information normally scattered throughout many other publications. This comprehensive book fills an important need as we rapidly advance into the 21st century.

Michael W. Chapman, MD
Professor and David Linn Chair of Orthopaedic Surgery
University of California, Davis

Acknowledgments

Many thanks to the efforts of Chris Pilarski, Josh Sankey, Adrienne Towsen, MD, Tom Garges and Lars Lanschwager, and the inspiration from Chris Evans, PhD, Freddie Fu, MD, and Albert B. Ferguson, Jr., MD.

Basic Science

Chapter 1

Orthopaedic Biomechanics

Donald D. Anderson, PhD

Outline

Generally defined, mechanics is that branch of the physical sciences concerned with describing the state of rest or motion of bodies that are subjected to the action of forces. Biomechanics represents a subset of mechanics in which the bodies studied are either living or are integrally related to living beings. Orthopaedics, as a medical subspecialty focused on the structural elements of the human body, is an especially logical area in which to apply the principles of biomechanics. The premise in coupling biomechanics and orthopaedics is that the theories and principles of mechanics, when suitably applied, provide a solid framework for understanding and developing sound orthopaedic practices. As motivation for this approach, one should ask, would I trust a bridge to be safe that was constructed without considering mechanics? Just as a solid foundation in mechanics is paramount to building a safe, reliable bridge, it is likewise crucial to practicing orthopaedics successfully. By the same token, biomechanics is not magic. Its principles must be applied only when it is beneficial to do so. The successful orthopaedic surgeon develops a strong intuition about mechanics that assists in making important surgical decisions.

Biomechanics is unique among the subspecialties of mechanics primarily because biological considerations share equal weight with mechanical considerations. For instance, the ideal form of fracture fixation must be strong enough to withstand the forces on fracture fragments without interfering with the biology of fracture healing. Such determinations require an understanding of biology and mechanics, and of how each is related to the other in the normal, diseased, and injured patient. This chapter is intended to introduce the orthopaedic resident to some of the basic considerations involved in biomechanics and to provide an overview of some specific applications of biomechanics to the practice of orthopaedics.

BASIC SCIENCE

The foundation of biomechanics is a set of terms and concepts; a shorthand used to describe a variety of ideas and physical phenomena. Before delving into the applications of biomechanics in orthopaedics, it is important to be familiar with several terms. Defining these terms helps us understand general mechanical concepts, which codify common sense observations about how bodies move and deform. The term body is intended in this context to have a broad, general meaning. A *body* might range in complexity from a single grain of sand to the space shuttle, or in orthopaedic terms, from a single osteocyte to the entire human body.

To discuss biomechanics, it is important to be familiar with the concept of a vector quantity. Certain physical phenomena, such as temperature, brightness, distance, or height, may be quantified with a single number, or *scalar* quantity. Other physical entities require additional information to fully describe them. For instance, the contribution of traction to reducing a fracture is best conveyed when both its magnitude and direction are known, for example, 50 pounds of traction was longitudinally applied across the fracture site. If that same weight were applied in a different direction, a very different situation would result. *Vector* quantities are used to measure phenomena requiring the additional descriptive information of magnitude and direction. The point at which a vector acts is another important piece of information to know when describing a vector. (Although beyond the scope of this text, yet more complex phenomena are neither scalar nor vector, but *tensor quantities*. Of relevance to mechanics, stress and strain are both tensor quantities. To describe tensor quantities one needs to state not only magnitude and direction, but also the surface on which they are defined to act.)

Scalar quantities can be added together just as can real numbers. If a 5-inch block is stacked on top of a 6-inch block that is resting on the ground, its top will be 11 inches off the ground (i.e., $6 + 5 = 11$). The addition of vector quantities is more complex unless the two vectors act in precisely the same direction. Geometry is used to add vectors. A vector can be represented by an arrow with length proportional to the vector's magnitude. The arrow points along the vector's direction, originating at its tail and pointing to its tip. The sum of two vectors can be obtained by connecting the arrows tip to tail and constructing a third vector from the tail of the first arrow to the tip of the second. This is the parallelogram rule

3

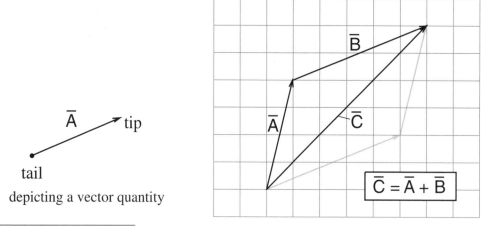

depicting a vector quantity

$$\overline{C} = \overline{A} + \overline{B}$$

Figure 1–1 Schematic representing the additive process for vectors $\overline{A}$ and $\overline{B}$, to produce their sum, vector $\overline{C}$.

of vector addition (Fig. 1–1). Vectors are labeled in this chapter by letters with a bar over the top. Subscripts are used in combination with the labels to further distinguish vectors (e.g., $\overline{F}_h$ and $\overline{F}_k$ could represent the force at the hip and at the knee, respectively).

> ## PEARL
>
> **The sum of two vectors can be obtained by connecting the arrows tip to tail and constructing a third vector from the tail of the first arrow to the tip of the second.**

Vectors may be described in shorthand by using an ordered combination of scalar values to represent magnitudes along a given set of directions. Most people deal with this daily. For instance, when someone gives street directions they will often use a vector shorthand: Go down this street 3 blocks, take a left, and then go 5 blocks down that street. In abbreviated notation this could be represented by the ordered pair (3, 5), with the basic understanding that the first number in the pair represents the number of blocks in a given direction along street x, and the second number represents the number of blocks in a given direction along street y. To label one of these two components, a vector label is enclosed in brackets and given a subscript denoting the component (e.g., x component of $\overline{F}_h$ is $\left[\overline{F}_h\right]_x$). The addition of vectors represented as ordered pairs involves simple scalar addition of, in turn, each of its components. In other words, $(3,5) + (4,8) = (7,13)$. In Figure 1–1, adding vectors $\overline{A}$ and $\overline{B}$ would be as simple as $(1,4) + (5,2) = (6,6)$, where the first number in each ordered pair is understood to be squares toward the right of the page, and the second squares toward the top of the page. [As a check, convince yourself that vector $\overline{C}$ can be accurately represented by the ordered pair (6,6).]

Force is an important vector quantity in biomechanics. A force acts along a given direction to move (displace) and/or deform a body, with the amount of displacement or deformation being dictated by the nature of the body. A body is deformed when its fully unloaded shape is changed, usually as a result of being subjected to a combination of forces. Forces can be supplied by a large variety of sources. The units in which force is measured are newtons (N), equivalent to 1 $kg \cdot m/s^2$. Forces are defined as compression if they act towards the inside of a body, and as tension if they act away from the inside of a body (Fig. 1–2). A person's weight is a force acting towards the center of the earth. The hip joint is routinely subjected to compressive forces with magnitudes greater than four times a person's weight. Shear forces act along a given surface of a body.

When a force displaces a body, that displacement is itself a vector quantity. The rate at which a body displaces with respect to time—its velocity—is likewise a vector quantity, as is the rate at which its velocity changes with respect to time—its acceleration. When a force acts on a body, the amount of displacement is dictated primarily by the body's inertia, and the amount of deformation is dictated by the stiffness of the material of which the body is constituted.

Having defined these simple mechanical terms, it is possible to introduce three powerful principles in mechanics, first published by Isaac Newton in 1686.

- Newton's first law of motion: *A body at rest or in motion resists a change in such state unless subject to an unbalanced force.* This innate resistance to a change in the state of rest or motion is defined as *inertia.*

- Newton's second law of motion: *A body subjected to an unbalanced force will accelerate in the direction of that force. The acceleration is directly proportional to the force and inversely proportional to the object's mass.* (Stated as an equation, this yields the familiar F = ma). Clearly, the mass of an object, a simple scalar measure of the amount of matter, is a very important quantity. Furthermore, mass and inertia are closely related.

- Newton's third law of motion: For every force acting on a body, that body exerts an equal, opposite, and collinear reactive force. This third law is the foundation of a branch of mechanics called statics. The concept follows directly from Newton's second law, given an acceleration of zero.

Compression   Tension   Shear

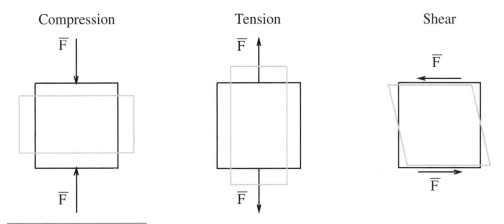

Figure 1–2 Forces can act to compress, elongate, or skew a given body. The solid lines denote the configuration of the bodies prior to force application, and the gray lines the configuration following force application.

Newton's laws of motion are simply statements conveying empirical observations regarding the mechanical behavior of the world around us. Their elegance lies in their precision and brevity. Many a scientist or orthopaedic surgeon could learn a great deal from this point! The powerful physical concept of equilibrium flows directly from Newton's second and third laws—that forces are balanced by opposing forces and/or accompanying accelerations. When a body is not moving, it is considered to be in *static equilibrium*.

The definitions and concepts introduced thus far might be incorrectly construed to be inherently linear in nature. This is not the case, as rotational analogs to these concepts are equally important in mechanics. For instance, a moment is directly analogous to a force in that it displaces and/or deforms bodies, but moments act to rotate and/or torque bodies about a given axis. Moments are vector quantities, with a moment's direction defined according to its axis. In simple terms, a *moment* can be thought of as a force acting at some distance from a point about which a body is constrained to rotate (Fig. 1–3). That distance is termed the

moment arm, and it dictates how strongly a given force contributes to developing a moment. Moments are prescribed units of force × distance, or N · m. Rotational or angular velocities and accelerations can also be defined, as can rotational inertia and stiffness.

In many instances, bodies are subjected to a combination of forces and moments that act to move and deform the body. The concepts put forth in Newton's laws of motion can be independently applied to forces and moments, allowing one to perform mechanical analyses of bodies by isolating these separate quantities and solving for their values. The nature and complexity of such analyses are dictated by the complexity of the mechanical problem being considered, and by the accuracy of the desired solution. In some cases, one wants to know precisely how fast a body is traveling and one is willing to exert all effort needed to obtain that precise answer. For the engineer (and generally the orthopaedic surgeon), simplifications are often made in the analysis to make an untenable solution feasible or to obtain a general idea of the mechanics involved.

When simplifying mechanical problems to obtain an acceptable solution, it is useful to differentiate several areas of mechanics based on important distinctions in the dominant feature one wishes to study. For instance, one can separate static problems in mechanics from dynamic ones. In the case of statics, no consideration is given to the time-varying characteristics of mechanical parameters. This is done because either (1) nothing is changing over time or (2) the rate at which things are changing is so slow that eliminating time from consideration has negligible influence on the accuracy of the predicted behaviors. The first instance is strictly considered a statics problem, and the second is a quasistatic problem. The implications of these distinctions in terms of the complexity and/or accuracy of a mechanical analysis can be substantial. In dynamics problems, in contrast to statics, time plays a central role in describing or predicting mechanical behavior. It takes the form of inertial terms contributing to the development of forces, time-dependent changes in physical properties, or changes in the driving forces that occur over time.

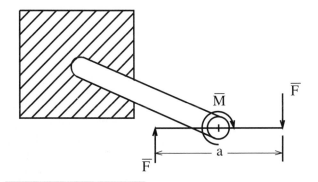

Figure 1–3 The moment, $\overline{M}$, acts to rotate the bar about its long axis. It is equivalent to two equal forces, $\overline{F}$, acting equidistant from the center of the bar. The magnitude of the moment is equal to the product of the force magnitude and its perpendicular distance from the axis about which it acts: $M = (F \times a/2) + (F \times a/2) = F \times a$.

These distinctions have direct implications in implant design. A plate applied to the clavicle is designed primarily to avoid static failure because the bones about it seldom move much relative to one another. In contrast, a compression hip screw is designed to accommodate the dynamic loads associated with walking, stair climbing, and rising from a chair.

Another important differentiation is between kinematics and kinetics. *Kinematics* is the study of the motion of a body without explicit consideration of the forces involved with those motions. *Kinetics*, in contrast, is study of forces and moments of bodies without explicit consideration of the motions associated with those forces and moments. Kinematic analysis involves careful observation and mathematical description of motion. Kinetics involves measurement of or deduction of the forces and moments at work in a system. Forward dynamics is the process whereby a kinetic analysis is used to provide estimates of motion. Inverse dynamics, in contrast, involves collecting kinematic data and extrapolating forces and moments that can not easily be measured. This extrapolation involves solving equations of motion for a simplified representation of the system being studied.

PEARL

Kinematics is the study of a body in motion, such as the positions of the femur and tibia during normal gait.

The study of mechanics may also be split into rigid and deformable body analysis. When a body, subjected to a set of forces, predominantly displaces rather than deforms, it can be considered a rigid body. For instance, in the human body, bones may be assumed to act as rigid bodies during gait and other activities. *Rigid body analysis* allows one to neglect the consideration of a very complex process, how a body deforms. Alternatively, when a body responds to force by not only displacing but also by deforming, it must be considered as a deformable body. Soft tissue, such as cartilage or ligaments, must be assumed to be a deformable body. The fundamental concept in deformable body analysis is that all structures may be considered a collection of springs. Together that collection of springs imparts a characteristic elastic stiffness, or resistance to deformation, to a given material or structure. In this respect, biomaterials and biomechanics are linked. Some materials exhibit *viscoelastic behavior*, meaning that their force/deformation response is influenced by the rate at which forces are applied to the material.

Free body diagrams can be a very helpful tool for understanding the rigid body mechanics acting on a single body or among multiple bodies. The basic concept is that a given body, or group of bodies, can be broken up into separate (free) bodies for the purpose of studying mechanics. Each of the bodies is carefully diagrammed, including representation of all the forces and moments acting upon it from either external sources or from the interactions among separate free bod-

ies. Regarding these latter forces of interaction, it is important to remember Newton's third law. Unknown forces or moments are determined by imposing static equilibrium through a set of equations, summing forces in a given direction and then moments, and setting each sum equal to zero. Remember Newton's second law, where the accelerations are equal to zero (static problem). The choice of how the free bodies are defined is dictated by the question to be solved.

Free body diagrams can be used to analyze combinations of bodies in a fully three-dimensional (3-D) sense. In practice, free body diagrams are often used to perform simplified planar analyses in which general 3-D forces and motions are considered only as they act within a single plane. Forces and motions acting out of the plane of analysis are neglected. This is useful in problems in which most motion occurs, and most forces act, within a single plane. For instance, the knee is often considered to act as a simple hinge, and sagittal plane analysis of the knee during flexion-extension is a classic example of planar analysis, where internal-external and varus-valgus rotations of the knee are neglected from consideration (Fig. 1–4).

As a second example of simplified planar analysis, let us consider dynamic compression plating. Free body diagram analysis helps us understand how the dynamic compression plate (DCP) delivers compression across a fracture site (Fig. 1–5). The DCP is applied in a tensioned state, and screws are placed to hold the plate in tension. In turn, the forces that the plate exerts on the screws are directed towards the fracture. Since the screws are being forced towards the fracture, they exert forces on the bone, thereby holding the bone in compression across the fracture site.

In a subset of mechanics problems, the available information allows solution of the equations of motion uniquely. That is, one solution is correct uniquely for the problem as it is posed. This is called a *determinate problem*, in which the number of equations is equal to the number of unknowns being solved. In the remainder of mechanics problems, and in a large number of problems in biomechanics, there are more unknowns than there are equations to solve for uniquely. This is called an *indeterminate problem*, and solving such problems involves making critical decisions about how bodies behave. In studying the human body, the analysis can be simplified by considering several muscles as a single muscle group. This may allow the formulation of a determinate problem. If one chooses to study the forces in each of these muscles separately, problems quickly become indeterminate. Although more complex, a number of techniques are available for solving such problems. Assumptions regarding the relative amount of force a muscle can generate based on its cross sectional area are often used to solve indeterminate problems.

Another powerful principle in mechanics is that mechanical energy is always conserved. Stated slightly differently, the amount of mechanical energy in a system subject to no external forces is constant. Mechanical energy is expressed in two general terms: kinetic energy and potential energy. *Kinetic energy* is a measure of energy being expended in motion; in its simplest case, equal to one half the product of the mass times the square of the velocity. *Potential energy* is a measure of

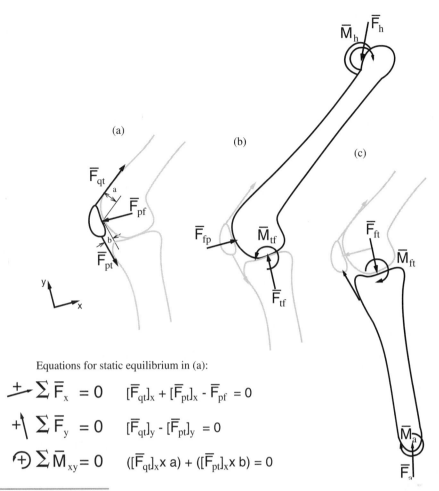

Equations for static equilibrium in (a):

$$\xrightarrow{+}\ \sum \overline{F}_x = 0 \qquad [\overline{F}_{qt}]_x + [\overline{F}_{pt}]_x - \overline{F}_{pf} = 0$$

$$+\!\!\uparrow\ \sum \overline{F}_y = 0 \qquad [\overline{F}_{qt}]_y - [\overline{F}_{pt}]_y = 0$$

$$\curvearrowright\!\!+\ \sum \overline{M}_{xy} = 0 \qquad ([\overline{F}_{qt}]_x \times a) + ([\overline{F}_{pt}]_x \times b) = 0$$

Figure 1–4   Static knee mechanics can be represented in a free body diagram by isolating, in turn: **(a)** the patella; **(b)** the femur; and **(c)** the tibia. Forces from the pull of the quadriceps, in the patellar tendon and in the quadriceps tendon, as well as patellofemoral contact force are included in **(a)**. In addition, forces representing flexion-extension knee moments and tibiofemoral contact force are included in **(b)** and **(c)**, as well as moments and forces on the femur and tibia from the hip and ankle.

stored energy; in its simplest case, a body's mass times the acceleration of gravity times the height above some reference plane. The motion of a ball thrown up in the air is dictated by the conversion of kinetic energy imparted to the ball when it is thrown into potential energy as it rises against gravity. As the ball travels, no external forces (other than gravity) act on it. At the top of its arc, all the energy in the system is stored as potential energy, which then converts back to kinetic energy as the ball accelerates back toward the ground.

Many of the concepts in mechanics revolve around the study of how energy is stored and transferred between bodies. These issues may be of greatest relevance to orthopaedics when considering the trauma caused by blunt impact or the differences in the nature of low and high velocity bullet wounds related to their different kinetic energies. When an external force acts on an object causing it to undergo dis-

placement, we say that work is being done by that force on the object. *Work* is a scalar quantity of energy, and in its simplest case it is the product of the magnitude of force times the distance traveled (W = fd), with units of N · m, or joules (J).

BIOMECHANICS IN ORTHOPAEDICS

With a basic understanding of the terms and concepts of biomechanics one can begin to apply biomechanics to help understand orthopaedics. In this section, more specific topics related to orthopaedics will be discussed: tissue type, joint biomechanics, and implant biomechanics.

Of the musculoskeletal tissues, bone is considered the most extensively in biomechanics. This is not surprising, as

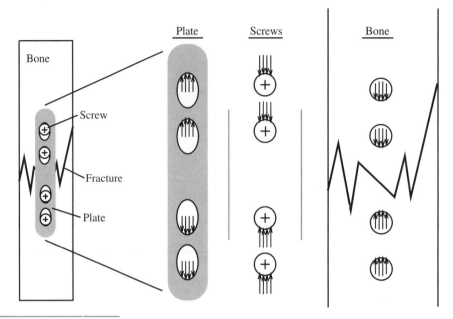

Figure 1–5 The entire fracture construct is diagrammatically broken into three separate components: the plate, the screws, and the fractured bone. By simply diagramming the action of forces, even without analyzing their magnitude, a better understanding of the dynamic compression plate can be achieved.

bone is the primary structural component on which the body is supported. Bone is a highly ordered, crystalline material, with organic and mineral phases. Compared with other tissues in the body, bone is very hard and strong.

A large branch of biomechanics, broadly termed *motion analysis*, is based on treating bones as rigid bodies. This involves tracking the motion of different body segments during activities of interest, such as gait, stair climbing, running, lifting, or jumping. The motion is most often tracked using video cameras, which record the motion of markers attached to body segments. Electromagnetic tracking systems are popular in motion measurement. These systems rely on a source that generates an electromagnetic field. The field is disturbed in a controlled fashion by sensors attached to body segments, and system electronics determine the location in space and orientations of the sensors, allowing sensor motion to be tracked. Muscle activity is often monitored concurrently using electromyogram, with electrodes attached to desired muscle groups. Using inverse dynamics, one is able to extrapolate joint forces and moments, difficult quantities to directly measure in a living person. Motion analysis has provided insight into how anterior cruciate ligament (ACL) sacrifice in total knee replacement impacts on biomechanics of the knee and other joints of the lower extremity. Likewise, it has helped to assess the biomechanical impact of choosing to reconstruct a ruptured ACL versus leaving it surgically untreated.

In certain instances, it becomes important to study the deformation of bone. Bones are most often considered as deformable bodies when one wishes to study bone fracture, fracture treatment, changes in bone over time, or other pathologies of the skeletal system.

Ligaments, as connective tissue, play an important role in dictating how bones move relative to one another. The structure of ligaments can range from narrow and cordlike to broad sheets of tissue. They provide static joint stability, as a passive system of constraint that maintains a stable, advantageous orientation of the bones in preparation for motion. The fibrous anatomy of ligaments, coupled with their broad, complex insertions into bone, allow them to play distinctly different roles depending on joint position. Along these lines, distinct fiber bundles can often be identified at a macroscopic level. Another important mechanical role of ligaments, which often places them at great risk of injury, is to check the relative motion of bones at the extremes of their range of motion. Ligaments are very strong and tough. In general, they fail not in midsubstance, but instead in a zone near the bone insertion, often with bony fragment avulsion.

Tendons govern how muscle contraction effects motion of the bones, by controlling where and along what direction the muscles pull on the bones. In so doing, tendons deliver a mechanical advantage to muscles, maximizing the moment arm thereby reducing the amount of force required to produce a given joint rotation. This can place great stress on the tendons; a stress they are prepared to handle due to a complex attachment to the muscles and insertion to the bone. Tendons also couple different actions motored by a given muscle, and they can cross one or more joints in so doing. In the hand, tendons make it possible for extrinsic muscles, located in the forearm, to effect motion of the finger joints (Fig. 1–6). Supporting structures such as the retinaculum and tendon sheath exert control over how the tendons are routed along their course and across joints by preventing bowstringing. The unsupported tendon lifts off the wrist during wrist extension. In doing so it loses its mechanical advantage.

Articular cartilage mechanics has received a great deal of attention during the past 20 years. Over that time, knowledge

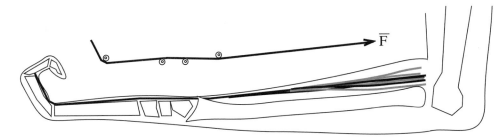

Figure 1–6 Tendons crossing the wrist, traveling along the metacarpal, and inserting on the middle phalanx allow extrinsic muscles of the forearm to effect flexion of the proximal interphalangeal joint. Tendon gliding is facilitated over its course by retinacular and ligamentous pulley structures.

of cartilage mechanical properties has greatly increased, including how cartilage deforms with time when subjected to a load. It has long been appreciated that cartilage, a highly porous, fluid-filled material, exhibits viscoelastic behavior. The interest in cartilage mechanics has been driven predominantly by the desire to better understand the complex mechanical changes accompanying the onset of arthritis and by attempts to identify new techniques to intervene in the disease process. For example, the inability of cartilage to heal full-thickness defects has stimulated new developments in cartilage transplantation.

The modern era of orthopaedic surgery has been dominated by the treatment of maladies of the articular joints. Biomechanics has played an important part in influencing the course of these treatments. Pain and stiffness in the joints can often be directly traced to a mechanical problem. Articular joints transmit forces across the spaces between bones while providing stability and flexibility. As loads cross the joint, articular cartilage deforms, joint articulations become more congruent, and loads are spread over a greater area. Muscles, tendons, and ligaments tighten to provide stability, protecting individual components from excessive forces. When this intricate yet robust system is disturbed, either through inflammation or trauma, pain and stiffness often follow.

Considerable effort has been invested in trying to determine the biomechanics of intact articular joints, and in designing implants to restore normal biomechanics. As one might expect, success in replacing joints varies. This is surely attributable to the varied complexities of different joints. Success in replacement of the hips and knees can be contrasted with less successful results in the ankle and the joints of the upper extremity.

The hip and the knee are constrained joints that experience large forces. At the ankle, similarly large forces are transmitted from the lower leg to the many bones of the foot, presenting a myriad of potential problems in replicating normal biomechanics. The joints of the upper extremity have designs that maximize motion, often at the expense of bony support. In the shoulder, the connective tissues about the joint bear the primary responsibility for providing support and stability, with heavy reliance on balance between muscles on opposing sides of the joint. A highly congruent and intricate bony articulation provides stability in the elbow. Difficulties also exist in replicating biomechanics of the wrist, with its myriad of interconnected bones and ligaments.

The spine, with its many coupled segments, presents a slew of unique orthopaedic problems. The spine is made especially complex by multiple structures (discs, facets, ligaments) connecting adjacent motion segments. Flexion of one motion segment can result in longitudinal distraction of an adjacent segment (the concept of coupled motion). When motions are coupled, the mechanical result of applying a given implant to reduce motion is difficult to predict. Fusion of one or more spinal segments to provide stability has been linked to increased forces on adjacent segments. This may lead to arthritis in these adjacent segments.

Against this backdrop of complex mechanics, implants and prosthetics are designed to provide stability and to restore pain-free motion. Some implants are designed for eventual removal, others are designed to remain indefinitely. Those intended for eventual removal are generally weaker and more likely to eventually fail if not removed. Those implants intended to be left in the body are designed to be more resilient over time because they will be subjected to millions of loading cycles during their service.

The majority of joint replacements involve disruption of substantial segments of the articular anatomy, including some stabilizing soft tissue elements. In total knee replacement, the preservation of cruciate function is considered an important design issue. In replacing the articulation of the knee, it is desirable to preserve the cruciate function. The cruciates help to control motion of the knee, especially during activities such as stair climbing and rising from a chair.

Biomechanical analysis of techniques in total hip replacement helped to identify failure of the bone cement mantle as an important factor in loosening and failure of femoral components. Second and third generation cementing techniques may improve long-term outcomes in hip replacement patients.

ORTHOPAEDIC CASE STUDIES

How does an orthopaedic surgeon use or benefit from biomechanics? A few case studies are presented to address this question.

An individual presents in the emergency department with a two-part femoral fracture. In relatively short order, the surgeon should be able to:

- understand the undisturbed biomechanical state of the femur in an isolated sense and within the context of the rest of the body.
- understand what mechanical factors caused the fracture, while keeping in mind other important biological factors, such as systemic metabolic or nutritional status.
- understand the altered mechanics resulting from the fracture and the implications on not only the femur but also on the rest of the body.
- assess whether it is possible, desirable, or feasible to restore the original biomechanics. This requires understanding the mechanics of surgical instrumentation as well as nonsurgical treatments. It also requires an understanding of the biology and the mechanics of fracture healing.

To a large degree, the success of treating the femoral fracture will depend upon a basic understanding of biomechanics.

Another case study illustrates surgical planning for an osteotomy. Consider a thirty-five-year-old patient with medial compartment arthritis of the knee. This individual is too young to be considered for a unicondylar or total knee arthroplasty. Pain may be alleviated with a high tibial osteotomy, where the geometry of the tibia is altered through a series of surgical cuts. The goal is to reorient the tibial surface to create a more equal distribution of forces between the two compartments (Fig. 1–7). Compressive forces cross the knee following two paths. The distribution is dictated by simple equations of equilibrium. As the surface of one compartment is altered by the ongoing arthritis the balance of moments at the knee dictate a shift in the distribution of forces. Ligaments and tendons about the knee carry tensile forces that stabilize the knee but also contribute to compressive forces across the joint surfaces. In the simplest cases, the osteotomy is a corrective procedure, restoring near-original anatomy. The angles of the cuts to be made are the answer to a simple mechanics problem, how to alter the geometry to evenly distribute the loads between the two compartments? In more complicated cases, multiple deformities of the lower limbs necessitate a much more involved determination of how to best redistribute forces through osteotomy.

A third case involves capsular procedures in the shoulder. A forty-four-year-old patient presents with anterior instability in the shoulder. Examination reveals laxity in the anterior

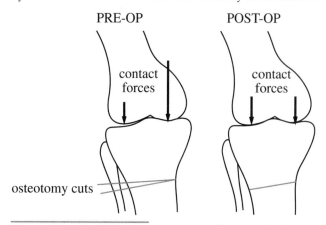

PRE-OP   POST-OP

contact forces   contact forces

osteotomy cuts

Figure 1–7 A tibial osteotomy can influence the biomechanics of the knee by altering the distribution of contact forces between the medial and lateral compartments.

stabilizing soft tissues of the shoulder. Surgical treatment is guided by a consideration of how best to restore balance of stabilizing soft tissues. If the anterior structures are tightened too much the relative positions of the bones is altered. This can lead to abnormal wearing of the glenoid and restricted motion. If the anterior structures are tightened too little there is a risk for recurrence of the anterior dislocation.

Learning from mistakes is an important part of biomechanics in orthopaedics. The concept of stress shielding represents an instance in which mechanics was given too much emphasis at the expense of biology. It has come to be recognized that implants which carry the majority of load will unload portions of the bone. Since bone is dependent upon continued loading to maintain mechanical integrity, this condition can compromise healing. Similarly, compromised vascularity beneath a highly conforming bone plate, negatively influencing bony healing, also demonstrates this point. In both instances, more careful attention to fundamental biomechanical principles has since produced more successful designs, such as load sharing implants and limited-contact bone plates.

SUMMARY

We live in exciting times in which technological and scientific advances have made possible new opportunities for applying biomechanics to orthopaedics. Recent research has centered on understanding how tissues in the body respond to stress and strain at the cellular level. These concepts lie at the interface between biology and mechanics, and they have far-reaching implications in terms of orthopaedic treatment and rehabilitation. Finite element analysis uses computer models that analyze surgical treatments and couple biomechanics with biochemistry to engineer protocols to augment soft tissue healing.

Researchers are subjecting bone, ligament, tendon, and cartilage cells, grown in petri dishes, to loading regimens and observing how cellular activity is altered by changes in the loadings. Many devices used to apply these loadings rely on diaphragms subjected to reciprocating pressure waveforms (Fig. 1–8). The results of this research could lead to implants that provide a greater stimulus to tissue healing.

Another area of research and development involves integrating computers more closely in preoperative surgical planning as well as in the actual surgery. Coupling 3-D computed tomography reconstructions of bony geometry with computer simulations of the associated mechanics may provide improved planning of surgical procedures. It also has the potential to deliver helpful cues to the surgeon in the operating room. This is worth mentioning in a discussion of biomechanics because decisions of a mechanical nature made during surgery are not always accurate, and the computer can be of great benefit in verifying intuition. This is especially true in the case of multibone fusions, such as those performed in the wrist. The human mind has a limited capacity to consider all the implications of a given change in mechanics.

Increasing the knowledge of the actions of biological agents, such as growth factors in musculoskeletal tissue healing, has opened new vistas for their therapeutic application in manipulating the body's normal healing process. This is

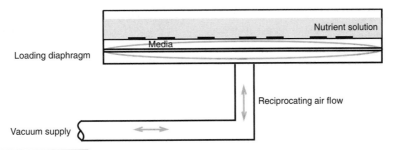

Figure 1–8 Schematic of generic cell-stretching device. Markers of biological activity are monitored as the cells are subjected to a variety of input loading profiles.

another area in which biomechanics is making contributions. Manipulating tissue healing is a problematic endeavor. Misjudgments can result in accelerated healing, but at the expense of a resulting decreased mechanical strength in the final healed tissues. Careful investigation coupling biochemistry and biomechanics using animal models is crucial in bringing to fruition these highly promising breakthroughs in treatment.

SELECTED BIBLIOGRAPHY

CHAFFIN D, ANDERSSON G, eds., *Occupational Biomechanics.* New York, NY: John Wiley & Sons Inc, 1984.

CROWNINSHIELD RD, BRAND RA, JOHNSTON RC, MILROY JC. The effect of femoral stem cross-sectional geometry on cement stresses in total hip reconstruction. *Clin Orthop.* 1980. 146:71–77.

HUISKES R. Failed innovation in total hip replacement: diagnosis and proposals for a cure. *Acta Orthop Scand.* 1993. 64:699–716.

MOW V, HAYES W, eds. *Basic Orthopaedic Biomechanics.* New York, NY: Raven Press, 1991.

MOW V, RATCLIFFE A, WOO S, eds. *Biomechanics of Diarthrodial Joints.* 2 Vols. New York, NY: Springer-Verlag, 1990.

NIGG B, HERZOG W, eds. *Biomechanics of the Musculoskeletal System.* West Sussex, England: John Wiley & Sons Ltd; 1994.

SIMON S, ed. *Orthopaedic Basic Science.* Chicago, Ill: American Academy of Orthopaedic Surgeons, 1994.

SOUDRY M, WALKER PS, REILLY DT, KUROSAWA H, SLEDGE CB. Effects of total knee replacement design on femoral-tibial contact conditions. *J Arthroplasty.* 1986. 1:35–45.

WHITE AA, PANJABI MM, eds. *Clinical Biomechanics of the Spine.* Philadelphia, PA: Lippincott, 1992.

SAMPLE QUESTIONS

1. A dynamic compression plate:
   (a) supplies compression across the fracture site because the plate is in compression
   (b) supplies compression across the fracture site because the plate is unloaded
   (c) can apply compression to a fracture site when screw heads place the plate in tension
   (d) applies a cyclic compressive loading across the fracture site
   (e) rigidly holds the fracture ends together

2. Inertia can be defined as:
   (a) the study of the motion of a body without explicit consideration of the forces involved
   (b) a body's innate resistance to a change in state of rest or motion
   (c) the resistance of a body to deformation
   (d) the rate at which a body moves through space
   (e) mechanical analysis in which bodies are considered to be rigid

3. In traditional motion analysis, bones are considered to be rigid bodies because:
   (a) bones do not deform during activities of daily living
   (b) it is convenient to assume that bones do not deform during motion of the human body
   (c) bone deformations during common motion are very small relative to other factors of interest
   (d) the analysis is focused on deformation of soft tissues
   (e) all of the above

4. A patients has a varus knee due to medial compartment arthritis. To relieve excessive force in the medial compartment, a tibial osteotomy should:
   (a) remove a wedge of bone such that a greater amount of bone is taken from the lateral side
   (b) remove a wedge of bone such that a greater amount of bone is taken from the medial side
   (c) remove a narrow slice of bone evenly across the tibia, decreasing the tibial height
   (d) preserve the anterior cruciate ligament
   (e) none of the above

5. Maximum forces across the intact hip and knee are generally:
   (a) equal to a person's body weight
   (b) roughly 85% of a person's body weight
   (c) twice a person's body weight
   (d) greater than four times a person's body weight
   (e) too large to reliably measure

Answers: 1) c; 2) b; 3) c; 4) a; 5) d

Chapter 2

Biomaterials

Joseph E. Hale, PhD

Outline

Biomaterials are a special class of biological and synthetic materials that exhibit biocompatibility when used on an intermittent or continuous basis to replace living tissue or augment tissue function. *Biocompatibility* refers to the failure of the material to elicit an adverse biological response as a result of such contact. Based on this definition, the study of biomaterials brings together aspects of a diverse set of disciplines including materials science, biology, and clinical medicine. This chapter is intended to familiarize the reader with some of the fundamental considerations involved in assessing the performance of biomaterials and to provide an overview of specific materials commonly used in orthopaedic applications. Terms that will be discussed in the text are introduced in Table 2–1.

TABLE 2–1 Biomaterials Terminology

Term	Definition
Load	Force applied to a material.
Stress	Load per unit area over which the load acts. Can be compressive, tensile (stretch), or shear
Strain	Change in length/original length in response to load
Elastic modulus	Response of material to compression or stretch
Elastic deformation	Material returns to original shape after being deformed by an applied load
Plastic deformation	Material remains permanently deformed following an applied load
Yeild point	Transition point between elastic and plastic regions of the stress-strain curve
Ultimate stress (Strength)	Maximum stress material can withstand before failure
Ductility	Capacity of a material to deform beyond its yield point; the opposite of brittle
Toughness	Energy expended in deforming a material to failure. Equal to the area under elastic and plastic portions of stress-strain curve
Creep	Deformation of material over time while under a constant load

MECHANICAL BEHAVIOR OF MATERIALS

Structural and Material Properties

Mechanical properties provide a measure of a material's ability to resist deformation when subjected to externally applied loads. The properties of a material are determined empirically by applying a compressive, tensile, or shear load at a constant rate and monitoring the displacement or deformation of the specimen. The relationship between the applied load and the observed displacement is dependent on two factors: the material being tested and the size and shape of the specimen. For example, a stainless steel Kirschner wire and a stainless steel intramedullary nail will exhibit dramatically different behavior when subjected to the same load even though they are made from the same material. Characteristics derived from the load-displacement data are therefore

Orthopaedic Surgery: The Essentials. Edited by M.E. Baratz, A.D. Watson, and J.E. Imbriglia. Thieme Medical Publishers, Inc., New York © 1999

referred to as *structural properties*. By scaling the load-displacement data to account for the geometry of the specimen, stress-strain data are obtained, from which the intrinsic properties of the material can be determined.

Stress-Strain Relationship

Stress is the internal reaction of a material to an externally applied load. For a uniformly distributed load, stress within a material is equal to the magnitude of the load divided by the cross-sectional area upon which it acts. Stress is expressed in units of newtons per square meter (N/m^2) or pascals (Pa). Three types of stress exist: compressive, tensile, and shear. A combination of two or more types of stress, such as occurs in bending, commonly act on a material.

Strain is the change in length of a material that has been subjected to a load divided by its original length (change in length/length). Strain values may be expressed as length per length (mm/mm) or as a percentage. By convention, increases and decreases in length are associated with positive and negative strains, respectively. For an elastic material having the same mechanical properties in all directions (i.e., isotropic), smaller strains of opposite sign occur orthogonal to the direction of loading. These changes are easily observed by stretching a rubberband and observing the decrease in its width (and thickness). The extent to which a material exhibits such behavior is characterized by the ratio of the transverse (lateral) strain to the longitudinal (axial) strain. The negative value of this ratio is referred to as Poisson's ratio and ranges between 0.0 for materials that exhibit maximal compressibility and 0.5 for materials that are incompressible, that is, they maintain a constant volume (Fig. 2–1).

Changes in the geometry of a material that occur during loading, such as narrowing or necking of a specimen being stretched, can affect calculations of stress and strain. Stress and strain values based on the unloaded cross-sectional area and length are referred to as "nominal" or "engineering" stress and strain. True stress accounts for these changes in geometry by normalizing the applied load to the instantaneous cross-sectional area over which it is distributed. True strain is equal to the ratio of the local change in cross-sectional area to the original cross-sectional area. For tensile loading, true stress and strain values are greater than the corresponding nominal stress and strain values. Although true stress and strain are arguably more representative of the stress state of a material at any point in time, they are considerably more difficult to determine in practice. For that reason, nominal stress and strain are typically reported.

The relationship between stress and strain is characterized by the shape of the stress-strain curve and is mathematically described by a constitutive equation (Fig. 2–2). Depending on the shape of the curve, more than one constitutive equation may be necessary to accurately describe the material's behavior over the entire range of stress. At low loads, most materials exhibit a linear or elastic response with stress simply related to strain by a proportionality constant. For compressive or tensile loading, that constant is referred to as the *elastic modulus* or Young's modulus and is equal to the slope of the stress-strain curve. Similarly, a *shear* modulus is defined for torsional loading. The magnitude of the modulus indicates the ability of the material to resist deformation; for a given stress, a material with a high elastic modulus deforms less than a material with a low modulus. Within the elastic region, unloading of the material proceeds back along the same curve produced by loading of the material. Any energy expended in producing deformation is fully recovered and the material returns to its original undeformed state.

PEARL

In the elastic region of a stress-strain curve a material that is stretched, compressed, or twisted will return to its original state when the deforming load is removed.

At higher loads, many materials exhibit a nonlinear response, requiring a higher-order constitutive equation to represent the stress-strain relationship. Because some degree of permanent or plastic deformation of the material persists following removal of the load, this portion of the stress-strain curve is referred to as the plastic region. Beginning at the point of highest stress, unloading typically follows a path parallel to the linear portion of the loading curve and intersects the strain axis (zero stress) at some nonzero value. Because part of the energy expended in producing deformation is consumed in rearranging the structure of the material, a net energy loss, equal to the difference in the area under the loading and unloading curves, occurs.

Yield and Ultimate Stress

The transition point between the elastic and plastic regions of the stress-strain curve is referred to as the *elastic limit*. Because it is difficult to pinpoint the end of the elastic region,

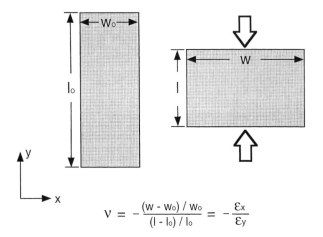

$$\nu = -\frac{(w - w_0)/w_0}{(l - l_0)/l_0} = -\frac{\varepsilon_x}{\varepsilon_y}$$

Figure 2–1 Uniaxial loading of a material specimen produces dimensional changes in both the longitudinal and transverse directions. The extent to which one dimension changes relative to the other is an intrinsic property of the material and is characterized by Poisson's ratio (ν).

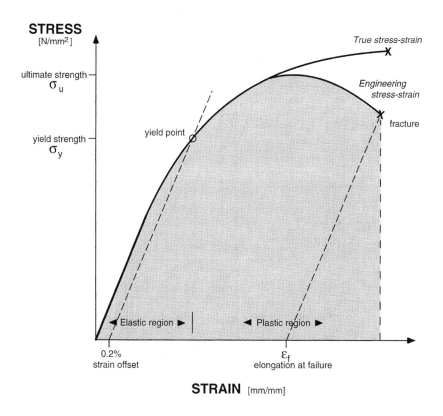

STRESS [N/mm²]

ultimate strength — σ_u

yield strength — σ_y

yield point

True stress-strain

Engineering stress-strain

fracture

◄ Elastic region ► | ◄ Plastic region ►

0.2% strain offset

ε_f elongation at failure

STRAIN [mm/mm]

Figure 2–2 The response of a material to an applied load can be described in terms of its stress-strain curve. Material properties correspond to specific features of the stress-strain curve and are independent of the size and shape of the specimen.

the proportional limit or yield point may be used instead. This point is determined by the intersection of the stress-strain curve and a line parallel to the linear portion of the curve with an arbitrarily defined strain offset, typically 0.2%. The stress value corresponding to the proportional limit is referred to as the (offset) *yield stress*.

> ## PEARL
>
> **If a material is loaded past the *yield point* of its stress-strain curve it enters the *plastic region* and will be permanently deformed.**

Ultimate stress or strength is defined as the maximum stress that a material is able to withstand prior to failure. The failure point corresponds to the stress value at which failure actually occurs. Depending on the material and the failure criteria imposed (and the definition of stress and strain), the failure point may coincide with the ultimate stress or may occur at a lower stress and higher strain than the ultimate stress. Because elastic recovery occurs following fracture, the elongation-at-failure is less than the maximum strain attained immediately prior to failure.

Toughness

Toughness is a measure of the energy expended in deforming a material to failure and is equal to the area under both the elastic and plastic portions of the stress-strain curve. Toughness has the dimensions of work or energy per unit volume (newton-meters per cubic meter = joules per cubic meter) and

is therefore also referred to as strain energy density. Although different materials may exhibit dramatically different behavior in response to the same applied load, the areas under their respective stress-strain curves may be similar (Fig. 2–3). For example, a ductile material such as ultra-high molecular weight polyethylene (UHMWPE), which fails at a relatively low stress (30 MPa) but undergoes very large strain (200%) may be as tough or tougher than a more brittle material such as stainless steel, which is able to withstand higher stresses (860 MPa) but fails at relatively low strain (10%).

Fatigue

Failure may be due to a single catastrophic loading event, as considered above, or may occur as a result of repeated or cyclic loading and unloading. Under the latter condition, it is possible for a material to fail at stress levels far below its ultimate strength as a result of accumulated microdamage. As the number of cycles increases, the stress required to produce failure decreases asymptotically. The fatigue or endurance limit represents the stress value below which the material could theoretically undergo an infinite number of loading cycles without experiencing failure. Given the cyclic demands associated with many daily activities, the choice of a material to be used as an orthopaedic implant along with a design that minimizes peak stresses is crucial to long-term survival.

Creep and Stress Relaxation

Our discussion of material characteristics thus far has assumed that stress and strain do not change as a function of time. Viscoelastic materials, including nearly all biological materials, possess characteristics that are time-dependent.

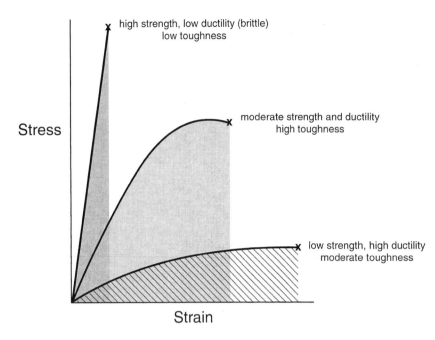

Figure 2–3 Material toughness corresponds to the area under the stress-strain curve. The relationship among strength, ductility, and toughness is illustrated for three different materials with widely varying properties.

This phenomenon can be analyzed experimentally using two approaches: creep and stress relaxation (Fig. 2–4). *Creep* describes plastic or permanent deformation that occurs over a period of time under a constant applied load. Although creep occurs in metals and ceramics at elevated temperatures, its occurrence in polymers at physiological temperatures is a potential source of implant degradation. Clinical procedures such as serial casting or bracing take advantage of this phenomenon in biological tissues to correct for example, joint confractures. The second experimental approach, *stress relaxation*, is defined as decreasing stress over a period of time under constant applied strain. Stress relaxation can also occur in polymers at physiological temperatures.

PEARL

Creep describes a permanent change in shape that occurs over time while a material is subjected to a constant load. The polyethylene cups used in total hip arthroplasty are subject to creep deformation.

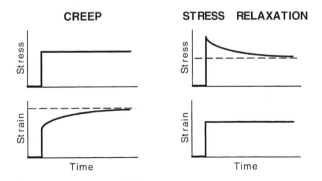

Figure 2–4 Viscoelastic materials exhibit changes in stress and strain as a function of time. The rate at which these quantities approach equilibrium is determined by a characteristic time constant of the material.

SPECIFIC MATERIALS FOR ORTHOPAEDIC APPLICATIONS

Classification of Materials

Clearly, the choice of a material must satisfy the mechanical requirements of its intended use. In addition, a biomaterial must also exhibit (bio)compatibility with the chemical, surface, and pharmacological properties of the environment in which it will function. This section focuses on the composition, mechanical characteristics, and biocompatibility of those materials that are most widely used in orthopaedic applications. Various means of categorizing materials are possible. Based on molecular composition and structure, four different types of materials will be considered: metals, ceramics and glasses, polymers, and composites. (Note: a fifth type of material, semiconductors, can be defined based on differences in atomic bonding, but are not of particular interest for orthopaedic applications.) Biological materials, despite differences such as metabolic activity and potential for repair compared with synthetic materials, can be considered as composite materials or, in some cases, as polymers.

Empirically determined values for mechanical properties, such as elastic modulus and ultimate strength, vary widely based on material composition, manufacturing processes, testing mode, the rate at which the load or displacement is applied, orientation of the material ultrastructure relative to the direction of loading, and homogeneity, among others (Fig. 2–5). Minimum standards for implant materials have been established by the American Society for Testing and Materials (ASTM). References to relevant standards are included in this chapter. In addition, standards also exist for methods of mechanical testing (ASTM E6–89) and assessment of biocompatibility (ASTM F981–93).

Metals

Because of their high strength, stiffness, and ductility, metals (and metal alloys) are particularly well-suited for hard tissue

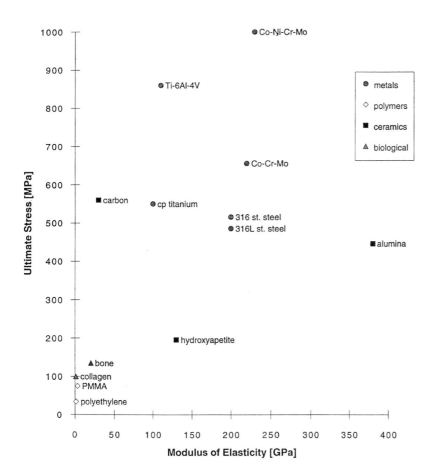

Figure 2–5 Typical values of ultimate strength and modulus of elasticity for some common orthopaedic biomaterials illustrate relative differences between and within material groups. Ultimate strength values are based on the American Society for Testing Materials minimum requirements where applicable and annealed condition for all metals except Co-Cr-Mo.

applications (e.g., joint replacements, plates, nails, and screws). These characteristics give metals the ability to resist plastic deformation under load and to provide an increased resistance to failure. As a result, failure of metal implants is uncommon and is almost always a result of fatigue.

Metal alloys are formed by the addition of other elements to pure metals. By selectively adding various elements, the mechanical properties and corrosion resistance of pure metals can be enhanced. Metal alloys that exhibit tensile strength greater than 1000 MPa at elevated temperature (above 1000°C) are referred to as *superalloys*.

Although well-suited to the demands of the loading environment in vivo, the properties of most metals greatly exceed those of bone, resulting in preferential load transfer through the implant when placed in parallel with bone. This condition, known as *stress-shielding*, decreases or eliminates the stimulus for bone remodeling and leads to bone resorption in regions of low stress (e.g., calcar region of femur with proximal femoral implant).

The biocompatibility of metals used for implantable devices is directly related to their ability to resist chemical degradation or corrosion. Compared with most other materials, metals are more susceptible to corrosion in the aqueous saline environment of the human body. Corrosion degrades the mechanical properties of the metal and releases potentially harmful metal ions into the surrounding tissues. Corrosion resistance can be improved by introducing other elements into the material matrix (alloying) and by passivation processes. *Passivation* consists of immersing an alloy in a strong nitric acid solution for 10 to 30 minutes (ASTM F86).

This process generates a thin, transparent but dense oxide film on the surface of the material.

PEARL

A corrosion-resistant film can be placed on a metal implant by immersing it in a nitric acid solution. This process is called *passivation*.

Metals and metal alloys most commonly used for orthopaedic applications include stainless steel, cobalt-chromium, and titanium. Other metals such as tantalum, platinum, gold, and silver, although extremely inert, have seen limited use as biomaterials due to their poor mechanical properties.

Stainless Steel

Stainless steel alloys designated for biomedical applications are commonly referred to by their American Institute of Steel and Iron (AISI) classification as types 316 and 316L. The composition of both types includes chromium (16–20 wt%) and molybdenum (2–4 wt%) as alloying elements. Type 316L is differentiated from type 316 by its lower carbon content (0.03% maximum vs. 0.08%, respectively). Material and manufacturing requirements are specified by ASTM standards F138, F139, and F621.

Although chromium is a reactive element, it can be passivated to provide excellent corrosion resistance in alloy form. The addition of chromium imparts a protective, self-regenerating oxide layer to stainless steel. The inclusion of molybdenum and nickel along with the decrease in carbon content further enhance corrosion properties. Although other stainless steel alloys are designated for use in surgical implants (ASTM F745, F1314), types 316 and 316L provide better resistance to corrosion than any other stainless steel alloy.

Nonetheless, stainless steel implants are still susceptible to corrosion. In multicomponent devices such as plate and screws, improper fit or differences in composition can produce crevice, fretting, or galvanic corrosion. The reader is referred to Shackelford (1996) or other materials science texts for a more in-depth discussion of corrosion mechanisms. Thus, stainless steel alloys are better suited for devices that are intended to remain in the body for a limited time and will be removed when they have served their purpose (e.g., fracture fixation).

Cobalt-Chromium Alloys

Although ASTM lists four types of cobalt-based alloys for biomedical applications, only two are used extensively for implant fabrication: cast cobalt-chromium-molybdenum (CoCrMo) alloy (ASTM F75) and wrought cobalt-nickel-chromium-molybdenum (CoNiCrMo) alloy (ASTM F562). As was the case for stainless steel, the addition of chromium (Cr) produces a highly resistant, passive film that contributes greatly to excellent corrosion resistance of both alloys. The addition of molybdenum (Mo) to CoCr alloys increases strength but decreases ductility of the material.

Differences in the composition of these two alloys are reflected in their mechanical properties. Wrought CoNiCrMo exhibits exceptional fatigue and ultimate tensile strength, making it particularly well-suited to the extreme mechanical demands associated with heavily loaded joints (e.g., femoral stems). However, despite having wear properties similar to that of CoCrMo, the inferior frictional properties of CoNiCrMo make it unsuitable for use as a bearing surface.

Titanium and Titanium Alloys

Unalloyed or commercially pure titanium (Ti) and titanium alloys are both used for implants (ASTM F67, F136, F620). Titanium's lower density (4.5 g/cm^3) compared with other metals (7.9, 8.3, and 9.2 g/cm^3 for 316L, CoCrMo, and CoNiCrMo, respectively) results in a higher specific strength (ratio of strength to density) than that of any other material. Pure titanium, although highly reactive, derives its corrosion resistance from a thin, adherent, solid oxide layer (TiO_2) that forms on the surface and effectively passivates the material. The corrosion resistance of Ti and its alloys greatly exceeds that of stainless steel and Co-Cr alloys.

Four grades of unalloyed or commercially pure titanium have been specified based on impurity content, with the maximum allowable weight percent established by ASTM F67-89. With increasing impurity content (increasing grade number), strength increases and ductility decreases. Both ductility and strength are strongly influenced by oxygen content.

Because of its low shear strength, commercially pure Ti is primarily used as a porous coating in Ti-based cementless prostheses and fiber-metal pads on arthroplasty components.

With the addition of alloying elements, the mechanical properties of titanium can vary over a wide range. The most commonly used Ti alloy for biomedical applications, Ti-6Al-4V, includes the addition of aluminum (5.5–6.5 wt%) and vanadium (3.5–4.5 wt%) as alloying elements. Heat treating or annealing of Ti-6Al-4V enhances its ductility. The lower stiffness of titanium compared with stainless steel and cobalt-chrome (approximately 110 GPa) has been reported to reduce the severity of stress-shielding and cortical osteoporosis associated with the use of more rigid materials for total joint arthroplasty components and fixation devices.

Polymers

Polymers are long-chain molecules formed from smaller molecules (monomers) by a polymerization reaction. Chains can be arranged in one of three ways: linearly, branched, or cross-linked. Cross-linking between chains creates a more ordered, three-dimensional arrangement within the material. The physical properties of polymers are influenced by their composition, molecular weight and length, degree of cross-linking, temperature, and loading rate, among other factors. Increasing chain length, molecular weight, size of side groups, and/or degree of cross-linking decreases the relative mobility of the chains within the polymer and generally results in higher strength. The long-chain molecular structure of polysaccharides and proteins places them in the category of biological polymers.

Polyethylene

Polyethylene is available commercially in five major grades based on density and molecular weight (ASTM F639, F755). Of those five, only UHMWPE (molecular weight $> 2 \times 10^6$ g/mol) is used extensively in orthopaedic implants. Due to its relatively low coefficient of friction, UHMWPE is particularly well-suited for bearing surface applications (e.g., acetabular cup, tibial plateau, and patellar surface). In bulk form, polyethylene is relatively inert and exhibits little or no environmental degradation. However, susceptibility to long-term wear and creep results in polyethylene wear particles that can, in turn, elicit an osteolytic host response.

Acrylic Polymers

Polymethylmethacrylate (PMMA; ASTM F451) is the most common type of acrylic polymer employed in orthopaedic applications. Widely referred to as bone cement, its uses include that of a grouting agent for fixation of joint prostheses within bone, a supplement to spinal fixation, and a filler for pathologic fractures. Although PMMA exhibits excellent biocompatibility in solid form, concerns arise because of its polymerization reaction. The exothermic nature of this reaction raises temperatures sufficiently to cause localized thermal necrosis of adjacent tissues. The peak reaction temperature is a function of both the thickness and the weight of the cement mass. In addition, a potentially toxic monomer that is not fully polymerized may be released into the surrounding tissue during or after polymerization.

The mechanical properties of PMMA also depend on polymerization conditions. If the material heats too quickly or becomes too hot as a result of the polymerization reaction, a decrease in mechanical properties results. PMMA characteristically exhibits higher strengths in compression than in tension or shear.

Biodegradable Polymers

Biodegradable polymers such as polyglycolic acid (PGA) differ from most other materials in that they are intended to be broken down and absorbed by the body over a period of time. Absorption of the material corresponds with a gradual decrease in the mechanical properties. Biodegradable polymers have been considered for use in fracture fixation as a means to increase load transmission within the bone and decrease load transmission through the fixation device as healing progresses. Implants fabricated from biodegradable polymers have the added advantage of not requiring surgical removal. However, the rate at which absorption occurs is difficult to control. Other potential applications include use as a temporary scaffold or support for tissue repair processes.

Ceramics

Ceramics are chemical compounds comprised of at least one metallic element and one of five nonmetallic elements: carbon, nitrogen, oxygen, phosphorus, or sulfur. Due to their insolubility and low chemical reactivity, these compounds display excellent biocompatibility. Ceramic materials possess high compressive strength and hardness, but they are especially susceptible to failure in tension. Tensile loading opens microcracks that tend to develop within ceramics, encouraging crack propagation and resulting in a lower tensile strength. Ceramics characteristically fail as a result of brittle fracture, with little or no plastic deformation. Ceramics possess a low coefficient of friction and exceptional wear resistance, making them well-suited for high wear applications (e.g., prosthetic femoral head). Ceramics used for biomedical applications fall into one of three categories based on their chemical reactivity with the host tissue: nonabsorbable, bioactive, or biodegradable.

Nonabsorbable ceramics such as alumina (Al_2O_3; ASTM F603) and carbon are relatively inert materials that maintain their physical and mechanical properties in the biological environment. Alumina implants exhibit extremely small surface roughness that is responsible for decreased friction and surface wear. Alumina has the lowest coefficient of friction μ of any synthetic bearing material in contact with itself (approx. 0.09 vs. 0.5 and 0.35 for steel and CoCr, respectively). Of the different carbon groups, only pyrolitic carbon is used for orthopaedic applications. Because of its excellent compatibility with tissue, carbon is used as a surface coating for implants. It is also employed as a reinforcing fiber in composite materials. Attempts to reconstruct ligaments using bundles of carbon fibers have been largely unsuccessful.

Bioactive or surface reactive ceramics are semi-inert materials designed to encourage bonding with the surrounding tissue and/or to be absorbed in vivo. Materials in this group include dense, polycrystalline glass-ceramics such as Bioglass

and Ceravital®. However, the same material formulation which ensures biocompatibility is also responsible for inferior mechanical properties. Because of their brittleness, bioactive ceramics are unsuitable for structural applications and are restricted to use as a filler for bony defects or a surface coating to enhance fixation of metal implants.

Biodegradable or resorbable ceramics are noninert materials that degrade in vivo and are replaced by endogenous tissues. Almost all biodegradable ceramics are variations of calcium phosphate (e.g., aluminum calcium phosphate; hydroxyapatite, ASTM F1185; and tricalcium phosphate, ASTM F1088). Hydroxyapatite is a crystallized form of calcium phosphate, with a chemical composition $[Ca_{10}(PO_4)_6(OH)_2]$ similar to that of the mineral phase of bone. Variations in composition, structure, and manufacturing processes result in a wide range of mechanical properties. Biodegradable ceramics are used to reinforce or replace bone and as a coating for other implant materials.

Composites

Any material comprising two or more distinct constituent materials or phases can be considered a composite material. In some cases (i.e., cellular solids such as cancellous bone and porous coatings), voids or empty spaces may be considered as one constituent. In contrast to metal alloys and ceramics, each constituent retains its chemical, structural, and mechanical identity. A composite material may have dramatically different physical properties than those of its individual constituents. The physical properties of the composite are dependent on a number of factors including the volume fraction of the constituents, the shape of the inclusions (e.g., fiber, particle, or lamina), the structure or arrangement of the constituents, and the strength of the interfacial bond between the constituents. Biocompatibility of the composite material demands that each of the constituent materials be biocompatible and the interface be resistant to environmental degradation.

By combining two or more of the material types discussed above, it is possible to custom design a material that is stronger and lighter than conventional materials, with physical properties that more closely approximate host tissues. Although composite materials are routinely used in other applications, most notably in the aerospace industry, their potential for biomedical applications has not yet been fully realized. Widespread use of composite materials in orthopaedics is currently limited to casting materials.

Biological and Tissue Engineered Materials

Most biological materials can be classified as composites. Musculoskeletal tissue such as bone, cartilage, and muscle consist of a complex mixture of organic fibers, inorganic matrix, and water; the properties of these tissues are dependent on the nature of that mixture, in much the same manner as those of synthetic composite materials. Biological materials are unique, however, in that they are living, metabolically active tissues that adapt to the demands of their mechanical environment and are capable of remodeling and repair. Tissue composition and mechanical properties are both influenced by changes in functional demands and vary considerably with anatomical location, orientation with respect to loading, biological age, etc. For a more detailed discussion of the material aspects of biological tissues, the reader is referred to Fung (1993).

Recent research efforts have focused on the development of "tissue engineered" materials. These new materials comprise a combination of biological tissues and engineering materials and are designed to be more efficacious in repairing or augmenting host tissues than either of the constituents alone. For example, a synthetic mesh may serve as a scaffold to which living cells can be attached and proliferate. Although synthetic materials used in this manner meet the definition of a biomaterial, the combination of synthetic and biological material effectively creates a composite biomaterial for successive use in other applications.

SELECTED BIBLIOGRAPHY

American Society for Testing and Materials. Section 13: Medical devices and services. In: *Annual Book of ASTM Standards*. Philadelphia, PA: ASTM; 1996.

BAJPAI PK and BILLOTTE WG. Ceramic biomaterials. In: Bronzino JD, ed. *The Biomedical Engineering Handbook*. Boca Raton, FL: CRC Press; 1995:552–580.

BLACK J. *Biological Performance of Materials*. 2nd ed. New York, NY: Dekker; 1992.

CALLAGHAN JJ. The clinical results and basic science of total hip arthroplasty with porous-coated prosthesis. *J Bone Jt Surg*. 1993;75A:299–310.

DUCHEYNE P, HASTINGS GW, eds. *Metal and Ceramic Biomaterials*. Boca Raton, FL; CRC Press; 1984.

FRIEDMAN RJ, BLACK J, GALANTE JO, JACOBS JJ, SKINNER HB. Current concepts in orthopaedic biomaterials and implant fixation. *J Bone Jt Surg*. 1993;75A:1086–1109.

FUNG YC. *Biomechanics: Mechanical Properties of Living Tissues*. 2nd ed. New York, NY: Springer-Verlag; 1993.

GIBSON LJ, ASHBY MF. *Cellular Solids: Structure and Properties*. Oxford, England: Pergammon Press; 1988.

LAKES R. Composite biomaterials. In: Bronzino JD, ed. *The Biomedical Engineering Handbook*. Boca Raton, FL: CRC Press; 1995:598–610.

LEE HB, KIM SS, KHANG G. Polymeric biomaterials. In: Bronzino JD, ed. *The Biomedical Engineering Handbook*. Boca Raton, FL: CRC Press; 1995:581–597.

MOONEY DJ, LANGER RS. Engineering biomaterials for tissue engineering: the 10–100 micron size scale. In: Bronzino JD, ed. *The Biomedical Engineering Handbook*. Boca Raton, FL: CRC Press; 1995: 1609–1618.

PARK JB. Metallic biomaterials. In: Bronzino JD, ed. *The Biomedical Engineering Handbook*. Boca Raton, FL: CRC Press; 1995:537–551.

PARK JB, LAKES RS. *Biomaterials: An Introduction*. 2nd ed. New York, NY: Plenum; 1992.

SHACKELFORD JF. *Introduction to Materials Science for Engineers*, 4th ed. Upper Saddle River, NJ: Prentice-Hall; 1996.

VON RECUM AF, ed. *Handbook of Biomaterials Evaluation*. New York, NY: Macmillan; 1986.

WRIGHT TM, GOODMAN SB, eds. *Implant Wear: The Future of Total Joint Replacement*. Rosemont, IL: American Academy of Orthopaedic Surgeons; 1996.

SAMPLE QUESTIONS

1. Compared with the properties of Co-Ni-Cr-Mo, Ti-6Al-4V alloy has a:
   (a) lower ultimate strength
   (b) lower elastic modulus
   (c) higher specific strength
   (d) all of the above

2. An elastic, isotropic material specimen with a rectangular cross-section (1 cm $\times$ 2 cm) and length of 10 cm is subjected to a uniaxial load of 5000 N, resulting in a longitudinal displacement of 1 mm. What is the elastic modulus for this material?
   (a) 2500 N/cm^2
   (b) 2.5 GPa
   (c) 5000 N/cm
   (d) 125 GPa

3. For a material with a Poisson's ratio of 0.5, which of the following is true:
   (a) longitudinal strain is less than transverse strain
   (b) true stress is equal to engineering stress (i.e., cross-sectional area remains constant)

   (c) volume of the specimen remains constant
   (d) volume of the specimen decreases by wdΔL cm^3, where w, d, and ΔL equal width, depth, and change in length of the specimen, respectively.

4. Which of the following are not material properties:
   (a) load-to-failure
   (b) elastic modulus
   (c) yield strength
   (d) cross-sectional area

5. A metal plate with a cross-sectional area of 100 mm^2 and an elastic modulus of 200 GPa is securely attached to the periosteal surface of a bone with a cross-sectional area of 500 mm^2 and an elastic modulus of 20 GPa. A compressive load of 1200 N is applied to the ends of the bone. In the region where the plate is attached, how much of the load is transferred through the bone? (Hint: Because the two materials are securely attached to each other, strain must be the same in both materials.)

(a) 120 N (10%)
(b) 400 N (33%)
(c) 600 N (50%)
(d) 1000 N (83%)

Solutions to Sample Questions

1. Referring to Figure 2–5:

	CoNiCrMo	Ti-6Al-4V
Ultimate strength	1000 MPa	860 MPa
Elastic modulus	220GPa	110 GPa

The lower density of Ti-6-4 compared with CoCrNiMo (4.5 vs 9.2 g/cm^3, respectively) results in a higher specific strength for titanium (i.e., ratio of strength to density). Therefore, the correct answer is (d).

2. Elastic modulus:

$E = \sigma/\varepsilon$.

$= (P/A)/(\Delta l/l)$, where $\sigma = P/A$ and $\varepsilon = \Delta l/l$

$= Pl/wh \Delta l$, where $A = wh$

Substituting known values:

$w = 1$ cm, $h = 2$ cm, $l = 10$ cm, $P = 5000$ N,

$\Delta l = 1$ mm.

$E = 2500$ N/mm^2

$= 2.5$ GPa

Note: 1 gigaPascal (GPa) $= 10^3$ megaPascals (MPa); 1 MPa $= 1$ N/mm^2. Therefore, the correct answer is (b).

3. Referring to Figure 2–1, Poisson's ratio $= -$ (transverse strain/longitudinal strain).
   (a) For $\nu < 1$, longitudinal strain must be $>$ transverse strain.
   (b) If the true stress equals the engineering stress, then the cross-sectional dimension and area must be constant. Thus, transverse strain $= 0$ and $\nu = 0$.
   (c) As defined in the text, materials with $\nu = 0.5$ are said to be incompressible.

(d) Any decrease in volume is inconsistent with the definition of an incompressible material.
Therefore, the correct answer is (c).

4. Material properties are independent of the geometry of the material specimen. Because load-to-failure and cross-sectional area are a function of the specimen, the correct answer is both (a) and (d).

5. Since both components are assumed to deform equally and share a 1200 N load:

$$\varepsilon 1 = \varepsilon 2 \qquad (1)$$

$$F_1 + F_2 = 1200 \text{ N} \qquad (2)$$

Where ε represents strain, F represents load, and subscripts 1 and 2 denote the plate and bone, respectively. Substituting for $= \varepsilon = \sigma/E = (F/A)/E = FA/E$ in equation (1):

$$F_1 A_1/E_1 = F_2 A_2/E_2$$

solving for F_2:

$$F_2 = F_1(E_2 A_2/E_1 A_1)$$

substituting for $F_2 =$ in equation (2):

$$F_1 + F_1(E_2 A_2/E_1 A_1) = 1200 \text{ N}$$

$$F_1 = 1200/(1 + E_2 A_2/E_1 A_1)$$

substituting given values for E_1, A_1, E_2, and A_2:

$$F_1 = 800 \text{ N}$$
$$F_2 = 1200 - 800 = 400 \text{ N}$$

Two thirds of the applied load is transferred through the metal plate and one third is transferred through the bone. Therefore, the correct answer is (b).

Chapter 3

Bone

Joseph M. Lane, MD

Outline

The structural integrity of the human musculoskeletal system depends on normal bone growth and development. Repetitive mechanical stress and occasional mechanical failure require a repair system to ensure skeletal integrity for locomotion. An understanding of the structure, development, metabolism, and healing of bone is essential for orthopaedic practice.

STRUCTURE, DEVELOPMENT, AND METABOLISM OF BONE

Bone is a well-organized, biphasic, composite tissue. The major organic component is type I collagen. Other peptides such as osteopontin, osteocalcin, bone sialoproteins, and growth factors including the bone morphogenetic proteins (BMPs) are present in lesser amounts. The predominant inorganic phase is hydroxyapatite.

Collagen provides tensile strength. It has a triple helix structure with overlapping hole zones. Hydroxyapatite provides compressive strength and is deposited adjacent to the collagen fibrils in the hole zones. The result is a ceramic and organic composite with tensile and compressive strength.

The ultrastructure of bone comprises cortical and cancellous bone. *Cortical bone* makes up the outer surface of a bone and is thickest in the diaphysis. Cortical bone is dense lamellar bone with limited spaces consisting largely of haversian canals and deeply buried osteocytes connected to the surface through a series of canaliculi. *Cancellous bone* is located within the bone and is most abundant in the epiphysis and metaphysis of bones. It has a trabecular structure with a large surface area. Cortical bone is significantly stronger than cancellous bone but is far less metabolically active.

Bone Cells

The predominant bone cells are osteoblasts, osteocytes, and osteoclasts. *Osteoblasts* are bone-forming cells that are bound to the surface of the cancellous trabeculae and endosteal cortex within haversian canals. Primitive mesenchymal cells differentiate into osteoblasts when stimulated by various growth factors including insulin-derived growth factor, platelet-derived growth factor, interleukins, and BMPs. Parathyroid hormone induces osteoblasts to become metabolically active. Active osteoblasts produce bone matrix consisting of type I collagen, osteocalcin, and various trace inorganic components. They also facilitate the mineralization of the matrix. Osteoblasts encapsulated within bone in lacunae are called osteocytes. *Osteocytes* are connected through canaliculi to each other and to the surfaces of bone. The total surface area of the canaliculi and osteocytes accounts for almost 90% of the total internal and external surface area of bone. Osteocytes are believed to have an important role in calcium flux.

Osteoclasts control bone resorption. These cells are derived from multiple macrophages that consolidate and bind to the surface of bone. Cell surface proteins called integrins bind osteoclasts to specific sites. The osteoclast forms a "ruffled border" adjacent to an area of bone resorption. The cell secretes acids to solubilize the calcium and phosphate and acid proteases to degrade the collagen matrix. The area of bone resorption microscopically resembles a pit and is called a Howship's lacuna (Fig. 3–1). Calcitonin directly activates osteoclasts. Parathyroid hormone (PTH) also increases osteoclastic bone resorption by stimulating osteoblasts to produce a local humoral factor that activates osteoclasts. Osteoclastic bone resorption and osteoblastic bone formation are coupled and reciprocal. Coordinated regulation of osteoblasts and osteoclasts results in constant bone turnover without net gain or loss of bone mass.

Orthopaedic Surgery: The Essentials. Edited by M.E. Baratz, A.D. Watson, and J.E. Imbriglia. Thieme Medical Publishers, Inc., New York © 1999

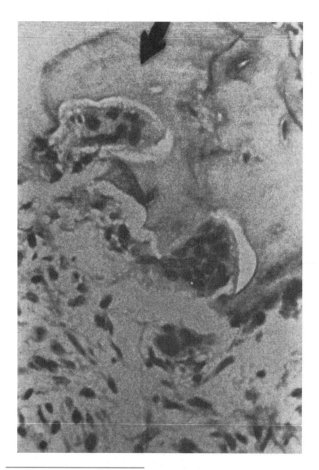

Figure 3–1 Howship's lacunae with multinucleated osteoclast marked by arrow. (Reprinted with permission from Form and Function of Bone by Frederick S et al. In Orthopaedic Basic Science, ed. S. R. Simon, 1994)

PEARL

Parathyroid hormone (PTH) stimulates osteoclasts indirectly by activating osteoblasts.

Embryonic Development and Bone Growth

Embryonic bone development can occur by intramembranous or enchondral bone formation. Intramembranous bone formation occurs with flat bones such as the scapulae and cranial bones. Long bones develop by enchondral bone formation.

Intramembranous bone formation is appositional. The periosteum of any bone comprises an inner cambrial layer and an outer adventitial layer. The cambrial layer generates organic matrix, which in turn is mineralized. Osteoblasts and osteoclasts remodel the bone to convert it from immature woven bone to mature lamellar bone.

The long bones are formed by enchondral bone development. The limb begins as a consolidation of primitive tissues that become a cartilage anlage. Growth and development of the diaphysis and metaphysis occur by chondrocyte proliferation and matrix production. Blood vessels invade the central portion of the cartilage anlage to establish the primary ossification center. A dominant longitudinal nutrient vessel establishes the marrow space. The nutrient vessel branches distally and proximally to its central entry point to become metaphyseal vessels. The vessels bring cells and substrates for mineralization of the matrix to form woven bone, which is remodeled by osteoblasts and osteoclasts into mature lamellar bone. Mineralization likewise begins centrally and progresses proximally and distally.

Nutrient vessels also enter the proximal and distal portions of the cartilage anlage, branch to become epiphyseal vessels, and establish the secondary ossification centers. The secondary ossification centers have peripheral avascular cartilage similar to the physeal cartilage. They undergo enchondral ossification as well to form the subchondral bone and overlying articular cartilage.

The metaphyseal and epiphyseal vessels do not anastomose. The avascular cartilage boundary that separates the metaphyseal and epiphyseal vessels forms the physis where longitudinal and metaphyseal radial growth occur. The fibrous tissue that encircles the physis is called the fibrous ring of LaCroix and is nourished by a third metaphyseal vessel.

Longitudinal growth occurs primarily at the physis. The physis is divided into a *reserve zone* of resting chondrocytes, a *proliferative zone* of dividing chondrocytes, a *hypertrophic zone* of metabolically active chondrocytes, and the *zone of calcification* where immature bone is formed and eventually remodeled.

The reserve zone of chondrocytes are minimally metabolically active. Oxygen tension is very low even though the epiphyseal vessels pass nearby. These chondrocytes store energy and produce proteoglycan matrix. The reserve zone occupies nearly 50% of the width of the physis. It does not contribute to the growth of the physeal plate and bone, but proteoglycans are produced that provide mechanical support.

The proliferative zone is subjacent to the reserve zone. Unlike the random arrangement of chondrocytes in the reserve zone, proliferative zone chondrocytes are arranged in columns. The epiphyseal vessels pass through the reserve zone and terminate at the first chondrocyte of the proliferative zone. These chondrocytes undergo a series of genetically programmed mitoses. The number of cell duplications determines the absolute length of the bone. The high oxygen tension in the proliferative zone permits aerobic metabolism that produces large amounts of adenosine triphosphate (ATP) to fuel matrix production. Cellular proliferation and matrix production together lead to linear growth.

Preparation of the cartilage for mineralization takes place in the hypertrophic zone, which is subjacent to the proliferative zone. The columnar arrangement of chondrocytes continues into the hypertrophic zone where the chondrocytes hypertrophy and prepare the matrix for mineralization and subsequent bone remodeling. The oxygen tension is lower in the hypertrophic zone and the glycogen stored by proliferative zone chondrocytes is expended in the hypertrophic zone to provide energy. In the portion of the hypertrophic zone immediately subjacent to the proliferative zone, the chondrocyte mitochondria absorb large volumes of calcium. As chondrocytes progress through the hypertrophic zone towards the bone metaphysis, they deplete their glycogen stores and the mitochondria release their stored calcium. Matrix vesicles bud from the chondrocytes in the hypertrophic zone and are most numerous near the metaphysis.

These vesicles contain enzymes necessary to initiate mineralization with hydroxyapatite. The vesicles absorb the calcium released from the mitochondria of the dying chondrocytes. The abundant proteoglycans in cartilage inhibit mineralization, therefore the matrix vesicles are essential to developing a local environment favorable for initiation of crystallization.

The calcified cartilage bars in the matrix between the chondrocyte columns constitute the zone of calcification and are the substrates for bone formation. Metaphyseal vessels between the calcified cartilage bars provide cellular and inorganic components necessary for transformation of the calcified cartilage bars to woven bone. The vessels also remove the dead hypertrophic chondrocytes. Once the bone is deposited in the matrix, it is remodeled to form lamellar bone by the coordinated activity of osteoblasts and osteoclasts.

The articular portion of the epiphysis grows and develops in a manner similar to physeal growth. The zone of calcification becomes the subchondral bone. Histologically, the "tide mark" represents the adult remnant of the zone of calcification.

PEARL

Longitudinal growth occurs primarily in the proliferative zone and is due to cell division and matrix production. Bone formation is initiated by mineralization in the hypertrophic zone.

The peripheral physis consists of the groove of Ranvier and the perichondral ring of LaCroix. The metabolically active groove of Ranvier produces latitudinal columns of chondrocytes that proliferate to increase radial growth of the physis. The perichondral ring of LaCroix is a fibrous membrane surrounding the physis that attaches to the epiphysis and metaphysis. It resists the lateral bulge of the physis that occurs with compressive load.

The biochemistry of the physis is complex. Type II collagen and proteoglycans are present throughout the physis and provide structural support. Type X collagen is found in the hypertrophic zone bordering the zone of calcification. It is believed to facilitate matrix mineralization. Oxygen tension is low in the reserve zone, high in the proliferative zone, and low again in the hypertrophic zone. Chondrocyte glycogen content is highest in the reserve zone and is gradually depleted as the chondrocytes progress through each zone until death in the zone of calcification. Mitochondria make ATP to fuel proliferation, matrix production, and calcium accumulation in the aerobic, glycogen-rich proliferative zone. Calcium is then released and used by the matrix vesicles to mineralize disaggregated matrix. Acid mucopolysaccharides facilitate proteoglycan disaggregation to permit mineralization. Type II collagen is degraded and replaced by Type I collagen as the woven bone is remodeled to lamellar bone.

PEARL

Type X collagen is found in the hypertrophic zone and is thought to facilitate mineralization.

Bone remodeling requires the coordinated activity of osteoclasts and osteoblasts. The process takes place continually in the routine maintenance of the skeleton, but it can be accelerated by trauma, metabolic disturbances, or growth. Both cancellous and cortical bone can be remodeled from the surface or by "cutting cones." Cutting cones consist of a group of osteoclasts that excavate bone to resemble a funnel and are followed by migrating osteoblasts that fill the funnel with new bone. Cutting cone remodeling is more common in cortical bone, and surface remodeling is more common in cancellous bone.

Physeal growth is a function of the number of divisions of the reserve zone chondrocytes that establish the chondrocyte columns in the proliferating zone. The number of divisions is genetically determined to assure symmetrical limb growth and is affected by hormones including growth hormone, thyroid hormone, estrogen, and testosterone. Primary or secondary deficiency of any may lead to dwarfing. Growth hormone stimulates growth, and the sex hormones accelerate growth. An excess of growth hormone and/or the sex hormones may cause early physeal closure and termination of growth.

Skeletal dysplasias are commonly physeal disorders. Achondroplastic dwarfism is due to a defect in the proliferative zone. Rickets is due to the failure of calcification in the hypertrophic zone and zone of calcification. Chondrocyte proliferation and hypertrophy occurs normally, but no mineralization takes place because of a vitamin D deficit. Osteopetrosis is the failure to remodel the calcified cartilage in the zone of calcification and metaphysis. Osteochondromas occur when proliferating latitudinal cell columns from the groove of Ranvier escape through the cambrial layer of the perichondral ring of LaCroix.

Bone Metabolism

Bone metabolism is under complex and strict hormonal control. Parathyroid hormone, calcitonin, and vitamin D are the hormonal regulators of bone metabolism. All three influence osteoblasts, osteocytes, and osteoclasts to regulate calcium and phosphate metabolism by way of bone turnover.

Parathyroid hormone is produced by the parathyroid glands. Low serum calcium increases serum parathyroid hormone levels. Direct actions of PTH to increase serum calcium include renal retention of calcium and excretion of phosphate. Indirectly, PTH increases serum calcium by converting 25-hydroxy-vitamin D to metabolically active 1,25-dihydroxy-vitamin D in the kidney. The 1,25-dihydroxy-vitamin D increases gut absorption of calcium. Osteoclastic bone resorption and liberation of calcium increases when PTH stimulates osteoblasts to produce an osteoclast-activating factor.

Vitamin D is synthesized from 7-dehydrocholesterol in the skin when stimulated by ultraviolet light. It is then converted to 25-hydroxy-vitamin D in the liver, and then to 1,25-dihydroxy-vitamin D in the kidney under the influence of PTH. The active form of vitamin D increases calcium absorption in the ileum by interacting with calcium binding protein on the surface of luminal cells. 1,25-dihydroxy-vitamin D also augments PTH recruitment of osteoclasts.

Calcitonin is produced by the parafollicular cells of the thyroid gland. High serum calcium levels increase serum calcitonin levels. Calcitonin directly decreases the number and activity of osteoclasts to decrease serum calcium. Indirectly, calcitonin is a diuretic that increases renal excretion of calcium.

Calcium requirements vary with age. Absorption becomes less efficient with age. Daily calcium requirements are 400 to 700 mg for children, 1300 mg for individuals aged 10 to 25, 500 mg for adults, 1500 mg for pregnant women, 2000 mg for lactating women, and 1500 mg for postmenopausal women. Individuals recovering from a major fracture require at least 1500 mg of calcium daily.

PEARL

The daily calcium requirement for post menopausal women is 1500 mg/day.

Calcium absorption is facilitated by low gastric pH, 1,25-dihydroxy-vitamin D, and a calcium to phosphorous ratio between 1:1 and 1:2. Inhibitors of calcium absorption include achlorhydria, vitamin D deficiency, malabsorptive disorders such as sprue or blind loop syndrome, renal disorders, non-thiazide diuretics, glucosuria, renal tubular acidosis, and high food content of phosphates, fats, phytates (tea), and oxalates (spinach).

Phosphate absorption occurs in the colon. It is excreted in the urine. The daily requirement is 1000 to 1500 mg. Phosphate absorption inhibitors include calcium, aluminum, and beryllium. Parathyroid hormone increases renal excretion.

FRACTURE HEALING, REMODELING, NONUNION, AND BONE GRAFTING

Fracture repair is a combination of healing and regeneration. Healing, by definition, involves inflammation and scar formation at the site of injury. No inflammation or scarring occur with regeneration—instead, new bone forms at the fracture site that incorporates with the bone on either side of the fracture.

Fracture of a bone disrupts the local microvascular structures. Bleeding creates a hematoma. Hematoma formation initiates the inflammatory process, which is mediated by cell-derived chemical messengers. The inflammatory process organizes the hematoma to provisionally stabilize the fracture and serve as a "scaffold" for further healing. Platelets release TGF-β, which stimulate macrophages to produce fibroblast growth factors that activate local angiogenesis.

Angiogenesis is essential for providing oxygen, nutrients, inflammatory cells, and stem cells to the healing fracture. Inflammatory cells modulate healing, stimulate collagen production by fibroblasts, and clear necrotic cells and debris. Cell proliferation continues and chemical mediators are produced that induce stem cells to differentiate into osteoblasts and osteoclasts. Local osteocytes and cambrial cells of the periosteum are induced to participate in fracture healing and bone regeneration.

Induction is a complex process that is initiated by physical and chemical stimuli. Initially, the oxygen tension and local pH are low in spite of angiogenesis. Lysosomal enzymes, kinins, growth factors, and TGF-β are abundant. This local environment fosters clearance of necrotic debris and formation of proteoglycan-rich chondroid. The induced cells produce proteoglycans on the collagen matrix made by the fibroblasts that were stimulated by the initial inflammatory response. Types I, II, III, and XI collagen constitute the matrix. There is little mineralization at this stage.

Enchondral ossification then occurs. Insulin-like growth factor and BMPs increase, and the pH normalizes. Proteoglycans and Type XI collagen are gradually degraded and replaced with type I collagen. The induced osteoblasts and osteocytes produce osteoid and mineralization increases. The cartilage is calcified and these calcified cartilage bars become woven bone. The remodeling process converts the woven bone to lamellar bone. Osteoclasts and osteoblasts are active in the remodeling process.

Physical stimuli also direct fracture healing. Failure of the bone at the time of fracture initiates the inflammatory process. The inflammatory process produces fibrous tissue at the fracture site that stabilizes the fracture and decreases the strain. Compression at the fracture site initiates cartilage formation at the fracture site. The cartilage further stabilizes the fracture. Enchondral ossification proceeds when the strain at the fracture site is less than 3%.

Motion at the fracture affects fracture healing. Rigid immobilization of the fracture leads to healing by "creeping substitution" with remodeling by cutting cones. Osteoclasts from one fragment resorb bone and migrate across the fracture site into the second fragment. Osteoblasts follow the osteoclasts to form bone that bridges the fracture site. Enchondral ossification does not take place.

Healing occurs by enchondral ossification and periosteal new bone formation if motion occurs at the fracture as occurs in a cast or after intramedullary nailing. Callus forms and increases the diameter of the bone at the fracture site. The increased diameter at the site of healing increases the strength of the injured bone because the strength of a rod increases with the square of its radius. As the callus remodels from woven bone to mechanically stronger lamellar bone, resorption decreases the diameter to that of the native bone.

PEARL

Healing by "creeping substitution" requires absolute contact and immobilization between the fracture fragments. Callus formation is capable of occurring when small gaps and incomplete immobilization are present.

Acute fracture care methods include cast immobilization, external fixation, internal fixation with plates and screws, and intramedullary nailing. Each method immobilizes fracture fragments to varying degrees. The fracture healing process with each method is a function of each method's inherent biomechanics.

Cast immobilization can control bending, translation, and rotation within the limits of the cast's ability to immobilize the fracture fragments. Fracture healing occurs by callus formation with cast immobilization. Cast immobilization is noninvasive, and no iatrogenic injury to the periosteal and endosteal blood supply occurs.

External fixation is minimally invasive, and improves immobilization by directly controlling the fracture fragments. Fracture healing occurs by callus formation because the immobilization is not rigid. Thermal or mechanical injury to the periosteal and endosteal blood supply may occur when the external fixator pins are drilled into the bone fragments.

Open reduction and internal fixation with plates and screws can achieve nearly complete immobilization through rigid fixation. Open reduction restores anatomic alignment, and internal fixation rigidly immobilizes the fracture fragments. Compression at the fracture site is essential because interlocking of the fracture fragments improves immobilization. Compression does not stimulate osteogenesis as is commonly thought. In fact, compression may cause local osteopenia from pressure necrosis, stress shielding, and decreased circulation under the plate. Stress shielding occurs because the plate is stiffer than bone, and bone forms in response to the stresses it receives. The stiffer plate absorbs most of the stress at the fracture site, and thus, osteoclast resorption exceeds osteoblast synthesis. The resulting bone resorption reduces the interlocking of the fragments, and compression and immobilization decrease. Therefore, bone healing is mostly by creeping substitution, but some callus forms as immobilization is lost. Internal fixation also injures the periosteal blood supply at the fracture site because the periosteum must be stripped off the bone to facilitate reduction and apply the plate.

Intramedullary devices are an "internal splint" that have adequate bending and torsional stiffness but do not provide rigid immobilization. These devices immobilize a fracture by maintaining close endosteal contact throughout the length of the bone. Interlocking screws are placed proximal and distal to the fracture site through the bone and the device control rotation. It is not possible to compress the fracture site with an intramedullary device. Therefore, rigid fixation and immobilization cannot be achieved, and fracture healing occurs by callus formation. The periosteal blood supply is not jeopardized if open reduction can be avoided, but injury to the endosteal blood supply occurs, especially if reaming of the medullary canal is performed prior to inserting the intramedullary device.

Nonunion

Nonunion occurs when fracture healing fails. Causes of nonunion include inadequate reduction or immobilization, soft tissue interposition, infection, and systemic disease. Anatomic reduction and rigid immobilization foster healing by creeping substitution. Fracture gap and/or fracture site mobility lead to healing by callus formation. However, callus is unable to bridge large gaps, and enchondral ossification cannot occur at the fracture site if the strain is greater than 3%. Infection and soft tissue injury compromise the local vascular supply. More severe open fractures have correspondingly higher nonunion rates because of significant soft tissue injury and the increased likelihood of infection.

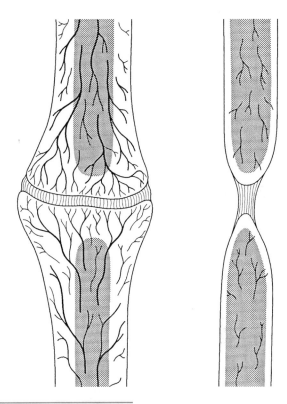

Figure 3–2 Hypertrophic nonunion (left) is distinguished by increased bone formation due to adequate healing process. Bone fragments resorb and fibrous tissue occupies fracture gap in atrophic nonunion (right).

Nonunions can be atrophic or hypertrophic (Fig. 3–2). A soft-tissue-filled gap between the fragments that consists of cartilage and fibrous tissue occurs in both. Bony resorption at the fracture site due to local vascular or nutritional compromise occurs in atrophic nonunions. The healing process is adequate in hypertrophic nonunions, but the fracture site is not mechanically stable. Therefore, hypertrophic nonunions simply require skeletal stabilization, but atrophic nonunions require biologic stimulation and skeletal stabilization. Biologic stimulation consists of debridement of the fibrous tissue and bone grafting.

Bone Grafting

Bone graft can be *autogenous*, *allogenic*, or *synthetic*. Autogenous and allogenic bone grafts can be cancellous, corticocancellous, or cortical. Vascularized bone grafts are another autogenous option. Synthetic bone grafts are typically ceramics of hydroxyapatite and, occasionally, collagen.

Incorporation of a bone graft depends on osteoconduction, osteoinduction, and osteogenesis. Not all bone grafts are capable of all three processes. A graft that provides a matrix environment conducive to bone formation is osteoconductive. Fibrillar collagen and hydroxyapatite are osteoconductive elements of all autogenic and allogenic bone grafts. A graft that contains materials that can initiate bone formation is osteoinductive. Bone marrow, hematoma, osteoprogenitor cells, and noncollagenous proteins such as growth factors and BMPs are osteoinductive elements. Grafts capable of osteogenesis contain growth factors and BMPs. Only autogenous bone grafts can be potentially osteoinductive and osteogenetic.

Autogenous cancellous bone graft is the most likely to be osteoconductive, osteoinductive, and osteogenetic; however, it does not have the structural properties of cortical bone graft. Cortical bone graft contains few osteoprogenitor cells and noncollagenous proteins, and thus, is poorly osteoinductive and osteogenetic. Corticocancellous graft may offer structural advantages without markedly compromising osteoinduction and osteogenesis.

Autogenous bone grafting can be complicated by wound infection and significant pain. It may be impossible to harvest sufficient autogenous bone graft. Allograft is an acceptable substitute, but it has no osteoinductive or osteogenetic properties. Potential complications of autologous bone grafting are disease transmission and inadequate durability.

Synthetic bone graft substitutes are another option; however they are expensive, lack osteoinductive and osteogenetic properties, and have no structural strength. Growth factors and BMPs are currently being evaluated as supplements for allografts and bone graft substitutes to provide osteoinductive and osteogenetic factors.

Vascularized, free bone graft transfers are osteoconductive, osteoinductive, and osteogenetic. Other advantages include immediate vascularization of the bone graft site and structural strength. Vascularized graft options include fibula, rib, and ilium. Harvest of a vascularized, free bone graft transfer entails significant morbidity and technical complexity, but the technique is useful for spanning large defects. The fracture rate for nonvascularized fibular grafts more than 12 cm in length is 58%, whereas the rate for vascularized fibular grafts more than 12 cm in length is 22%.

METABOLIC BONE DISEASE

Hyperparathyroidism

Primary hyperparathyroidism occurs when the parathyroid glands produce excessive PTH regardless of the serum calcium. Secondary hyperparathryoidism occurs when the parathyroid glands function normally but produce high levels of PTH in response to low serum calcium levels. The most common cause of secondary hyperparathyroidism is renal failure. The diseased kidney is unable to retain calcium or convert 25-hydroxy-vitamin D to metabolically active 1,25-dihydroxy-vitamin D.

The most common clinical manifestations of hyperparathyroidism include bone pain and pathologic fractures. Symptoms of hypercalcemia due to primary hyperparathyroidism can include neuromuscular and/or emotional depression and renal calculi.

Radiographic findings in hyperparathyroidism include brown tumors, which are lytic lesions with a ground glass appearance; osteopenia; osteosclerosis; diaphyseal scalloping of the phalanges; erosion of the distal phalangeal tuft or distal clavicle; and soft tissue calcification. Serum calcium and PTH are high, serum phosphate is low, and urine calcium is high in primary hyperparathyroidism. Serum calcium is low or normal, serum PTH is high, serum phosphate is very high, and urine calcium is high in secondary hyperparathyroidism.

Histologic bony changes in primary hyperparathyroidism include active turnover with abundant osteoclasts and osteoblasts, multiple cement lines, and peritrabecular fibrosis. Similar findings occur in secondary hyperparathyroidism, but osteomalacia manifested by unmineralized osteoid predominates.

Rickets and Osteomalacia

Rickets and osteomalacia are both disorders where there is failure to mineralize physeal cartilage and osteoid. Rickets occurs in children who are unable to mineralize the hypertrophic zone of the physis adjacent to the metaphysis. Children with rickets and adults with osteomalacia are also unable to mineralize osteoid produced as part of normal bone turnover.

The most common causes of osteomalacia include primary vitamin D deficiency, malabsorption syndromes, renal osteodystrophy, and hypophosphatemic vitamin D-resistant rickets. Malabsorption syndromes cause vitamin D deficiency in spite of adequate dietary intake. Renal failure causes phosphate retention and inadequate synthesis of 1,25-dihydroxy-vitamin D in renal osteodystrophy. Hypophosphatemic vitamin D-resistant osteomalacia is hereditary and is characterized by defective renal phosphate reabsorption.

Osteomalacia can be difficult to diagnose because the signs and symptoms are frequently vague, nonspecific, and nonlocalizing. Bone pain, which may or may not be localized, is often the only presenting symptom. Muscle weakness may accompany the pain. Physical examination is often normal.

Radiographic findings of osteomalacia include stress fractures and Looser's lines (Looser's transformation zones). These are radiolucencies that represent unmineralized osteoid that was deposited to heal a stress fracture. Angulatory deformity in weight-bearing bones may develop over time with repeated stress fractures.

Diagnosis of osteomalacia requires clinical suspicion, laboratory studies, and transilial bone biopsy. Serum calcium is low or normal, serum phosphate is low, PTH is high, and 1,25-dihydroxy-vitamin D is low in Vitamin D deficiency due to inadequate dietary intake or malabsorption. Serum calcium is low or normal, serum phosphate is high, PTH is very high, and 1,25-dihydroxy-vitamin D is low in renal osteodystrophy. Serum calcium, PTH, and 1,25-dihydroxy-vitamin D are normal with profoundly decreased phosphate in vitamin D-resistant osteomalacia.

Transilial bone biopsy reveals widespread unmineralized osteoid with wide seams indicating multiple cycles of osteoid formation without mineralization. Tetracycline labeling may reveal a decreased mineralization rate manifested by indiscrete layers of labeled bone. Aluminum staining should be considered in patients on renal dialysis and will reveal aluminum deposition at the mineralization front.

Treatment of osteomalacia depends on the etiology. Primary vitamin D deficiency requires dietary supplementation of vitamin D. Vitamin D and 25-hydroxy-vitamin D supplementation are necessary in malabsorptive deficiency. Treatment of renal osteodystrophy includes low phosphate diet, 1,25-dihydroxy-vitamin D, and possibly phosphate binders. Desferoxamine to chelate aluminum may be necessary in patients on long-term renal dialysis. High dose 1,25-dihydroxy-vitamin D, phosphate supplementation, and bicarbonate are necessary to treat hypophosphatemic vitamin D-resistant osteomalacia.

The differential diagnosis of rickets is the same as that for osteomalacia; however, vitamin D deficiency is the usual cause. The modern incidence of rickets is quite low because of dietary supplementation. Patients with rickets are often short for their age, apathetic, and irritable. Frontal bossing and angulatory deformities of the lower extremities are common. Gower's sign may be present.

Radiographic findings in rickets include those of osteomalacia as well as a widened physis with cupping of the epiphysis over the metaphysis and an indistinct border between the metaphysis and physis. Histologically, the zone of provisional calcification is indistinct and the physis is wide.

Treatment of rickets, like osteomalacia, depends on the etiology. Serum levels of calcium, phosphate, PTH, and 1,25-dihydroxy-vitamin D will determine the cause; treatment guidelines for each etiology are the same as they are for osteomalacia. Bracing and possibly corrective osteotomies during adolescence may be necessary to correct angulatory deformities.

Osteoporosis

Decreased density of normal bone defines osteoporosis. Unlike osteomalacia, mineralization is normal in osteoporosis. Osteoporosis can be divided into two groups. Type I osteoporosis occurs during the immediate postmenopausal period, affects only women, and most frequently affects cancellous bone. It is due to acute estrogen deficiency. Type II osteoporosis occurs in elderly individuals with a male to female ratio of 1:2. It is believed to be due to aging and long-term calcium deficiency. It affects cancellous and cortical bone.

Men and women achieve peak bone mass at the approximate age of 25 and undergo gradual decrease thereafter. Women may have increased deficiency while pregnant and lactating if the increased calcium requirements are not met.

Bone mass markedly decreases in the immediate postmenopausal period and continues to decrease at a slower rate with age. Additional risk factors for osteoporosis include Northern European ancestry, hypothyroidism, anticonvulsant medication, and sedentary lifestyle with inadequate weight-bearing exercise such as frequent walks.

Pathologic fractures are the most common manifestation of osteoporosis. Vertebral body, proximal femur, proximal humerus, lateral tibial plateau, and distal radius fractures are the most common because of the predominance of cancellous bone in these areas. Cummings et al (1995) identified risk factors for fracture. They include maternal hip fracture, tall height and no weight gain with age, poor health, thyroid replacement, anticonvulsant medications, infrequent weight-bearing activities such as standing and walking, high resting pulse rate, benzodiazepene use, history of previous fracture after age 50, bone mass greater than 2 standard deviations less than normal, and inability to arise from a chair without using hands. The fracture rate in elderly patients is 1 per 1000 in individuals with two or fewer risk factors and 27 per 1000 in individuals with five or more risk fractures.

Unlike osteomalacia, in which patients present with generalized bone pain, patients with osteoporosis present either incidentally or when they sustain a fracture. Radiographic findings of osteoporosis include osteopenia, loss of vertebral body horizontal trabecula, and loss of the trabecular lines of the proximal femur. Radiographically evident osteopenia is not apparent until there has been at least 30% decrease in bone mass.

Laboratory studies are used to rule out a primary pathologic process resulting in osteopenia. The differential diagnoses of osteopenia includes osteomalacia, hyperparathyroidism, renal failure, bone marrow malignancy, and various endocrine disorders. Table 3–1 summarizes the differences between osteoporosis and osteomalacia. Evaluation should at least include a complete blood count, serum electrolytes, blood urea nitrogen and creatinine, calcium, phosphorous, and alkaline phosphatase. The levels of pyridinoline and

TABLE 3–1 Differences between Osteoporosis and Osteomalacia

	Osteomalacia	Osteoporosis
Definition	Normal or decreased bone mass Deficient mineralization	Decreased bone mass Normal mineralization
Etiology	Vitamin D deficiency Malabsorption Renal failure Hypophosphatemia	Post-menopausal Age-related
Symptoms	Generalized bone pain Pathologic fractures	Asymptomatic Pathologic fractures
Radiographs	Osteopenia Looser's lines	Osteopenia
Laboratory	Varies with etiology but always abnormal	Normal
Bone biopsy	Unmineralized osteoid "Blurred" tetracycline labeling	Decreased bone mass Normal tetracycline labeling

deoxypyridinoline in a 24-hour urine collection are sensitive indicators of bone resorption. Urine osteocalcin measures bone formation and turnover. It is secreted exclusively by osteoblasts.

PITFALL

Osteoporosis is a diagnosis of exclusion. It is imperative to rule out other causes of osteopenia. Osteomalacia is often confused with osteoporosis, but it is medically correctable and easily diagnosed with laboratory methods.

Early identification and treatment of osteoporosis should decrease the incidence of fractures in the elderly. Bone densitometry testing may be a useful screen to detect early osteoporosis. Currently used techniques include single- and dual-energy X-ray densitometry (SXA or DEXA), quantitative computed tomography (QCT), and radiographic absorptiometry. SXA and DEXA require special equipment, but are easily performed with minimal radiation. Quantitative CT requires a special imaging technique, is more costly, and uses more radiation than SXA or DEXA, although less than a typical CT scan. Radiographic absorptiometry can be performed with standard radiographic techniques, but analysis is done at a central location to which the x-rays must be sent.

The treatment goal in osteoporosis is to decrease fracture risk. Treatment includes exercise, adequate dietary calcium, and medical management. Weight-bearing exercise such as walking is essential because repetitive compressive stresses stimulate bone formation. Strenuous activity is not essential. Guided conditioning and balance training may be useful in deconditioned, elderly patients at risk for falls. Calcium intake should be 1500 mg per day. Nutritional evaluation may be used to determine if supplementation is necessary.

Estrogen replacement is effective in maintaining and increasing bone mass after menopause. The fracture rate is decreased in individuals on estrogen replacement therapy. Other benefits of estrogen replacement include decreased cardiac risk, improved cholesterol profile, and relief of other postmenopausal symptoms. Estrogen replacement alone increases the risk of uterine cancer; however, combining estrogen with progesterone eliminates the increased risk. Some authors have reported an increased risk of breast cancer when estrogen has been used for more than 5 years before age 65, but other studies have been inconclusive.

Bisphosphonates such as etidronate and allendronate are pyrophosphate analogues that bind to bone and act as a shield to interfere with osteoclast resorption. Allendronate increases bone mass in the spine and hip. The incidence of spine and hip fracture in patients treated with allendronate is approximately half that in patients treated with placebo. The major complication of allendronate is gastrointestinal intolerance. This side effect may be minimized by slowly increasing the dosage to the recommended dose.

Calcitonin is used for treating high turnover osteoporosis because it inhibits osteoclasts. It increases spine bone mass

but not proximal femur bone mass. It also has analgesic properties that are believed to be due to endorphin release. Nasal or injectable methods of administration are available. Nasal administration is more convenient but is associated with nasal irritation.

Paget's Disease of Bone

Paget's disease is a bone remodeling disorder. A childhood infection with an unidentified slow virus has been theorized as the etiology because paramyxovirus nucleocapsids in the nuclei and cytoplasm of osteoclasts have been identified in the bone. These nucleocapsids are absent from osteoclasts in normal bone.

Paget's disease is most common in England, Western Europe, the United States, Austria and New Zealand. It is uncommon in Scandinavian countries, China, Japan, and India. The mean age at diagnosis is 58. The prevalence in individuals less than 40 years old is less than 1%; it is 3 to 5% in individuals between ages 50 and 70, and 10% in individuals older than 80. Eighty percent of those afflicted are asymptomatic and are diagnosed incidentally on radiographs performed for other reasons.

Symptomatic individuals complain of bone and/or joint pain, swelling, warmth, tenderness, and occasionally fracture. Symptoms may occur in only one (monostotic) or multiple bones (polyostotic). The most commonly affected bones include the pelvis, femur, spine, skull, and tibia. Physical findings are nonspecific and include bone tenderness, painful joint motion, deformity, swelling, warmth, and tenderness.

Radiographic manifestations of Paget's disease include a "front" of osteolysis in the diaphysis or metaphysis followed by sclerosis and bony enlargement. Radiographic osteolysis predominates in early Paget's disease, progresses to a mixture of osteolysis and osteosclerosis, and eventually has a disorganized medullary architecture from the waves of accelerated bone turnover and disordered remodeling (Fig. 3–3). This latter radiographic stage is often referred to as "burnt out" Paget's disease.

Alkaline phosphatase levels are increased due to increased bone formation and increased urinary excretion of hydroxyproline due to increased bone resorption. Urine pyrodinoline and N-telopeptide levels may be more sensitive for Paget's disease. Calcium metabolism and renal function are normal in Paget's disease.

PEARL

Serum alkaline phosphatase levels are a simple, reliable, and objective method of following the clinical course and effectiveness of medical management in Paget's disease.

Complications of Paget's disease include high-output heart failure, neurologic compromise, pathologic fractures,

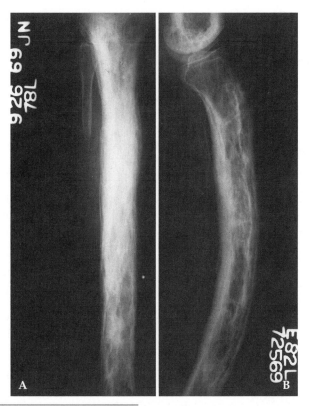

Figure 3–3 Radiograph of tibia with Paget's disease of bone illustrating disorganized bone turnover (**A**) and remodeling manifested by coexistent lysis and sclerosis (**B**).

arthritis, and sarcomatous degeneration. The accelerated bone turnover increases cardiac demand, which can lead to high-output heart failure. Bony deformities in the spine can cause spinal stenosis and neurologic compromise. Failure of remodeling compromises the structural properties of bone and predisposes involved bones to fracture. Deformities may cause altered weight-bearing that leads to degenerative arthritis in joints adjacent to the involved bone. The incidence of sarcomatous degeneration is less than 1% and tends to occur in polyostotic disease. A discrete lytic lesion in pagetic bone should raise the suspicion for sarcomatous degeneration.

PEARL

Remember the <u>FACTS</u> about Paget's disease: it can lead to <u>f</u>racture, <u>a</u>rthritis, <u>c</u>ardiac failure, <u>t</u>umor, and <u>s</u>pinal stenosis.

Indications for treatment of Paget's disease include bone pain, joint pain, neurologic compromise, and high-output heart failure. Bisphosphonates and calcitonin are useful.

Medical treatment is continued until symptoms have improved and alkaline phosphatase and urine hydroxyproline levels have normalized.

Surgical treatment is necessary for pathologic fracture, disabling degenerative joint disease, deformity, and sarcomatous degeneration. Pathologic fractures are most common in the femur and tibia and require internal fixation. Intramedullary devices are preferred because screws and plates may not achieve sufficient purchase in the pathologic bone. Simultaneous realignment osteotomies may be necessary to achieve intramedullary fixation. Fracture healing takes longer in pagetic bone than in normal bone.

Disabling deformities are amenable to realignment osteotomies with intramedullary fixation. Healing is often delayed. Total joint arthroplasty is useful for degenerative joint disease but is rarely necessary. Despite anecdotal reports, increased blood loss does not occur in patients with Paget's disease who undergo surgery.

Sarcomatous degeneration requires wide excision and adjuvant chemotherapy. The cure rate for appendicular sarcomatous degeneration of Paget's disease approaches 30%, whereas the axial cure rate is extremely low. It remains unclear whether long-term medical treatment of Paget's disease will decrease the risk of sarcomatous degeneration.

SUMMARY

Bone is a complex tissue that undergoes continuous remodeling in response to mechanical stresses and the metabolic environment. Coordinated osteoblast and osteoclast function are essential for bone maintenance. Calcium metabolism and bone formation are under hormonal influence but also depend on diet, liver, and kidney function.

Bone growth occurs at the physis, a complex but orderly cartilage structure that grows by chondrocyte apposition and that is converted to bone by gradual calcification and remodeling. Bone injury initiates an inflammatory response that in turn directs bone healing. Fracture healing usually occurs by enchondral ossification similar to physeal growth. Anatomic reduction and rigid fixation lead to primary bone healing by creeping substitution. The ideal bone graft is osteoinductive, osteoconductive, and osteogenic. Autografts can be all three, whereas allografts and synthetic graft substitutes are usually only osteoconductive. Growth factors are being developed that may be able to supplement grafts and provide osteoinduction and osteogenesis.

Common metabolic bone diseases include hyperparathyroidism, osteomalacia, osteoporosis, and Paget's disease. Hyperparathyroidism is a disorder of calcium metabolism with implications for bone turnover. Osteomalacia is a disorder of mineralization; whereas osteoporosis is a disorder of decreased bone mass and density. Both compromise bone's structural integrity and can have disabling complications. Paget's disease is a disorder of accelerated bone turnover with disordered remodeling. It is usually asymptomatic, but fractures, deformity, and degenerative arthritis are common complications.

SELECTED BIBLIOGRAPHY

BUCKWALTER JA, GLIMCHER MJ, COOPER RR, RECKER R. Bone biology; Part II: formation, form, modeling, remodeling, regulation of cell function. *Inst. Course Lect* 1996; 45:387–399.

BUCKWALTER JA, WOO SLY. Effects of repetitive motion on the musculoskeletal tissues. In: DELEE JC, DREZ D, eds. *Orthopaedic Sports Medicine.* Philadelphia, PA: WB Saunders; 1994;60–72.

COOPER RR, MILGRAM JW, ROBINSON RA. Morphology of the osteon. *J Bone Jt Surg* 1966;48A:1239–1271.

CUMMINGS SR, NEVITT MC, BROWNER WS, STONE K, FOX KM, ENSRUD KE, CAULEY J. BLACK D, and VOGT TM. Study of Osteoporotic Fractures Research Group: Risk factors for hip fracture in white women. Study of Osteoporotic fractures Research Group. *New Engl J Med.* 1995;332:767–773.

EINHORN TA, SIMON G, DEVLIN VJ, WARMAN J, SIDHU SPS, VIGORITA VJ. The osteogenic response to distal skeletal injury. *J Bone Jt Surg.* 1990;72A:1374–1378.

FRIEDLAENDER GE. Bone grafts: the basic science rationale for clinical applications. *J Bone Jt Surg.* 1987;69A:786–790.

GABEL GT, RAND JA, SIM FH. Total knee arthroplasty for osteoarthritis in paitents who have Paget's disease of bone at the knee. *J Bone Jt Surg.* 1991;73A:739–744.

GOODSHIP AE, LANYON LE, McFIE H. Functional adaptation of bone to increased stress. *J Bone Jt Surg.* 979;61A:539–546.

KAPLAN FS, SINGER FR. Paget's disease of bone: pathophysiology, diagnosis, and management. *J Am Acad Orthop Surg.* 1995;3:336–344.

LANE JM, RILEY EH, WIRGANOWICZ PZ. Osteoporosis: diagnosis and treatment. *J Bone Jt Surg* 1996;78A:618–632.

LINDSAY R. Hormone replacement therapy for prevention and treatment of osteoporosis. *Am J Med.* 1993;95:37S–39S.

PERREN SM. Physical and biological aspects of fracture healing with special reference to internal fixation. *Clin Orthop.* 1979;138:175–196.

SERET P, BASLE MF, REBEL A, RENIER JC, SAINT-ANDRE JP, BERTRANS G, AUDRAN M. Sarcomatous degeneration in Paget's bone disease. *J Can Res Clin Oncol.* 1987;113: 392–399.

SAMPLE QUESTIONS

1. Osteoblasts and osteoclasts are respectively derived from:
   (a) macrophages, platelets
   (b) mesenchymal cells, platelets
   (c) mesenchymal cells, macrophages
   (d) macrophages, endothelial cells
   (e) endothelial cells, mesenchymal cells

2. Mitochondria store calcium for physeal mineralization in the:
   (a) reserve zone
   (b) proliferative zone
   (c) hypertrophic zone
   (d) groove of Ranvier
   (e) epiphysis

3. Which pathway describes the synthesis of metabolically active vitamin D:
   (a) liver - skin - kidney
   (b) gut - kidney - liver
   (c) kidney - liver - skin
   (d) skin - liver - kidney
   (e) gut - skin - kidney

4. Which of the following are properties of cancellous allograft:
   (a) osteoinductive
   (b) osteoconductive
   (c) osteogenetic
   (d) structurally strong
   (e) b and d

5. Which of the following are characteristics of osteomalacia?
   (a) diffuse bone pain
   (b) normal mineralization of osteoid
   (c) decreased bone mass
   (d) a and c
   (e) none of the above

Chapter 4

Cartilage and Synovium

Christopher H. Evans, PhD, DSc, FRCPath

Outline

All intra-articular surfaces are synovial or cartilaginous in nature. This fact alone demonstrates the importance of understanding the biology of synovium and cartilage. Indeed, a thorough appreciation of the structure and physiology of diarthrodial joints in health and disease depends upon it. This chapter reviews these matters from the orthopaedic perspective and highlights active research areas where progress may be expected to impinge upon orthopaedic practice in the next century.

CARTILAGE

Cartilage is among the body's most unusual tissues. In nearly all instances, cartilage is aneural, alymphatic, and avascular. Indeed, the L5-S1 disc is the largest avascular structure in the body. Cartilage possesses an unusually high ratio of extracellular matrix to cells and contains types of collagen and proteoglycans that are absent from most, and in some cases all, other organs. Chondrocytes, the cells that populate cartilage, are themselves atypical in that they are able to grow in culture under so-called anchorage independent conditions, a property normally associated with tumor cells. Because cartilage lacks a blood supply, chondrocytes are called on to perform under anoxic, acidotic conditions that would disable most other cell types. Cartilage clearly has much to teach the biologist and orthopaedist. Although there exists a variety of cartilaginous tissues, including the intervertebral discs and

the elastic cartilage of the ears, this section is restricted to the types of cartilage found in diarthrodial joints, namely articular and meniscal cartilage.

Articular Cartilage Histology

A histological section through articular cartilage (Fig. 4–1) reveals a tissue that lacks blood vessels, nerves, and lymphatics, but which contains an abundant extracellular matrix. Within this matrix exist the cartilage cells, or chondrocytes. Beneath the articular cartilage lies the subchondral bone.

Articular cartilage is not the homogeneous tissue that it is sometimes assumed to be. Indeed, it can be divided into four zones, based upon the morphology and arrangement of the chondrocytes and the staining properties of the matrix. The deepest zone of the cartilage, zone IV, is mineralized. This is signaled by an abrupt change in the staining behavior of the tissue, which leads to a line of demarcation known as the tide mark. The different zones of articular cartilage also vary in their precise biochemical composition, water content, and orientation of their collagen fibrils.

Most stains used in the histological analysis of cartilage, such as Alcian blue, toluidine blue, and safranin O, are cationic (positively charged) and bind to proteoglycans present in the matrix that, are strongly anionic (negatively charged). During injury and disease, there is often a depletion of proteoglycans which leads to loss of staining.

Articular Cartilage Biochemistry

Articular cartilage covers the ends of the long bones and provides elastic, resilient surfaces that articulate with exceptionally low friction; the co-efficient of friction of cartilage on cartilage is one fifth of that of ice on ice. The mechanical, and to some degree rheological, properties of articular cartilage are largely determined by the biochemistry of its matrix. The major components of this matrix are water, proteoglycans, and collagens (Table 4–1).

It has been known for many years that articular cartilage is a highly hydrated tissue, with water accounting for approximately 65 to 75% of its mass. The reason for this lies with its high concentration of proteoglycans. Cartilage contains a variety of proteoglycans, all of which share a basic biochemical arrangement where glycosaminoglycan (GAG) chains are covalently attached to a so-called core protein. GAGs are

Orthopaedic Surgery: The Essentials. Edited by M.E. Baratz, A.D. Watson, and J.E. Imbriglia. Thieme Medical Publishers, Inc., New York © 1999

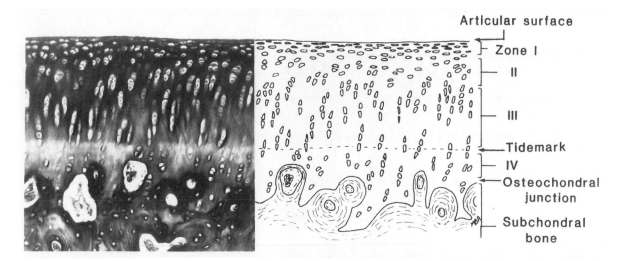

Figure 4–1 Section through the articular surface of canine femoral condyle (left) with explanatory diagram (right). Reproduced with permission from Aydelotte MB, Kuettner KE. Heterogeneity of articular chondrocytes and cartilage matrix. In: Woessner JF, Howell DS, eds. *Joint Cartilage Degradation: Basic and Clinical Aspects.* New York, NY: Marcel Dekker Inc; 1993: 37–63.

TABLE 4–1 Approximate Composition of Adult Articular Cartilage

Component	Approximate Percentage (by Mass)
Water	65–75
Proteoglycan	5–10
Collagen	10–20
Noncollagenous proteins	5–10
Minerals	1–2
Cells	2–5

themselves large sugar molecules consisting of repeating disaccharide units. The GAGs most commonly found in cartilage are chondroitin sulfate and keratan sulfate, with minor amounts of dermatan sulfate and heparan sulfate. Keratan sulfate is worth noting, because it is not found in structures other than cartilage and the cornea of the eye. Because of this, there is interest in measuring concentrations of keratan sulfate in various body fluids as a convenient, specific marker of cartilage breakdown. Take care not to confuse *keratan* with *keratin*; the latter is the major protein in hair and nails. The individual sugar molecules present in GAGs are acidic, due to the presence of either a carboxyl group (COO^-), a sulfate group, ($-O\text{-}SO_3^-$) or both. It is the high number of negative charges on the GAG chains that give proteoglycans their high affinity for water and, as described in the previous section, cationic dyes. Because proteoglycans are so abundant in cartilage, they hydrate the entire tissue. This property is important in understanding the mechanical behavior of cartilage.

Discussion of the material properties of cartilage lies outside the scope of this chapter; interested readers can refer to the references given in the bibliography.

Aggrecan is gravimetrically the most abundant proteoglycan in articular cartilage. It is a huge molecule. The core protein has a molecular weight of approximately 240 kDa. To this core are added up to 100 chains of chondroitin sulfate and up to 50 chains of keratan sulfate as well as a smaller number of polysaccharide chains. These substitutions provide an aggrecan molecule (or monomer) with a molecular weight of approximately 10^6 Da. The GAGs are covalently bound to the core protein at discrete chondroitin sulfate and keratan sulfate binding domains. As shown in Fig. 4–2, there are three other globular domains to the core protein, known as G1, G2, and G3 ("G" stands for globular). The functions of the G2 and G3 domains are unknown; an additional puzzle is provided by the observation that about a half of the aggrecan molecules extracted from articular cartilage lack the G3 domain. The G1 domain, in contrast, has a well defined and extremely important role in binding to hyaluronic acid (hyaluronan). The latter is itself a huge GAG with a molecular weight of more than 10^6 Da; unlike chondroitin, keratan, and dermatan sulfates, it is not covalently attached to a core protein. Instead it binds noncovalently to the G1 domain of the aggrecan monomer. This interaction is further stabilized by noncovalent interactions with a 45 kDa protein, called link protein, which binds both to hyaluronan and the G1 domain. Link protein has considerable homology to the G1 domain of aggrecan core protein. Large numbers of aggrecan molecules can associate in this manner with a single hyaluronan molecule thus forming enormous aggregates (hence the name aggrecan) of 10^8 Da or more in mass (Fig. 4–3). This is important because it is the extremely large size of the aggregate,

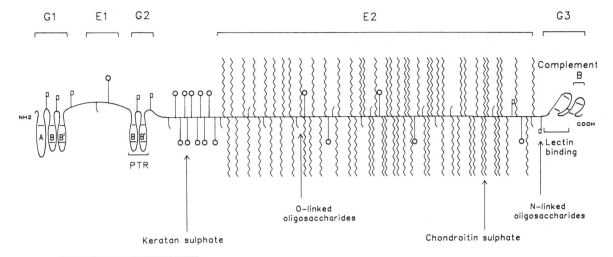

Figure 4–2 The aggrecan monomer, showing its domain structure. G1, G2, and G3 are three globular domains. E1 and E2 are two extended domains. The G3 domain has homology to lectin and complement, as indicated. Reproduced with permission from Hardingham T, Bayliss M. Proteoglycans of articular cartilage: changes in aging and in joint disease. *Sem Arth Rheum.* 1990; 20:12–33.

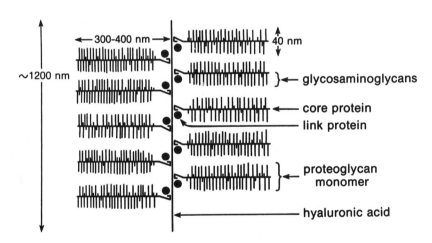

Proteoglycan aggregate

Figure 4–3 Aggregate structure formed by the interaction between aggrecan and hyaluronan. Aggrecan monomers bind to hyaluronan via the G1 domains. The stability of this association is increased by link protein.

not any covalent bonding, that traps aggrecan within the cartilaginous matrix. This has major implications for the way in which aggrecan is lost from the cartilaginous matrix because it means that even limited proteolysis of the core protein will disengage the proteoglycan monomer from the aggregate and enable it to diffuse from the matrix.

Much less is known of the so-called minor proteoglycans in cartilage. These include decorin, biglycan, fibromodulin, syndecan, lumican, and perlecan (Table 4–2). Unlike aggrecan, several of these are concentrated in the pericellular domain of the chondrocytes, along the surfaces of collagen fibrils, or near the articular surface. Little is known of their function, but despite their relatively low *gravimetric* concen-

trations in cartilage, their *molar* concentrations are equivalent to those of aggrecan in certain cases.

Collagen constitutes the other major class of structural macromolecule within the matrix of articular cartilage. Several of these collagens are unique to articular cartilage and, like keratan sulfate, are under investigation as markers of cartilage breakdown. At the time of writing, 20 different types of collagen have been identified. All are large glycoproteins with at least one triple helical domain. This domain contains a characteristic repeating tripeptide sequence with glycine at every third residue. One of the other two residues is frequently proline or hydroxyproline. The latter amino acid is rarely found in proteins other than collagen.

TABLE 4–2 The Proteoglycans of Cartilage

Name	GAGs	Core Protein Molecular Weight (Da)
Aggrecan	Chondroitin Sulfate Keratan Sulfate	240,000
Decorin	Chondroitin Sulfate Dermatan Sulfate	35,000
Biglycan	Chondroitin Sulfate Dermatan Sulfate	36,000
Fibromodulin	Keratan Sulfate	37,000
Syndecan	Heparan Sulfate	30,000
Lumican	Keratan Sulfate	38,000
Perlecan	Heparan Sulfate	466,000

Type II collagen accounts for approximately 95% of the collagen in articular cartilage. It is a so-called fibrillar collagen, which means that the individual triple-helical collagen molecules are able to align spontaneously in the extracellular space after synthesis and secretion to form fibrils. Fig. 4–4

summarizes the steps in the synthesis, secretion, and extracellular events in the formation of fibrillar collagens. Each collagen molecule is a trimer of three α chains. These are synthesized as separate proteins that undergo extensive post-translational modification, including hydroxylation and glycosylation as a prelude to their annealing intracellularly to form trimeric triple helical structures known as procollagen. At this stage they are secreted from the cell, as specific proteolytic processing enzymes cleave small, nonhelical extensions from both ends of the molecule. This process converts procollagen molecules into collagen molecules, which polymerize into collagen fibrils, as indicated in Fig. 4–4. The molecules within these fibrils are staggered (Fig. 4–4), an arrangement which gives collagen fibrils a characteristic banding pattern when examined by transmission electron microscopy. Individual fibrils come together to form large collagen fibers, whose interaction is further stabilized by the formation of covalent, intermolecular cross-links. In addition to type II collagen, cartilage contains several minor types of collagen (Table 4–3), with types IX, X, and XI being found only in articular cartilage. Type X is usually thought of as being restricted to the deep, calcified zone of cartilage below the tidemark (Fig. 1), although recent research has identified it in the surface layer of articular cartilage (Rucklidge et al., 1996). It is also present in the growth plate of immature cartilage, and it seems to be associated with cartilaginous tissues that mineralize. Type IX collagen is interesting because it contains a covalently attached chondroitin sulfate chain. It is found on the surfaces of the type II collagen fibers (Fig. 4–5).

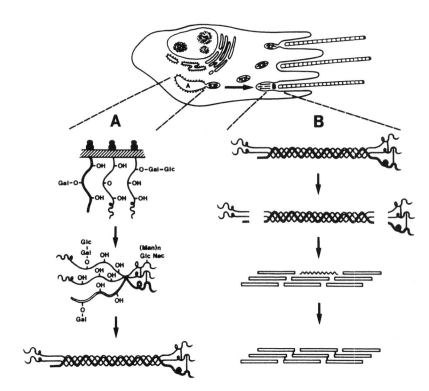

Figure 4–4 Collagen synthesis and assembly. **(A)** intracellular; **(B)** extracellular. Reproduced with permission from Prockop DJ, Kivirikko KI. Heritable diseases of collagen. *New Engl J Med.* 1984; 311:376–386.

TABLE 4–3   The Collagens of Articular Cartilage

Collagen Type	Percentage of Total Collagen	Comment
II	90–95	
IX	1–2	Contains a chondroitin sulfate chain
XI	1–2	Copolymerizes with type II collagen
V	1–2	Pericellular
VI	1–2	Pericellular
X	<1	Restricted to calcified and, possibly, surface zones
XIV	?	Predominantly found in surface layers

Types II, IX, X, and XI are unique to cartilaginous tissues.

Type XI collagen is able to copolymerize with type II collagen, forming hybrid fibers. Types V and VI collagen, in contrast, are localized to the pericellular environment of chondrocytes where they may participate in cell-matrix interactions. The presence of type XIV collagen in the surface layer (zone I) of articular cartilage has just been reported.

A number of noncollagenous proteins exist within the extracellular matrix of articular cartilage (Table 4). These are less well characterized and their functions are thus difficult to ascribe. Fibronectin is a cell adhesion molecule that may be involved in the interactions between chondrocytes and their surrounding matrix. A related molecule, chondronectin,

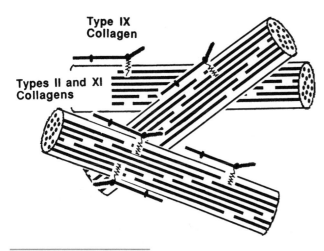

Figure 4–5   Fibrillar structure of cartilage collagens showing the interactions between collagen types II, IX, and XI.

TABLE 4–4   Examples of Noncollagenous Proteins Found in the Cartilaginous Matrix (excluding proteoglycan core proteins)

Protein	Molecular Weight (Da)
Fibronectin	555,000 (dimer)
Chondronectin	176,000 (trimer)
Comp	524,000 (pentamer)
Tenascin	1,900,000 (hexamer)
Thrombospondin	382,000 (trimer)
GP39	39,000
Link Protein	45,000

which may be unique to cartilage, has also been identified. Among the other noncollagenous proteins of cartilage, mention should be made of cartilage oligomeric protein, (COMP), a pentameric molecule with a molecular weight of 524,000 kDa. COMP is another molecule of interest in the search for quantifiable markers of cartilage breakdown.

Chondrocytes, Chondrons, and Matrix Metabolism

The metabolic duties of the chondrocytes are large in proportion to their low numbers. Because other types of cells are absent chondrocytes are responsible for all aspects of the metabolism of cartilage. This includes the coordinated synthesis and breakdown of various matrix components during normal turnover, as well as repair synthesis following injury. Under certain pathological conditions, the chondrocytes mediate the destruction of their own matrix.

Chondrocytes exist singly within the matrix, and thus, unlike the cells of most other solid tissues, do not form extensive intercellular contacts. They are further isolated by existing within a sort of cocoon, known as the chondron (Fig. 4–6), which contains various matrix components including collagen types II, VI, and IX; proteoglycans, and fibronectin. The plasma membrane of the chondrocyte contains a number of receptors with which the chondrocyte binds to various components of its immediate pericellular matrix. Such receptors include CD44, various integrins, annexin, anchorin, and others. Chondrocytes are also known to possess a flagellum, but its role remains to be determined.

Not all chondrocytes are equal. In particular, recent research has shown that the flattened, superficial cells lying close to the joint surface are quite different from the rounded, deeper cells. These morphological differences can be seen by electron microscopy in Fig. 4–7 and by light microscopy in Figures 4–1 and 4–7. Chondrocytes from different zones can

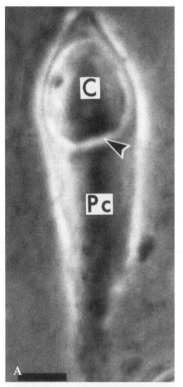

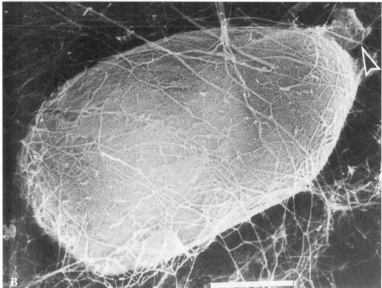

Figure 4–6   Chondrons isolated from canine articular cartilage. **(A)** Phase contrast light image of a single chondron showing chondrocyte (C), its pericellular matrix (arrow), and pericellular capsule (Pc). **(B)** Scanning electron microscopic image of a single chondron. Arrow points to extension at one pole of the chondron (Bar - 4 μm). Reproduced with permission from Poole CA, Flint MH, Beaumont BW. Chondrons extracted from canine tibial cartilage: preliminary report on their isolation and structure. *J Orthop Res*. 1988; 6:408–419.

be distinguished not only by their shapes but also by the types and amounts of proteoglycans and collagens that they synthesize, as well as by their responses to cytokines such as interleukin- 1 (IL-1). There is also evidence that metabolic differences exist between the chondrocytes present in the weight bearing areas and nonweight bearing areas of cartilage. Furthermore, there are, in addition, differences between the chondrocytes of different joints. Such variations may help explain why some joints are more susceptible than others to osteoarthritis.

The various matrix components of cartilage turn over at different rates. Collagen taken as a whole, for instance, barely turns over, whereas the various proteoglycans turnover with half-lives of days to months. The breakdown of the cartilaginous matrix is largely proteolytic and involves a variety of proteinases.

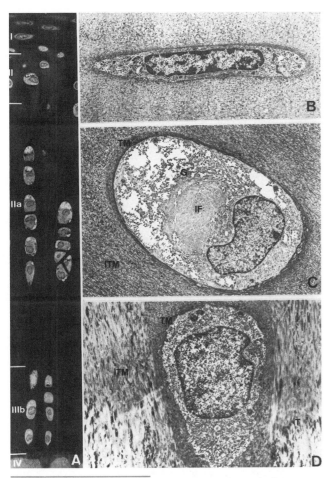

Figure 4–7   Light micrograph of section through the articular cartilage of an adult rabbit (**A**, left), with electron micrographs of individual chondrocytes from different zones (**B–D**, right). In the micrograph, zone III has been sub-divided into zone IIIa and IIIb. **B**: chondrocyte from zone I; **C**: chondrocyte from zone IIIa; **D**: chondrocyte from zone IIIb, near the tide-mark; ITM: interterritorial matrix; TM: territorial matrix; IF: intermediate filament; G: glycogen. Reproduced with permission from Schenk RK, Eggli PS, Hunziker EB. Articular cartilage morphology. In: Kuettner KE, Shleyerbach R, Hascall VC, eds. Articular Cartilage Biochemistry. New York, NY: Raven Press; 1986; 3–22.

Chondrocyte metabolism is largely anaerobic, and glycolytic activity is high. This partly reflects the low oxygen tension of cartilage, but it also seems to be an intrinsic property of the cells because they continue to favor glycolysis over oxidative phosphorylation under tissue culture conditions where oxygen is abundantly available. The high rates of glycolysis mean that large amounts of lactic acid are produced. This implies that the pericellular environment of the chondrocyte is acidic. Technical limitations have precluded direct measurement of the pericellular pH in articular cartilage, but it is possible to insert a pH probe into the intervertebral disc, where values as low as 6.5 have been recorded.

Cartilage Injury and Repair

Orthopaedic surgeons, especially those in sports medicine, frequently encounter circumstances where injury has produced a symptomatic lesion in the articular cartilage. These are not to be confused with the ulcerations that occur in an osteoarthritic joint, where an underlying disease process exists. The repair of cartilaginous lesions is not only clinically challenging, but also highly controversial as abrasion arthroplasty, subchondral drilling, and autologous chondrocyte transfer vie for utilization.

It is frequently stated that articular cartilage has no ability for intrinsic repair. This is not strictly true. In the absence of other insult, chondrocytes are, for example, quite capable of regenerating lost proteoglycan and restoring a fully functional articular surface. It is widely held that chondrocytes cannot replace or repair damaged collagen. This may well be so, although experimental evidence is lacking. What is clear, however, is that cartilage cannot repair partial-thickness defects. This deficiency has been blamed on the lack of a blood supply, but things are not that simple. Even when injuries penetrate the subchondral bone and there is bleeding followed by clot formation in the defect, healing is incomplete. Although the defect becomes filled with a white tissue which looks superficially cartilaginous, repair tissue is biochemically and anatomically aberrant and ultimately fails. Before failure occurs there may be clinical improvement. This is the process and typical course of abrasion arthroplasty and subchondral drilling.

Much activity and controversy presently surrounds the practice of autologous chondrocyte transfers to treat isolated, symptomatic defects in the knee. This procedure begins with the arthroscopic removal of healthy cartilage from a non-weight bearing area of the femoral condyle. This serves as a source of autologous chondrocytes, whose numbers are expanded 5 to 10 fold by in vitro cell culture. The cells are then surgically re-implanted into the defect and held in place by a periosteal flap.

The initial clinical results were quite encouraging. Their publication in the *New England Journal of Medicine* (Brittberg et al, 1994), followed by the rapid, aggressive commercialization of the process has led to enormous controversy which, at the time of writing, is in full flood. At issue are a whole raft of concerns ranging from the design of the *NEJM* study, the preclinical data, and the rapid drive to widespread clinical implementation to the marketing techniques used to profit from this procedure.

Often overlooked in the above debate is that chondrocyte transfers, both as allo- and autografts, have been attempted in experimental animals for decades. Had the data warranted, human trials could have begun years ago; that they did not do so reflects the preclinical findings. In nearly all cases, a promising early result was followed after a year or so by degeneration of the repair tissue. This result has been most recently confirmed in a prominent study of autologous chondrocyte transfers in dogs.

As we learn more about cartilage and chondrocytes, there are increasing numbers of reasons for questioning the procedure on biological grounds. It is well known that chondrocytes rapidly undergo phenotypic modulation, loosely called dedifferentiation, when propagated as monolayers through several generations in vitro. The degree to which these cells recover their original phenotype after re-implantation is unknown. Such considerations are complicated by the heterogeneity that exists among chondrocytes. As we have seen, the cells from the surface layers are different from the deeper cells. The cell culture techniques used as part of autologous transfer not only jumble up these different cells but may encourage selective growth of cells of one particular subtype. It is not known whether this mixture of cells, following re-implantation, has the ability to reform the zonal distinctiveness of the cartilage. Can cells recovered from the deep zones function as superficial cells following re-implantation, and vice versa? This is simply not known. The answer is not merely academic; the integrity of the articular surface is crucial to the performance of articular cartilage. Related to these issues is the exquisite microarchitecture of articular cartilage. It is not merely a jumble of type II collagen, aggrecan, and miscellaneous other molecules. It is, in contrast, a highly ordered and structured tissue. Whether this can be regenerated by a mixture of dedifferentiated, ecotopic, adult cells is unknown. Additional problems concern the ability of the newly formed tissue to fuse with the surrounding intact cartilage and the subchondral bone. Despite these biological concerns, the procedure is in widespread clinical use as a result of a single, uncontrolled, unblinded, human trial. This partly reflects the orthopaedic "herding instinct" and the absence of FDA guidelines on such procedures. The FDA has now established guidelines retrospectively. As the rules now stand, the commercial use of autologous chondrocyte transfers would not be allowed to continue, but the present procedure is grandfathered. As controlled, multicentered trials are now in progress we will eventually learn how autologous chondrocyte transfer compares with other methods for treating cartilaginous defects, and what place it might take in the orthopaedic surgical armamentarium.

As an alternative to the transfer of cells derived from adult articular cartilage, there is the prospect of repairing lesions by the transfer of chondroprogenitor cells. Such cells may exist in the bone marrow, periosteum and, perhaps, the synovium. The term *mesenchymal stem cell* has been applied to bone marrow cells with the potential to develop into, among other things, chondrocytes. Because of their differentiational plasticity, progenitor cells have a greater potential to regenerate authentic articular cartilage than the committed cells obtained from adult tissue. Data from studies in rabbits suggest that this may indeed be the case.

The efficacy of cell-based healing may be augmented by one or more growth factors that stimulate growth, differentiation and matrix synthesis of chondrocytes and chondroprogenitor cells. Examples include, but are not limited to, transforming growth factor-β, insulinlike growth factors, bone morphogenetic proteins and fibroblast growth factors.

These factors are proteins and may be added to the cells during cell culture or introduced at the time of re-implantation. Because of the short in vivo half-lives of these factors, they may need to be added in conjunction with some sort of slow release device. As these can be problematic, we have suggested transferring growth factor genes to the cells so that they manufacture their own growth factors following re-implantation. Preliminary from our laboratory data support the feasibility of this gene therapy approach.

Cartilage Loss in Arthritis

Cartilage loss is a prominent feature of most forms of arthritis. In general terms, there are two ways to lose cartilage: reduced synthesis and increased breakdown. In rheumatoid arthritis there is probably a general inhibition of matrix synthesis. In osteoarthritis the picture is more complicated. Researchers have long puzzled over the paradox that during the early and middle stages of osteoarthritis, matrix synthesis is increased at a time of net matrix depletion. The standard explanation has been to propose that matrix breakdown is occurring at an even higher rate. This may be so, but recent data indicate that matrix synthesis is strongly suppressed in the superficial, but not the deeper, cells of cartilage in osteoarthritis. Increased hydration is another prominent change in early osteoarthritis. This is thought to reflect proteolysis of the collagenous network, which permits the proteoglycans to swell and imbibe water.

Elevated breakdown of the matrix is thought to occur in both rheumatoid and osteoarthritis. Much of this catabolic activity is mediated by the chondrocytes, in a process which has been called *chondrocytic chondrolysis*. A variety of proteinases have been implicated in matrix destruction including secreted matrix metalloproteinases (MMPs), membrane bound metalloproteinases (MT-MMPs), cysteine proteinases, serine proteinases and members of a newly identified group of enzymes known as the A disintegrin and metalloproteinase (ADAMS) family. Most attention over the past decade has focused on the MMPs. This consists of a large and growing family of proteinases which require Ca^{2+} for activity and contain Zn at the active site of the enzyme. Some relevant members are listed in Table 4–5. The activities of these proteinases is regulated biologically by both general proteinase inhibitors, such as α_2-macroglobulin and inhibitors that are specific for certain enzymes or groups of enzymes. The best studied example of the latter is tissue inhibitor of metalloproteinases (TIMP), which exists in four forms: TIMP-1, -2, -3, and -4. Another activity that deserves mention is *aggrecanase*. Study of the fragments released by the breakdown of the core protein of aggrecan led to the surprising conclusion that no presently characterized proteinase could account for these products. The existence of a novel proteinase, aggrecanase, was postulated. Several years of intense research activity failed to isolate or identify this putative enzyme, and its existence has been questioned. Nevertheless, there is a strong rumor among the orthopaedic research community that aggrecanase has finally been identified and cloned. It is to be hoped that this information will be rapidly disseminated. Inhibitors of the enzymes that degrade cartilage may

TABLE 4–5 Matrix Metalloproteinases of Relevance to Cartilage Matrix Breakdown

Enzyme	Number	Predominant Substrate
Interstitial collagenase	MMP-1	Collagen types II and XI
Neutrophil collagenase	MMP-8	Collagen types II and XI
Collagenase-3	MMP-13	Collagen types II and XI
72 kDa Gelatinase (Gelatinase A)	MMP-2	Denatured collagen (gelatin), intact type X collagen
92 kDa Gelatinase (Gelatinase B)	MMP-9	Denatured collagen (gelatin), intact type XI collagen
Stromelysin-1	MMP-3	Proteoglycan
Stromelysin-2	MMP-10	Proteoglycan

protect the matrix from breakdown and thus act as *chondroprotective* agents in arthritis. Synthetic MMP inhibitors are about to enter clinical trials in this regard.

Although there is a net loss of matrix in arthritis, not all matrix components are lost at an equal rate and there are also qualitative changes in matrix macromolecules. Loss of proteoglycans, for example, precedes that of collagen, although there is evidence that subtle "clipping" of the collagenous meshwork precedes this. In the matrix of cartilage in osteoarthritis, there is an increase in fibronectin, and type X collagen becomes much more abundant. Type III collagen, which is normally absent from articular cartilage, also starts to appear in osteoarthritis.

What provokes these changes in the turnover of matrix metabolism in arthritis? In osteoarthritis, the answers have been traditionally sought in the area of biomechanics. Although the old-fashioned "wear and tear" hypothesis is now defunct, mechanical influences may still be important as a means of modulating chondrocyte metabolism. When articular cartilage is loaded, the shapes of the chondrocytes are changed and the cells experience, in addition to direct mechanical load, shear forces and streaming potentials, as well as changes in the local fixed charge density and pH. All of these have the potential to influence chondrocyte physiology. Laboratory data suggest that both the under- and overloading of cartilage reduce matrix synthesis and lead to matrix depletion. Static loading is particularly harmful in this regard. Intermittent loading of the appropriate magnitude and frequency, in contrast, greatly increases matrix synthesis and reduces breakdown.

Although mechanical forces help explain why osteoarthritis primarily affects weight bearing joints such as the hips and knees, they do not explain why the ankles are spared. Observations such as this point to the growing appreciation that biological factors are important to the etiopathogenesis of osteoarthritis. What these factors might be is presently the subject of much research. Particular attention has been paid to cytokines, particularly IL-1, which both inhibits matrix synthesis and accelerates matrix loss. Of particular relevance are recent findings that superficial chondrocytes are much more responsive to IL-1 than deeper cells, and that knee cartilage is much more responsive to IL-1 than ankle cartilage from the same individual. These observations may help explain why matrix synthesis is selectively suppressed in the superficial zone of osteoarthritis cartilage, and why osteoarthritis is more prevalent in knees than ankles.

Nitric oxide is another mediator of interest. This free radical is induced by IL-1 and certain other stimuli, and inhibits the synthesis of both proteoglycans and collagen by articular cartilage. Chondrocytes are a particularly rich source of nitric oxide. They also produce prostaglandins, particularly PGE_2, whose effects on matrix turnover are surprisingly poorly studied. Of clinical importance are observations suggesting that nonsteroidal anti-inflammatory drugs, which inhibit prostaglandin synthesis and are used to treat arthritis, may accelerate cartilage loss.

The probability that cartilage loss in osteoarthritis has an important biological dimension permits optimism about future treatment. In particular, manipulation of IL-1 or other cytokines may prove helpful. Indeed, a naturally occurring protein called the interleukin-1 receptor antagonist (IL-1Ra) has proved effective in preventing early osteoarthritic changes in dogs. Growth factors may be useful agents with which to promote matrix deposition, although osteoarthritic chondrocytes are unresponsive to insulinlike growth factor-1. This illustrates the point that the chondrocytes within an osteoarthritic joint are not normal, and may thus perform poorly when used as autologous grafts into areas of cartilage loss. I raise this issue because it is often assumed that the autologous chondrocyte transfers used to treat post-traumatic cartilaginous lesions in otherwise healthy joints will be effective in osteoarthritis. This is unlikely to be the case.

In certain patients suffering from familial osteoarthritis, the cause of the disease almost certainly lies with mutations in the structural macromolecules of the cartilaginous matrix. Mutations in the gene encoding the α chain of type II collagen have been particularly well characterized, but changes in genes encoding other components of the matrix are also likely to cause arthritis in certain patients. It is not yet clear how the mutations result in disease, but it is assumed that the matrix is biomechanically abnormal. The ultimate treatment for such patients would be gene therapy, but this will be extremely difficult to achieve for a number of reasons, including the transdominant nature of the mutation and the serious problems associated with targeting genes to chondrocytes.

In rheumatoid arthritis there is generalized suppression of matrix synthesis in response to cytokines, particularly IL-1, secreted by the rheumatoid synovium. Increased breakdown of the matrix is mediated both by the chondrocytes in response to synovial cytokines, and by direct invasion by pannus. In both cases, proteinases of the types discussed earlier in this section are thought to be responsible for digesting the matrix.

There is presently much interest in developing better ways to monitor cartilage breakdown and repair. These are needed to improve monitoring of patients with arthritis and, in particular, to evaluate responses to chondroprotective drugs. Present methods include x-rays, which are extremely insensitive, and magnetic resonance imaging, which is very expensive and also imprecise. Among the more promising approaches are those that measure in various body fluids the presence of specific substances released from the cartilage as it is degraded or as it regenerates. Various markers, such as keratan sulfate, COMP, type II collagen, and collagen crosslinks are under investigation in this regard. In the future, it may be possible for orthopaedic surgeons to monitor the condition of their patients' cartilage by a simple blood test.

Meniscus

Like articular cartilage, meniscal cartilage contains relatively few cells embedded in an abundant extracellular matrix. However, much less is known about the matrix and cells of the meniscus. When grown in culture, cells derived from the meniscus may be fibroblastic or rounded, depending on the culture conditions. Some cultures contain a mixed population of cells with these two morphologies, while cells with an intermediate morphology have also been noted. The word "fibrochondrocytes" has been coined, but it is still not clear whether there exists within meniscus a single cell type which can adapt its phenotype according to the cell culture conditions, or whether there pre-exist within meniscus both fibroblastic and rounded cells.

The meniscal matrix (Table 4–6) contains far less proteoglycan than the matrix of articular cartilage. Meniscus is primarily a collagenous tissue, a circumstance that reflects its primary role as a structure that transmits load. Unlike articular cartilage, the meniscus has type I collagen as its predominant type of collagen, accounting for more that 90% of the total collagen. Small amounts of types II, III, V, and VI collagen are also present. The distribution of the different collagens is not uniform throughout the matrix of the meniscus. In the surface layer of the meniscus, the type I collagen fibers are oriented parallel to the surface, while in the bulk tissue the fibers are orient circumferentially. These orientations

TABLE 4–6 Composition of Meniscal Cartilage

Substance	Approximate Percentage by Weight
Water	75
Collagen	20
Proteoglycan	1
Noncollagenous proteins	2
Cells	1

enable the meniscus to withstand the compressive forces imposed by the femoral condyles and tibial plateau.

Analysis of meniscal proteoglycans is less complete than that of their counterparts in articular cartilage. However, there is evidence for the presence of aggrecan, perlecan, and several of the small proteoglycans listed in Table 4–2. Non-collagenous proteins found in meniscus include elastin, thrombospondin, and fibronectin.

The outer one third of the meniscus is vascularized and is able to repair following injury. The inner two thirds, in contrast, the so-called white meniscus, lacks a blood supply and has poor healing capacity. Strategies for enhancing meniscal healing mirror those for articular cartilage and include the introduction of cells and growth factors, or growth factor genes, into the lesion. None of these strategies are yet in clinical use.

SYNOVIUM

Normal Synovium

Synovium is a thin, weak, deformable tissue whose main function is to help regulate the intra-articular biochemical environment. Strictly speaking, the synovium is defined anatomically as the intimal layer of the joint space. It is normally only 2 to 3 cells in depth. Clearly, the average surgical synovectomy removes much more than synovium, even allowing for the increased thickness of the rheumatoid tissue. Immediately beneath the intimal layer lies a subsynovium, which may be areolar, fibrous, or adipose, depending upon the region of the joint (Fig. 4–8). The tissue beneath the synovial intima is richly innervated, highly vascularized, and contains lymphatics. Underlying the subsynovium is the joint capsule.

The joint space is unique among body cavities in not being lined by a basement membrane. Instead, the synovium is a loose, connective tissue where both cells and matrix are in direct contact with the joint cavity. Defining the cells of the synovium, the *synoviocytes*, has proved problematic, but most commentators now agree that there are two types: type A and type B synoviocytes (Fig. 4–9). The type A cells closely resemble macrophages and may be considered as the resident macrophages of the synovium analogous to the Kupffer cells of the liver. The type B cells are fibroblastic and secrete large amounts of hyaluronan into the synovial fluid. This accumulates to a concentrations of approximately 3 mg/ml, giving synovial fluid its characteristically high viscosity. Little is known of the biology of these cells. It has been estimated that synoviocytes turnover every 20 weeks, but there are few hard data on this matter. The type A cells are derived from the bone marrow and probably do not divide. The type B cells have the capacity to divide in vitro, but it has been difficult to confirm the presence of mitoses in vivo. It is thus possible that the type B cells, assuming that they turnover, are not replenished by local cell division, but by immigration of cells from some other location.

The matrix of synovium is largely collagenous, with types I, III, IV, V, and VI having been identified. Other proteins found in synovium include fibronectin and tenascin;

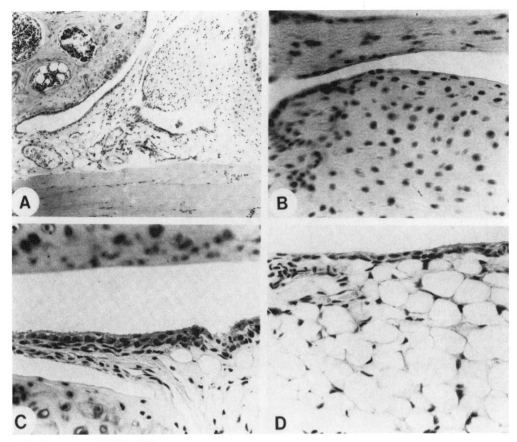

Figure 4–8 Histological sections through the normal synovial lining of the mouse knee joint demonstrating the three types of subintimal tissue. **(A)** Section showing the three types of subintima (original magnification 100×). **(B)** Fibrous subintima (original magnification 400×). **(C)** Areolar subintima (original magnification 400×). **(D)** Adipose subintima (original magnification 400×). Reproduced with permission from Henderson B, Pettipher ER. The synovial lining cell: biology and pathology. *Sem Arth Rheum.*, 1985; 15:1–32.

hyaluronan is also present. Proteoglycans, including perlecan, are present in small amounts, but their characterization is incomplete.

Synovium regulates the intra-articular biochemical environment in two ways: by acting as a diffusional barrier to the trans-synovial flow of materials from the synovial capillaries and by the metabolic activities of the synoviocytes which add and remove materials to and from the synovial fluid (Fig. 4–10). Within approximately 25 μm of the joint space lies an exceeding rich subsynovial capillary network. These capillaries are fenestrated, with their fenestrations orientated towards the joint space. This arrangement facilitates the diffusion of plasma from the capillaries via the synovium into the joint space. The vessel wall and the synovium exert a sieving effect, such that large molecules are impeded in their progress. As shown in Table 4–7, the protein concentration of normal, human synovial fluid is only 28% of that in the serum. When the concentrations of individual proteins are examined in relation to their molecular weights, it is evident that the larger the protein, the lower its representation in the synovial fluid compared with the serum (see Table 4–7). Synovial fluid can be considered as an ultrafiltrate of plasma to which synoviocytes have added hyaluronan. An important plasma protein excluded from synovial fluid is fibrinogen. This means that synovial fluid does not clot. Hyaluronan provides synovial fluid with its high viscosity and is widely assumed to be the major lubricant in the joint, but this is not so. Lubrication is instead provided by a large glycoprotein called lubricin, secreted by synoviocytes.

Although proteins enter the joint by diffusion from the subsynovial capillaries, they leave the joint via the synovial lymphatics (see Fig. 4–10). Unlike diffusional entry, exit through the lymphatics does not discriminate among molecules of different sizes. It is also much more efficient. Indeed, it is thought to impose a slight negative pressure upon the joint, which has been estimated as 4 mm Hg in the normal human knee. This contributes to the stability of the joint.

Synovial Changes in Arthritis

Most forms of arthritis are associated with some degree of synovial inflammation (synovitis) and thickening. These changes are seen at their largest extent in the rheumatoid joint.

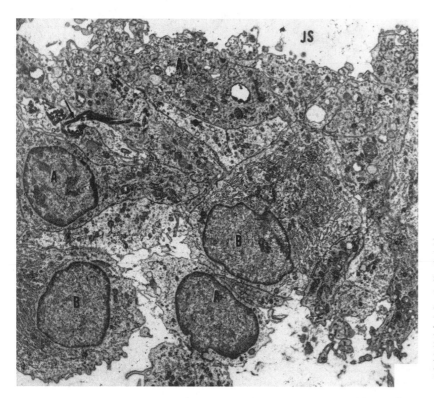

Figure 4–9 Electron micrograph of a transverse section through human synovial membrane, showing type A and type B synoviocytes. Labels "A" and "B" designate the types A and B synoviocytes. JS = joint space. Reproduced with permission from Barland P, Novikoff AB, Hamerman D. Electron microscopy of the human synovial membrane. *J Cell Biol.* 1962; 14:207–220.

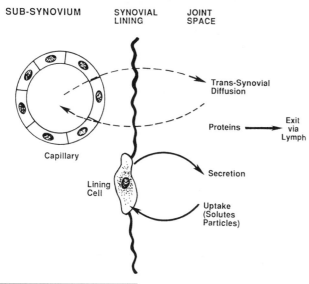

Figure 4–10 Major routes by which synovium regulates the intra-articular biochemical environment. Reproduced with permission from Evans CH. Response of synovium to mechanical injury. In: Finerman GAM, Noyes FR, eds. *Biology and Biomechanics of the Traumatized Synovial Joint: The Knee as a Model.* Rosemont, IL: American Academy of Orthopaedic Surgeons; 1992; 17–26.

The thickening of the synovium results from a combination increased matrix deposition (hypertrophy) and increased cellularity. The increase in cell number reflects both an increase in the number of synoviocytes (hyperplasia) and colonization of the synovium by infiltrating leukocytes. In acute inflammation, the predominant type of leukocyte is the neutrophil. In chronic inflammation, macrophages and lymphocytes predominate. Mast cells are also common in the inflamed synovium. There are a number of reports indicating the presence of giant cells in the synovia of arthritic joints, where they are often associated with cartilaginous or osseous wear debris.

It has been widely assumed that the increase in type B synoviocytes noted in the rheumatoid joint reflects local proliferation of the resident cells. However, ex vivo analysis of the tissue has failed to provide convincing evidence of this. As a particularly intriguing explanation of this paradox, it has been postulated that the increase in synovial cell number occurs not by increased cell division, but by decreased cell death. In particular, a form of programmed cell death known as apoptosis is claimed to be defective in the rheumatoid joint. If true, this has important implications for the understanding and, possibly, treatment of rheumatoid arthritis.

Synoviocytes are altered qualitatively, as well as quantitatively, in the inflamed joint. In particular, there occurs an unusual stellate cell with long dendritic processes. The nature and origins of this type of cell have been the subject of much discussion. Present opinion favors the notion that this is a type B synoviocyte which has undergone phenotypic change in response to the ambient inflammatory environment. Recent observations suggest that the cells in the rheumatoid pannus are different from both synoviocytes and chondrocytes and may thus represent a novel type of cell within the joint. These cells, about which little is presently known, have been called pannocytes.

Both the resident synoviocytes and the infiltrating leukocytes within the inflamed synovium, as well as activated chondrocytes, secrete a variety of mediators that amplify and perpetuate the inflamed condition and that lead to cartilage breakdown. Among these mediators are cytokines such as IL-1, 6, 8, 12, 15, and 17; tumor necrosis factor α (TNF-α); and various colony stimulating factors, free radicals such as NO and superoxide ($^{\bullet}O_2^{-}$) and arachadonic acid derivatives such

TABLE 4–7   Concentrations of Proteins in Synovial Fluid of Normal and Rheumatoid Human Knees

Protein	Molecular Weight (kDa)	Synovial Fluid Concentration (mg/ml)		Synovial Fluid Plasma Ratio	
		Normal	RA	Normal	RA
Total	—	19.0	50.0	0.28	0.71
α_1-globulins	$\approx$44	1.3	2.5	0.32	0.63
Albumin	69	12.0	19.1	0.37	0.65
γ-globulins	$\approx$160	2.4	11.0	0.21	0.65
α_2-globulins	100–800	1.1	3.2	0.14	0.46
α_2-macroglobulin	900	0	1.2	0	0.35

RA = Rheumatoid arthritis.
Data From: Levick JR. Permeability of rheumatoid and normal human synovium to specific plasma proteins. *Arthritis Rheum*. 1981; 24:1550–1560.

as prostaglandins and leukotrienes. Resolution of inflammatory conditions is associated with the local production of anti-inflammatory cytokines such as IL-10 and IL-1Ra, as well as soluble forms of the cell surface receptors for IL-1 and TNF-α.

Inflammation is also associated with neovascularization, and the inflamed synovium is hyperemic. However, there is evidence that in chronic inflammation the rate of collagen deposition exceeds that of neovascularization so that the concentration of vessels within the synovium falls, and the capillaries lie deeper below the joint surface. This might explain why synovial fluid aspirated from joints with established rheumatoid arthritis is acidotic, hypoxic, and rich in lactic acid. These unfavorable physical conditions may contribute to the pathology of the disease.

Changes also occur in the permeability of the vascular wall. Because the capillaries of the inflamed synovium are more "leaky," the volume of synovial fluid increases considerably, and large proteins are now able to enter the synovial fluid. The protein content of synovial fluid increases in both absolute terms and relative to the serum (see Table 4–7). Larger proteins are less restricted in their access to the synovial fluid, and very large proteins, such as α_2-macroglobulin, now appear intraarticularly (see Table 4–7).

A secondary effect of this increase in ingress is to eliminate the negative pressure existing within the normal joint; instead, the joint experiences a positive pressure. This not only leads to pain, but also destabilizes the joint.

Treatment of the rheumatoid joint has traditionally been almost entirely by the systemic delivery of anti-inflammatory drugs. These may provide symptomatic relief, but they fail to protect the articular cartilage and are associated with serious side effects. The discovery of naturally occurring anti-inflammatory and chondroprotective proteins, such as IL-10 and IL-1Ra mentioned earlier in this section, offer novel opportunities for treating joint diseases biologically. Proteins, however, make poor drugs in chronic disease because there is no good way to deliver them. Gene delivery offers an attractive and elegant solution to this problem. Nine patients with rheumatoid arthritis have been treated with a gene encoding

IL-1Ra in the first human trial of gene therapy for arthritis. Results are pending.

FUTURE HORIZONS

Early in the next century, medical records will begin including patients' DNA sequences. These will have been automatically scanned for the presence of sequences that are not only diagnostic for specific genetic diseases, such as osteogenesis imperfecta, but that also indicate susceptibility to complex, multifactorial conditions, such as arthritis. The patients' genetic information will also predict the susceptibility of their musculoskeletal systems to injury and their capacities for repair. The information will be of considerable clinical utility to the orthopaedic surgeon.

Individuals with genetic polymorphisms consistent with mechanically weak menisci, cartilage, or ligaments, for instance, might be counseled to avoid contact sports or long distance running. Patients at risk of osteoarthritis might additionally be monitored at frequent intervals for early signs of cartilage degeneration. This could take the form of a simple blood test to measure levels of one or more matrix components.

Cell and molecular biology will have provided the orthopaedist with powerful new therapies to use once injury or disease has occurred, and treatments will be selected to suit the individual patient's genetic predispositions. If, for example, there is a likelihood of delayed or nonunion, the healing of a fracture will be promoted by the use of a suitable growth factor or combination of growth factors. Gene transfer may well be employed as a way of achieving a sustained, local synthesis of the appropriate factors. Cartilaginous lesions and arthritis will be treated by cell therapy, gene therapy, or a combination of the two. Orally active, chondroprotective drugs that inhibit the proteinases that degrade cartilage will also be available. Monogenic genetic diseases, such as osteogenesis imperfecta and familial osteoarthritis will be treated by gene therapy. Assuming that the appropriate ethical issues can be satisfactorily addressed, such diseases may be eradicated by in utero and, ultimately, germline gene therapy.

If even some of these predictions come true, they will dramatically alter the practice of orthopaedic surgery. There will be a greater emphasis on the preventative aspects of musculoskeletal disease, and treatments will become far more biological and individualized. Although much of the carpentry will have been removed from the discipline, practitioners will be rewarded by a happier patient population.

SELECTED BIBLIOGRAPHY

Articular Cartilage Biochemistry

KUETTNER KE. Biochemistry of articular cartilage in health and disease. *Clin Biochem.* 1992; 25:155–163.

MAYNE R. BREWTON RG. Extracellular matrix of cartilage: Collagen. In: Woessner JF, Howell DS, eds. *Joint Cartilage Degradation: Basic and Clinical Aspects.* New York, NY: Marcel Dekker Inc; 1993: 81–108.

MOLLENHAUER J. KUETTNER KE. Articular cartilage. In: Dee R, ed. *Principles of Orthopaedic Practice.* 2nd ed. New York, NY: McGraw-Hill, 1997:85–98.

NEAME PJ. Extracellular matrix of cartilage: Proteoglycans. In: Woessner JF, Howell DS, eds. *Joint Cartilage Degradation: Basic and Clinical Aspects.* New York, NY: Marcel Dekker Inc; 1993:109–138.

POOLE CA. Chondrons: The chondrocyte and its pericellular microenvironment. In: Kuettner KE, Schleyerbach R, Peyron JG, Hascall VC, eds. *Articular Cartilage and Osteoarthritis.* New York, NY: Academic Press; 1992.

POOLE CA. The structure and function of articular cartilage matrices. In: Woessner JF, Howell DS, eds. *Joint Cartilage Degradation: Basic and Clinical Aspects.* New York, NY: Marcel Dekker Inc; 1993:1–36.

RUCKLIDGE GJ, MILNE G, ROBINS SP. Collagen type X: A component of the surface of normal human, pig, and rat articular cartilage. *Biochem Biophys Res Commun* 1996; 224:297–302.

Cartilage Breakdown

AIGNER T, VORNEHM SI, ZEILER G, DUDHIA J, VON DER MARK K, BAYLISS MT. Suppression of cartilage matrix gene expression in upper zone chondrocytes of osteoarthritic cartilage. *Arthritis Rheum.* 1997; 40:562–569.

SANDY JD, FLANNERY CR, NEAME PJ, LOHMANDER LS. The structure of aggrecan fragments in human synovial fluid: evidence for the involvement in osteoarthritis of a novel proteinase which cleaves the Glm 373-Ala 374 bond on the interglobular domain. *J Clin Invest.* 1992; 89:1512–1516.

WOESSNER JF. Matrix metalloproteinases and their inhibition in connective tissue remodeling. *FASEB J.* 1991; 5:2145–2154.

Meniscus

McDEVITT CA, WEBBER RJ. The ultrastructure and biochemistry of meniscal cartilage. *Clin Orthop Rel Res.* 1990; 252:8–18.

Cartilage Repair

BRITTBERG M, LINDAHL A, NILSSON A, OHLSSON C, ISAKSSON O, PETERSON L. Treatment of deep cartilage defects in the knee with autologous chondrocyte transplantation. *New Eng J Med.* 1994; 331:889–895.

HUNZIKER EB, ROSENBERG LC. Repair of partial-thickness defects in articular cartilage: cell recruitment from the synovial membrane. *J Bone Jt Surg.* 1996; 78A:721–733.

WAKITANI S, GOTO T, PINEDA SJ, YOUNG RG, MANSOW JM, CAPLAN AI, GOLDBERG VM. Mesenchymal cell-based repair of large, full-thickness defects in articular cartilage. *J Bone Jt Surg.* 1994; 76A:579–592.

Nitric Oxide

EVANS CH, STEFANOVIC-RACIC M LANCASTER J. Nitric oxide and its role in orthopaedic disease. *Clin Orthop Rel Res.* 1995; 312:275–294.

Cytokines

FELDMAN M, BRENNAN FM, MAINI RN. Role of cytokines in rheumatoid arthritis. *Ann Rev Immunol.* 1996; 14:397–440.

TRIPPLE SB, COUTTS RD, EINHORN TA, MUNDY GR, ROSENFELD RG. Growth factors as therapeutic agents. *J Bone Jt Surg.* 1996; 78A:1272–1286.

Synovium

EVANS CH. Synovial Membrane. In: Dee R, ed. Principles of Orthopaedic Practice. 2nd New York, NY: McGraw-Hill; 1997:99–108.

HENDERSON B, PETTIPHER ER. The synovial lining cell: biology and pathobiology. *Sem Arth Rheum.* 1985; 15:1–32.

HUNG GL, EVANS CH. Synovium In: F. Fu, C. Harner, K.G. Vince, *Knee Surgery,* pp. 141–145, Williams and Wilkins, Baltimore, MD, 1994.

SIMKIN PA. Physiology of normal and abnormal synovium. *Sem Arth Rheum.* 1991; 21:179–183.

Gene Therapy

EVANS CH, ROBBINS PD. Possible orthopaedic applications of gene therapy. *J Bone Jt Surg.* 1995; 77A:1103–1114.

EVANS CH. ROBBINS PD, Ghivizzani SC, et al: Clinical trial to assess the safety, feasibility and efficacy of transferring a potentially anti-arthritic cytokine gene to human joints with rheumatoid arthritis. *Human Gene Ther.* 1996; 7:1261–1280.

Human Genome Project

JAFFURS D, EVANS CH. Orthopaedic implications of the human genome project. *J AAOS.* 1998; 6:1–14.

SAMPLE QUESTIONS

The following questions were collected from recent orthopaedic in-training examinations.

1. In hyaline cartilage, the proteoglycans are attached to hyaluronic acid via:
   (a) chondroitin sulfate
   (b) keratan sulfate
   (c) link protein
   (d) peptide bonds
   (e) disulfide bonds

2. The early changes in articular cartilage in degenerative joint disease of the knee include:
   (a) decreased cartilage hydration, increased breakdown of matrix framework, and decreased proteoglycan synthesis
   (b) decreased cartilage hydration, increased breakdown of matrix framework, and increased proteoglycan synthesis
   (c) increased cartilage hydration, increased breakdown of matrix framework, and decreased proteoglycan synthesis
   (d) increased cartilage hydration, increased breakdown of matrix framework, and increased proteoglycan synthesis
   (e) increased cartilage hydration, decreased breakdown of matrix framework, and decreased proteoglycan synthesis

3. Which of the following collagen types is most closely associated with the calcification of cartilage?
   (a) I
   (b) II
   (c) III
   (d) IX
   (e) X

4. Which of the following is the most prevalent glycosaminoglycan [sic] in cartilage proteoglycans?
   (a) chondroitin sulfate
   (b) dermatan sulfate
   (c) keratan sulfate
   (d) hyaluronate
   (e) fibronectin

Answers: 1) c; 2) d; 3) e; 4) a.

Chapter 5

Musculoskeletal Soft Tissues

Joseph A. Buckwalter, MD

Outline

Although they share a common origin from undifferentiated mesenchymal cells (Fig. 5–1), the musculoskeletal soft tissues—skeletal muscle, tendon, ligament, joint capsule, menisci, and intervertebral disc differ in structure, composition, vascularity, innervation, aging changes, and capacity for repair. Understanding diseases and injuries of the musculoskeletal system and their treatment requires a knowledge of these tissues. Failure to consider their biological properties, aging and capacity for repair can lead to misinterpretation of diagnostic information, suboptimal treatment decisions, and undesirable results of treatment. Furthermore, future advances in the diagnosis and treatment of musculoskeletal problems will depend on increased knowledge of the cell and matrix biology of these musculoskeletal tissues.

This chapter reviews current understanding of the structure, composition, vascular supply, innervation, age-related changes, and injury and repair of skeletal muscle, tendon, ligament, joint capsule, menisci, and intervertebral disc.

SKELETAL MUSCLE

Skeletal muscle contraction produces joint motion and stabilizes joints against resistance. Performance of these functions depends not only on the structure and composition of the muscle cells, but on the muscle, nerves, and blood vessels, as well as the organization of the tissue and the attachment of muscle cells to tendons. Age-related changes in skeletal muscle produce profound alterations in strength, mobility, and risk of injury. Injuries to skeletal muscle vary considerably in extent and type of tissue damage and the potential for restoration of function. Some injuries allow full recovery of function while others permanently compromise the function of the musculoskeletal system.

Structure

The muscle cells that produce muscle contraction (myofibers or muscle fibers) cluster into bundles or fascicles (Fig. 5–2). Aggregates of fascicles combined with their extracellular matrix (ECM) form named muscles (Fig. 5–2B). In addition to the myofibers responsible for muscle contraction, muscles contain neuromuscular spindles: fusiform sensory end organs that detect passive stretch of the surrounding muscle tissue. They contain from 3 to 10 striated muscle fibers (intrafusal fibers), which are much smaller than regular myofibers and are separated from them by a capsule that encloses the muscle spindle. Although the ECM makes up only a small fraction of muscle volume, it is critical for normal muscle function, maintenance of muscle structure, and healing. A basal lamina containing collagens, noncollagenous proteins, and muscle-specific proteoglycans surrounds each myofiber. The basal lamina (Fig. 5–3) together with the surrounding irregularly arranged fine, collagen fibers form the endomysium. A thicker matrix sheath composed primarily of collagen fibers and elastic fibers (the perimysium) covers muscle fasciculi (see Fig. 5–2). The epimysium, a more dense peripheral sheath of connective tissue, covers the entire muscle and

Orthopaedic Surgery: The Essentials. Edited by M.E. Baratz, A.D. Watson, and J.E. Imbriglia. Thieme Medical Publishers, Inc., New York © 1999

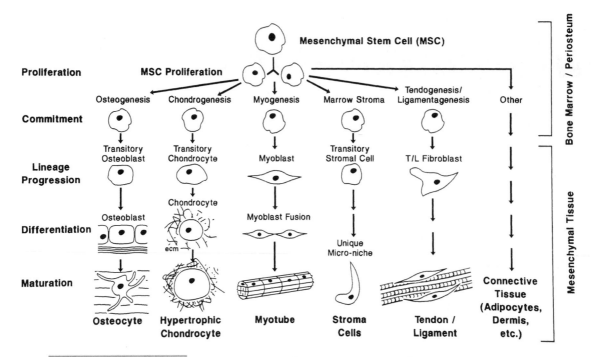

Figure 5–1 A diagrammatic representation of the potential of mesenchymal stem cells to proliferate and differentiate into specialized musculoskeletal tissue cells, including skeletal muscle cells (myoblasts fuse to form myofibers or myotubes) and fibroblasts of tendon, ligament, and joint capsule. Reproduced with permission from Buckwalter JA, Einhorn TA, Bolander ME, Cruess RL. Healing of the musculoskeletal tissues. In: Rockwood CA, Green DP, Bucholz RW, Heckman JD, eds. *Fractures*. 4th ed. Philadelphia, PA: Lippincott; 1996:261–304. Provided by Arnold Caplan.

usually joins with the fascia overlying the muscle and with the muscle tendon junction (Figs. 5–2 and 5–4).

> ## PEARL
>
> Actin + Myosin = Sarcomere.
> $(Sarcomere)^n$ = Myo<u>fibril</u>.
> Myofibril + Sarcomplasmic Reticulum +
> Multiple Nuclei = Muscle Cell (Myo<u>fiber</u>)

Composition

Muscle contains connective tissue cells, endothelial cells of blood vessels and nerve cell processes, but most of the tissue consists of large highly differentiated muscle cells (Fig. 5–2). Each muscle cell, (or myofiber or myotube) contains multiple nuclei, a unique form of endoplasmic reticulum called the sarcoplasmic reticulum, and contractile protein filaments (actin and myosin) organized into contractile cylindrical organelles called myofibrils. Each myofibril consists of regular repeating units, called sarcomeres, that consist primarily of actin and myosin filaments and that give skeletal muscle its cross-striated appearance. These myofibrils fill most of the cell volume: They have a diameter of about 1 μm, but they often extend through the entire length of the cell (Fig. 5–2a). Flattened vesicles of sarcoplasmic reticulum surround the myofibrils, and a series of invaginations of the cell mem-

brane, called transverse tubules, extend from the cell surface to lie next to each myofibril and the membranes of the sarcoplasmic reticulum. The interfibrillar sarcoplasm contains mitochondria, lysosomes, and ribosomes. Myofibers (myotubes), form by fusion of multiple small mesenchymal cells called myoblasts (Fig. 5–1). In mature individuals, some myoblasts remain next to myofibers, and following muscle injury they can proliferate and fuse to form new muscle cells. Myofibers cannot proliferate; therefore, increase in muscle mass occurs through cell enlargment. The basal lamina that covers the surface of each myofiber contain laminin (a noncollagenous protein that forms part of basement membranes), types IV and V collagen, and heparan sulfate proteoglycan. The outer connective tissue envelops of muscle consist primarily of type I collagen fibrils (Fig. 5–2b).

Blood Supply and Innervation

Skeletal muscle has elaborate networks of blood vessels and sensory and motor nerves. Large numbers of blood vessels penetrate the epimysium passing between muscle fasciculi within the muscle connective tissue matrix (Fig. 5–2b). They then enter the muscle fascicles to form rich capillary networks around individual myofibrils. In contracted muscle, the capillary networks surrounding myofibers assume a coiled form and then straighten with muscle extension. Nerves that sense muscle tension terminate on the intrafusal fibers of muscle spindles and golgi tendon organs. Three types of motor neurons supply myofibers: (1) alpha motor

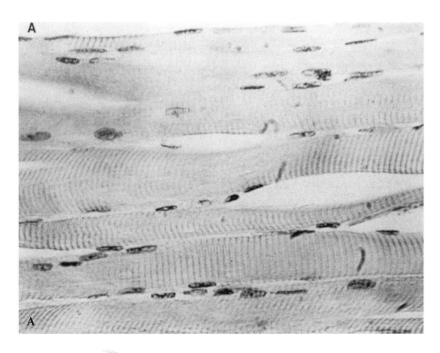

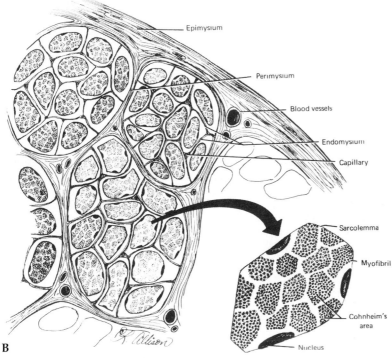

Figure 5–2 Skeletal muscle. **(A)** Light micrograph showing the myofibers or myotubes that form the bulk skeletal muscle. Notice the tubular shape of the myofibers, the prominent cross striations, and the multiple nuclei within each myofiber. **(B)** Diagram of cross section of skeletal muscle showing the organization of myofibers into bundles or fasicles. Notice the connective tissue matrix of the muscle: Endomysium surrounds each myofiber, perimysium surrounds and separates bundles of myofibers, and the epimysium covers the suface of the muscle. Blood vessels pass through the connective tissue framework to form capillary networks around each myofiber. Reproduced with permission from Buckwalter JA. Musculoskeletal tissues and the musculoskeletal system. In: Weinstein SL, Buckwalter JA, eds. *Turek's Orthopaedics: Principles and Their Application.* Philadelphia, PA: Lippincott; 1994:48–49.

neurons innervating extrafusal myofibers, (2) beta motor neurons innervating both extrafusal and intrafusal myofibers, and (3) gamma motor neurons innervating intrafusal myofibers. One motor neuron innervates each myofiber, but each motor neuron generally innervates more than one myofiber. A motor unit consists of the motor neuron and the muscle fibers it innervates. Motor nerves attach to myofibers through neuromuscular junctions that transmit signals from the motor nerves to limited regions of the myofibers. Release of neurotransmitters from a motor nerves terminal creates an action potential in the muscle cell membrane that extends into folds in the cell membrane to the sarcoplamic reticulum. The

sarcoplasmic reticulum releases calcium ions, and the rapid increase in intracellular calcium triggers simultaneous contraction of myofibers throughout the cell.

PEARL

In response to an action potential, the sarcoplasmic reticulum releases calcium ions to a field of myofibers through its extensive irrigating system: the transverse tubules.

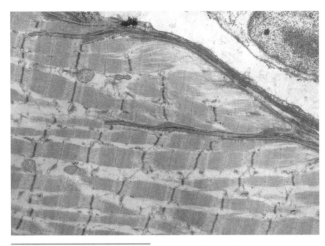

Figure 5–3 Electron micrograph of myofiber at a muscle tendon junction. Notice the highly ordered myofibrils, the mitochondria and the interdigitation of the myofiber cell membrane with the basal lamina. The myofibrils consisting primarily of actin and myosin filaments extend throughout the length of the myofiber or muscle cell.

Age-related Changes

Beginning in middle age or earlier, most individuals notice a progressive decline in strength. Loss of muscle mass resulting from decreases in the number and size of muscle cells appears to be the major cause of this age-related decline in strength. In addition to decreasing strength, loss of muscle mass may lower body temperature and increase the risk of hypothermia during cold stress. Factors that contribute to the loss of muscle mass with age include decreased exercise, especially fewer contractions against high loads; decreases in hormonal levels including growth hormone, testosterone, and thyroxin; and neuromuscular changes, including structural and functional changes in spinal motor neurons and neuromuscular junctions. In addition to the decrease in strength, the ability of some muscles to provide sustained power during repeated contractions declines with age, and age-related changes in skeletal muscle may increase the probability of muscle injury and decrease the ability of muscle to heal. The combination of increased vulnerability to injury and slower healing may contribute to the increased weakness and fatiguability of older muscles.

Although loss of skeletal muscle mass and declining strength and endurance with age appear to be inevitable, a number of interventions can slow these changes. Hormone supplementation or replacement therapy, including growth hormone and testosterone, can have beneficial effects in some individuals, but these therapies also have a variety of potential complications. Exercise increases the strength of older individuals by increasing muscle mass, cross-sectional areas, contractile proteins, motor unit recruitment, and oxidative capacity. However, minor musculoskeletal injuries and pain with exercise, primarily joint and back pain, occur more commonly in older people, especially with aerobic training. These problems occur less frequently with lower intensity strength and flexibility training programs, and usually respond quickly to conservative treatment.

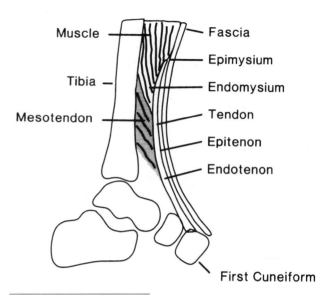

Figure 5–4 Diagram showing a muscle tendon unit (schematic representation of the tibialis anterior): muscle, muscle tendon junction, tendon insertion, and the surrounding connective tissue structures. The muscle-tendon juction extends well into the muscle, and the epimysium and endomysium pass into epitenon and the endotenon. The mesotendon extends from the surrounding tissues to the tendon and provides blood vessels for the tendon substance. (Reproduced with permission from Buckwalter JA, Maynard JA, Vailas A: Skeletal fibrous tissues. In: Albright JA, Brand RA, eds. *The Scientific Basis of Orthopaedics*. Norwalk, CT: Appleton-Lange; 1987;387–405.

PEARL

Excercise increases the strength of older individuals by increasing muscle mass, cross-sectional areas, contractile proteins, motor unit recruitment, and oxidative capacity.

Injury and Repair

Damage to myofibers initiates inflammation, which includes migration of inflammatory cells into the injured muscle and, in most injuries, hemorrhage and formation of a hematoma. An important part of the inflammatory process in skeletal muscle is the removal of damaged muscle fibers by phagocytic inflammatory cells that penetrate and fragment necrotic myofibers (Fig. 5–5). After they enter damaged muscle fibers these cells ingest bundles of contractile filaments and other cytoplasmic debris. This macrophage activity not only removes damaged cell organelles, it may have an important role in stimulating regeneration of myofibers.

As macrophages remove damaged or necrotic myofibers, spindle-shaped myoblasts appear and begin to proliferate and fuse with one another to form long myotubes with chains of central nuclei (Figs. 5–1 and 5–5). Frequently, several of these early regenerating myotubes form within the basement membrane tube of a single necrotic muscle fiber. As they

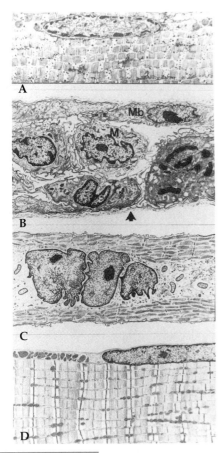

Figure 5–5 Injury and repair of a myofiber. **(A)** Immediately after injury, the nucleus shows evidence of chromatic clumping, and the myofrils are degenerating. **(B)** Macrophages (M) enter the injured myofiber and remove myofilaments and other cytoplasmic debris. Next to the basal lamina (arrow), myoblasts (Mb) line up to form new myofibers. **(C)** Myoblasts fuse to form a new myofiber that contains newly formed myofilaments. **(D)** The regenerated myofiber has peripheral nuclei and well-formed myofilaments. Reproduced with permission from Skeletal muscle. In: Woo SL, Buckwalter JA, eds. *Injury and Repair of the Musculoskeletal Soft Tissues.* Park Ridge, IL: American Academy of Orthopaedic Surgeons; 1988.

enlarge, the myotubes form a sarcoplasmic reticulum and begin to assemble organized bundles of contractile filaments. The central chains of nuclei break up and migrate to the periphery of the myotube, completing the transition of the myotube into a muscle fiber (see Fig. 5–5). Contractile proteins continue to accumulate and form myofibrils. To become functional, a regenerating muscle fiber must be innervated, including formation of a neuromuscular junction.

At the same time myotubes are regenerating, fibroblasts are producing granulation tissue that is necessary to repair the matrix of the muscle. However, this granulation tissue can interfere with the orderly regeneration of the myofibers producing a disorganized mass of scar and partially regenerated myofibers. This type of tissue may restore the continuity of the muscle, but not its contractile function. Therefore, the optimal results of muscle healing require a balance

between myofiber regeneration and synthesis of new matrix and appropriate organization and orientation of these two components of the healing muscle. Once muscle fibers have appeared, the ECM continues to remodel. If excessive scar formation can be avoided and the muscle cells are innervated, controlled muscle contraction and loading increases the strength of the injured muscle. In addition to the muscle cell and fibrous tissue repair responses, muscle injury occasionally stimulates bone formation (i.e., myositis ossificans). The new bone can be contiguous with periosteum or lie entirely within muscle, free of any connection with underlying bone.

Classifying muscle injuries by the severity and mechanism of injury makes it possible to predict the potential for restoration of muscle function. A type I muscle injury damages muscle fibers but leaves the ECM, blood vessels, and nerve supply intact. Blunt trauma, including surgical trauma, mild stretching injuries, and temporary ischemia can cause a type I injury. The muscle fibers will be damaged but the basal lamina and other components of the extracellular matrix, the blood supply, and the nerve supply remain intact. These injuries occur frequently and can heal through spontaneous muscle fiber regeneration that restores the original structure, composition, and function of the muscle (see Fig. 5–5). A type II muscle injury damages the nerve supply and may include damage to the myofibers, but it leaves the ECM and blood supply intact. Type II injuries may result from isolated peripheral nerve damage, blunt trauma, or stretching of nerve and muscle. Because the matrix maintains the muscle structure, if regenerating nerve fibers reach intact neuromuscular junctions, the potential for restoration of function exists. A type III muscle injury causes loss or necrosis of all muscle tissue components, including myofibers and ECM and/or prolonged loss of blood and nerve supply. Type III injuries result from severe blunt trauma, tearing, or penetrating trauma. If the vascular supply remains intact, the inflammatory response can remove the necrotic tissue, but some type III injuries compromise the blood supply, and the necrotic muscle is not removed and must be surgically debrided. If the necrotic tissue is removed, repair can begin. Cells capable of differentiating into myoblasts survive even severe injuries or migrate into the injury site. However, the lack of an ECM to guide regeneration of myofibers usually prevents formation of organized muscle tissue. Even if such tissue forms, lack of guidance for reinnervation prevents regenerated myofibers from regaining function. For these reasons, the usual result of a type III muscle injury is healing by scar formation with scattered myoblasts attempting to form myofibers.

TENDON, LIGAMENT, AND JOINT CAPSULE

The specialized musculoskeletal dense fibrous tissues—tendon, ligament and joint capsule, have a major role in providing the stability and mobility of the musculoskeletal system. These tissues differ in shape and location and vary slightly in structure, composition, and function, but they have in common their insertion into bone and their ability to resist large tensile loads with minimal deformation. Tendon transmits the muscle forces to bone that produce joint movement;

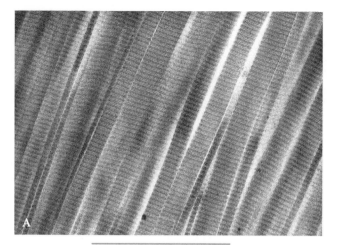
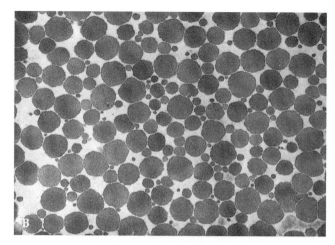

Figure 5–6   Electron micrographs of the densely packed collagen fibrils consisting primarily of type I collagen forming a ligament. **(A)** Longitudinal section. **(B)** Transverse section.

ligaments and joint capsule stabilize joints and the relationships between adjacent bones while allowing and guiding joint movement. Age-related degeneration or injuries that affect these tissues can destabilize joints or lead to loss of muscle function.

Structure

Tendon, ligament, and joint capsule take the form of tough yet flexible and pliant fibrous sheets, bands, and cords that consist of highly oriented dense fibrous tissue. The high degree of matrix organization and density of the matrix (reflecting a high concentration of collagen) distinguish these tissues from irregular dense fibrous tissues and loose fibrous tissues (Fig. 5–6).

Tendon

Tendons vary in shape and size from the small fibrous strings that form the tendons of the lumbrical muscles to the large fibrous cords that form the Achilles tendons. But in any shape or size, they unite muscle with bone and transmit the force of muscle contraction to bone. They consist of three parts: the substance of the tendon itself, the muscle tendon junction, and the bone insertion (Fig. 5–4). Connective tissues surrounding tendons allow low-friction gliding and access for blood vessels to the tendon substance. Many tendons have a well developed mesotendon, a structure that attaches the tendon to the surrounding connective tissue and consists of loose, elastic connective tissue that can stretch and recoil with the tendon and provide a blood supply to the tendon substance (Fig. 5–4). In certain locations, the surrounding connective tissue forms sheaths that enclose the tendon (Fig. 5–7) and specialized pulleys of dense fibrous tissue that influence the line of tendon action.

Multiple fascicles or bundles, consisting of fibroblasts and dense linear arrays of collagen fibrils, form the tendon substance and give tendons their fibrous appearance. The endotendon, a less dense connective tissue containing fibroblasts, blood vessels, nerves, and lymphatics, surrounds individual tendon fascicles (Fig. 5–7). The separation of tendon fascicles by endotendon may allow small gliding movements between adjacent tendon bundles. The endotendon tissue continues to

form the epitenon, a thin layer of connective tissue that covers the surface of the tendon. Where the tendon joins the muscle, the fibrous tissue of the epitenon continues as the thin fibrous covering of the attached muscle called the epimysium (Fig. 5–4).

Muscle-tendon junctions must efficiently transmit the force of muscle contraction to the tendon (Fig. 5–4). The attachment of muscle to tendon occurs through continuation of the collagen fibrils of the fibrous tissue layers of muscle (epimysium, perimysium, and endomysium) into the collagen fibrils of the tendon and through elaborate interdigitation of the muscle cell membrane with the collagen fibrils of

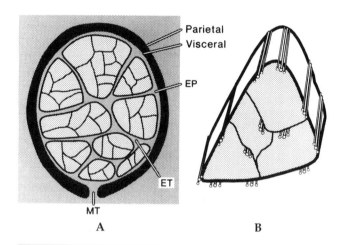

Figure 5–7   Diagram showing a sheathed segment of tendon. **(A)** The mesotendon (MT) extends from the sheath to the tendon substance and contains blood vessels. The epitenon covers the collagen bundles that form the tendon and the endotenon (ET) passes between the collagen fiber bundles. The visceral and parietal layers of the tendon sheath form the opposing gliding surfaces. **(B)** The internal blood supply of the tendon consists of parallel arrays of vessels in the epitenon and endotenon. Reproduced with permission from Buckwalter JA, Maynard JA, Vailas A. In: Albright JA, Brand RA, eds. Skeletal fibrous tissues. *The Scientific Basis of Orthopaedics.* Norwalk, CT: Appleton-Lange; 1987;387–405.

the tendon. This interconnecting of muscle cell and tendon has the appearance of interlocking fingers when examined by electron microscopy, and it provides a strong bond between the muscle cell and the tendon collagen. Collagen fibrils do not enter the muscle cells, but lie next to their basement membranes. The muscle-cell plasma membrane thickens at the muscle tendon junction, and muscle myofilaments extend directly to it.

PEARL

The musculotendinous junction is fortified through two connections:

1. **collagen fibrils spanning the muscles' fibrous envelopes and the tendon.**
2. **interdigitation of muscle cell membrane with collagen fibrils of the tendon.**

Normal tendon gliding, efficient transmission of muscle forces to move joints, and tendon nutrition depend on the peritendinous connective tissue structures sometimes called peritenon. These structures range from loose connective tissue to elaborate, well-defined mesotendons (Fig. 5–4), sheaths (Fig. 5–7) and pulleys. Where tendons follow a straight course, the surrounding tissue usually consists of loose areolar tissue. In some locations, this tissue must stretch several centimeters and then recoil without tearing or disrupting the tendon blood supply. The tissue consists of an interlacing meshwork of thin collagen fibrils and elastic fibers filled with abundant soft, almost fluid ground substance. Where tendons change course between their muscle attachment and their bone insertion, often as they cross or near a joint, the surrounding connective tissue may form a bursa or a discrete tendon sheath. These structures allow low-friction movement between the tendon and adjacent bone, joint capsule, tendon, ligament, fibrous tissue retinacula, or fibrous tissue pulleys. Tendon bursae and sheaths consist of flattened synovial-lined sacks that usually cover only a portion of the tendon circumference. Tendon sheaths and bursae resemble synovial joints in that they consist of cavities lined with synovial-like cells, they contain synovial-like fluid, and they facilitate low-friction gliding between two surfaces (Fig. 5–7). Mesotenons generally attach to one surface of a tendon within a tendon sheath and provide the blood supply to this portion of the tendon (Figs. 5–4 and 5–7).

Distinct dense, fibrous tissue retinacula, pulleys, or fascial slings lie over the outer surface of some regions of tendon sheaths. These firm, fibrous structures direct the line of tendon movement and prevent displacement or "bowstringing" of the tendon that would decrease the efficiency of the muscle tendon unit. For example, the dense fibrous tissue extensor tendon retinacula of the wrist keep the wrist and digital extensor tendons from displacing dorsally when the fingers are extended and the wrist is in dorsiflexion. The flexor tendons of the fingers and thumb pass through a more elaborate series of pulleys and sheaths that make possible efficient finger flexion.

Joint Capsule and Ligament

Joint capsule and ligament have similar structures and functions, and in some regions ligament and capsule form a continuous structure. Like tendon, both of them consist primarily of highly oriented, densely packed collagen fibrils (Fig. 5–6). Unlike tendon, they more often assume the form of layered sheets or lamellae. Both ligament and capsule attach to adjacent bones and cross synovial joints, yet allow at least some motion between the bones. Ligament has the primary function of restraining abnormal motion between adjacent bones. Joint capsule also restrains abnormal joint motion or displacement of articular surfaces, but usually to a lesser extent. Both capsule and ligament consist of a proximal bone insertion, ligament or capsular substance, and a distal bone insertion, and both contain nerves that may sense joint motion and displacement.

A joint capsule forms a fibrous tissue cuff around a synovial joint. A synovial membrane lines the interior of the joint capsule and loose areolar connective tissue covers the exterior. This loose tissue often contains plexes of small blood vessels that supply the capsule. Nerves and blood vessels from this loose connective tissue penetrate the fibrous capsule to supply the capsule and outer later of synovium. Each end of the capsule attaches in a continuous line around the articular surface of the bones forming the joint, usually near the periphery of the articular cartilage surface. Tendon and ligament reinforce some regions of joint capsule. For example, the glenohumeral ligaments form part of the glenohumeral joint capsule and the expansion of the semimembranosus tendon contributes to the posterior oblique ligament of the knee and part of the knee joint capsule.

Unlike joint capsule, ligament varies in its anatomic relationship to synovial joints. This variability separates ligament into three types: intra-articular or intracapsular ligament, articular or capsular ligament, and extra-articular or extracapsular ligament. Intra-articular ligaments, including the cruciate ligaments of the knee, have the form of distinct separate structures. In contrast, capsular ligaments, such as the glenohumeral ligaments, appear as thickenings of joint capsule. Extra-articular ligaments, such as the coracoacromial ligament, lie at a distance from a synovial joint. Despite these differences in relationship to joints, the function of the three ligament types remains that of stabilizing adjacent bones or restraining abnormal joint motion.

Composition

Individual tendons, ligaments, and capsules differ slightly in cell and matrix composition; but they all contain the same basic cell types, share similar patterns of vascular supply and innervation, and have the same primary matrix macromolecule, type I collagen.

Cells

Fibroblasts form the predominant cell of tendon, ligament and joint capsule. The endothelial cells of blood vessels, and in some locations nerve cell processes, exist within tendon, ligament and joint capsule, but they form only a small part of the tissue. The fibroblasts surround themselves with a dense fibrous tissue matrix and throughout life continue to maintain the matrix. They vary in shape, activity, and density among ligaments, tendons, and joint capsules and among regions of the same structure. Most dense fibrous tissue fibroblasts have long small diameter cell processes that extend between collagen fibrils throughout the matrix.

Matrix

Tissue fluid contributes 60% or more of the wet weight of most dense fibrous tissues, and the matrix macromolecules contribute the other 40%. Collagens, elastin, proteoglycans, and noncollagenous proteins combine to form the macromolecular framework of the dense fibrous tissues. Collagens, the major component of the dense fibrous tissue molecular framework, contribute 70 to 80% of the dry weight of many dense fibrous tissues. Type I collagen commonly forms more than 90% of the tissue collagen. Type III collagen also occurs within the dense fibrous tissues, in some tissues it forms about 10% of the total collagen, and other collagen types may also be present in small amounts. Most dense fibrous tissues have some elastin, less than 5% of their dry weight.

Some ligaments, in particular the nuchal ligament and ligamentum flavum, have higher elastin concentrations, up to 75% of the tissue dry weight. Proteoglycans usually contribute less than 1% of the dry weight of dense fibrous tissues, but they may have important roles in organizing the ECM and interacting with the tissue fluid. Most dense fibrous tissues appear to contain both large aggregating proteoglycans and small nonaggregating proteoglycans. The large proteoglycans presumably occupy the interfibrillar regions of the matrix, and the small proteoglycans lie directly on or near the surface of collagen fibrils. Noncollagenous proteins also form a critical part of the dense fibrous tissue matrix even though they contribute only a few percent to the dry weight of most of the tissues. Fibronectin occurs in all dense fibrous tissue.

Other noncollagenous proteins also contribute to the structure of these tissues, but their composition, structure, and function have not been well-defined.

Insertions into Bone

The bony insertions of tendon, ligament, and joint capsule attach the flexible, dense fibrous tissue securely to rigid bone, yet they allow motion between the bone and the dense fibrous tissue without damage to the dense fibrous tissue. Despite their small size, insertions have a more complex and variable structure than the substance of the tissue, and they have different mechanical properties. They vary in size, strength, and the angle of their collagen fiber bundles relative to the bone and in the proportion of their collagen fibers that penetrate directly into bone. Based on differences in the angle between the collagen fibers of the dense fibrous tissue structure and the bone and on the proportion of collagen fibrils that penetrate directly into bone, dense fibrous tissue insertions can be separated into two types: direct insertions (insertions where many collagen fibrils pass directly into bone), and indirect or periosteal insertions (insertions where only a few the collagen fibrils pass directly into bone) (Fig. 5–8).

Direct insertions, such as the insertion of the medial collateral ligament of the knee into the femur, consist of sharply defined regions where the ligament joins the bone; only a thin layer of the substance of the ligament, tendon, or capsule joins the fibrous layer of the periosteum (Fig. 5–8a). Most of the collagen fibrils at the insertion pass directly from the substance of the tendon, ligament, or joint capsule into the bone cortex, usually entering at a right angle to the bone surface. These fibrils then mingle with the collagen fibrils of the organic matrix of bone, creating a strong bond between the tendon, ligament, or capsule and the bone matrix. The deeper collagen fibers that enter the bone pass through four zones

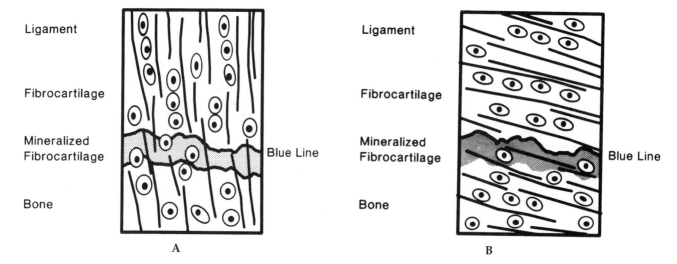

Figure 5–8   Diagrams of ligament insertions. **(A)** Direct insertion, the majority of the ligament collagen fibrils pass directly into bone. **(B)** Indirect insertion, the majority of the ligament collagen fibrils pass into the periosteum. Reproduced with permission from Buckwalter JA, Maynard JA, Vailas A. In: Albright JA, Brand RA, eds. Skeletal fibrous tissues. *In The Scientific Basis of Orthopaedics.* Norwalk, CT: Appleton-Lange; 1987;387–405.

of increasing stiffness: the substance of the dense fibrous tissue structure, fibrocartilage, mineralized fibrocartilage, and bone. In the fibrocartilage zone, the cells are larger than the fibroblasts of the tendon, joint capsule, or ligament, and they are more spherical. A sharp border of unmineralized matrix separates the zone of fibrocartilage from the mineralized fibrocartilage zone.

The less common indirect insertions, like the insertion of the medial collateral ligament of the knee into the tibia, usually cover more bone surface area than direct insertions because a larger proportion of their collagen fibrils join the periosteum (Fig. 5–8b). Like direct insertions, indirect insertions have superficial and deep collagen fibrils, but most of their collagen fibrils form the superficial layer that joins the fibrous layer of the periosteum. The deep collagen fibrils enter the bone cortex, but they generally do not pass through sharply defined zones of mineralized and unmineralized fibrocartilage.

Blood Supply and Innervation

Most dense fibrous tissues have well developed networks of blood vessels extending throughout their substance. Generally, these vascular systems follow the longitudinal pattern of the collagenous matrix (Fig. 5–7), but they may have multiple anastomoses between parallel vessels. Some blood vessels in tendon, ligament, and joint capsule insertions enter the bone. In addition to nerve cell processes next to blood vessels, dense fibrous tissues have specialized nerve endings that lie on the surface or within the substance of the tissue. Presumably, the nerve fibers in the dense fibrous tissues function as pain receptors, vasomotor efferents, and mechanoreceptors sensitive to stretch or distortion. The mechanoreceptors presumably sense joint position, muscle tension, and loads applied to ligaments, capsules, and tendons. In tendon, they can adjust muscle tension. In ligament and capsule, they may have a role in initiating protective reflexes that oppose potentially damaging joint movements.

Age-related Changes

Age-related degenerative changes in dense fibrous tissues may result in spontaneous or low-energy-level ruptures of the shoulder rotator cuff, the long head of the biceps, the tibialis posterior, the patellar and the Achilles tendons, and sprains and ruptures of joint capsules and ligaments including those of the spine and wrist. It is likely that chronic activity-related musculoskeletal pain or at least some of the soreness following physical activity in people middle aged and older results from injuries to the fibrous components of muscle-tendon junctions or to tendon, ligament, and joint capsule insertions into bone.

The tensile mechanical properties of at least some dense fibrous tissue-bone complexes, including stiffness and strength, deteriorate significantly with age. The tissue changes responsible for the age-related decline in the properties of dense fibrous tissues have not been clearly identified. In at least some locations, including the rotator cuff, the nutrition of dense fibrous tissue cells may decrease with age due to decreased vascular perfusion. The resulting decline in cell function may lead to tissue degeneration. Changes in the cell function, matrix composition, and organization of the

matrix macromolecules that occur independently of alterations in nutrition may also contribute to the decline in mechanical properties. Aging fibroblasts flatten and elongate, lose most of their rough endoplasmic reticulum and Golgi membranes, and undergo a decrease in metabolic and biosynthetic activity. Although biochemical analyses have not shown dramatic age-related changes in tendon or ligament matrix composition, the collagen and water concentration of these tissues may decline slightly with age as the labile reducible collagen cross-links decrease and the more stable nonreducible cross-links increase. The properties of the tissues could also be affected by alterations in the organization and molecular structure of the collagens. Post-translational modifications of the collagens may also contribute to the age-related decline in mechanical properties.

Injury and Repair

Although the specialized forms of dense fibrous tissue follow the same general pattern of healing, because of the differences in their structure and function tendon, ligament, and joint capsule healing present different clinical problems. All three tendon components may suffer acute traumatic injuries. Tears of the muscle-tendon junction are the most common injuries. Avulsions or fractures through tendon insertions, lacerations of tendon substance or complete avulsions of the tendon from the muscle-tendon junction occur less frequently. Complete disruption of any part of the muscle-tendon unit allows the muscle to retract, increasing the gap at the injury site. If the injury is left untreated, scar tissue may eventually fill the gap, but it will leave the muscle-tendon unit longer than before injury and may bind the tendon to the surrounding tissues. Without restoration of normal tendon length and gliding, the function of the muscle-tendon unit will be poor. For this reason restoration of muscle-tendon unit function following a complete disruption usually requires a surgical repair that re-establishes normal tendon length and has sufficient strength to allow immediate motion of the tendon relative to the surrounding tissues.

Achieving healing of lacerated digital flexor tendons within tendon sheaths while preserving the pulleys and the tendon motion presents a unique problem in the treatment of musculoskeletal injuries. The cut tendon ends can be sutured and will heal, but if the repair tissue scars the tendon to the sheath or the pulleys, tendon motion will be restricted and may cause joint contracture. Tendons without sheaths do not usually present this problem because scarring of their repair tissue to surrounding loose areolar tissue often will not severely restrict motion.

Tendon healing following an acute laceration or tear, including tears of the muscle-tendon junction, begins with hematoma formation followed by inflammatory cell, capillary, and fibroblast migration into the site of injury. Granulation tissue proliferates around the injury site and between the ends of the tendon, and fibroblasts in the granulation tissue form a new matrix with randomly oriented collagen fibrils. The density of fibroblasts increases up to 3 weeks after injury when granulation tissue fills and surrounds the repaired area. If the tendon has been sutured, the suture material holds the tendon ends together until the fibroblasts have produced sufficient collagen to form a "tendon callus." The tensile strength of the repaired tendon depends on the collagen concentration and the orientation of the collagen fibrils. The collagen fibrils become longitudinally oriented by about 4 weeks, and during the next 2 to 3 months the repair tissue remodels until it resembles normal tendon. The amount and density of the scar tissue adhesions between the tendon injury site and surrounding tissues depend on the intensity, extent, and duration of the inflammatory and repair phases of healing and the mobility of the tendon during repair.

Early controlled mobilization of a repaired tendon can reduce scar adhesions between the tendon injury site and the surrounding tissue and facilitate healing, but excessive loading may disrupt the repair tissue. Thus, optimal tendon healing depends on surgical apposition and mechanical stabilization of the tendon ends without excessive soft tissue damage and on creating the optimal mechanical environment for healing. This mechanical environment includes sufficient tendon mobility to prevent adhesions and sufficient loading to stimulate remodeling of the repair tissue matrix along the lines of stress, but the loads applied to the tendon must not exceed the strength of the surgical repair.

Disruption of tendon insertions into bone often involves a fracture or avulsion of a bone fragment at the site of injury. These injuries usually can be treated by surgically reducing and stabilizing the fracture or re-inserting the tendon into the bone and stabilizing the insertion. Healing occurs either by bony union or by union of the bone to the tendon substance.

Partial muscle-tendon junction injuries usually will heal successfully if further injury can be prevented, but complete or nearly complete avulsions or tears can present difficult problems because attempts to suture to tendon muscle tissue consisting primarily of muscle cells is unlikely to produce a predictable result. Optimal healing of these injuries depends on approximation of the avulsed tendon and any remnants of the tendon remaining attached to the muscle or, when available, muscle fascia. Although it may appear that muscles attach to tendons over a small area, in many muscles thin extensions of their tendons penetrate long distances within the muscle bellies. Identification of these thin bands of tendon within muscle may make it possible to suture them to an avulsed or partially avulsed tendon in the proximal and distal thirds of many muscles and as far as the middle third of some muscles. If this can be accomplished, the tendon-muscle injury site must then be stabilized for a sufficient time to allow repair of the muscle-tendon junction with scar tissue.

Ligament and joint capsule substance healing follows the sequence described for healing of tendon substance. Also as in tendon healing, early motion and loading of injured ligaments can stimulate healing. Because controlled normal motion of a joint does not necessarily cause large forces in the ligaments and joint capsule, limited motion will not necessarily disrupt the repair of the tissue.

MENISCI

Menisci perform important mechanical functions in synovial joints including load bearing, shock absorption, and participation in joint lubrication. They may also contribute to joint stability. Menisci and meniscus like structures consist of dense fibrous tissue or fibrocartilage and project from the margins of synovial joints to interpose themselves between

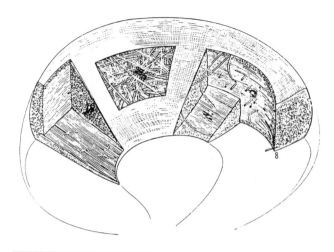

Figure 5–9 Schematic diagram of a knee meniscus showing the collagen fibril organization. Reproduced with permission from Bullough PG. Munuera L. Murphy J. Weinstein AM. The strength of the menisci of the knee as it relates to their fine structure. *J Bone Jt Surg* 1970;52B:564–567.

articular cartilage surfaces. They include the knee menisci (two C-shaped menisci that lie on the tibial plateaus and form part of the knee joint) (Fig. 5–9), the articular discs of the sternoclavicular and acromioclavicular joints, the triangular fibrocartilage that binds the distal ends of the ulna and radius together and forms part of the wrist joint, and the labra found in some joints such as the hip and shoulder.

Structure

Within the knee, menisci collagen fibril diameter and orientation and cell morphology vary from the surface to the deeper central regions (Fig. 5–9). The superficial regions that lie against articular cartilage usually consist of a mesh of fine fibrils. Immediately deep to these fine fibrils, small-diameter collagen fibrils with a radial orientation relative to the body of the meniscus form a thicker subsurface layer. The flattened ellipsoid-shaped cells of this layer orient their maximum diameter roughly parallel to the articular surface. In the deeper central or middle region, making up the bulk of the meniscus, large-diameter collagen fibril bundles surround larger cells with a more spherical shape. The deeper collagen fibril bundles follow the curve of the menisci, and smaller radially oriented fibril bundles weave among the circumferential fibril bundles (Fig. 5–9). The circumferential arrangement of the large collagen bundles gives the menisci great tensile strength for loads applied parallel to the orientation of the fibers. The radial fibers may resist the development and propagation of longitudinal tears between the larger circumferential collagen fiber bundles.

Composition
Cells

Meniscal cells closely resemble articular cartilage chondrocytes in their appearance and have been referred to as meniscal fibrochondrocytes. Like chondrocytes, they lack cell-to-cell contacts and attach their membranes to specific matrix macromolecules. Fibrochondrocytes have the primary function of maintaining the surrounding matrix. Most of them lie at a distance from blood vessels and, therefore, rely on diffusion through the matrix for transport of nutrients and metabolites.

Matrix

Water contributes 60 to 75% of the total wet weight of the meniscus. As in the other musculoskeletal tissues, the interactions between the matrix fluid and the macromolecular framework significantly influence the mechanical properties of menisci. The macromolecular framework of the meniscus contributes 25 to 40% of the meniscus wet weight and consists of collagens, noncollagenous proteins, proteoglycans, and elastin. The collagens give menisci their form and tensile strength and contribute approximately 75% of the dry weight of the tissue. Type I collagen makes up more than 90% of the total tissue collagen. Type II collagen, type V collagen, and type VI collagen each contribute 1 to 2% of the total tissue collagen. Noncollagenous proteins, including fibronectin and other noncollagenous proteins, contribute 8 to 13% of the dry weight. Large aggregating proteoglycans and smaller nonaggregating proteoglycans together contribute about 2% of meniscal dry weight. Presumably they have functions similar to those of the proteoglycans found in other dense fibrous tissues. Elastin forms less than 1% of the tissue dry weight. This small amount of elastin probably does not significantly influence the organization of the matrix or the mechanical properties.

Blood Supply and Innervation

Most menisci and meniscal-like structures have blood vessels and some nerve endings, at least in their more peripheral regions. Branches from the geniculate arteries form a capillary plexus along the peripheral borders of the knee menisci. Small radial branches project from the circumferential parameniscal vessels into the meniscal substance. In adults, these vessels penetrate into 10 to 30% of the width of the medial meniscus and 10 to 25% of the width of the lateral meniscus. As a result, the cells of the inner portions of menisci depend on diffusion of nutrients and metabolites. Nerves lie on the peripheral surface of the knee menisci and other meniscal-like structures. Although these nerves enter the more superficial regions of some parts of the tissue, they generally do not penetrate into the central regions. The functions of these nerve endings have not been clearly defined, but they may contribute to joint proprioception.

PEARL

At birth, radial branches of the parameniscal vessels extend to the inner margins of the menisci. By adulthood, they retreat to the peripheral 10 to 30%.

Age-related Changes

With increasing age, some meniscal tissues develop degenerative changes that include fibrillation or even erosion of the tissue surfaces. Alterations in the tissue structure composition and mechanical properties presumably lead to "degenerative tears" of menisci. Despite the clinical importance of these age-related alterations in menisci, the aging changes in meniscal cells and matrix have not been extensively studied, although they probably closely resemble the changes seen in dense fibrous tissues.

Injury and Repair

The response of meniscal tissue to tears depends on whether the tear occurs through a vascular or an avascular portion of the meniscus. The vascular regions respond to injury like other vascularized dense fibrous tissues. This response can heal a meniscal injury and restore the tissue structure and function if the torn edges remain apposed and if the repair tissue is not disrupted in the early stages of healing. The avascular regions of meniscal tissue do not repair significant tissue defects. Cells in the region of the injury may proliferate and synthesize new matrix, but there is no evidence that the cells migrate into the defect site or produce new matrix that can fill the defect site.

INTERVERTEBRAL DISC

Normal function of the spine depends greatly on the intervertebral discs. Throughout the spine, they contribute to stability while allowing movement between vertebrae and absorbing compressive loads. With age, the gross and microscopic appearance, cell content, and matrix composition of disc tissues change more than any other tissues.

Structure

Human intervertebral disc consist of four tissues: hyaline cartilage end plate, annulus fibrosis, transition zone, and nucleus pulposus.

Cartilage End Plate

Hyaline cartilage end plate covers the superior and inferior surfaces of each disc and separate the other disc tissues from the vertebral bone. Grossly and microscopically end plate closely resembles other hyaline cartilages. The dense collagen fibers of the annulus fibrosis pass through the outer edges of the end plate into the vertebral bodies. With age, the cartilage plate mineralizes and eventually cannot be identified as a distinct structure.

Annulus Fibrosis

The annulus fibrosis consists primarily of densely packed collagen fibers formed into two components: the outer circumferential rings of collagen lamellae or layers and an inner larger fibrocartilagenous component. The collagen lamellae that form the outer concentric rings of the annulus have a high degree of orientation: Collagen fibrils within a layer lie parallel to each other; collagen fibrils within adjacent layers lie at 40 to 70 degree angles to the collagen fibers within layers on either side. In the fibrocartilagenous component of the annulus, collagen fibrils run concentrically and vertically but lack the high degree of orientation found in the outer concentric rings.

Transition Zone

When the intervertebral disc first forms, the nucleus pulposus and annulus fibrosus have a sharp boundary where the gelatinous nucleus pulposus lies directly against the fibrous annulus. With growth, a transition zone appears that lies between the fibrocartilagenous component of the annulus fibrosis and the nucleus pulposus.

Nucleus Pulposus

In newborns and young individuals, the soft gelatinous nucleus pulposus tissue has a translucent appearance. It contains relatively few collagen fibers and they lack any apparent orientation. With age, the nucleus pulposus becomes more

fibrous making it increasingly difficult to separate the nucleus pulposus from the transition zone and the fibrocartilagenous part of the annulus fibrosus.

Composition

Intervertebral disc tissues consist of water, cells, and matrix macromolecules. The composition of the hyaline cartilage plate has not been extensively studied, but it appears to resemble other hyaline cartilage. The annulus, like other dense fibrous tissues, has water concentration of 60 to 70% throughout life. In contrast, the water concentration of the nucleus pulposus declines from about 80 to 90% at birth to about 70% in adults.

Cells

Intervertebral discs contain two principal cell types: notochordal cells and connective tissue cells (Fig. 5–10). Notochordal cells (Fig. 5–10a) form the nucleus pulposus in the fetus. With growth, development, and aging they gradually disappear, and the cells found in the nucleus of older indi-

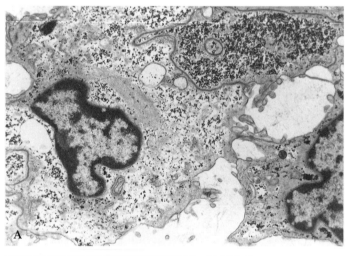

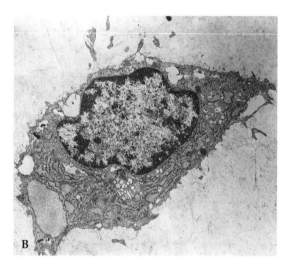

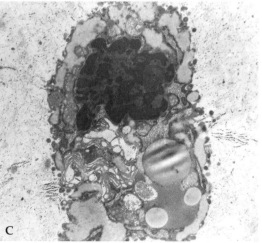

Figure 5–10 Electron micrographs of human intervertebral disc cells. **(A)** Notochordal cells from human infant nucleus pulposus. Notice the interdigitation of the cell membranes and the granular glycogen deposits. **(B)** Viable connective tissue cell from adolescent human nucleus pulposus. **(C)** Degenerating connective tissue cell from adult nucleus pulposus.

viduals have the appearance of connective tissue cells, often resembling chondrocytes (Fig. 5–10b). The connective tissue cells of the outer annulus have the appearance of fibroblasts, like those found in other dense fibrous tissues. The connective tissue cells of the inner regions of the annulus and other disc components have a more spherical form, like chondrocytes. The cells of the cartilage end plate tissue have the shape and organelles of hyaline cartilage chondrocytes.

Clusters and cords of large irregular notochordal cells populate the nucleus pulposus of the newborn human intervertebral disc. These cells contain endoplasmic reticulum, golgi membranes, mitochondria, glycogen, and bundles of microfilaments. Unlike mesenchymal cells, notochordal cells form multiple specialized junctions with other cells, and their membranes form elaborate interdigitations with those of other cells (Fig. 5–10a). During skeletal growth the notochordal cell clusters, or cords, disappear, and the glycogen content of the cells declines. In some regions, they retain cell to cell contact by elongated cell processes. With aging, the density of notochordal cells declines further.

In the outer annulus the fibroblasts lie with their long axes parallel to the collagen fibrils. In the inner fibrocartilagenous region of the annulus more of the cells assume a spherical form like those seen in other fibrocartilages. In the nucleus pulposus, connective tissue cells have oval nuclei and slightly elongated form, but most have a more spherical shape. The proportion of viable nucleus pulposus cells declines with age, but even in discs from elderly people some viable connective tissue cells survive.

Matrix

The matrix macromolecular framework of the human intervertebral disc forms from collagens, elastin, proteoglycans, and noncollagenous proteins. The concentrations and specific types of these molecules vary among the disc tissues. The collagens, including fibrillar and short chain collagens, give the disc its form and tensile strength. The concentration of collagen decreases progressively from the outer annulus to the most central portion of the nucleus. In the adult disc, the contribution of collagen to the tissue dry weight declines from 60 to 70% in the outer rim of the annulus to 10 to 20% in the most central part of the nucleus.

The annulus fibrosus contains fibrillar and short chain collagens. The fibrillar collagens found in the annulus fibrosis include type I, type II, type III and type V. The concentration of type I collagen declines from about 80% of the total collagen in the outer rim of the annulus to zero in the transition zone and nucleus. The concentration of type II collagen follows the opposite pattern. It increases from zero to 80% of the total collagen from the outer rim of the annulus to the transition zone and nucleus. Type III collagen occurs in trace amounts, and Type V collagen contributes about 3% of the total collagen of the annulus fibrosus. The short chain collagens found in annulus fibrosus include type VI and IX. Type IX collagen forms only about 1% of annulus fibrosus collagen, but type VI occurs in unusually high concentrations, it forms about 10% of total annulus fibrosis collagen.

Fibrillar and short chain collagens also form part of the matrix of the nucleus pulposus. It contains at least three fibril

forming collagens: type II, type III and type XI. Type II is the predominant collagen contributing about 80% of the total nucleus pulposus collagen. Type III occurs in trace amounts, and type XI contributes about 3% of the total collagen of the nucleus. Nucleus pulposus short chain collagens include type VI and type IX. As in the annulus fibrosis type IX forms only about 1% of the total collagen, but type VI contributes even more to the nucleus than to the annulus, forming about 14 to 20% of the total collagen. The reason for the unusually high concentration of type VI collagen in the annulus and nucleus remains unknown. This short chain collagen forms banded fibrillar aggregates of longitudinal fibrils about 5 nm in diameter with alternating transverse bands consisting of two 15-nm-wide dark bands separated by a 15-nm-wide lucent strip. These fibrillar aggregates occur most frequently in the matrix immediately surrounding cells. They may have a role in resisting tensile loads on the matrix or may provide a loose fibrillar network that helps organize other matrix molecules.

Aggregating and nonaggregating proteoglycans form a significant part of the disc macromolecular framework and help give the disc stiffness to compression and resiliency. Their concentration increases from the periphery of the disc to the center. They contribute about 10 to 20% of the dry weight of the outer annulus and as much as 50% of the dry weight of the central nucleus. Annulus fibrosus and nucleus pulposus proteoglycans differ from those found in hyaline cartilages such as disc cartilage end plate, articular cartilage, or epiphyseal or growth plate cartilage. The proteoglycan populations found in annulus fibrosus and nucleus pulposus include fewer aggregates, smaller aggregates, and smaller more variable aggrecans. Aggregated and nonaggregated disc proteoglycan aggrecans have shorter protein core filaments, vary more in size, and have less chondroitin sulfate and more keratan sulfate than those found in hyaline cartilages. The high concentration of these small variable aggrecans in the nucleus pulposus suggests that fragments of degraded aggrecans accumulate in the central regions of the disc.

Elastin occurs in trace amounts in annulus fibrosis and nucleus pulposus. In the annulus, elastin appears as fusiform or cylindrical fibers lying parallel to the collagen fibrils. In the nucleus, elastin assumes irregular lobular shapes without apparent relationship to collagen fibrils. The contribution of elastin to disc mechanical properties remains unclear.

As in other musculoskeletal tissues, noncollagenous proteins appear to help organize and stabilize the ECM of intervertebral disc and may facilitate adhesion of cell membranes to other matrix macromolecules. The concentration of disc noncollagenous proteins increases with age. In the annulus, the proportion of tissue dry weight contributed by noncollagenous proteins increases from 5 to 25% with increasing age, and in the nucleus it increases from 20 to 45% of the dry weight. Some of the increasing concentration of noncollagenous proteins may be due to accumulation of degraded molecules.

Blood Supply and Innervation

Small blood vessels and plexes of vessels lie on the surface on the annulus fibrosis, and occasional small vessels penetrate a short distance into the outer layers of the annulus. The intra-osseous blood vessels of the vertebrae contact but do not penetrate the cartilage end plate. This arrangement of blood vessels leaves the central disc as the largest avascular structure in the body. The cells must rely on diffusion of nutrients and metabolites through a large volume of matrix. Mineralization of the end plate with increasing age may further compromise diffusion of nutrients to the central regions of the disc. Perivascular and free nerve endings lie on the outer surface of the annulus and some of these nerve cell processes penetrate the outer most collagen lamellae. Despite multiple investigations of disc innervation, no nerves have been identified deep to the outer annular layers.

Age-related Changes

Growth, maturation, and aging dramatically alter disc tissues, especially the nucleus pulposus (Fig. 5–11). The four tissue components of the disc are easily identified in the newborn. A clear gelatinous nucleus fills almost half the disc and consists almost entirely of notochordal tissue. A narrow transition zone and larger ring of annulus fibrocartilage surround the nucleus. The outermost layers of the annulus encircle the annular fibrocartilage. As the disc grows and matures during childhood, the nucleus gradually becomes opaque. The decreasing water concentration makes it dense, firm, and difficult to separate from the fibrocartilage and transition zones. The annular fibrocartilage ring increases in size as the proportion of the disc occupied by the nucleus decreases. In the elderly, the components of the disc inside the outer annular layers consist almost entirely of fibrocartilage and clefts and fissures appear in the central parts of the disc.

The disk cells also change with age. Viable notochordal cells fill most of the fetal nucleus pulposus. With growth and maturation, their numerical density progressively decreases, and cells with the morphologic features of connective tissue cells appear in the nucleus pulposus (Fig. 5–10b). In adults, few if any notochordal cells remain and the percentage of necrotic cells in the nucleus increases from about 2% in the fetus to about 50% in adults (Fig. 5–10c). In the adult and in the elderly, a dense pericellular matrix forms around most cells in the nucleus pulposus and the inner annulus fibrosus, possibly because of accumulation of cell products and metabolites. In the elderly, less than 20% of the nucleus cells remain viable. The causes of these age changes remain unclear. They may result from decreased nutrition of central disc cells due to increased disc volume, decreased diffusion of nutrients into the disc following mineralization of the cartilage end plate, and accumulation of cell products and metabolites in the matrix.

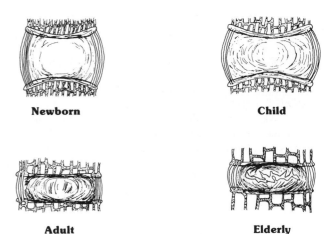

Newborn　　　　　　**Child**

Adult　　　　　　　**Elderly**

Figure 5–11 The age-related changes in human intervertebral disc.

Injury and Repair

The injury and repair of human intervertebral disc has not been extensively studied and information from studies of animal disc has limited value because of the multiple differences between human and most animal disc. The available information indicates that acute tears or ruptures of the outer regions of the annulus fibrosus lead to invasion of the normally avascular regions of the disc by granulation tissue. This tissue may mature into fibrous scar or remain as poorly organized loose vascular fibrous tissue. In most instances, once the disc has been torn the repair process does not restore the structural and mechanical integrity of the tissue.

ACKNOWLEDGMENT

This chapter includes revised and updated information that was previously published by the author and that is reprinted with permission from Buckwalter JA. Musculoskeletal tissues and the musculoskeletal system. In: Weinstein SL, Buckwalter JA, eds. *Turek's Orthopaedics: Principles and Their Application.* Philadelphia, PA: Lippincott; 1994:13–67; Buckwalter JA, Einhorn TA, Bolander ME, Cruess RL. Healing of the musculoskeletal tissues. In: Rockwood CA; Green DP, Bucholz RW, Heckman JD, eds. *Fractures.* 4th ed. Philadelphia, PA: Lippincott; 1996:261–304; and Buckwalter JA, Woo SL-Y, Goldberg VM, Hadley EC, Booth F, Oegema TR, Eyre DR. Soft tissue aging and musculoskeletal function. *J Bone Jt Surg* 1993; 75A:1533–1548.

PEARL

The aging nucleous pulposus loses water and viable notochordal cells while accumulating noncollagenous proteins.

SELECTED BIBLIOGRAPHY

BUCKWALTER JA. Fine structural studies of human intervertebral disc. In: White AA, Gordon SL, eds. *Proceedings of the Workshop on Idiopathic Low Back Pain*. St. Louis, CV Mosby; MO:1982:108–143.

BUCKWALTER JA. Musculoskeletal tissues and the musculoskeletal system. In: Weinstein SL, Buckwalter JA, eds. *Turek's Orthopaedics: Principles and Their Application*. Philadelphia, PA: Lippincott; 1994:13–67.

BUCKWALTER JA. Effects of early motion on healing of musculoskeletal tissues. *Hand Clinics*. 1996; 12:13–24.

BUCKWALTER JA, Cooper RR. The cells and matrices of skeletal connective tissues. In: Albright JA, Brand RA, eds. *The Scientific Basis of Orthopaedics*, Norwalk, CT: Appleton-Lange; 1987:1–29.

BUCKWALTER JA, EINHORN TA, BOLANDER ME, CRUESS RL. Healing of the musculoskeletal tissues. In: Rockwood CA, Green DP, Bucholz RW, Heckman JD, eds. *Fractures*. 4th ed. Philadelphia, PA: Lippincott; 1996:261–304.

BUCKWALTER JA, GOLDBERG V, WOO S-LY, eds. *Musculoskeletal Soft-tissue Aging: Impact on Mobility*. Rosemont IL: American Academy of Orthopaedic Surgeons; 1993.

BUCKWALTER JA, MARTIN JA. Intervertebral disc degeneration and back pain. In: Weinstein JW, Gordon SL, eds. *New Approaches to Low Back Pain*. Rosemont, IL: American Academy of Orthopaedic Surgeons; 1996:607–623.

BUCKWALTER JA, MAYNARD JA, VAILAS A. Skeletal fibrous tissues. In: Albright JA, Brand RA, eds. *The Scientific Basis of Orthopaedics*. Norwalk, CT: Appleton-Lange; 1987:387–405.

BUCKWALTER JA, WOO SL-Y, GOLDBERG VM, HADLEY EC, BOOTH F, OEGEMA TR, EYRE DR: Soft tissue aging and musculoskeletal function. *J Bone Jt Surg*. 1993; 75A:1533–1548.

SIMON SR, ed. *Orthopaedic Basic Science*. American Academy of Orthopaedic Surgeons; 1994.

WOO SL, BUCKWALTER JA, eds. *Injury and Repair of the Musculoskeletal Soft Tissues*. Park Ridge, IL: American Academy of Orthopaedic Surgeons; 1988.

SAMPLE QUESTIONS

1. The basal lamina of myofibers consists primarily of:
   (a) fibronectin and types I and II collagen
   (b) chondroitin sulfate and types I and II collagen
   (c) keratan sulfate and types II and V collagen
   (d) laminin and types IV and V collagen
   (e) laminin and types I and II collagen

2. Following most injuries to myofibers that leave their ECM intact, the myofibers:
   (a) are invaded by capillaries and fibroblasts
   (b) are replaced by fibrous tissue
   (c) are degraded by white cell enzymes
   (d) regenerate by proliferation and fusion of myoblasts
   (e) remain as aggregations of degraded actin and myosin filaments

3. Proteoglycans contribute about what percentage of the dry weight of tendons and ligaments:
   (a) 1%
   (b) 10%
   (c) 25%
   (d) 40%
   (e) 60%

4. The collagen fibrils of the tibial insertion of the medial collateral ligament of the knee insert primarily into:
   (a) subchondral bone
   (b) cortical bone
   (c) the cambium layer of the periosteum
   (d) the fibrous layer of periosteum
   (e) the calcified cartilage of the insertion

5. The known age-related changes in the properties of ligaments include:
   (a) increased stiffness and elastic modulus
   (b) decreased stiffness and elastic modulus
   (c) decreased stiffness and strength
   (d) increased stiffness and decreased strength
   (e) decreased stiffness and increased elastic modulus

6. Optimal healing of lacerated tendons within tendon sheaths occurs with apposition and stabilization of the tendon ends and:
   (a) intermittant compression loading and motion before tendon healing occurs
   (b) immobilization until tendon healing occurs
   (c) intermittant tensile loading and motion before tendon healing occurs
   (d) intermittant tensile loading and immobilzation until tendon healing occurs
   (e) continuous tensile loading and immobilization until healing occurs

7. The following collagens make up about 90% of the total collagen in menisci:
   (a) type I and type V
   (b) type II and type V
   (c) type V and type VI
   (d) type III and type VI
   (e) type III and type IX

8. The percent of the width of the adult human medial meniscus that has a blood supply is:
   (a) less than 5%
   (b) 10 to 30%
   (c) 30 to 50%
   (d) 50 to 70%
   (e) more than 70%

9. The percent of the width of adult human intervertebral disc that has a blood supply is:
   (a) less than 5%
   (b) 10 to 30%
   (c) 30 to 50%
   (d) 50 to 70%
   (e) more than 70%

10. The primary age-related changes in the human nucleus pulposus include:
    (a) increased water concentration and increased cell density
    (b) increased water concentration and decreased cell density
    (c) decreased water concentration and decreased collagen concentration
    (d) decreased water concentration and increased non-collagenous protein concentration
    (e) decreased water concentration and decreased non-collagenous protein concentration

Chapter 6

Genetic Aspects of Orthopaedic Disorders

Reed E. Pyeritz, MD, PhD, FACP, FACMG

THE ROLES GENES PLAY IN HEALTH AND DISEASE

Typically, when physicians think of the importance of genes in diseases, rare conditions caused by gross aberrations of chromosomes or mutations in single genes come to mind. A number of factors are forcing a much broader—and more accurate—view of the many and varied roles genes play in the etiology and pathogenesis of every human disorder. More than any other single issue, the Human Genome Project, to be completed early in the 21st century, has brought this fact home. This international effort has already provided the tools (panels of DNA markers for genetic linkage and banks of defined "pieces" of DNA for physical mapping) necessary for determining which gene or genes are most important in any given disease. Next to come is the complete sequence of all 3 billion nucleotide base-pairs in the haploid set of human chromosomes. Having the complete sequence available—and the informatics and computational abilities to store and analyze the data—will enable the identification of all of the estimated 70,000 genes. How many of these genes directly participate in the embryology, growth, function, and repair of the musculoskeletal system is unclear, but extrapolation from current crude estimates places the number at about 10% of the total.

For students and practitioners, an appreciation of the broad principles of human and medical genetics is of fundamental importance. A number of comprehensive texts can be recommended (see Selected Bibliography). For the specialist, the standards of care are shifting toward the expectation that a patient's family history will be obtained in sufficient detail to uncover genetic predispositions to disease and to susceptibilities that might affect management choices or adverse responses to certain treatments. Furthermore, when a genetic factor is identified, counseling must be provided about the implications to a patient's health and future, and about the same implications for the patient's close relatives.

Etiology, the study of causation of disease, must include consideration of genes. However, all diseases have both genetic and environmental components, and pathogenesis involves interaction of both sets to produce the condition and to effect its resolution. Disorders due primarily to mutations in single genes are usually inherited, as Mendel predicted for traits in the garden pea, and the principles of autosomal dominant, autosomal recessive, and X-linked inheritance are well known and straightforward. But recent investigations show that life is never as simple as it first appears. Mutant human genes do not always behave in families as Mendel would have predicted. Phenomena such as imprinting, uniparental disomy, anticipation, and somatic mutation all introduce clinically important variations from Mendelian expectations. The genes found on the mitochondrial chromosome are inherited only from the mother and are important in a number of disorders of skeletal muscle metabolism.

GENES OF SPECIAL IMPORTANCE IN ORTHOPAEDIC DISORDERS

One approach to identifying genes that function in a specific tissue or organ is to isolate messenger RNA from the tissue of interest at different stages of life. From the mRNA, complementary DNA (cDNA) is synthesized by reverse transcription. The cDNA, which represents only the coding sequences (exons) of the gene, and not the regulatory or spacer (intron) regions, may represent only a small fraction of the nucleotide sequence that constitutes the entire gene. Nonetheless, the cDNA is the crucial information in functional terms, and the cDNA can be mapped to a specific chromosome, even though the actual function of the protein that is encoded by that cDNA is completely unknown. In this way and others, a great many (more than 1000) genes have been mapped and identified as being expressed in skeletal muscle, bone, supporting structures, or the extracellular matrix (ECM). These sequences are accessible in on-line, public databases. As the Human Genome Project winds down, the next phases begin

Orthopaedic Surgery: The Essentials. Edited by M.E. Baratz, A.D. Watson, and J.E. Imbriglia. Thieme Medical Publishers, Inc., New York © 1999

to build, one of which has been termed *functional genomics*, which subsumes investigating the function and dysfunction of all of the genes in a given system.

For the student and practitioner of orthopaedics, considerable interest focuses on the ECM. Not only is the ECM the principal component of bone, cartilage, ligament, and tendon, but all of embryogenesis takes place over and through ECMs of various types. Inflammation intrinsically affects all types of ECM, and all repair and healing involves ECMs. General classes of constituents of the ECM of the skeletal system include: growth factors and cytokines and their receptors; fibrous elements, such as collagen and elastic fibers; ground substance, including proteoglycans of many types; integrins that establish specific links and communications with the cells; and proteinases. Hundreds of constituents make up the ECM, and the composition varies from tissue to tissue and at different stages of development.

More than 40 years ago, Victor McKusick introduced the term *heritable disorder of connective tissue*. The first edition of his monograph bearing that name described six specific conditions that were inherited as Mendelian traits. The list of heritable disorders of connective tissue now numbers more than 200. Some are relatively common (e.g., Stickler syndrome, Marfan syndrome, familial mitral valve prolapse), and some are exceedingly rare. Many fall in the broad range of "relatively rare," with prevalences of 1 to 10 per 100,000. But because most of these individuals develop problems with their skeletons at some point in their lives, it is incumbent on orthopaedists and rheumatologists to understand the biology and pathobiology of the ECM. The magnitude of these tasks cannot be overestimated. Among proteins called collagens there are 19 distinct entities, encoded by more than 30 genes. More than 300 mutations in these genes have been associated with several dozen clinically distinct disorders. Several of the more common and instructive disorders will be discussed.

LESSONS FROM HERITABLE DISORDERS OF CONNECTIVE TISSUE

Marfan Syndrome

This autosomal dominant condition is relatively common (1-3 per 5,000) and a challenge for medical specialists in many areas. Even though the cause is now well established, the diagnosis remains based on clinical findings. Mutations in the gene encoding the major constituent of the extracellular microfibril, fibrillin-1, is the cause of Marfan syndrome, as well as less severe variants of the condition, such as familial tall stature. Thus, testing the fibrillin-1 (*FBN1*) gene on chromosome 15 is appropriate primarily to use the information within a family with clinically documented Marfan syndrome, such as for prenatal diagnosis.

The diagnosis is established by examining carefully the organ systems most often affected: skeletal; ocular; cardiovascular; pulmonary; and integument (Table 6–1). One fundamental observation, the pathogenesis for which is not understood, is overgrowth of tubular bones. As a result, the excessive stature is disproportionate, with particularly long arms and legs. A hallmark of the heritable disorders of connective tissue is variability, and this feature is well illustrated by Marfan syndrome. A patient can have joint hypermobility,

congenital contractures, or both. Two affected brothers can differ markedly, one with a deep pectus excavatum and the other a prominent pectus carinatum. One facet of variability is age dependency. Many of the features develop with time, including scoliosis, anterior chest deformity, and dental crowding due to a narrow palate. Some skeletal changes are secondary to other pathology; lumbosacral vertebrae become eroded and deformed by the pressure of an expanding dural sac, so-called dural ectasia. Other skeletal changes have been under-recognized because of the shortened life-expectancy that was so common until the past 20 years. Thus, patients who survive because of aggressive management of their cardiovascular problems are likely to develop degenerative osteoarthritis at a relatively early age because of both bony deformity and joint laxity. One joint particularly at risk is the hip because of a high prevalence of protrusio acetabulae. Another is the thumb carpometacarpal joint. A recent controlled survey of consecutive patients seen in a specialty clinic revealed that patients with Marfan syndrome of all ages had much more chronic discomfort at multiple joints and in their backs than did age-matched controls.

PEARL

A patient with Marfan syndrome can have joint hypermobility, congenital contractures, or both.

Most patients with Marfan syndrome can expect nearly normal life expectancy when they receive medications to reduce the risk of aortic dissection, and when they undergo prophylactic repair of their dilated ascending aorta. Thus, orthopaedists can expect to see more such patients in the future. The long-term outlook for the musculoskeletal system will be improved if appropriate orthopaedic evaluation and management begins early in life, including counseling to avoid unnecessary wear and tear, bracing for developing scoliosis, and physical therapy to foster muscular stabilization of lax joints.

Achondroplasia

This condition is the most common cause of disproportionate short stature. Achondroplasia is characterized by rhizomelic dwarfism, (meaning the proximal limb segments are disproportionately affected), relative macrocephaly with mid-face hypoplasia, and typical radiographic changes on a skeletal survey including: Legs are often bowed due to overgrowth of the fibulae and knee laxity; tubular bones are short and thick with flared metaphyses; vertebrae have relatively normal height but progressive caudal narrowing of the interpediculate distances and shortened spinal processes; and the foramen magnum is small. Achondroplasia is an autosomal dominant condition. In past decades, most cases were sporadic, meaning both parents were of average stature; the mutation causing the skeletal dysplasia was thought to arise in either the ovum or the sperm of the child's conception. Now, as people with achondroplasia have entered the mainstream due to both better socialization and improved medical care, many are having their own families, with the 50–50 chance that any child will be affected. The

TABLE 6–1   Diagnosis of the Marfan Syndrome.

Family History

Major criteria
- having a parent, child, or sibling who meets these diagnostic criteria independently
- presence of a mutation in fibrillin-1 (*FBN1*) known to cause the Marfan syndrome
- presence of a haplotype around *FBN1*, inherited by descent, known to be associated with unequivocally diagnosed Marfan syndrome in the family

Minor criteria
- none

For the family history to be contributory, one of the major criteria must be present.

Skeletal System

Major criteria. Presence of at least four of the following manifestations.
- pectus carinatum
- pectus excavatum requiring surgery
- reduced upper to lower segment ratio or arm span to height ratio (> 1.05)
- positive wrist and thumb signs
- scoliosis of $\geqq 20°$ or spondylolithesis
- reduced extension of the elbows ($< 170°$)
- medial displacement of the medial malleolus causing pes planus
- protrusio acetabulae of any degree (ascertained on radiographic imaging)

Minor criteria
- pectus excavatum of moderate severity
- joint hypermobility
- highly arched palate with crowding of teeth
- facial appearance (dolicocephaly, malar hypoplasia, enophthalmos, retrognathia, down-slanting palpebral fissures)

For the skeletal system to be involved, at least two of the components comprising the major criteria or one component comprising the major criteria plus two of the minor criteria must be present.

Ocular System

Major criterion
- ectopia lentis

Minor criteria
- abnormally flat cornea (as measured by keratometry)
- increased axial length of globe (as measured by ultrasound)
- hypoplastic iris or hypoplastic ciliary muscle causing a decreased miosis

For the ocular system to be involved, at least two of the minor criteria must be present.

Cardiovascular System

Major criteria
- dilatation of the ascending aorta with or without aortic regurgitation and involving at least the sinuses of Valsalva
- dissection of the ascending aorta

Minor criteria
- mitral valve prolapse with or without mitral valve regurgitation
- dilatation of main pulmonary artery, in absence of valvular or peripheral pulmonic stenosis or any other obvious cause, below the age of 40 years
- calcification of the mitral annulus below the age of 40 years
- dilatation or dissection of the descending thoracic or abdominal aorta below the age of 50 years

For the cardiovascular system to be involved a major criterion or only one of the minor criteria must be present.

(continued)

TABLE 6–1   *(continued)*   Diagnosis of the Marfan syndrome.

<table>
<tr><td colspan="2" align="center">**Pulmonary System**</td></tr>
<tr><td>**Major criteria**
• none</td><td>**Minor criteria**
• spontaneous pneumothorax
• apical blebs (ascertained by chest radiography)</td></tr>
<tr><td colspan="2">For the pulmonary system to be involved one of the minor criteria must be present.</td></tr>
<tr><td colspan="2" align="center">**Skin and Integument**</td></tr>
<tr><td>**Major criterion**
• none</td><td>**Minor criteria**
• striae atrophicae (stretch marks) not associated with marked weight changes, pregnancy or repetitive stress
• recurrent or incisional herniae</td></tr>
<tr><td colspan="2">For the skin and integument to be involved one of the minor criteria must be present.</td></tr>
<tr><td colspan="2" align="center">**Dura**</td></tr>
<tr><td>**Major criterion**
• lumbosacral dural ectasia by computed tomography or magnetic resonance imaging</td><td>**Minor criteria**
• none</td></tr>
<tr><td colspan="2">For the dura to be involved, the major criterion must be present.</td></tr>
<tr><td colspan="2" align="center">**Requirements of the Diagnosis of the Marfan Syndrome**</td></tr>
<tr><td>**For the index case**
• major criteria in at least two different organ systems and involvement of a third organ system</td><td>**For a family member**
• presence of a major criterion in the family history and one major criterion in an organ system and involvement of a second organ system</td></tr>
</table>

* Hall, et al, 1984.
Reproduced with permission from DePaepe A, Deitz HC, Devereny RB, Hennekem R, Pyeritz RE. Revised diagnostic criteria for the Marfan Syndrome. *Am J Med Genet.* 1996;62:417–426.

cause of achondroplasia is mutations in a gene encoding one of the receptors for fibroblast growth factor, *FGFR3*. Most surprisingly, only one mutation in FGFR3 accounts for 95% of cases of achondroplasia. This is in striking contrast to all of the other conditions discussed here, and most Mendelian disorders generally, in which many different mutations in the same gene cause a given condition.

PEARL

A single mutation in a gene encoding one of the receptors for fibroblast growth factor accounts for 95% of cases of achondroplasia.

Management of people with achondroplasia varies with age. In infancy, efforts are directed toward identifying the 10% or so who have severe obstruction of the craniocervical junction and are at risk of central apnea, quadriparesis, and sudden death. In childhood, progressive ventriculomegaly from obstruction of cerebrospinal fluid circulation must be detected and shunting performed if needed. Also, attention must be paid to bowing of the legs, with osteotomies needed in some, and progressive thoracolumbar kyphosis. In adulthood, a syndrome of neurogenic claudication due to compression of the spinal cord, cauda equina, or roots is quite common and often insidious. This must be managed by wide decompression before permanent neurologic sequelae occur.

PEARL

Narrowing of the cervical spinal canal in achondroplasia can cause apnea, quadriparesis or even death in childhood. Progressive narrowing of the lumbosacral canal can cause neurogenic claudication in the adult.

Multiple Epiphyseal Dyslpasia

Patients with any of the individual variants of this autosomal dominant syndrome typically present in childhood or early adolescence because of short stature, joint pain, or joint "stiffness." In the most common type (Fairbank), radiographs show: relative shortening of all tubular bones; irregular, small, and fragmented epiphyses, especially in the legs; delayed appearance of secondary ossification centers and absences of ossification of the cuboids; and relative sparing of the skull and vertebrae. Marked involvement of the spine suggests the diagnosis should be one of the spondyloepiphyseal dysplasias. The diagnosis should be suspected in any adult with precocious osteoarthritis of the hips and a family history of degenerative joint disease or short stature.

The cause of this form of multiple epiphyseal dyslpasia (MED) is mutation of the gene encoding cartilage oligomeric matrix protein (COMP), which maps to human chromosome 19p13. Mutations in this gene also cause a clinically and radiographically distinct skeletal dysplasia, pseudoachondroplastic spondyloepiphyseal dysplasia. Other varieties of MED exist. The Ribbing variant also is caused by mutations in COMP.

Management is supportive. Parents and affected children must be counseled about the cause of a child's short stature and the lack of any effective treatment. Many patients eventually require joint replacement, especially of the hips.

Mucopolysaccharidosis IV (Morquio Syndrome)

The Morquio syndrome was first defined in 1929 and for years was the diagnosis of any patient with "short-trunk" dwarfism (in distinction to achondroplasia, in which the trunk is relatively spared). Now, of course, a wide variety of osteochondrodysplasias are know to affect the spine, either with or without marked involvement of the limbs. Mucopolysaccharidosis (MPS) IV must be reserved for individuals with a documented defect in one of two lysosomal enzymes. MPS IVA is due to deficiency of N-acetyl-galactosamine-6-sulfate sulfatase, while type IVB is due to deficiency of (β-galactosidase. Both are autosomal recessive conditions in which catabolism of proteoglycan is blocked and the intermediate metabolites accumulate in lysosomes of certain cells. In MPS IV, accumulation is most marked in the skeleton, cornea, airways, and heart. In some other mucopolysaccharidoses, accumulation occurs in nervous tissue and causes mental retardation. Patients with MPS IV, however, are of normal intelligence.

Patients are short at birth and develop progressive bony deformity. The typical radiographic changes of the other MPS disorders are called dysostosis multiplex, but the changes in MPS IV are distinctive. All of the vertebral bodies are short (platyspondyly), and often have a central, anterior beak. Notable by its absence or marked hypoplasia, is the odontoid.

PEARL

In Morquio syndrome there is a defect in proteoglycan catabolism leading to an accumulation of proteglycan metabolites in the cellular lysosomes of bone, the cornea, respiratory system, and heart.

The ribs flare and a pectus carinatum is typical. The pelvis is often diagnostic, with constricted iliac wings, steeply sloped roof of the acetabulum, coxa valga, and aseptic necrosis of the femoral head. The major clinical problem, potentially dating from childhood, is atlantoaxial instability and cervical myelopathy. Craniocervical fusion is generally required. Stenosis and regurgitation of cardiac valves, especially the aortic, and progressive restrictive pulmonary disease are later complications that result in reduced life expectancy. Because of narrowing of the middle airways, and atlantoaxial instability (if fusion has not been performed) or immobility of the neck (if fusion has been performed), intubation is difficult and even life threatening. No patient with an MPS disorder should be administered general anesthesia without the benefit of a detailed anesthesia consultation, an assessment of the cervical spine, and the availability of a pediatric flexible bronchoscope to assist placement of the endotracheal tube.

Ehlers-Danlos Syndrome

This heterogeneous group of disorders often proves frustrating to the physician because of its complexity, to the orthopaedist because surgical results to stabilize joints are often less than ideal, and to patients because they may be prone to life-long discomfort and disability without benefit of definitive therapy. To qualify for a diagnosis of Ehlers-Danlos syndrome (EDS), an individual should have both abnormal skin and hyperextensibility of joints. Nine types (Table 6–2) are distinguishable clinically, and, increasingly,

TABLE 6–2 Ehlers-Danlos Syndrome

Type	Inheritance	Skeletal Features	Other Features	Basic Defect
I	AD	Marked joint hypermobility	Skin hyperextensibility and fragility	some ⇓ type V collagen
II	AD	Less severe than type I	Less severe skin changes than type I	some ⇓ type V collagen
III	AD	Marked joint hypermobility	Mild skin changes	?
IV	AD, AR	Hypermobile digits	Arterial and bowel rupture	⇓ type III collagen
V	X-L	Similar to type II	Similar to type II	?
VI	AR	Marked joint hypermobility	Rupture of globe	⇓ lysyl hydroxylase
VII	AD, AR	Marked joint hypermobility and dislocations; short stature	Minimal skin change	defect in procollagen I cleavage
VIII	AD	Variable joint hypermobility	Peridontitis	? some with deficient type III collagen
X	AD	Mild joint hypermobility	Mild skin changes; MVP	? defect in fibronectin

by molecular diagnosis. However, it remains a truism of clinical genetics that about one half of all patients who have EDS-like findings cannot be placed with assurity into one of the defined types.

The "classic" form is EDS I, in which the skin is extremely elastic, such that it can be pulled painlessly away from the body and returns immediately to its original position (as opposed to cutis laxa, in which the skin droops). The skin is also prone to bruising and minimal trauma produces gaping wounds. The skin holds sutures poorly, and patients typically develop wide, atrophic ("cigarette paper") scars despite prompt and competent medical attention. The joints are markedly hyperextensible but usually do not dislocate. Nonetheless, the degree of laxity is associated with perceived "weakness" in many physical activities, joint trauma from physical activities, and chronic joint pain, often without inflammation.

Fortunately, patients and families with EDS I are rare. In some, a defect in type V collagen has been discovered. In this autosomal dominant condition, an affected parent has a 50-50 chance of having an affected offspring at each conception. Because the gestational membranes are fetal in origin, a pregnancy carrying an affected child often suffers premature rupture of the membranes and a precipitous delivery.

PEARL

The ligamentous laxity seen in patients with Ehlers-Danlos syndrome is due to a defect or deficiency in collagen.

EDS IV is the one form that is potentially lethal. Due to deficiency of type III collagen, the walls of arteries, the gut, and the uterus are fragile and subject to spontaneous rupture. Unfortunately, no therapy is preventive, and surgery is particularly hazardous because of the friability of the tissues.

THE IMPORTANCE OF GENETIC FACTORS IN COMMON DISEASES

Commonly, multiple members of a family develop osteoporosis or osteoarthritis. Given the frequency of these disorders, this is likely to happen by chance alone. But many studies have demonstrated some families with unusually high prevalence of these disorders of maturity, often occurring at younger than expected ages. Defects in cartilage collagen (i.e., types II, IX and X) have been suggested to predispose to osteoarthritis, and defects of bone collagen (type I especially) have been found in some families with early osteoporosis. How general these relations will be is undetermined. Systematic screening of collagen genes for mutations is not trivial or cheap, and is clearly not indicated clinically as yet. However, the time will likely come when, just as we now contemplate screening patients for mutations that predispose to certain cancers, testing for ECM mutations that predispose to arthritis and osteoporosis will be feasible.

ACKNOWLEDGMENT

Supported in part by NIH grant HL 35877.

SELECTED BIBLIOGRAPHY

General

BEIGHTON P, ed. *McKusick's Heritable Disorders of Connective Tissue.* 5th ed. St. Louis, MO: CV Mosby; 1993.

BEIGHTON P, GRAHAME R, BIRD H. *Hypermobility of Joints.* 2nd ed. New York, NY: Springer-Verlag; 1989.

BYERS PH. Disorders of collagen biosynthesis and structure. In: Scriver CR, Beaudet AL, Sly WS, Valle D, eds. *Metabolic and Molecular Bases of Inherited Disease.* 7th Ed. New York, NY: McGraw-Hill; 1995:4029–4078.

MCKUSICK, VA. On-line Mendelian Inheritance in Man. Center for Medical Genetics, Johns Hopkins University, Baltimore, MD and National Center for Biotechnology Information. Bethesda, MD: National Library of Medicine, 1995. Available from http://www3.ncbi.nlm.nih.gov/omim/; INTERNET.

PYERITZ RE. Heritable and developmental disorders of connective tissues and bone. In: Koopman WJ, ed. *Arthritis and Allied Conditions.* 13th ed. Philadelphia, PA: Lea and Febiger; 1997:1719–1750.

RIMOIN DL, CONNER JM, PYERITZ RE, eds. *Principles and Practice of Medical Genetics.* 3rd ed. New York, NY: Churchill Livingstone; 1997.

ROYCE PM, STEINMANN B, eds. *Connective Tissue and Its Heritable Disorders: Molecular, Genetic and Medical Aspects.* New York, NY: Wiley-Liss; 1993.

Sequences and Genomics

BOGUSKI MS, SCHULER GD. Establishing a human transcript map. *Nature Genet.* 1995;10:369–371.

ADAMS MD, et al. Initial assessment of human gene diversity and expression patterns based upon 83 million nucleotides of cDNA sequences. *Nature.* 1995;377:3–174. Available from http://www.tigr.org/; INTERNET.

ADAMS MD. KERLAVAGE AR. FLEISCHMANN RD. FULDNER RA. BULT CJ. LEE NH. KIRKNESS EF. WEINSTOCK KG. GOCAYNE JD. WHITE O. et al. Initial assessment of human gene diversity and expression patterns based upon 83 million nucleotides of cDNA sequence. Nature. 377(6547 Suppl): 3–174, 1995 Sep 28.

Marfan Syndrome

BALLO R. BRIGGS MD. COHN DH. KNOWLTON RG. BEIGHTON PH. RAMESAR RS. Multiple epiphyseal dysplasia, ribbing type: a novel point mutation in the COMP gene in a South African family. *American Journal of Medical Genetics.* 68:396–400, 1997 Feb 11.

DEPAEPE A, DEITZ HC, DEVEREUX RB, HENNEKEM R, PYERITZ RE. Revised diagnostic criteria for the Marfan syndrome. *Am J Med Genet.* 1996;62:417–426.

DIETZ HC, PYERITZ RE. Mutations in the human gene for fibrillin-1 (*FBN1*) in the Marfan syndrome and related disorders. *Hum Molec Genet.* 1995;4:1799–1809.

GRAHAME R, PYERITZ RE. Marfan syndrome: joint and skin manifestations are prevalent and correlated. *Br J Rheum.* 1995;34:126–131.

MAGID D, PYERITZ RE, FISHMAN EK. Musculoskeletal manifestations of the Marfan syndrome. *AJR.* 1990;155:99–104.

PYERITZ RE. Marfan syndrome and other disorders fibrillin. In: Rimoin DL, Connor JM, Pyeritz RE, eds. *Principles and Practice of Medical Genetics.* 3rd ed. New York, NY: Churchill Livingstone; 1997;1027–1066.

RAI A. WORDSWORTH P. COPPOCK JS. ZAPHIROPOULOS GC. STRUTHERS GR. Hereditary arthro-ophthalmopathy (Stickler syndrome): a diagnosis to consider in familial premature osteoarthritis. *British Journal of Rheumatology.* 33:1175–80, 1994.

SCHERER LR, ARN PH, DRESSEL D, PYERITZ RE, HALLER JA Jr. Surgical management of children and young adults with the Marfan syndrome and pectus excavatum. *J Pediatr Surg.* 1988;23:1169–1172.

SHIANG R. THOMPSON LM. ZHU YZ. CHURCH DM. FIELDER TJ. BOCIAN M. WINOKUR ST. WASMUTH JJ. Mutations in the transmembrane domain of FGFR3 cause the most common genetic form of dwarfism, achondroplasia. Cell. 78(2):335–42, 1994.

SPONSELLER PD, HOBBS W, RILEY LH III, PYERITZ RE. The thoracolumbar spine in Marfan syndrome. *J Bone Jt Surg.* 1995;77A:867–876.

Achondroplasia

PYERITZ RE, SACK GH Jr, UDVARHELYI GB. Thoracolumbosacral laminectomy in achondroplasia: long-term results in 22 patients. *Am J Med Genet.* 1987;28:433–444.

RIMOIN DL, LACHMAN RS. Chondrodysplasias. In: Rimoin DL, Conner JM, Pyeritz RE, eds. Principles and Practice of Medical Genetics. 3rd ed. New York, NY: Churchill Livingstone; 1997:2779–2815.

SHIANG R, et al. Mutations in the transmembrane domain of FGFR3 cause the most common genetic form of dwarfism, achondroplasia. *Cell.* 1994;78:335–342.

Mutiple Ephyiseal Dysplasia

BALLO R, et al. Multiple epiphyseal dysplasia, Ribbing type: a novel point mutation in the COMP gene in a South African family. *Am J Med Genet.* 1997;68:396–400.

DEERE M, et al. Genetic heterogeneity in multiple epiphyseal dysplasia. *Am J Hum Genet.* 1995;56:698–704.

Mucopolysaccharidoses

NEUFELD EF, MUENZER J. The mucopolysaccharidoses. In: Scriver CR, Beaudet AL, Sly WS, Valle D, eds. *Metabolic and Molecular Bases of Inherited Disease.* 7th ed. New York, NY: McGraw-Hill; 1995:2465–2494.

SEMENZA GL, PYERITZ RE. Respiratory complications of the mucopolysaccharide storage disorders. *Medicine.* 1988;67:209–219.

SPRANGER J. Mucopolysaccharidoses. In: Rimoin DL, Conner JM, Pyeritz RE, eds. *Principles and Practice of Medical Genetics.* 3rd ed. New York, NY: Churchill Livingstone; 1997:2071–2079.

Ehlers-Danlos Syndrome

BYERS P. Ehlers-Danlos syndrome. In: Rimoin DL, Conner JM, Pyeritz RE, eds. *Principles and Practice of Medical Genetics.* 3rd ed. New York, NY: Churchill Livingstone; 1997:1067–1082.

Common Disorders of Connective Tissue

HORTON WA. Connective tissue biology and common skeletal disorders. In: King RA, Rotter JI, Motulsky AG, eds. *The Genetic Basis of Common Diseases.* New York, NY: Oxford Univ Press; 1992:625–640.

RAI A, et al. Hereditary arthro-ophthalmopathy (Stickler syndrome): a diagnosis to consider in familial premature osteoarthritis. *Br J Rheum.* 1994;33:1175–1180.

SAMPLE QUESTIONS

1. Which of the following statements is false:
   (a) There are more than 200 heritable disorders of connective tissue.
   (b) The prevalence of most heritable disorders of connective tissue is 1 to 10 per 100,000.
   (c) cDNA is a copy of the entire nucleotide sequence of a gene.
   (d) The untranslated regions of a gene are believed to perform regulatory funtions in RNA synthesis.
   (e) The exon region is the coding sequence, that portion of the DNA transcribed into RNA.

2. The following characteristic(s) are consistent with the diagnosis of Marfan syndrome:

   (a) a defect in the fibrillin-1 gene on chromosome 15
   (b) scoliosis
   (c) dilitation of the ascending aorta
   (d) a sister with Marfan syndrome
   (e) all of the above

3. Which statement is false:
   (a) Marfan syndrome is inherited as an autosomal dominant trait.
   (b) Achondroplasia is inherited as an autosomal recessive trait with variable penetrance.
   (c) MED is inherited as an autosomal dominant trait.

(d) Morquio syndrome is inherited as an autosomal recessive trait.

(e) The most common form of inheritance for the various types of EDS is autosomal dominant.

4. True or false: Most forms of EDS are the result of a defect in collagens type III or V.

(a) true

(b) false

5. True or false: Achondroplastic adults are at risk to develop neurogenic claudication.

(a) true

(b) false

Chapter 7

Joint Pathology

Vincent J. Vigorita, MD

Outline

ARTHRITIS

Degenerative Joint Disease (Osteoarthritis)

Osteoarthritis is been estimated to affect 10% of the population over age 60. While the etiology is unknown, osteoarthritis remains a convenient term for a broad range of disorders. These disorders have in common subtle synovial changes, loss of articular cartilage, and remodeling of bone. Inspection of the synovium from the osteoarthritic joint reveals minimal inflammation, leading some clinicians to prefer the term *osteoarthosis*.

Pathogenesis

It is believed that the integrity of the joint requires an even distribution of load across the joint. Therefore, proper alignment of joint structures and the resiliency of the subchondral bone and cartilage is essential. Abnormalities of alignment (e.g., trauma, acromegaly), subchondral bone (e.g., Paget's disease), and integrity of associated tissues (e.g., ochronosis,

calcium pyrophosphate crystal deposition diseases) may lead to the development of degenerative joint disease(DJD). In addition, an association between osteoarthritis of the knee and obesity has been established.

Cartilage is composed of water, proteoglycans, type II collagen, and glycoproteins, such as chondronectin and fibronectin. The negatively charged proteogylcans and glycoproteins draw water into the collagenous mesh. Both aging and degenerative joint disease have been associated with changes in water content, proteoglycan type, size, and aggregation. In degenerative joint disease (DJD), these changes have been postulated to lead to water retention, proteoglycan dilution, and proteoglycan loss by diffusion. In addition, synovial cells and chondrocytes may produce enzymes that degrade collagen and proteoglycans. Eventually, cartilage is unable to withstand transarthrodial forces.

Theories about the pathogenesis of DJD can be summarized as those beginning in cartilage, the subchondral bone, or the synovium. In cartilage, a change in the microenvironment of chondrocytes may be the culprit. De novo influences of cartilage degeneration in acromegaly is an example. A change in the stiffness of the subchondral plate has been postulated to initiate joint degeneration. The change in the stiffness could arise from stress fractures due to repetitive trauma or through changes in bone turnover as is seen in Paget's disease. Synovial tissue may also be activated by a broad range of both clinical and subclinical insults. Once activated, synovium may digest protein cores of proteoglycan moieties.

Recently, the role of cytokines, proteases, and growth factors in the pathogenesis of osteoarthritis have received considerable attention. Of these, interleukin 1-β (IL-1β) has been identified as an inflammatory cytokine that may induce the breakdown of proteoglycans. It stimulates the synthesis of metalloproteases; plasminogen activator inhibits proteoglycan synthesis and decreases the synthesis of type II and type XI collagen. Tumor necrosis factor α, a cytokine, may help produce and be synergistic with IL-1β. Stromelysin, a metalloprotease, degrades proteoglycans and collagen and is activated by plasminogen activator. Fibronectin, an extracellular glycoprotein, binds cells, collagen, and proteoglycans. It is greatly elevated in osteoarthritic cartilage.

Other causes of joint degeneration include microvascular disease with associated bone damage due to osteonecrosis. It is likely that the cause of osteoarthritis is multifactorial.

Orthopaedic Surgery: The Essentials. Edited by M.E. Baratz, A.D. Watson, and J.E. Imbriglia. Thieme Medical Publishers, Inc., New York © 1999

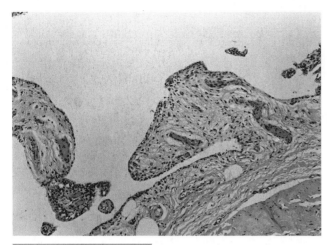

Figure 7–1 Degenerative joint disease (DJD), synovium. The characteristic synovial appearance in DJD is subtle alteration of the normal mild villous architecture. Inflammation, if present at all, is mild and scattered.

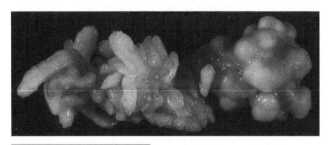

Figure 7–2 Synovial chondromatosis. Most commonly resulting from metaplastic synovium in DJD or trauma, direct transformation from synovium to cartilage is observed.

Synovium

Normally the synovium consists of a discrete layer of intimal lining cells beneath a richly vascular layer of loose connective tissue. The presence of hyperplastic synovium in osteoarthritis varies within any given joint and from patient to patient. When seen it is characterized by increased villous folds and villous hypertrophy (Fig. 7–1). Inflammatory cells may be present but never to the extent seen in rheumatoid arthritis (RA). The inflammatory infiltrate usually consists of scattered mononuclear cells such as lymphocytes.

Osteocartilaginous loose bodies often form in the joint in the osteoarthritic joint. Although other mechanisms may contribute, they are usually the result of synovial metaplasia (Fig. 7–2 and Fig. 7–3).

Articular Cartilage

Hyaline cartilage is an avascular structure composed of water, collagen, proteoglycan, and chondrocytes. It is sparsely cellular at its joint surface (the lamina splendens), with increasing cellularity toward the subchondral bone. The site of calcification is a wavy, basophilic junction at the base of the articular cartilage. This is called the mineralization front or tidemark.

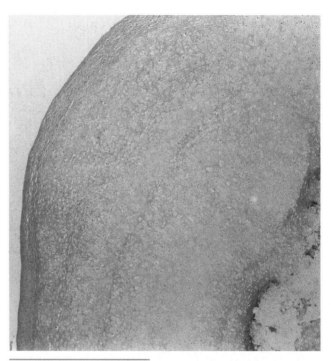

Figure 7–3 Synovial chondromatosis. Usually, a secondary phenomenon, the growth, calcification, and eventual ossification of loose bodies is often seen as a concentric, ringlike process.

Changes seen in degenerative joint disease include erosions and fibrillation of the surface (Fig. 7–4). The cartilage becomes thin, and fissures or clefts form. Fissures are both vertical and horizontal in orientation. Often chondrocyte proliferation occurs adjacent to the fissures. These cartilage clones may represent an attempt by the cartilage to repair itself. Microscopically, there is a marked variation in cellularity and intensity of the proteoglycan matrix when examined with stains such as Alcian blue and safranin O (Fig. 7–5). At the base of the articular cartilage, vascular penetration is visible originating from the underlying subchondral bone, with duplication and marked irregularity to the tidemark.

Eventually the cartilage is denuded (eburnation) (Fig. 7–6) Mesenchymal proliferation ensues, with endochondral ossification similar to that seen at the growth plate resulting, eventually, in a discernible region of new articular bone—the osteophyte.

Osteophytes

Osteophytes are the growth of new bone in osteoarthritic joints. Usually they are found at the margins of osteoarthritic cartilage and form by endochondral ossification. (Figs. 7–7 and 7–8).

Subchondral Bone

The bone underlying the degenerating cartilage is characterized by a hypermetabolic state. This marked increased

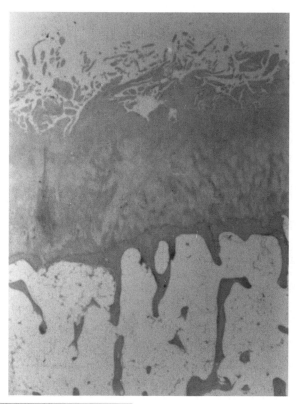

Figure 7–4 Degenerative joint disease. Microscopic early changes include thinning of cartilage layer, fibrillation, and cleft formation.

remodeling results in both the development of cysts, as well as a focal thickening of the bone (subchondral sclerosis).

Fibrocartilage

Degenerative joint disease affects fibrocartilaginous tissue, such as the triangular fibrocartilage complex in the wrist and the menisci in the knee. Fibrocartilage ligament changes in DJD include myxoid degeneration, microcyst formation, chondroid metaplasia, and even crystal deposition.

Repair of Articular Cartilage

Once lost, articular cartilage has limited regenerative capacity. However, the new tissue is more fibrous. It derives from subchondral tissue and may actually resurface parts of the joint (Figs. 7–9 and 7–10).

Natural History of Degenerative Joint Disease

The natural history of osteoarthritis is variable. The disease may stabilize or progress. Although joint replacement has been a major advance in bypassing crippling arthritis at a severely involved joint, no current treatment is known to alter the course of the disorder. Recently, cultured autologous chondrocytes have been used to repair deep cartilage defects in the knee joint, suggesting the reparative process may be successfully manipulated.

Variants of osteoarthritis include rapidly destructive degenerative joint disease or "analgesic joint" and erosive osteoarthritis.

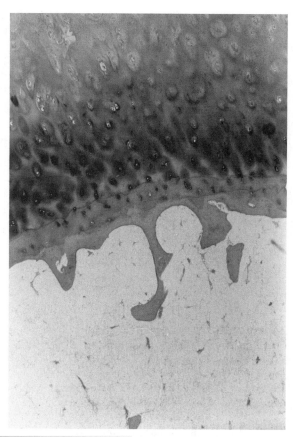

Figure 7–5 Degenerative joint disease. Microscopic changes at the cartilage bone interface in early DJD include staining alterations reflecting early proteoglycan change, cartilage cloning, and duplication of the tidemark (the basophilic linear border between cartilage and calcified cartilage).

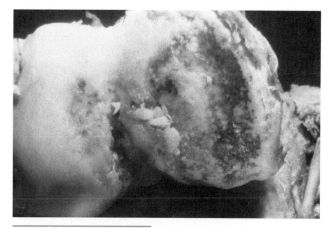

Figure 7–6 Degenerative joint disease, femoral condyles, knee. One condyle is nearly completely eburnated with loss of cartilage and exposure of sclerotic subchondral bone.

Rapidly Destruction Degenerative Joint Disease

Rapidly destructive arthropathy is a syndrome characterized by the rapid destruction of a joint. Within months, the joint is

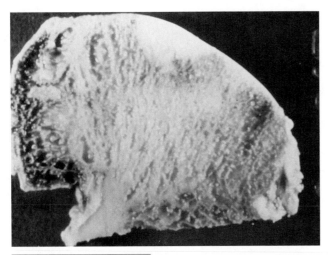

Figure 7–7 Degenerative joint disease. Coronal section femoral head with sclerotic subchondral bone and large marginal osteophyte.

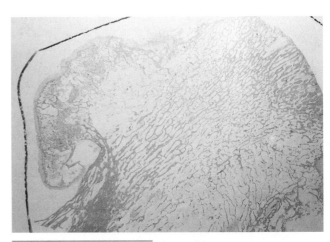

Figure 7–8 Degenerative joint disease. Coronal section femoral head with eburnated bone surface, sclerotic subchondral bone, and large marginal osteophyte. Bone density in the head reflects remodelling forces.

destroyed with a notable paucity of osteophytes. Histologically, there may be changes suggestive of DJD or avascular necrosis. There are fewer inflammatory cells than seen in rheumatoid arthritis. In some cases, prostaglandins, cytokines, and metalloproteinases are present in greater concentrations than seen in osteoarthritis.

Erosive Osteoarthritis

Erosive osteoarthritis is an unusual presentation of DJD which involves mainly middle-aged women. These patients present with severe, acute pain and swollen joints. The clinical presentation can be confused with inflammatory type arthritides such as RA.

Radiographically, erosive osteoarthritis is a condition usually seen in small joints of the hand. Both the distal interphalangeal joints and proximal interphalangeal joints are involved. These joints are narrowed with small osteophytes

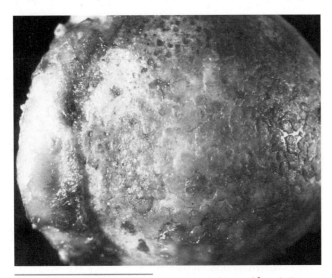

Figure 7–9 Degenerative joint disease, femoral head. Reparative phase. Eburnated osteoarthritic head demonstrating surface regrowth of fibrocartilaginous tufts giving the surface a roughened appearance.

and an irregular subchondral surface. In some cases erosive osteoarthritis can lead to joint fusion.

RHEUMATOID ARTHRITIS

Rheumatoid arthritis is a self-perpetuating, inflammatory process. It is initially characterized clinically by joint swelling and stiffness lasting several weeks. Serological studies, such as the rheumatoid factor, erythrocyte sedimentation rate, and acute phase reactants, may be elevated in RA. However, none are pathognomonic, and the diagnosis rests on clinical and radiographic findings and, where appropriate, histopathologic correlation. A diagnosis of RA should be made only after excluding conditions that can mimic the disorder, that is, the so-called rheumatoid variants or serum negative spondyloarthropathies.

Although initially the small joints and feet are most often involved, any joint may be affected. In 1987, the American College of Rheumatology refined its criteria for the diagnosis of RA. Patients with RA experience morning stiffness in and around joints for at least one hour before significant improvement. Joint swelling is noted in at least three joints. Simultaneous and bilateral involvement is typical, as are subcutaneous rheumatoid nodules. Demonstration of rheumatoid factor in serum and roentgenographic changes of articular erosions and osteopenia in x-rays of the hand and wrist complete recently defined criteria for diagnosis. The course of RA is variable and ranges from mild and relapsing to a more progressive, severely debilitating condition.

Epidemiology

Rheumatoid arthritis has been been diagnosed worldwide and affects all racial and ethnic groups. Its prevalence in the United States has been estimated to be at least 0.5% of the population. Higher incidences, such as 5.8% estimated in the Black Feet and Pima Indians in the United States, have been recorded. Although onset can occur at any age, there appears to be a steady occurrence with increasing age. A female predominance is noted particularly in young patients.

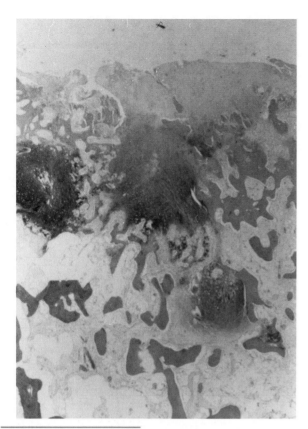

Figure 7–10 Degenerative joint disease, femoral head. Reparative phase with fibrocartilaginous tissue forming in the subchondral marrow and protruding up into and over the newly resurfacing eburnated bone.

The prevalence in women has led to investigations of the roles of endogenous and exogenous sex hormones, including oral contraceptive medications. Pregnancy has been known to be associated with remission, and nulliparity with an independent risk factor. Oral contraceptives may modify the course of the disease.

Many microbial infections are known to be followed by arthritis, but none have been unequivocally shown to lead to the development of RA. Agents that have been studied extensively include bacteria such as streptococci, mycoplasmas, and mycobacteria. A group of children who had been followed for juvenile RA were subsequently diagnosed as having been infected with the spirochete *Borrelia burgdorferi*, the causative bacterial organism in Lyme disease.

A genetic predisposition in RA is now clearly established. Monozygotic twins show a higher concordance for RA (32%) than dizygotic twins (9%). Most significant, is the association of RA with the human leukocyte (HLA) antigen HLA-DR4, a genetically determined allele of the major histocompatibility complex MHC located on the short arm of chromosome 6. The relative risk of developing RA is approximately 8 times greater in HLA-DR4 positive individuals. Although the biological role for HLA-DR genes is not known, HLA molecules regulate T-cell responses by selectively binding antigenic fragments in specialized grooves. This complex formed by the HLA molecule and the antigenic fragment may then be recognized by the appropriate T-cell receptor, leading to activation of an antigen specific T-cell.

Pathogenesis

Although the etiology of RA is unknown, examples of infection- triggered arthritis mimicking RA suggests an infectious origin. Whatever the initial event, RA is characterized by a striking and destructive immune reaction.

Initially, macrophages in the synovial membrane process and present foreign protein antigen to helper T-lymphocytes. The T-lymphocytes stimulate the production of B-lymphocytes which mature into antibody-secreting plasma cells. As mentioned, there is evidence of a genetic component in that the receptors on the cells processing the antigen are on a major histocompatibility complex locus. Therefore, there may be susceptibility to RA by some patients who carry a specific genetic molecule.

The early events of antigen processing and T-cell activation are clinically silent. Symptoms begin with the secondary changes of this inflammatory process, including synovial hyperplasia, synovial vascular proliferation, and ongoing inflammation involving polymorphonuclear leukocytes. The production of cytokines, proteins produced by a broad array of cells including lymphocytes, macrophages, and fibroblasts, augment the inflammatory process by attracting other cells, including lymphocytes. Although T-helper lymphocytes predominate, B-lymphocytes also proliferate and produce the antibody-producing plasma cells, the latter responsible for the production of immunoglobulins such as IgM and IgG. The IgG will bind to the IgM creating a complex called rheumatoid factor. Rheumatoid factor (RF) is usually significantly higher in RA than other conditions in which it may be present. Rheumatoid factor may be present in infections, renal disease, myocardial infarction, malignancy, thyroid disease and the so-called collagen-vascular disorders such as lupus, scleroderma, polyarteritis nodosa, Sjögren's syndrome and Felty's syndrome.

The pathology of RA can be described in four basic stages. In the first stage, an unknown antigen reaches the synovial membrane and initiates a local immune response. In the second stage, a chronic synovial inflammation ensues with numerous cellular infiltrates and cytokines. In the third stage, pannus develops leading to a final fourth stage of bone and cartilage destruction.

Gross and Histological Changes

In the early stage of RA there is synovial cell hypertrophy and hyperplasia that is mild, as well as vascular proliferation (Fig. 7–11). With time, the inflammation leads to significant lymphoid infiltration with aggregates, with and without plasma cells. These aggregates eventually form germinal centers with pericentral plasma cells (Fig. 7–12). There is fibrin deposition and stromal edema where the subsynovium thickens and protrudes into the joint as villous hypertrophy. Numerous synovial villi engulfed with lymphocytes and plasma cells develop with dramatic synovial hyperplasia and hypertrophy (Figs. 7–13 and 7–14). This synovial hyperplasia is often greater than 10 layers in thickness, and hypertrophied cells include large peculiar giant cells called Grimley-Sokoloff giant cells. "Rice bodies," or fibrinous aggregates of synovial exudate, accumulate and fill the joint.

On gross examination the synovium transforms from its slender, smooth, and glistening appearance to prominent,

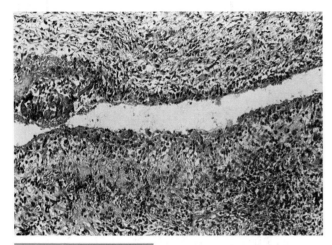

Figure 7–11   Rheumatoid arthritis (RA), synovium. Hyperplasia and hypertrophy of both synovial intimal lining cells and subsynovial cells. The surface exudes the fibrinous exudate which can clump and form soft, tan "rice bodies" filling the joint.

edematous villi protruding into the joint space. There is a loss of lustre with an irregular grainy appearance and often a reddish hue indicating vascular congestion. Color may vary depending on fibrinous and inflammatory changes with the synovium appearing yellowish or even gray. With hemorrhage, extravasated red blood cells and areas of necrosis, a brown staining, may be evident.

Articular cartilage also loses its lustre and becomes engulfed by the invading synovial pannus. Eventually, cartilage breaks down into fragmented cartilage debris. Denuded bone surfaces are exposed. The underlying subchondral bone appears rough, pitted from erosive destruction, and reddish, belying the underlying vascular congestion, marrow hyperplasia, invading granulation tissue of the pannus, and tissue breakdown (Fig. 7–15) It is as if the surface was removed and the underlying inflamed and hyperplastic marrow exposed to view.

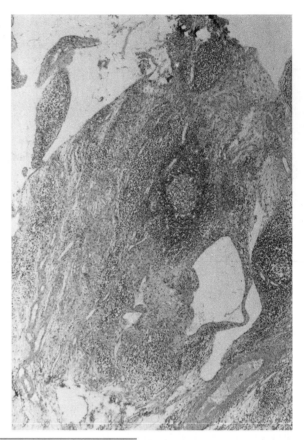

Figure 7–12   Rheumatoid arthritis synovium. Germinal centers mimicking the organization of lymph tissue in lymph nodes may be observed.

The synovial fluid is characterized by a decreased viscosity, and it is often translucent, with a greenish hue. There is an elevated white count, the range may be from 2,000 to 75,000 mm. Other features include identification of rice bodies, cytoplasmic inclusions from distended phagocytic vacuoles, and relatively low glucose and complement. There may be synovial fluid in the immune complexes composed of both IgG and IgM RF.

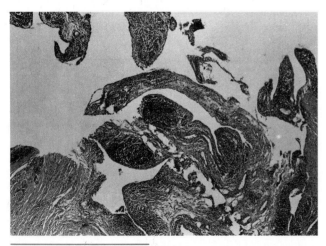

Figure 7–13   Rheumatoid arthritis, synovium. In contrast to DJD synovium, RA synovium shows hyperplastic villous hypertrophy with villi engorged with inflammatory cells. Here in the chronic state, tissue shows nodular aggregates of lymphocytes.

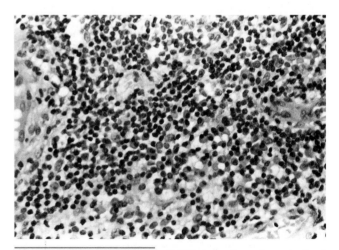

Figure 7–14   Rheumatoid arthritis synovium characterized by leukocytosis in the synovial fluid is characterized in tissue by aggregates of lymphocytes and plasma cells.

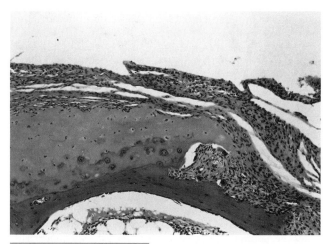

Figure 7–15   Rheumatoid pannus. The inflamed synovium aggressively proliferates and encroaches upon the articular cartilage enveloping it causing chondrolysis and destructive arthropathy.

Key Pathological Elements in Rhematoid Arthritis and Their Significance

1. polymorphonuclear leukocytes (neutrophils) in synovial fluid
2. nodular lymphocytosis with germinal center formation and plasma cell cuffing
3. Grimley-Sokoloff synovial giant cells
4. vascular proliferation
5. rice bodies (fibrin)
6. pannus factors
7. chondrolysis
8. bone and cartilage debris (detritus)
9. osteopenia

Polymorphonuclear Leukocytes

Polymorphonuclear leukocytes (PMNs) are abundant in the synovial fluid. Damage is done when the PMNs degranulate, stimulate cytokines, produce reactive oxidants, arachidonic acid, and other metabolites that breakdown hyaluronic acid, a major constituent of articular cartilage. Other substances lead to fibrinolysis and clotting irregularities, producing fibrin clots (rice bodies) that cover the synovial membrane.

Lymphocytosis

The lymphocytosis of RA is seen early in the disease and can be identified by the predilection to form nodules of lymphoid aggregates. There is perinodular cuffing with plasma cells. Nodular lymphocytosis initially occurs just below the synovial intimal lining cells and eventually fills the synovial villi causing gross engorgement and enlargement. In its full blown expression, nodular lymphocytosis may show germinal centers mimicking the architecture of a lymph node.

Grimley-Sokoloff Synovial Giant Cells

The hyperplasia and hypertrophy of both intimal and subintimal synovial lining cells is dramatic in RA. Grimley and

Sokoloff (1981) described Langhans-type giant cells with nuclei situated in a peripheral horseshoe-type arrangement and located very superficially in the synovial tissue. When seen, 25 to 100 mm below the synovial surface, they are considered specific for RA.

Vascular Proliferation

Extensive vascular proliferation, or angiogenesis, accompanies RA. Hypervascularity may lead to breakdown with microscopic hemarthrosis. In fact, hemosiderin deposition is often noted in RA and can give rise to a grossly visible tan or brown synovium.

Rice Bodies

One end result of synovial proliferation and degeneration is the production of collagen cell debris and fibrin (rice bodies). Grossly, this appears as small, tan and mushy loose bodies filling and coating joint structures. Histologically, the fibrinous exudate is seen loose or attached by inflammatory granulation stalks to the underlying synovium or pannus.

Pannus

Pannus is neoplasticlike growth of inflamed synovial tissue, the presence of which leads to destruction of joint structures. (Fig. 7–15) It is initially a granulation tissue consisting of blood vessels, inflammatory cells, and proliferating fibroblasts that invades and overruns the articular cartilage. The articular cartilage at pannus interfaces appears to undergo chondrolysis or direct phagocytic resorption.

Chondrolysis

Chondrolysis is a characteristic finding in RA and is evidenced by pallor of staining and enlarged lacunae around chondrocytes. In RA the cartilage appears to melt away. Although this phenomenon is more dramatic when cartilage is enveloped by invading pannus, chondrolysis occurs in areas remote from the pannus. This is most likely the result of collagenase and other destructive enzymes released by synovial cells into the synovial fluid. It is also possible that activated chondrocytes play a role in chondrolysis.

Bone and Cartilage Debris

The destructive activity brought on by the active inflammatory rheumatoid pannus leads to resorption and fragmentation of articular structures including fibrocartilaginous tissue such as the meniscus in the knee, articular cartilage, and bone. These fragments are irregular pieces of tissue lying in surrounding tissue. Often these pieces of debris are engulfed by phagocytic cells.

Osteopenia

The bone is adversely affected in RA from both without and within. The destruction by invading pannus leads to direct macrophage-like resorption. In addition, destructive enzymes, cytokines, and other mediators from the cyclical inflammation eventually destroy bone. The bone marrow may show a relative plasmacytosis; plasma cells are known producers of local tissue resorbing factors. When the RA is treated with steroids, adverse effects are confounded because known effects of these compounds include osteoporosis and osteonecrosis.

In summary, the constellation of histologic changes that best characterize RA includes synovial cell hypertrophy and hyperplasia; mononuclear cell inflammation, particularly with perivascular lymphocyte and plasma cell aggregates; chondrolysis, and vessel thrombosis leading to rice bodies. A near pathognomonic group of findings in the identification of RA comprises the collective presence of germinal centers within nodules of lymphocytosis, Grimly-Sokoloff giant cells, rheumatoid nodules, and fibrinous rice bodies.

Extra-articular Manifestations

The most obvious manifestations of extra-articular disease are constitutional symptoms, including fatigue, fever, myalgias, lymphadenopathy, anemia, and, occasionally, thrombocytopenia due to Felty's syndrome. Approximately 20% of patients develop subcutaneous nodules. Nodules are most commonly seen over the olecranon process of the ulna, but they may also be seen on the extensor aspects of the finger joints, about the Achilles tendon, or even in the occiput.

In RA, tendons, ligaments, and other periarticular structures may be involved, the process usually one of nonspecific, chronic inflammation.

Peripheral neuropathies and other Lesions of the peripheral nerve and arteries have also been described..., but they are nonspecific in nature. Myelopathies due to cervical vertebral subluxation and entrapment neuropathies including ulnar, median (carpal tunnel syndrome), and tibial (tarsal tunnel syndrome) nerves are not uncommon. Other lesions include rheumatic heart disease, pericarditis, interstitial myocarditis, aortic insufficiency, granulomatous aortitis, and coronary arteritis. In the lungs, chronic pulmonary diseases, such as Caplan's syndrome, granulomatous lesions, interstitial pneumonia, pulmonary fibrosis, pulmonary arteritis, and obliterative bronchiolitis, have also been described. Enlargement of regional lymph nodes, as well as splenomegaly (Felty's syndrome), can occur. Bone marrow changes are nonspecific and may show an increase in plasma cell production. Renal proteinuria, amyloidosis, mesangial nephritis, and, less commonly, glomerulonephritis, have been described. Ocular manifestations include episcleritis, scleritis, corneal ulcerations, and keratoconjunctivitis secondary to Sjögren's syndrome.

MISCELLANEOUS JOINT CONDITIONS

Iron in tissue is usually seen in the form of hemosiderin, visible as granular brown pigments in an intracytoplasmic localization. The presence of hemosiderin can be seen in a broad variety of conditions. A somewhat incidental finding of iron can be seen in association with fracture hemorrhage. Iron can be a contributing factor to the pathophysiology of disorders such as hemophilic arthropathy and the transfusional hemosiderosis of thalassemia. Deposition of iron at the mineralization front, causing osteoporosis or even osteomalacia can be seen in primary or secondary hemochromatosis. The term "pigmented" in pigmented villonodular synovitis (PVSN)

refers to the brown pigmentation caused by iron deposition in the synovial tissue.

Incidental hemosiderin deposition seen in association with microscopic or macroscopic hemorrhage is usually of little pathophysiologic consequence. However, iron has been linked directly to several important hemosiderin-driven osteoarticular pathologies: trauma-related hemosiderotic synovitis, hemophilic arthropathy, and the osteoarticular iron osteopathy in hemochromatosis.

The most commonly encountered iron related injury in orthopaedic pathology is that related to hemorrhage into the joint. Considering the rich vascularity of the subintimal layer of the synovium, microscopic bleeds from normal daily use of the joint may be expected. In fact, a few red blood cells are considered normal in joint fluid analysis. Trauma to the knee, however, is often accompanied by significant hemarthrosis; an important association because the iron released from the blood cells stimulates significant synovial changes, characterized clinically by pain and swelling.

In chronic hemarthrosis, iron will accumulate in the synovium. Grossly, the synovium may attain a "rusty" appearance (Fig. 7–16). Histopathologic hemosiderin is visible in the synovial intimal cells and the histiocytic cells of the subintimal zone (Fig. 7–17).

Hemosiderotic Synovitis

Hemorrhages that occur within the synovium eventually disintegrate via phagocytosis by histiocytes. The hemoglobin is broken down and processed into hemosiderin. It is the hemosiderin that is so characteristically seen as a brown, granular substance in cells of the synovium. Hemosiderin may be noted either intracellularly or extracellularly. The gross appearance of the joint with chronic hemarthrosis is that of a rusty pigmentation, although more acute bleeding may be demonstrable as a blackish-green discoloration.

The response of the human joint to bleeding is the formation of a hyperplastic vascular synovium. There is a proliferation of the synovial cells and other subsynovial lining cell connective-tissue elements including inflammatory cells. (Fig.

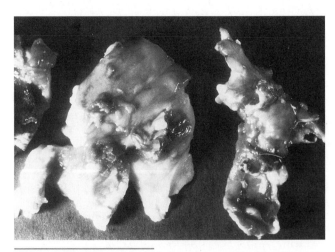

Figure 7–16 Hemosiderin induced synovitis. Bleeding into the joint leads to a tan discoloration of synovium, the result of hemosiderin accumulation originating in red blood cells.

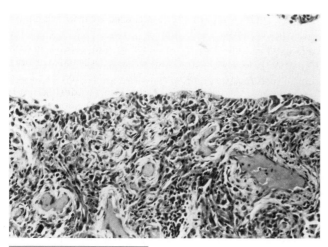

Figure 7–17 Hemosiderin changes may be minimal with accumulation in synovial lining cells or subintimal cellular tissue.

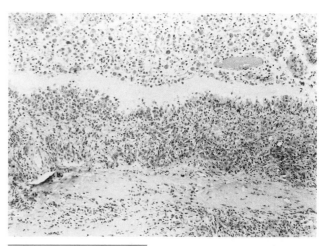

Figure 7–18 Hemosiderin synovitis. Hyperplasia and hypertrophy can be extensive and lead to a pannus-like inflammatory proliferation with resultant joint destruction.

7–18) Under the electron microscope, iron-containing electron dense particles that are membrane bound, called siderosomes, are noted within the synovial cells and subsynovial macrophages.

In addition to trauma, hemosiderotic synovitis may result from the use of oral anticoagulant therapies, the breakdown of synovial hemangiomas, or as a secondary phenomenon in conditions such as RA, PVNS, scurvy, and sickle cell anemia.

With bleeding into the joint, two pathways may lead to damage. As mentioned, the red blood cells may break down causing macrophage activation. Intracellular hemosiderin precipitates the release of leukocyte and synovial-derived chondrolytic enzymes. In the second pathway, iron deposition into tissues such as the meniscus may be severe enough to cause mechanical dysfunction and degenerative changes.

Hemophilic Arthropathy

The adverse effect of chronic hemorrhage has been extensively studied in the joints of hemophiliacs. There is hyperplasia of the synovial lining cells with abundant intracytoplasmic hemosiderin granule accumulation. In tissue cultures of hemophilic synovium, pigment-laden fibroblast cells have been shown to proliferate and secrete large amounts of collagenase and neutral proteinases.

Iron is known to accumulate in cartilage as well. It has been localized to superficial chondrocytes suggesting chondrocytic uptake triggering a degradative enzyme release similar to that described in synovial cells.

Hemophilia

Hemophilia A is the most common hereditary coagulation disorder. It occurs in 20 per 100,000 male births due to the deficiency, absence, or malfunction of coagulation factor VIII.

Hemophilia A is a heterogeneous disorder ranging from mild disease (1–4% deficiency) to severe disease. The disorder may not be recognized in patients with mild or moderate disease unless a significant traumatic event precipitates bleed-

ing. Excessive bleeding during surgery may be the first clue. Therapy centers around replacement of factor VIII. One unit of Factor VIII increases plasma activity by 0.024 U/mL. Because 0.3 U/mL are usually needed to treat a mild bleeding episode, the physician should prescribe greater than this amount.

Most commonly involved are the knees and elbows, followed by the ankles, shoulders and hips. Childhood signs include discomfort and joint limitation. Pain and swelling follow. Numerous damaging microhemarthroses have transpired before the initial clinical symtoms, unfortunately delaying diagnosis.

Roentgenographically, joint space narrowing, loss of articular cartilage, cystic remodeling of bone, and hemophilic "pseudotumors" characterize the illness. Adhering to maintenance of factor VIII levels to prevent spontaneous hemorrhage has been associated with significantly decreased morbidity.

Intra-articular, intrabursal, and soft tissue bleeding in hemophilia may result in painless masses called pseudotumors. These consist of spongy coagula of partially clotted blood encapsulated by thick fibrous membranes. Complications due to these pseudotumors include muscle and bone damage, infection, and neuropathy. Surgical removal is not without danger. Pseudotumors occur in 1 to 2% of hemophiliacs, mostly in the lower extremity and pelvis.

Prior to 1970, hemophilia A was associated with severe disability and even death at a young age. Median life expectancy has grown throughout the 20th century from 11.4 years to 68 years in carefully followed populations. However, the transfusion of blood products, including factor VIII concentrates, has led to transfusion-related acquired immunodeficiency virus (AIDS). Approximately two thirds of hemophiliacs with positive test results for human immunodeficiency virus (HIV) have eventually died of AIDS.

Now factor VIII concentrates are sterilized with heat treatment or solvent cleaning. Genetically engineered products are now available and being tested for complications.

Surgeons have accrued knowledge and experience with both total knee and total hip arthroplasty in hemophilic arthropathy. With proper surgical technique and factor replacement, excellent results can be expected with total knee arthroplasty. With hip replacement, rates of lossening are higher. In addition, a high rate of deep infection in HIV-positive patients has been noted.

Synovial Chondromatosis

Loose bodies may occur in any joint and may vary in size and number. They may be asymptomatic or cause pain and result in limited motion, locking, and, in extreme cases, subluxation.

Primary Synovial Chondromatosis

The synovium is capable of undergoing metaplasia to form cartilaginous and chondro-osseous nodules. The nodules may dislodge from the synovium and become, free loose bodies ranging in number from a few to hundreds (Fig. 7–19).

Synovial chondromatosis is a monoarticular condition of the third through fifth decades of life, with predilection for the knee, elbow, ankle, hip and shoulder. Rarely, the wrists, fingers, or temporomandibular joints may be involved.

The condition is usually associated with swelling, pain, limited motion, and, occasionally, clicking or locking. Radiographically synovial chondromatosis is easily recognized if the cartilaginous bodies have undergone calcification or ossification. The numerous radiopaque densities range in size from a millimeter to centimeters, varying considerably in the extent of calcification and size. Arthrography is useful in diagnosing the noncalcified bodies.

Grossly, the synovium shows flake-like bodies; or it may possess an irregular nodular contour. Whitish or translucent bluish-gray nodules, ranging in size and shape, may be attached on the membrane or floating in the joint space. Histopathologic differences of these bodies have supported a distinction between a secondary synovial chondromatosis associated with DJD and a primary synovial chondromatosis

not associated with any underlying disorder. The loose bodies in the secondary synovial chondromatosis show more organized cellular growth, often in concentric rings. Transformation between cartilage and bone may be abrupt. In the typical case, orderly zones of transformation from fibrocartilage to hyaline-type cartilage through endochondral ossification to bone may be noted.

PEARL

If synovial chondromatosis is not related to trauma or an obvious arthritic process, think primary (i.e., tumorous) synovial chondromatosis.

In primary synovial chondromatosis, a more disorganized growth of cartilage cells is often apparent (Fig. 7–20). There are increased chondrocytes, often crowded and irregular in spatial distribution. Nuclei vary and binucleate cells may be seen. Calcification may be patchy or diffuse.

Surgical removal of all the nodules is important in preventing recurrence. If the chondro-osseous bodies are free within the joint, a thorough "cleaning" of the joint may suffice. However, the disorder may involve chondro-osseous change within the synovial subintimal connective tissue, a fact that may require total synovectomy to prevent recurrence.

Secondary Chondromatosis

Cartilaginous or osseous loose bodies can result from DJD, neuropathic joint diseases (Charcot's joint), osteochondritis dissecans, meniscal tears, or other trauma. These cartilage segments (with or without underlying bone) may dislodge

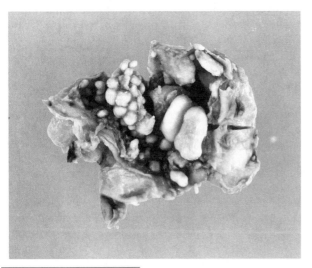

Figure 7–19 Synovial chondromatosis. Loose bodies are often multiple, varying in size and shape and in degree of calcification and/or ossification.

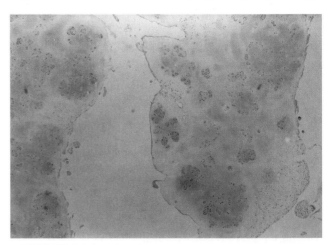

Figure 7–20 Primary synovial chondromatosis. Cartilage may proliferate in a tumorous fashion and in such cases differs from secondary synovial chondromatosis in its irregular lobular growth pattern. Cellularity and cellular morphology mimics primary cartilage tumors.

and continue to grow with the synovial fluid acting as a culture media. Villi formed in patients with PVNS can twist, infarct, and form a loose body.

Synovial Chondrosarcoma

A malignant tumor arising within the joint is extremely rare. However, chondrosarcomas may arise in the setting of synovial chondromatosis. This condition can be suspected when there is evidence of aggressive growth, such as invasion into adjacent extra-articular tissues. The clinical behavior of these neoplasms varies from that of low-grade neoplasm, with a propensity to recur locally, to those that may metastasize.

Pigmented Villonodular Synovitis

Pigmented villonodular synovitis is usually a monoarticular process that is found in synovial joints and tendon sheaths. Common locations include the knee and the tendon sheaths of the digits of the hand (giant-cell tumors of tendon sheath). Three forms have been identified: an isolated lesion involving tendon sheaths (giant-cell tumor of tendon sheath); a solitary intra-articular nodule (localized nodular synovitis); and a diffuse, often villous and pigmented process involving the synovial tissue (PVNS). The lesion is rarely polyarticular and does not metastasize, but it may invade bone locally. The localized tenosynovial and diffuse pigmented synovia lesions do not appear to be separate entities, judging from their similar histologic characteristics and biological behavior. Solitary tenosynovial nodules in the digits of the hand have been reported to recur in 7 to 45% of patients, and diffuse processes (PVNS) of the knee have been reported to recur in as many as 45% of patients. The peak incidence for knee lesions is the third decade; finger or thumb lesions occur with the greatest frequency in the sixth decade.

Jaffe et al., in their classic description of this lesion in 1941, suggested that it is an inflammatory process. However, it may be neoplastic, although the cell of origin remains obscure.

Clinical presentations depend on the site. In joint lesions, swelling, stiffness, or discomfort is common. Torsion of a pedunculated nodular form of PVNS has been associated with the unusual clinical presentation of acute pain.

Joint fluid ranges in color from normal, that is clear, to brownish-red. The synovium may appear pigmented due to hemosiderin from microscopic synovial hemorrhage (brown) and aggregations of lipid-laden macrophages (yellow) in the periphery of expanding nodules (Fig. 7–21).

At least five clinical types of PVNS are identified in the knee: (1) loose body, (2) a localized nodule (pedunculated or embedded in the synovium), (3) aggregates of nodules confined to one compartment, (4) a diffuse involvement of the synovium, and (5) synovial PVNS extending into bursa. Localized nodular and nodular aggregate types are the most common types of PVNS.

The radiological findings are dependent on the anatomy of the involved joint. Articulations with close apposition of the capsule of the joint to the underlying bone, such as the hip,

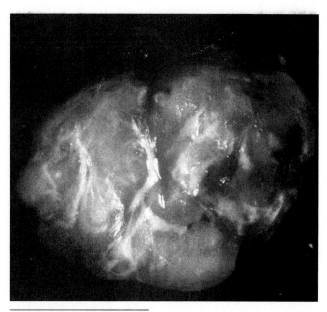

Figure 7–21 Pigmented villonodular synovitis (PVNS). Cut section of a solitary nodule. Note silk color, lobular growth, and peripheral zones of clear (lipid macrophages) and dark (hemosiderin accumulation from bleeding) color.

develop bone erosions. The erosions are well defined, with minimal sclerosis. The erosions are most often located in the bare areas of bone but can be located in subchondral surfaces. Pigmented villonodular synovitis does not calcify. The joint space is usually preserved because articular cartilage most of the times is not eroded. The hip represents an unusual situation because often these patients can first present with narrowing of the joint space. The most common x-ray findings in the knee are soft tissue swelling. Arthrograms may demonstrate the nodules as discrete pitting defects. Bone changes are less frequent but may include erosions and degenerative changes. Magnetic resonance imaging reveals an isointense or low signal intensity compared with muscle on T1- and T2-weighted images. However, findings are variable depending on the amount of hemosiderin, lipid, cellularity, and fibrosis.

> ### PEARL
> The "apple core" lesion is typical of PVNS. The femoral or humeral neck is eroded, with preservation of the head giving the appearance of a partially eaten apple.

Grossly, the lesions are usually categorized as nodular or villonodular. Solitary nodules or aggregates of confluent nodules are designated nodular (see Fig. 7–21). Poorly delineated

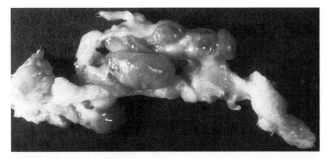

Figure 7–22 Pigmented villonodular synovitis. Often multinodular along tendon sheath, the 30% recurrence rate can be attributed to surgically missed nodules.

lesions characterized by plump synovial villi and by small unencapsulated nodules, not necessarily contiguous to one another and often blending into the surrounding tissue, are designated villonodular (Figs. 7–22 and 7–23).

The hallmark histopathologic findings required to establish the diagnosis of PVNS are proliferating fibroblasts and histiocytes, with occasional giant cells and abundant collagen production (Fig. 7–24). Based on ultrastructural findings, a giant-cell tumor of tendon sheath can be considered a tumorous proliferation of fibroblasts and histiocytes, that is, a benign fibrous histiocytoma. Others clinicians have suggested a synovial cell derivation.

The differential diagnosis for PVNS includes any soft tissue mass that causes erosions of adjacent bones such as gout, rheumatoid nodules, tuberculous arthritis, or juxtacortical chondromas. The absence of osteoporosis, joint space narrowing, or calcifications are helpful in making the diagnosis of PVNS. Histologically, PVNS must be distinguished from both benign and neoplastic conditions. Hemosiderotic synovitis, as is seen in hemophilia, and the chronic synovitis caused by either RA or trauma, do not have a distinct submembranous nodule or nodules composed of proliferating mononuclear and giant cells. Monophasic synovial sarcoma is differentiated by its characteristic increased cellularity, cellular pleomorphism, lack of fibrosis, and high mitotic counts. Other rare lesions such as angioma, hemangiopericytoma, histiocytoma, and fibroma are morphologically homogeneous and, therefore, histologically distinct.

PEARL
Pigmented villonodular synovitis does not calcify. Pigmented villonodular synovitis recurs in one third of cases.

The treatment of PVNS is surgical. If an isolated loose body or nodule is confirmed, arthroscopic surgical excision may be attempted. However, the propensity of the lesions to recur (in up to one third of cases) requires careful examination of the joint to exclude multiple foci. The diffuse form of PVNS requires total synovectomy.

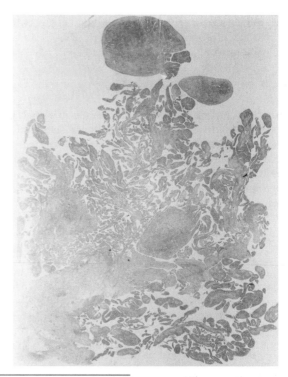

Figure 7–23 Pigmented villonodular synovitis. Diffuse or villonodular PVNS, a rare form of PVNS, is characterized by villous hyperplasia interspersed with fibrohistiocytic nodules of varying size.

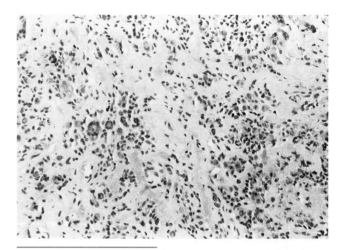

Figure 7–24 Pigmented villonodular synovitis. Microscopically, mononuclear and giant-cell histiocytes and fibroblasts proliferate and produce an abundant collagen matrix.

SELECTED BIBLIOGRAPHY

Osteoarthritis

Brittberg M, Lindahl A, Nilsson A, Ohlsson C, Isaksson O, Peterson L. Treatment of deep cartilage defects in the knee with autologous chondrocyte transplantation. *N Engl J Med*. 1994;331:889–895.

Felson DT, Anderson JJ, Naimark A, Walker AM, Meenan RF. Obesity and knee osteoarthritis: the Framingham study. *Ann Int Med*. 1988;109:18–24.

Hamerman D. The biology of osteoarthritis. *N Engl J Med*. 1989;320:1322–1330.

Hannan N, Ghosh P, Bellenger C, Taylor T. Systemic administration of glycosaminoglycan polysulphate (Arteparon) provides partial protection of articular cartilage from damage produced by meniscectomy in the canine. *J Orthop Res*. 1987;5:47–59.

Healey JH, Vigorita VJ, Lane JM. The coexistence and characteristics of osteoarthritis and osteoporosis. *J Bone Jt Surg*. 1985;67-A:586–592.

Kindynis P, Haller J, Kang HS, Resnick D, Sartoris DJ, Trudell D, Tyson R. Osteophytosis of the knee: anatomic, radiologic, and pathologic investigation. *Radiology*. 1990;174:841–846.

Kleinbart FA, Bryk E, Evangelista J, Scott WN, Vigorita VJ. Histologic comparison of posterior cruciate ligaments from arthritic and age-matched knee specimens. *J Arthroplasty*. 1996;11:726–731.

Komiya S, Inoue A, Ssaguri Y, Minimitani K, Morimatsu M. Rapidly destructive arthropathy of the hip: studies on bone resorptive factors in joint with a theory of pathogenesis. *Clin Orthop*. 1992;284:273–282.

Lawrance JAL, Athanasou NA. Rapidly destructive hip disease. *Skeletal Radiol*. 1995;24:639–641.

Mankin HJ, Dorman H, Lippiello L, Zarins A. Biochemical and metabolic abnormalities in articular cartilage from osteo-arthritic human hips. II: correlation of morphology with biochemical and metabolic data. *J Bone Jt Surg*. 1971;53-A:523–537.

Mankin HJ, Brandt KD, Shulman LE. Workshop on etiopathogenesis of osteoarthritis. Proceedings and recommendations. *J Rheum*. 1986;13:1130–116.

Williams JM, Ongchi DR, Thonar EJ-MA. Repair of articular cartilage injury following intra-articular chymopapain-induced matrix proteoglycan loss. *J Orthop Res*. 1993;11:705–716.

Rheumatoid Arthritis

Allard SA, Muirden KD, Maini RN. Correlation of histopathological features of pannus with patterns of damage in different joints in rheumatoid arthritis. *Ann Rheum Dis*. 1991;50:278–283.

Bresnihan B. Synovial histology in rheumatoid arthritis: clues for the clinician. *J Rheum*. 1988;15:885–887. Editorial.

Caruso I, Santandrea S, Puttini PS, Boccassini L, Montrone F, Cazzola M, Azzolini V, Segre D. Clinical, laboratory, and radiographic features in early rheumatoid arthritis. *J Rheum*. 1990;17:1263–1267.

Haraqui B, Pelletier JP, Cloutier JM, Faure MP, Martel-Pelletier J. Synovial membrane histology and immunopathology in rheumatoid arthritis and osteoarthritis. *Arthritis Rheum*. 1991;34:153–163.

Harris ED. Rheumatoid arthritis: pathophysiology and implications for therapy. *N Engl J Med*. 1990;322:1277–1289.

Persselin JE. Diagnosis of rheumatoid arthritis: medical and laboratory aspects. *Clin Orthop*. 1991;265:73–82.

Soren A and Waugh TR: The Giant Cells in the Synovial Membrane. *Ann Rheum dis*. 1981; 40:496–500.

Ziff M. The rheumatoid nodule. *Arthritis Rheum*. 1990;33:761–765.

Wilder RL, Crofford LJ. Do infectious agents cause rheumatoid arthritis? *Clin Orthop*. 1995;265:36–41.

Hemosiderin

Arnold WD, Hilgartner MW. Hemophilic arthropathy: current concepts of pathogenesis and management. *J Bone Jt Surg*. 1977;59-A:287–305.

Maffulli N, Binfield PM, King JB, Good CJ. Acute haemarthrosis of the knee in athletes: a prospective study of 106 cases. *J Bone Jt Surg*. 1993;75B:945–949.

Mainardi CL, Levine PH, Werb Z, Harris ed Jr. Proliferative synovitis in hemophilia: biochemical and morphological observations. *Arthritis Rheum*. 1978;21:137–144.

Phelps K, Vigorita V, Bansal M, Einhorn T. Histochemical demonstration of iron but not aluminum in a case of dialysis-associated osteomalacia. *Am J Med*. 1988;84:775–780.

Safran MR, Johnston-Jones K, Kabo JM, Meals RA. The effect of experimental hemarthrosis on joint stiffness and synovial histology in a rabbit model. *Clin Orthop*. 1994;303:280–288.

Synovial Chondromatosis

Milgram JW. Synovial osteochondromatosis: a histopathologic study of 30 cases. *J Bone Jt Surg Am*. 1977;59-A:792–801.

Villacin AB, Brigham LN, Bullough PG. Primary and secondary synovial chondrometaplasia: histopathologic and clinicoradiologic differences. *Human Pathol*. 1979;20:439–451.

Pigmented Villonodular Synovitis

Cotten A, Flipo R-M, Chastanet P, Desvigne-Noiulet M-C, Duquesnoy B, Delcambre B. Pigmented villonodular synovitis of the hip: review of radiographic features in 58 patients. *Skeletal Radiol*. 1995;24:1–6.

COTTEN A, FLIPO R-M, MESTDAGH H, CHASTANET P. Diffuse pigmented villonodular synovitis of the shoulder. *Skeletal Radiol.* 1995;24:311–313

HUGHES TH, SARTORIS DJ, SCHWEITZER ME, RESNICK DL. Pigmented villonodular synovitis: MRI characteristics. *Skeletal Radiol.* 1995;24:7–12.

JAFFE HL, LICHTENSTEIN L, SUTRO CJ. Pigmented villonodular synovitis, bursitis, and tenosynovitis: a discussion of the synovial and bursal equivalents of the tenosynovial lesions commonly denoted as xanthanoma, xanthogranuloma, giant cell tumor, or myeloplaxoma of the tendon sheath, with some considerations of this tendon sheath lesion itself. *Arch Pathol.* 1941;31:731–765.

RAO S, VIGORITA VJ. Pigmented villonodular synovitis (giant-cell tumor of the tendon sheath and synovial membrane): a review of 81 cases. *J Bone Jt Surg.* 1984;66A:76–94.

SAMPLE QUESTIONS

1. Which of the following is correct:
   (a) Blood in the joint is harmless.
   (b) Iron can localize in synovial cells and mineralization fronts of bone.
   (c) Blood injected into animal joints creates PVNS.

2. Which of the following is false; osteoarthritis:
   (a) is primarily an inflammatory process.
   (b) is associated with cartilage degradation and repair.
   (c) is multifactorial but often age related.
   (d) may be precipitated by changes in the biochemical constituents of articular cartilage.

3. Which of the following is false; PVNS:
   (a) is most common in the knee.
   (b) recurs ~ 30% of the time.
   (c) is an inflammatory lesion.
   (d) is usually monoarticular

4. Which of the following is false; synovial chondromatosis:
   (a) frequently progresses to synovial chondrosarcoma.
   (b) rises from metaplastic synovium.
   (c) does not metastasize.
   (d) may or may not calcify or ossify.

5. Which of the following is false: rheumatoid arthritis:
   (a) it has a proven infectious etiology.
   (b) has an autoimmune component.
   (c) is an inflammatory disease dominated by T-lymphocyte-mediated events.
   (d) is associated with genetic predisposition.

Answers: 1) b; 2) a; 3) b; 4) a; 5) a

The Scientific Method

Anthony D. Watson, MD

Clinical and basic science research are essential to the improvement of orthopaedic care. The purpose of research is to advance the science of musculoskeletal care. Rigorous study design minimizes errors that can degrade the strength of the data and thus decrease the confidence investigators have in their conclusions.

Statistical analysis is an important research tool. Statistics summarize vast amounts of data, and hypothesis testing tries to determine the significance and predictive power of the data. Statistical analysis does not prove any hypothesis. Statistics try to quantify the amount of confidence investigators can have that the hypothesis is confirmed or refuted by the data.

Investigators and clinicians have a responsibility to ensure that research advances the science of orthopaedic care. Investigators must design rigorous studies and collect and analyze the data appropriately. Clinicians who review orthopaedic research must be able to critically evaluate study design and statistical analysis before accepting the investigators' conclusions.

There has been great progress in study design in the recent biomedical literature; however, approximately 40% of recent clinical studies use incorrect statistical testing methods. The objectives of this chapter are: (1) define and describe study design techniques, (2) describe sources of error in data gathering, analysis, and statistical testing, (3) define statistical terms, (4) describe the basic types of statistical tests and their applications, and (5) describe and discuss evolving techniques such as outcomes analysis, decision-analysis, and cost-effectiveness analysis.

RESEARCH DESIGN

Definitions

Performing a clinical or basic science study consists of seven basic steps. First, the investigators must ask a question to define the problem. Second, the investigators must guess the answer or define a hypothesis. The third step is the most difficult: defining the materials and methods of study. Once defined, data must be gathered and analyzed. The researchers must then determine whether the data supports or refutes the hypothesis. Finally, the relevance of the conclusions must be explained.

An essential element of study design is defining the materials and methods. The *population* must be defined so that readers of the study can determine for which patients the results are relevant. The study conclusions are based on *observations*, or measurements, of the *variables* determined to be important by the investigators. The observations are collected from a *sample* that is a subset of the population that is available to the investigator. For example, a study is designed to determine the incidence of deep venous thrombosis (DVT) after total hip arthroplasty (THA). It is impractical for investigators to study every patient in the country who has undergone a THA. Therefore, the investigators define a sample that reflects the population of patients who have had a THA and collects observations of the variable, DVT. If the sample is representative of the population, the conclusions are *generalizable*.

> **PITFALL**
>
> One can only generalize the conclusions of a study to the population implied by the investigators' definition of the sample.

There are three types of observations and each requires a different method of data collection and analysis. *Ordinal* and *nominal* variables are categorical variables that have no arithmetic relationship and therefore require nonparametric data analysis techniques. Ordinal variables consist of categories that can be ranked in order such as "excellent/good/fair/poor." Nominal variables comprise categories with no inherent rank order such as gender and race. The third observation

Orthopaedic Surgery: The Essentials. Edited by M.E. Baratz, A.D. Watson, and J.E. Imbriglia. Thieme Medical Publishers, Inc., New York © 1999

type comprises *continuous* data that is numeric with constant, defined, and equal intervals between each data point. Examples include temperature, height, weight, and range of motion.

Precision and *accuracy* describe the robustness of data collection. Precision describes how closely each observation resembles the other observations. Accuracy describes how closely each observation resembles the true value. Thus, precision is a measure of the quality of the technique used to collect data. Accuracy measures the similarity of the sample to the population from which it is proposed to be drawn. Observations can be precise without being accurate and accurate without being precise, but ideally they are both accurate and precise (Fig. 8–1).

Types of Studies

Orthopaedic research can involve basic science or clinical studies. Basic science studies can be *descriptive* or *comparative*. Examples of descriptive studies include histological and anatomic studies. The investigators ask, What does this structure look like? and hypothesizes the characteristics given an understanding of related structures and the function of the structure. Observations are made and summarized to either confirm or refute the hypothesis. Simple, descriptive statistics may be helpful. An explanation of the relevance of the observed pattern(s) of characteristics completes the study.

Biomechanical, biomaterial, biochemical, and physiologic properties are commonly evaluated in comparative basic science studies. These studies attempt to distinguish a difference between two or more implants, biologic materials, or pharmaceuticals. The investigators ask the question, Which of these is better? then hypothesize which may be better on the basis of prior knowledge. The testing is performed, data collected and analyzed, and statistics are used to determine whether the data confirm the hypothesis. The investigators must explain the clinical relevance of the conclusions.

Clinical studies include *case reports*, *retrospective* studies, and *prospective* studies. Well-designed prospective studies are the most scientifically robust, but they are difficult to perform in clinical practice. Retrospective studies are more easily performed and are less robust, but they provide useful information if designed and executed well.

Case reports are descriptive studies of a rare and unusual pathologic process, clinical intervention, or outcome. Conclusions can rarely be generalized, but they do help raise awareness of the rare and unusual.

Retrospective studies review the results of one or more interventions at a specified time period after the intervention(s). A typical retrospective study would evaluate the outcome of THA after 10 to 15 years. The key feature of a retrospective study is that the *follow-up* population and sample are defined first, and *then* the observations are collected and analyzed. Retrospective studies that evaluate one group's outcomes are experiential whereas comparative retrospective studies evaluate for differences between two or more groups.

Prospective studies define a study population and sample *prior* to initiating treatment and collect observations over a defined follow-up period. During the course of follow-up in any study, a patient's data may vary from the average course. Because this patient was defined to be included prior to follow-up in a prospective study, the patient will not be lost from the study. The variation from the average course may cause the patient to be "missed" in a retrospective study. Robustness of follow-up strengthens prospective studies.

Prospective studies are the only type of clinical study that can be randomized and blinded. Patient selection occurs before a retrospective study is initiated. A prospective study defines patient selection because the study is designed and

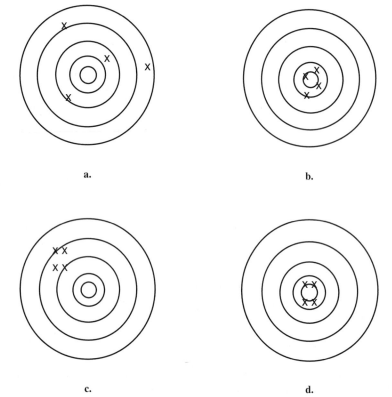

a.   b.

c.   d.

Figure 8–1 Measurement precision and accuracy are analogous to shooting a target. (**a**) neither precise nor accurate; (**b**) accurate but not precise; (**c**) precise but not accurate; (**d**) precise and accurate.

the population and sample defined prior to patient enrollment. For greatest strength, selection should be random, and data collection should be double-blind, where neither the investigators nor the patients know what treatment has been rendered. This is rarely possible in modern orthopaedics.

There are two types of prospective studies: cohort and case-control. Cohort studies prospectively evaluate a single sample over time. Natural history studies are a common type of cohort study. Case-control studies are typically randomized, double-blind prospective studies that compare a treatment group (case) to a group that does not receive treatment (control). The control group may receive placebo, "sham" surgery, or withholding of treatment. Case-control studies have the greatest strength, but they are costly and can present ethical dilemmas.

BASIC STATISTICAL METHODS

Definitions

Data must be summarized after collection to simplify analysis. However, the descriptive and analytic statistics are meaningless unless the method of data collection is *valid*, *reliable*, and minimizes *error*.

The variables must measure what the study proposes to measure. This is known as *validity*. To maximize validity in the previously mentioned DVT after THA study, the investigators must perform venography of every THA patient enrolled in the study. Simply evaluating for the presence or absence of calf swelling measures only the incidence of calf swelling and not necessarily the incidence of DVT.

The measurements must also be *reliable*. That is, the observations should be reproducible. *Inter-observer reliability* describes the degree of similarity between observations made by independent observers. *Intra-observer reliability* measures the similarity of observations made repeatedly by the same observer. For example, intra-observer reliability is high when a spine surgeon measures a scoliosis film on a number of different occasions and arrives at the same Cobb angle without knowing what the measurement was the last time. Inter-observer reliability is high when the residents and attending in the spine clinic all measure the same Cobb angle on a scoliosis film without knowledge of each others' measurement.

Error degrades precision and accuracy. Error is the difference between an observation and its true value. Error arises from a variety of sources. *Random* error is due to naturally occurring variations about the true value. An observation may be greater than or less than the true value. With enough observations, random errors tend to cancel each other out.

Bias is a form of error that occurs unidirectionally. That is, a measured value that is biased is either always greater than or always less than the true value. By definition, it is not random. *Systematic bias* occurs when the bias is introduced by the design of the study or the measurement technique. A classic example would be a butcher who puts a thumb on the scale when weighing a purchase. Less obvious would be a study that proposes to determine how long it takes to achieve radiographic union of a femur fracture. In one variation of such a study, radiographs are performed at 2, 4, 6, 12, and 24 weeks, and the average time to union is found to be 10 weeks. In another variation, x-rays are performed at 2, 4, 6, 10, and 24

weeks, and the average time to union is found to be 8 weeks. This difference occurs because fractures that may have been healed at 7 weeks are recorded as healing at 12 weeks in the first study. This in turn artificially increases, or biases, the mean. Redesigning the study, as in the second variation, reduces, but does not eliminate, this systematic bias.

Careful definition of sample inclusion and exclusion criteria are essential to minimize *selection bias*. For example, two studies propose to determine the incidence of wound complications after total knee arthroplasty (TKA). The first study is done at a university hospital, has an 8% wound complication rate, and includes patients with osteoarthritis (72%) and rheumatoid arthritis (28%). The second study is done at a large, suburban community hospital, has a 1% wound complication rate, and includes no patients with rheumatoid arthritis. The patient selection has biased the result in one or both of these studies. The first study has more patients with rheumatoid arthritis who may have been on corticosteroids and/or methotrexate. The patients at the university hospital may also have been more likely to have comorbidities that could compromise wound healing. Thus, it is imperative to determine whether or not selection bias is present before interpreting and generalizing the results of a study.

Descriptive statistics include the *mean, range, variance, standard deviation*, and *standard error of the mean*. The mean represents the central tendency of a *distribution* of observations. It is the value that emerges as random errors cancel each other out. The mean presumably approximates the true value. A plot of all the observations by their frequency is a *frequency distribution*. The *normal distribution* is one type of frequency distribution that is assumed to resemble the distribution of observations of most naturally occurring populations. Basic and clinical science research usually assumes a normal distribution when analyzing the data.

PEARL

The mean is the central value in a normal distribution. The values on either side of the mean are distributed equally because each differs from the mean by varying amounts of random error. These random errors cancel each other out to yield the mean.

The *range* is the interval between the smallest and largest measurements. The range indicates the limits of the observations and roughly implies the variability and precision. The *variance* (Var), however, is a more useful measure of the variability and measures the range as well as how tightly "packed" the observations are about the mean. (Fig. 8–2) illustrates the usefulness of variance when summarizing data. *Standard deviation* (SD) also measures variability like the variance and is the square root of variance. It is used more often because its units are the same as the mean. Assuming a normal distribution, two thirds of the observations can be expected to fall within an interval between 1 SD less than the mean and 1 SD greater than the mean. Ninety-five percent of the observations can be expected to fall within 2 SDs of the

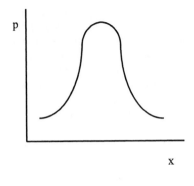

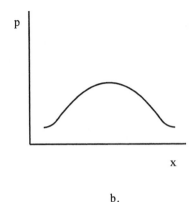

Figure 8–2 The observations are tightly "packed" about the relatively apparent central tendency or mean in distributions with a small variance as in (**a**). The observations are more widely scattered with a less apparent mean with a large variance as in (**b**).

mean, and 99% within 3 SDs of the mean. The standard deviation is thus used to define *confidence intervals*. In a sample of bone densities with a mean of 32 and a SD of 8, for example, 67% of the patients can be expected to have a bone density between 24 and 40.

Standard error of the mean (SE) is equal to the standard deviation divided by the number of observations (n). It is useful for comparing the means of two samples that differ in size. To fully understand a sample, it is important to know the mean, range, and standard deviation.

It is imperative to remember that these descriptive statistics can only be applied to continuous data where the interval between any two measurements is defined, measurable, and constant. Categorical data must be summarized and analyzed by frequency analysis where *contingency tables* (Fig. 8–3) are created.

Recently, outcome instruments, such as the SF-36 and the American Academy of Orthopaedic Surgeons (AAOS) Outcome Assessment Scales, have garnered attention in the orthopaedic community. These are questionnaires that attempt to standardize subjective measurements to improve reliability. Most have been shown to be valid instruments and are quite useful. The purpose of the instrument is to generate a score for each patient that reflects the impact that their disease has on their life. It is not uncommon for investigators to calculate standard summary statistics with the scores;

however, these scores are numeric ordinal data. It is incorrect to calculate a mean with these scores because the interval between any two scores is not defined, objectively measurable, and constant. Instead, the scores are arbitrarily assigned. For example, different levels of pain may be assigned scores of 40, 30, 20, and 0. There are no in-between values. Thus, the "scores" are merely numeric rankings and not continuous data.

Numeric ordinal data can nevertheless be summarized with the median and range. The *median* is the value below which half of the measurements are found and above which half of the measurements are found. The investigators may specify the upper limit of the range of values that includes one fourth of the measurements greater than the median and the lower limit of the range of values that includes one fourth of the measurements less than the median. These are called the second and third quartiles, respectively, and indicate the "spread" of the values around the median.

Hypothesis Testing

Statistical analysis is performed to test whether the measured data supports or refutes the investigators' hypothesis. The general technique is to form a hypothesis and then specify a null hypothesis. The null hypothesis is the contradiction of the hypothesis. Examples of hypotheses and corresponding null hypotheses include:

1. *Hypothesis*: Individuals with achondroplasia are shorter than normal individuals.
   Null hypothesis: There is no difference in height between normal individuals and individuals with achondroplasia.
2. *Hypothesis*: Bone mineral density decreases with age.
   Null hypothesis: There is no association between age and bone mineral density.
3. *Hypothesis*: Outcomes are better with intramedullary nailing of grade II open tibia fractures than with cast treatment.
   Null hypothesis: There is no difference in outcomes between intramedullary nailing of grade II open tibia fractures and cast treatment.

A statistical test is then performed to determine how confident the researcher can be that the null hypothesis is false and the proposed hypothesis is true. All of the standard statistical

	FUSION	NO FUSION
SATISFIED	88	42
NOT SATISFIED	7	28

Figure 8–3 Contingency tables tabulate frequencies of categorical data as in this example wherein 95 patients underwent fusion with 88 satisfied outcomes; 70 patients did not have fusion of which 42 were satisfied. It can also be stated from this table that of 130 satisfied patients, 88 had fusion and 42 did not; of 35 unsatisfied patients, 7 had fusion and 28 did not.

tests consist of calculating a "test statistic." From this, the researcher estimates the probability of randomly selecting another test statistic from the relevant test statistic distribution that is larger than the calculated test statistic. The lower the likelihood of randomly selecting a larger test statistic, the greater the statistical significance. For example, investigators measure the heights of 50 "normal" individuals and 50 individuals with achondroplasia. The investigators then calculate a mean and standard deviation for each group. The "normal" individuals have a greater mean height than the individuals with achondroplasia. The investigators wonder if this is due to random error or if the difference is real. The investigators need to determine how confident they can be that the difference in mean height is not due to chance and random error.

The investigators decide to perform a two-sample t-test. They calculates a test statistic (t_o) with the means and variances of the two groups. The probability of randomly selecting a test statistic (t') greater than the calculated test statistic (t_o) is then reported on a table that has been prepared from the t-distribution. This probability is also known as the p-value. (Fig. 8–4) illustrates this procedure. The procedure is the same for all the different statistical tests, but each test has its own specific test statistic distribution.

A difference between two groups is less likely to be due to chance when the test statistic (t_o) is large. A large difference between the means, a small standard deviation, and little overlap of the distributions of the observations all increase the test statistic as illustrated in (Fig. 8–5).

The p-value measures the probability that a difference between two groups is due to chance and thus measures *statistical significance*. Typically, investigators report that a difference is statistically significant at $p<0.01$ or $p<0.05$. This means that they have arbitrarily decided that a difference is not due to chance, the null hypothesis is incorrect, and the hypothesis is correct if the p-value is less than 0.01 or 0.05. It also means that the investigator is 99 or 95% confident that the measured difference is not due to chance. This critical p-value is known as *alpha*.

Alpha (α) is the probability of making a *type I error*. Type I error occurs when the investigators incorrectly reject the null hypothesis. That is, the investigators state that a statistically significant difference exists, when in fact none does. A type I error is a false positive result of a statistical test. A critical p-value of 0.05 implies that there is a 1% chance that a statistically significant difference is erroneous. Thus, it seems that the smallest critical p-value should always be used.

Choosing a small critical p-value decreases power, however. *Power* measures the ability to detect a difference between two groups. A difference is more likely to be significant when the critical p-value is larger. For example, a spine surgeon compares the nonunion rates of lumbar fusions with and without internal fixation. With internal fixation, the nonunion rate is 6%, and without internal fixation it is 9%. A χ^2 test yields a p-value of 0.018. If the surgeon selected 0.05 as the critical p-value, then the difference is significant. If 0.01 is selected as the critical p-value, then the difference is not significant.

Power is a function of *beta* (β), which is the probability of committing *type II error*. Type II error occurs when the investigators incorrectly accept the null hypothesis and conclude that any difference that appears to exist is due only to chance. Mathematically, power is equal to $1-\beta$. Therefore, β must be minimized to maximize power. The probability of committing type II error increases as the criteria for significance becomes stricter. That is, β increases as α decreases.

Recall the lumbar fusion investigation. If the difference in nonunion rate is due to chance and random error, and the critical p-value (α) is 0.05, then type I error is committed with a test p-value of 0.018. This is because the test p-value is less than the critical p-value. The investigators conclude that the difference is not due to chance and incorrectly reject the null hypothesis. If, on the other hand, the difference in nonunion rate is not due to chance and random error, and the critical p-value (α) is 0.01, then type II error is committed with a test p-value of 0.018 because the test p-value is greater than the critical p-value and the investigators have concluded that the difference is due to chance and incorrectly accepts the null hypothesis. The investigators have sacrificed significance for power in the first instance and power for significance in the second instance.

A large sample size, a large difference between groups, and small standard deviations all increase power while a small α decreases it. A power analysis mathematically determines the sample size necessary to achieve a defined level of power given the difference to be tested, the standard deviations, and the critical p-value (α).

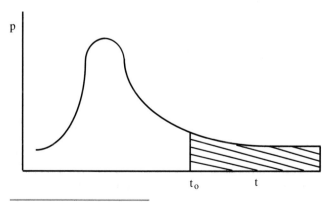

Figure 8–4 This example of Student's t-distribution plots values of the test statistic (t) on the x-axis and the corresponding frequency (p) of each t on the y-axis. The shaded area represents all values of t greater than the test statistic (t_0). The p-value of t_0 equals the fraction of the area under the curve occupied by the shaded area and represents the probability of randomly generating a test statistic greater than t_0.

PEARL

There is an inherent trade-off between power and significance. Increasing one decreases the other. However, it is possible to increase both by increasing the number of subjects in the sample.

The appropriate level of power ($1-\beta$) and significance (α) depend on the nature of the investigation. For example, it

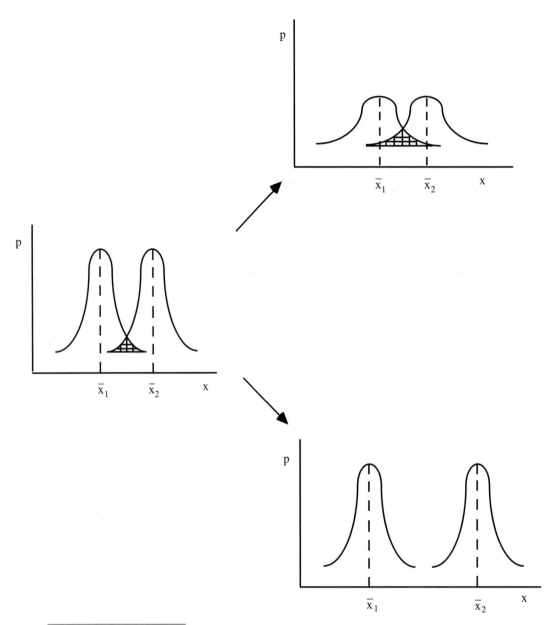

Figure 8–5   The significance of a difference between two samples is a function of the overlap of the two sample distributions. The overlap is a function of the difference in the means (as illustrated by the lower graph on the right) and the variance of the distributions (as illustrated by the upper graph on the right). A large difference between the means decreases the overlap and a large variance increases the overlap.

would be preferable to sacrifice significance for power when testing for differences in the incidence of side effects of various medications. That is, it is important to err towards concluding that the difference in the incidence of side effects is "real" by choosing a critical *p*-value of 0.05 to increase power but decrease significance. On the other hand, investigators would want to sacrifice power for significance when testing for differences in benefits of various medications so that only a "very real" difference would be statistically significant. The investigators should choose a critical *p*-value of 0.01 to

increase significance at the expense of decreasing power. Put another way, the investigators are willing to accept type I error in order to minimize type II error in the first case, and they are willing to accept type II error in order to minimize type I error in the second case.

Statistical Tests

There are three basic methods of statistical testing, each with its own application. The first method is to test for a difference between groups. Examples include *t*-test, analysis of variance (ANOVA), and Wilcoxon signed rank test. The second method is regression and correlation. It is applicable when an association between two or more variables is hypothesized. The third method is goodness-of-fit analysis and is applied to categorical variables. The χ^2 test and Fisher's Exact test are examples of goodness-of-fit tests.

There are *parametric* and *nonparametric* versions of each of these statistical tests. Parametric statistical tests are applicable for continuous data with a normal distribution. Nonparametric statistical tests are applicable for any other kind of data such as categorical (nominal or ordinal) data, continuous data with a *non*-normal distribution, or continuous data with a small sample size.

Parametric statistical tests for comparing two groups include the Student's *t*-test, ANOVA, and regression/correlation. Student's *t*-test evaluates differences between the means of two groups. A two-sample Student's *t*-test compares the mean of one group to the mean of another. A test statistic is generated and the *p*-value of the test statistic is derived from the Student's *t*-test distribution.

A paired Student's *t*-test is used when the two groups consist of matched pairs of subjects. The observation for subject 1 in Group A is subtracted from the observation for subject 1 in Group B to yield a paired difference. This is repeated for each pair. A test statistic is then generated to compare the mean of the paired differences to 0. Zero is used because the assumption is that the mean of the paired differences should approximate 0 if there is no difference between groups. The Student's *t*-test distribution is then used to determine the *p*-value for the test statistic. (Fig. 8–6) illustrates an example of a paired *t*-test.

Analysis of variance is similar to a *t*-test but compares the variances of groups instead of the means. Variances for each group are calculated and averaged. This is the "between-groups variance." Next a "pooled" variance of all the observations collectively as one group is calculated. This is the "within-groups variance." The F-statistic is then calculated as the ratio of "between-groups variance" to "within-groups variance" and the *p*-value is obtained from the F-distribution.

The probability of statistical significance decreases as the ratio approaches 1.

Analysis of variance is more flexible than a *t*-test because it can be used to compare more than two groups. Multiway ANOVA is useful when comparing two or more groups on two or more variables simultaneously. Repeated measures ANOVA is useful when a subject undergoes a series of interventions. For instance, investigators may propose to determine the effect of a bisphosphonate in osteoporosis. The investigators may perform bone mineral density scanning before initiating treatment and repeat the scan after concluding treatment. Nested ANOVA evaluates two or more groups on two or more variables where the subsequent variables are partially or wholly dependent on the first. For example, investigators wish to determine whether a thigh tourniquet influences the incidence of DVT after TKA and then which anticoagulant, warfarin or aspirin, reduces the incidence of DVT in the tourniquet and nontourniquet groups. The anticoagulant variable is nested within the tourniquet variable.

Regression analysis evaluates for an association between two variables. It is commonly referred to as *correlation*. Each observation of a variable is plotted against its corresponding observation for the second variable to create a *scatter plot*. The least squares method is used to fit an equation to the observed data. Mathematically, this consists of deriving an equation for a regression line that minimizes the sum of the squared differences between the observed data points and the corresponding data points on the hypothetical regression line. Regression analysis is most commonly linear but can be geometric or polynomial as well.

Careful interpretation of linear regression is essential. (Fig. 8–7) illustrates common misinterpretations of linear regression, which include extrapolating values beyond the range of the scatter plot, interpolating values between two clusters of scatter plots, assuming a linear function when a geometric or polynomial function fits better, and inferring a relationship when the regression fits the data but the regression is not statistically significant. The first two misinterpretations can be prevented by evaluating the range of the observations when

SUBJECTS	GROUP A	GROUP B	DIFFERENCE (B-A)
1	20	17	-3
2	18	15	-3
3	16	18	2
4	17	21	4
5	23	20	-3
6	19	17	-2
7	18	14	-4
8	18	12	-6
9	17	22	5
10	14	11	-3

Figure 8–6 The paired *t*-test generates a test statistic from the arithmetic difference between an observation in one group and its matched observation in a second group. The difference is calculated the same way for each pair regardless of which value is larger. The mean of the differences (B-A) is compared to 0 when generating the test statistic.

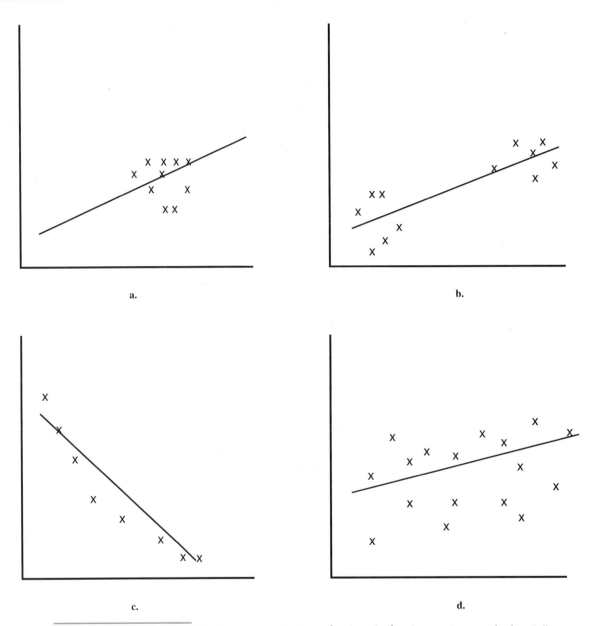

Figure 8–7   (**a**) through (**d**) illustrate regression lines that best fit the observations marked as "x" in the scatter plots. Common errors when interpreting linear regression include: (**a**) extrapolating a relationship beyond the scatter plot; (**b**) interpolating a relationship between two scatter plots; (**c**) fitting a linear regression model when a geometric regression model is more appropriate; and (**d**) inferring a relationship from a linear regression model that fits but is not statistically significant.

evaluating the regression model. Rigorous testing of various regression models may be necessary to ensure that a linear function is indeed appropriate. Finally, the regression model can undergo hypothesis testing by using the null hypothesis that there is no relationship and then calculating a test statistic in a manner similar to ANOVA.

Nonparametric statistical tests are necessary whenever the data do not meet the criteria for a parametric test. Nonparametric tests include the Mann-Whitney rank sum test, the Wilcoxon signed rank test, the Kruskal-Wallis test, the Spearman rank correlation test, and the χ^2 goodness-of-fit test. The χ^2 test is a frequency analysis of a contingency table of categorical data. The other tests are essentially parametric tests of ranks assigned to each observation.

The basic method of performing a rank-based nonparametric statistical test is to rank order the observations and then calculate a test statistic from the ranks instead of the actual observations. The *p*-value is then derived from the appropriate test distribution. Each test has an analogous parametric test. The Mann-Whitney rank sum test is the nonparametric version of the two-sample Student's *t*-test. The Wilcoxon signed rank test is analogous to the paired Student *t*-test. The nonparametric ANOVA analog is the Kruskal-Wallis test. The Spearman rank correlation test is used for nonparametric correlation.

The χ^2 test is frequently applicable in orthopaedic research. The method consists of constructing a contingency table of the observed frequencies of each combination as illustrated in Figure 8–3. A second contingency table is then created with the expected frequencies assuming a random distribution. The χ^2 test statistic is calculated from the differences between the observed and expected frequencies. The corresponding p-value is obtained from the χ^2 distribution.

OUTCOMES ANALYSIS

Outcomes analysis is gaining increasing popularity in orthopaedic clinical science literature. All clinical studies are outcomes studies in that the outcomes, or results, of some treatment are presented and discussed. Only recently, however, have investigators attempted to quantify outcomes to assign objective values to subjective results.

The most common method of functional outcomes analysis is to assign scores to patients based on various subjective and objective criteria. Health measurement scales have been developed for this purpose and include examples such as the SF-36, the Harris hip score, and the HSS knee score. Scores can be used to compare preoperative and postoperative status, the outcomes of a given operation, or to compare the results of surgery in different populations or by different surgeons.

Health measurement scales can be general or specific. Generic scales measure the global effect of a disease or condition on a patient, whereas specific scales focus on the particular part. Specific scales may include some global items when they are relevant. The argument for using specific scales is that they do not measure irrelevant aspects of a patient's outcome. For example, bowel function or cognition have little to do with the outcome of bunion surgery. The advantage of generic scales is that no component of an outcome goes unmeasured.

Whatever scale is used, it must be valid, reliable and sensitive. A *valid* scale actually measures what it proposes to measure. A scale has *face validity* when the scale items appear to measure what they are meant to measure. In other words, there are no "trick questions" or "poorly worded questions" when a scale has high face validity. *Content validity* refers to the entire scale measuring what it proposes to measure. All the items on the scale must be relevant to the outcomes of interest, and all relevant items must be included.

The measurements taken with a scale must be reproducible for the scale to be *reliable*. Two common measurements to evaluate reliability include *Internal consistency* and *stability*. Internal consistency can be measured by including multiple items that measure the same attribute on the scale. Similar scores for these multiple items indicate high internal consistency and thus high reliability.

The stability of a scale can be measured with interobserver reliability, intra-observer reliability, and/or test-retest reliability. All three methods use correlation to measure reliability. Interobserver reliability requires agreement between multiple observers or administrators of the scale. No observer can be aware of another observer's results. The observer can administer the scale to the same subjects on multiple occasions to assess intra-observer reliability. The observer must not be aware of the previous results. Finally, the subjects can undergo testing with the scale on multiple occasions separated by a time interval to assess test-retest reliability. The time interval should be long enough so that subjects cannot recall their responses, but not so long that the condition being assessed has changed significantly.

A scale must be *sensitive* so that changes or differences in outcome are reflected by score differences. The magnitude of the interval between two scores should indicate the approximate magnitude of the difference between two outcomes or statuses. The scale must also be sensitive enough to discriminate a difference between two similar outcomes or statuses.

Valid, reliable, and sensitive scales are very useful in clinical research because they help standardize the results and can be used to compare the results of various investigators or the results of a given intervention for different conditions. A common mistake made with these scales is to assume that results can be quantified by numbers that can be summarized with quantitative techniques and analyzed with parametric hypothesis testing. The "scores" that result from the scales are ordinal data, and thus can only be summarized with a median, percentiles, and range and analyzed with nonparametric hypothesis testing.

For example, the American Orthopaedic Foot and Ankle Society (AOFAS) hindfoot-ankle scale has a subscale for pain wherein the score for no pain is 40; minor pain, 30; moderate pain, 20; and severe pain, 0. There are no possible interval values. Furthermore, moderate pain has different meanings for different patients. Therefore, the corresponding score of 20 is not defined or constant, and therefore, the numeric scores do not fulfill the definition of continuous data.

PITFALL

It is inappropriate to calculate a mean and standard deviation for scores obtained with an outcome instrument or health measurement scale. Furthermore, the scales cannot be analyzed with parametric hypothesis testing techniques. Nonparametric methods should be used.

COST-EFFECTIVENESS ANALYSIS

Cost-effectiveness has become more important in clinical orthopaedic practice as the health care environment continues to evolve. Studies that propose to measure cost-effectiveness are beginning to appear in the orthopaedic literature. It is important to understand the definition and measurement of cost-effectiveness to be able to practically apply the results of cost-effectiveness analysis studies.

Cost-effectiveness and cost-benefit ratios are frequently confused. A cost-benefit ratio measures how much benefit can be achieved per unit of cost spent. Cost-effectiveness compares the cost-benefit ratios of multiple interventions or compares the cost-benefit ratio of an intervention with doing nothing at all.

Average cost and marginal cost must be understood to understand cost-effectiveness analysis. Average cost is calculated with cost as the denominator and the benefit as the numerator. For example, the average cost of healing a tibia fracture is calculated by dividing the union rate in a sample of patients with tibia fractures by the total cost of care for *all* the patients in the sample. The average cost of treatment must not be confused with the average cost of the outcome. For example, investigators study a sample of 100 patients with tibia fractures treated with intramedullary nailing. Ninety-eight of the fractures heal. The total amount of money spent on the 100 patients is $800,000. Thus, the average cost of treatment is $800,000/100 = $8000. The average cost of *union*, however, is $800,000/98 = $8163. Marginal cost is the theoretical cost of increasing the benefit by one unit. In the tibia fracture example, the marginal cost would be the cost required to improve the union rate by one tibia. It is calculated as follows:

$$\text{marginal cost} = \text{cost difference}/\text{benefit difference}$$

For example, an investigator wishes to compare intramedullary nailing and cast treatment of displaced tibia fractures. As determined above, the average cost of *union* with intramedullary nailing is $8163. The total cost of cast treatment is $200,000 and 70 of 100 fractures heal. Thus, the average cost of *union* with cast treatment is $200,000/70 = $2857. The marginal cost of union with intramedullary nailing is ($8163 − $2857)/(0.98 − 0.70) = $18,950. In other words, to get one more fracture to heal with intramedullary nailing instead of cast treatment would theoretically cost $18,950. The average cost of union with cast treatment is $2857, which is far less than the marginal cost of intramedullary nailing. Intramedullary nailing dramatically improves the union rate, but does so at great cost.

The results of cost-effectiveness analysis are a function of the definition of the outcome. Redefining the outcome in the tibia fracture example as "return to work" requires other costs to be considered such as lost wages, additional intervention for malunion or nonunion, and care of complications. More patients get back to work sooner with intramedullary nailing than with cast treatment because union takes longer with cast treatment and the nonunion rate is higher with cast treatment.

By redefining the outcome in the tibia fracture model, the total cost of intramedullary nailing is $1,083,800, and the total cost of cast treatment is $1,132,000, assuming all patients eventually get back to work. The total cost of cast treatment is higher because the higher nonunion rate delays the return to work for more patients in this group. The average cost of return to work is $10,838 for intramedullary nailing and $11,320 for the cast treatment group. The marginal cost cannot be calculated in this example because the benefit, return to work, is equal in both groups. Thus, the denominator, which is the benefit difference, would be 0. Therefore, the intervention with the lower average cost is more cost-effective.

In another example, investigators decide to measure "return to work *and* activity" as the outcome. Again, all patients return to work, but 90% and 64% return to their normal preinjury activity in the intramedullary and cast groups, respectively. Furthermore, the average cost for the outcome is $9384 and $8756 in the two groups, respectively. Therefore, the marginal cost of return to work and activity for the intramedullary nail is ($9384 − $8756)/(0.90 − 0.64) = $2415. The intramedullary nail improves the outcome, but at a higher cost. However, the marginal cost of the improved income is less than the average cost of the alternative. Therefore, the additional cost of improving the outcome could be justified. Cost-effectiveness analysis is not a simple matter of collecting costs and outcomes and determining which is cheaper. Careful and thorough definition of the outcomes and *all* associated costs is imperative. Average and marginal costs must both be calculated to determine cost-effectiveness, but cost-effectiveness decisions are ultimately a function of value-based decisions regarding how much benefit is appropriate and necessary, and what resources are available to achieve an outcome.

SUMMARY

Orthopaedic basic science and clinical research is essential to advance the practice of orthopaedics. Clinically useful knowledge develops from the conclusions of well-designed research studies. Careful and thorough definition of the population, sample, data collection, and analysis techniques are imperative to minimize both bias and random error.

The type of data being collected and analyzed must be defined so that appropriate statistical methods are used. A common error in orthopaedic clinical research is to use parametric statistical techniques to analyze categorical data. Nonparametric statistical techniques are frequently necessary to analyze continuous data as well.

Statistical analysis consists of hypothesis testing. The investigators establish a hypothesis and a null hypothesis. The investigators next generate a test statistic from the data with the appropriate statistical method. The test statistic corresponds to a probability that the null hypothesis is true. In general, a larger difference between two or more groups yields a larger test statistic, which in turn implies a smaller probability that the null hypothesis is true. Significance is a function of this probability.

Power measures the investigator's ability detect a difference between two or more groups. Either power or significance can be increased at the expense of decreasing the other. However, increasing sample size can increase both power and significance simultaneously. Evolving research methods in orthopaedics include health measurement scales and cost-effectiveness analysis. Both are useful tools when understood and used correctly. Health measurement scales help standardize the evaluation of orthopaedic outcomes and may be useful for cost-effectiveness analysis. Cost-effectiveness analysis compares benefits and costs, requires careful and thorough definition of variables, and may entail value judgments.

SELECTED BIBLIOGRAPHY

Dawson-Saunders B, Tratt RG. *Basic and Clinical Biostatistics.* 2nd ed. Norwalk, CI: Appleton-Lange; 1994.

Deyo RA, Patrick DL. Barriers to the use of health status measures in clinical investigation, patient care, and policy research. *Med Care.* 1989;27:S254–S268.

Glantz SA. *Primer of Biostatistics.* 4th ed. New York, NY: McGraw-Hill; 1997.

Petitti DB. *Meta-Analysis, Decision-Analysis, and Cost-effective Analysis: Methods for Quantitative Synthesis in Medicine.* New York, NY: Oxford Univ Press; 1994.

Ratain JS, Hochberg MC. Clinical trials: a guide to understanding methodology and interpreting results. *Arthritis Rheum.* 1990;33:131–139.

Sackett DL. How to read clinical journals, I: why to read them and how to start reading them critically. *Can Med Assoc J.* 1981;124:555–558.

Streiner DL, Norman GR. *Health Measurement Scales: A Practical Guide to Their Development and Use.* 2nd ed. New York, NY: Oxford Univ Press; 1995.

Weinstein MC, Fineberg HV. *Clinical Decision-Analysis.* Philadelphia, PA: WB Saunders; 1980.

SAMPLE QUESTIONS

1. Investigators evaluate the long-term results of total elbow arthroplasty by asking patients whether they are satisfied, satisfied with reservation, or unsatisfied. A co-investigator asks each patient to fill out a validated functional outcome questionnaire. Eighty percent of the patients are satisfied. Fifty-eight percent of the patients have a satisfactory functional outcome score. This difference is statistically significant. This difference is likely due to:
   (a) poor interobserver reliability
   (b) random error
   (c) poor test-retest reliability
   (d) systematic bias
   (e) a and c

2. Factors that increase power include:
   (a) large sample size
   (b) high significance (small α)
   (c) large difference to be detected
   (d) large standard deviation of one sample
   (e) a and c

3. The most appropriate statistical test to evaluate the relationship between age at onset of back pain and Minnesota multiphasic personality inventory score is:
   (a) two-sample Student t-test
   (b) linear regression correlation
   (c) χ^2 test
   (d) Wilcoxon signed rank test

   (e) Spearman rank correlation

4. Investigators devise a knee scale and obtain scores from a group of 100 patients with osteoarthritis of the knee preoperatively and again 2 years after TKA. The investigators also ask the patients to report their pain relief and functional activity after surgery. Ninety-two percent report good or excellent pain relief and 84% report increased activity after surgery. There is no statistically significant correlation between the preoperative and postoperative scores, for example, some patients' scores went up while others went down. Which of the following is (are) most true of the investigators' outcome instrument:
   (a) construct validity is high
   (b) sensitivity is low
   (c) intra-observer reliability is high
   (d) test re-test reliability is low
   (e) b and d

5. Which of the following is (are) true of the p-value?
   (a) It is the probability of randomly generating a test statistic lower than that generated by the statistical test.
   (b) It is equal to the probability of committing type II error.
   (c) It is equal to the probability of incorrectly rejecting the null hypothesis.
   (d) It is equal to power α.
   (e) b and d

Answers: 1) d; 2) e; 3) e; 4) e; 5) c

Diagnostic Studies

Chapter 9

Nonimaging Diagnostic Studies

Betsy W. Blazek-O'Neill, MD

Outline

Most musculoskeletal conditions are diagnosed on the basis of a history, physical examination, and imaging studies, with laboratory studies playing a less important role. However, there are a few tests of particular interest to the orthopaedist because of their importance in the diagnosis of musculoskeletal disorders.

LABORATORY TESTS

Erythrocyte Sedimentation Rate

The erythrocyte sedimentation rate (ESR) may be elevated in any type of inflammatory condition, and is, therefore, a nonspecific test. The ESR may be increased in malignancy, infection, inflammatory arthritic conditions, conditions that involve tissue necrosis (including myocardial infarction), anemia, and a variety of miscellaneous disorders. However, a normal ESR does not rule out any of these conditions. For example, up to 5% of rheumatoid arthritis and systemic lupus erythematosis patients may have a normal ESR.

The ESR may be useful to monitor the course of disease or the response to treatment in conditions such as polymyalgia rheumatica, rheumatoid arthritis, and systemic lupus erythematosis. The Westergren method for ESR is more sensitive and usually more clinically relevant in following the course of disease activity. Expected elevations of ESR usually do not occur in the conditions noted if there is concomitant polycythemia, sickle cell anemia, spherocytosis, or hypofibrinogenemia.

Rheumatoid Factor

Rheumatoid factor assays test for circulating IgM and IgG autoantibodies, which bind to IgG to form immune complexes. Rheumatoid factor is found in rheumatoid arthritis, systemic lupus erythematosis, Sjögren's syndrome, Wegener's granulomatosis, scleroderma, dermatomyositis, Waldenström's disease, sarcoidosis, mycobacterioses (including tuberculosis), liver disease, and in some healthy subjects. Approximately 75% of rheumatoid arthritis patients have positive rheumatoid factor tests. The highest titers are seen in those with severe, active disease and multiple rheumatoid nodules. Titers of 1:80 or less are sometimes found in elderly patients, patients with infectious mononucleosis, and in acute inflammation.

Antinuclear Antibody

A positive antinuclear antibody (ANA) test can be seen in a number of clinical conditions, most notably in various connective tissue disorders. Ninety-five percent of systemic lupus erythematosis patients will have a positive ANA titer, and many of the remaining 5% will test positive for one of several ANA subtypes. Other conditions associated with positive ANA titers include rheumatoid arthritis, progressive systemic sclerosis, mixed connective tissue disease, Sjögren's syndrome, polymyositis, thyroid disease, chronic liver disease, and advancing age. Up to 10% of normal individuals will have a positive ANA titer, usually 1:80 or less. Positive titers are also seen in individuals with a family history of connective tissue disease.

If a specific connective tissue disease is suspected on clinical grounds, an ANA titer and titers for specific subtypes of nuclear proteins may be measured to provide confirmatory evidence. When the clinical situation is less clear, but a connective tissue disorder is suspected, most clinicians recommend testing for ANA positivity first and then selecting various ANA subtypes for further investigation.

HLA-B27 Antigen

Human leukocyte (HLA) antigens are the histocompatability antigens used for matching transplant patients. Certain HLA

Orthopaedic Surgery: The Essentials. Edited by M.E. Baratz, A.D. Watson, and J.E. Imbriglia. Thieme Medical Publishers, Inc., New York © 1999

antigen types have been associated with disease states. HLA-B27 antigen has been associated with an increased incidence of various spondyloarthropathies, including ankylosing spondylitis, psoriatic arthritis, Reiter's syndrome, and arthritis associated with inflammatory bowel disease. Not all individuals with HLA-B27 antigen develop disease, and not all individuals with spondyloarthropathy have the antigen. However, HLA-B27 antigen testing is positive in 80 to 90% of individuals with ankylosing spondylitis.

VENOUS STUDIES

Deep venous thrombosis (DVT) is common in hospitalized and surgical patients (Table 9–1). While DVT itself is a benign condition, it can lead to significant morbidity and mortality in the forms of pulmonary embolism and postphlebitis syndrome. Clinical assessment for DVT can be difficult. As many as 50% of all cases of DVT occur without symptoms; only 30 to 50% of persons with clinical signs and symptoms consistent with DVT have the condition. Clinical usefulness of diagnostic tests for DVT depends on the probability of disease.

PITFALL

Patients with bilateral lower extremity symptoms are extremely unlikely to have DVT. Alternative causes for the patient's condition should be evaluated before testing for DVT is considered.

Diagnostic Testing for Deep Venous Thrombosis

Tools available for evaluation of the patient with suspected DVT include untrasonography, venography, and impedance plethysmography. At present, some type of ultrasonography protocol constitutes the first (and often definitive) approach.

TABLE 9–1 Risk Factors for Deep Venous Thrombosis.

Orthopedic surgery hip/knee	Stroke
	Brain injury
Trauma	Intracranial bleed
Immobilization	Spinal cord injury
Malignancy	Neurosurgical
Sepsis	procedures
General anesthesia	Abdominal/pelvic
Male gender	surgery
Previous DVT	Increasing age
Lower extremity fractures	Hypercoagulable states
	Intravenous procedures

Ultrasonography

The most useful ultrasound technique to diagnoses DVT is B-mode compression ultrasound. B-mode ultrasound technology allows direct visualization of the vein but cannot by itself distinguish a clot. Compression is applied through the ultrasound transducer to demonstrate the collapsibility of normal veins; visualization of a venous structure that fails to collapse suggests the presence of clot at that site. Compression ultrasonography is equally effective as a screening tool for patients at high risk for DVT and to evaluate suspected cases. This technique has the advantages of being noninvasive, inexpensive, highly sensitive and specific (93% and 99%, respectively, for clot above the popliteal bifurcation compared with venography), and easily repeatable without risk to the patient. In addition, ultrasonography will detect other abnormalities in the involved area that may be responsible for the signs and symptoms noted, including pseudoaneurysms, Baker's cysts, cellulitis, some cases of superficial phlebitis, lymph nodes, hematomas, arteriovenous fistulae, and Lymphoceles. Most clinical centers consider compression ultrasonography the new "gold standard" for diagnosis of DVT in the lower extremity. This technique is the first diagnostic tool to choose in the evaluation of suspected DVT in most patients.

Compression ultrasonography examinations generally involve visualization of the femoral veins, the popliteal veins, and the take-off of the tibial and peroneal veins. Assessment of the calf veins considerably lengthens the time and cost of the exam, and the results in this area are less accurate. For these reasons, complete assessment of calf veins is usually not pursued. Clinicians recommend that patients with persistent or worsening signs and symptoms of DVT following negative above-knee compression ultrasonography be restudied in 3 to 5 days. Studies suggest that calf vein DVT is a benign disease, but approximately 20% of calf vein thromboses will eventually propagate above the knee, and of these, a significant number are suspected of going on to cause pulmonary emboli.

In less than 5% of cases, compression ultrasonography fails to confirm or exclude DVT. Equivocal results may be seen when there has been a previous DVT, with atypical venous anatomy, or when there is a known pelvic mass complicating compressibility of proximal veins. Regular or color Doppler studies, which evaluate for the presence of normal flow patterns in venous structures, may be helpful in some difficult cases. Color Doppler examination may also be helpful in evaluating the calf veins. It is particularly useful in upper extremity assessment, where compression of proximal veins is usually impossible. Duplex ultrasound testing is not employed routinely because of excessive cost, and is reserved for difficult cases. In some cases of equivocal ultrasonography results, venography may be necessary.

Venography

Long considered the gold standard for diagnosis of DVT, venography is now used less often because of expense, complications, and availability. During venography, contrast material is injected into a superficial vein in the foot and radiographs are taken as contrast passes proximally through the

PITFALL

Be aware that thrombosed veins recanalize slowly. After DVT, compression ultrasound may remain abnormal for several months, even in the absence of recurrent thrombosis.

venous system. Venography will demonstrate clot with a higher degree of anatomic accuracy than ultrasound techniques, but studies have demonstrated at least a 10% nondiagnosis or misdiagnosis rate. This is related to interpreter variability or technical problems. Therefore, the sensitivity and specificity of venography is essentially equivalent to, and not superior to, ultrasonography techniques. Venography is more expensive than noninvasive techniques, carries a small risk of infection and contrast reaction, and is not as readily available or convenient as ultrasonography. Venography is not appropriate for use as a screening tool, and serial studies cannot be recommended because of its invasive nature. Venography is usually reserved for difficult cases that cannot be resolved with the use of noninvasive techniques.

Impedence Plethysmography

Impedence plethysmography is a relatively inexpensive, noninvasive technique that has been used in some settings to detect DVT. It attempts to measure changes in venous capacitance during physiologic maneuvers to detect signs of thrombosis. Normal capacitance changes associated with respiration are monitored with skin electrodes; absence or blunting of such responses is consistent with the presence of clot. Sensitivity results for impedance plethysmography have generally been in the range of 70% for detection of DVT above the knee, with extremely poor results noted in the calf. More recent studies have indicated that actual sensitivity may be higher, but the success of ultrasonography techniques makes the use of impedance plethysmography unnecessary in most settings.

ELECTRODIAGNOSTIC TESTING

Electrodiagnostic tests allow measurement of the electrophysiological function of nerve and muscle. Nerve conduction studies provide information regarding the status of peripheral nerve axons and myelin sheaths. Electromyography (EMG), or needle examination of muscle, provides information regarding the status of muscle fibers, which can be affected by peripheral nerve lesions, primary muscle diseases and central nervous system lesions. For the purpose of this chapter, we will focus on the use of electrodiagnostic studies to evaluate peripheral nerve lesions.

Questions that may be answered through electrodiagnostic testing comprise:

1. Is there a peripheral nerve lesion?
2. Where is the lesion located?
3. How severe is the lesion?
4. What is the prognosis for recovery?

Types of Nerve Lesions

Neuropraxia

Loss of conduction occurs without damage to nerve axons, usually as a result of demyelination. Demyelination most commonly results from compression. Symptoms range from parethesias in mild or early cases to paralysis in severe or late cases. Recovery usually occurs within days to weeks after removal of the cause (time for remyelination).

Axonotmesis

Axonal damage occurs with most of the surrounding connective tissue elements of the nerve intact. This type of nerve damage is seen in compression, trauma, and in metabolic derangements. With injury, there is a conduction block at the site, but distal conduction initially remains normal. Wallerian degeneration of the distal segment 5–7 days following injury will result in loss of conduction over the distal segment. Muscle fibers will begin to show signs of denervation recognizable with EMG techniques within 1 to 3 weeks after the insult. Recovery after injury depends on the integrity of the connective tissue supports, such as the epineurium.

Neurotmesis

Significant disruption of nerve and connective tissue elements usually occurs related to trauma. Again, one sees conduction block at the injury site initially, but preservation of distal segment conduction continues until Wallerian degeneration occurs. Recovery depends on the type of injury and age of the patient, among other factors.

PEARL

Timing of electrodiagnostic studies is important. Nerve conduction studies immediately following an injury will not distinguish between conduction block and axonal loss; this cannot be done until at least 5 to 7 days after the injury. Muscle fibers will not display EMG signs of denervation until a minimum of 1 week following injury; most electrodiagnosticians recommend waiting 2 to 3 weeks to increase the yield of test results. In some clinical situations, early studies may be helpful to localize a nerve lesion, with subsequent studies giving more information regarding the type of injury and prognosis.

Nerve Conduction Studies

Electrical stimuli are applied through the skin to peripheral nerves. The responses generated are measured, through the skin at a point further down the limb. Standardized procedures are used to measure conduction along important nerve branches, and the results are compared with expected normal values. Techniques and machine settings can be manip-

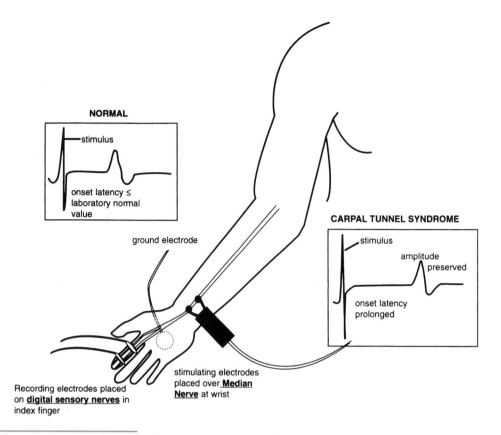

Figure 9–1 Examples of median sensory nerve conductions in a normal individual and in the presence of carpal tunnel syndrome.

ulated to highlight sensory, motor, or mixed nerve responses. Information gathered includes latency of responses, amplitude of responses, and conduction velocity (Fig. 9–1).

Latency

This is the time required for an electrical stimulus applied to a peripheral nerve to traverse a segment of that nerve, recorded in milliseconds. Latency values reflect the health of the myelin sheath and can be affected by significant loss of fast-conducting axons. Increased latency implies a slowing of conduction over that segment. These results are most important across potential sites of nerve compression. Sensory responses tend to show slowing earlier than motor responses in many compressive neuropathies.

Amplitude

This is the size of the response obtained at the recording site when a supramaximal electrical stimulus is applied to a peripheral nerve. It reflects the number of axons firing or the degree of conduction over that segment. Decreases in amplitude seen with stimulation both proximal and distal to the injury site imply axonal loss, if performed at least 5 to 7 days after the injury. A decrease in proximal amplitude compared to distal amplitude implies partial conduction block between the proximal and distal stimulation sites. Amplitude is expressed in millivolts or microvolts.

Conduction Velocity

This is the velocity with which an applied electrical stimulus travels over a motor nerve segment, measured in meters per second. Decreased conduction velocity most often reflects a widespread neuropathic process as seen in metabolic disorders such as diabetic polyneuropathy. Decreased conduction velocity will occasionally be seen with significant focal nerve lesions such as ulnar neuropathy at the elbow.

PEARL

Increased latencies in a widespread pattern may be consistent with peripheral neuropathy, a finding that complicates the electrodiagnostic assessment of superimposed entrapment or injury-related nerve lesions.

Electromyography

A recording electrode is placed in specific muscle locations and acts as an antenna to receive transmitted electrical activity from each muscle site. Normal muscle fibers will demonstrate electrical silence at rest, and will generate normal-appearing motor units with contraction. Denervated muscle

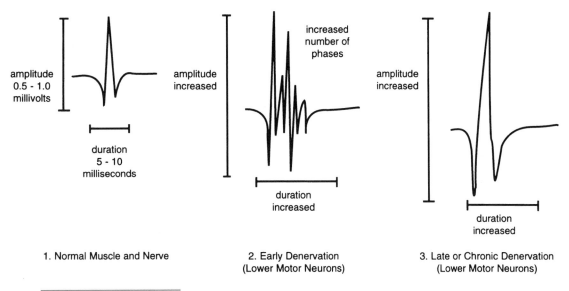

Figure 9–2 Examples of muscle motor unit action potentials in normal and disease states.

fibers emit characteristic electrical abnormalities; the presence of abnormalities in specific muscles will often allow localization of a motor nerve lesion. The electromyographer looks for signs of abnormal spontaneous activity, notes the configuration of motor unit action potentials, and assesses recruitment of fibers during muscle contraction (Fig. 9–2).

> ### PEARL
>
> **Lesions affecting only the sensory component of the nerve will not demonstrate abnormalities on electromyography (EMG). This is often the case in early or mild compressive nerve lesions.**

Abnormal Spontaneous Activity

There are several electrical signs of abnormal spontaneous muscle fiber firing seen in denervating conditions. These findings are usually graded from 0 to 4 based on the frequency of their appearance in a sampled muscle, with higher grades of spontaneous activity generally correlating to greater severity of nerve injury. Fibrillations and positive sharp waves are typically seen in lower motor neuron disorders such as anterior horn cell diseases, radiculopathies, plexopathies, and axonal mono- or polyneuropathies. These abnormal responses are usually seen together and imply axonal loss. They may also be seen in myopathic conditions. Fasciculations result from spontaneous discharges of an entire motor unit or part of a motor unit, and they may be visible as muscle twitches. An occasional fasciculation will be seen in normal muscle, but grouped fasciculations from multiple locations are most commonly seen in motorneuron disease (e.g., amyotrophic lateral sclerosis).

Configuration of Motor Unit Action Potentials

During voluntary muscle contraction, motor unit action potentials will be generated that have characteristic features

similar to the wave forms generated by cardiac muscle as measured with an electrocardiogram. An increase in polyphasic units tends to be seen in acute denervating processes, whereas very large, long duration motor units are seen in longstanding neuropathic conditions or following reinnervation.

Recruitment Pattern

During voluntary muscle contraction, motor units will be recruited as the force of contraction increases, in a regular pattern. A decrease in the number of motor unit action potentials recruited with full contraction, or recruitment of high numbers of motor units at low levels of contraction (as surviving units fire early and rapidly to compensate for the loss of available motor units) indicate axonal loss in the tested muscle.

Prognosis
Conduction Block vs. Axonal Loss

Nerve recovery is usually complete when partial demyelination has occured due to nerve compression. When there has been axonal loss, full recovery is less likely. In general, the patient with abnormal nerve conduction studies but normal EMG has a more favorable prognosis than a patient with an abnormal EMG.

Amount of Axon Loss

Significant amplitude reductions during nerve conduction testing (in a pattern suggestive of axon loss rather than partial conduction block) imply a more severe lesion. Large amounts of spontaneous activity along with significantly decreased numbers of motor units and recruitment of motor units during EMG indicate a more severe peripheral nerve lesion.

Site of the Lesion

Recovery from proximal peripheral nerve lesions may be less than that from more distal lesions if there is significant axonal loss. The presence of intact sensory nerve conduction in the face of clinical paralysis, if tested after an appropriate time delay from injury, has a particularly bad prognosis. These findings suggest a lesion proximal to the dorsal root ganglion, such as a nerve root avulsion.

Changes in Study Results Over Time

Increasing numbers of motor unit potentials and improved recruitment seen during EMG on sequential studies implies reinnervation.

SUMMARY

These comments are intended to give the orthopaedist a general understanding of electrodiagnostic studies. There are innumerable elements of this complex diagnostic art that are beyond the scope of this chapter. Electrodiagnostic tests are interpreted visually and through sound as they occur, and the information presented in report form does not represent raw data. The reader is therefore advised to seek out a highly skilled electrodiagnostician with which he or she can build a relationship. Electrodiagnosticians should serve as consultants regarding the appropriateness and timing of testing. They should be available to discuss the significance and relevance of the results to the clinical situation.

SELECTED BIBLIOGRAPHY

Laboratory Results

McCARTY DJ. *Arthritis and Allied Conditions*. Philadelphia, PA: Lea and Febiger; 1989.

TIETZ NW. *Clinical Guide to Laboratory Tests*. Philadelphia, PA: WB Saunders; 1995.

Venous Studies

CRONAN JJ. Contemporary venous imaging. *Cardiovasc Interven Radiol*. 1991;14:87–97.

DORFMAN GS, CRONAN JJ. *Seminars Intervent Radiol* 1990;7:9–18.

KRISTO DA, PERRY ME, KOLLEF MH. Comparison of venography, duplex imaging, and bilateral impedance plethysmography for diagnosis of lower extremity deep vein thrombosis. *South Med J*. 1994;87:55–60.

PEARSON SD, POLAK UL, CARTWRIGHT S. et al. A critical pathway to evaluate suspected deep vein thrombosis. *Arch Intern Med*. 1995;155:1773–1778.

WEINMANN EE, SALZMAN EW. Deep vein thrombosis. *N Eng J Med*. 1994;331:1630–1641.

WHEELER HB, HIRSCH J, WELLS P, ANDERSON FA. Diagnostic tests for deep vein thrombosis. *Arch Intern Med*. 1994;154:1921–1928.

Electrodiagnostic Studies

KIMURA J. *Electrodiagnosis in Disease of Nerve and Muscle. Principles and Practice*. Philadelphia, PA: FA Davis; 1989.

SAMPLE QUESTIONS

1. Which of the following statements is true:
   (a) Five percent of rheumatoid arthritis and systemic lupus erythematosis patients may have a normal ESR.
   (b) Seventy-five percent of rheumatoid arthritis patients have positive rheumatoid factor tests.
   (c) Ten percent of normal individuals may have a positive ANA titer.
   (d) Eighty to ninety percent of individuals with ankylosing spondylitis test positive for HLA-B27 antigen.
   (e) all of the above

2. The most appropriate first step in the evaluation of most patients with suspected deep vein thrombosis of the lower extremity is:
   (a) venography
   (b) impedance plethysmography
   (c) color Doppler flow studies
   (d) B-mode compression ultrasound
   (e) duplex ultrasound examination

3. Advantages of compression ultrasonography testing as compared with venography include:
   (a) more sensitive for calf vein clot
   (b) more sensitive for thigh vein clot
   (c) easily repeatable without risk to the patient
   (d) more technically appropriate for upper extremity examinations
   (e) better anatomic resolution

4. Muscle fibers will begin to show electrical signs of denervation demonstrable with electrodiagnostic testing techniques at what point in time following peripheral nerve injury:
   (a) immediately
   (b) 1 to 2 days
   (c) 1 to 2 weeks
   (d) 1 month
   (e) 2 months

5. Which of the following electrodiagnostic test findings would you expect to see in a patient with mild compressive neuropathy at the carpal tunnel:
   (a) 3+ positive sharp waves and fibrillation potentials in the abductor pollicus brevis
   (b) decreased median sensory and mixed nerve latencies across the wrist segment
   (c) decreased median nerve conduction velocity
   (d) increased median sensory and mixed nerve latencies across the wrist segment
   (e) 2+ fasciculations in the abductor pollicus brevis

Answers: 1) e; 2) d; 3) c; 4) c; 5) d

Chapter 10

Musculoskeletal Imaging

Richard H. Daffner, MD, FACR

Medical imaging began with humble origins just more than a century ago on November 8, 1895. Wilhelm Konrad Röentgen, a Dutch physicist was experimenting with cathode ray tubes and studying their behavior in a completely darkened room. When the tube was operating, he observed a faint glow on the table of his laboratory. He discovered that the glow was caused by a fluorescent plate that had been inadvertently left on the bench. His experiments over the next few weeks revealed that this new form of unknown radiation, which he called "X-strahlen" (x-rays) were invisible, could penetrate objects, and could cause fluorescence. Röentgen published his finding on December 28, 1895, and entitled the paper, "On a New Kind of Rays" in the *Sitzungberichte der Physikalisch-Medizinischen Gesellschaftz zu Würzburg*, the publication of the Würzburg Physical Medical Society. On January 23, 1896, Röentgen first demonstrated his new rays before the Society. At that demonstration, he made a radiograph of the hand of the famed Swiss anatomist, von Kölliker. The first clinical radiographs made in North America were made simultaneously at McGill University in Montreal, Canada, and at Dartmouth College in Hanover, New Hampshire, on February 3,

1896, by professors John Cox and Edwin B. Frost, respectively. Cox successfully localized a bullet in the leg of a patient who had been shot. Frost demonstrated the radiographic findings of a Colles-type fracture of the distal radius and ulna. It is not surprising that both of these radiographs involve orthopaedic problems.

In the seventy-five years that followed Röentgen's discovery, there have been many advances in radiologic technology that have improved its efficiency and safety for diagnosis. However, the last quarter century has seen developments that have far surpassed those made prior to that time. These advances include computed tomography (CT) and magnetic resonance imaging (MRI) have revolutionized medical diagnosis. It is now possible to image areas of the body previously accessible only to the surgeon's knife or to pathologists. In addition, the ability to accurately identify these areas now makes it possible for interventional and biopsy procedures to be performed using fluoroscopy, CT, or ultrasound guidance. Musculoskeletal imaging employs all the diagnostic modalities, either individually or in combination. While plain film radiography is the mainstay for evaluation of the musculoskeletal system, CT, MRI, nuclear radiology, and diagnostic ultrasound all have their places. Invasive techniques such as arthrography and biopsy also fall within the realm of use to the diagnostic radiologist evaluating the musculoskeletal system. A brief introduction to each of these modalities is necessary to fully understand how each type of examination may be used for clinical problem solving.

TECHNICAL ASPECTS

Plain Film Radiography

X-rays or roentgen rays are a form of electromagnetic energy or radiation of extremely short wavelengths. As a rule, the shorter the wavelength of an electromagnetic radiation form, the greater its energy and the greater its ability to penetrate various materials. X-rays are often described in terms of packs of energy called *photons*. Photons travel at the speed of light, and the amount of energy carried by each depends on its wavelength. The energy is measured in electron volts (the amount of energy an electron gains as it is accelerated through a potential of 1 volt). Atoms are ionized when they lose an electron. Any photon with 15 or more electron volts of energy is capable of producing ionization in atoms and molecules (*ionizing radiation*).

107

Orthopaedic Surgery: The Essentials. Edited by M.E. Baratz, A.D. Watson, and J.E. Imbriglia. Thieme Medical Publishers, Inc., New York © 1999

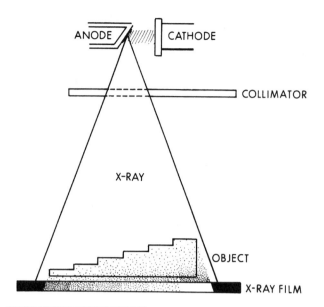

Figure 10–1 Relationship between density and absorption of x-rays. The denser a material is, the greater its ability to absorb x-rays and the less darkening of the film. The reverse is true for less dense materials. Reproduced with permission from Daffner RH. *Clinical Radiology: The Essentials.* Baltimore, MD: Williams and Wilkins; 1993.

The x-rays used in diagnostic radiology are produced when there is a high potential difference between a cathode and an anode in a vacuum. In the basic x-ray tube, electrons boil off the cathode (filament) when it is heated to extremely high temperatures. In order to produce x-rays, a high potential of up to 125,000 volts (125 kV) is used to move the electrons toward the anode. When the accelerated electrons strike the tungsten anode, x-rays are produced.

When x-rays pass through objects, some are removed from the primary beam through absorption and scatter. This process is called *attenuation.* In general, materials of high density (measured in grams per cubic centimeter) have a greater ability to absorb or scatter x-rays (Fig. 10–1). Dense structures such as bone or metallic implants produce greater attenuation, and, as a result of that, there is less blackening of the film since fewer x-rays strike the film. Conversely, less dense structures such as muscle or fat remove fewer of the x-rays, and this results in a greater blackening of the film as more x-rays strike it (Fig. 10–2). Image production by x-ray results from this process.

The type of density described is physical density. A physician is likely to hear the term *density* when discussing radiographs with radiologists or other colleagues. *Radiographic density* refers to the degree of blackness on a radiograph. *Radiographic contrast* is the difference in radiographic densities on a radiograph. The radiographic density of any substance is inversely related to its physical density, that is structures of high physical density result in a lesser degree of radiographic density and vice versa. Any structure that produces more blackening on a film is referred to as being *radiolucent.* Air-filled structures and fatty structures are in this category. Those that produces less blackening such as bone or metallic implants are referred to as being *radiodense* or *radiopaque.* In

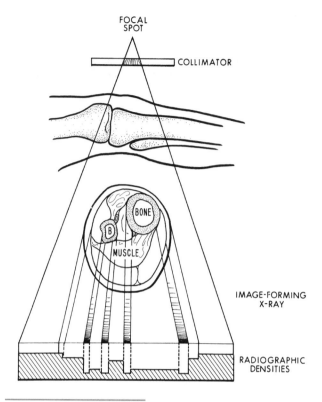

Figure 10–2 Differential absorption of x-rays. Denser tissue absorbs more of the x-ray beam; less dense tissues transmit more of the beam. The resultant image is essentially a "shadowgram." Reproduced with permission from Daffner RH. *Clinical Radiology: The Essentials.* Baltimore, MD: Williams and Wilkins; 1993.

summary, there are four types of radiographic densities: gas (air), fat, water, and bone (metal), which radiographically appear as black, gray-black, gray, and white, respectively.

The most common and familiar type of recording media is x-ray film. This basically consists of a plastic sheet coated with a thin emulsion of silver halides. The emulsion is sensitive to light and radiation. Light or ionizing radiation produces chemical changes within the emulsion resulting in the deposition of metallic silver, which is black. Thus, the amount of blackening in a film is dependent entirely upon the amount of radiation reaching that film, and therefore, on the amount attenuated from the beam by the subject. There are other recording media including fluoroscopic screen-image intensification systems, photoelectric detector crystals, xenon detector systems, and computer-linked detectors that measure actual attenuation. The radiology department of the future will be entirely filmless with images recorded directly onto computer-linked detectors with subsequent digitization and storage, as is found in the current picture archiving and communications systems (PACS). The images thus obtained may be transferred electronically from computer work station to computer work station. There will no longer be the problems of film loss or film sign-out that often occurs in radiology departments within hospitals. Any person with a computer work station linked to the central computer in the radiology department will be able to access the images at will.

Computed tomography (CT) scanners and digital radiographic units utilize electronic sensors that actually measure the amount of attenuation that occurs in tissues when an x-ray beam passes through. These sophisticated machines convert the mathematic value to digitize a shade of gray. A computer then plots the location of each of these measurements that produce the image.

There are several physical and geometric factors that affect the radiographic image. These include the thickness of the part being examined, motion, scatter, magnification, and distortion. The thickness (and thus physical density) of the part determines how much of the beam is attenuated. Obese patients require more x-rays for adequate penetration than do thin patients. Bone requires more x-rays for penetration than the surrounding muscle as do limbs in casts. Motion results in blurred, nondiagnostic images, but it can be overcome by shortening the exposure time or by enhancing the effectiveness of the recording system. This is done by using intensifying screens. In addition to reducing motion, intensifying screens also reduce the amount of radiation required to produce an image of a given radiographic density.

Scatter occurs when some of the primary radiation is deflected as it passes through the object being examined, producing "fog" on a film, which is undesirable. Scatter is controlled by using grids that have alternating angled slats of very thin, radiolucent material combined with thin, lead strips. This removes most of the scatter. The grid is moved to prevent the lead strips from casting their own shadows as they absorb the radiation. The grid system is known as the Bucky-Potter system.

A radiographic image is a two-dimensional representation of three-dimensional structures. Some structures will be farther from the film than others. Since x-rays physically behave similar to light, there will be magnification of objects that are some distance from the film. The closer the object is to the film, the less the magnification; the farther the object is from the film, the greater the magnification (Fig. 10–3). The best way to reduce the undesirable effects of magnification is to have the part of greatest interest *closest* to the film. This will produce the truest image of the region of interest. Distortion occurs when an object is not perpendicular to the x-ray beam. Remember, the radiographic image of any object is dependent on the sum of the shadows produced by that object. Changes in the relationship of that object to the x-ray beam may distort its radiographic image (Fig. 10–4). Therefore, it is best to have the part of major interest not only as close to the film, but also as perpendicular to the film, as possible.

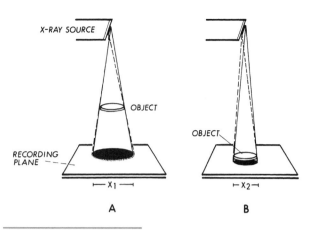

Figure 10–3 Magnification and image sharpness. **(A)** The object is farther from the film, resulting in a larger image whose margin is not as distinct as in **B. (B)** The object is closer to the film resulting in a smaller and sharper image than in A. Reproduced with permission from Daffner RH. *Clinical Radiology: The Essentials.* Baltimore, MD: Williams and Wilkins, 1993.

Conventional Tomography

Conventional tomography is a form of radiography in which the x-ray tube and film move in concert to deliberately produce a blurred image. Any structures within the focal plane, or fulcrum, of that motion remain in sharp focus (Fig. 10–5). The premise of tomography is that unwanted structures are blurred while the object of interest is kept in clear focus. Many orthopaedic surgeons prefer conventional tomography for evaluating complex fractures. However, in most major institutions, conventional tomography is being replaced by CT because of the advantages of this latter modality, which

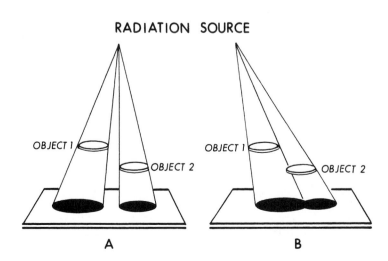

Figure 10–4 Distortion. The shape of an object on a radiograph depends on the angle at which the radiographic beam strikes it. **(A)** Two objects of similar size cast distinct images with the x-ray beam nearly perpendicular. There is a size difference as the result of magnification. **(B)** Angling the x-ray beam while the objects remain in the same relationship to one another produces an overlapping image that is not a true representation of the axial objects. This frequently occurs on radiographs of bones. Reproduced with permission from Daffner RH. *Clinical Radiology: The Essentials.* Baltimore, MD: Williams and Wilkins; 1993.

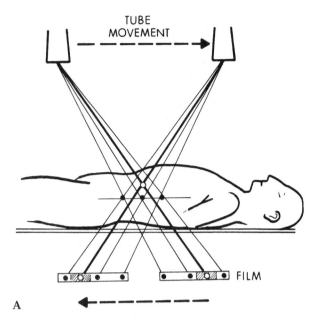

A

Figure 10–5 Conventional tomography. **(A)** The x-ray tube and the film move in opposite directions. The focal point (open circle) remains in sharp focus; the other images are blurred. Reproduced with permission from Daffner RH. *Clinical Radiology: The Essentials.* Baltimore, MD: Williams and Wilkins; 1993. Segond fracture of the lateral tibia **(B)–(D)**: **(B)** Frontal radiograph shows an avulsed fragment off the lateral aspect of the proximal tibia (arrow). Bony debris in the central portion of the joint is obscured. **(C)** Frontal tomogram shows fractures of the central intercondylar tibial spines. **(D)** Lateral tomogram shows the avulsed fragments (arrow) at the insertion point of the anterior cruciate ligament.

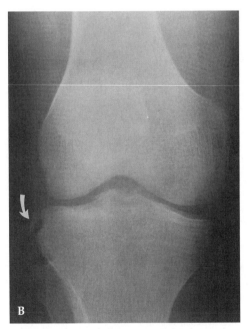

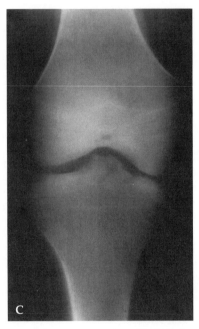

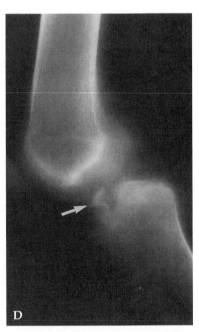

will be discussed in the next section. At the present time, none of the major manufacturers of radiographic equipment are making conventional tomographic units. Once the parts for the existing units are no longer available, conventional tomography will be added to the list of imaging procedures no longer performed.

Computed Tomography

Computed tomography (CT), as previously mentioned, revolutionized medical imaging. While the fleshy organs of the body such as the heart, kidneys, liver, and muscle are considered to be of uniform water radiographic density, these tissues vary significantly in their chemical properties. Thus, it is possible using computer enhancing techniques to measure the differences, to magnify them, and to display them in various shades of gray or in color. In CT (Fig. 10–6), an x-ray

beam and a detector system move through an arc of 360 degrees irradiating a narrow area of the body with a highly collimated (restricted) beam. Modern CT scanners now employ a helical or spiral motion as the patient rapidly passes through the beam. This results in images of extreme clarity. Most significantly, however, is the fact that helical scans require only a fraction of the time that was previously necessary to study the same body parts. Data may be obtained on tissue sections as thin as 1 mm. New computer algorithms allow this data to be portrayed not only in the plane being scanned (usually axial), but also allow multiplanar tomographic reconstruction in sagittal, coronal, or occasionally oblique planes. In addition, three-dimensional reconstruction is now possible (Fig. 10–7). The multiplanar tomographic capability of CT is rapidly replacing conventional tomography in most large medical centers. The information gleaned from the CT examination is just as diagnostic as that obtained

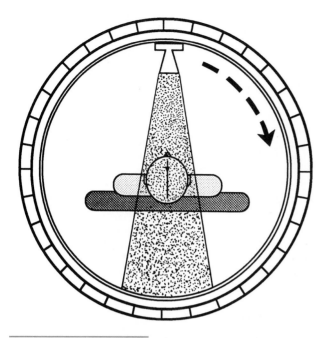

Figure 10–6 Principle of computed tomography (CT). The x-ray tube rotates within the gantry. Instead of film, detectors measure the amount of radiation removed from the x-ray beam. Reproduced with permission from Daffner RH. *Clinical Radiology: The Essentials*. Baltimore, MD: Williams and Wilkins; 1993.

from conventional tomography. The big difference is that the CT images are obtained without having to move the patient from a supine to a lateral position, with less radiation, and in a fraction of the time.

PEARL

Conventional and computed tomography (CT) are very useful for defining fragment size and orientation in intra-articular fractures.

Nuclear Imaging

Nuclear imaging relies on the principle that certain compounds have selective uptake by different body organs. Thus, these compounds may be labeled with a radioactive substance with sufficient energy level to allow its detection outside the body. The ideal isotope is therefore one that may be administered in low doses, is relatively nontoxic, has a short half-life, is readily incorporated into "physiologic" compounds, and is relatively inexpensive. For nuclear imaging of the skeleton, technetium 99m methylene diphosphonate fulfills most of these requirements. The substance is readily incorporated into areas of active bone metabolism (either osteoclastic or osteoblastic activity).

Radionuclide bone scanning is used primarily to detect metastatic lesions (Fig. 10–8), to detect fractures (Fig. 10–9),

and to detect areas of osteomyelitis. It is not particularly useful in patients with multiple myeloma since the isotope is frequently not incorporated into the areas of abnormal bone.

PEARL

Bone scans are often "cold" in patients with multiple myeloma.

Magnetic Resonance Imaging

Magnetic resonance imaging (MRI) is a noninvasive procedure that uses no ionizing radiation. In addition, the magnet strengths used for medical imaging (0.2–2.0 Tesla [T]), have no significant health hazards. Magnetic resonance imaging was originally used to evaluate chemical characteristics of matter on a molecular level. Bloch and Purcell, the original investigators of this technique, were awarded the Nobel Prize for physics in 1982. In 1991, Damadian began investigating the possibilities of using MRI for medical imaging. The computer imaging algorithms developed for CT, accelerated the adaptation of MRI for medical diagnosis.

Magnetic resonance imaging makes use of radiofrequency (RF) radiation in the presence of a high magnetic field. The principle is based on the fact that the nuclei of any atoms with an odd number of protons and neutrons behave like weak magnets and will align themselves within a strong magnetic field (Figs. 10–10a and 10–10b). When a specific RF signal is employed, the nucleus that is being studied is deflected in its orientation (Fig. 10–10c). This is known as *excitation*. Once the RF signal is turned off, the nuclei will return to their magnetized state, and will generate a radiosignal of their own having the same frequency as the signal that initially disrupted it (Fig. 10–10d). This signal may then be amplified and recorded, and using the same computer algorithms developed for CT, the exact location of the nuclei causing that signal can be plotted in space. Although many nuclei may be used for MRI, the most common is hydrogen because of its abundance in tissue (as water) and because of its sensitivity to the phenomenon of magnetic resonance.

Magnetic resonance imaging has the ability to display structures in virtually any plane. This is a distinct advantage over CT, which is limited, by and large, to transverse or axial planes. The most common positions employed for MRI are sagittal, coronal, and axial planes. An additional advantage is the ability of MRI to emphasize the pathologic changes in different tissues through contrast manipulation. This may be accomplished through a number of scanning techniques by altering the pattern of RF pulses in any study. The magnetic resonance (MR) image, therefore, reflects the strength or intensity of the RF signal received from the sample. This signal intensity depends upon several factors, the most important of which are hydrogen density, and two magnetic relaxation times, T1 and T2. The greater the hydrogen density, the more intense or brighter will be the MR signal. Tissues that are low in hydrogen density such as cortical bone, flowing blood, and air-filled lungs, generate little or no MR signal and appear black. Tissues high in hydrogen, such as fat, have high signal intensity and appear white.

A detailed explanation of T1 and T2 is complicated and goes beyond the scope of this text. In simple terms, however,

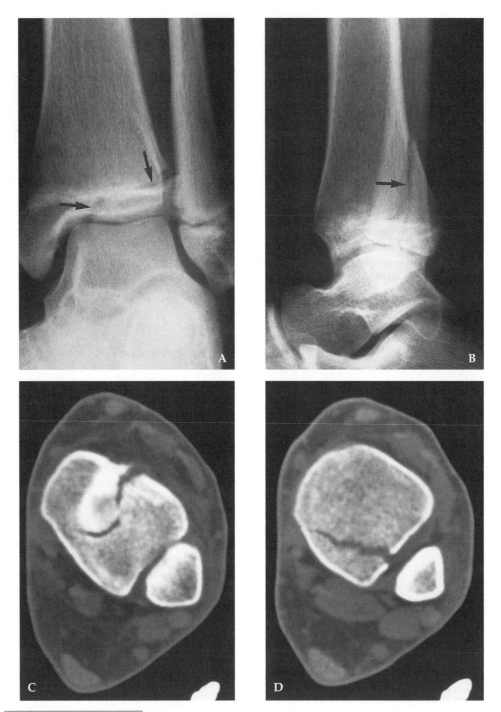

Figure 10–7   The utility of CT in a patient with a triplane fracture. **(A)** Frontal and **(B)** Lateral radiographs demonstrate fractures through the epiphysis, lateral physis, and posterior metaphysis of the tibia (arrows). **(C–D)** Axial CT images show fractures through the epiphysis and posterior metaphysis, respectively.

these two measurements reflect quantitative alterations in the MR signal strength as the result of interactions of the nuclei being studied. Briefly, T1 is the rate at which nuclei align themselves with the external magnetic field following RF stimulation; T2 is the rate at which the RF signal emitted by the nuclei decreases following stimulation. You will hear and see other terms used in both the literature and in reports of studies on your patients. There are a variety of acronyms

(STIR, FLASH, GRASS, SPGR, FISP, GRE) used to describe various fast scanning parameters, and from a practical standpoint, they are of no consequence to the practicing orthopaedist. They are more important to the radiologist who has performed the studies. It is imperative, however, that the referring orthopaedic surgeon fully define the clinical problem and state the information desired from the study. Furthermore, plain radiographs should always accompany an

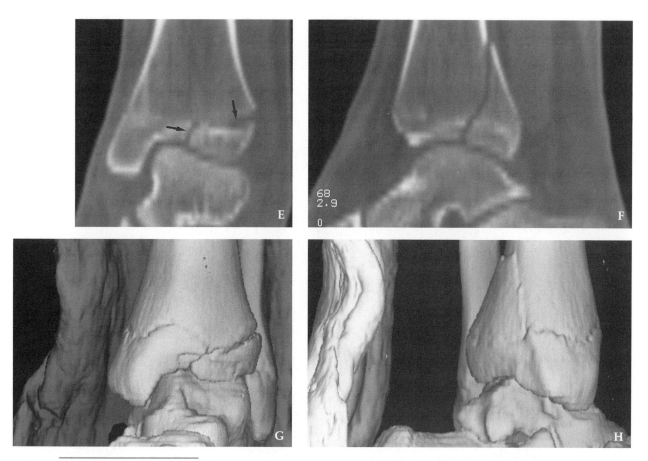

Figure 10–7 *(continued)* **(E)** Coronal tomographic reconstruction shows the epiphyseal and lateral physeal fractures (arrows). **(F)** Sagittal tomographic reconstruction shows the metaphyseal fracture extends down to the joint line. **(G–H)** Three-dimensional reconstructions in frontal and lateral planes show the fractures in a different perspective.

MR study since it is impossible to make a diagnosis of a bone lesion from the MR study itself. In that way, the radiologist can adjust the scanning times and the techniques to best serve your needs as well as those of the patient.

At present, the most commonly used MR examinations are of the central nervous system (brain and spinal cord). Orthopaedic applications constitute the second most common usages. MRI is particularly useful for defining abnormalities of joints (Figs. 10–11 and Figs. 10–12); for evaluating tumors (Fig. 10–13), of either bone or soft tissues; for infections (Fig. 10–14); and for various tendon tears (Fig. 10–15). In addition, MRI is useful for herniation of intervertebral discs (Fig. 10–16) that are, on occasion, managed by orthopaedic surgeons.

PEARL

Magnetic resonance imaging (MRI) is the technique of choice for viewing the bone marrow and most soft-tissue abnormalities in the musculoskeletal system.

Ultrasound

Diagnostic ultrasound is being used with greater frequency today for the diagnosis of a variety of soft tissue abnormali-

ties involving the musculoskeletal system. Areas under study at present include the rotator cuff, Baker cysts, and ganglion cysts (Fig. 10–17), and for tendon ruptures of the Achilles, quadriceps, or patellar tendons. Ultrasound is extremely operator-dependent. However, it does not make use of ionizing radiation. In addition, aspiration of cystic lesions may be performed under ultrasonic guidance.

Arthrography

Arthrography is a diagnostic study where a positive contrast, without or with air, is injected directly into the joint space. In the past it was used to evaluate the knee for meniscal and ligamentous tears, as well as the shoulder for detect tears of the rotator cuff (Fig. 10–18) and the wrist for ligamentous tears, and to evaluate patients with painful joint prostheses. Many arthrographic studies have been replaced, for the most part, by MR. Magnetic resonance arthrography, however, is being used for some knee and shoulder disorders. For this type of study, dilute solutions of gadolinium compounds are injected directly into the joints.

Biopsy

The biopsy of suspected bone or soft tissue lesions may now be made in a radiology department under fluoroscopic or CT

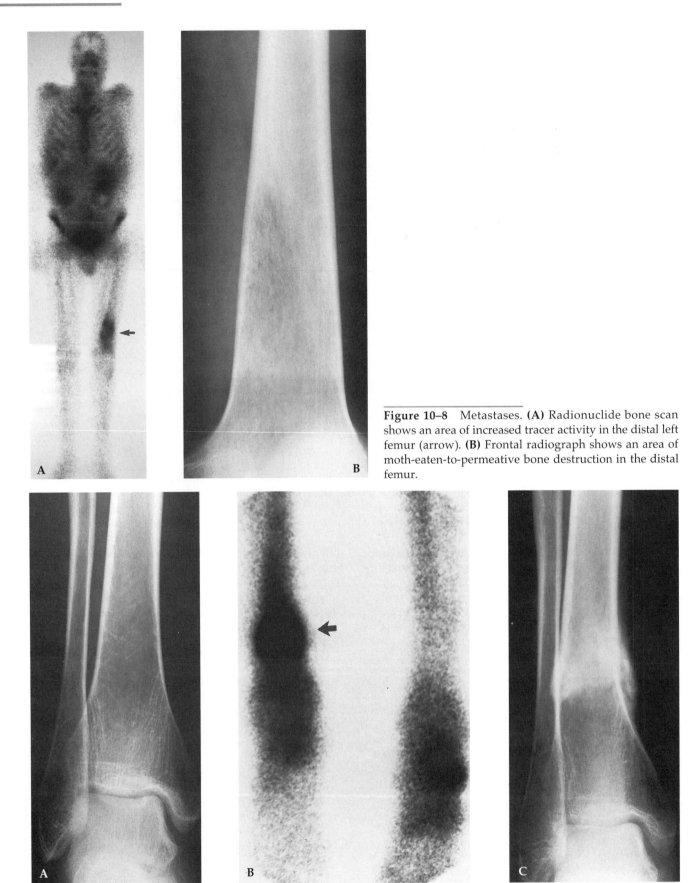

Figure 10–8 Metastases. **(A)** Radionuclide bone scan shows an area of increased tracer activity in the distal left femur (arrow). **(B)** Frontal radiograph shows an area of moth-eaten-to-permeative bone destruction in the distal femur.

Figure 10–9 Use of bone scan to detect an occult insufficiency stress fracture. **(A)** Frontal radiograph of the distal tibia shows osteopenia. There is no evidence of fracture. **(B)** Bone scan made several days later shows increased tracer activity in the distal tibia (arrow). **(C)** Radiograph one month after A shows a healing insufficiency stress fracture of the tibia.

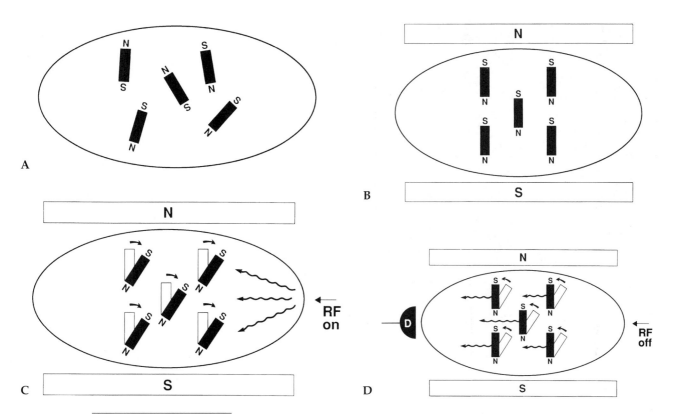

Figure 10–10   Principles of magnetic resonance imaging (MRI). **(A)** Resting state. The molecules in the body behave like small bar magnets and are arranged in a random fashion. **(B)** Magnetization. The molecules align themselves along the plane of magnetization. **(C)** Excitation. A pulsed radiofrequency (RF) beam deflects the molecules as they absorb the energy from that beam. **(D)** Relaxation. When the RF beam is switched off, the molecules return to their pre-excitation position, emitting the energy they absorb, which is measured with a detector **(D)**. Reproduced with permission from Daffner RH. *Clinical Radiology: The Essentials*. Baltimore, MD: Williams and Wilkins; 1993.

guidance. Performing biopsies in this manner eliminates the need for general anesthesia and operating room time and decreases the morbidity associated with the procedure. Percutaneous biopsy is generally considered a radiologic procedure. Instruments used include small, aspirating (22 G) needles increasing in size to the large Craig needle system. Performing the procedure under CT guidance adds an element of accuracy in exact localization. It also reduces cost by eliminating operating room fees.

The Imaging Restaurant

The imaging modalities described above represent a large variety of studies available to the clinician to solve a variety of problems. Thus, a physician has a large "menu" of studies that are available for evaluating a patient. A clinician must choose one of three approaches to take toward this evaluation: the "*shotgun*," the *algorithmic*, or the *directed*. The shotgun approach, is, unfortunately, one that is all too often employed. Little thought is given when a battery of diagnostic laboratory and imaging studies are ordered for each patient in the hope that one or more of these studies will provide the important diagnostic information sought. An example is the clinician who orders both conventional tomography and CT on virtually every fracture encountered.

The algorithmic approach follows a more orderly selection of studies based on the specific problem with which the patient presents. Thought is required by the clinician, and it often possible to be selective in ordering examinations. However, what most often occurs is that unnecessary studies are performed just because they are in the protocol for evaluating patients with a particular complaint. A good example is the patient with an acute back strain of nontraumatic etiology, who usually needs no radiographs initially and may be treated conservatively. All too often, such a patient receives a complete radiographic series of the lumbar vertebrae.

The directed approach is a well-conceived process in which the clinician has taken a careful history and performed a thorough physical examination, and only then considers the diagnostic possibilities for that patient. The physician chooses the appropriate diagnostic imaging studies based primarily

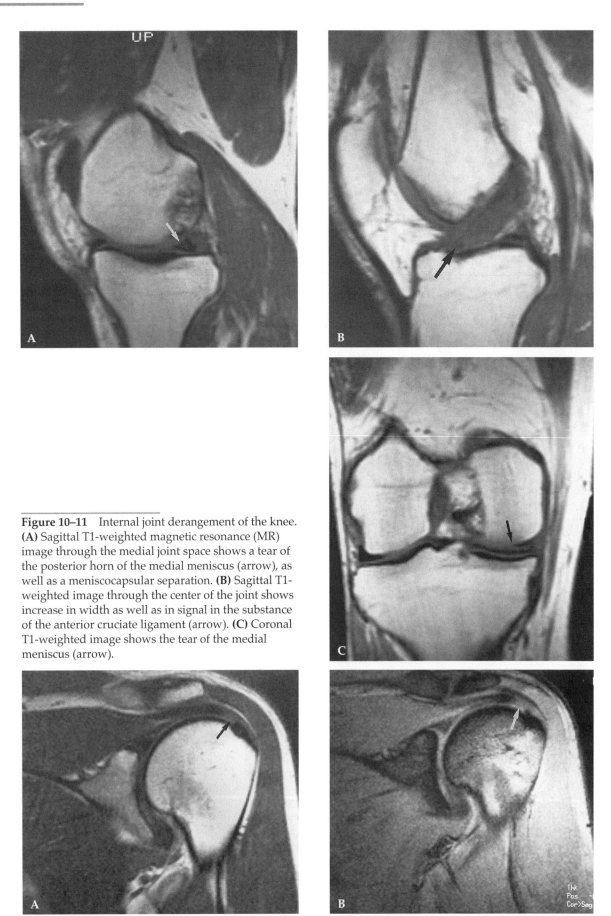

Figure 10–11   Internal joint derangement of the knee. **(A)** Sagittal T1-weighted magnetic resonance (MR) image through the medial joint space shows a tear of the posterior horn of the medial meniscus (arrow), as well as a meniscocapsular separation. **(B)** Sagittal T1-weighted image through the center of the joint shows increase in width as well as in signal in the substance of the anterior cruciate ligament (arrow). **(C)** Coronal T1-weighted image shows the tear of the medial meniscus (arrow).

Figure 10–12   Rotator cuff tear. **(A)** T1-weighted and **(B)** gradient echo coronal oblique images show the tear near the insertion point onto the greater tuberosity (arrows).

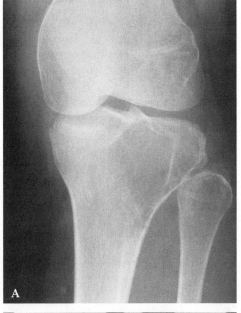

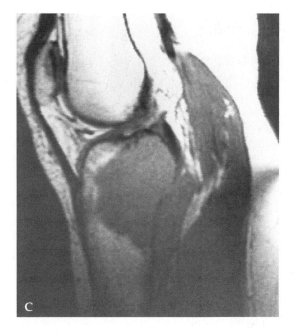

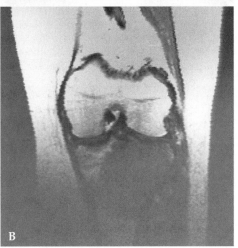

Figure 10–13 Giant-cell tumor of the proximal lateral tibia. **(A)** Frontal radiograph shows a lytic destructive lesion of the lateral tibial plateau and proximal tibia. **(B)** Coronal and **(C)** sagittal T1-weighed images show the extent of the lesion within the marrow space.

on the *probability of diagnostic yield*. Secondary considerations include *safety, radiation dose, cost,* and *medical/legal aspects*. I personally prefer this approach and stress it in my consultation with orthopaedic surgeons and other clinicians. In an era of cost containment and limiting of medical resources, it is incumbent upon all medical practitioners to see that the patient gets as much "bang for the buck" as possible.

The Radiologist and the Orthopaedic Surgeon

In many instances, orthopaedic surgeons view radiologists as an unnecessary middle person in the evaluation process of their patients. Where poor radiologic consultative service is provided, this certainly may be considered true. Furthermore, although most orthopaedic surgeons are very good in interpreting radiographs of the skeleton, particularly for fractures, they continue to have difficulty with more complicated bone disorders such as dysplasias or even tumors. A radiologist who is interested in musculoskeletal imaging can aid orthopaedic surgeons by advising them on the best methods

to solve specific diagnostic problems. The radiologist can tailor an examination to the exact needs of the patient as well as to the surgeon. This will save time as well as money, and may shorten the hospital stay.

One of the greatest values that a radiologist has in dealing with any clinician is the fact that he or she has no vested interest in the patient, nor in the ego process of the referring physician. Thus, a patient coming to an orthopaedist with low back pain, may, in fact, have lumbar spondylosis, which the surgeon easily sees on a radiograph. Because the patient complained of back pain, and because a skeletal disorder that might explain the back pain was found, the surgeon may be satisfied. Unfortunately, the focus has been entirely on the lumbar vertebral column. What may easily be missed is the hypernephroma off the lower pole of a kidney that the radiologist would see due to a focus on the *entire* study.

Finally, in the era of cost containment, the radiologist may be able to be of assistance. There is little benefit in ordering expensive studies that duplicate the diagnostic information. If clinicians don't govern their own practices, outsiders will do it for them. The radiologist can help in that process. Thus,

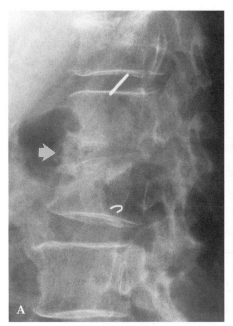
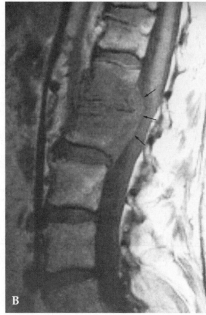
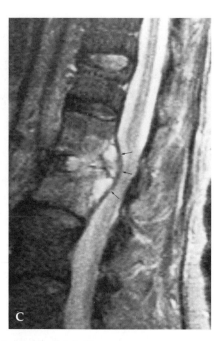

Figure 10–14 Epidural abscess. **(A)** Lateral radiograph shows destruction of the L1-2 disc space (arrow). **(B)** Sagittal T1-weighted image shows low signal material in L-1 and L-2, disc space destruction, and an epidural abscess compressing the thecal sac (arrows). **(C)** Sagittal T2-weighted image shows the abscess to advantage (arrows). Note the posterior displacement of the conus.

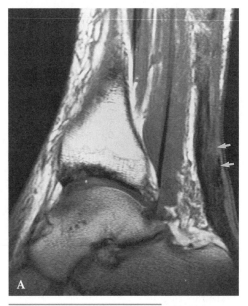
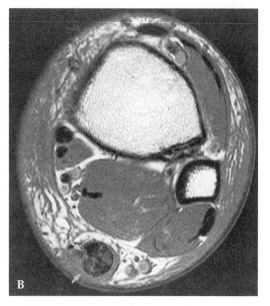

Figure 10–15 Acute tear of Achilles' tendon. **(A)** Direct sagittal T1-weighted image of the ankle shows shredding of the normally black and solid Achilles' tendon, with areas of increased signal within the substance (arrows). **(B)** Axial T1-weighted image shows increased signal within the Achilles' tendon (arrows). Note the soft tissue edema represented as gray material in the subcutaneous soft tissues.

consultation with the radiologist is as important for helping your patient as consulting with any other specialist.

ANATOMIC ASPECTS

The key to an understanding of radiographic abnormalities of bone is founded on a thorough understanding of skeletal anatomy. While many of the anatomic parts of bone may not hold any clinical significance to the orthopaedic surgeon, their radiographic appearance may, on occasion, cause some consternation. "*Daffner's First Law of Radiographics*" states that if you understand the gross anatomy of a structure, you will have no difficulty predicting its radiographic appearance. Thus, one should have a thorough knowledge of the anatomy of each bone being studied.

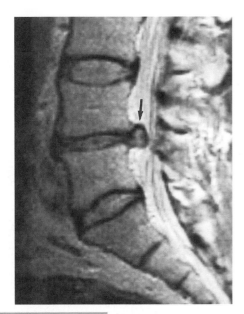

Figure 10–16 Herniated intervertebral disc (arrow) at L-4. Note narrowing of the L-4 disc space.

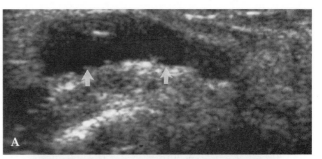

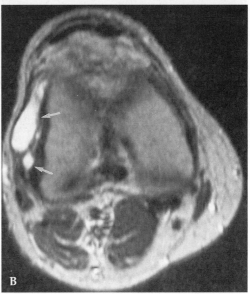

Figure 10–17 Ganglion cyst of the lateral aspect of the knee. **(A)** Ultrasound study shows an echo-free zone (arrows) representing the cyst. **(B)** Axial T2-weighed CT image shows the multilocular cyst (arrows).

As we will discuss later, certain bone diseases have a predilection for particular kinds of bone. From a purely anatomic standpoint, there are five types of bones based on their shapes:

1. long bones characterized by two ends and a shaft (this category also includes phalanges, metacarpals, and metatarsals)
2. short bones characterized by six sides (carpals and tarsals)
3. flat bones (calvaria, ribs, sternum)
4. irregular bones characterized by many sides (vertebrae)
5. sesamoid bones that are located within tendons

In addition, there are two architectural types of bone: compact (dense), generally present where strength is necessary; and cancellous (spongy) designed for distributing weight over a greater area. All bones contain three parts: the epiphysis and physis (growth center); the metaphysis, an area that lies just beneath the physis or growth plate; and the diaphysis or shaft. Although flat bones, such as those that form the pelvis, do not have these three areas as distinctly as long bones, they do have analogs to the long bones. For example, the region adjacent to the triradiate cartilage in the acetabulum is considered a *metaphyseal equivalent*. It is not surprising that diseases that are commonly found in the metaphyses of long bones may also be found in the metaphyseal equivalent areas of flat bones. As will be discussed later, such locations have importance in predicting the nature of many bone lesions.

PATHOLOGIC ASPECTS

Plain film radiography is the cornerstone for the diagnosis of diseases of the musculosketal system. Thus, it is mandatory to obtain conventional radiographs prior to ordering more sophisticated studies since the plain film serves as the "road map" for further investigation and diagnosis. Many lesions

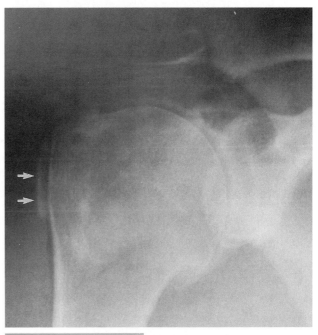

Figure 10–18 Rotator cuff tear. External rotation view of an arthrogram shows contrast extravasated laterally into the subdeltoid bursa (arrows).

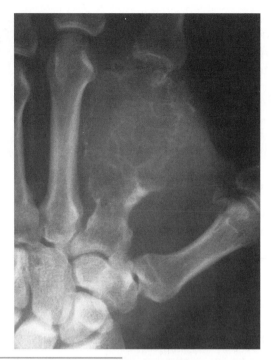

Figure 10–19 Aneurysmal bone cyst of the second metacarpal. An expanded bubbly lesion extends to the joint line but has not crossed. This appearance is considered pathognomonic of aneursymal bone cyst.

have a radiographic appearance characteristic enough to allow confident and accurate pathologic diagnosis, particularly when combined with pertinent clinical and/or laboratory findings (Fig. 10–19). Other lesions, unfortunately, will have an indeterminate appearance that may require obtaining tissue for a diagnosis. The goal of radiologic diagnosis of bone lesions, therefore, is to establish one of four management categories:

1. definitely benign, the "leave me alone" lesion
2. benign symptomatic, in which elective biopsy or removal is needed
3. definitely malignant (or aggressive) in which biopsy is needed to confirm the diagnosis and to plan therapy
4. The "I don't know" lesion, which also requires a biopsy.

The author uses the acronym ABCS for analyzing bone and joint lesions:

A: **A**natomic appearance and **A**lignment abnormalities
B: **B**ony mineralization and texture abnormalities
C: **C**artilage (joint space) abnormalities
S: **S**oft tissue abnormalities

Each radiograph is analyzed for each of the components. Using this analysis, combined with a group of *"predictor variables"* (discussed below), allows a confident diagnosis to be made in most instances.

> **PEARL**
>
> Never, ever forget to examine the entire film, including the edges. The margin may include a finding that holds the key to the diagnosis.

Distribution

One may obtain important clues to the nature of a bone or joint lesion by observing its distribution. Lesions may be monostotic or monoarticular, polyostotic or polyarticular, or diffuse, involving virtually every bone or joint. Combining the distribution with six basic pathologic categories—congenital, inflammatory, metabolic, neoplastic, traumatic, and vascular—one may narrow the diagnostic possibilities down to one or two categories. For example, diffuse involvement of bones or joints occurs only in metabolic or neoplastic conditions.

> **PEARL**
>
> Common diseases occur more commonly; even in unusual locations. Common diseases in an usual location still look like the original entity.

Table 10–1 shows the relationship of distribution of certain diseases to the pathologic category.

TABLE 10–1   Distribution of bone disease by pathologic category

Category	Monostotic/Articular	Polyostotic/Articular	Diffuse
Congenital	Cervical rib	Cleidocranial dysostosis	
Inflammatory	Osteomyelitis, gout	Congenital lues, rheumatoid arthritis	
Neoplastic	Any primary bone tumor	Myeloma	Metastasis
Metabolic	(Paget's disease)	(Paget's disease, fibrous dysplasia)	Osteopetrosis, hyperparathyroidism
Traumatic	Single fracture	Multiple fractures, battered child	
Vascular	Perthes' disease	Perthes' disease	

Predictor Variables

Predictor variables are a group of radiologic appearances that may be applied to any bone or joint lesion to aid in making the correct diagnosis. These include the behavior of the lesion; which specific bone or joint is involved; the location within a bone or joint; the age, gender, and race of the patient; the margin and shape of the lesion; the involvement or crossing of a joint; bony reaction (if any); matrix production by the lesion (if any); soft tissue changes; and a history of trauma or surgery. Table 10–2 expands upon these diagnostic parameters.

Many of the variables apply specifically to the diagnosis of bone tumors. Indeed, they were originally developed for that purpose. Keep in mind, however, that primary bone tumors, exclusive of myeloma, are rare lesions. One should also remember that it still may not be possible to make a specific diagnosis even after all of the variables have been condensed. In these situations, this process should be used to determine whether a lesion is agressive or nonaggressive; that is, whether or not a lesion needs to have a biopsy performed.

TABLE 10–2 Predictor Variables for Bone and Joint Lesions

1. *Behavior of the Lesion*
     Osteolytic
     Osteoblastic
     Mixed
2. *Bone or Joint Involved*
3. *Locus within a Bone*
     Epiphysis (apophysis)
     Metaphysis (or equivalent)
     Diaphysis
4. *Age, Gender, and Race of Patient*
5. *Margin of Lesion*
     Sharply defined
     Poorly defined
6. *Shape of Lesion*
     Longer than wide
     Wider than long
       Cortical breakthrough
       No breakthrough
7. *Joint Space Crossed*
8. *Bony Reaction (If Any)*
     Periosteal
       Solid
       Laminated ("onion-skin")
       Spiculated, sunburst, "hair-on-end"
       Codman's triangle
     Sclerosis
     Buttressing
9. *Matrix Production*
     Osteoid
     Chondroid
     Mixed
10. *Soft Tissue Changes*
11. *History of Trauma or Surgery*

Reproduced with permission from: Daffner RH. *Clinical Radiology: The Essentials.* Baltimore, MD: Williams and Wilkins; 1993.

Behavior of the Lesion

Bone lesions generally fall into three behavioral categories: Primary osteolytic (osteoclastic or bone destroying); osteoblastic (bone forming, reactive, or reparative); or mixed, demonstrating features of both. Joint lesions, similarly, may be primarily lytic or proliferative. Three types of osteolytic bone destruction have been identified: *geographic* (Fig. 10–20), *moth-eaten* (Fig. 10–21), and *permeative* (Fig. 10–22). Geographic destruction is the term that indicates that large areas of bone have been destroyed and are easily visible with the unaided eye (Fig. 10–20). Of the three types of bone destruction, it is generally considered to be the least aggressive. A moth-eaten appearance occurs when the lesion has produced many discrete small holes throughout the bone. This appearance suggests a more aggressive lesion (Fig. 10–21). A permeative pattern indicates an extremely aggressive disease process. There is fine bone destruction that represents the lesion diffusely infiltrating throughout the haversian system. In many instances, a magnifying lens may be required to actually see the bone destruction (Fig. 10–22) of the bone or joint involved.

Bone or Joint Involved

Many diseases have a predilection for certain bones or joints (Fig. 10–23), a fact that is useful for establishing a diagnosis of many lesions. For example, rheumatoid arthritis commonly

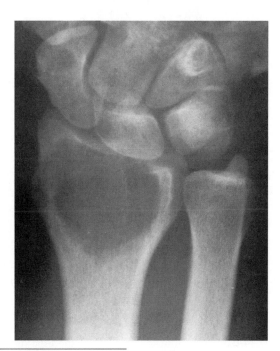

Figure 10–20 Giant-cell tumor of the distal radius demonstrating geographic bone destruction.

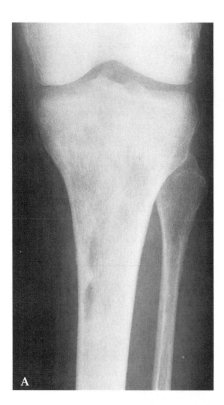

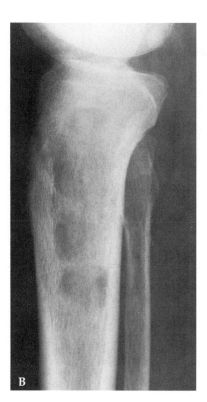

Figure 10–21 Osteomyelitis of the proximal tibia demonstrating moth-eaten bone destruction.

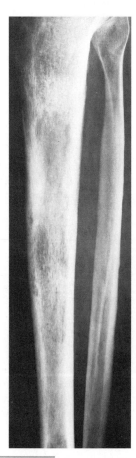

Figure 10–22 Reticulum cell sarcoma of the tibia demonstrating permeative bone destruction along with some areas of moth-eaten destruction.

affects the hands and feet; hyperparathyroidism the skull, distal clavicles, and bones of the hands and feet; Paget's disease the pelvis, skull, and vertebral column (while sparing the fibula); chondrosarcomas the pelvis; and enchondromas the phalanges and metacarpals.

PEARL
If it looks like nothing you've seen before, think of fibrous dysplasia.

Locus Within a Bone or Joint

The location of a lesion within a bone or joint is another clue to the etiology. Some bone lesions occur often in the epiphysis, the metaphysis, or the diaphysis. Among the common bone tumors, chondroblastoma frequently is found in the epiphysis in the skeletally immature patient. Round-cell tumors (Ewing's, myeloma, malignant lymphoma) occur often in the diaphysis. All of the other major neoplasms are commonly found in the metaphysis. Some lesions, such as a giant-cell tumor (Fig. 10–20), will extend to the epiphysis once complete bone growth has occurred.

Nonneoplastic lesions also occur often in certain areas of bones or joints. Osteoarthritis, for example, is found in the weight-bearing surfaces of the large joints, whereas rheumatoid arthritis affects the entire surface of the same joint. Osteomyelitis frequently occurs in the diametaphyseal region where red marrow is prevalent. This is also a common location for eosinophilic granuloma. Further selection may be seen in the location of certain of the arthritides. For example,

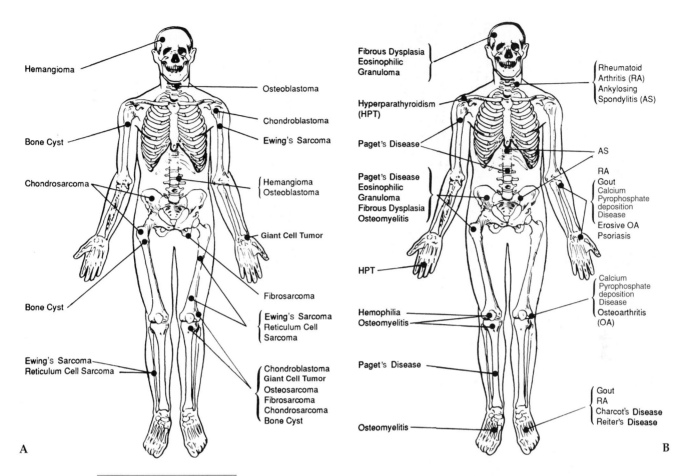

Figure 10–23 Common locations for bone lesions. **(A)** Neoplastic conditions. **(B)** Nonneoplastic conditions. Reproduced with permission from Daffner RH. *Clinical Radiology: The Essentials*. Baltimore, MD: Williams and Wilkins; 1993.

rheumatoid arthritis and osteoarthritis attack the cartilaginous surface of a joint (Fig. 10–24). Conversely, conditions such as gout or psoriatic arthritis affect the so-called bare, or para-articular, areas around the joint, sparing the articular surfaces until late in the disease (Fig. 10–25).

Age, Gender, and Race

The patient's age is an important factor in the occurrence of many diseases. For example, a skeletally immature patient with a permeative lesion in the shaft of a long bone is more likely to have an Ewing's tumor (Fig. 10–26). A similarly appearing lesion in an older patient should suggest malignant lymphoma of bone or perhaps myeloma. As a rule, one may confidently predict the type of a malignant bone neoplasm based solely on the patient's age. For example, neuroblastoma is the most common type of tumor encountered under age 1. Ewing tumor of long bones is common in the first decade. Between ages 10 and 30, osteosarcoma and Ewing's tumor of flat bones are common. Between ages 30 and 40, most of the malignant sarcomas are encountered. Over age 40, metastatic carcinoma, along with multiple myeloma and chondrosarcoma, are encountered.

Age also is a factor in benign lesions. Paget's disease, for example, is almost never found in patients under 40 years of

age. Similarly, infantile cortical hyperostosis (Caffey's disease) is not seen in patients over 1 year of age.

> **PEARL**
>
> With lytic lesions in a patient over age 50, 99% will be metastases.

> **PEARL**
>
> With odd-looking lesions in a child, think of eosinophilic granuloma.

Many diseases have a gender distribution. Paget's disease occurs more commonly in males; rheumatoid arthritis and fibrous dysplasia are found more commonly in females. Lastly, there is often racial heredity in some diseases, particularly sickle cell anemia and thalassemia.

Margin of the Lesion

The appearance of the margin of the lesion, that is, the zone of transition between normal and abnormal bone, is important

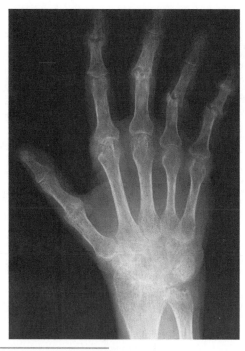

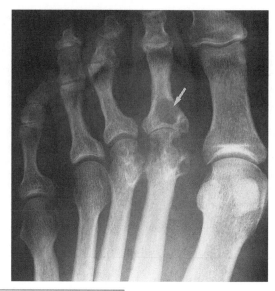

Figure 10–25   Gout. There are para-articular erosions of the distal ends of the second and third metatarsals. An intra-osseous lesion is present in the base of the proximal phalanx of the second toe (arrow). The articular surfaces are generally spared. Compare with Figure 10–24.

Figure 10–24   Advanced rheumatoid arthritis. Virtually all of the joints are involved with severe erosions. There is pronounced osteoporosis. The central portions of the joints are the primary targets. Compare with Figure 10–25.

in establishing the etiology of a particular bone lesion. As a rule, a sharp transition zone appearing as a dense zone of sclerosis between normal and abnormal bone or as a thin, well-defined line (Fig. 10–27) indicates a nonaggressive or benign process. Conversely, a wide or broad, poorly defined transition zone between normal and abnormal bone indicates

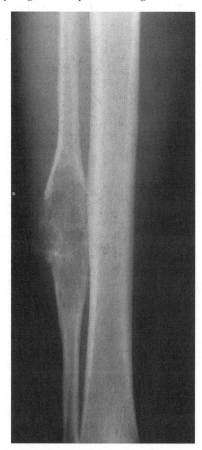

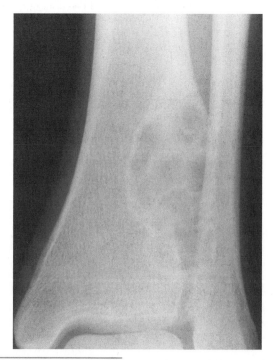

Figure 10–26   Ewing's tumor of the mid shaft of the fibula of a 9-year-old boy. An aggressive lesion in this location in a young child is highly suggestive of this entity.

Figure 10–27   Benign fibrocystic lesion of the distal tibia (fibroxanthoma, nonossifying fibroma). This bubbly lesion is longer than it is wide and has a sharp transition zone.

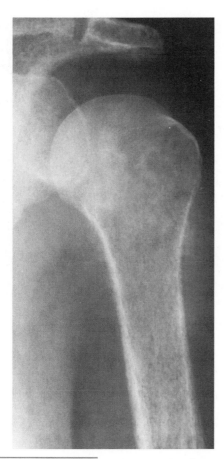

Figure 10–28 Metastases of the proximal humerus. This lesion diffusely infiltrates the proximal humerus. There is moth-eaten-to-permeative destruction and cortical break-through laterally, where a "hair-on-end" appearance is evident. Benign lesions do not behave like this.

a more aggressive lesion (Fig. 10–28). The appearance of the transition zone is directly related to the growth rates of each type of lesion. A slow-growing, benign lesion, such as a nonossifying fibroma, progresses at a rate sufficiently slow to allow the bone to react in an attempt to contain the lesion. Aggressive lesions, on the other hand, such as osteomyelitis or malignant tumor, progress at such a rapid rate that the bone is unable to adequately respond.

Shape of the Lesion

Assessing the shape of a bone lesion also helps in the same way as evaluating the margin. Any lesion that is longer than it is wide and that is oriented with the shaft of the bone is more likely to be a nonaggressive benign process (Fig. 10–27). On the other hand, lesions that are wider than bone, have broken out of the bone, and extend into the soft tissues are more aggressive (Fig. 10–29). The actual confirmation of the lesion extending through the bone into the soft tissues may have to be done using CT or MRI.

Joint Space Involvement

As a rule, any lesion that crosses a joint space is most likely either of an inflammatory nature (Fig. 10–30) or is due to a

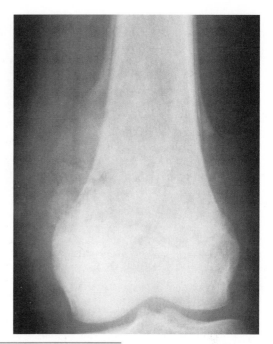

Figure 10–29 Osteogenic sarcoma of the distal femur showing cortical breakthrough medially and laterally. Note the extension of tumor into the soft tissues adjacent to the bone.

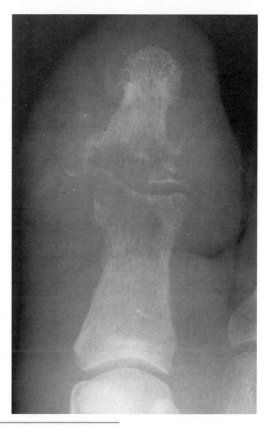

Figure 10–30 Osteomyelitis and joint space infection of the great toe in a diabetic. The lesion has extended to both sides of the joint. This identifies it as inflammatory in nature.

primary joint disorder such as arthritis or pigmented villon-odular synovitis (Fig. 10–31). This rule generally remains

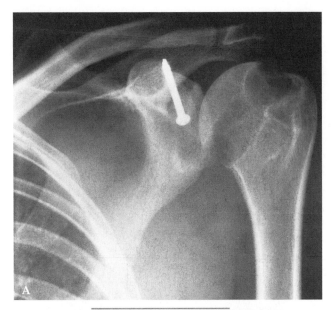

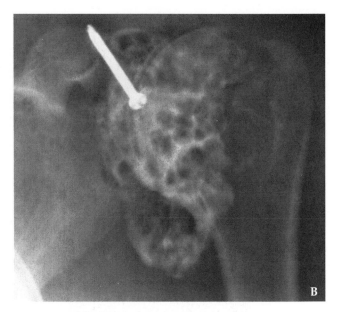

Figure 10–31   Pigmented villonodular synovitis. **(A)** Radiograph shows erosions involving the humeral head and inferior glenoid. A surgical screw is present. **(B)** Arthrogram shows the grape-like hypertrophied synovial tissue.

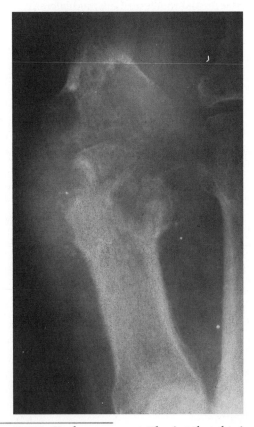

Figure 10–32   Tophaceous gout. The fact that this lesion is on both sides of the metatarsal phalangeal joint of the great toe indicates an inflammatory lesion rather than a neoplasm despite its aggressive appearance.

valid, no matter how aggressive the process may appear otherwise (Fig. 10–32). *Infections cross joints; tumors do not.* Those tumors that have a predilection for the ends of bones, such as chrondroblastoma and giant-cell tumor (Fig. 10–33),

extend to the joint but do not cross it. As a rule, even the most malignant bone tumors respect the cartilage of the joint as well as of the physis (Fig. 10–34). Abnormalities found on both sides of a joint with intact cortical margins would suggest a polyostotic disorder rather than an arthropathy.

PEARL

Infection can look like anything. Tuberculosis is not rare. Tuberculosis and eosinophilic granuloma are great imitators.

Bony Reaction

There are three reactions of bone to any insult: periosteal reaction, sclerosis, and buttressing. Periosteal reaction occurs in four varieties: solid, laminated (onion skin), spiculated (sunburst or "hair-on-end"), or Codman's triangle. Solid, uninterrupted periosteal reaction indicates a benign process. This is most often encountered in osteomyelitis and fracture healing. A laminated or onion-skin type of periosteal reaction indicates repetitive insults to the bone (Fig. 10–35). The nature of the lamination should be determined by the thickness. Thin, irregular, or disorganized lamination with many interruptions indicate an aggressive process such as an Ewing's tumor (Fig. 10–36). Benign processes have laminations that are uninterrupted between the layers (Fig. 10–35). A spiculated, sunburst, or hair-on-end appearance periosteal reaction is almost always associated with a malignant bone lesion, usually an osteogenic sarcoma (Fig. 10–37). This type of periosteal reaction is the result of a neoplastic process breaking through a layer of periosteal new bone, followed by additional periosteal osseous deposition and subsequent breakthrough. The Codman's triangle represents a triangular ossification of an area of periosteum that has been elevated

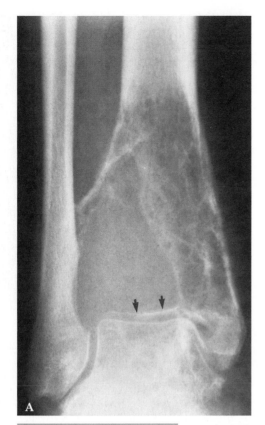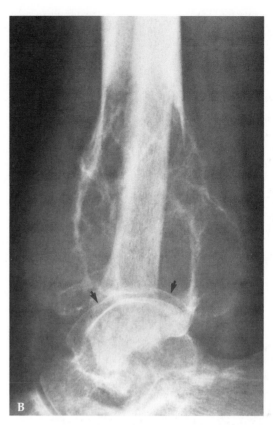

Figure 10–33 Giant-cell tumor of the distal tibia. This lesion extends to the joint surface but has not crossed. Note the thin rim of preserved cortical bone along the tibial articular surface (arrows).

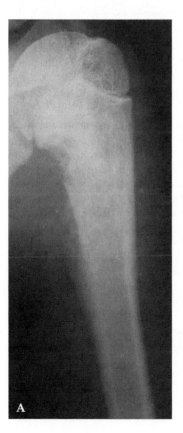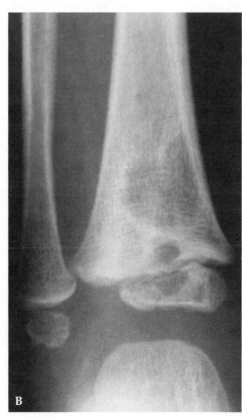

Figure 10–34 Physeal barrier. **(A)** Osteosarcoma of the proximal humerus involves the metaphysis and proximal shaft. The physis and epiphysis are spared in this patient. **(B)** Tuberculosis of the distal tibia. The metaphyseal lesion has extended across the physis into the epiphysis.

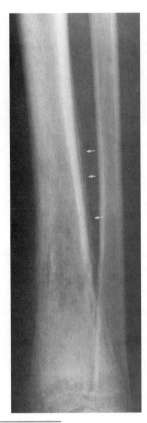

Figure 10–35 Solid laminated periosteal reaction of the distal tibia (arrows) in a patient with osteomyelitis.

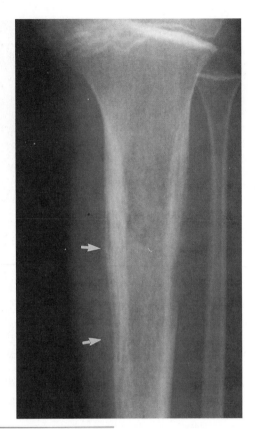

Figure 10–36 Irregular periosteal lamination (arrows) in a patient with an Ewing's tumor. Compare with Figure 10–35.

from the bone. This occurs in a variety of benign and malignant conditions and should not be considered pathognomonic of any particular lesion.

PEARL
In expanded lytic lesions in older patients, don't forget brown tumors.

Sclerosis and buttressing are additional attempts by bone or joint to wall off an area of disease. They generally indicate a nonaggressive process. Buttressing typically occurs around the joint. Osteophytes or syndesmophytes are examples.

Matrix Production

Certain bone tumors produce a substance termed *matrix* that may be cartilaginous (chondroid), bony (osteoid), or occasionally mixed. Chondroid matrix may be identified as fine, stippled, calcification, or as multiple popcornlike calcification arranged in groups of "Cs" or "Os" (Fig. 10–38). Osteoid matrix is dense and is found most often in osteogenic sarcoma (Fig. 10–39), but also may be seen in the benign ossifying condition, myositis ossificans.

Soft Tissue Changes

Changes in soft tissue often reveal important clues regarding an underlying injury, disease process, or specific bone lesion. For example, diffuse muscle wasting is frequently seen with

PEARL
A fracture is a soft tissue injury in which a bone is broken. With any fracture, look for the soft tissue component. It may be more significant than the bony component!

chronic debilitating diseases such as disseminated neoplasm, acquired immunodificiency syndrome, or paralysis. Soft tissue swelling may be due to a mass, hemorrhage, inflammation, or edema. Displacement or loss of normally appearing fat lines is also an indication of adjacent abnormality. The obliteration of the pronator quadratus fat line in the wrist frequently accompanies a fracture about that joint. Elevation or displacement of the elbow fat pad indicates a joint effusion, usually the result of trauma (Fig. 10–40). Sometimes it may be found in inflammatory conditions such as rheumatoid or septic arthritis. Horizontal radiographs of the knee in patients with tibial plateau fractures frequently show a lipohemarthrosis manifested as a fat-fluid level (Fig. 10–41).

PEARL
In patients with knee trauma, look carefully at the lateral view for effusion. No effusion virtually guarantees no significant injury.

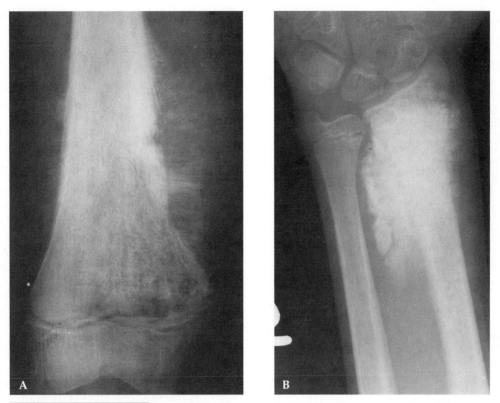

Figure 10–37 **(A–B)** Hair-on-end periosteal reaction in two patients with osteogenic sarcoma. Note the variability of the appearance of this reactive tissue medially and laterally.

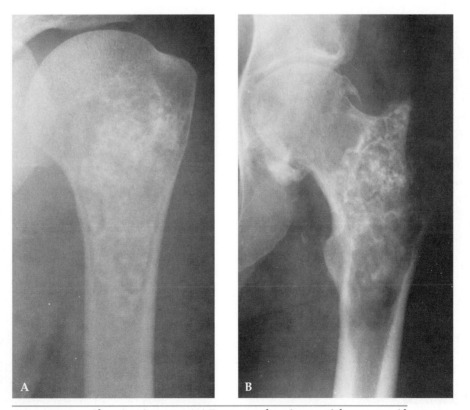

Figure 10–38 Chondroid matrix. **(A)** Benign enchondroma of the proximal humerus. **(B)** Chondrosarcoma of the proximal femur. Note how the matrix is better organized and is more confined in A.

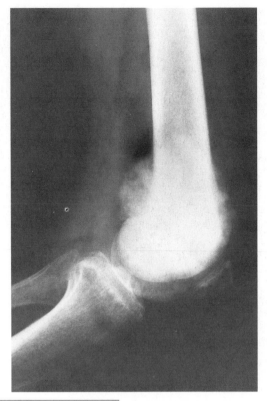

Figure 10–39   Osteoid matrix in an osteogenic sarcoma of the distal femur. Compare with Figure 10–38.

Soft tissues should also be evaluated for the presence of calcification, either alone or within a mass (Fig. 10–42). Streaky calcifications within soft tissues may be indicative of myositis ossificans or, on occasion, a parasitic disease.

Gas in the soft tissues is frequently the result of open trauma or gas gangrene. Other soft tissue findings include the presence of foreign bodies, vascular calcifications, abdominal aortic aneurysm, or renal calculi in patients being evaluated for back pain.

History of Trauma or Surgery

Trauma constitutes the most common bone disorder encountered. It is, therefore, important to elicit a history of it whenever possible. The traumatic event that caused the abnormality may be deemed trivial by the patient but should be actively sought. In addition, the history of activities that may predispose to certain traumatic conditions such as stress fractures should also be actively sought. On occasion, one will encounter situations where the history of trauma is deliberately withheld. This is frequently found in the case of the battered child or of the child or adult who is engaged in some prohibited or illegal activity.

In addition, it is important to know whether the patient has undergone surgery. Healing surgical sites, particularly those used for bone graft donation (Fig. 10–43), may be easily misinterpreted as a more ominous lesion if the history is not obtained. It is, therefore, incumbent that a complete surgical history also be obtained.

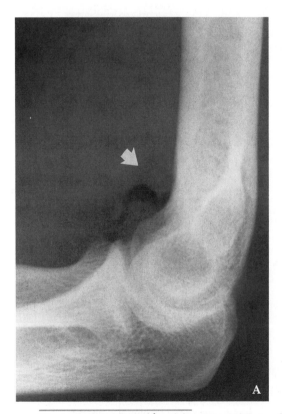

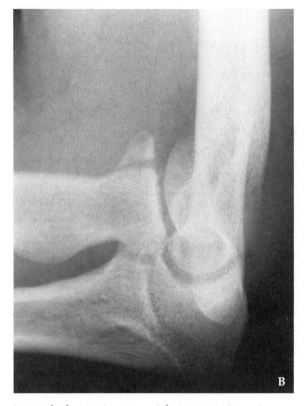

Figure 10–40   Radial head fracture. **(A)** Lateral radiograph shows elevation of the anterior fat pad (arrow). No fracture can be identified. **(B)** Tilt view shows the fracture of the radial head.

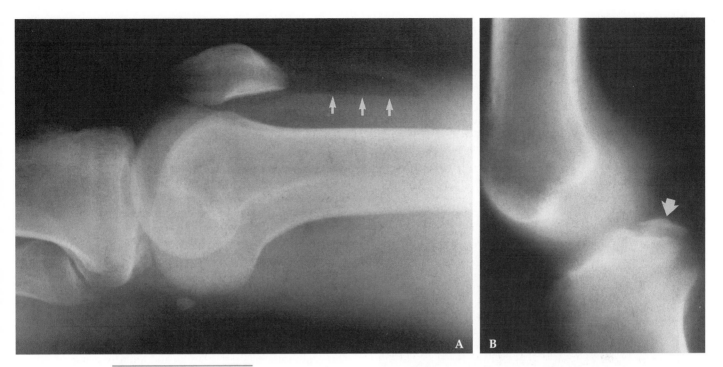

Figure 10–41   Lipohemarthrosis of the knee. **(A)** Lateral horizontal beam radiograph shows the fat-fluid level (arrows). **(B)** Lateral tomogram shows fracture of the posterior aspect of the central tibial plateau (arrow).

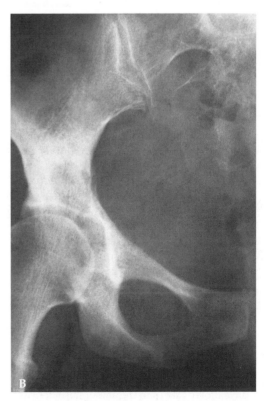

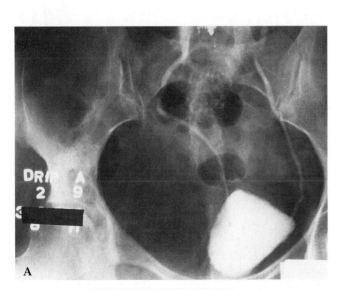

Figure 10–42   Chondrosarcoma of the pelvis. **(A)** Soft tissue mass displaces the contrast-filled ureter and bladder to the left. **(B)** A detail view shows faint calcification within the mass. Note the bony destruction above the right acetabulum.

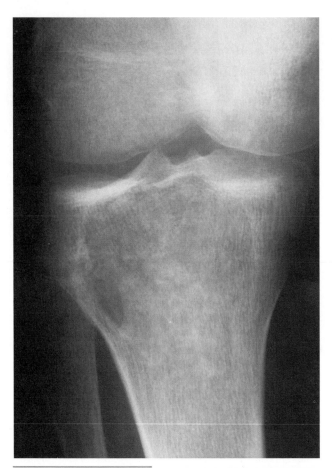

Figure 10–43   Bone graft donor site of the proximal tibia. Without a history of previous trauma, this lytic lesion could easily be misinterpreted as representing a giant-cell tumor.

Additional Observations

Abnormalities of Bony Anatomy and/or Alignment

Bony deformity generally indicates either congenital abnormality or the sequelae of previous trauma. In addition, there are two types of malalignment that occur in joints: *subluxations* and *dislocations*. Subluxation is a partial loss of continuity between articulating surfaces; dislocation is complete loss of continuity at that joint space.

PEARL

Any trauma view of the cervical spine that "looks odd," isn't. Look for signs of unilateral jumped and locked facet.

Abnormalities of Bony Mineralization or Texture

The degree of bony mineralization is directly related to the patient's age, physiologic state, and the amount of activity or stress being placed on that bone. The texture of the bony trabeculae (thin, delicate, coarsened, smudged) also tells something about the patient's general state of health. Osteoporosis is the most common metabolic bone disease. It is most frequently found in the elderly, and in particular, in post-

menopausal women. An acute form of osteoporosis may occur, however, following limb mobilization. Diminished mineralization (osteopenia) is also a common manifestation of certain diseases such as rheumatoid arthritis, scurvy, and renal osteodystrophy. Renal osteodystrophy is a complex of several metabolic conditions in which there are four prominent radiographic manifestations: osteoporosis, coarsening of bony trabeculae, osteomalacia, and hyperparathyroidism. One is most likely to encounter this in patients with chronic renal failure who are undergoing dialysis. Any one of the four components may be featured more prominently than the others on a radiograph. However, as a rule, the radiographic image represents a combination of all four findings. Features of osteomalacia include osteoporosis; trabeculae that are smudged and indistinct, bony resorption about the physes in skeletally immature patients; and a classic appearance of the vertebral column where there are horizontal alternating bands of osteoporosis centrally with osteosclerosis along the disc end plates, termed "rugger jersey spine" (Fig. 10–44). Hyperparathyroidism classically produces osteoporosis; subperiosteal resorption along the radial borders of phalanges; the tufts of the distal phalanges; resorption about the distal clavicles and other symphyseal joints, as well as along entheses (tendinous insertion points); and an interesting mixed pattern of osteoporosis and fluffy sclerosis in the calvarium referred to as "salt and pepper skull" (Fig. 10–45).

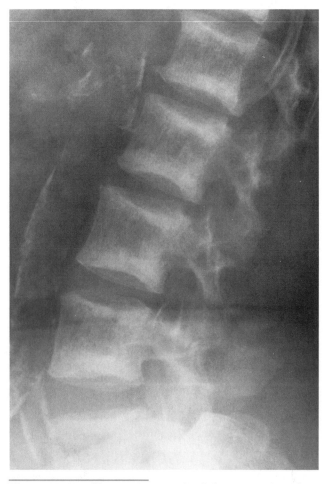

Figure 10–44   "Rugger jersey spine" demonstrating alternating areas of osteosclerosis and osteoporosis in this patient with chronic renal failure.

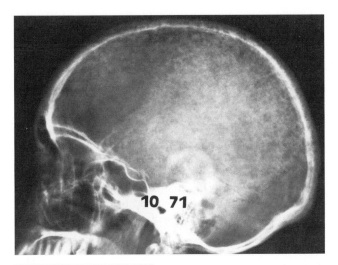

Figure 10–45 "Salt and pepper" skull in a patient with primary hyperparathyroidism.

In many instances, severe osteoporosis is difficult to differentiate from a permeative bone destruction on either plain films or CT. This is particularly troublesome in elderly patients who have suffered vertebral compression fractures. Magnetic resonance imaging is the procedures of choice to aid in making the differentiation. On T1-weighted images, osteoporosis shows fatty replacement of marrow that is high in signal (Fig. 10–46). Infiltrative disorders, on the other hand, produce low signal in the marrow spaces on T1-weighted studies (Fig. 10–47). In addition, recent osteoporotic vertebral

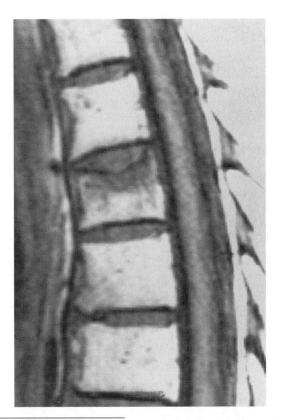

Figure 10–46 Osteoporotic vertebral collapse. Sagittal T1-weighted image demonstrates collapse of a thoracic vertebra with low marrow signal in a linear fashion. Compare this with Figure 10–47.

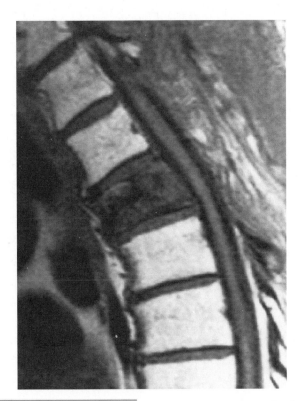

Figure 10–47 Metastatic infiltration and collapse of the thoracic vertebra. The signal in the entire vertebra is low. Compare with Figure 10–46. Metastases were demonstrated elsewhere in the vertebral column in this patient.

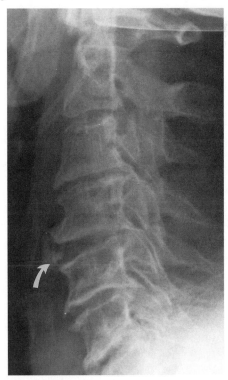

Figure 10–48 Hyperextension sprain. Lateral cervical radiograph demonstrates widening of the C–4 disc space (arrow). There is also retrolisthesis of C–4 on C–5. The patient is quadriplegic.

fractures have more of a linear distribution of abnormal signal than do those of an infiltrative disorder.

Joint Changes

The width of the joint space and the appearance of the distal ends of articulating bones are important in the diagnosis of traumatic and arthritic disorders. While joint space narrowing is typically found in degenerative conditions, widening of a joint space is often indicative of associated trauma (Fig. 10–48).

The distribution, location, and erosive pattern (cartilage surface vs. "bare areas") produced by the various arthritides allow one considerable accuracy in establishing a radiographic diagnosis, particularly when correlated with clinical and laboratory findings.

SUMMARY

This chapter briefly reviewed types of examinations available for the imaging diagnosis of bone and joint disorders. Most musculoskeletal lesions fall into one of six basic pathologic categories: congenital, inflammatory, metabolic, neoplastic, traumatic, or vascular. Recognition of patterns of destruction, distribution of lesions, and application of a series of predictor variables make it possible to reduce the complexity of skeletal diseases to a workable format. Radiographs of the skeleton should be evaluated using the "ABCS approach" wherein abnormalities of bony anatomy and alignment, bony mineralization and texture, cartilage, and soft tissue changes are evaluated.

SELECTED BIBLIOGRAPHY

BERQUIST TH. *MRI of the Musculoskeletal System*. 3rd ed. Philadelphia, PA: Lippincott-Raven; 1996.

BLOEM JL, SARTORIS DJ. *MRI and CT of the Musculoskeletal System: A Text-Atlas*. Baltimore, MD: Williams and Wilkins; 1991.

DAFFNER RH. *Clinical Radiology: The Essentials* 2nd Ed. Baltimore, MD: Williams and Wilkins; 1999.

EDEIKEN J, DALINKA MJ, KARASICK D. *Edeiken's Roentgen Diagnosis of Diseases of Bone*. 4th ed. Baltimore, MD: Williams and Wilkins; 1989.

GREENFIELD GD. *Radiology of Bone Diseases*. 5th ed. Philadelphia, PA: Lippincott-Raven; 1995.

RESNICK D. *Diagnosis of Bone and Joint Disorders*. 3rd ed. Philadelphia, PA: WB Saunders; 1994.

SAMPLE QUESTIONS

1. Defining the size and position of fracture fragments in an intra-articular fracture is best achieved with:
   (a) MRI
   (b) plain radiographs
   (c) ultrasound
   (d) conventional or computed tomography
   (e) radionuclide bone scan

2. True or false: A permeative pattern of bone destruction is consistent with a benign disease process.
   (a) true
   (b) false

3. The following lesion(s) tend to form in the epiphysis of the bone.
   (a) round cell tumors
   (b) osteosarcoma
   (c) chondroblastoma
   (d) fibrous dysplasia
   (e) aneurysmal bone cyst

4. True or false: A Codman's triangle is pathognomonic for osteogenic sarcoma.
   (a) true
   (b) false

5. Which of the following is not a characteristic radiographic finding in hyperparathyroidism:
   (a) osteopenia
   (b) subperiosteal resorption of the radial border of the phalanges
   (c) resorption of the end of the distal clavicle
   (d) salt and pepper skull
   (e) thickened cortex in the diaphysis of long bones

Answers: 1) d; 2) b; 3) c; 4) b; 5) e

Chapter 11

Anesthesia for Orthopaedic Procedures

Mark R. LoDico, MD

Outline

Due to the great strides that have been made in reducing the risk of perioperative mortality specifically attributable to the administration of anesthesia, physicians and patients fail to appreciate the risks involved in performing "just a nerve block" or simply having the patient "go off to sleep." It has been estimated that the risk of death due to anesthesia may now be as low as 1:200,000, but a more conservative estimate of 1:10,000 is generally accepted. Given an average of 24 million surgical operations per year, there may be 2400 deaths per year primarily due to anesthesia. Anesthesiologists may believe that the risk of death is near zero because, on average, 5 or 10 years of practice may result in no deaths. Nonfatal complications constitute additional risk. These include minor complications such as sore throat, nausea and vomiting, ileus, peripheral nerve injury, and dental injury, as well as major complications such as cardiac arrest, myocardial infarction, cerebrovascular accident, aspiration pneumonitis, acute renal failure, hepatitis, and hepatic necrosis. Some studies estimate the cumulative risk of anesthetic morbidity at 18% or higher.

The selection of an anesthetic technique depends upon five factors:

1. the condition of the patient,
2. the site and type of surgery to be performed,
3. the physiologic effects of the anesthetic (general vs. regional, mechanical vs. spontaneous ventilation),
4. the experience of the person administering the anesthetic (anesthesiologist-administered vs. supervised vs. unsupervised, level of skill at various techniques), and
5. the experience of the surgeon (faster vs. slower, greater vs. less blood loss, use of cement).

Selection of an anesthetic based on the above five factors will result in maximal patient safety. Care should be taken to avoid prejudicing the patient for or against a particular technique before consulting the anesthesiologist. It does not serve the patient to be led to expect a certain anesthetic technique only to be informed by the anesthesiologist that an alternative approach would bring better success. Surgical or anesthetic convenience should not play a significant role. Time pressures recently amplified by the cost restrictions of managed care and capitation should be managed over the entire hospitalization of the patient. Ten minutes saved by the induction of general anesthesia instead of allowing a peripheral nerve block to completely "set up" may be more than squandered in the operating room by the cost of additional medications and supplies, or in the recovery room by ventilatory assistance and lag time to adequate postoperative analgesia.

PREOPERATIVE EVALUATION

The goal of a preoperative evaluation is to reduce the morbidity and mortality associated with the planned surgery. Preoperative assessment identifies the need for treatment to optimize patient health perioperatively. This improves surgical outcome. Data that support this claim have been collected over four decades and repeatedly demonstrate that the patient's preoperative condition is a significant predictor of intra-operative and postoperative morbidity.

Ideally, the anesthiologist should have access to the patient far enough in advance to allow implementation of recommendations. This is facilitated by a preoperative clinic staffed by anesthesiologists. Many hospitals and outpatient surgery centers utilize this concept and find it both efficient and cost effective. The traditional arrangement of seeing the patient the night before has become an infrequent occurrence. More than 60% of all operations are performed on an outpatient basis, and up to 30% of patients are admitted as inpatients the morning of surgery. Meeting the patient for the first time in the preoperative holding area causes unnecessary delays. Given the increasing age at which surgeries are offered, and the resultant increase in associated medical problems, the evaluator is likely to require consultation or additional tests. The surgeon can prevent delays by ordering appropriate consultations and tests in advance and having the results available the day of surgery. The surgeon should develop a working relationship with the anesthesiologist to

Orthopaedic Surgery: The Essentials. Edited by M.E. Baratz, A.D. Watson, and J.E. Imbriglia. Thieme Medical Publishers, Inc., New York © 1999

learn which records, tests, or consultations are required when a patient has a complex medical history. Simply requesting "clearance for surgery" from a primary care physician or specialist managing the patient may not provide all the necessary information for a safe anesthetic.

Guidelines considering risk for patients with cardiovascular disease undergoing noncardiac surgery have been formulated. Patient factors have been stratified into minor, intermediate, and major predictors of perioperative myocardial infarction, congestive heart failure, and death. Characteristics of the surgical procedure anticipated have been stratified into low, intermediate, and high risk of perioperative fatal and nonfatal myocardial infarction. Including all the above-mentioned considerations, an algorithm has been constructed to guide cardiologists and anesthesiologists in their evaluation of the patient with known or suspected coronary artery disease. Further work-up, such as stress testing with exercise and pharmacologic agents or coronary angiography, may be requested if the patient and surgical factors predict a significant incidence of morbidity and mortality. If these risk factors aren't addressed before the patient is interviewed in the preoperative holding area, a delay of nonemergency surgery may be recommended to allow for interventions such as antidysrhythmics, antihypertensives, and even transluminal or operative angioplasty.

Cardiovascular disease must be considered within the framework of comorbid diseases. Pulmonary disease, diabetes with renal impairment, and hematologic disorders, such as anemia, polycythemia, and coagulopathies, all heighten the patient's already increased risk of cardiac complication.

Emergency surgery poses unique risks. Is the patient in a life-threatening condition that can be reduced by the surgery? Are there other conditions which require medical management before surgery, such as cardiac or pulmonary contusion, hypotension, or intra-abdominal bleeding? These may be addressed in the immediate preoperative period or even during the operation by placement of a pulmonary artery catheter, insertion of a chest tube, or peritoneal lavage.

A frequent point of misunderstanding between surgeon and anesthesiologist is the issue of NPO (nothing per orum [nothing by mouth]) status as it relates to emergency surgery. All patients undergoing elective or urgent surgery should be kept NPO for at least 6 hours, or as much of it as possible, to reduce the risk of aspiration pneumonitis. Nothing per orum reduces the volume of stomach contents by allowing the gastric emptying function to pass food and drink distal to the pyloric sphincter, into the duodenum. The two factors found to correlate with the severity of aspiration pneumonitis following vomiting are (1) volume of 25 ml or greater and (2) acidity of pH 2.5 or less. In the case of an emergency, the anesthesiologist is obligated to establish that it is the surgeon's opinion to proceed without delay to prevent the loss of life or limb, justifying the additional risk of aspiration. The patient must then be considered to have a full stomach, and measures must be taken to reduce the additional risk. The patient is asked to drink a nonparticulate antacid, such as sodium bicitrate, to increase the pH of the stomach contents. A regional anesthetic may then be performed, or if a general anesthetic is planned, an awake intubation may be used to leave the patient's own protective mechanisms intact during the airway manipulation. A rapid sequence induction may also be employed to provide the fastest time to optimal intubating conditions. Pressure on the cricoid cartilage helps to prevent passive regurgitation and omits positive pressure mask ventilation with the risk of regurgitation by insufflating gas into the stomach. An H2 blocker such as cimetidine or ranitidine can raise the pH and reduce the volume of the stomach contents. Metoclopramide has also been used to increase gastric emptying by antidopaminergic and cholinergic effects, but it requires time to produce this effect. These medications are more likely to be used in urgent situations than for emergencies.

PEARL

The risk of aspiration pneumonitis in a patient with a full stomach can be minimized by reducing the acidity of the stomach contents with sodium bicitrate or H2 blockers; reducing the volume of stomach contents with metoclopramide; or by reducing the risk of regurgitation by regional anethesia, awake intubation, or rapid sequence induction of general anesthesia.

ANESTHETIC TECHNIQUES

Neuraxis Blocks

Neuraxically applied local anesthetics produce perfect operating conditions via sensory, motor, and sympathetic blockade. Surgery on the lower extremities and procedures on the trunk are regularly performed under subarachnoid and epidural anesthesia. A subarachnoid block (SAB) often referred to as a "spinal" can reliably produce anesthesia up to a T4 dermatomal level, from an injection performed at the lumbar level below L2 where the cord ends. The duration of the block can be as little as 30 minutes or as long as 6 hours depending on the choice of local anesthetic and the dose used. Epidural anesthesia can be tailored to the level of the surgery by single injection or catheter placement in the lumbar, thoracic, and cervical levels. Analgesia is maintained for up to a week. Both neuraxial techniques involve delivering local anesthetic to the spinal cord, the former by injecting directly into the subarachnoid space, and the latter by injecting into the epidural space, relying on transdural passage to the cord.

Advantages of both subarachnoid and epidural blocks include superior postoperative pain relief by both preemptive analgesia and continuous infusions, avoidance of airway manipulation and it's risk of aspiration and other pulmonary complications, and obliteration of the stress response elicited by surgery which inhibits wound healing. The neuroendocrine and metabolic stress responses are mediated by hormones and other humoral factors that produce increased catabolism, hyperglycemia, and sodium and water retention. General anesthesia does not prevent the afferent input from reaching the hypothalamus and therefore results in pituitary initiation of the catabolic cascade. Local anesthetics block these afferent fibers at the spinal cord level. Neuraxial blockade can also decrease the patients risk for nausea and vomiting by avoiding the higher doses of certain drugs necessary for general anesthesia. Several studies have demonstrated a 50% reduction in thromboembolic complications in the lower extremities of patients receiving a neuraxial block for total hip arthroplasty, as well as reductions in blood loss. The mechanism is likely the combined effects of individually documented physiologic changes in blood flow, vessel walls, and coagulation/fibrinolysis.

Despite the many advantages and safety of neuraxial anesthesia, patients frequently express fear over the prospect of receiving a needle in the spine. Patients can be given perspective by informing them of the large number of surgeries performed safely under neuraxial blockade today. Patients also express concern about lying awake, staring at the ceiling, while listening to hammering and drilling. They can be reassured by advising them that they will be sedated and will likely fall asleep without anxiety and remember little.

Historically, subarachnoid blocks carried a relatively high risk for postdural puncture headaches. When it was found that dural puncture could be avoided by injecting a larger dose of local anesthetic into the epidural space, this newer technique became quite popular. Development of thinner, fiber splitting spinal needles has decreased the incidence of postdural puncture headaches to about 1%.

Epidurals require a period of 15 to 30 minutes to produce the dense sensory blockade necessary for surgical anesthesia compared to the almost immediate onset of subarachnoid blocks. Anesthesiologists initially saw this as an advantage because the slower onset provided a greater opportunity to administer drugs and fluids necessary to compensate for the hypotension associated with the accompanying sympathectomy. In practice, the rate, severity, and time to successful compensation of hypotension are no different. Severe hypotension can be prevented by the administration of fluids and medications.

Contraindications to subarachnoid and epidural techniques relate to the injection site and the physiologic effects of the block. Infection at the site of injection, gross coagulopathy, and uncorrected hypovolemia are therefore the obvious absolute contraindications. Increased intracranial pressure must also be included because it leaves the medullary vasomotor and respiratory centers vulnerable to herniation if the spinal pressure is released. Relative contraindications include congenital or surgical deformities of the spine at the site of injection, minor coagulation abnormalities, including "mini dose" heparin, and failure to place the needle after multiple attempts.

Extremity Blocks

Due to improvements made in the safety and efficacy of general anesthetic techniques in the 1940s and 1950s, the use of regional techniques waned as anesthesiologists sought a simplified approach to extremity surgery. Today, plexus and peripheral nerve blockade enjoy a rejuvenation, facilitated by studies documenting their benefits. Surgeons performing reimplantations or neurovascular repairs are aware of the improved blood flow and prophylaxis against pain provided by regional techniques, and they typically request prolonged plexus blocks and catheter infusions for continuous postoperative analgesia and sympathectomy. Regional anesthesia limits the anesthetic to the area of surgery leaving other vital centers intact. This places less stress on the high risk patient. Other advantages include early ambulation, reduced risk of aspiration in patients with a full stomach, decreased nursing demands, and operating conditions tailored to a surgeon's requirements. In addition, by weakening the motor block, the patient can cooperate with specific movements; or complete paralysis can be produced. Patients with rheumatoid arthritis benefit from regional anesthesia by maintaining consciousness and monitoring their own position. This helps prevent neuropraxias, joint injury, and other complications of positioning in this high risk group. Regional techniques are usually supplemented with some level of sedation, titrated to individual patient requirements.

One technical consideration in performing regional blocks is "eliciting a paresthesia." Many regional techniques require this to reliably produce adequate anesthesia, but there is a small risk of nerve injury associated with it. Nerve damage can be minimized by using a short bevel needle, which is less likely to sever the nerve fibers. The short bevel needle is also more likely to prevent intraneural placement by both pushing the nerve ahead of it and producing a paresthesia before entering the nerve. Damage by inadvertent intraneural injection can be avoided by recognizing the signs of intraneural needle placement: inability to easily inject the local anesthetic and excruciating pain with each attempt to inject. This is easily distinguished from the pressure paresthesia produced by perineural injection. This necessitates a conscious, albeit a sedated and amnestic patient.

Anesthesia of the upper extremity can be produced by injection of local anesthetic into the brachial plexus, the peripheral nerves, and the cervical plexus. The most common of these is the axillary block. The brachial plexus is formed by the anterior primary rami of C5 through T1 with an occasional contribution from C4. When injected from the axillary approach, the plexus has already formed the median, radial, and ulnar nerves. The needle can be redirected to reach the musculocutaneous nerve in the belly of the coracobrachialis and subcutaneously to block the intercostobrachial and medial antebrachial cutaneous nerves, allowing for surgery on the radial aspect of the forearm and application of a tourniquet above the elbow. A Bier block produces a similar distribution of anesthesia by intravenous injection into an exsanguinated arm.

The interscalene approach to the brachial plexus produces anesthesia of the proximal arm and shoulder by a more proximal spread to the roots of not only the brachial plexus, but also those of the cervical plexus, C2 to C4. This block is particularly advantageous for patients undergoing shoulder surgery and those who are unable to abduct their arm for an axillary approach. The lower roots are occasionally spared, but the ulnar nerve can be blocked with a supplemental injection at the elbow. If surgery is limited to one or two peripheral nerve distributions such as a finger or palmar aspect of the hand, these may be injected individually. A note of caution: Epinephrine containing solutions should never be used for digital nerve blockade owing to vasoconstriction and subsequent prolonged ischemia.

There is far less enthusiasm for plexus and peripheral nerve blocks of the lower extremity due to the frequent need to inject at more than one site and the availability of the simpler neuraxial blocks. Nevertheless, patients who have contraindications to a neuraxial block may be candidates for regional anesthesia. The nerve supply to the lower extremity is composed of the lumbar and sacral plexuses, L1 to L4 and L4 to S3, respectively. Owing to the lack of a good approach to the sacral plexus and the accessibility of the sciatic nerve, which receives the bulk of it, the lower extremity is best anesthetized by a combination of a lumbar plexus and a sciatic nerve block. The lumbar plexus is reached by injecting a 30 ml volume of local anesthetic into the femoral neurovascular bundle at the level of the inguinal ligament while maintaining distal pressure to force flow proximally to the lumbar roots. The sciatic nerve can be approached anteriorly at the level of the lesser trochanter. A needle is advanced to the femur and walked off medially until a paresthesia is obtained. The sciatic nerve may also be approached posteriorly with the patient in a lithotomy or prone position. The anterior and lithotomy approaches are convenient when combining this block with a femoral paravascular injection since the patient is already in the supine position. This combination has resulted in excellent anesthesia for total knee arthroplasties and surgery on the lower leg.

Although peripheral nerves can be injected at many levels of the lower extremity, such as the tibial and common peroneal at the level of the knee, the ankle block is the only other commonly used regional technique of the leg. This entails infiltrating local anesthetic around the terminal branches of the sciatic nerve, the posterior tibial, the deep and superficial peroneal, and the sural nerves, and the termination of the femoral nerve, the saphenous. These are individually injected in the same cross-sectional plane immediately superior to the malleoli.

General Anesthesia

General anesthesia is an option for most patients and surgical procedures. The patient is induced into unconsciousness and provided with agents that render him analgesic, immobile, amnestic, and hemodynamically stable. Any one of these parameters may be difficult to manage in a particular patient and may limit the overall effectiveness of a general anesthetic. The patient must be continuously monitored to assure maintenance of hemodynamic stability since anesthetic agents can induce hypotension. The airway usually requires support and may be manipulated and protected with a device, most commonly an endotracheal tube. Many patients and physicians perceive general anesthesia as simply a state of sleep from which one awakens easily, and they fail to recognize the complexity of physiologic effects and the management required to provide this type of anesthetic safely and effectively.

INTRA-OPERATIVE CONSIDERATIONS

Blood transfusions continue to be a significant consideration during major orthopaedic procedures. There is considerable debate as to what amount of intra-operative blood loss can be tolerated by patients of various ages and conditions. In healthy patients undergoing elective surgery such as joint replacement, some studies suggest hemoglobin concentrations as low as 5 or 6 mg/dL are tolerable and safe. Preoperative donation of the patients own blood, hemodilution, induced hypotension, and cell savers can reduce the need for transfusion. Orthopaedic procedures that result in significant blood loss and massive fluid shifts require close, usually invasive, hemodynamic monitoring.

The use of methyl methacrylate has resulted in hypotension, cardiac arrest, and death. The mechanism of action is thought to be the toxic effects of the methyl methacrylate monomer. Insertion of a prosthesis into the femoral canal may produce pulmonary emboli of air and fat, introduced into the blood by the pressure gradient produced during the insertion of the femoral component.

POSTOPERATIVE PAIN

Treatment of postoperative pain is provided to relieve suffering and to reduce the neuroendocrine, metabolic, and autonomic effects of the surgical stresses induced by nociception, which interfere with safe and efficient recovery of organ systems. These include pulmonary, cardiovascular, gastrointestinal, and urinary dysfunction, as well as muscle metabolism, immunosuppression, and interference with would healing. Immune system suppression induced by surgical stress may be prevented by epidural analgesia, which has been shown to improve monocyte chemotaxis and lytic function during hip surgery. Most physicians treat postoperative pain in the recovery room and thereafter, but the pain and its consequences can be addressed more effectively beforehand. Surgical stimulation causes release of algesic substances such as prostaglandins, histamine, serotonin, bradykinin, and substance P, which generate afferent impulses transduced by nociceptors and transmitted by A-delta and C nerve fibers to the neuraxis where a complex system of modulation occurs. A sensitization occurs at the spinal cord level and higher that result in a functional change, sometimes called "wind up" of the central nervous system. Regional anesthesia, neuraxial opioids, and even systemic opioids and nonsteroidals administered prior to surgery can prevent this and have been reported to reduce postoperative pain for up to 10 days. This decrease in sensitization may explain the apparent decreased incidence of phantom limb pain in patients who have undergone amputation under neuraxial anesthesia.

Local infiltration of the surgical site and neural blockade may be continued into the postoperative period for safe and effective analgesia. Long-acting local anesthetics and vasoconstrictors around a peripheral nerve or plexus can produce total analgesia for up to 24 hours after a single injection. In outpatient surgery, a local anesthetic is frequently chosen considering the duration of the surgery alone with an aim to reduce recovery room time. Many hospitals and outpatient surgery centers have a policy of discharging patients only after complete resolution of the block. Selected patients have successfully managed an anesthetized limb for a few hours at home and were able to benefit from the 24 hours of analgesia because of a longer acting agent. For the hospitalized patient, constant infusions and intermittent boluses via catheters in the brachial plexus, lumbar plexus, and epidural spaces have also provided complete comfort, and sympathetic blockade when desirable, as with nerve and vascular repair. Neuraxially applied opioids in single shot spinals have kept patients pain free for up to 24 hours. Opiods injected epidurally, alone and in combination with dilute local anesthetics, have facilitated continuous passive range of motion following knee arthroplasty, enabled early ambulation, improved bowel function, and reduced pulmonary complications. Severe respiratory depression is an infrequent but dangerous complication of neuraxially applied opioids. This requires close postoperative observation. With protocols for monitoring respiratory depression, neuraxial narcotics can be provided on orthopaedic wards. Ventilatory rate alone may not be sensitive enough to monitor for hypercarbia and hypoxemia. Level of consciousness should also be assessed, and any patient who becomes obtunded should be considered in respiratory distress until proven otherwise and treated appropriately. Equipment to support ventilation should be kept on the ward for these occurrences and the opiod antagonist naloxone should be kept at the bedside.

In the past, postoperative pain was addressed with intermittent boluses of systemically administered opioids. Concerns over adverse effects such as respiratory depression, sedation, abuse, and urinary retention often limited the use of opiods and resulted in inadequate pain control. Advances in the administration of systemic opioids culminated in patient-controlled analgesia (PCA), where the patient controls the titratation of small doses of opioids administered intravenously to meet analgesic needs. This system allows the matching of medication intake to pain. This analgesic regimen is simple and has been used successfully in patients as young as 5 years old. The concept of a "therapeutic blood level" is a dynamic one and is not likely to be achieved by a bolus dose at fixed intervals or a constant infusion. A programmable pump is used to provide safeguards such as dose and interval limits. When this system fails to provide enough medication for analgesia, it is usually due to the use of limits arbitrarily arrived at and ordered by the inexperienced physician who adheres to doses he or she believes "should take care of the pain." Dose-response curves that demonstrate the pharmacokinetics and pharmacodynamics of opioids in individual patients vary as much as seven fold. These observations have lead to the tailoring of PCA dosing, which requires that the physician continually reassess the analgesic requirement and take cues from the patient. There is no rationale for avoiding an increase in the medication out of concern for abuse by the patient. The postoperative patient in pain is at no particular risk for new onset addiction or exacerbation of an addictive disorder. In fact, in patients with a history of substance abuse inadequate analgesia may create drug craving for pain relief, anxiety, frustration, and anger, all of which feed addiction. The issue is frequently encountered on the orthopaedic service, as the prevalence of addictive disease is 40 to 60% in trauma patients. Even patients with no history of addiction who experience fear and anxiety may attempt, and usually fail, to treat this "pain" with PCA. Careful assessment of the patient will reveal such mislabeling and the physician can guide treatment with reassurance and benzodiazepines.

Combining analgesic regimen has the potential to take advantage of additive and synergistic effects and thereby reduce individual doses and their dose-dependent side effects. Nonsteroidal anti-inflammatory drugs in combination with systemic opioids provide superior analgesia and reduce the opioid requirement and its side effects. Nonsteroidal anti-inflammatory drugs have also been combined with epidural infusions of local anesthetic and opioids with greater efficiency than either regimen alone.

SELECTED BIBLIOGRAPHY

American College of Cardiology and American Heart Association Task Force. ACC/AHA guidelines for perioperative cardiovascular evaluation for noncardiac surgery. *J Circulation*. 1996; 93:1280–1317.

BRIDENBAUGH LD. The upper extremity: Somatic blockade. In: Cousins MJ, Bridenbaugh LD, eds. *Neural Blockade in Clinical Anesthesia and Management of Pain*. Philadelphia, PA: Lippincott; 1988:387–416.

BRIDENBAUGH PO, GREENE NM. Spinal (subarachnoid) neural blockade. In: Cousins MJ, Bridenbaugh LD, eds. *Neural Blockade in Clinical Anesthesia and Management of Pain*. Philadelphia, PA: Lippincott; 1988:213–251.

BROWN DL. Spinal, epidural, and caudal anesthesia. In: Miller R, ed. *Anesthesia*. New York, NY: Churchhill Livingstone; 1994:1505–1533.

COUSINS MJ, BROMAGE PR. Epidural neural blockade. In: Cousins MJ, Bridenbaugh LD, eds. *Neural Blockade in Clinical Anesthesia and Management of Pain*. Philadelphia, PA: Lippincott; 1988:253–360.

GIBBS CP, MODELL JH. Pulmonary aspiration of gastric contents: Pathophysiology, prevention, and management. In:

Miller R, ed. *Anesthesia*. New York, NY: Churchhill Livingstone; 1994:1437–1464.

GREENE NM. Anesthesia. In: Schwartz S, ed. *Principles of Surgery*. New York, NY: McGraw-Hill; 1984:435–453.

KATZ J. *Atlas of Regional Anesthesia*. Dorwalk, CT: Appleton-Lange; 1985.

KEHLET H. Modification of responses to surgery by neural blockade: Clinical implications. In: Cousins MJ, Bridenbaugh LD, eds. *Neural Blockade in Clinical Anesthesia and Management of Pain*. Philadelphia, PA: Lippincott; 1988: 145–188.

KEHLET H. The value of "multimodal" or "balanced analgesia" in postoperative pain treatment. *J Anesth Analg*. 1993;77:1048–1056.

READY LB. Acute postoperative pain. In: Miller ed. *Anesthesia*. New York, NY: Churchhill Livingstone, 1994: 2327–2341.

ROIZEN MF. Preoperative evaluation. In: Miller R, ed. *Anesthesia*. New York, NY: Churchhill Livingstone; 1994: 827–882.

ROSS AF, TINKER JH. Anesthesia risk. In:Miller R, ed. *Anesthesia*. New York, NY: Churchhill Livingstone; 1994: 791–825.

SAVAGE S. Treatment of acute pain, cancer pain, and chronic pain in addiction. In: Miller N, ed. *Principles of Addiction* *Medicine*. Washington, DC: American Society of Addiction Medicine; 1994.

SAMPLE QUESTIONS

1. The convention of keeping the patient NPO for at least six hours reduces the risk of aspiration pneumonitis by which mechanism(s):
   (a) reducing gastric acidity
   (b) reducing gastric volume
   (c) reduces nausea and vomiting
   (d) a and b
   (e) all of the above

2. Benefits of neuraxial (subarachnoid or epidural) blocks for lower extremity surgery include:
   (a) reduced blood loss
   (b) reduced thromboembolic risk
   (c) prevention of catabolic cascade
   (d) a and b
   (e) all of the above

3. Signs of intraneural needle placement during peripheral nerve blockades include:
   (a) resistance to injecting
   (b) pain during needle placement
   (c) parasthesia while injecting
   (d) a and b
   (e) all of the above

4. True statements about opioids include:
   (a) interpatient differences in dose-response curves may be as high as sevenfold
   (b) addiction risk in the immediate postoperative period is very low
   (c) epidural opioids and local anesthetics produce decreased bowel function
   (d) a and b
   (e) all of the above

5. Inadequately treated postoperative pain results in:
   (a) no change in pulmonary complications
   (b) no change in bowel function
   (c) inhibition of wound healing
   (d) a and b
   (e) all of the above

Answers: 1) b; 2) e; 3) a; 4) d; 5) c

Trauma

Chapter 12

Approach
to Multiply Injured Patients

Michael A. Miranda, MD and Kelly L. Welsh, RN

Orthopaedic management of the polytrauma patient is performed "to protect the patient from systemic problems—not to promote fracture healing." Sigvard Hansen, 1991

Careful orthopaedic management will positively impact both the short and long term outcome of the trauma patient. The orthopaedist managing multitrauma patients should focus on assisting the trauma team in the prevention of parenchymal damage to tissues. Conceptually, this transcends fracture care and is best done within the context of a trauma center. This chapter will review the issues surrounding the care of the trauma patient.

INITIAL MANAGEMENT

The key to initial care of injuries is treatment in the order of their life-threatening potential. The priorities in management have been established by the American College of Surgeons and have been characterized by the acronym of ABCs: Airway, Breathing, and Circulation.

Airway

Irreversible brain injury can occur after 3 minutes of anoxia. Therefore, the first priority in management is to ensure an open airway, adequate ventilation, and oxygenation. Airway management should be performed with the assumption of a cervical spine injury. While maintaining the head in neutral position, a jaw thrust and chin lift should be performed. Mechanical clearance of the oropharynx is often necessary in establishing an airway. Should the airway need to be cleared a full log roll position should be performed. With insertion of a nasal or oropharyngeal airway, a clear passageway can be maintained. Should this fail to establish an airway, endotracheal intubation should be performed. Indications for intubation are listed in Table 12–1. In the patient with documented cervical spine injury, nasotracheal intubation should be considered. In a patient with facial trauma, nasotracheal intubation should be avoided. In a patient with the unfortunate combination of C-spine and facial injuries, fiberoptic techniques are available. Ultimately, if these techniques fail in obtaining direct control of the airway, cricothyroidotomy should be performed.

Breathing

Once an airway is established, ventilating the patient is the next priority. High-flow oxygen (10L/min) should be administered with mechanical ventilation if necessary. Arterial blood gases and a pulse oximeter will help assess the quality of ventilation. Agitation is a sign of hypoxia while obtundation is a sign of hypercarbia. Failure to oxygenate should prompt observation and auscultation (look and listen) of neck and chest for venous distention, tracheal deviation, paradoxical chest movement, and unilateral breath sounds. These findings can be seen with the three most common causes of failure to oxygenate in the trauma patient: tension pneumothorax, open pneumothorax, and a flail chest. Rapid treatment with large bore catheter in the fifth intercostal space on the side of decreased breath sounds will eliminate the tension pneumothorax. This should be further treated with a

TABLE 12–1 Indications for Intubation

Inadequate or Labored Ventilation
Flail Chest
Unconscious Patient
Multiple Facial Fractures
Deteriorating Blood Oxygenation
Multitrauma
Pulmonary Contusion

Orthopaedic Surgery: The Essentials. Edited by M.E. Baratz, A.D. Watson, and J.E. Imbriglia. Thieme Medical Publishers, Inc., New York © 1999

chest tube on the affected side. Placement of an occlusive dressing over the open pneumothorax will aid in the restoration of negative intrathorax pressure and allow lung expansion. A flail chest should be treated with positive pressure ventilary support and judicious fluid resuscitation to avoid overhydration.

Circulation

Hypotension in the multiply traumatized patient is usually due to blood loss. Rapid establishment of two large bore intravenous catheters and fluid challenge of Ringer's lactate (2-L in adults; 30 mL/kg in children) should be the first response. Hemorrhage from open wounds should be controlled by direct pressure. Tissue perfusion can be evaluated by urine output and by capillary refill in the fingertips. More than 2 seconds to refill the fingertip indicates poor perfusion.

If the hypotension responds to the initial challenge, crystalloid should be maintained until fully matched type-specific blood is available. If little or no response is seen, a further 2-L challenge is given. Then, type specific or noncrossmatched universal donor O negative blood should be given immediately. Vasopressors should not be employed in hypovolemic shock.

PEARL

Hypotension and tachycardia are present after a 30 to 40% loss of blood volume.

Hemorrhage classification can aid in estimating blood loss. There are four classes of hemorrhage (Table 12–2). Class I indicates less than 15% loss, approximately 800 mL. These patients are usually asymptomatic. Class II represents a 15 to 30% loss or 800 to 1500 mL. Tachycardia as well as slow capillary refill can be noted. One can also appreciate slight decrease in urinary output. Class III hemorrhage represents 30 to 40% loss of circulating blood volume and results in hypotension and tachycardia. Tachypnea may also be appreciated. Class IV represents greater than 40% loss of circulating blood with profound hypotension, marked tachycardia, and extremis.

In the trauma patient, blood pressure may be gauged by evaluation of the radial pulse which, if present, represents roughly 80 mm Hg. The more central femoral pulse represents 70 mm Hg and if only the carotid pulse is palpable, 60 mm Hg of systolic blood pressure is present. Delayed capillary refill at the nail bed for more than 2 seconds is indicative of hypotension. More specific monitoring methods require a Foley catheter to monitor urine output (>30 mL/hr) and an arterial line for evaluation of mean arterial pressure. Assuming traumatic hypovolemia, these will gauge fluid status. This may be confirmed by central venous catheters showing pressure measure units less than 5 mLH$_2$O.

PEARL

If a radial pulse is palpable the injured patient has a systolic pressure of at least 80 mm Hg. With a palpable carotid pulse the systolic pressure is at least 60 mm Hg.

Failure to control hypotension may be combated by application of medical anti-shock trousers (MAST) in the extreme situation. It is notable that increased periods of hypovolemic shock are associated with increased rates of adult respiratory distress syndrome (ARDS) and increased infection rates. Class III and IV hemorrhage are also associated with increased coagulopathy.

Neurologic Injury

Evaluation for neurologic injury should begin with prompt neurologic examination. Assessment of the patient's level of consciousness, papillary response, sensation, and motor activity in extremities are essential. Performance of Glasgow coma scale will provide a measure of neurologic disability and predicted recovery. (Table 12–3)

FURTHER EVALUATION

Evaluation, throughout this process, should be performed by electrocardiogram monitoring of the heart as well as radiographic evaluation of the cervical spine, chest, and pelvis.

Following stabilization of the patient, a thorough physical exam should be performed. Throughout this entire process, great care should be made to avoid decreasing core temperature. Hypothermia can cause arrhythmias, coagulopathies, and acid-base abnormalities. Hypothermia is best treated by prevention, however, rapid rewarming with warmed intravenous fluids, heated respiratory gases and external warming devices are indicated in the hypothermic patient.

Prior to transport of the patient for further diagnostic or treatment measures, appropriate splinting of extremity fractures should be performed.

TABLE 12–2   Hemorrhage

	Loss (%)	Loss (mL)	Symptoms
Class I	<15	<800	0
Class II	15-25	800–1500	tachycardia, slight hypotension
Class III	25-35	1500–2500	tachycardia, hypotension, tachypnea
Class IV	>40	>2500	extremis, profound hypotension

TABLE 12–3 Glasgow coma scale

Eye Opening	
Spontaneous	4
To command	3
To pain	2
Nil	1
Best Motor Response	
Obeys	6
Localizes	5
Withdraws	4
Flexion	3
Extension	2
Nil	1
Verbal Response	
Oriented	5
Confused	4
Inappropriate	3
Incomprehensible	2
Nil	1

TREATMENT

Five phases of care for the multiply injured patient have been identified by Ruedi et al (1985).

1. resuscitation
2. emergency procedures
3. stabilization
4. delayed operative procedures
5. rehabilitation

We have briefly discussed resuscitation. Adjunctive diagnostic studies in a stable patient may include head and abdominal computed tomography to rule out occult injuries. In the unstable patient, failure of resuscitation would demand immediate or life-saving operations. Note that in the trauma patient, hypovolemic shock is assumed. Other causes of shock include cardiogenic shock (pump failure), neurogenic shock, and sepsis. Prior to transport to the operating room, these should be considered. If a hemothorax is noted on chest tube placement, thoracotomy for aortic, vena cava, or pulmonary vessel injuries would be indicated. Laparotomy after positive diagnostic peritoneal lavage may address splenic, liver, or possibly renal parenchymal injuries. Neurosurgical attention for ongoing mass lesions or depressed skull fractures would also be indicated during this phase.

Stabilization of pelvic fractures may be indicated in the face of ongoing hypotension. Strong consideration for fixation of femoral shaft fractures should be given during this initial anesthesia. In the literature, there is sufficient evidence to indicate that prompt stabilization of the pelvis and femur can decrease damage to pulmonary as well as other parenchymal tissues.

At this critical stage of treatment, knowledge of the patient's age, injury severity and premorbid medical condition will help in prioritizing management. The injury severity score and other scoring systems such as the mangled extremity severity score (MESS) may help in identifying treatment algorithms for patients.

Stabilization

This phase is a natural extension of the resuscitation phase with the goal of stable hemodynamics and adequate organ profusion. Preparation of the patient for further operative intervention usually requires placement of central venous catheters, including triple lumens, for monitoring pulmonary artery capillary wedge pressures and cardiac output. The early use of positive end expiratory pressure mechanical ventilation is helpful in preventing pulmonary failure.

In the traumatic setting, bleeding disorders are uniformly due to hemodilution. For every 8 to 10 units of blood transfused, 6 units of platelets should be administered. Fresh frozen plasma use should be limited to prolonged prothrombin time and partial thromboplastin times. Adequate resuscitation and stabilization have been realized when normal cardiac output, normal mixed venous oxygen, and normal A-a gradient is established. Other considerations prior to proceeding with delayed procedures (4–24 hr(s) post injury) include a stable neurologic condition and assurance of normal clotting mechanism.

Operative treatment of major fractures in patients with severe head injuries remains a hotly debated area. Hofman and Goris (1991) retrospectively reviewed 58 patients with a Glasgow coma scale rating of less than 7 and found no negative influence on mortality or outcome in the patients who had aggressive early fixation of their fractures. Chapman (1992) has proposed a reasonable algorithm: In the patient with a head injury who has a focal lesion, neurosurgery should decompress first, followed by orthopaedic stabilization of the long bone fractures, open fractures, and dislocations. In patients with diffuse head injury, treatment with hyperventilation and intracranial monitoring for prompt recognition of a diffuse process localizing or lateralizing is reasonable. Given that 31% of patients with severe head injuries (Glasgow coma scale < 10) have a major skeletal injury, as well as the fact that early stabilization of fractures clearly benefits the patient's overall well being, prompt stabilization of this severe subset of musculoskeletal injuries is indicated.

Long Bone Management

Early stabilization of long bone fractures in the multitraumatized patient has been studied extensively. Riska and Myllymen (1982) found an 18% reduction in fat emboli in operative versus nonoperatively treated patients. Riska and Myllymen went on to change their protocol to include early stabilization in these multitraumatized patients and found the fat emboli rate decreased to 1.4%. Goris et al (1982) retrospectively studied 58 patients, all of whom received positive end expiratory pressure ventilation, and compared those stabilized by early fixation and those stabilized late. With age and injury severity score controlled, Gore et al found that mortality reduced by 45% and ARDS dropped from 82%

down to 26%. Johnson et al (1985) retrospectively reviewed a series of 132 patients with 511 fractures. All patients had an injury severity score greater than 18. Using a stepwise logistical regression analysis, the researchers found that early stabilization versus the late stabilization resulted in a 5-fold difference in the incidence of ARDS. The most convincing study comes from Bone et al (1989), who performed a prospective study with randomization of multiple trauma patients into early versus late groups and compared data with isolated femur fractures. Bone and his colleagues found that the group stabilized late had an increased number of days on the ventilator; increased intensive care unit stay; increased hospital stay; and increased rate of ARDS, as well as other pulmonary complications, 6 and 19-fold, respectively. There was also a significant cost savings for the early treatment group. Given this data, it is clear that long bone stabilization has a significant enough impact on overall morbidity and mortality that unless the patient is in extremis, femur fractures should be stabilized during the initial anesthetic.

The method of stabilization depends on the circumstances and the surgeon's experience. The vast majority of patients can and should be stabilized with reamed, locked intramedullary nails. Worldwide experience has shown a union rate greater than 95% with an extremely low infection rate. Recent concerns have been raised about employing a reamed technique in the patient with a pulmonary injury. In this small subset of patients, unreamed techniques or plate fixation may be employed safely. In grade III open femur fractures, external fixation would be the initial procedure of choice with repeated debridement and early exchange with an intramedullary nail.

Pelvic Fracture Management

Pelvic fractures have a 10% mortality rate. Riemer et al (1994) demonstrated that early stabilization of pelvic fractures in the multitrauma patient decreases mortality. In general, emergent treatment of pelvic fractures reflects on two issues: that of hemodynamic instability and ease of transport. These may both be addressed by application of the two-pin external fixators "resuscitation frame" or newer devices, which are called pelvic "clamps." These second-generation external fixators, either the Ganz antishock clamp (Synthes, Paoli, PA) or Browner's pelvic stabilizer (Ace Medical; Los Angeles, CA) have been shown in preliminary studies to close down the pelvic ring and decrease blood requirements. The relative ease of application makes them ideal for use in the emergency department. Delayed internal fixation and substitution for the pelvic external fixation may be performed when the patient is more stable. Should application of the clamp or external fixator fail to control hemorrhage, angiography should be considered. Slatis et al (1972) have shown that the majority of hemorrhage emanates from low pressure bleeding in the posterior aspect of the pelvis. Arterial involvement occurs roughly 10% of the time. In recognition of this, angiography in the hemodynamically unstable patient without prior application of external fixation is strongly discouraged.

In the acute setting, application of external fixation in treatment of pelvic fractures is limited to the following indications: (1) hemodynamically unstable patient with a pelvic ring disruption, (2) the rotationally unstable pelvis, (3) in conjunction with traction for the vertically unstable pelvis.

The surgeon treating multiply traumatized patients should be aware of the Young classification. Its importance in predicting associated injuries has been established. It also provides a predictive index for resuscitative requirements. This information helps in minimizing morbidity and mortality.

The Young classification is a modification of the original Pennal classification. It is modified so as to include subsets as well as a combined mechanism category. Dalal et al (1989) found that with lateral compression injuries, a high incidence of brain and visceral injuries were found. Shock was not as common in lateral compression injuries as it was in anterior and posterior compression injuries. Anterior and posterior compression injuries have increased incidence of shock, sepsis, ARDS and death, in direct proportion to the severity of the fracture. Volume requirements directly reflected the severity of the anterior and posterior injuries. A review of this paper is recommended to the reader.

Open Fracture Mangement

The goal of open fracture management is prevention of infection promoting, fracture healing, and restoring of function. Fracture stabilization is a priority because it facilitates healing of both bone and soft tissues. The classification of open fractures established by Gustilo et al (1990) is commonly used (Table 12–4).

Open fractures are surgical emergencies. Emergency department treatment should include application of sterile bandages with minimal wound exploration until the patient is in the operating room. This approach has decreased infection rates three- to four-fold. Administration of first generation cephalosporins are indicated in Gustilo types I and II. Aminoglycosides can be added in grade III fractures. For farm injuries, 4 to 5 million units of penicillin G is administered at 4- to 6-hour intervals.

Antibiotics should be maintained for 72 hours. After 72 hours, the antibiotics should be discontinued or adjusted so as to match culture results. Treatment with tetanus toxoid is the best method to avoid clostridial infections.

Prompt stabilization and meticulous debridements are the keys to operative management. To paraphrase Gustilo, et al (1990) the type of device employed for stabilization is indicated by the anatomic site, the wound, the degree of comminution and the expertise of the surgeon. Repeat debridements are usually necessary in type II and type III fractures.

External fixators have become standard for treating severe open fractures. In less severe fractures, their use has been less frequent due to advances with other techniques. When properly applied, external fixators allow for rapid immobilization of fracture fragments and may be applied at varying distances to the wound without harming the soft tissues. One can anticipate 30 to 40% of patients will develop pin-tract infections. Bach and Hansen (1989) found that external fixators have a higher malunion rate when compared with plates. Thus, in fractures with minimal soft tissue injuries, other devices may be employed with less complications. Late exchange of an external fixator for an intramedullary device has been noted to have a high infection rate. By nailing within 30 days of the

TABLE 12–4 Classification of open fractures

Type	Wound Size	Energy	Bone Injury
Grade I	<1 cm inside out	Low	Simple
Grade II	>1 cm	Minimal–Moderate	Min Comminution
Grade III	>1 cm Extensive soft tissue swelling		
Grade IIIA	>1 cm Adequate bone covering	High	Comminuted/ Segmental
Grade IIIB	>1 cm Periosteal stripping Contamination	High	Comminuted/ Segmental
Grade IIIC	Requires vascular repair		

initial injury in patients without evidence of soft tissue pin-tract infection, a low infection rate can be achieved. The use of perioperative antibiotics is also mandated.

The use of plates in upper extremity open fractures has been shown to have acceptable infection rates. This has not been the case in the lower extremity where Bach and Hansen (1989) found an increased infection rate (35% vs. 13%) as well as an increased osteomyelitis rate (19% vs. 3%) when comparing plating with external fixation. Plate fixation for low extremity fractures is best reserved for metaphyseal and intra-articular fractures.

Intramedullary nailing of grades I, II, and III-A open fractures has been noted to have acceptable infection rates. Using unreamed nails with an interlocking technique allow for excellent wound access, early mobilization, and decreased problems with malunion. Reimer et al (1993) noted a 30 to 35% re-operation rate using locked unreamed nails in open tibia fractures. This may be addressed by early dynamization and bone grafting in the rehabilitation phase of management.

Soft tissue coverage of open fractures is key to maintaining a sterile environment. Delayed primary closure is feasible for most grade I, II and some grade III-A open wounds. In grade III-B and III-C fractures, microvascular free flaps or rotational flaps may be employed. Whenever possible, open fractures should be covered within a week before the wound is colonized with bacteria. Split-thickness skin grafts are ideal for covering large skin defects or for covering viable tissue such as muscle.

Compartmental Syndrome

Compartmental syndrome occurs when interstitial pressure rises above that of the capillary bed. Local ischemia of nervous and muscle tissue then occurs. Prolonged ischemia ultimately results in necrosis. Compartmental syndrome usually develops over a period of several hours and may not be present on patient arrival to the trauma center. It can occur as a result of closed or open fractures, the use of MAST, or in a delayed fashion after crush injuries or restoration of blood

flow to a previously ischemic extremity. The signs and symptoms are pain on passive stretch of the involved muscles and marked swelling. Delayed signs are that of decreased sensation, weakness, or paralysis. It is notable that the presence or absence of pulses distally will not aid in the diagnosis. While intercompartmental measurements greater than 35 to 45 mm Hg suggest impaired capillary blood flow, the diagnosis is a clinical one, made by history and physical exam. In the multitrauma patient who is often head-injured or chemically obtunded, a high index of suspicion should be maintained and prompt fasciotomies should be performed.

Spinal fractures

Multiply injured patients with head injuries should be assumed to have a spine fracture until proven otherwise. Cervical collars and backboards should be employed for transport. Initial screening exam should include a lateral cervical spine radiograph to the C7-T1 interspace. For the thoracic and lumbar spine, a lateral radiograph will be adequate for 85% of fractures. The patient should be logrolled until the spine has been fully cleared.

The patient with a spinal cord injury will require increased fluid replacement due to autonomic dysreflexia. Prompt neurosurgical consultation should be performed.

For those patients with spine injuries, use of rotokinetic beds can be helpful in maintaining skin integrity. General principles of treatment of spine fractures reflect, for the large part, those of long bones. Early stabilization facilitates mobilization and a timely rehabilitation. In the incomplete spinal lesion, the use of corticosteroids and early fusion is generally endorsed.

Operative Management

In the multitraumatized patient, rapid management of orthopaedic issues is required. Chapman (1992) encourages the following general principles: routine placement of patients on radiolucent tables; liberal use of fluoroscopy; use of double or triple teams; use of separate surgical set-ups, and use of cell saver or tourniquets to minimize blood loss. The surgical team should avoid cross contamination, preoperatively plan with the entire team and most importantly, simplify the procedure as much as possible.

SELECTED BIBLIOGRAPHY

American College of Surgeons. *Advanced Trauma Life Support Manual.* 5th ed. Chicago, IL: American College of Surgeons; 1993.

Bach AW. Hansen ST Jr. Plates versus external fixation in severe open tibial shaft fractures. A randomized trial. *Clinical Orthopaedics and Related Research.* 1989;(241):89–94.

Baker SP. O'Neill B. Haddon W Jr. Long WB. The injury severity score: a method for describing patients with multiple injuries and evaluating emergency care. *Journal of Trauma.* 1974;14(3):187–96.

Bone L, Chapman, M. American Academy of Orthopaedic Surgeons management of the multiply injured patient. April 9–11, 1992; Baltimore, MD.

Bone LB, Johnson, KD, Weigelt J, Scheinberg R. Early versus delayed stabilization of femoral fractures. *J Bone Jt Surg.* 1989;71A:336–340.

Burgess AR. Eastridge BJ. Young JW. Ellison TS. Ellison PS Jr. Poka A. Bathon GH. Brumback RJ. Pelvic ring disruptions: effective classification system and treatment protocols. *Journal of Trauma.* 1990;30(7):848–56.

Chapman, NW. Multiply injured patient. Instructional course lecture 212. Presented at the Annual Meeting of the American Academy of Orthopaedic Surgeons; February 12, 1989; Las Vegas, NV.

Dalal SA. Burgess AR. Siegel JH. Young JW. Brumback RJ. Poka A. Dunham CM. Gens D. Bathon H. Pelvic fracture in multiple trauma: classification by mechanism is key to pattern of organ injury, resuscitative requirements, and outcome. *Journal of Trauma.* 29(7):981–1000; discussion 1000–2, 1989 Jul.

Failinger M. McGanity P. Unstable fractures of the pelvic ring. *J Bone J Surg.* 1992;74A:783–791.

Goris RJ. Gimbrere JS. *van Niekerk* JL. Schoots FJ. Boey LH. Early osteosynthesis and prophylactic mechanical ventilation in the multitrauma patient. *Journal of Trauma.* 22(11):895–903, 1982 Nov.

Gregory P. DiCicco J. Karpik K. DiPasquale T. Herscovici D. Sanders R. Ipsilateral fractures of the femur and tibia: treatment with retrograde femoral nailing and unreamed tibial nailing. *Journal of Orthopaedic Trauma.* 1996;10(5):309–16.

Gustilo RB, Merkow RL, and Templeman, D: The Management of open Fractures. *J Bone Jt Surg.* 1990;72A:229–303.

Hofman PA. Goris RJ. Timing of osteosynthesis of major fractures in patients with severe brain injury. *Journal of Trauma.* 1991;31(2):261–3.

Johnson EE, Simpson LA, Helfet DL. Delayed intramedullary nailing after failed external fixation of the tibia. *CORR.* 1990;253:251–259.

Johnson KD et al. Incidence of adult respiratory distress syndrome in patients with multiple skeletal injuries: effect of early operative stabilization of fractures. *J Trauma.* 1985;25:375–384.

Patzakis MF, Wilkins J, Moore. Considerations in reducing the infection rate in open tibia fractures. *CORR.* 1983;176:36–41.

Peltier LF. An appraisal of the problems of fat emboli. *Surg Gynecol Obstet.* 1957;104:313–324.

Pennal GF, Tile M, Waddell, JP et al. Pelvic disruption: assessment in classification. *Clin Orthop.* 1980;151:12–21.

Phillips TF, Contreras, DM. Timing of operative treatment in patients who have multiple injuries. *J Bone Jt Surg.* 1990;72A:784–789.

Riemer BL, Butterfield SL, Diamond DL, Young JC, Raves, JJ, Cottington, E, Kislam K. Acute mortality associated with injuries to the pelvic ring: the role of early patient stabilization and external fixation. *J Trauma.* 1993;35:671–677.

Riemer BL, Foglesong, ME, Miranda MA. Femoral plating. Orthop Clin North Am. 1994;25:625–633.

Riemer BL. Miranda MA. Butterfield SL. Burke CJ 3rd. Non-reamed nailing of closed and minor open tibial fractures in patients with blunt polytrauma. *Clinical Orthopaedics and Related Research.* 1995;(320):119–24.

Riska EB, Myllymen P. Fat embolism in patients with multiple injuries. *J Trauma.* 1982;22:891–894.

Ruedi's Reference: Hevl. Chir. Acta 52:331–335, 1985. Priorities in the management of multiple trauma. Anonymous. Priorities of care in the multiple trauma patient. *Helvetica Chirurgica Acta.* 1985;52(2):329–44.

Slatis P. Huittinen VM. Double vertical fractures of the pelvis. A report on 163 patients. *Acta Chirurgica Scandinavica.* 1972;138(8):799–807.

Slauterbeck JR. Britton C. Moneim MS. Clevenger FW. Mangled extremity severity score: an accurate guide to treatment of the severely injured upper extremity. *Journal of Orthopaedic Trauma.* 1994;8:282–5

Tscherne H, Gotzen L. *Fractures With Soft Tissue Injuries.* New York, NY: Springer-Verlag; 1984.

Wolff G. Dittmann M. Ruedi T. Buchmann B. M. Prevention of posttraumatic respiratory insufficiency by coordination of surgery and intensive care (author's transl). *Unfallheilkunde.* 1978;81(6):425–42.

SAMPLE QUESTIONS

1. Management of a patient with a suspected cervical spine fracture requires:
   (a) logrolling the patient to inspect the back
   (b) a lateral radiograph that includes vertebrae C-1 through C-6
   (c) fluid replacement for hypotension due to autonomic dysreflexia from a spinal cord injury
   (d) a, b, and c
   (e) a and c

2. True or false: Plating of open fractures is associated with a similarly high rate of infection in fractures of both the upper and lower extremities.
   (a) true
   (b) false

3. External fixation of acute pelvic fractures is indicated for all of the following except:
   (a) diastasis of the pubic symphasis
   (b) pelvic ring disruption and hemodynamic instability
   (c) vertically unstable pelvis in conjunction with traction
   (d) rotationally unstable pelvis

4. Early stabilization of femurs seems to accomplish all of the following except:
   (a) reduced number of days on a ventilator
   (b) increased rate of ARDS
   (c) reduced pulmonary complications
   (d) decreased hospital stay
   (e) early mobilization

5. All of the following are true regarding blood loss except:
   (a) A palpable radial pulse usually indicates a minimum systolic pressure of 80 mm Hg.
   (b) Loss of 30% of the blood volume will result in marked hypotension and death.
   (c) The first therapeutic measure for hypotension due to blood loss is a fluid challenge with 2 liters of lactated Ringer's solution.
   (d) If the patient's hypotension does not improve following a fluid challenge, the patient should receive a transfusion of unmatched O negative blood.
   (e) A palpable carotid pulse usually indicates a minimum systolic pressure of 60 mm Hg.

Answers: 1) e; 2) b; 3) a; 4) b; 5) b

Soft Tissue Coverage

Chapter 13

Soft Tissue Coverage of the Upper Extremity

Guy Foucher, MD, David J. Smith Jr., MD, and Paul S. Cederna, MD

ETIOLOGY

The fingers and hand are frequently exposed to trauma, but trauma is not the only situation in which the surgeon must consider options for skin coverage. Etiology is fundamental in the decision making for skin coverage. Burns, Dupuytren's disease, a malignant tumor, or a congenital deficiency presents unique problems to the surgeon. A clean cut is simple to treat, while a deep structure injury, a burn, a crush, an avulsion, or a blast needs more careful attention.

RELEVANT ANATOMY

Knowledge of the vascularization of the skin of the upper extremity is the key for the use of local and regional axial flaps and free flaps. One of the great advances of microsurgery has been to stimulate clinicians to study vascular anatomy. The clinical distinction between a "random" pattern flap (having strict shape, length, and width due to absence of axial vessels) and the axial pattern flap was stressed by McGregor and Jackson in 1972. This was followed by the description of muscle and musculocutaneous flaps by McCraw (1980) and the fasciocutaneous flap by Ponten (1981).

Different types of flaps are available for the upper extremity. The random pattern flap needs to respect a ratio between width and length (from 1:1 to 1:2). An axial pattern flap contains a dominant vessel, and the ratio of length to width can be much larger (5:1) depending on the length of the dominant vessel. Vascularization can come through the muscles. Mathes and Nahai (1981) have separated the musculocutaneous flap into different types:

- Type 1 has only one pedicle (anconeus).
- Type 2 has a dominant pedicle closed to muscle origin (brachioradialis).
- Type 3 has a dominant pedicle plus segmental vascularization (latissimus dorsi).

This classification combines three points that help define a flap: its nature (skin, fat, aponeurosis, muscle, composite, etc.), its vascularization (random or axial pattern, arterial or venous, reverse or direct flow), and its surgical technique (local, regional, distant, pedicled, island, free).

Some vessels are worth mentioning to illustrate certain useful flaps for coverage of the upper extremity. Around the lateral aspect of the elbow exists an arterial circle supplied proximally by the division of the profunda brachii artery separating in two branches. The posterior radial collateral artery feeds the lateral arm flap, and anastomoses with the posterior interosseous recurrent artery and the radial recurrent artery. This circle allows the lateral arm flap to be used either as a free- or a reverse-flow flap (island or distally pedicled as described by Maruyama (1987)). According to Martin (1995), a reverse-flow flap, with an extended Y-V pedicle based on a posterior branch of the posterior radial collateral artery (after severing the profunda brachii artery), is possible in half the dissections, giving a long pedicle allowing the flap to join the distal third of the forearm. On a branch of the radial recurrent artery, a muscle or musculocutaneous flap of the brachioradialis could be used.

At the forearm level, a knowledge of the anatomy of the interosseous arteries is useful (Fig. 13–1). The anterior (AIOA) and posterior interosseous (PIOA) arteries come from a common trunk in 85% of specimens; in the remaining cases, they come separately from the ulnar artery. A direct distal anastomosis at the radioulnar joint is found in most cases. The communication with the carpal arcades is variable. Anastomosis has been found in the middle forearm in 20% of cases by Pahl

Orthopaedic Surgery: The Essentials. Edited by M.E. Baratz, A.D. Watson, and J.E. Imbriglia. Thieme Medical Publishers, Inc., New York © 1999

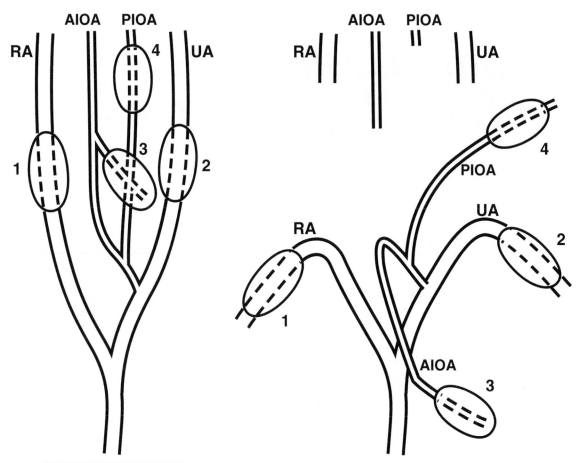

Figure 13–1 Reverse flow flaps based on the radial artery (RA-1), the ulnar artery (UA-2), the posterior branch of the anterior interosseous artery (AIOA-3), and the posterior interosseous artery (PIOA-4). (They could be direct or reverse flow).

and Schmidt (1994). The AIOA has two distal posterior branches, the more proximal branch permits harvesting a reverse flow posterior forearm flap with a 10-cm long pedicle formed by the distal segment of the AIOA and the proximal dorsal branch (after severing the AIOA, using the Y-V lengthening procedure described by Martin [1995]). The AIOA also vascularizes the pronator quadratus, allowing a direct- or reverse-flow muscular flap. The PIOA has 7 to 14 perforating branches, the most relevant being 8.5 cm from the lateral epicondyle. The posterior interosseous flap (Zancolli and Angrigiani, 1988, Masquelet 1987) with either a direct- or a reverse-flow is based on this anatomy. The radial artery has many perforating branches for the forearm skin (9 to 17 according to Timmons, 1986), less in the proximal area, but bigger and longer. A constant branch arises 2 to 4 cm proximal to the radiostyloid process (corresponding to the nutrient artery of the Goffin flap). Proximally, a branch has been described by Cormack and Lamberty (1985), perforating between the brachioradialis and the pronator teres, which allows harvesting an island or free antecubital fasciocutaneous flap.

The ulnar artery has fewer perforating branches than the radial artery, and they are concentrated in the middle and distal forearm. At 2 to 5 cm from the pisiform, the ulnar artery gives off a dorsoulnar branch of a few centimeters, which separates into three branches, the ascending one allowing a medial flap described by Becker (1990).

Recently, the constant presence of two digital arteries in each finger has been challenged by Brunelli (1993), who has found a 10% absence of the radial artery in the index and ulnar artery in the auricular. The dominant artery is close to the axis of the hand, which means that the ulnar artery of the index and the radial collateral artery of the small finger are dominant. Communication occurs between the two digital arteries mainly through retrotendinous arcades at the metaphyseal levels of the phalanges and through distal pulp arcades.

On the dorsum of the hand, the intermetacarpal arteries are more constant in the first two spaces than in the last two ones, providing the possibility of lifting metacarpal flaps either with direct or reverse flow.

EVALUATION

A major step in the treatment of traumatic loss of skin is debridement. At present, no method of assessing skin viability has reached daily clinical use. Toluidine blue has been tried in the past but found to be of little clinical use. Fluorescein is more complicated to use. The two methods that are of clinical value are to (1) release the tourniquet during the debridement or (2) "shave" the surrounding skin by harvesting a split-thickness graft to assess the vascularity of the deep surface.

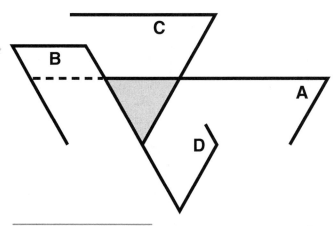

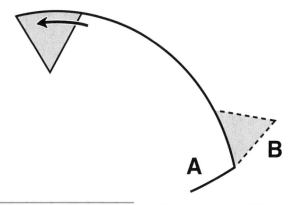

Figure 13–3   Rotation flap. **(A)** Classical design. **(B)** Excision of a Burrow's triangle.

Figure 13–2   Transposition flaps. **(A)** Classical design with a critical line twice as long as one side of the triangle. **(B and C)** The flap is made longer to facilitate the transposition. **(D)** Use of a "back-cut" for the same purpose.

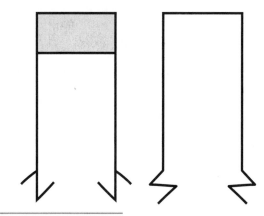

Figure 13–4   Advancement flap. To facilitate the advancement of the distal border of the flap, a proximal Z-plasty can be drawn on each lateral side of the flap.

TREATMENT

Spontaneous Healing

Spontaneous healing remains the simplest technique when applicable. It is not a way of neglecting the wound but of allowing healing by secondary intention. Some retraction is unavoidable. This method, reserved for many years for fingertip loss in children, can be applied to any age. Indications are skin loss without exposure of major structures such as bone, tendon, nerve and vessels.

Skin Grafts

Skin grafting is a simple method with advantages and drawbacks. The advantages include: simplicity, concealment of the donor site (e.g., the groin area), and good sensibility (in children). Grafting takes more easily when thin (split-thickness graft). A skin graft needs a bed with low contamination and good vascularization such as the periosteum, peritenon, or perimysium. Bare bone, denuded tendons, cartilage, or nerves should not be skin grafted. Skin grafts placed over an arterial repair may take, but we have avoided using skin grafts over nerve and vessel repairs. Shortcomings to skin grafts include: limited return of sensation in adults, retraction inversely proportionate to thickness, and disparate pigmentation. Many donor sites are available: the ulnar border of the hand for small defects and the buttock or thigh for larger defects. The inner arm or the groin is available for full-thickness grafts. In children, it is important to remain on the lateral aspect of the groin to avoid hair growth on the graft at puberty. Some sites are to be avoided—the flexion of the wrist crease will create a scar that looks like a self-inflicted injury. The elbow flexion crease can create a hypertrophic scar.

Local Flaps

Local flaps remain the best source of "like skin" when available. They are constructed on three models: transposition, rotation, or advancement (Lisk 1988).

PEARL

Skin graft taken from the groin crease in children should be harvested as laterally as possible to avoid hair growth on the graft at puberty.

In the transposition flap, the skin deficit is shaped in an equilateral triangle (Fig. 13–2); a parallelogram is then cut extending one side of the triangle (A in Fig. 13–2). After rotation around the pivot point, a deficit identical to the triangle is created. Other ways to facilitate migration are: The flap could be made longer (B and C in Fig. 13–2) or a "back cut" could be made (D in Fig. 13–2) if the vascularization allows it as in the hand.

Rotation flaps have no special geometry and take advantage of the skin's elasticity. The skin deficit is first triangulated and one side opposite to the apex is extended in a gentle curve (A in Fig. 13–3). All the incisions can usually be closed. A back cut can also be used with this flap if necessary.

Advancement flaps (Fig. 13–4) are popular for fingertip losses. An example is the V-Y advancement flap where a triangular palmar flap is designed and advanced distally creating a Y.

Local flaps have the advantage of good sensibility and the presence of a corneous layer. They are contra-indicated in cases of crush injury, vascular disease, or heavy contamination. In secondary reconstruction, their use has been enhanced by using skin expansion techniques.

Regional Flaps

Regional flaps have certain advantages: They can be used in a scarred area and can provide coverage of very large defects. However, a donor site is required with additional morbidity (such as the cross-finger flap), and a second procedure may be necessary for separation of the flap.

The concept of island flaps with normal- or reverse-arterial flow taken from the forearm has revolutionized the coverage of large losses of the hand and elbow. These flaps have an independent blood supply, their recipient site can be sealed, and they can be harvested with other tissues (such as bone, fascia, or tendons) or without the skin (fascial flap). The radial forearm flap, based on the radial artery, is one of the most popular. With normal flow, it can cover any area of the elbow. It can be shifted laterally on a neighboring forearm defect. Based on a reverse flow, it can cover virtually any defect in the hand. It is a simple, versatile, and reliable flap; but it sacrifices a major artery. It is frequently thick and hairy and leaves a quite conspicuous forearm scar (even when used as a facial flap). The ulnar flap shares the same advantages and drawbacks, except that the donor area is easier to conceal. Other forearm island flaps are available at present, avoiding the sacrifice of a major vessel. The posterior interosseous flap based on the posterior interosseous artery is useful for both the elbow and the hand. Other flaps are used only for hand coverage: the radial flap based on a constant branch arising at the styloid process, the ulnar flap based on the ulnodorsal artery, or the anterior interosseous flap based on the posterior branch of the anterior interosseous artery.

Distant Pedicle Flaps

The indications for random flaps taken from the chest or other areas have decreased, whereas axial pattern flaps such as the groin flap remain useful due to the large area of skin available, the technical simplicity and reliability of the flap, the use of a long pedicle to allow early motion, and the easily concealed donor scar.

However, distant pedicle flaps are performed under general anesthesia. Two operations (or more in the case of secondary defatting) are necessary, and the position of the hand is awkward while the flap is healing.

Free Flaps

Free flaps in the upper extremity are less frequently performed than in the lower limbs, due to the possibility of moving the hand to a donor site and the availability of numerous forearm island flaps. Free flaps in the arm are indicated only when a local or island flap cannot be used.

One of the main indications for a free flap is complete loss of pulp in a finger used in fine pinch (such as the thumb or the index). The pulp of the great toe provides young, well-motivated patients with tissue of the same structure and texture and good sensibility. In compound losses, a piece of vascularized bone, a nail bed flap, or the nail complex can be simultaneously transferred, improving cosmesis and function.

Among the numerous free flaps available, some have enjoyed popularity in the past, such as the dorsalis pedis flap; but due to the problems at the donor site, they have been given up by the majority of surgeons. Other flaps, have come back into favor, such as the free groin flap, despite the technical difficulty and variable pedicle due to a nonconspicuous donor site. The lateral arm flap continues to be popular despite its often tiny vessels, frequent thickness, and conspicuous scar. The flap can be harvested under regional anesthesia and tourniquet, and its shape can be tailored to match the defect. Each flap, such as the temporofascia flap and the scapular or parascapular flap, has its own advantages and drawbacks. Only a few among a hundred potential donor sites have been mentioned. Free muscle or musculocutaneous flaps are indicated in large defects of the upper extremity and can simultaneously restore a cover and a functional muscle. The three most frequently used are the latissimus dorsi, the gracilis, and the serratus anterior.

Fingertip Reconstruction

Although Bunnel (1994) stated that the fingertips may be considered as the "eyes" of the hand, one must note the important added functions of durability and pseudomotor activity that, together with sensibility, give the fingertip its unique function.

When treatment by simple methods, such as secondary healing or closure after shortening, is insufficient or undesirable, a regional flap should be considered. The primary indications for a regional flap are the need to maintain finger length, the depth of tissue loss exposing tendon or bone, or the wish to preserve the nail. Mobility is very important in the consideration of any particular flap. Knowledge of the limitations, complications, and expected outcomes of each flap in this regard is crucial.

In the management of the injured digit, the surgeon must consider the physiological and vascular age of the patient. Island flaps, free-pulp transfer, and neurotization of islands by the recipient digital nerve are all ill-advised procedures in the older patient. Associated pathology (smoking, diabetes, atherosclerosis, Raynaud's disease, etc.) as well as long-term medications (e.g., corticosteroids) play a significant role in the decision. Professional and leisure activities should be considered. One may not propose the same management for the index of a manual laborer as one would for a violinist.

Among the local flaps, the V-Y flap is useful in moderate loss. The Tranquilli Leali (1935) flap popularized by Atasoy (1970) (A in Fig. 13–5) has replaced the Kutler (1947) flaps. It provides only a moderate advancement of 0.5 cm, thus limiting the indications to distal transverse amputations. This flap requires a meticulous technique if sufficient advancement is to be obtained. A fine needle inserted through the distal edge of the flap, skewering the skin to the distal phalanx, helps maintain the flap's position without traction on the nail bed. The needle obviates the need for skin suture, which can compromise the vascularity of the flap.

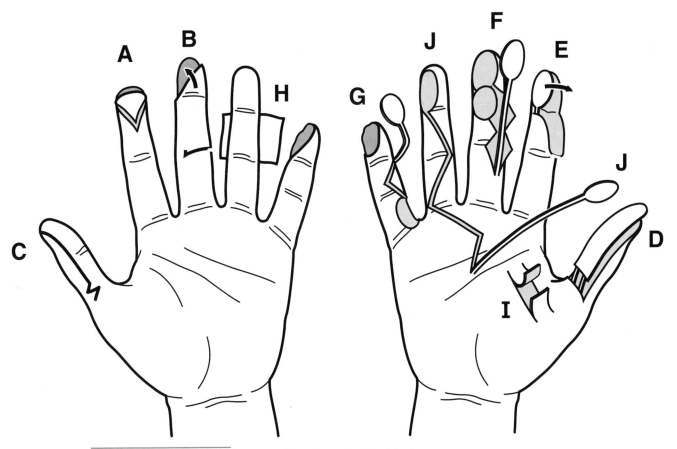

Figure 13–5 Drawing of different palmar flaps described in the text.

An advancement of approximately 0.8 cm is provided by the Hueston's flap (B) shown in Figure 13–5. This flap is useful for reconstruction of transverse guillotine amputations as well as oblique defects. The "L" incision, with the horizontal limb at the proximal interphalangeal (PIP) joint crease, allows lifting of the flap, incorporating one neurovascular bundle. For an advancement of 1 cm, the Moberg flap (C in Fig. 13–5) was initially intended for use in the thumb; used on other fingers (Snow's flap), it carries the risk of a dorsal skin necrosis if one dorsal artery is not saved during the dissection. The original technique involved raising a volar flap by longitudinal, medial, and lateral incisions with advancement on both neurovascular pedicles. With slight interphalangeal (IP) joint flexion, the flap is advanced to cover the distal defect. A number of modifications have since been proposed. Two Z-plasties proximally will improve advancement and lessen the requirement for joint flexion.

More mobility is given through homodigital island flaps. Listed in order of increasing potential for advancement are the flaps of O'Brien (1968), Venkataswami (1980), and Glicenstein (1988). Retention of sensibility is particularly good in the O'Brien and Venkataswami flaps. O'Brien (D in Fig. 13–5) has modified the technique of Moberg by adding a proximal transverse incision with dissection of both pedicles, converting the flap into a homodigital bipedicled island.

The principle of pulp exchange has been well enunciated by Littler (1956). The design has been modified (E in Fig. 13–5) by transferring a true island. In cases with scarred, nonsensate pulp on the dominant aspect of the index (where the distal digital nerve is destroyed), the design is altered to avoid sacrificing healthy skin. In the young, the aim is to prevent cortical reorientation problems by suturing the flap's digital nerve to the recipient nerve. The stump of the donor nerve should be transected proximally and translocated into the interosseous space.

The advancement island flap (F in Fig. 13–5) is an ideal technique for major loss of finger tip coverage. The most significant advancement (maximum 22 mm) by "medialization" of the pedicle has been obtained in the index. The major complication of this flap is a residual extension deficit at the PIP joint. This can be prevented by immobilization of the digit in full metacarpal phalangeal (MP) joint flexion with the IP joints and by extension night splinting after the 10th postoperative day. A recently described island flap has retrograde flow (Glicenstein, 1988) based on the same principle as the radial forearm flap. The flap is raised on the palmar aspect of the proximal phalanx (G in Fig. 13–5). The nutrient artery is ligated at the proximal border. The vessel is then dissected distally to the midpoint of the middle phalanx. The retrotendinous diaphyseal and epiphyseal vessels are preserved to nourish the island. Brunelli (1993) has proposed a modification to render the flap sensate; the nerve is sectioned with the artery and connected distally to the contralateral nerve.

Regional flaps are relied on when local flaps are contraindicated or unavailable. One of the most popular is the cross-finger flap. In a variation of the standard cross-finger flap, two flaps with opposite hinges are fastened to replace the epidermis on the donor digit and a reversed de-epithelialized flap is moved to the recipient finger (H in Fig. 13–5). Meissl and Berger (1980) have suggested innervating the flap through neurotization of the dorsal nerve branches. At the thumb, numerous surgeons have used a cross-finger flap from the dorsum of the index with translocation of sensory radial branches from the dorsum of the index finger.

The thenar flap (I in Fig. 13–5) is raised on the thenar eminence and is based proximally or distally. The donor site is either sutured directly or grafted, and the flap is inset to the defect. The pedicle is divided after 12 to 21 days, and final adjustment is frequently indicated at a later stage. A good deal of criticism has been leveled at this flap because of poor sensory quality, tenderness at the donor site, and, most notably, flexion contracture of the recipient digit. To prevent the latter two problems, it has been suggested that the flap be designed so as to lie in the proximal thumb crease and be based radially. This lessens the PIP flexion of the recipient digit.

The heterodigital island flap as described in 1956 by Littler (E in Fig. 13–5) has been utilized to resurface distal digital skin losses. There are several problems associated with the use of this flap. Most surgeons agree that there is no true cortical reintegration with the heterodigital island flap. In a series of 38 patients, we found that 22% had cross sensibility, 39% exhibited a combination of cross and integrated sensibility, and 39% exhibited complete integration. Neurotization of the nerve by the recipient nerve in the young subject (average age 26 years) has avoided problems with cortical reintegration without altering two-point discrimination (average 6.8 mm). Cold intolerance in the donor digit was recorded in 83% of our cases. The main indication for neurotization is a combined injury of two fingers, one with a huge pulp loss and the other requiring shortening, thus providing an undamaged area of skin with a neurovascular pedicle.

A local flap is the first choice, and a regional flap is to be considered when the local flap is inappropriate. The distal flap is a last resort. Few things are less appealing, esthetically or functionally, than the abdominal or buttock flap on the thumb! The "socklike" mobility and poor sensibility render pinch difficult. Use of a distant flap is indicated for extensive tissue loss on the thumb and in cases of extensive distal skin loss in multiple digits. The distant flap is only the first step. The second stage provides sensibility either through a local-advancement flap or a free-pulp flap.

The ipsilateral great toe for thumb defects and the contralateral great toe for the index provide ample vascularized, sensate coverage. This flap provides a large pulp surface, which has excellent sensibility in the young subject. Composite tissues may be transferred to replace the missing distal tissues in a "custom-made" way. In addition to pulp, one may transfer vascularized bone, part of the nail bed, or the entire nail complex. The vascularization of the bony segment

prevents resorption and the development of a hook nail deformity. Painful neuromas are not a contraindication. Repair of the involved digital nerve to the donor flap nerve appears to prevent recurrent neuroma formation.

Many options are available to treat fingertip injuries, and the use of flaps provides a powerful tool. A number of techniques may produce a satisfactory outcome. The surgeon is obliged to select that method which is the simplest and most effective for the treatment of a specific digit in any given patient. It is also important to take into account the socioeconomic impact of the injury and its treatment during the decision-making process.

Dorsum of Finger and Hand

The quality of the dorsal skin is peculiar. To allow full finger and wrist motion elasticity extra skin is mandatory. When deciding to replace this skin, keep in mind that it is the exposed part of the hand and try to minimize the amount of scar.

At the finger level, many local flaps are available when the loss is moderate. The oblique flap as designed by Flint and Siegle (1994) (A in Fig. 13–6) is useful to cover the distal interphalangeal (DIP) joint. The Smith rotation flap (B in Fig. 13–6), cut on the three sides of a rectangle, has been commonly used for loss at the PIP joint. When the loss is more than 1 square

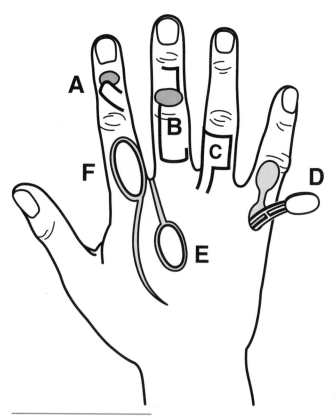

Figure 13–6   Drawing of some dorsal skin flaps described in the text.

centimeter, it is combined with a similar flap designed on the middle phalanx. In more extensive losses, a regional flap could be used, such as the cross-finger flap for the second and third phalanges or the flag flap (Vilain) for the proximal phalanx (C in Fig. 13–6). A proximal phalanx limited by loss can be covered by a venous island flap called the neutral flap (D in Fig. 13–6). A more extensive loss might require a reverse-flow metacarpal flap (E in Fig. 13–6). For dorsal losses on the thumb, the island kite flap (F in Fig. 13–6) based on the first dorsal metacarpal artery remains very useful.

On the dorsum of the hand, skin losses are frequently extensive and combined with extensor tendon injuries. A simple skin graft combined with early splinting in extension can result in mobile tissue able to provide acceptable extension when the extensors are covered with paratenon. Engel (1977) has used silastic rods under skin grafts to prepare for a flap that allows secondary grafting or tendon transfer. A compound flap can be isolated on the radial artery (free or as an island), incorporating the palmaris longus and the brachioradialis tendon. Another free compound flap for dorsal hand coverage is the dorsalis pedis with the toe extensor mechanism.

Palmar Skin

The skin of the palm is very thick and protects the volar structures. It is firmly anchored to the deep fascia, facilitating a stable grip. These qualities explain the difficulty in finding a good flap for this area.

Local flaps are not frequently indicated due to the unusual blood supply of palmar skin, as well as its poor mobility and elasticity. Some muscular flaps can be useful. The first interosseous, a lumbrical, or the abductor minimi can be used for local coverage. Distant flaps for large defects are disappointing due to socklike mobility and thickness, which can impede full flexion. An alternative is a fascial flap, such as the temporal artery free flap, the anterior interosseous, or the radial forearm fascia flap.

Forearm and Elbow

In the forearm, flaps such as the direct-flow radial, ulnar, and posterior interosseous flaps, can be used. More frequently, a distant flap is necessary. Free flaps are preferred to random thoracic flaps for the proximal aspect of the forearm. The distal forearm can be covered with a pedicled groin flap. In large palmar or dorsal losses, a muscular flap has the advantage of providing good coverage and can also compensate for missing flexor or extensor function. In such cases, the latissimus dorsi is preferred to the gracilis. In the elbow and proximal forearm, two other useful island flaps need special mention: the brachioradialis and the reverse-flow or classical lateral arm flap. If the vessels to these flaps have been injured, a free flap may be necessary.

CONCLUSION

We did not try to perform a comprehensive overview of all the flaps available for the elbow, the forearm, or the hand. A thorough knowledge of the possible choices is mandatory. It is necessary to select the simplest, but the best, flap for each case. Always consider function, morbidity, and cosmesis.

SELECTED BIBLIOGRAPHY

Atasoy E, Ioakimidis E, Kasdan ML, Kutz JE, Kleinert HE. Reconstruction of the amputated fingertip with a triangular volar flap. *J. Bone Jt Surg* 1970;52A; 921–926.

Becker C. Lambeau antébrachial des branches distales de l'artére cubitale. In: Gilbert A. Les lambeaux artériels pédicurés du membre supérieur. Paris: *Expansion Scientifique.* 1990;102–106.

Brunelli F. Dorsoulnar thumb flap. *Ann Chir Main.* 1993; 12:105–114.

Cormack GC, Lamberty BGH Fasciocutaneous vessels in the upper arm: application to the design of new fasciocutaneous flaps. *Plast Reconstru Surg.* 1984;74(2):244–250.

Cormack GC, Lamberty BGH. *The Arterial Anatomy of Skin Flaps.* London: Churchill-Livingstone. 1985.

Engel J. Stur C, Horoshowsky H. Dosal silicone rods in the primary care of war injuries. *The Hand* 1977;9:153–156.

Flint I.D., Siegle R.J. The bipedicle flap revisited. *Journ of Dermatologic Surg and Oncology.* 1994;20(6):394–400.

Foucher G. *Fingertip Injuries.* London: Churchill-Livingstone. 1991:151.

Foucher G. Second toe to finger transfers in hand mutilations. *Clinical Ortho.* 1995;314:8–12.

Foucher G., Citron N. Hoang P. Techniques and applications of the forearm flap in surgery of the hand. *Microsurgery for Major Limb Reconstruction.* Mosby. 1984;239–263.

Foucher G., Smith D. Free Vascularized Toe Transfer in Posttraumatic Hand Reconstruction In *Surgery of the Hand and Upper Extremity.* New York: McGraw-Hill. 1995:1911–1917.

Foucher G, Smith D, Citron, N. Homodigital neurovascular island flap for digital pulp loss. *J Hand Surgery.* 1989;14B: 204–208.

Glicenstein J. Island flaps in hand surgery: introduction. *Ann Chir Main.* 1988;7(2):120–121.

Goffin D, Brunelli F, Galbiatti A, Sammut D, Gilbert A. A new flap based on the distal branches of the radial artery. *Ann Chir Main.* 1984;74(2):244–250.

Guimberteau JC., et al. The ulnar reverse forearm flap: about 54 cases. *Plast Reconstr Surg.* 1988;925–932.

Katsaros J., et al. The lateral forearm flap: anatomy and clinical applications. *Ann Plastic Surgery.* 1984;489–500.

KUTLER W. A new method for fingertip amputations. *J Am Med Ass* 1947;133:29–30.

LISTER G. Local flaps to the hand. *Hand Clinics*. 1985;1:623–640.

LITTLER, JS "Neurovascular Pedicle Transfer of Tissue in Reconstructive Surgery of the Hand." *J of Bone Jt Surgery*. 1956;38A:917–920.

MARTIN D. Evolution des techniques de transfert. Nouvelles autoplasties décrites pendant cette periode. *Ann Chir Plast Esth* 1995;40:527–582.

MARUYAMA Y, ONISHI K., IWAHIRA Y. The ulnar recurrent fasciocutaneous island flap: reverse medial arm flap. *Plastic and Reconstructive Surgery*. 1987;79(3):381–388.

MASQUELET AC., PENTEADO CV., The posterior interosseous flap. *Ann Chir Main*. 1987;6(2):131–139.

MATHES SJ, NAHAI F. Classification of the vascular anatomy of muscles: experimental and clinical correlation. *Plastic and Reconstr Surg*. 1981;67(2):177–187.

McGRAW JB The recent history of myocutaneous flaps. *Clinics in Plastic Surgery*. 1980;7(1):3–7.

MEISSL G, BERGER A. Surgical restoration of sensitivity in childhood. *Zeitschrift fur Kinderchirurgie und Grenzgebiete*. 1980;30:160–162.

MOBERT E. Aspects of sensation is reconstructive surgery of the upper extremity. *J Bone Jt Surg*. 1964;46A:817–825.

O'BRIEN B. Neurovascular island pedicle flaps for terminal amputations and digital scars. *British J of Plastic Surg*. 1968;21:258–261.

PAHL S, SCHMIDT HM. Clinical anatomy of the interosseous arteries of the forearm. *Handchirurgie, Mikrochirurgie, Plastiche Chirurgie*. 1994;26(5):246–250.

PONTEN B. The fasciocutaneous flap: its use in soft tissue defects of the lower leg. *British J of Plastic Surg*. 1981;34(2):215–220.

STICE RC, WOOD MB, Neurovascular island skin flaps in the hand: functional evaluation. *Microsurgery*. 1987;8:162–167.

TIMMONS MJ. The vascular basis of the radial forearm flap. *Plast Reconstr Surg*. 1986;77(1):80–92.

TRANQUILI-LEALI E. Ricostruzione dell'apice delle falangi ungueali mediante autoplastica volare pedundolata per scorrimento. *Infort Trauma Lavoro* 1935;1;186–193.

VENKATASWAMI R. SUBRAMANIAN N. Oblique triangular flap: a new method of repair for oblique amputation of the fingertip and thumb. *Plast Reconstr Surg*. 1980;66:296–300.

ZANCOLLI EA, ANGRIGIANI C. Posterior interosseous island forearm flap. *J Hand Surg*. 1988;13B:130–135.

SAMPLE QUESTIONS

1. A random pattern flap has a ratio between length and width from:
   (a) 1:3 to 1:4
   (b) 1:5 to 1:6
   (c) 1:1 to 1:2
   (d) The ratio is of no concern.
   (e) 1:4 to 1:5

2. Skin viability is best assessed with:
   (a) fluoroscein and Wood's lamp
   (b) toluidine blue
   (c) direct visualization with the tourniquet down
   (d) "shave" the skin (e.g., harvest a split-thickness skin graft)
   (e) c and d

3. Which of the following is false:
   (a) The posterior radial collateral artery supplies the lateral arm flap.
   (b) The anterior interosseous artery supplies the distal posterior interosseous flap.
   (c) The radial forearm flap is supplied by the ulnar artery.
   (d) The digital arteries supply the reverse metacarpal flaps.
   (e) none of the above

4. Which of the following is not an acceptable surface for a skin graft:
   (a) exposed paratendon
   (b) exposed bone
   (c) exposed muscle
   (d) granulation tissue
   (e) exposed vessels

5. Sensate, durable coverage for the thumb with exposed bone on the palmar tip can be achieved with all of the following except:
   (a) neurovascular island flap
   (b) full-thickness skin graft
   (c) moberg advancement flap
   (d) innervated cross-finger flap
   (e) healing by secondary intention in a child

Chapter 14

Soft Tissue Coverage of the Lower Extremity

Enrico B. Robotti, MD and William M. Swartz, MD

Outline

Methods for closure of soft tissue defects of the lower extremity have evolved from simple relaxing calf incisions, local random flaps and cross-leg pedicle flaps, to more robust local muscle and myocutaneous flaps, fasciocutaneous flaps, and microvascular free flaps. Treatment has historically focused on the traumatized extremity. However, many of the same principles are applicable to defects from other etiologies, including tumor resection. Soft tissue reconstruction of the lower extremity is a vast topic that can hardly be condensed into a few pages. Technical details of flap dissection and mobilization, usually performed by the plastic surgeon, cannot be covered here except for a few major flaps. This chapter has been designed to function as a concise review of the topic. The material should be supplemented with further reading, especially regarding the less frequently used coverage options. The selected bibliography is limited to the key papers and texts relevant to each issue.

BASIC CONCEPTS IN RECONSTRUCTION AFTER TRAUMA

The Purpose of Reconstruction

Reconstruction of any wound aims to restore function and form. Because the primary function of the lower extremity is

weight-bearing, an adequate reconstruction consists of well vascularized soft tissue coverage with padding of weight-bearing bony prominences and re-establishment of at least protective sensation. An acceptable contour should also be provided. In this respect, reconstruction of the lower extremity is simpler than that of the upper extremity, where many more complex functional issues need to be addressed. There are, however, problems peculiar to the lower limb: Venous stasis, deep vein thrombosis and persistent edema due to the effect of dependency, and arterial atherosclerosis. Also, the main weight-bearing bone of the leg, the tibia, is located subcutaneously for much of its surface, which predisposes it to nonunion and infection in open trauma. Autologous tissue transfer to the lower extremity should take all these factors into account.

Trauma

Lower extremity reconstruction is closely linked with trauma. Historically, most advances in reconstructive techniques parallel war surgery endeavors.

The outcome of severe compound lower extremity injuries (Gustilo's types IIIB and IIIC, and Byrd's type III and IV) (Table 14–1) has been traditionally poor. Now there is indisputable evidence that early coverage with well-vascularized soft tissue, preferably muscle, greatly improves the prognosis of these injuries and significantly reduces the incidence of complications. The importance of close interspecialty management providing bony fixation and flap coverage of these injuries cannot be overstressed. Key steps are: assessment, debridement, stable fixation, soft tissue coverage, and bone reconstruction, with appropriate timing of and between each one of these steps.

Assessment

Initial examination involves the neurovascular status. If the leg has been devascularized, urgent revascularization is required. Fasciotomy is performed in the presence of increased compartment pressure. Extreme energy forces with crush or degloving, associated with neurovascular injury, may contraindicate heroic salvage attempts. Realistic expectations of outcome in this situation may be so poor that primary amputation should be considered.

161

TABLE 14–1 Classification* of tibial fractures according to energy expended and soft tissue injury

Type	Description
I	An open fracture with a cutaneous wound less than 1 cm in length
II	An open fracture characterized by extensive soft tissue damage
IIA	Adequate soft tissue coverage of a fractured bone despite extensive soft tissue laceration or flaps, or high-energy trauma irrespective of the size of the wound
IIIB	Extensive soft tissue injury loss with periosteal stripping and bone exposure, usually associated with massive contamination
IIIC	Open fracture associated with arterial injury requiring repair

* Classification after Gustilo et al 1984

Gustilo RB, Mendoza RM, Williams DN: Problems in the management of type III (severe) open fractures: a new classification of type III open fractures. Journal of Trauma. 24:742, 1984

Debridement

The importance of debridement cannot be overstressed. Thorough debridement of devitalized tissue is the single most important step in the management of extremity trauma. Although broad spectrum antibiotics should be administered after injury, they are ineffective in the absence of adequate debridement. Debridement must be performed without concern about reconstruction. Pressurized irrigation is employed. Exposed nerves and vessels that are still viable are preserved and marked with sutures if reconstruction is to be delayed. Exposed tendons, especially in the distal third of the leg, are covered with moist dressings to prevent dessication. Skin from full-thickness degloved flaps can be used for split-thickness skin grafts (STSGs) harvested with an electric dermatome. Large bone fragments with wide, soft tissue attachments are preserved, while small, free fragments are excised.

PEARL

Thorough resection to bleeding soft tissue and bleeding bone represents the end point of debridement.

PITFALL

Attempts to reposition degloved full-thickness flaps in the lower extremity are generally unsuccessful, resulting in necrosis of the flaps and infection of underlying tissues.

Stable Fixation

Appropriate fixation must precede soft tissue closure. Together with appropriate blood supply, stabilization is the essential element for healing of fractures. Although intramedullary rods or AO compression plates can be employed, external fixation is usually preferred in more severe cases. External fixation is associated with a lower infection rate and avoids the risk of further devascularization due to periosteal stripping. External fixation provides rigid stability to the fracture and maintains overall bone length when a segment of bone is missing. External fixation is obligatory in cases of severe comminution and segmental bone loss. Newer fixators allow compression or distraction of fragments and three-dimensional positioning of bone. The orthopaedic and plastic surgeon should consult about the type of frame to be applied and the position of the pins, to allow unimpeded flap placement. Another recent option is limb shortening at the site of injury and use of the Ilizarov technique to transfer both bony and soft tissue elements. This allows significant reduction in the initial soft tissue defect but requires subsequent prolonged transport time.

Soft Tissue Coverage

Soft tissue coverage with adequate blood supply, when provided within the first 5 to 7 days after injury, results in the fewest complications (less time to bone union and reduced rates of osteomyelitis, nonunion, and amputation) and the shortest hospitalization time. Immediate coverage is advisable only if the level of debridement is sufficient, and a clean surgical wound has been created. Multiple debridements at 24- to 48-hour intervals may be necessary when it is difficult to assess the zone of injury. All devitalized tissue must be debrided before wound coverage is attempted.

Byrd and colleagues advocate radical bone and soft tissue debridement and muscle flap coverage in the acute phase, the first 5 to 6 days after type III and IV injuries. When treatment is withheld, fractures enter a subacute, infected phase extending from 1 to 6 weeks after injury. Flap coverage is avoided in this phase, because of the difficulty in establishing appropriate borders for bony debridement. After the subacute phase, a chronic phase begins, with a granulating wound, adherent soft tissue, and persistent areas of localized infection. Limits for debridement become well demarcated, and flap coverage is again safe. Other authors, such as Yaremchuck and colleagues (1987), believe that flap coverage poses no additional risk in the subacute phase. The main difference between these two attitudes is in the extent of debridement of all bone fragments. Obviously, complete removal of all bone fragments lowers the infection rate and allows coverage even in the infected subacute phase. In the event of comminuted intermediate fragments or type IV fractures, total bony debridement is preferable. However, many type III fractures with a large intermediate segment proceed to uncomplicated bone union while avoiding a discontinuity defect.

Appropriate guidelines in clinical practice supported by most authors comprise:

1. muscle flap coverage within the first 5 to 7 days of injury, before wound colonization
2. accurate debridement of all small, free, bone fragments

3. large intermediate bone segments are retained and covered by the muscle flap

Muscle obliterates dead space and fills the debridement cavity. Muscle also provides a well-vascularized soft tissue cuff for proper bone healing or for later cancellous bone grafting, and it restores contour. In weight-bearing areas, muscle will withstand ambulation and allow the wearing of shoes. Muscle has a well-proven salutary effect in the resolution of deep wound infections, including chronic osteomyelitis, as well as a superior resistance to bacterial inoculation as compared with conventional "skin" flaps. Microscopically, muscle provides increased blood supply with improved oxygen tension and enhanced delivery of leukocytes and other immunologic mediators, including complement and immunoglobulins.

PEARL

There is evidence to support the use of muscle to eliminate infection at the fracture site and to promote bony union.

Bone Reconstruction

Skeletal continuity is generally restored after soft tissue coverage has healed. Cancellous bone grafts are performed in a secondary operation. Bead spacers can be used in the interim to preserve the length of the diaphyseal defect. Many believe in cancellous bone grafting at an average of 8 weeks after soft tissue coverage. Vascularized bone (fibula, iliac crest, and scapula) can be used for long bone gaps (usually > 8 cm). The iliac crest is typically used when the defect is 10 cm or less, while the fibula is preferred for longer defects. When bone grafting beneath a free or pedicled flap, prior consultation with the plastic surgeon will avoid the risk of severing the pedicle and losing the flap during soft tissue elevation.

Reconstruction for segmental defects can also be performed with osseous-bearing composite free flaps or simply with cancellous bone grafts beneath vascularized muscle flaps at the time of soft tissue coverage. Another alternative in secondary bone reconstruction is distraction osteogenesis via the Ilizarov technique. Many believe the distraction technique to be safer and more effective than secondary vascularized bone transfer. Further details on bone defect reconstruction are beyond the scope of this chapter.

RATIONALE FOR COVERAGE OPTIONS

In deciding how to provide soft tissue coverage to a lower extremity wound, the surgeon should consider possible methods in order from simple to complex. The simplest method that adequately meets the reconstructive goal should be preferred. In increasing order of complexity, the available options, arranged on the "reconstructive ladder" are: primary closure, skin graft, local flap (muscle, myocutaneous, or fasciocutaneous), and free tissue transfer.

The recent advances in local flaps and in microvascular techniques have modified the way a reconstructive procedure is chosen. One is no longer forced to close a wound with the simplest available technique, which may not be the optimal solution for function or form. The best technique for a particular defect, rather than the most simple and expeditious, should be elected on the basis of the quality of the anticipated result. Oftentimes, microvascular free flaps are the first choice for coverage.

Skin Grafts

Split-thickness skin grafts from the thigh or buttock require a well vascularized bed. They cannot be used on exposed tendon or bone. Meshed STSGs provide adequate permanent coverage over exposed muscle or subcutaneous tissue. Centripetal contracture of the graft usually improves the local contour and texture over time. Skin grafts are also useful when a temporary measure is chosen to close a complex wound, provided paratenon or periosteum is preserved. As mentioned, STSGs are indicated in degloving injuries of the lower extremity.

Flaps

Modern reconstructive options for the lower extremity include local flaps and free flaps. These include: muscle (muscle flap), muscle and overlying skin (musculocutaneous flap), or fascia with or without the overlying skin (fascial or fasciocutaneous flaps). Muscle flaps have been classified by Mathes and Nahai (1982) into five types depending on the pattern of their vascular pedicle (Fig. 14–1). This classification is extremely important in planning the appropriate pedicled or free muscle transfer.

Pedicled distant flaps, (i.e., transferred from distant sites in multiple stages) employing the "delay" phenomenon and complex "waltzing" modalities, are mostly of historical interest. However, a technique that still has occasional indications is the cross-leg flap. The standard cross-leg flap was the workhorse for distal lower extremity reconstruction until its recent replacement by free flaps. The design of the flap has been changed to a longitudinal fasciocutaneous flap on an axial blood supply, which permits a longer length-to-width ratio and allows the procedure to be performed without a delay procedure. The cross-leg flap may still have a place for distal leg coverage when free flaps and local fasciocutaneous flaps have failed (Fig. 14–2).

Local Muscle and Musculocutaneous Flaps

A precise understanding of the type of blood supply to different muscles and the point where the vascular pedicle enters the muscle is essential in planning the flap transfer. This point represents the pivot point for a muscle rotation flap. Additional length to the arc of rotation may be achieved by dividing the muscle origin and mobilizing the vascular pedicle (e.g., the gastrocnemius muscle for knee coverage). Muscle flap elevation is a simple matter, easily performed between muscle planes.

Muscle flaps are chosen to minimize the functional deficit. For example, both soleus and gastrocnemius contribute to plantar flexion, and the use of either does not result in a functional deficit. Portions of the muscle can be used to preserve most of the muscle function. Local muscle flaps are used for soft tissue coverage of important structures, such as the knee

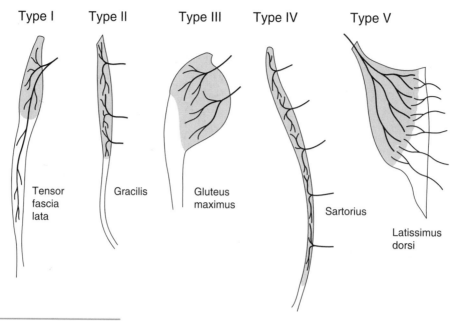

Figure 14–1 Patterns of vascular anatomy of muscle: Type I, one vascular pedicle; Type II, dominant pedicle(s) and minor pedicle(s); Type III, two dominant pedicles; Type IV, segmental vascular pedicles; Type V, one major pedicle and secondary segmental pedicles. Reproduced with permission From Mathes SJ, Nahai, F. Classification of the vascular anatomy of muscles: experimental and clinical correlation. *Plast Reconstr Surg.* 1981;67:177.

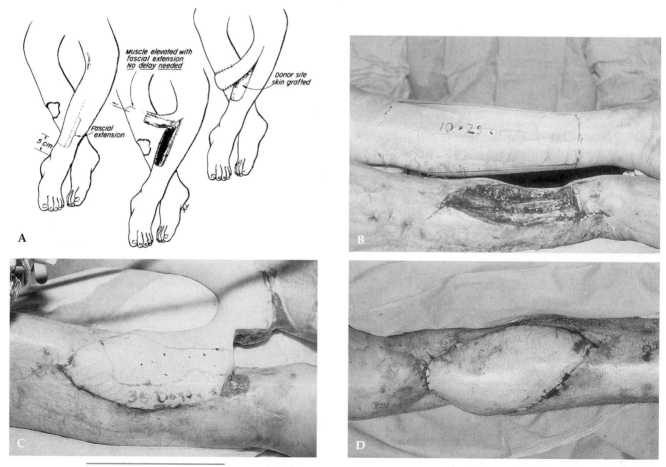

Figure 14–2 Gastrocnemius cross-leg flap as undelayed procedure. This flap is useful in salvage situations where free tissue transfers have failed. **(A)**. Diagrammatic representation of undelayed gastrocnemius myocutaneous cross-leg flap. **(B)** Open wound of right leg following unsuccessful free tissue transfer. **(C)** Division of cross-leg flap in stages due to robust blood supply from gastrocnemius muscle. **(D)** Completed flap transfer following division and inset.

joint or exposed tibia. Muscle flaps provide excellent contour and minimal bulk when covered with skin grafts.

The use of local muscle flaps for lower extremity coverage is still an excellent choice that should not be overshadowed by the excitement over free flaps, particularly in the proximal two thirds of the lower leg. However, local muscle flaps should not be considered in extensive crush injuries because muscle damage usually extends further than is immediately apparent, and vascular compromise is likely. In high-energy injuries, vascular trauma in the region of the major blood supply to the muscle will contraindicate the muscle transfer. The judicious use of arteriography is recommended in trauma cases before selecting a treatment option.

Both local and free muscle flaps will undergo some atrophy in time, due to denervation. Thus, flaps that are initially bulky settle into an acceptable contour. Split-thickness grafts over muscle are durable and provide a better contour than the cutaneous island of a myocutaneous flap. This is because skin and subcutaneous tissue do not undergo the same atrophy as grafted muscle and frequently require secondary defatting. Also, STSGs are often required on myocutaneous flaps donor sites, thus adding significant donor site deformity.

Local Fasciocutaneous Flaps

In the early 1980s, a number of studies described the blood supply of the deep fascia and established the landmark concept of axiality of the fascial plexus. First introduced by Ponten in 1981, many fasciocutaneous flaps were subsequently reported for the lower extremity. Fasciocutaneous flaps are vascularized by musculocutaneous perforators, septocutaneous perforating vessels running in the intermuscular septa, and axial vessels (Fig. 14–3). All three flaps, after piercing the deep fascia of the leg, contribute to a rich plexus just superficial to the deep fascia that supplies the overlying skin. This plexus has a longitudinal orientation, which allows for the design of long flaps, based on perforators of the posterior tibial, peroneal, and anterior tibial vessels, with a high length-to-width ratio, along the axis of the leg. The respective fasciocutaneous flaps are based on the medial, posterolateral, and anterolateral groups of septocutaneous perforators. On the lower leg, these flaps can be raised medially (most commonly), laterally, or posteriorly. There is a positive correlation between the size of a fasciocutaneous perforator and the size of its largest fascial branch, thus providing further rationale for using large perforators in clinical practice. Fasciocutaneous flaps based on the sural artery (posterolaterally) and saphenous artery (medially) have also been described. In this case, such axial vessels strongly contribute to the suprafascial plexus (Figs. 14–4 and 14–5).

Fasciocutaneous flaps are traditionally proximally based. However, new distally based flaps have been introduced in recent years. In these flaps, based on distal septocutaneous perforators of the posterior tibial and peroneal vessels, the proximal-to-distal flow is reversed, and coverage of distal defects, including the foot, is provided. Distally based, fasciocutaneous flaps require a second-stage procedure of cutting the bridge and insetting the flap, unless raised as fascia only (Fig. 14–6). Ease of dissection, versatility in positioning, and short operating time are the most significant advantages of fasciocutaneous flaps. Preoperative Doppler assessment is

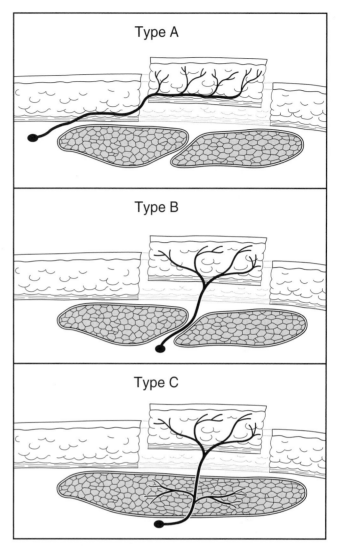

Figure 14–3 Classification of fasciocutaneous flaps by their pattern of blood supply. Type A demonstrates an axial blood supply into the flap from an artery that comes from beneath the fascia. Type B shows a septocutaneous perforator that comes through intermuscular septum to penetrate the overlying skin. In type C, the blood supply is derived from a musculocutaneous perforating vessel. Reproduced with permission from Mathes SJ, Nahai F. Classification of the vascular anatomy of muscles. Experimental and clinical correlation. *Plast Reconstr Surg.* 1981;67:8.

necessary, especially for distally based flaps. Fasciocutaneous flaps are not appropriate for deep defects with bone loss, where free muscle transfer is preferable. Well-vascularized muscle provides a better healing milieu to the chronic or infected wound.

Free Flaps

Free flaps are mandatory in all high energy or crushing injuries with associated vascular injury (Gustilo type IIIB and IIIC or Byrd type IV), where salvage of the limb is still possible. This is because the vascularity of the remaining local tissues is so precarious that local flap mobilization may result in flap necrosis. The gastrocnemius and soleus muscles are often

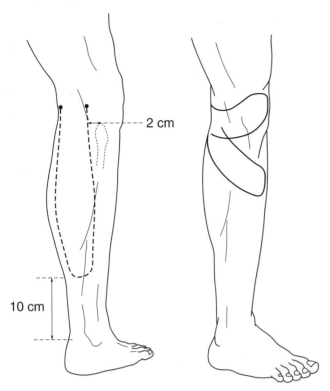

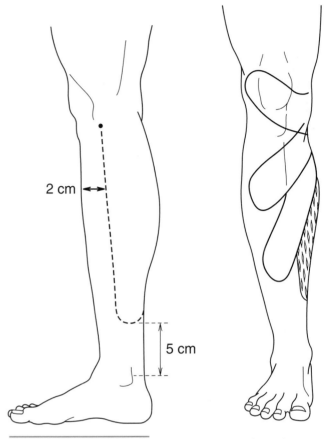

Figure 14–4   Fasciocutaneous flap of the lower extremity based on the sural artery. The sural artery supplies skin of the posterior lateral aspect of the leg as a type A fasciocutaneous flap. The flap is elevated to include the posterior fascia and provides an arc of rotation that covers the proximal lateral tibia and knee.

Figure 14–5   A fasciocutaneous flap based on the saphenous artery and vein. This subfascial vessel penetrates the subcutaneous tissues proximal to the knee and supplies the skin of the medial leg to within 5 cm of the medial malleolus. This fascia and skin flap provide coverage for proximal and middle tibial defects.

involved in the injury zone of high-energy trauma, and thus, are unsuitable for local transfer. Free muscle provides an unlimited supply of undamaged, well-vascularized tissue.

Microvascular tissue transfer has progressed to the point that it is often the first choice for coverage of complex lower extremity wounds, even when other alternative methods could be considered. The lack of reliable local flaps for distal leg coverage has actually simplified the decision-making process. Thus, indications for free tissue transfer include most distal and middle third tibial wounds, weight-bearing foot wounds, high-velocity injuries, radiation damage, osteomyelitis, tumor resections, and all instances where simultaneous bone reconstruction is required. Free flaps have been shown to shorten hospitalization (usually 5 to 7 days for most lower extremity reconstructions) and reduce the number of operative procedures when compared with conventional techniques. Although many free flaps have been described, only a handful of reliable transfers are needed in everyday practice. These include mostly muscle flaps, such as rectus abdominis, latissimus dorsi, serratus anterior and gracilis, all with STSGs. Less frequently, fasciocutaneous or fascial free flaps, such as scapular, radial forearm and temporoparietal fascia, are used.

Free muscle flaps will mold to the irregular geometry of lower extremity wounds. They have long, vascular pedicles

of large caliber and are easily dissected. They have acceptable donor morbidity and provide ample well-vascularized tissue to the ischemic and often infected defect.

Essential guidelines for free flaps to the lower extremity are:

1. *The microvascular anastomosis should be made outside the zone of injury.* In the severely traumatized lower limb, major distal vessels may be enclosed in fibrotic tissue and undergo severe vasospasm during dissection. Anastomoses must be carried out to vessels free of fibrosis and scarring, even if this requires the use of vein grafts. Pulsatile flow in the recipient artery is an absolute prerequisite in vessel assessment. A long, vascular pedicle, such as for the latissimus dorsi, usually permits placement of the vascular anastomoses well away from the zone of injury.

2. *End-to-side arterial anastomoses should be used.* Major distal vessels may be injured in severe trauma, and circulation to the leg may depend on a single vessel. It is mandatory to prevent the sacrifice of these vessels. Arteriography is essential in planning these procedures. End-to-side anastomoses are reliable and justified in the single vessel extremity.

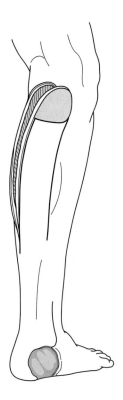
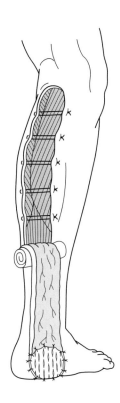
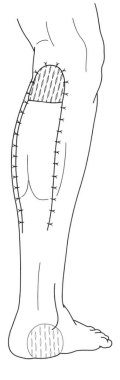
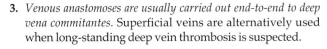

Figure 14–6 Distally based pedicle fasciocutaneous flaps derive their blood supply to the subfascial plexus through perforating vessels of the posterior tibial and peroneal arteries. With this reversed blood flow coverage of distal defects of the foot and ankle are possible. A second staged division of the flap is required. The donor site must be skin grafted.

3. *Venous anastomoses are usually carried out end-to-end to deep vena commitantes.* Superficial veins are alternatively used when long-standing deep vein thrombosis is suspected.

Thrombosis at the anastomotic site is usually the result of technical errors (inadequate resection of the injured vessel segment, elevation of an intimal flap in preexisting vascular disease, or improper placement of sutures) and is most likely in the first 24 to 48 hours following surgery. Heparin or dextran are not routinely administered. Rather, attention is kept on maintaining the patient normothermic and normotensive, especially after the anastomosis is completed. If platelet thrombi form intra-operatively, a full anticoagulant dose of intervenous heparin is administered. Flaps are monitored postoperatively with attention to the venous signal. An implantable Doppler venous probe, providing monitoring for 4 to 5 days postoperatively, is routinely used. This method has proved to be accurate in early detection of thrombosis at the anastomotic site. Alternatively, transcutaneous Doppler monitoring of flap vessels or flap color, temperature, and capillary refill are used.

The magnitude of the traumatic insult is considered to be the most significant factor associated with anastomotic failure. In the review by Khouri and Shaw (1989) of the NYU-Bellevue experience of 304 lower extremity wounds treated with free flaps, the rate of thrombosis doubled in the presence of vascular trauma, increased threefold in the presence of large bony defects, and increased fivefold when vein grafts were needed.

Contrary to widespread belief, microvascular tissue transfer is not contraindicated in elderly patients. The length of the surgical procedure does not influence the operative risk in patients of any age. Obviously, specific medical problems, more frequent in the elderly population, need to be considered.

PEARL

Only a recipient vessel with pulsatile flow is acceptable for microvascular anastomosis.

PITFALL

In the operative sequence, it is sound practice to identify the recipient vascular bundle and decide whether it is acceptable for free flap transfer *before* dissecting the flap and *before* thorough debridement of the recipient defect.

RECONSTRUCTIVE OPTIONS BY REGION

Although a multitude of flaps have been described for lower extremity reconstruction, relatively few are used frequently. Robust flaps that have withstood the test of time are presented.

Thigh

Skin grafts are applied if no bone or vital structures are exposed. Flap reconstruction is reserved for deep-space obliteration following removal of infected hip prostheses or for coverage of the femoral artery and nerves following tumor resection. Many regional muscle flaps are available for defects associated with exposure of vascular prostheses, postradiation wounds, or large tumor resection. In the upper thigh and groin, these include inferior rectus abdominis, gracilis, sartorius, tensor fasciae latae, vastus lateralis, and rectus femoris muscle flaps. In the distal thigh the muscle flaps include: extended rectus abdominis myocutaneous flaps/gastrocnemius muscle with fascial scoring/distally based gracilis and free flaps.

Gracilis and sartorius muscle units are occasionally used for proximal thigh defects to cover vascular prostheses and are best used as a turn-over flap. In the groin, the segmental (type IV) pattern of circulation of the sartorius limits its rotation. Tensor fasciae latae, better known for trochanteric pressure sores coverage, is occasionally used for posterior thigh or groin defects. Vastus lateralis and medialis can be useful to cover the middle thigh. Each of these flaps is based on the medial femoral circumflex artery (Fig. 14–7).

The rectus abdominis muscle, or myocutaneous flap, deserves some attention: Supplied by the deep inferior epigastric artery, the flap can reach the groin, hip, and midthigh. When including an extended skin paddle on a fully mobilized vascular pedicle, it can reach the distal femur. This flap is useful for obliterating hip wounds from infected prostheses (Fig. 14–8). The skin paddle can also be de-epithelialized and

employed to fill dead space. In women, a useful design is the "flag flap," which uses a transverse island of skin and fat on the ipsilateral rectus muscle. Morbidity is minimal if care is taken in closure of the fascial layers of the abdominal wall. Management of the stiff, fibrosed hip wound following failed total hip prostheses precludes use of local muscle flaps for dead space management. In these cases, we have used a latissimus free muscle flap with vascular anastomoses to the femoral artery and saphenous vein.

Knee

Knee reconstruction options include: medial or lateral gastrocnemius muscle flap, distally based, vastus lateralis flap; and free tissue transfer.

Although skin grafts are the method of choice when the joint capsule is intact, the orthopaedic surgeon is often faced with an open knee joint following trauma or exposed prosthesis. The increased frequency of knee arthroplasty has

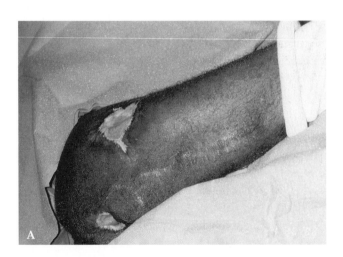

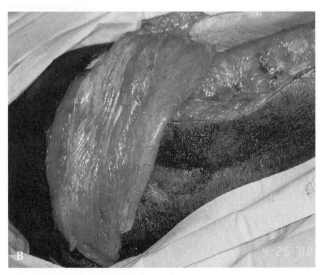

Figure 14–7 Use of the vastus lateralis muscle for coverage of infected hip wound and girdle-stone procedure. **(A)** Preoperative wound showing chronic opening over the greater trochanter and ischial pressure sore of the right leg. **(B)** The vastus lateralis muscle is elevated on the descending branch of the lateral femoral circumflex artery. The arc of rotation permits passage of the muscle into the hip cavity. **(C)** Healed wound approximately 6 weeks after surgery. The muscle flap fills the cavity resulting from a girdle-stone resection of the proximal femur.

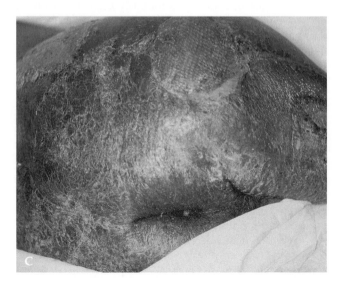

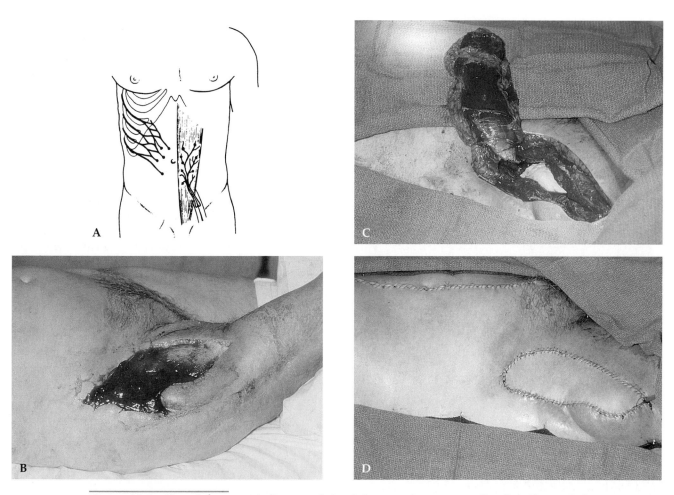

Figure 14–8 Use of the extended rectus abdominis musculocutaneous flap for coverage of infected hip wound. **(A)** Diagrammatic representation of the rectus abdominis flap based on the deep inferior epigastric artery and vein. The skin island may be extended on the ipsilateral side to include intercostal perforating vessels. **(B)** Patient with open wound of the hip following complication after total hip arthroplasty. **(C)** Elevation of rectus abdominis musculocutaneous flap. The infected hip wound was debrided and filled with antibiotic impregnated methyl metracrylate. **(D)** Hip wound closed with musculocutaneous flap.

resulted in an increased number of patients with exposed prostheses. Total knee arthroplasty has a 5% rate of deep infection and wound failure. Rheumatoid arthritis and steroid use are predisposing factors to the development of deep infection.

In most instances of wound breakdown with exposure of the prosthesis, *early soft tissue coverage is required*. Failure to act promptly may result in loss of the prosthesis. The preferred flap is the medial or lateral head of the gastrocnemius, depending on the size of the defect and its location. In most cases, even lateral defects can be closed by the use of the medial flap, which is larger, more robust and more mobile (Fig. 14–9). Free muscle flaps, usually the latissimus dorsi with STSG, are used when the prosthesis is exposed and a large area of tissue is required for coverage. The free, latissimus dorsi flap is large and has a long, vascular pedicle. When innervated, it can be used to provide extension of the knee through reconstruction of the quadriceps muscle.

Microvascular anastomoses are usually performed to the popliteal artery and saphenous vein, well outside the area of fibrosis (Fig. 14–10).

Another application for gastrocnemius local flaps and latissimus dorsi free flaps is limb-sparing surgery for sarcoma around the knee.

When injury to the popliteal precludes the use of the gastrocnemius muscle, a vastus lateralis muscle flap can be used for knee coverage. The vastus lateralis, based on its distal blood supply from the superior lateral geniculate artery, will reach upper lateral knee defects if the main proximal vascular pedicle is divided from the lateral femoral circumflex artery. Superficial muscle necrosis, managed by subsequent STSG, is a frequently seen complication.

The gastrocnemius has a type I pattern of circulation, with its medial and lateral head each receiving a single pedicle from the popliteal artery, the sural artery, which enters the deep surface of the muscle within the popliteal fossa. The

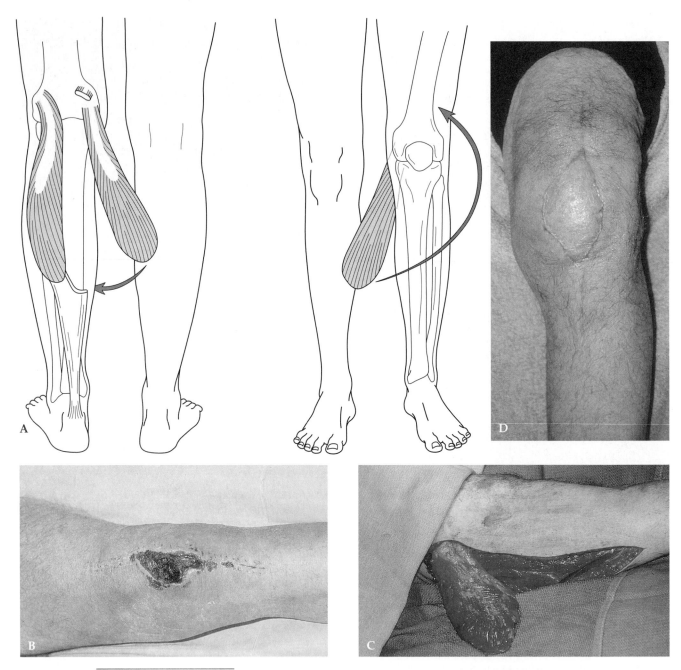

Figure 14–9   Use of the medial gastrocnemius muscle flap for knee coverage. **(A)** Diagrammatic representation of the blood supply and arc of rotation of the gastrocnemius muscle flap. The medial gastrocnemius muscle is somewhat longer than the lateral head. **(B)** Skin necrosis of anterior knee following total knee prosthesis. **(C)** Elevation of a medial gastrocnemius muscle flap through a midlateral approach. The distal portion of the gastrocnemius muscle is separated from the Achilles' tendon and the medial half remains functional. **(D)** Late result showing complete healing of the knee wound with preservation of knee prosthesis.

PEARL

The gastrocnemius muscle flap is an excellent salvage procedure when a knee prosthesis becomes exposed and should always be considered before deciding on removal of the prosthesis.

medial gastrocnemius is larger and longer than the lateral gastrocnemius, and has a wider arc of rotation (Fig. 14–9a). Although the flap may include a large, skin paddle extending distally to the muscle, (see middle third leg coverage below) this provides excessively bulky coverage and creates an unsightly donor defect. Muscle with a meshed STSG is preferred. The myocutaneous version should be reserved only for extensive defects about the knee.

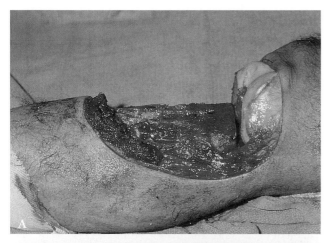

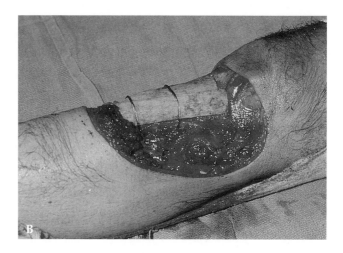

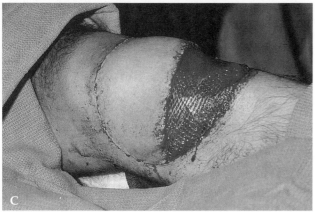

Figure 14–10 Use of latissimus dorsi free flap for coverage of extensive knee wound following tumor reconstruction. **(A)** Defect of proximal tibia following resection of osteosarcoma and surrounding soft tissues of the tibia. **(B)** Knee fusion was performed with prosthesis and allograft bone. **(C)** Coverage of the defect was provided with a latissimus dorsi musculocutaneous free flap. The muscle portion is skin grafted. Vascular anastomosis was performed using the popliteal artery and vein through a medial approach.

Technique

The medial gastrocnemius is exposed through a medial longitudinal incision from the knee to the ankle, 2 cm posterior to the medial edge of the tibia. After bluntly separating gastrocnemius and soleus in the upper third of the leg, the medial head is divided from the lateral head on the deep surface of the muscle. Usually, a midline raphe is apparent at this level. The dissection proceeds distally, with separation from the medial half of the soleus, until the tendinous junction with the medial Achilles' tendon is completely divided. Rotation of the muscle doesn't require direct visualization of the pedicle. After transposition into the defect, the muscle is covered by a meshed STSG, and the donor site is closed directly.

Elevation of the lateral gastrocnemius is similar, through a lateral longitudinal incision 2 cm posterior to the fibula. The peroneal nerve is encountered at the head of the fibula and must be protected when rotating the flap anteriorly.

For extensive knee defects, both medial and lateral heads can be elevated by a posterior midline "stocking seam" incision. No functional deficit results if the soleus is intact.

Below-knee Amputation Stump

A frequent problem in patients with a below-knee amputation is breakdown of the skin overlying bone. When shortening the bone is undesirable, coverage options include V-to-Y advancement of the remnant of the gastrocnemius muscles or free tissue transfer. Division of the origin of the gastrocnemius from the femoral condyles will allow distal advance-

---

PEARL

Linear incisions (scoring) or excision of the thick, posterior fascia on the underside of the gastrocnemius will allow expansion of the muscle and increase the area of coverage. Better "fit" of the muscle into defects of irregular depth is also achieved. The same technique is used for the soleus. A rim of fascia is preserved to facilitate suture placement while insetting the flap.

PITFALL

When raising a lateral gastrocnemius muscle flap, injury to the common peroneal nerve must be avoided.

---

ment of muscle and sensate skin approximately 3 cm. The popliteal donor site is closed in a V-Y fashion, and the wound below the pressure area is closed directly. The latissimus muscle or myocutaneous flap is usually used if a free flap is necessary because it provides ample soft tissue coverage with a long vascular pedicle, allowing anastomosis in the popliteal fossa. The skin over the free flap will be insensate. The patient must be careful to avoid pressure ulceration (Fig. 14–11).

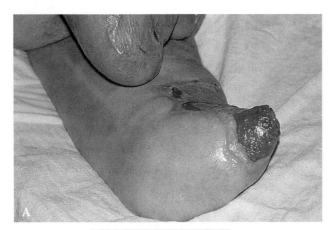
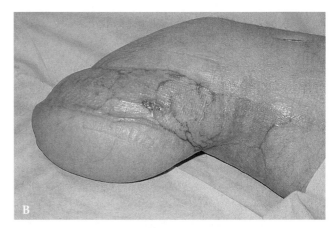

Figure 14–11 Free latissimus dorsi flap for preservation of below knee amputation stump. **(A)** Traumatic below-knee amputation with inadequate soft tissue for preservation of proximal tibial stump. **(B)** Use of latissimus dorsi muscle in a free tissue transfer. The skin and subcutaneous tissues provide excellent padding. The flap, however, is not sensate, and requires vigilance in the use of prosthetic application.

Leg

There are different options for soft tissue coverage of upper, middle, and distal thirds of the leg. Local muscle flaps or fasciocutaneous flaps are used for coverage of the proximal and middle third defects when their blood supply is intact. Free tissue transfer is generally the best option for distal third defects.

Upper Third

The available muscles for covering defects of the upper third of the tibia in decreasing order of preference are: (1) the medial head of the gastrocnemius, (2) the lateral head of the gastrocnemius, (3) the proximally based soleus, and (4) the bipedicled tibialis anterior (lower part).

Medial or lateral gastrocnemius muscle flaps with STSG are the method of choice for coverage of exposed bone. The medial head is ideal because of its single proximal vascular pedicle and broad belly. It is usually the first choice when all options are open. The lateral gastrocnemius is smaller and will resurface most of the anterior aspect of the knee except for the medial surface. These flaps can also be elevated as undelayed musculocutaneous flaps as described above for cross-leg flaps (Fig. 14–2). When the origin of either muscle is freed from the condyle of the femur, mobilization of the neurovascular pedicle will increase the reach of the flap. The medial gastrocnemius can be advanced distally an additional 5 cm to cover defects of the mid tibia or proximally to provide better coverage for defects up to 10 cm above the knee joint.

The proximally based soleus may reach upper third defects with extensive dissection, but is best for middle third defects. When the sural pedicles to the gastrocnemius are damaged due to the injury, there is a high likelihood of the proximal blood supply to the soleus being damaged also. A free flap is required in such cases.

The tibialis anterior muscle is best used as a pull-over bipedicled flap, preserving its origin and insertion, and thus preserving muscle function. The tibialis anterior is the main dorsiflexor of the foot and shouldn't be sacrificed. Dissection requires separating the muscle from its dense anterior tibial connections and transposing it to small tibial defects while retaining the segmental blood supply from the anterior tibial artery. Another possibility is to split the tibialis anterior through an external longitudinal incision and turn the medial portion of the muscle over as an anteriorly hinged flap. In each option, innervation and muscle function are maintained.

Fasciocutaneous flaps, based on perforators from the deep arterial system, are another good option for both upper and middle third defects, although muscle is preferred to cover exposed hardware and infected bone. Also, transfer of large fasciocutaneous flaps will cause a significant, grafted donor site deformity. Preoperative Doppler assessment of the location of the main perforators is prudent; the posteromedial saphenous flap (on perforators from the saphenous artery) and the sural flap (on perforators from the medial superficial sural artery). When the sural nerve is harvested with the sural flap, this becomes a neurosensory flap. (Figs. 14–5 and 14–6)

Finally, free flaps can be employed when there is a large area of exposed bone or when the gastrocnemius vascular pedicle has been damaged.

Middle Third

The available muscles for covering defects of the middle third of the tibia in decreasing order of preference are: (1) the soleus muscle, proximally based; (2) the medial gastrocnemius muscle or myocutaneous flap (with division of the muscle origin); (3) the tibialis anterior; and (4) other local muscles (extensor digitorum longus, flexor digitorum longus, extensor hallucis longus, and flexor hallucis longus muscle for the lower portion of the middle third).

The most useful muscle for coverage of soft tissue defects in the middle third is the soleus. The soleus muscle, based proximally, can be reliably carried anteriorly to a point approximately 5 cm above its tendinous insertion (Fig. 14–12). In evaluating a lower extremity wound, the status of the soleus needs to be ascertained. An angiogram is essential whenever integrity of the proximal vascular pedicles to the muscle is in doubt. The soleus has a type II pattern of circu-

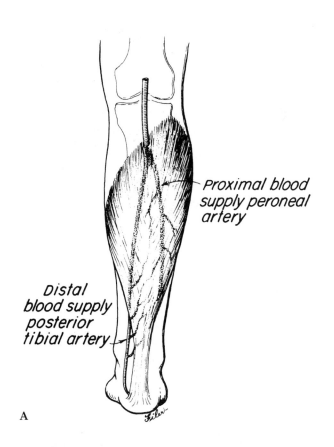

Proximal blood supply peroneal artery

Distal blood supply posterior tibial artery

A

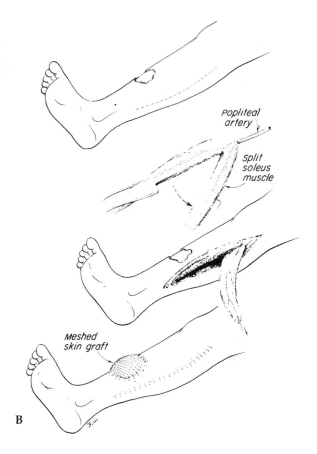

Popliteal artery

split soleus muscle

Meshed skin graft

B

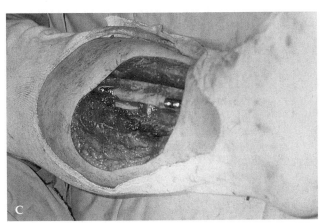

C

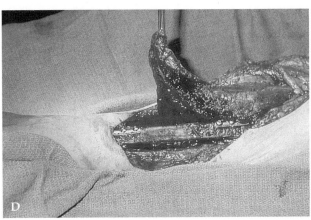

D

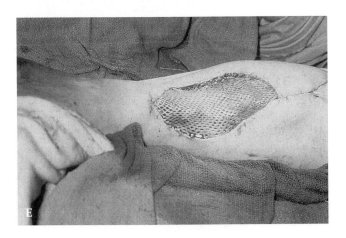

E

Figure 14–12 **(A)** Blood supply to the soleus muscle. The proximal portion of the soleus is supplied by the peroneal artery and popliteal artery. The distal portion is supplied by branches of the posterior tibial artery. **(B)** The soleus muscle is detached from the Achilles' tendon and rotated to cover middle third tibial defects. Rotation of the entire muscle is preferred. **(C)** Use of the soleus muscle flap for coverage of middle third tibial defect following radical resection for malignant fibrohystiocytoma. **(D)** The soleus muscle is elevated based on its proximal blood supply and rotated to cover the reconstructed tibia. **(E)** Closure of wound with skin graft over soleus muscle.

lation, with dominant vessels to the muscle from the popliteal, posterior tibial, and peroneal artery in its proximal portion and minor pedicles from the posterior tibial artery in its distal portion. The most important perforators are located in the proximal third. Dissection can usually be stopped well before this point, still allowing adequate rotation to cover the tibial defect. All the soleus or the medial half can be used, leaving the lateral muscle in continuity with the Achilles tendon. No functional defect is noted if the soleus muscle is utilized leaving both heads of the gastrocnemius intact. The soleus is responsible for the venous pump phenomenon and aids in posture stabilization and slow gait. Although its action is not missed after transfer, there may be long-term effects on the venous return of the lower extremity. Some authors even describe taking both soleus and one of the heads of the gastrocnemius without significant functional morbidity. We would prefer a free flap for such an extensive deformity.

Technique

The soleus is exposed through the same midline medial incision used for the medial gastrocnemius. After blunt separation of soleus from gastrocnemius in the intermuscular plane proximally, the soleus is divided from its junction with the Achilles tendon from midcalf distally. The deep surface of the muscle is separated from the flexor digitorum longus, and the soleus is elevated proximally, dividing minor distal vascular pedicles to allow anterior rotation of the muscle. Once elevation of the flap reaches the midcalf level, no vascular pedicle is divided unless its release is obligatory to increase flap length. After transposition into the defect, the exposed muscle is covered by a meshed STSG. The donor site is closed directly.

PEARL

It is good practice to take as much of the soleus as possible distally because the muscle often extends more distally than is commonly appreciated. Although the vascularity of this distal portion needs to be assessed at the time of surgery, it is often found that the soleus will cover even the more proximal portion of distal third defects.

PITFALL

Although the medial half of the soleus can be used, in practice it is often best to take the whole muscle. This avoids the risk of leaving the main blood supply behind.

The medial gastrocnemius muscle flap with division of its origin from the femoral condyle has been already described. When taken with a skin island extending to within 5 cm from the medial malleolus, the reach of the flap is extended distally, at the expense of a grafted donor site. The fascia underlying the skin island is included in the flap because the blood supply to the skin is from fasciocutaneous vessels derived

from the most distal perforators through the muscle. Another option is the bipedicled myocutaneous gastrocnemius flap transposed anteriorly to cover the tibial defect (Fig. 14–13).

Lesser-used options for middle third defects are smaller muscle flaps including tibialis anterior, flexor and extensor digitorum longus, and flexor and extensor hallucis longus. These muscles are seldom used because of functional considerations and because of their small size and tenuous blood supply (type IV). Extensive mobilization of these muscles in the traumatized extremity frequently leads to muscle necrosis. The flexor digitorum longus can be transferred without significant functional loss, but the lack of bulk in the muscle belly limits it to small defects or as an adjunct to other flaps. Its function in toe flexion is probably not missed because of its attachment to the flexor hallucis longus, and because it is also supplemented by the action of the flexor digitorum brevis. The extensor digitorum longus should be used only by separating a portion of the muscle belly from the tendon, otherwise permanent loss of toe extension results. Also, the superficial peroneal nerve must be protected during dissection. The extensor hallucis longus extends almost to the level of the lateral malleolus, but its belly is so narrow that it can only be used in small defects or to augment other flaps. To prevent drop of the great toe the distal tendon should be attached to the extensor digitorum communis when dividing the muscle for transfer. The flexor hallucis longus muscle is larger than the adjacent flexor digitorum communis, but its primary function of providing push off for the great toe should contraindicate its use, particularly in athletic individuals (Fig. 14–14).

Fasciocutaneous flaps are another option for middle third defects. Ponten's medial flap based on perforators from the posterior tibial artery and lateral flap based on perforators from the peroneal and anterior tibial artery are reliable "super flaps." Actually, most fasciocutaneous flaps for the middle third of the leg can be designed without identifying a specific perforating artery. They are "random pattern" fasciocutaneous flaps, whose length-to-width ratio can be 3:1; double that of random cutaneous flaps (1.5:1). However, preoperative Doppler assessment of the location of the main perforators is prudent.

Finally, free flaps should be employed for large areas of exposed bone or when the proximal pedicles to the soleus have been damaged.

Lower Third

Most distal leg wounds are best reconstructed with free tissue transfer. Local muscle flaps are useful for small defects of exposed tibia. Potentially useful muscles include the flexor hallucis longus, flexor digitorum longus, tibialis anterior, and abductor hallucis for medial lower third injuries and the peroneus tertius and peroneus brevis muscles for lateral lower third injuries.

Distally based muscle flaps offer an advantageous arc of rotation, but their use is associated with high failure rates, especially acutely when the tissue around the fracture site is damaged. The distally based soleus, on its pedicles from the posterior tibial artery, may be a useful alternative, especially in children, for coverage of larger defects of the distal lower third. However, this flap is considered unreliable by many

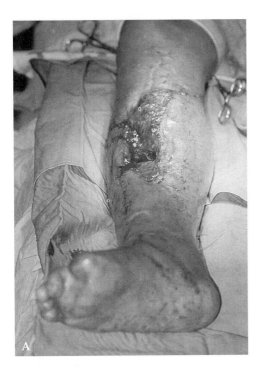

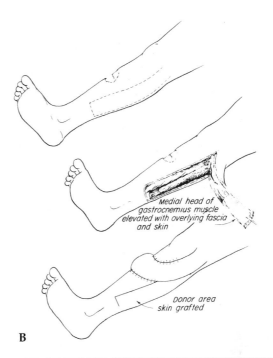

Medial head of
gastrocnemius muscle
elevated with overlying fascia
and skin

Donor area
skin grafted

B

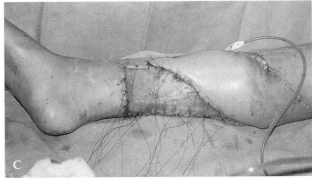

C

Figure 14–13 Use of the gastrocnemius undelayed myocutaneous flap with fascia extension for middle third defect. **(A)** Middle third tibial wound following traumatic crush injury to the middle third of the tibia. **(B)** Diagram of gastrocnemius myocutaneous flap with fascial extension. A skin flap can be elevated in conjunction with the medial gastrocnemius muscle to within 5 cm of the medial malleolus. **(C)** The skin flap is rotated anteriorly and a donor site covered with a skin graft.

authors. Tissue losses of this magnitude are better treated with free flaps.

Distally based fasciocutaneous flaps have been described in recent years. These reverse-flow flaps are perfused by distal septocutaneous perforators from the posterior tibial (medially), peroneal (posterolaterally), and anterior tibial vessels (anterolaterally), while preserving all the main arterial flows to the extremity. Reverse-flow island flaps on the peroneal artery, anterior tibial artery, and posterior tibial artery have also been employed. They are simple, versatile, and can easily cover in one stage distal third and foot defects; however, they all involve the sacrifice of an important artery of the leg. Free tissue transfer is preferred (Fig. 14–15).

Free tissue transfer is the primary option for distal third coverage of the tibia, an open ankle joint, or extensive soft tissue defects. Muscle flaps covered by a meshed STSG provide the best contour after subsequent shrinkage of muscle. For large defects, the tailored latissimus dorsi flap has the additional advantage that its vascular pedicle is long enough to allow anastomosis well proximal to the zone of injury. For smaller defects, such as around the ankle and very distal tibia, the gracilis flap, based on the medial femoral circumflex artery, is convenient and reliable. The rectus abdominis muscle, on the deep inferior epigastric artery, is very useful

for intermediate-sized or long-and-narrow defects. The pedicle is long, and dissection is easily accomplished through a transverse suprapubic incision. These flaps are reliable workhorses for microsurgical transfer, In experienced hands their success rate is greater than 95% (Fig. 14–16).

Finally, when a free flap is not possible or has failed, the time honored cross-leg flap remains a useful option despite its significant morbidity. The flap should be designed on a longitudinal axis, as a proper medial fasciocutaneous flap. The medial gastrocnemius muscle can be included in the flap (see Fig. 14–2). A Hoffman external fixator device provides better immobilization than the conventional plaster and cross-brace technique.

Foot

Split-thickness or full-thickness skin graft coverage of all non–weight-bearing areas of the foot is perfectly adequate and remains the method of choice when bone, cartilage, or tendons are not exposed. If the weight-bearing bony surface has adequate pad, but there is deficient local cutaneous cover, a skin graft is also appropriate, although hyperkeratosis and ulceration can subsequently be seen. Defects on weight-

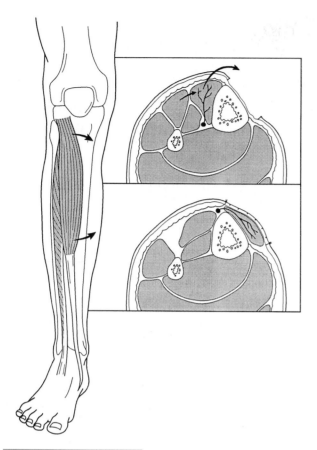

Figure 14–14 Use of the tibialis anterior and extensor digitorum longus for middle third tibial coverage. The muscle is split with preservation of the tendon integrity and turned over small defects of the middle third of the tibia. The muscle is then skin grafted.

bearing surfaces where adequate soft tissue padding is missing should instead be covered with similar plantar tissue, local muscle flaps, or free tissue transfer. Similar plantar tissue, provided by the non–weight-bearing midsole "instep" area, is the ideal solution because it replaces the defect with the same specialized dermal-epidermal histology and with the same "padding" architecture of sparse subcutaneous tissue adhering by robust septi to the underlying fascia.

For practical purposes, it is useful to classify the foot into four different zones: ankle, dorsum, proximal plantar area, and distal plantar area. For each of these, different flaps are available.

Ankle (malleoli, Achilles' tendon and non–weight-bearing heel)

- lateral calcaneal artery flap (medial malleolus)
- lateral supramalleolar flap
- extensor digitorum brevis muscle island flap
- dorsalis pedis island flap
- distally based fasciocutaneous flaps
- free flaps

The lateral calcaneal artery fasciocutaneous flap is a sensory flap based on the lateral calcaneal artery, which runs with the

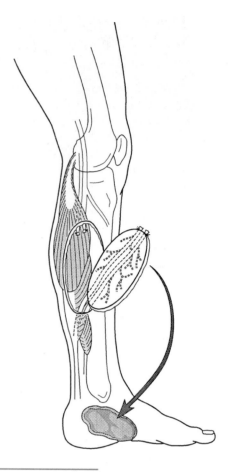

Figure 14–15 Distally based fasciocutaneous flaps based on perforators of the posterior tibial or anterior tibial arteries. Reverse-flow flaps may be elevated to include the major artery of the leg. This does require sacrifice of a major inflow vessel. The donor site is skin grafted; however, secondary division of the pedicle is not required.

lesser saphenous vein and the sural nerve and originates from the peroneal artery. It can be employed either as a transposition flap or as an island flap to cover defects up to 3 cm of the Achilles' tendon and posterior heel. The donor site is skin grafted. Doppler examination or arteriography is indicated whenever trauma, atherosclerotic disease, or diabetes may cause doubt about the integrity of the lateral calcaneal artery (Fig. 14–17).

The lateral supramalleolar flap, described by Masquelet in 1988, is a fasciocutaneous flap supplied by a cutaneous branch from the constant perforator of the peroneal artery located 5 cm above the lateral malleolus. Its arc of rotation allows coverage of the dorsal, lateral, and plantar aspects of the foot and posterior heel, as well as the lower medial portion of the leg. Advantages of the flap are its large size, long pedicle, a distal pivot point, and the fact that a main arterial pedicle need not be sacrificed. Potential problems include venous insufficiency and painful neuroma of the superficial peroneal nerve (Fig. 14–18).

The extensor digitorum brevis muscle island flap is an excellent option for defects of the malleoli and the Achilles' tendon. Based on the lateral tarsal artery and dorsalis pedis

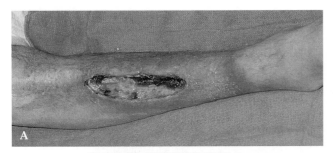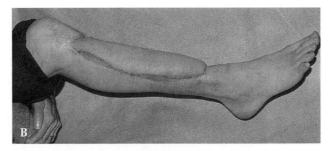

Figure 14–16   Use of latissimus dorsi free flap for extensive defect of the middle third of the tibia. **(A)** Radiation necrosis of middle third of the tibia with exposed bone. **(B)** Resolution of wound with large latissimus dorsi myocutaneous flap. Microvascular anastomoses were performed to the distal anterior tibial artery and vein.

artery and elevated by a plane of dissection near the bone to preserve the entire blood supply, it has a very large arc of rotation after distal transection of the four tendons and dorsalis pedis artery. A medial incision on the dorsum of the foot allows minimal donor site morbidity.

The dorsalis pedis island flap and the first-toe web space island flap are occasionally used options for coverage of the medial and lateral malleoli. To reach the malleoli, the dorsalis pedis flap requires dissection of its vascular pedicle through the extensor retinaculum onto the anterior tibial artery. The grafted donor site on the dorsum of the foot may represent a significant morbidity. The first-toe web space transfer is an innervated flap that includes the peroneal nerve and is based on the first dorsal metatarsal artery, a continuation of the dorsalis pedis artery. The donor defect is sufficiently distal on the foot that the skin graft used to resurface it is not on a friction point when shoes are worn. In patients with vascular insufficiency, sacrifice of the dorsalis pedis system is contraindicated.

Distally based fasciocutaneous flaps, described previously, are used occasionally for coverage of the ankle and proximal foot.

Free muscle flaps or fascia flaps are the first option where there is an open joint or fracture. The temporoparietal fascia free flap with STSG provides ideal, thin cover over the Achilles' tendon (Fig. 14–19).

PEARL

In general, the usefulness of local muscle flaps for Achilles' tendon and malleolar coverage has been overestimated in the past. Small, free flaps provide a much better solution.

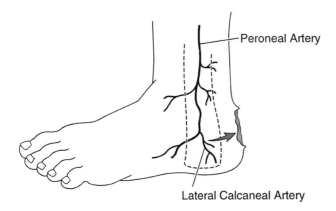

Figure 14–17   Use of the lateral calcaneal artery flap for coverage of posterior heel defects. The lateral calcaneal artery fasciocutaneous flap is supplied by terminal extensions of the saphenous vein, sural nerve, and arterial supply emanating from the peroneal artery. This flap can be elevated and rotated posteriorly to cover non–weight-bearing heel defects. The donor site must be skin grafted.

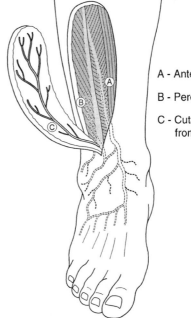

A - Anterior tibial artery
B - Peroneal artery
C - Cutaneous branch derived from distal peroneal artery

Figure 14–18   Lateral supramalleolar flap based on a perforator of the peroneal artery located 5 cm above the lateral malleolus. The flap's arc of rotation allows coverage of the dorsal, lateral, and plantar aspects of the foot and posterior heel. The donor site must be skin grafted, and a major artery of the leg is not sacrificed.

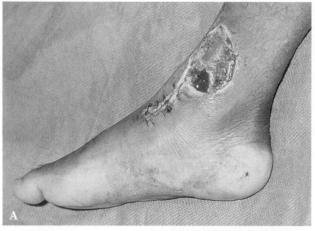

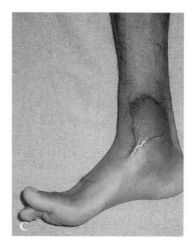

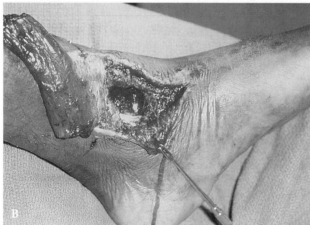

Figure 14–19 Use of a gracilis muscle free flap for coverage of ankle wound including osteomyelitis of the distal tibia. **(A)** Soft tissue loss and open wound of the tibia following distal tibial fracture. **(B)** Gracilis muscle used to obliterate cavity of distal tibia. Vascular anastomoses were performed through the posterior tibial artery and vein. **(C)** Healed wound at one year with resolution of distal tibial osteomyelitis.

Dorsum

- skin grafts
- free muscle flaps plus STSG
- free temporoparietal fascia flap

Skin grafts are first choice where intact paratenon is left over the extensor tendons. Large defects with bone/tendon exposure are best treated with free muscle transfer. Properly contoured rectus, latissimus, and serratus flaps provide bulky coverage useful for obliteration of dead space and prevention of chronic osteomyelitis. These muscles may remain thick and bulky, however, due to dependent venous stasis. The free temporoparietal fascia flap is thin, permits the use of normal footwear, and has an inconspicuous donor site. Its filmy areolar surface permits easy gliding of the extensor tendons beneath it. When extensive surgery is to be avoided, the extensor tendons of the toes can be excised and the underlying interosseii muscles skin grafted.

Proximal Plantar Area and Weight-bearing Heel

- proximal plantar subcutaneous plexus rotation flaps
- medial plantar flap

- lateral plantar flap
- flexor digitorum brevis muscle flap
- free muscle flaps plus STSG

Instep flaps from the non–weight-bearing skin of the plantar arch provide ideal characteristics for sole reconstruction. Sensate suprafascial subcutaneous rotation flaps are based medially, so as to include the medial calcaneal nerve. They are broad-based and capture the subcutaneous plexus of arteries and veins above the deep fascia. The plantar arteries are not sacrificed, nor is any damage caused to the sensory innervation of the distal foot. Flaps of this design are the first choice for resurfacing small defects on the weight-bearing heel. The flap is designed contiguous with the defect and rotated posteriorly, and the donor site is skin grafted (Fig. 14–20).

The medial plantar flap carries the instep of the foot as an axial pattern fasciocutaneous island flap based on the medial plantar vessels. It is a first choice for reconstruction of medium-sized heel defects. Sensation is supplied by branches of the medial plantar nerve identified by intraneural dissection. Good light touch sensitivity and adequate two-point discrimination is provided. This flap will not reach the Achilles area satisfactorily, due to its stiffness and short arc of rotation. The donor site on the instep is skin grafted (Fig. 14–21).

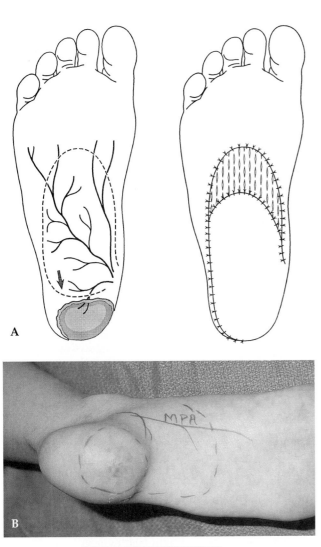

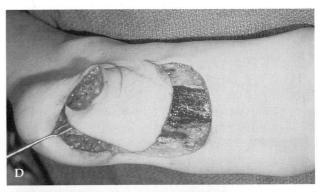

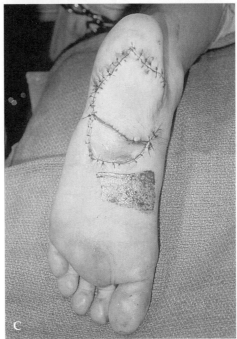

Figure 14–20 **(A)** Reconstruction of weight-bearing heel with plantar subcutaneous rotation flap. The subfascial plexus of the foot permits rotation of plantar instep flaps elevated above the plantar fascia. The plantar arteries are not sacrificed, and the flap remains sensate from branches of the medial calcaneal nerve. The donor site may require skin graft for larger defects. **(B)** Extensive A-V malformation of the weight-bearing heel. **(C)** Rotation of instep flap, which includes medial calcaneal nerve and plantar fascia. **(D)** Inset of flap with skin graft of donor site. Skin graft was harvested from the instep of the foot.

Technique

After making a transverse incision proximal to the weight-bearing area over the metatarsal heads, the medial plantar neurovascular bundle is identified distally between the abductor hallucis and flexor digitorum brevis muscles deep to the plantar fascia. The medial plantar artery and vein are divided distally and included in the flap as the flap is raised proximally. The entire non–weight-bearing portion of the midfoot can thus be raised to reconstruct the soft tissue over the heel. The flap may also be transferred as a free flap on the medial plantar artery.

The lateral plantar flap is a lesser used option that carries the instep of the foot on the lateral plantar vessels. The third choice for coverage of heel defects is a local turnover flexor digitorum brevis muscle flap and STSG. The muscle is

exposed through a midline plantar incision and folded posteriorly on itself after division of its four distal tendons. If mobilized to its neurovascular pedicle, the flexor digitorum brevis can cover the plantar surface of the heel. The muscle can also be included in a lateral plantar artery instep flap (Fig. 14–22).

Distal Plantar Area

- toe fillet
- V–Y flaps
- plantar digital web-space island flaps
- reverse medial plantar artery fasciocutaneous island flap
- free muscle flaps plus STSG

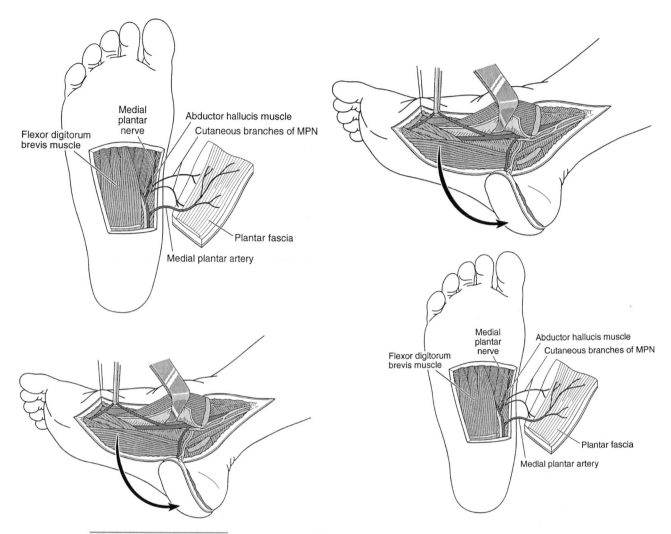

Figure 14–21 The medial plantar flap is used for coverage of extensive weight-bearing heel defects. This flap is based on the medial calcaneal artery and vein and a branch of the posterior tibial nerve. Dissection of this vascular pedicle is tedious and requires magnification. The instep of the foot requires skin grafting.

PEARL

The medial plantar artery instep flap, usually taken as an island, is an excellent choice for heel coverage.

PITFALL

Although the abductor hallucis and abductor digiti minimi muscles may reach their respective malleoli, these muscles are too small and are not usually recommended for coverage.

The principal indication for reconstruction of the forefoot is ulceration over the metatarsal heads due to diabetes. Infections involving the joint itself may be dealt with by joint resection and secondary closure. Flap coverage is required when the metatarsal head can be preserved. A good, time-honored technique for resurfacing defects in the weight-bearing aspect of the forefoot makes use of tissues obtained in toe fillet. A toe can be filleted and the bone discarded to allow transfer of the cutaneous coverage with its neurovascular supply to cover lesions over the metatarsal heads. The skin is well vascularized and innervation is maintained. The donor toe is not missed unless the great toe is filleted. The great toe, however, is sufficiently large to provide transfer of lateral tissue without sacrificing the whole toe.

Single or double V-Y flaps, based upon the plantar fascia perforators to the skin, are easily mobilized by division of the plantar fascia. They can be employed for coverage of any metatarsal head defect. Large flaps are designed to insure capture of the small perforators.

Plantar digital web space neurovascular island flaps can be useful for metatarsal head defects. The donor defect is advantageously placed in a non–weight-bearing area.

Another option for distal plantar defects is a distally based medial artery fasciocutaneous flap, based, via the plantar

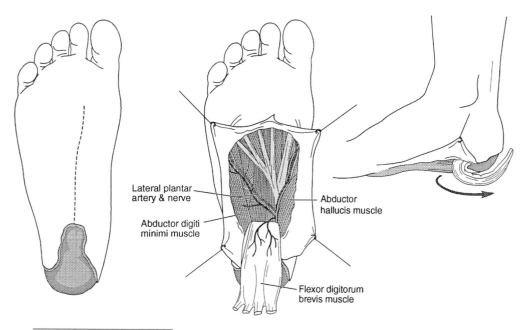

Figure 14–22 The flexor digitorum brevis muscle flap for coverage of weight-bearing heel defects. This expendable muscle is supplied by a branch of the medial or lateral plantar artery and as such can be elevated from distal to proximal through a midplantar incision. The muscle is turned over and skin grafted for posterior heel defects.

arch, on reverse flow from the lateral plantar artery. Each of these flaps is tedious to dissect and depends on accurate preoperative assessment of the intended vascular supply.

Free Tissue Flaps

Free tissue transfer is most useful in large defects, anterior defects, instances where local flaps are not available or have failed, and in deep defects with significant dead space after bony debridement.

Free muscle flaps covered by STSG can be precisely contoured to the defect, and, after shrinkage, eventually allow the patient to use normal footwear. Precise insetting of the flap without redundancy is simplified by preserving the muscle fascia and using it to tie the inset under some tension. Such flaps are superior in the presence of chronic wound infection or osteomyelitis, and remain durable. Patients bear weight directly on the grafted muscle, with deep pressure sensation present in the area, as has been shown in a series of gait analysis studies. Weight-bearing forces are well withstood because there are two "shear planes" in such flaps, one between STSG and muscle, and the other between muscle and bone. Latissimus, serratus, rectus, and gracilis are all useful for plantar resurfacing depending on size and pedicle length needs (Fig. 14–23).

> ## PEARL
>
> **Large defects of the weight-bearing heel and sole are best treated with free tissue transfer.**

OTHER ISSUES IN LOWER EXTREMITY RECONSTRUCTION

Osteomyelitis

Chronic post-traumatic osteomyelitis typically complicates Byrd type III and IV open tibial fractures. It is often due to multiple and/or highly resistant organisms and is frequently associated with bone loss. Major causes are retained necrotic or infected bone, avascular scar, dead space, and inadequate soft tissue cover. Practically, osteomyelitis of the lower extremity is now considered a chronic ischemic wound occurring in the least favorable anatomic site. Thus, the currently accepted principles of treatment are aggressive debridement, muscle flap coverage with dead space obliteration, and culture-specific intravenous antibiotic therapy.

Radical excision of all pathologic and poorly vascularized tissue is the mainstay of treatment. Although many tissue-staining methods, as well as imaging scans, may facilitate the differentiation of nonviable bone, in practice, any bone of questionable viability should be debrided to punctate bleeding from healthy bone. The vast majority of even long-term recurrences of osteomyelitis can be attributed to inadequate debridement. If debridement has compromised bone stability, rigid fixation must be performed. Traditionally, external fixators have been the preferred method, but the Ilizarov device is gaining popularity for segmental defects. Although the technical difficulty of muscle flaps is increased because of the circumferential bars, the potential for later limb lengthening can obviate the need for secondary bone grafting.

Muscle flap coverage with STSG should be done immediately if debridement is adequate. Local or free muscle flaps

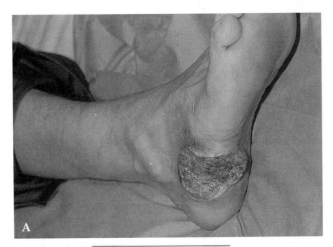
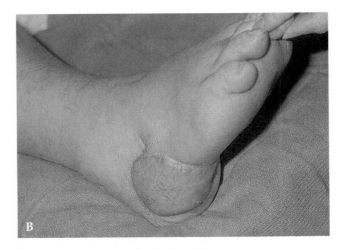

Figure 14–23 Use of free tissue transfer for weight-bearing portion of the heel. **(A)** Extensive squamous cell carcinoma of the foot and heel requiring radical resection. **(B)** Use of lateral arm flap for reconstruction of lateral and plantar surface of the heel. Vascular anastomoses were performed to the dorsalis pedis artery through a subcutaneous tunnel.

are selected depending upon the availability of local muscle and the site and extent of the zone of injury adjacent to the osteomyelitis.

Although they may cover defects in those areas, fasciocutaneous flaps are generally avoided. The fascial surface is stiff and won't easily fill in the debridement cavity, and these flaps have been found to be inferior to muscle flaps in treating infected wounds.

When secondary cancellous bone grafting or vascularized bone transfer is required, it should be delayed at least 6 weeks after the debridement and muscle flap procedure, so as to allow stable and well-revascularized wound coverage.

Finally, for particularly difficult wounds where complete debridement may not be possible (osteomyelitis involving joints or long segments of the medullary canal), the supplementary use of gentamicin beads, of implantable antibiotic pumps, or of continuous irrigation catheters should be considered.

Soft Tissue Expansion

Although the concept of recruiting tissue by expansion is an attractive one, there is no place for the use of soft tissue expansion in the acute and subacute stage of trauma to the lower extremity. The primary application of skin expansion in the lower extremity is to resurface areas of chronically unstable soft tissue or unsightly scar. Infection rates, however, range between 5 and 30%. Soft tissue expansion is definitely more difficult in the lower extremity than in other parts of the body. While expansion in the thigh is generally successful, only about 50% of expanders at or below the knee will be ultimately successful. The ankle and foot, in particular, are not suited to soft tissue expansion.

Replantation

There have been very few reports of successful outcome following replantation of the lower extremity. The degree of recovery of the peripheral nerves is generally poor, and thus a replanted lower limb may end up in technical success without restoration of function. Thus, the outcome of replantation should always be graded in terms of function as compared with a well-designed and well-fitting prosthesis. For the lower extremity, "function" should be defined as a well-vascularized limb, a well-healed wound, stable bone and joints, and protective sensibility without pain, enabling the patient unassisted ambulation.

In practice, replantation should probably be reserved to the most ideal situation, a young patient and a sharp guillotine-type amputation located in the distal third of the leg. These ideal conditions are unfortunately rarely met in clinical practice, where traumatic detachment of the extremity is usually associated with the dissipation of a tremendous force creating a wide zone of injury.

Other candidates in which a special effort to replantation should be considered are bilateral amputees, in whom sensibility of the replanted limb would be a definite advantage over two insensate prostheses.

Sensation

Free flaps and many local flaps to the lower extremity are insensate flaps. This would appear to be a problem, especially when insensate flaps are transferred to the weight-bearing portion of the foot. Neurosensory or neurotized flaps have been advocated to prevent breakdown after resurfacing the sole. However, the importance of sensibility in plantar resurfacing is overestimated. Innervated flaps to the sole of the foot do not correlate with greater soft tissue stability. They do not usually provide normal sensibility and can still break down. There is no evidence that innervated flaps provide a greater level of sensibility than their noninnervated counterparts. Many flaps with very poor sensibility have excellent durability despite this lack of sensation. For free flaps in particular, there seems to be no correlation between the sensibility and soft-tissue stability of the reconstruction.

Nonneurovascular and nonneurotized free flaps will eventually develop some sensibility to deep pressure. One can postulate that some recovery of protective sensibility occurs through some degree of reinnervation from the recipient bed and/or the periphery.

The most important reason for recurrent breakdowns after reconstruction is high pressure points in the sole. Pressure points caused by traumatic changes in bony foot architecture should be identified preoperatively and corrected at the reconstructive operation. Patient education in proper foot care and customized footware to reduce the load on the reconstruction are essential in preventing breakdown and must be provided by gait and pressure-point analysis.

SELECTED BIBLIOGRAPHY

General Overview of Lower Extremity Reconstruction

Byrd HS. Lower extremity reconstruction. *Select Read Plast Surg.* 1992;6.

Reconstructive Surgery of the lower extremity. In: McCarthy JG, ed. *Plastic Surgery.* Vol 6. Philadelphia, PA: WB Saunders; 1990:4029–4093.

Swartz WM, Jones NF. Soft tissue coverage of the lower extremity. *Curr Probl Surg.* 1985;22:1–59.

Basic Concepts in Reconstruction after Trauma

Aldea PA, Shaw WW. The evolution of the surgical management of severe lower extremity trauma. *Clin Plast Surg.* 1986;13:549–569.

Arnez ZM. Immediate reconstruction of the lower extremity. an update. *Clin Plast Surg.* 1991;18:449–457.

Byrd HS, Cierny G, Tebbetts JB. The management of open tibial fractures with associated soft-tissue loss: external pin fixation with early flap coverage. *Plast Reconstr Surg.* 1981;68:73–82.

Byrd HS, Spicer TE, Cierny G III. Management of open tibial fractures. *Plast Reconstr Surg.* 1985;76:719–730.

Cierny G III, Zorn KE, Nahai F. Bony reconstruction in the lower extremity. *Clin Plast Surg.* 1992;19:905–916.

Francel TJ et al. Microvascular soft-tissue transplantation for reconstruction of acute open tibial fractures. timing of coverage and long-term functional results. *Plast Reconstr Surg.* 1992;89:478–487.

Godina M. Early microsurgical reconstruction of complex trauma of the extremities. *Plast Reconstr Surg.* 1986;78:285–292.

Gustilo RB, Anderson JT. Prevention of infection in the treatment of 1025 open fractures of long bones. *J Bone Surg.* 1976;58A:453–458.

Hansen ST. The type IIIC tibial fracture: salvage or amputation. *J Bone Jt Surg.* 1987;69A:799–800.

Hidalgo DA. Lower extremity avulsion injuries. *Clin Plast Surg.* 1986;13:701–710.

Khouri RK, Shaw WW. Reconstruction of the lower extremity with microvascular free flaps. a 10-year experience with 304 consecutive cases. *J Trauma.* 1989:29:1086–1094.

May JW Jr, Gallico GG III, Lukash FN. Microvascular transfer of free tissue for closure of bone wounds of the distal lower extremity. *N Eng J Med.* 1982;306:253–257.

Meyer M, Evans J. Joint orthopaedic and plastic surgery management of types III and IV lower limb injuries. *Br J Plast Surg.* 1990;43:692–694.

Naggar L, Chevalley F, Blanc CH, Livio JJ. Treatment of large bone defects with the Ilizarov technique. *J Trauma.* 1993;34:390–393.

Serafin D, Voci VE. Reconstruction of the lower extremity. microsurgical composite tissue transplantation. *Clin Plast Surg.* 1983;10:55–72.

Taylor GI. The current status of free vascularized bone grafts. *Clin Plast Surg.* 1983;10:185–209.

Vasconez HC and Nicholls PJ. Management of extremity injuries with external fixator or Ilizarov devices. cooperative effort between orthopedic and plastic surgeons. *Clin Plast Surg.* 1991;18:505–513.

Weiland AJ, Moore JR, and Daniel RK. Vascularized bone autografts: experience with 41 cases. *Clin Orthop.* 1983;174:87–95.

Yaremchuk MJ et al: Acute and definitive management of traumatic osteocutaneous defects of the lower extremity. *Plast Reconstr Surg.* 1987;80:1–14.

Coverage Rationale Options

Banis JC, Werker PMN, Abul-Hassan HS, Derr JW. Cutaneous free flaps, In: GS Georgiade, R Riefkohl, Scott Levin L, eds. *Plastic, Maxillofacial, and Reconstructive Surgery.* 3rd ed. Baltimore, MD: Williams and Wilkins; 1996;911–949

Batchelor JS, Moss ALH. The relationship between fasciocutaneous perforators and their fascial branches. an anatomical study in human cadaver lower legs. *Plast Reconstr Surg.* 1995;95:629–633.

Calderon W, Chang KN, Mathes SJ. Comparison of the effect of bacterial inoculation in musculocutaneous and fasciocutaneous flaps. *Plast Reconstr Surg.* 1986;77:785–794.

Carriquiry C, Costa MA, Vasconez LO. An anatomic study of the septocutaneous vessels of the leg. *Plast Reconstr Surg.* 1985;76:354–363.

Chang KN, Mathes SJ. Comparison of the effect of bacterial inoculation in musculocutaneous and random pattern flaps. *Plast Reconstr Surg.* 1981;70:1–10.

Cordeiro PC, Neves RI, Hidalgo DA. The role of free tissue transfer following oncologic resection in the lower extremity. *Ann Plast Surg.* 1994;33:9–16.

Levin LS. Free muscle and musculocutaneous flaps, In: *Plastic, Maxillofacial, and Reconstructive Surgery.*

Goldberg JA, Goldberg BS, Lineaweaver WC, Buncke HJ. Microvascular reconstruction of the lower extremity in the elderly. *Clin Plast Surg.* 1991;18:459–465.

Grotting JC. Prevention of complications and correction of postoperative problems in microsurgery of the lower extremity. *Clin Plast Surg.* 1991;18:485–489.

Guzman-Stein G, Fix RJ, Vasconez LO. Muscle flap coverage for the lower extremity. *Clin Plast Surg.* 1991;18:545–552.

Haertsch P. The blood supply to the skin of the leg. a post-mortem investigation. *Br J Plast Surg.* 1981;34:470–477.

Hallock GG. Complications of 100 consecutive local fasciocutaneous flaps. *Plast Reconstr Surg.* 1991;88:264–268.

Hallock, GG ed. *Fasciocutaneous Flaps.* Boston, MA: Blackwell; 1992.

Hidalgo DA, Carrasquillo IM. The treatment of lower extremity sarcomas with wide excision, radiotherapy, and free-flap reconstrucfion. *Plast Reconstr Surg.*1992; 89:96–101.

Mathes SJ, Nahai F. *Clinical Atlas of Muscle and Musculocutaneous flaps.* St. Louis, MO: CV Mosby; 1979.

Mathes SJ, Nahai F. Classification of the vascular anatomy of muscle: experimental and clinical correlation. *Plast Reconstr Surg.* 1981;67:177–189.

Mathes SJ, Nahai F. *Clinical Applications for Muscle and Musculocutaneous Flaps".* St. Louis, MO: CV Mosby; 1982.

May JW, Jupiter JB, Gallico GG et al. Treatment of chronic traumatic bone wounds: microvascular free tissue transfer. a 13-year experience in 96 patients. *Ann Surg.* 1991;214:241–250.

McCraw JB, Arnold PG. *McCraw and Arnold's Atlas of Muscle and Musculocutaneous Flaps.* Norfolk, VA: Hampton Press; 1986.

Muscle and musculocutaneous flaps. In: GS Georgiade, R Riefkohl, Scott Levin L, eds. *Plastic, Maxillofacial and Reconstructive Surgery.* Baltimore,MD: Williams and Wilkins; 1996;29–34.

Ponten B. The fasciocutaneous flap. its use in soft tissue defects of the lower leg. *Br J Plast Surg.* 1981;34:215–220.

Principles and physiology of skin flap surgery. In: McCarthy JG ed. *Plastic Surgery.* Vol 1. Philadelphia, PA: WB Saunders; 1990;275–329.

O'Brien BM, Morrison WA, Gumley GJ. Principles and techniques of microvascular surgery. In: McCarthy JG, ed. *Plastic Surgery.* Vol 1. Philadelphia, PA: WB Saunders; 1990;412–475.

O'Brien BM, Morrison WA, Gumley GJ. Principles and techniques of microvascular surgery. Skin grafts. In: McCarthy JG, ed. *Plastic Surgery.* Vol 1. Philadelphia, PA: WB Saunders; 1990;221–275.

Wei FC, Gammal TA. Free vascularized bone grafts, and osteocutaneous flaps, In: *Plastic, Maxillofacial, and Reconstructive Surgery.*

Reconstructive Options by Region

Amarante J, Costa H, Reis J, Soares R. A new distally based fasciocutaneous flap of the leg. *Br J Plast Surg.* 1986;39: 338–390.

Asko-Seljavaara S et al. Comparison of latissimus dorsi and rectus abdominis free flaps. *Br J Plast Surg.* 1987;40: 620–628.

Bailey BN, Godfrey AM. Latissimus dorsi muscle free flaps. *Br J Plast Surg.* 1982;35:47–52.

Banic A, Wulff K, Latissimus dorsi free fiaps for total repair of extensive lower leg injuries in children. *Plast Reconstr Surg.* 1987;79:765–775.

Barclay TL, Cardoso E, Sharpe DT, Crockett DJ. Repair of lower leg injuries with fascio-cutaneous flaps. *Br J Plast Surg.* 1982;35:127–132.

Barclay TL, Sharpe DT, Chisholm EM. Cross-leg fasciocutaneous flaps. *Plast Reconstr Surg.* 1983;72:843–847.

Barford B, Pers M. Gastrocnemius-plasty for primary closure of compound injuries of the knee. *J Bone Jt Surg.* 1970; 528:124–127.

Bunkis J, Walton RL, Mathes SJ. The rectus abdominis free flap for lower extremity reconstruction. *Ann Plast Surg.* 1983; 11:377–380.

Colen LB, Replogle SL, Mathes SJ. The V-Y plantar flap for reconstruction of the forefoot. *Plast Reconstr Surg.* 1988; 81:220–228.

Dawson RLG. Complications of the cross-leg flap operation. *Proc R Soc Med.* 1972;65:626–629.

Dibbell DG, Edstrom LE. The gastrocnemius myocutaneous flap. *Clin Plast Surg.* 1980;7:45–50.

Donski PK, Fogdestam I. Distally based fasciocutaneous flap from the sural region: a preliminary report. *Scand J Plast Reconstr Surg.* 1983;17:191–196.

Ferreira MC, Gabbianelli G, Alonso N, Fontana C. The distal pedicle fascia flap of the leg. *Scand J Plast Reconst Surg.* 1986;20:133–136.

Fix RJ, Vasconez LO. Fasciocutaneous flaps in reconstruction of the lower extremity. *Clin Plast Surg.* 1991;18:571–582.

Gang RK. Reconstruction of soft-tissue defects of the posterior heel with a lateral calcaneal artery island flap. *Plast Reconstr Surg.* 1987;79:415–421.

Gallico GG, Ehrlichman RJ, Jupiter J. et al. Free flaps to preserve below knee amputation stumps: long-term evaluation. *Plast Reconstr Surg.* 1987;79:871–878.

Ger R. The technique of muscle transposition and the operative treatment of traumatic and ulcerative lesions. *J Trauma.* 1971;2:502–510.

Grabb WC, Argenta LC. The lateral calcaneal artery skin flap (the lateral calcaneal artery, lesser saphenous vein, and sural nerve skin flap). *Plast Reconstr Surg.* 1981; 68:723–730.

Granick MS. The plantar digital web space island flop for reconstruction of the distal sole. *Ann Plast Surg* 1987; 19:68–74.

Gumener R, Zbrodowski A, Montandon D. The reversed fasciosubcutaneous flap in the leg. *Plast Reconstr Surg.* 1991;88:1042–1043.

Hartrampf CR, Scheflan M, Bostwick J III. The flexor digitorum brevis muscle island pedicle flap. A new dimension in heel reconstruction. *Plast Reconstr Surg.* 1980; 66:264–270.

Heckler F. Gracilis myocutaneous and muscle flaps. *Clin Plast Surg.* 1980;7:27–44.

Hirshowitz B, Mascoma R, Kaufman T, Har-Shai Y. External longitudinal splitting of the tibialis anterior muscle for coverage of compound fractures of the middle third of the tibia. *Plast Reconstr Surg.* 1987;79:407–414.

Hong G, Steffens K, Wang FB. Reconstruction of the lower leg and foot with the reverse pedicled posterior tibial fasciocutaneous flap. *Br J Plast Surg.* 1989;42:512–516.

Laing JHE, Hancock K, Harrison DH. The exposed total knee replacement prosthesis: a new classification and treatment algorithm. *Br J Plast Surg.* 1992;45:66–69.

Landi A, Soragni O, and Monteleone M. The extensor digitorum brevis muscle island flap for soft-tissue loss around the ankle. *Plast Reconstr Surg.* 1985;75:892–897.

LESAVOY MA, DUBROW JJ, WACKYM PA, Eckardt JJ. Muscle-flap coverage of exposed endoprostheses. *Plast Reconstr Surg.* 1989;83:90–99.

LONG CD, GRANICK MS, SOLOMON MP. The cross-leg flap revisited. *Ann Plast Surg.* 1993;30:560–563.

MASQUELET AC, BEVERIDGE J, ROMANA C, GERBER C. The lateral supramalleolar flap. *Plast Reconstr Surg.* 1988;81:74–81.

MAY JW, GALLICO GG, JUPITED J, SAVAGE RC. Free latissimus dorsi muscle flap with skin graft for treatment of traumatic chronic bony wounds. *Plast Reconstr Surg.* 1984;73:641–651.

MAY JW, HOLLS MJ, SIMON SR. Free microvascular muscle flaps with skin graft reconstruction of extensive defects of the foot. a clinical and gait analysis study. *Plast Reconstr Surg.* 1985;75:627–641.

MAY JW, ROHRICH Rl. Foot reconstruction using free microvascular muscle flaps with skin grafts. *Clin Plast Surg.* 1986;13:681–689.

MIYAMOTO Y, IKUTA Y, SHIGETI S, YAMURA M. Current concepts of instep island flap. *Ann Plast Surg.* 1987;19:97–102.

MOLLER-LARSEN F, PETERSEN NC. Longitudinal split anterior tibial muscle flap with preserved function. *Plast Reconstr Surg.* 1984;74:398–401.

REATH DB, TAYLOR JW. The segmental rectus abdominis free flap for ankle and foot reconstruction. *Plast Reconstr Surg.* 1991;88:829–830.

RECALDE ROCHA JF GILBERT A, MASQUELET A, YOUSIF NJ, SANGER JR, MATLOUB HS. The anterior tibial artery flap. Anatomic study and clinical application. *Plast Reconstr Surg.* 1987;79:396–406.

REIFFEL RS, MCCARTHY JG. Coverage of heel and sole defects: a new subfascial arterialized flap. *Plast Reconstr Surg.* 1980;66:250–260.

SANDERS R, O'NEILL T. The gastrocnemius myocutaneous flap used as a cover for the exposed knee prosthesis. *J Bone Jt Surg.* 1981;63B:383–386.

SCHEFLAN M, NAHAI F, HARTRAMPF CR. Surgical management of heel ulcers: a comprehensive approach. *Ann Plast Surg.* 1981;7:385–406

SHANAHAN RE, GINGRASS RP. Medial plantar sensory flap for coverage of heel defects. *Plast Reconstr Surg.* 1979; 64:295–298.

SHAW WW, HIDALGO DA. Anatomic basis of plantar flap design. clinical applications. *Plast Reconstr Surg.* 1986; 78:637–649.

SNYDER GB, EDGERTON MT. The principle of the island neurovascular flap in the management of ulcerated anesthetic weight-bearing areas of the lower extremity (toe fillet). *Plast Reconstr Surg.* 1965;36:518–528.

SOMMERLAD BC, MCCROUTHER DA. Resurfacing the sole. long-term follow-up and comparison of techniques. *Br J Plast Surg.* 1978;31:107–116.

STEVENSON TR and MATHES SJ. Management of foot injuries with free-muscle flaps. *Plast Reconstr Surg.* 1986; 78:665–671.

SWARTZ WM RAMASASTRY SS, MCGILL JR, NOOMAN JD. Distally based vastus lateralis muscle flap for coverage of wounds about the knee. *Plast Reconstr Surg.* 1987; 80:255–265.

TOBIN G. Hemisoleus and reversed hemisoleus flaps. *Plast Reconstr Surg.* 1985;76:87–96.

WHITNEY TM et al. The serratus anterior free-muscle flap: experience with 100 consecutive cases. *Plast Reconstr Surg.* 1990;86:481–490.

YOSHIMURA M et al. Peroneal island flap for skin defects in the lower extremity. *J Bone Jt Surg.* 1985;67A:935–941.

Other Issues in Lower Extremity Reconstruction

ANTHONY JP, MATHES SJ, ALPERT BS. The muscle flap in the treatment of chronic lower extremity osteomyelitis. Results in patients over 5 years after treatment. *Plast Reconstr Surg.* 1991;88:311–318.

BORGES FILHO PT, NEVES RI, GEMPERLI R et al. Soft-tissue expansion in lower extremity reconstruction. *Clin Plast Surg.* 1991;18:593–599.

DAMHOLT WV. Treatment of chronic osteomyelitis: a prospective study of 55 cases treated with radical surgery and primary wound closure. *Acta Orthop Scand.* 1982; 53:715–720.

GAYLE LB, LINEAWEAVER WC, BUNCKE GM et al. Lower Extremity Replantation. *Clin Plast Surg.* 1991;437–447.

LEVIN LS, SERAFIN D. Plantar skin coverage. *Problems Plast Reconstr Surg.* 1991;1:156.

MANDERS EK, OAKS TE, AU UK et al. Soft-tissue expansion in the lower extremities. *Plast Reconstr Surg.* 1988;81:208–219.

MATHES SJ, ALPERT BS, CHANG N. Use of the muscle flap in chronic osteomyelitis: experimental and clinical correlation. *Plast Reconstr Surg.* 1982;69:815–829.

RAUTIO J. Resurfacing and sensory recovery of the sole. *Clin Plast Surg.* 1991;18:615–626.

VECSEI V, BARQUET A. Treatment of chronic osteomyelitis by necrectomy and gentamicin-PMMA beads. *Clin Orthop.* 1981;159:201–207.

WEILAND AJ, MOORE JR, DANIEL RK. The efficacy of free tissue transfer in the treatment of osteomyelitis. *J Bone Jt Surg.* 1984;66:181–193.

SAMPLE QUESTIONS

1. Degloving injuries of the lower extremity are best managed by:

   (a) careful repositioning and postoperative limb elevation

   (b) excision of degloved flaps and local or free flap coverage

   (c) coverage by split-thickness skin grafts harvested from the excised degloved flaps

2. When should soft tissue coverage of salvageable type III and IV lower extremity injuries usually be carried out:

(a) immediately following debridement, stable fixation, and bone reconstruction

(b) immediately after single-stage adequate debridement and stable fixation or after staged multiple debridements and stable fixation but before bone reconstruction

(c) after the "chronic" phase of the injury is past

3. An exposed knee prosthesis should be managed by:

(a) intravenous antibiotic coverage, constant antibiotic irrigations, and flap coverage after improvement of local wound conditions

(b) immediate removal of the prosthesis, wound closure, and subsequent replacement of the prosthesis after wound healing

(c) joint debridement leaving the prosthesis in situ and rotation flap closure

(d) joint debridement leaving the prosthesis in situ and muscle flap closure

(e) removal of the prosthesis, joint debridement, and arthrodesis

4. A traumatic, contaminated, middle third lower extremity defect with exposed tibia is preferably managed, after debridement, by:

(a) a proximally based medial or lateral fasciocutaneous flap

(b) a soleus muscle flap, after arteriography

(c) a medial gastrocnemius myocutaneous flap with extended skin paddle

(d) a widely mobilized medial gastrocnemius muscle flap with division of the muscle origin

(e) a tibialis anterior bipedicled muscle flap

5. A post-traumatic weight-bearing heel defect exposing the calcaneum (measuring 3 x 4 cm) is best managed by:

(a) split-thickness skin grafting

(b) a gracilis or rectus free muscle flap

(c) a flexor digitorum brevis muscle turnover flap

(d) a medial plantar artery flap

(e) a distally based fasciocutaneous flap

Answers: 1) c; 2) b; 3) d; 4) d; 5) d

Spine

Chapter 15

Traumatic and Degenerative Conditions of the Cervical Spine

James D. Kang, MD and Lars Gilbertson, PhD

Outline

ETIOLOGY

The etiology of cervical spine injuries involves both traumatic and degenerative conditions. Traumatic conditions can result in upper cervical spine injuries from occiput - C2 or subaxial injuries from C3-C7. The mechanism of injury can be neck hyperextension, rotation or axial load. Each may act as an isolated incident or as a combination of two or more forces. The degenerative conditions result from degeneration of the disc or formation of bone spurs. This can lead to compression of the cord, referred to as cervical myelopathy, or compression of nerve roots described as radiculopathy.

Rheumatoid arthritis creates dysfunction in the cervical spine due to erosion of supporting ligaments and softening of the bony elements. Common problems include C1-2 instability, basilar invagination or subaxial subluxation.

Traumatic Conditions: Fractures and/or Dislocations

Upper Cervical Spine Injuries (Occiput-C2)
Subaxial Injuries (C3-7)

Degenerative Conditions

Cervical Radiculopathy
Cervical Myelopathy

Rheumatoid Arthritis

C1-2 Instability
Basilar Invagination
Subaxial Subluxation

Disorders of the cervical spine may encompass clinical diagnoses from acute traumatic fractures and dislocations to chronic degenerative or inflammatory conditions. Due to potential catastrophic neurological complications, the treatment of these conditions requires that the physician have a thorough understanding of the pathophysiology as well as the appropriate steps towards diagnosing and managing these patients. This chapter outlines the basic fundamentals in diagnosing and treating some of the more common conditions affecting the cervical spine.

BASIC SCIENCE

Biomechanics of the Cervical Spine

The human cervical spine is a complex mechanical system as well as a biologically active system in which the passive structures (discs, ligaments, facet joints) and active elements (the muscles) normally function together to enable the cervical spine to maneuver and bear load while protecting the spinal cord and nerve roots. Biomechanical studies of the cervical spine have been helpful in improving understanding of (a)

Orthopaedic Surgery: The Essentials. Edited by M.E. Baratz, A.D. Watson, and J.E. Imbriglia. Thieme Medical Publishers, Inc., New York © 1999

the kinematics and load-motion characteristics (kinetics) of the entire cervical spine and its individual segments; (b) the functional role of the discs, ligaments, facet joints, and other structures (such as Luschka's joints); (c) mechanisms of cervical spine injury; (d) in vivo injured behavior (e.g., "stability/instability"); and (e) the mechanical effects of surgical and nonsurgical procedures and devices (including implants and spinal orthoses). A few selected concepts and relevant biomechanical studies are described in the following paragraphs.

Range of Motion

Range of motion (ROM) is a clinically useful concept defining the physiological limits of joint motion beyond which injury can occur. White and Panjabi (1990) have compiled tables of representative values for motion of spinal segments within the cervical spine. In axial rotation, approximately 60% of the overall motion takes place in the upper cervical spine (i.e., within the occipito-atlanto-axial or C0-C1-C2 complex), with the remaining motion occurring in the lower cervical spine (C3-T1). In flexion/extension, approximately 33% of the motion occurs in the upper cervical spine, and in lateral bending, 16%.

PEARL

The articulations of the upper cervical spine (C0-C1-C2) are responsible for 60% of axial rotation and 33% of the flexion/extension that take place in the entire cervical spine.

Due to the disproportionately large contributions of the upper cervical spine to overall mobility in axial rotation and in flexion/extension, certain clinical entities (such as degeneration or surgical fusion) may affect the patient's function more adversely if the region of involvement is the upper cervical spine rather than the lower cervical spine. Additionally, it is important to recognize that the activities of daily living often involve combined movements, for example, flexion/extension combined with axial rotation. While estimates of overall loss of motion in the cervical spine following surgical fusion can be made for single degrees of freedom (e.g., flexion/extension rotation alone), the effect of fusion on combined motion is less predictable. This is due to the coupling between the degrees of freedom (e.g., axial rotation influences flexion/extension and vice-versa).

Biomechanics of Spinal Injuries

Cervical spinal injury constitutes a spectrum of hard and soft tissue injuries, with or without facet dislocation or subluxation. Hard and soft tissue injuries can occur separately or together. Examples include:

1. disruptions in the normal continuity (i.e., fracture) of vertebral bone
2. stretch, rupture, or pull-out (bony avulsion) of the spinal ligaments
3. disruptions to intervertebral discs

It is widely accepted that the mechanical loading conditions (i.e., forces and moments) strongly influence what type of injury will occur. A large number of biomechanical studies, experimental as well as analytical, have been carried out to try to elucidate the mechanisms of injury of the cervical spine. In the upper cervical spine, mechanisms of injury have been well established for these injury types: posterior arch fractures of C-1, Jefferson's fracture (comminuted ring fracture of C-1), odontoid process fractures, and "hangman's fracture." In the lower cervical spine, mechanisms of injury are well established for compression fracture (including the "tear-drop" fracture), certain flexion and extension injuries, and "clay shoveler's fracture." Injuries that are unique to a particular portion of the cervical spine are due to differences in anatomy and forces unique to that particular level. The different injuries pose different risks to the neural structures. Assessment of this risk is an area of ongoing refinement and controversy.

The evaluation of the spinal "stability" or "instability" marks a critical decision point in the treatment algorithms of any clinician. If the condition being treated is deemed to have created instability, then some form of surgical stabilization is implemented. Stable conditions generally merit more conservative treatment such as bedrest or an orthotic. One area of the ongoing debate has to do with what constitutes an "unstable" spine because this determination often means the difference between surgery or no surgery. White and Panjabi (1990) define instability as "the loss of the ability of the spine under physiologic loads to limit patterns of displacement so that there is no initial or additional neurological deficit, no major deformity, and no incapacitating pain." They also devised criteria for evaluating instability of the upper and lower cervical spine regions. Clinical instability in the upper cervical spine (C0-C1-C2) is based largely on the review of radiographs. Instability is defined by any of the following seven criteria:

1. axial rotation C0-C1 greater than 8 degrees to one side
2. an increase of more than 1 mm in the distance (usually 4–5 mm) between the basion of the occiput and the top of the dens
3. total left and right overhang C1-C2 greater than 7 mm
4. axial rotation C1-C2 greater than 45 degrees to one side
5. distance between the anterior border of the dens and the posterior border of the ring of C1 greater than 4 mm
6. distance between the posterior margin of the dens and the anterior cortex of the posterior ring of C1 less than 13 mm
7. avulsed transverse ligament.
   Clinical instability in the lower cervical spine is based on a point scale: Different indications are assigned a point value, and if the total is 5 points or more, the spine is diagnosed as clinically unstable.

Abnormal disc narrowing, developmentally narrow spinal canal (sagittal diameter <13 mm or Pavlov's ratio <0.8), nerve root damage and dangerous loading anticipated are each assigned a point value of 1. Anterior elements destroyed or unable to function, posterior elements destroyed or unable to function, positive stretch test, and spinal cord damage are each assigned a point value of 2. The positive stretch test is a clinical test whereby the examiner applies manual traction to the head, and the patient experiences some neurological symptoms. Radiographic criteria are assigned up to 4 points: 2 points each for sagittal plane translation >3.5 mm (or 20%) and sagittal plane rotation >20 degrees in flexion/extension x-rays or 2 points each for sagittal plane translation >3.5 mm (or 20%) and relative sagittal plane angulation >11 degrees in resting x-rays. Although these are arguably the most comprehensive stability/instability scales devised to date and are strongly supported by relevant biomechanical studies, work is ongoing in trying to define new, clinically relevant concepts of spinal stability/instability. One interesting new concept has to do with the "neutral zone"—the region of least resistance within the range of motion in which a large displacement of a vertebra relative to another can occur with application of a small load.

Degenerative Disc Disease

Cervical spondylosis is progressive degeneration of the intervertebral discs. This condition is usually an age-related phenomena that occurs naturally in most human beings. Age-related biochemical changes within the intervertebral discs are due to progressive loss of proteogylcan matrix within the nucleus pulposis, which results in a less hydrated disc. The ability of the degenerating disc to withstand normal biomechanical forces is diminished, which may result in progressive narrowing of the disc space.

The natural aging phenomena may become pathological if certain conditions arise that compromise the spinal canal and cause neural compression. The degenerating disc may herniate into the spinal canal or neural foramen leading to radiculopathy with neurologic deficits. Cervical radiculopathy may also manifest in patients who develop progressive narrowing of the neural foramen due to uncovertebral spurs and hypertrophic facet joints. With further degeneration, patients may develop chondro-osseous spurs or "spondylotic bars," which encroach into the spinal canal and compress the spinal cord (Fig. 15–1). These patients may develop the syndrome of cervical spondylotic myelopathy (dysfunction of the spinal cord).

The sagittal diameter of the spinal canal plays an important role in the pathophysiology of cervical radiculopathy and myelopathy. Based on lateral radiographs of the cervical spine, the average subaxial canal diameter in the normal population is approximately 17 to 18 mm. Patients with a sagittal diameter of less than 12 to 13 mm are considered to have congenital cervical stenosis and are predisposed to developing early cervical radiculopathy or myelopathy.

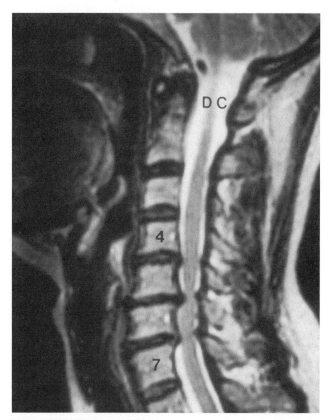

Figure 15–1 Magnetic resonance imaging (MRI) scan of a patient with cervical stenosis and myelopathy due to degenerative disc disease and progressive compression of the spinal cord.

"stabilize" the cervical spine. The proliferating synovial tissue (pannus) may destroy the transverse, alar, and apical ligaments as well as the osteochondral bone of the atlanto-axial and atlanto-odontoid joints. This ultimately leads to progressive subluxation and instability of the C1-2 complex, with the risk of neurologic complications (Fig. 15–2). With progressive destruction of the lateral pillars of the atlas, the odontoid may migrate into the foramen magnum (cranial settling). The odontoid may compress the medulla leading to paralysis or death. The pannus may also destroy the subaxial facet joints, which may lead to subaxial (C3-7) subluxation and spinal cord compression.

RELEVANT ANATOMY AND SURGICAL APPROACHES

The Upper Cervical Spine (Occiput-C2)

Relevant Anatomy

The occipito-atlantal-axial complex is a specialized articulation that provides for a large range of motion between the head and torso. There are no intervertebral discs in this region, and the articulations are all synovial joints. The first cervical vertebrae has no true spinous process. The occipito-atlantal joint is a shallow ball-and-socket joint that allows for the greatest degree of flexion/extension of any cervical articulation.

> ### PEARL
>
> Congenital cervical stenosis is defined as a sagittal diameter of the spinal canal less than 12 to 13 mm.

Rheumatoid Arthritis

The cervical spine is a common focus of destruction and pathology in patients with rheumatoid arthritis. Instabilities that occur in the cervical spine are secondary to the destruction of articular and ligamentous structures that normally

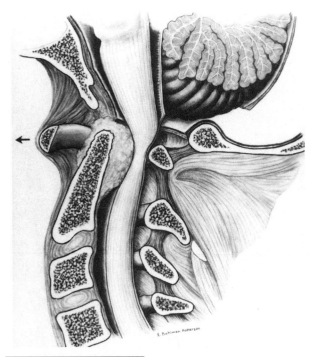

Figure 15–2 Illustration demonstrating the pathologic pannus in patients with C1-2 instability. The destructive pannus erodes the normal stabilizing ligaments and bony architecture producing clinical instability. Reproduced with permission from Boden SD, Dodge LD, Bohlman HH, Rechtine GR. Rheumatoid arthritis of the cervical spine. A long-term analysis with predictors of paralysis and recovery. *J Bone Jt Surg.* 1993;75A:1286.

The vertebral artery is an important structure that courses from the transverse foramen of the atlas to a point approximately 2 cm from the midline on the posterior, superior aspect of the atlas. This is important to realize when performing posterior fusions because careless dissection beyond 2 cm from the middle may injure the vertebral artery.

PITFALL

During a posterior exposure of C-1 (atlas), dissection 2 cm beyond the midline risks injury to the vertebral artery.

The second cervical vertebra (axis) is also a unique structure and serves as a transition between the upper and lower cervical vertebrae. The odontoid process (dens) extends upward and articulates with the anterior ring of the atlas and acts as a pivot between the first and second vertebrae, permitting the greatest degree of axial rotation (45 degrees). The relative stability of the C1-2 complex almost completely relies on the ligaments in this region. Within the spinal canal and posterior to the dens, there are a number of ligaments that firmly bond the odontoid to the anterior ring of the atlas and the occiput. These ligaments include the cruciform ligament, the transverse ligament, the alar ligaments, and the apical odontoid ligament (Fig. 15–3). Injuries or inflammatory processes that destroy these ligaments may render the upper cervical spine unstable.

The spinal cord in the upper cervical spine is housed in the spinal canal anterior to the odontoid process. Unlike the

---

Figure 15–3 Axial view of atlanto-axial (C1-2) articulation (**A**). Posterior view of atlanto-axial (C1-2) articulation (**B**).

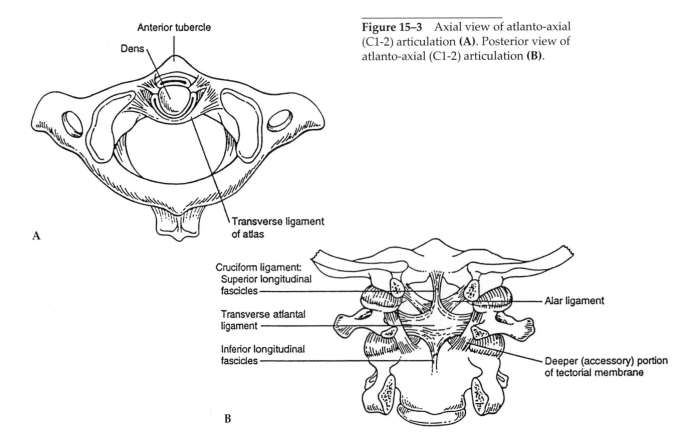

subaxial spine, the space available for the cord is rather capacious. Within the atlas ring, the "Steele's rule of thirds" refers to the fact that the first third of the space is occupied by the odontoid, the second third by free space, and the final third by the spinal cord. Due to the relatively large spinal canal in the C1-2 complex, fractures in this region are rarely associated with spinal cord injury.

Surgical Approaches

The type of preoperative and intra-operative immobilization of the head and neck is important when performing surgical procedures on the cervical spine. In traumatic and in degenerative conditions, the spinal cord may be at risk for iatrogenic injury if appropriate steps are not taken to immobilize the cervical spine. Positioning and preparing the patient prior to the surgical incision may pose the greatest danger to the spinal cord. The use of Gardner-Wells or Mayfield tongs for immobilization and traction, as well as the use of a rotating Stryker bed, is crucial in minimizing the risk of spinal cord injury.

Transoral Anterior Approach

This approach was traditionally used to drain infections of the upper cervical spine and was historically associated with high complication rates. With the advent of modern antibiotics, it is being used more frequently with fewer complications. This is a useful approach for procedures such as odontoid resections in rheumatoid arthritis patients with basilar invagination.

With the use of a microscope, a midline longitudinal incision is made through the pharyngeal membrane. Dissection is carried down to the pathological region of the upper cervical spine. Because this is a transoral approach, wide exposure is usually not feasible.

Extrapharyngeal Anterior Approaches

Three types of extrapharyngeal approaches have been described:

1. the lateral extrapharyngeal approach described by Whitesides, which approaches the upper cervical spine lateral to the carotid sheath
2. the anteromedial retropharyngeal approach, originally described by DeAndrade and MacNab
3. the anteromedial retropharyngeal approach modified by Riley and MacAfee

Both anteromedial approaches gain access to the C1-2 region medial to the carotid sheath. These extrapharyngeal approaches are used for resecting tumors or treating late complications or deformities of the upper cervical spine. Most acute traumatic injuries and degenerative conditions will not require these technically demanding approaches.

Posterior Approach To C1-2

The posterior approach is the most frequently utilized approach when treating traumatic and degenerative conditions of the upper cervical spine. The patient's head must be immobilized (usually with Mayfield or Gardner-Wells tongs) when turning the patient into, and maintaining the patient in, a stable prone position. Depending on the clinical situation, a halo brace may be applied preoperatively and the surgical procedure performed through the halo brace posteri-

orly. Exposure is made from the occiput to the third spinous process through the midline avascular raphe. Straying from the midline raphe may cause excessive bleeding from the muscle's venous plexus. Bony prominences of the occiput and the C-2 spinous process are dissected subperiosteally. Care must be taken when dissecting the posterior arch of C-1 because this structure is often thin and easily fractured. In addition, the exposure of the C-1 ring should not be carried out more than 2 cm lateral to the midline due to the proximity of the vertebral artery. This exposure allows for fusion surgery of the occiput to C-2 articulations (Fig. 15–4).

The Lower Cervical Spine (C3-7)
Relevant Anatomy

The lower (subaxial) cervical vertebrae (C3-7) and their articulations are similar to one another. The vertebral bodies are separated anteriorly by the intervertebral discs. The upper portions of the vertebral body are shaped like a cup that cradles the vertebral body above. This is due to the important uncovertebral joints (joints of Luschka), which articulate (nonsynovial) with the posterolateral aspect of the vertebral body above. The uncovertebral joint is the anterior anatomical border of the neural foramen, and therefore, degenerative bone spurs in this area may cause nerve root compression. The transverse process of the subaxial spine extends laterally from the vertebral body and uncovertebral joint and forms a gutter supporting the nerve roots as they leave the neural foramina. The transverse processes of the first six cervical vertebrae also contains a foramen through which the vertebral arteries ascend into the head. The transverse process of the sixth cervical vertebra is where the vertebral artery enters the transverse foramen. In most patients, this is the most prominent tubercle and can be palpated. It has been named the carotid or Chassaignac's tubercle.

Posteriorly, the facet joints are angled 45 degrees in the coronal plane. This permits easy gliding between the articular surfaces during flexion/extension as well as during lateral bending. More medially, the lamina forms the posterior border of the spinal canal. In the midline, the spinous processes of the second through the sixth cervical vertebrae are usually bifid. The seventh spinous process (the largest) is not bifid.

The ligaments of the subaxial spine also play important roles in the dynamic and static stability of the cervical spine. The anterior longitudinal ligament is usually thin and adherent to the vertebral bodies and the intervertebral discs. The posterior longitudinal ligament is a thick band of dense, fibrous tissue running over the posterior vertebral bodies (anterior to the spinal cord). Posteriorly, the supraspinous and interspinous ligaments, the ligamentum flavum, and the facet joint capsules provide the static soft tissue stability.

The cervical musculature can be divided into a superficial layer and a deep layer. The superficial layer consists of the platysma and sternocleidomastoid muscles, along with the infrahyoid muscles of the neck. The platysma is a thin broad plate, which lies directly beneath the skin between the lower portion of the face and the upper thorax. The sternocleidomastoid muscle originates with two heads from the sternum and clavicle. It courses upward and across the lateral surface of the neck where it inserts into the mastoid process and superior nuchal line. It is supplied by the accessory nerve that

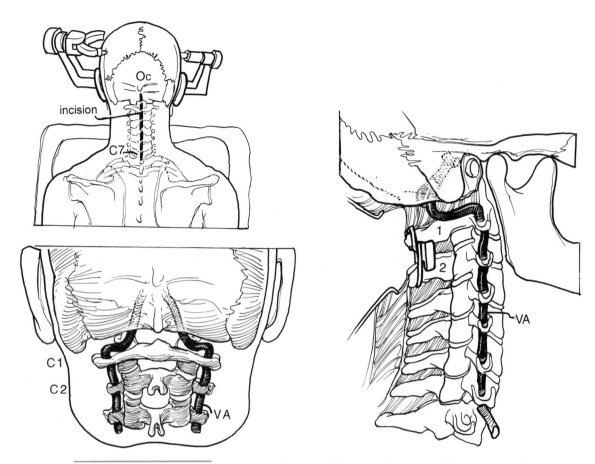

Figure 15–4 Illustration demonstrating the normal bony architecture of the upper cervical spine during a posterior approach. Note the course of the vertebral artery with relation to the posterior C-1 ring. Reproduced with permission from Wertheim SB, Bohlman HH. Occipitocervical fusion. Indications, techniques, and long-term results in thirteen patients. *J Bone Jt Surg* 1987;69A:834

enters the muscle from the lower side between the cranial and middle third (Fig. 15–5).

The scalene muscles of the deep layer are innervated by the ventral branch of the spinal nerve. The anterior scalene muscle originates at the transverse process of C3-6 and inserts at the scalene tubercle of the first rib. The middle scalene muscle arises at the transverse processes of C2-7 and inserts at the first rib dorsolateral to the subclavian groove. The posterior scalene muscle originates at the transverse processes of C4-6 and attaches to the superior border of the second rib. The longus colli muscle connects the vertebral bodies of C2-5 with the bodies of the lower cervical and three upper thoracic vertebrae (Fig. 15–6).

Cervical fascia is a collective term for connective tissue layers that enclose muscles and nerves in the cervical region. The superficial layer lies below the platysma and encloses the sternocleidomastoid and trapezius muscle. It attaches at the anterior surface of the manubrium sterni), clavicle, and lower margin of the mandible. The middle, or pretracheal layer, lies between the two omohyoid muscles and attaches to the dorsal border of the manubrium and clavicle. The deep prevertebral layer lies between the vertebral column and pharyngeal constrictors and esophagus. It covers the scalenes and contains the sympathetic trunks and phrenic nerves. The carotid sheath is connective tissue derived from the pretracheal lamina and envelops the neurovascular bundle, including the carotid artery, jugular vein and vagus nerve (Fig. 15–7).

Surgical Approaches

Acute traumatic and chronic degenerative conditions of the cervical spine most frequently involve the subaxial region. A thorough understanding of the anterior and posterior approaches to the lower cervical spine is critical in managing problems involving the subaxial spine.

Anterior Approach (Robinson Technique)

This anteromedial approach allows for exposure of the anterior cervical spine from C-3 to C-7. The approach can be made from either the right or the left side. The rationale for approaching from the left side is that the recurrent laryngeal nerve is less likely to be injured.

PEARL

Performing the anterior approach to C3-7 through the left side avoids the recurrent laryngeal nerve on the right.

A transverse incision is made at the level of the pathology. A longitudinal incision can be made if exposure of more than 3 intervertebral disc levels is needed. The platysma muscle is divided near the medial margin of the sternocleidomastoid muscle. The superficial layer of the deep cervical fascia is

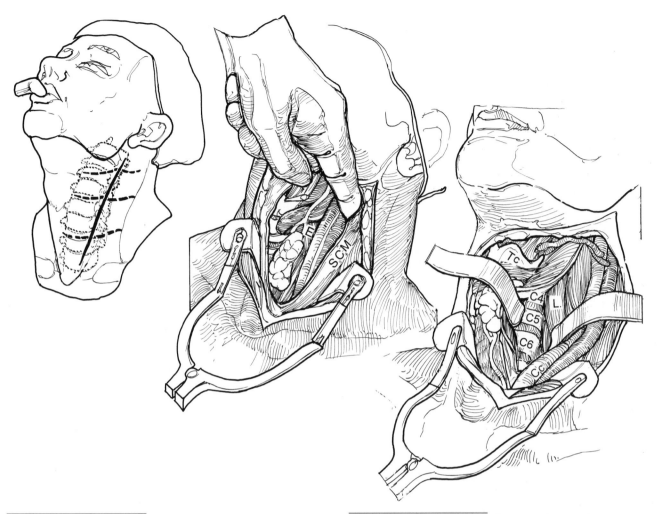

Figure 15–5   Superficial layer of the cervical musculature.

Figure 15–6   Deep layer of the cervical musculature.

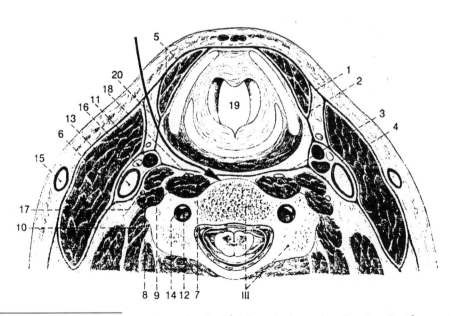

Figure 15–7   Anatomic cross-section at level of third cervical vertebra. Reprinted with permission from Bauer R, Kershbaumer F, Poisel S. *Operative approaches in orthopaedic Surgery and Traumatology*. Thieme, NY 1989;8.

transversely incised. Dissection proceeds proximally and distally along the medial border of the sternocleidomastoid muscle. Care must be taken to protect the anterior and external jugular veins.

Palpation deep to the sternocleidomastoid muscle will identify the carotid sheath, which is then retracted laterally. The trachea and esophagus are retracted medially, allowing for direct exposure of the pretracheal and prevertebral fascia. These layers are sharply dissected. The anterior aspect of the cervical spine is exposed along with the longus colli muscles. The longus colli muscle is dissected laterally over the disc spaces to fully expose the entire anterior aspect of the cervical spine. Injuries to the sympathetic chain, as well as to the vertebral artery, can be avoided by not dissecting too far laterally during this approach (Fig. 15–8). This approach allows for anterior discectomies, corpectomies, and fusions, with and without instrumentation.

Posterior Approach

Exposure of the lower cervical spine is initiated by palpating the spinous processes of the C-2 and C-7 vertebrae. A longitudinal incision is made and dissection is carried through the midline raphe to the bifid spinous processes. The laminae and the lateral facet joints are exposed subperiosteally with a

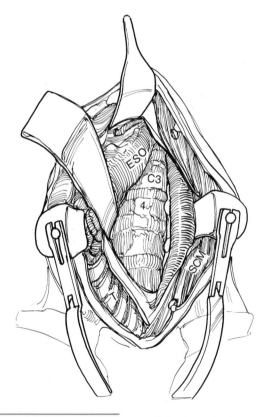

Figure 15–8 Operative approach to the anterior cervical spine. Through a transverse incision, dissection is carried between the carotid sheath and the trachea and esophagus to expose the anterior spine. Reproduced with permission from Zdeblick TA, Bohlman HH. Cervical kyphosis and myelopathy. Treatment by anterior corpectomy and strut-grafting. *J Bone Jt Surg.* 1989;71A:178.

Cobb elevator and electrocautery. Unless indicated, the muscles inserting or originating on the C-2 spinous process should not be detached. This preserves stability of the upper cervical spine. A lateral radiograph should always be taken to ensure the appropriate level of dissection and fusion. A wider exposure over the facet joints is necessary if posterior instrumentation with lateral mass plates is contemplated.

EXAMINATION

History

A thorough clinical history is of great importance in the evaluation of a patient with cervical spine pathology. Following trauma, the mechanism of injury should be determined. A history of a flexion injury versus an extension injury may establish the diagnosis. Any history of transient paralysis should be elicited because this may suggest an "unstable" cervical spinal injury.

Patients that complain of "neck pain" following a trauma should be evaluated for a cervical spine injury prior to discontinuing cervical immobilization.

When evaluating patients with degenerative conditions of the cervical spine, it is important to ascertain whether there is a component of radiculopathy or pain that radiates into the upper extremity. The distribution of the pain along a dermatome will usually point to the level of pathology. Patients with an acute cervical disc herniation may get pain relief by abducting their arm over their head (abducting sign). In elderly patients, a history of gait disturbance or loss of coordination may herald the onset of myelopathy. However, be aware that myelopathy may progress slowly so that the patient does not recognize the neurological deterioration. Bladder or bowel dysfunction are rare and occur only in advanced myelopathy.

Patients with a long history of rheumatoid arthritis should undergo periodic examination of their cervical spine. These patients may have significant instability of their upper cervical spine as measured by radiographic criteria but may be totally asymptomatic. If a patient with rheumatoid arthritis complains of "neck pain," instability must be excluded, especially if the patient is contemplating a major operative procedure. In severe cases, patients may complain of an "electrical shock" into their extremities with forward bending of the neck (Lhermitte's sign). This sign implies significant instability with impending neurological injury. Unless the clinician has a high index of suspicion and carefully monitors these patients, the first sign of cervical instability may be death due to respiratory compromise. Although rare, these patients will die in their sleep due to compromise of the cervicomedullary junction of the spinal cord (Ondine's curse).

Physical Examination

A physical examination in patients with cervical spine pathology should begin with inspection. In the trauma patient, cranial injuries and facial lacerations may point to a cervical spinal injury. In a patient with altered consciousness, a thorough examination may not be possible, but spontaneous movements in the extremities should be noted. In an awake and alert patient, palpation of the cervical spine may elicit pain; a harbinger of a significant injury. In degenerative conditions of the cervical spine, motion in all planes should be assessed. Pain that radiates into the arm suggests compression of a cervical nerve root.

Whether a patient presents with an acute injury or a chronic pain syndrome, a neurological exam is critical. The examiner must have a grasp of the normal motor and sensory distribution of all the cervical nerve roots, as well as the appropriate reflexes (Table 15–1). The exam begins with evaluation of gait. Patients with myelopathy may have a wide-based gait with difficulty performing toe-to-toe walking. A motor and sensory exam will often identify the cervical nerve root lesion in a patient with radiculopathy. Patients with advanced myelopathy will often display upper motor neuron signs such as hyperreflexia, clonus, Babinski's sign, Hoffmann's sign, spasticity, and generalized quadiparesis. In patients with an acute spinal cord injury, documentation of the motor and sensory level is extremely important because this may change within the first 24 to 72 hours following injury. A rectal exam is a key component of the neurological exam. Patients that have perianal sensation may have "sacral sparing." This implies an incomplete spinal cord injury and a better prognosis for neurological recovery. The bulbocavernosis reflex should also be elicited because the presence of this reflex signals the end of "spinal shock (a short period of paralysis, insensibility, and absence of reflex activity following any severe traumatic injury to the spinal cord)." The reflex is present when there is a reflex contraction of the anal sphicter following stimulation of the glans penis. It can also be elicited in a patient who has a Foley catheter by pulling on the catheter.

PEARL

Return of the bulbocavernosus reflex signals the end of spinal shock.

Prior to the return of this reflex, one cannot adequately determine the final neurologic diagnosis with reference to whether there is a complete or an incomplete spinal cord injury.

AIDS TO DIAGNOSIS
Plain Radiographs

Initial diagnostic studies should include plain anteroposterior and lateral radiographs of the cervical spine showing all seven vertebra. In trauma, an open-mouth odontoid view, trauma oblique views, and a swimmer's view may also be required. A fracture or dislocation of the cervical spine will, in most instances, be visible on these plain radiographic studies. Some diagnostic difficulties may arise in elderly patients with pre-existing degenerative disc disease. There may be subtle subluxation due to degeneration, which can be mistaken for an acute injury. Correlation of radiographs with the history and examination is required in these instances.

Flexion-extension lateral radiographs may aid in the diagnosis of ligamentous injuries of the cervical spine. One must use caution in performing this examination. It must be done in an alert patient with the physician guiding the patient. The main indication for flexion-extension studies is to determine whether a ligamentous injury is present in a patient with neck pain and normal radiographs. Sagittal translation of greater than 3.5 mm or 11 degrees of angulation is considered to be an unstable cervical spine.

PEARL

Sagittal translation of 3.5 mm or angulation of greater than 11 degrees on a flexion-extension lateral radiograph of the cervical spine indicates ligamentous instability.

These same radiographic studies will aid in the diagnosis of degenerative and inflammatory spinal disorders. In patients with degenerative cervical radiculopathy or myelopathy, the space available for spinal cord (SAC) on the lateral radiograph may help diagnose cervical spinal stenosis. A diameter of less than 13 mm is considered to be congenitally narrow (Fig. 15–9). A flexion-extension lateral radiograph of the upper cervical spine is also useful in evaluating patients with long-standing rheumatoid arthritis. Abnormal

TABLE 15–1   Cervical and lumbar nerve roots by their physical assessment

Root Level	Motor	Reflex	Sensation
C-5	Deltoid/biceps	Biceps	Lateral upper arm
C-6	Wrist extension	Brachioradialis	Thumb/index
C-7	Triceps	Triceps	Middle finger
C-8	Finger flexion	None	Ring/little finger
T-1	Hand intrinsic	None	Axilla
L-3	Quads	Knee jerk	Medial knee
L-4	Quads/tib ant	Knee jerk	Medial foot
L-5	Extensor hallucis Longus (EHL)	Post tib	Dorsum foot
S-1	Gastrocnemius	Ankle jerk	Lateral foot

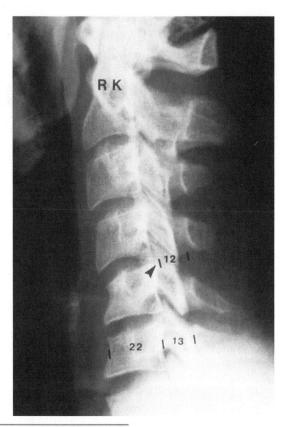

Figure 15–9 A lateral radiograph demonstrating the sagittal measurements of the cervical spine. Note the space available for the cord measures 12 to 13 mm, consistent with congenital cervical stenosis. Reproduced with permission from Kang JD, Figgie MP, Bohlman HH. Sagittal measurements of the cervical spine in subaxial fractures and dislocations. An analysis of two hundred and eighty-eight patients with and without neurological deficits. *J Bone Jt Surg.* 1994;76A:1618.

atlanto-axial motion, odontoid invagination, and subaxial subluxation may be diagnosed with plain radiographs. An anterior atlanto-dental interval of greater than 3.5 mm, a posterior SAC of less than 14 mm, or abnormal motion greater than 6 to 7 mm all signify an unstable C1-2 complex. There are numerous "lines" described to assess the amount of basilar invagination, but the most commonly used is the McGregor's line (drawn from the hard palate to the posterior aspect of the basiocciput). If the tip of the odontoid process is greater than 4.5 mm above this line, the patient has radiographic evidence of basilar invagination.

Computed Tomography Scans/Sagittal Reconstructions

Computed tomography (CT) is a useful adjunct in assessing patients with traumatic injuries. It may provide a greater understanding of the "anatomy of the fracture." Subtle fractures not seen on plain radiographs may be identified by CT scans. Image reconstructions help evaluate the cervical thoracic junction where plain radiographs may provide insufficient visualization of the problem.

Magnetic Resonance Imaging

Magnetic resonance imaging (MRI) is currently the diagnostic tool of choice when evaluating patients with neurological dysfunction. This includes patients with acute spinal cord or nerve root injuries as well as patients with chronic degenerative conditions causing radiculopathy or myelopathy. The degree of neural compression by fracture fragments, the intervertebral disc, or degenerative osteophytes can be readily assessed with MRI. The MRI does not have the bony resolution of the CT scan. Therefore, those conditions requiring careful evaluation of the bony elements may be better assessed using a CT/myelogram.

When dealing with patients with acute cervical trauma, clinical judgment should be used when an MRI is ordered. In most institutions, an MRI scan may take up to 2 to 3 hours to complete (especially in the middle of the night). An MRI should be only used if the information will change the course of treatment. In a multiply injured patient with several long bone fractures, it may not be feasible to obtain an MRI scan.

Myelogram/Computed Tomography Scan

A myelogram/CT scan is not used as frequently as in the past due to the development of the MRI scan. This is especially true in the acutely injured patient. It can be extremely valuable in degenerative conditions such as spinal stenosis due to its superior bony resolution. In these cases, it may be more helpful than the MRI in preoperatively planning for surgical decompression.

Electrodiagnostic Studies

Electromyograms and nerve conduction studies are of little value in trauma situations but may be of value in patients with cervical radiculopathy. Although not routinely used, they may be useful in patients with diabetes or other chronic conditions in which peripheral neuropathy must be distinguished from radiculopathy. Somatosensory evoked potentials (SSEPS) may show early changes in patients with severe myelopathy, but currently, such a study is of limited use as an aid to diagnosis. SSEPs are more often used intraoperatively to monitor the spinal cord during decompression surgery.

PEARL

Somatosensory evoked potentials can be used to monitor the spinal cord during surgical decompression of the spine.

SPECIFIC CONDITIONS: TREATMENT AND OUTCOME

Upper Cervical Trauma
Occiput-C1 Dislocation

Occipitocervical dislocations are extremely rare injuries that occur with forceful rotation of the C-1 lateral mass on the occipital condyles. Most patients with such dislocations die at the time of the injury, but there have been case reports of patients with normal neurological function. The diagnosis may not be obvious using plain radiographs unless the index of suspicion is high. Computed tomography scans may be needed to confirm the diagnosis. The treatment for this extremely unstable injury is a posterior occiput to C-2 fusion with wire stabilization. The fusion should be protected with a halo orthosis for 3 months. A solid arthrodesis in a patient who survives this injury will usually result in a stable, painless spine.

Jefferson's Fracture

The Jefferson's fracture is a burst fracture of the ring of C-1, usually due to an axial load to the spine. Because the atlas (C-1) is a bony ring, multiple fracture lines are seen with lateral displacement or spreading of the fracture fragments. An anterioposterior radiograph will generally show widening of the distance between the odontoid and the lateral mass. If the overhang of the lateral masses on either side totals 7 mm or more, there is a high likelihood that the transverse ligament is disrupted. The significance of a rupture of the transverse ligament is that the patient may develop C1-2 instability requiring a posterior fusion. Lateral radiographs may show edema anterior to the anterior portion of the ring. Computed tomography scan has made diagnosis and follow-up of the healing process easier and more accurate. Levine (1989) has reported on a series of atlas fractures detailing three types of fractures with treatment tailored to the type of injury.

Jefferson's fractures rarely require surgical intervention. If the fracture is nondisplaced, a rigid cervical orthosis for 6 weeks can result in uneventful healing. If the fracture is displaced, a more rigid halo-jacket orthosis may be required for up to 3 months. In rare instances, patients may develop a delayed union or post-traumatic degenerative arthritis necessitating a posterior occiput to C-2 fusion.

A combination of Jefferson's fracture and odontoid fracture is not an uncommon clinical situation. The traditional treatment consists of a halo-jacket orthosis, which allows the fractures to heal.

PEARL

When using a halo-jacket orthosis, the anterior halo pins should be placed slightly above the brow line and the posterior pins slightly above and posterior to the superior tip of the ear.

PITFALL

Never overtighten halo pins in the presence of a pin-tract infection.

In the traditional treatment, if the odontoid fracture does not heal, a posterior arthrodesis of C1-2 is performed, but the use of an odontoid screw to acutely stabilize the dens fracture has become popular for this particular situation, especially if the dens fracture is displaced (Fig. 15–10).

PEARL

Intraoperative biplanar flouroscopic imaging is absolutely mandatory during odontoid screw fixation.

Odontoid Fractures

Three distinct types of odontoid fractures have been described by Anderson and D'Alonzo (1974).

Type I fractures have an oblique fracture line through the upper part of the odontoid process and probably represent an avulsion fracture at the alar ligament attachment.

Type II is a fracture occurring at the junction of the odontoid and the body of the axis.

Type III fractures extend down into the cancellous bone of the body of the axis. Open-mouth odontoid views, lateral tomograms, and/or sagittal CT reconstructions will help in the diagnosis of these fractures.

Type I fractures are extremely rare and usually stable injuries with a good prognosis. They require minimal support with a soft collar. Type II injuries tend to be more unstable and have been shown to have a high rate of nonunion (up to 30%) when treated in a halo brace. Minimally displaced Type II fractures may be initially treated in a halo. If significant displacement ensues, surgical stabilization is indicated. Prognostic indicators for nonunion of type II odontoid fractures include greater than 5 mm of displacement (especially posteriorly), age greater then 50, and smoking. Surgical options include posterior C1-2 fusion with various techniques of wire fixation. If the patient has a posteriorly displaced fracture, a traditional Gallie fusion may further displace the fracture as the wires are tightened (Fig. 15–11). In these instances, a Brook's sublaminar fusion with an intervening bone block may be more appropriate (Fig. 15–12). Magerl has popularized placement of a transarticular screw in the lateral mass to rigidly fuse the C1-2 complex (Fig. 15–13). The advantage of this fixation is that the patient may be spared the halo brace. The disadvantage is the risk of injury to the vertebral artery as well as neurological injury. Others have advocated the use of an odontoid screw to treat type II fractures in order to avoid fusing the C1-2 motion segment. This form of fracture fixation clearly has its advantages, but is technically demanding and carries the risk of neurological complications. Type III fractures, because of their large cancellous surfaces, tend to heal well with treatment using a halo brace.

Hangman's Fractures

Levine and Edwards (1985) have classified injuries of the C-2 posterior elements into four types. Type I fractures have a fracture through the neural arch with no angulation and up to 3 mm of displacement. Type II fractures have significant angulation and/or displacement greater than 3 mm. Type IIA fractures show minimal displacement but severe angulation

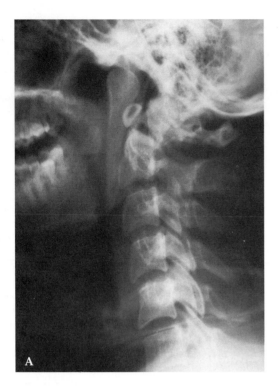

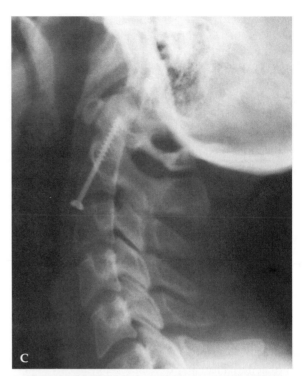

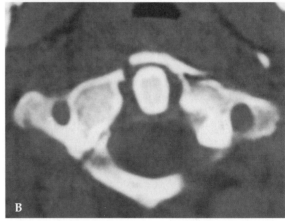

Figure 15–10 Lateral radiograph of a patient with an odontoid fracture that is posteriorly displaced (**A**). A computed tomography (CT) scan, however, also demonstrates a concomitant Jefferson's fracture of the atlas (**B**). The patient underwent an anatomic closed reduction and application of a halo vest, but the odontoid fracture was redisplaced. Due to persistent displacement in a halo, the patient underwent an anterior odontoid screw fixation, which allowed for complete healing of the odontoid in an anatomically reduced position (**C**).

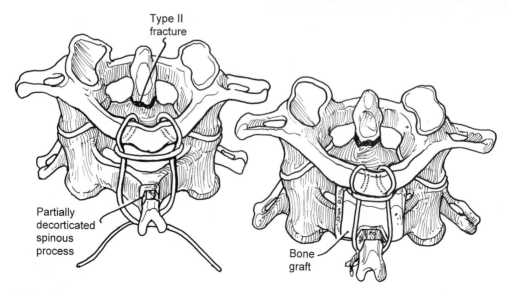

Figure 15–11 Technique of modified Gallie fusion. Redrawn with permission from Meyer PR Jr. ed. *Surgery of Spine Trauma*. New York, NY: Churchill Livingston, 1989. Redrawn by Tony Pazos.

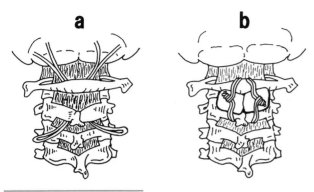

Figure 15–12 Technique of Brook's fusion.

deformity. Finally, Type III fractures combine bilateral facet dislocation of C2-3 with a fracture through the neural arch.

Type I fractures are relatively stable injuries and may be treated with a cervical collar. Most Type II injuries require reduction with the patient in halo traction, followed by halo brace immobilization. Type IIA injuries show increased displacement with traction. They are best treated with gentle extension and immobilization in compression with a halo

brace. Type III injuries are very unstable and usually require a posterior fusion. Hangman's fractures are rarely associated with neurological injuries. In most instances, these are "decompressive" fractures in which the spinal canal enlarges following fracture. These fractures heal extremely well (Fig. 15–14). In those rare cases of a symptomatic nonunion, an anterior C2-3 fusion or a posterior C1-3 fusion can be contemplated.

Lower Cervical Trauma
Unilateral Facet Fractures/Dislocations

The diagnosis of a unilateral facet injury is usually made on a lateral radiograph when there is 25% anterior translation of one vertebral body on another. This finding may be due to either a facet fracture or a unilateral facet dislocation. When a facet is fractured unilaterally (either the superior or the inferior facet), the bony buttress is lost resulting in rotatory instability. This differs from a pure unilateral dislocation in which the inferior articular facet has "locked" in a displaced position anterior to the superior articular facet. The initial treatment for either of these injuries depends on the patient's neurological condition. If the patient has a normal neurological

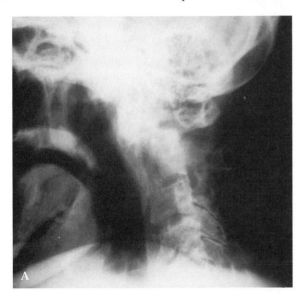

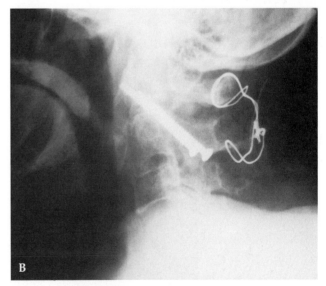

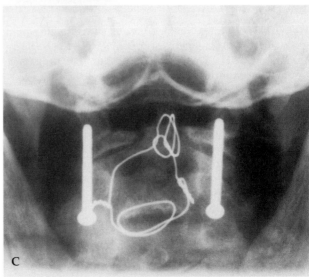

Figure 15–13 Lateral radiograph showing a grossly unstable type II odontoid fracture (**A**). The patient underwent a posterior C1-2 fusion using the Magerl trans-articular screw fixation with excellent clinical results (**B–C**). Halo vest immobilization was not required.

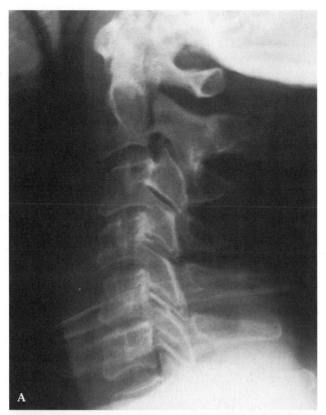

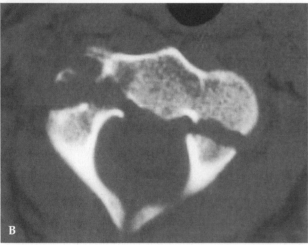

Figure 15–14 Lateral radiograph of a patient with a minimally displaced Hangman's fracture (**A**) which can be clearly seen on the axial CT scan (**B**). The fracture line propagates through the posterior pedicles.

exam or has a root or an incomplete spinal cord lesion, an MRI should be done "prereduction" to determine whether there is a traumatic disc herniation that could potentially produce an iatrogenic injury with a reduction maneuver. If the MRI scan is negative, a closed reduction of the dislocation can be attempted with Gardner-Wells tongs while the patient is awake. A unilateral facet fracture injury will reduce fairly easily using this technique. The final treatment of these injuries is controversial. Although the initial treatment may be a halo vest (if the reduction is maintained), most patients will require a posterior fusion due to the tendency of this injury to redisplace in a halo vest. Immediate surgical fusion

should probably be performed on all patients that present with a neurological deficit (Fig. 15–15).

In contrast, patients with a unilateral facet dislocation with associated fracture have a purely ligamentous injury. These are often difficult to reduce with tong traction. Closed reduction is only successful in 50% of cases. If successful, the neck is immobilized in a halo vest. Fusion is recommended for late instability. If closed reduction is not successful, an open reduction should be contemplated after a prereduction MRI scan. If the MRI does not show a traumatic disc herniation, a open reduction and fusion through a posterior approach can be performed under SSEP monitoring. If the MRI demonstrates a disc herniation, a posterior open reduction may be dangerous. In these situations, an anterior decompression followed by an anterior or a posterior fusion may be more appropriate.

PEARL

Prior to reducing a facet dislocation in a neurologically normal patient, an MRI scan should be used to determine whether a traumatic disc herniation is present.

The potential pitfalls are numerous when treating patients with facet injuries. The goal is to prevent further neurological injury. No one algorithm for treatment will ensure and prevent an iatrogenic injury. Each patient should be treated individually to optimize the safety of the spinal cord. This will be facilitated by keeping in mind the general guidelines and rationale for treatment mentioned above.

Bilateral Facet Fracture/Dislocations

Bilateral facet injuries are produced with severe cervical flexion and distraction. They are often associated with neurological deficits. Similar to the unilateral injuries, these bifacet injuries can be either fractures, pure ligamentous dislocations, or a combined injury. The typical finding on a lateral radiograph is one vertebral body displaced more than 50% anterior to the vertebrae below. These are extremely unstable injuries, often with associated spinal cord injury. All require surgical stabilization following reduction. These injuries can have associated disc herniations. The guidelines for treatment should follow those outlined above for patients with unilateral facet injuries, especially if the patient has a normal neurological exam or an incomplete spinal cord injury (Fig. 15–16).

Because a majority of these patients will present to the emergency room with a complete spinal cord injury, a closed or an open reduction should be performed followed by a posterior spinal fusion. An MRI scan can be obtained following the reduction and fusion to determine whether any residual cord compression exists. If present, a delayed anterior decompression may allow for greater "root recovery" and enhance function in quadriplegic patients.

Burst Fractures

Vertebral body burst fractures are produced by severe axial loading and neck flexion. This causes failure of the anterior

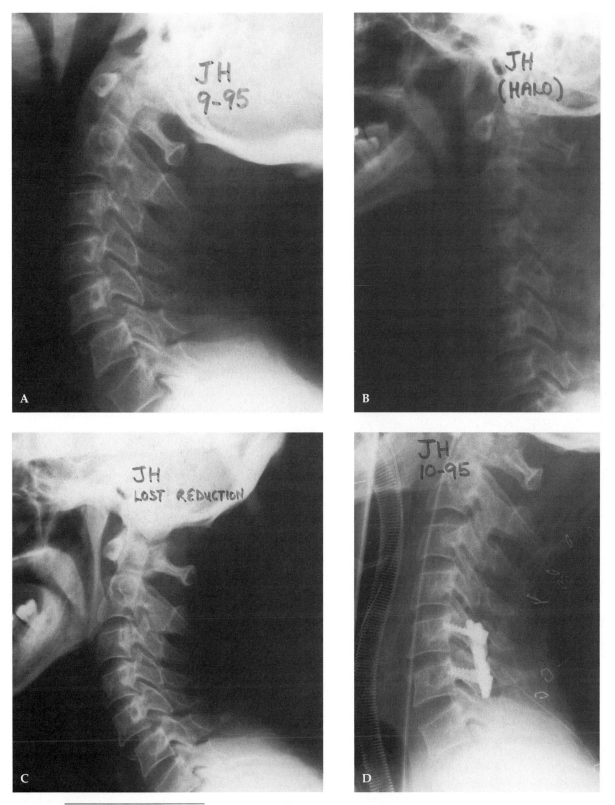

Figure 15–15   Lateral radiograph of a patient with a unilateral facet fracture/dislocation at the C5-6 level (**A**). The patient presented with a right C-6 root weakness. He underwent a closed reduction with minimal traction and was placed in a halo vest (**B**). However, the reduction was lost once the patient became ambulatory (**C**). Due to recurrent instablility, the patient required a rigid posterior fusion of C5-6 using posterior plate and lateral mass screw fixation (**D**).

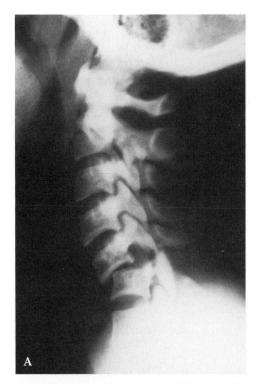

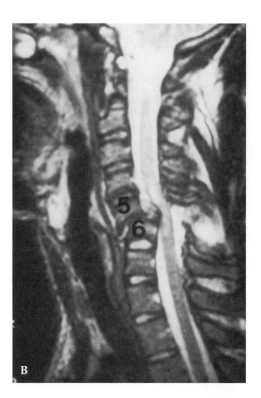

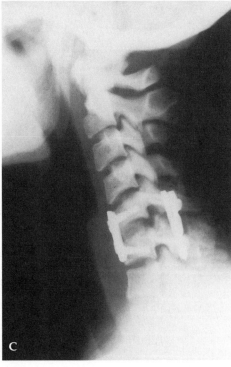

Figure 15–16 Lateral radiograph demonstrating a bilateral facet dislocation in a patient with an incomplete spinal cord injury (**A**). An MRI demonstrated a traumatic herniation of the C5-6 disc (**B**), which could potentially produce further neurologic injury if open reduction is contemplated. A closed reduction was attempted but was unsuccessful. Due to the large disc herniation, an anterior decompression and fusion was performed prior to posterior stabilization (**C**).

and middle column with bony retropulsion into the spinal canal and the potential for spinal cord injury. In a neurologically normal patient, an awake closed reduction with longitudinal traction followed by a halo vest may be the definitive treatment. However, these patients are prone to develop late kyphosis due to loss of the anterior column support. If kyphosis occurs, a late anterior strut fusion may be required.

In a neurologically injured patient, closed reduction with longitudinal traction followed by a posterior fusion may suffice if the anterior column is reasonably realigned.

PEARL

In most burst injuries, the anterior column has been disrupted. This often necessitates an anterior fusion with strut graft.

In addition, if the spinal cord is still compromised following a closed reduction, an anterior decompression and strut graft fusion is usually the better course of treatment. The anterior fusion may have to be augmented with a posterior fusion if there has been a disruption of the posterior ligaments.

Teardrop Fracture/Dislocation

Teardrop fractures of the cervical spine generally have a complex instability pattern. This injury should be differentiated from the anterior avulsion fracture seen in stable hyperextension injuries. In contrast, the true teardrop fracture/dislocation is due to a combination of flexion, axial load, and rotation. The inferior tip of the upper body is driven down into the lower body by compression and flexion. A fracture line proceeds from superior to inferior and exits through the disc space, totally disrupting the disc as well as the posterior elements. By definition, these are unstable injuries that are associated with severe neurological deficits. Addressing these injuries with only anterior or posterior fusions has been met with numerous complications. With the advent of more rigid anterior and posterior spinal instrumentation, rigid stabilization of these injuries both anteriorly and posteriorly is recommended (Fig. 15–17).

PEARL

During posterior plate instrumentation, the lateral mass screws should be angled in a cephalad direction by approximately 45 degrees and out laterally by 10 to 15 degrees.

PITFALL

Lateral mass screws not appropriately angled can injure the exiting nerve roots or the vertebral artery.

Degenerative Conditions of the Cervical Spine

Cervical Radiculopathy

Cervical radiculopathy, or pain that radiates in a dermatomal distribution of the upper extremity, is usually due to an inflammatory process brought on by mechanical compression of a cervical nerve root. In patients who suddenly develop radicular arm pain, the etiology is usually due to a soft herniated disc. In patients who present with a chronic, insidious onset of arm pain, the cause is usually foraminal stenosis from enlarged uncovertebral spurs, bulging hard discs, and hypertrophic facets.

Nonoperative treatment of patients with neck pain and radiculopathy should be instituted for a minimum of 6 to 8 weeks prior to surgical intervention. This includes anti-inflammatory medications, cervical traction, collar immobilization, and physical therapy. The majority of patients will respond to nonoperative treatment. Those patients who have persistent, disabling arm pain with neurological deficits are candidates for surgical treatment. The Robinson anterior disectomy and fusion using a tricortical iliac crest bone graft is

the "tried and true" procedure of choice. Bohlman (1993) and colleagues have shown that patients have excellent long-term results using this procedure to treat cervical radiculopathy (Fig. 15–18).

Although the Robinson anterior cervical disectomy and fusion is the most popular surgical procedure for radiculopathy, an anterior disectomy without a fusion, and a posterior foraminotomy are advocated by some surgeons as options to avoid the morbidity of a fusion. Overall results appear to be comparable, but, to date, no good prospective studies exist.

PEARL

During a Robinson anterior disectomy and fusion, the structural bone graft should be placed in compression. This is accomplished by distracting the disc space 2 to 3 mm prior to placement of the graft.

Cervical Stenosis with Myelopathy

Cervical spondylotic myelopathy is an entity characterized by a dysfunctioning spinal cord. The cord is gradually compressed by degenerative spondylotic processes including the discs, uncovertebral spurs, a thickened ligamentum flavum and lamina, and hypertrophic facets. Patients who develop profound myelopathy before age 50 usually have a congenitally narrow spinal canal (sagittal diameter less than 13 mm). These patients may also develop a dynamic component to their myelopathy; a hypermobile segment above a stiff spondylotic segment. When a patient displays the signs and symptoms of cervical myelopathy, surgical decompression can substantially improve the clinical course. The goals of surgery are to halt the progression of the myelopathy and recover neurological deficits due to chronic cord compression.

In most instances, cervical myelopathy is due to compression of the spinal cord from the anterior side of the spine. A direct anterior decompression and fusion addresses the static as well as the dynamic compression of the cord. Radically decompressing the spinal cord by performing disectomies and corpectomies of the involved levels followed by an iliac crest or fibular strut fusion is in most patients the treatment of choice (Fig. 15–19 and Fig. 15–20). Neurological outcome in patients treated in this manner depends on the preoperative level of involvement. Patients with advanced myelopathy will have less return of function compared with those with lesser myelopathy. This is probably due to the intrinsic changes that occur within the spinal cord (i.e., gliosis) in those patients with longstanding advanced spinal cord compression.

Japanese surgeons have popularized the posterior laminoplasty to treat multilevel cervical stenosis. This procedure is technically more simple to perform and involves less morbidity for the patient. The entire posterior laminae and spinous processes are hinged open either centrally or unilaterally to enlarge the space available for the cord. The theoretical advantage of this procedure is that it causes less instability than a complete laminectomy, which can lead to late kyphosis. However, any posterior procedure must have one impor-

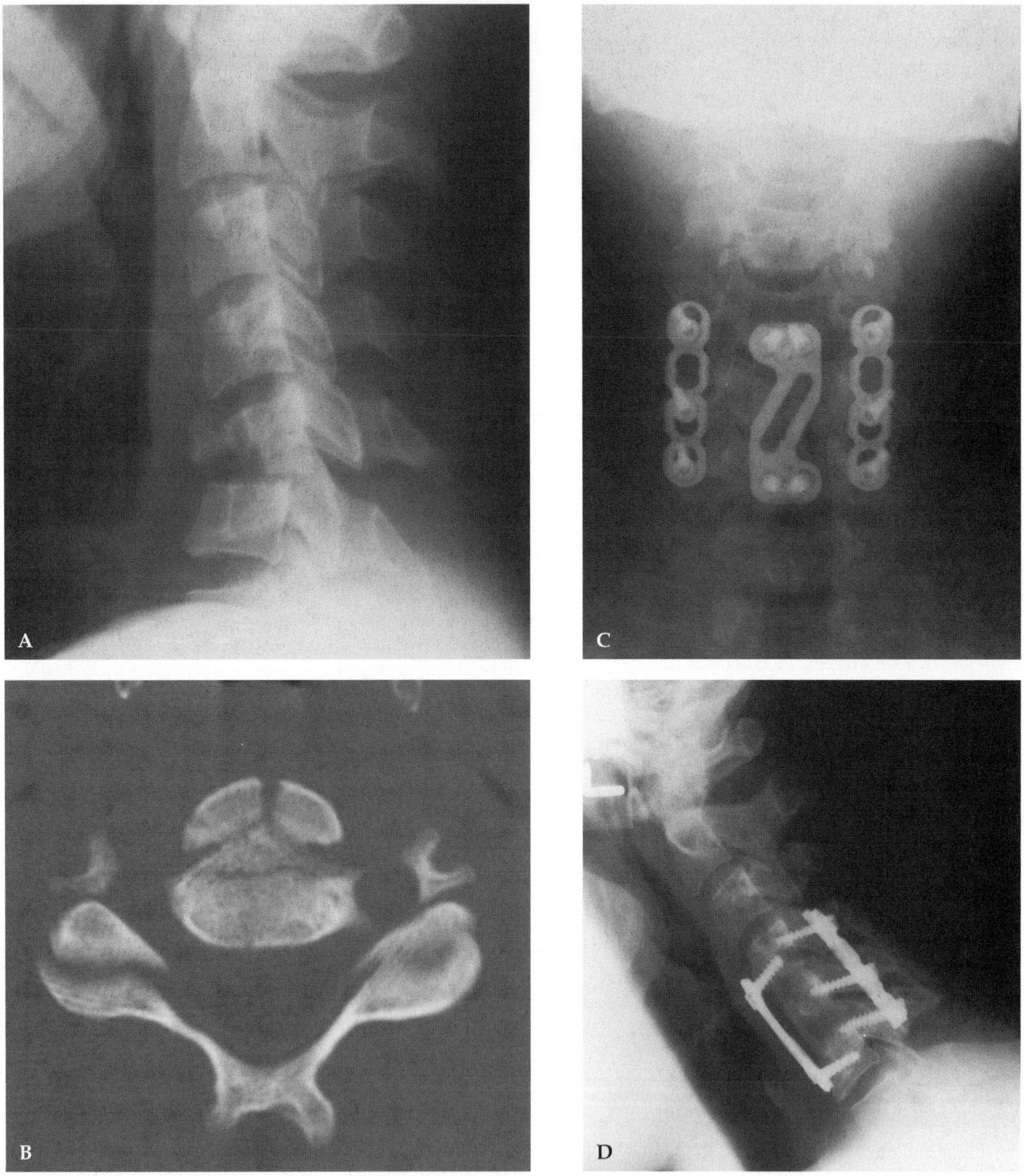

Figure 15–17   Lateral radiograph of a patient with a classic teardrop fracture/dislocation. Note the posteriorly displaced C-5 body relative to the C-6 body with the anterior body fracture of C-5 (**A**). The CT scan demonstrates the complex fracture pattern, which includes a sagittal split fracture (**B**). The patient underwent an anterior corpectomy and fusion followed by a posterior fusion (**C–D**).

tant prerequisite. The patient must have a relatively normal cervical lordosis to allow the spinal cord to drift away from the anterior spondylotic compression. A cervical lamino-plasty is contraindicated in patients with any kyphosis (Fig. 15–21). It is currently unknown whether patients have a better outcome with anterior or posterior techniques.

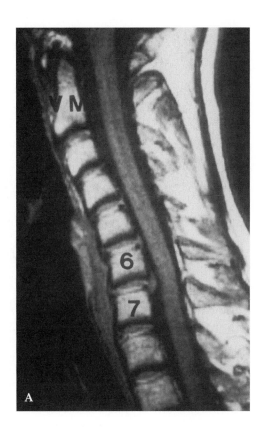

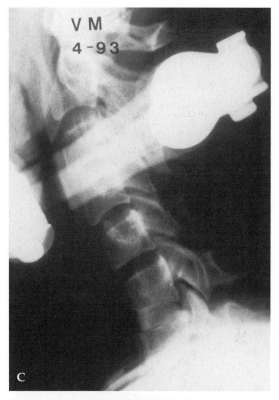

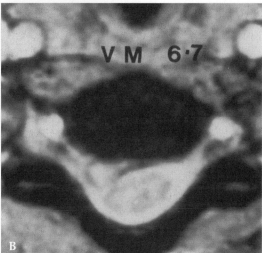

Figure 15–18   Lateral MRI scan of a patient presenting with severe right C-7 radiculopathy (**A**). The axilla view demonstrates a large extruded disc herniation compressing the right exiting C-7 nerve root (**B**). The patient underwent a successful anterior disectomy and fusion with complete relief of her symptoms (**C**).

Rheumatoid Arthritis

C1-2 Instability

Atlanto-axial instability is the most common cervical spine abnormality in patients with rheumatoid arthritis. It is the result of erosive synovitis in the atlanto-axial, atlanto-odontoid, and atlanto-occipital joints. The spinal cord is at risk for compression as the C-1 ring slides anteriorly during neck flexion. In this position the spinal cord is compressed between the posterior portion of the C-1 ring and the odontoid process. Due to the varying degrees of instability in patients with rheumatoid arthritis, there is controversy about

when to fuse the necks of patients who have radiographic evidence of C1-2 instability.

Most would agree that patients with any sign of cord compromise and those with suboccipital neck pain and radiographic evidence of C1-2 instability should undergo a posterior fusion. There is controversy concerning the management of asymptomatic patients with radiographic evidence of instability.

Boden et al. (1993) established radiographic guidelines based on clinical outcomes of patients with rheumatoid arthritis of the cervical spine. The guidelines recommend performing fusions on any patient who has a posterior atlanto-

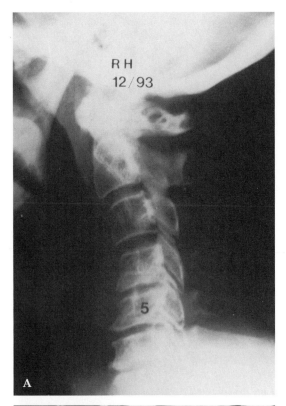

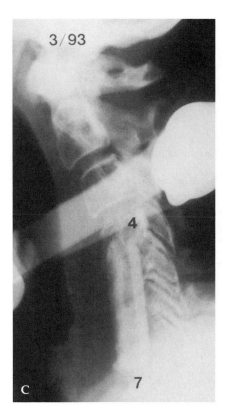

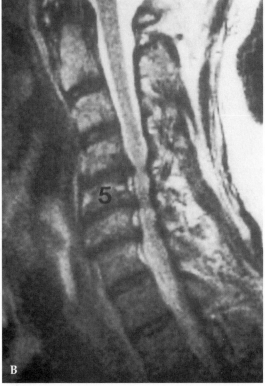

Figure 15–19   Lateral radiograph of a patient presenting with cervical myelopathy. Note the congenitally narrow spinal canal and relative kyphosis (**A**). The MRI scan demonstrates severe spinal cord compression due to degenerative spondylotic segments at C4-7 (**B**). The patient underwent an anterior corpectomy of C-5 and C-6 with a fibular strut graft fusion from C4-7 with complete resolution of myelopathic symptoms (**C**).

dental interval or space available for the cord of less than 14 mm (Fig. 15–22).

A posterior C1-2 arthrodesis can be accomplished by a number of techniques, most being variations of the classic Gallie procedure. When the C1-2 subluxation is fixed and cannot be reduced by preoperative traction or extension, removal of the posterior C-1 ring and fusion to the occiput is necessary to adequately decompress the spinal cord.

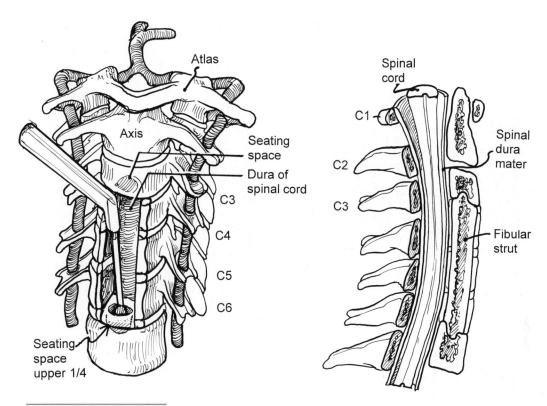

Figure 15–20   Schematic illustrating technique for placement of fibular strut graft. Illustrated by Tony Pazos.

Basilar Invagination

Basilar invagination in a patient with rheumatoid arthritis is a dangerous condition due to the potential neurological consequences. Invagination results from destruction of the lateral masses of the C-1 ring. This allows the skull to "settle" onto the odontoid process. Basilar invagination can be detected by lateral radiographs. Use of the McGregor's line (Fig. 15–23) is recommended with the criteria that the tip of the odontoid process should not project more than 4.5 mm above this line.

Patients with basilar invagination require a posterior fusion from the occiput to C-2 to prevent progression and neurological deterioration. If patients present with quadriparesis, immobilization and halo traction prior to fusion may improve spinal cord function. Various techniques have been described for occipito-cervical fusions. The authors favor the triple wire method of Bohlman, which has been shown to be very effective in achieving a high rate of fusion (Fig. 15–24 and Fig. 15–25).

Subaxial Subluxation

Subaxial subluxations are the result of destructive changes in the facet, interspinous ligaments, and intervertebral discs. Patients present with neck pain and myelopathy when there is significant subluxation and cord compression. If the posterior space available for the spinal cord is less than 14 mm, there is a high risk for neurological impairment. In this instance, most orthopaedic surgeons would recommend a posterior fusion. The Bohlman triple wire technique is recommended because it provides fairly rigid stabilization with a high fusion rate.

PEARL
The drill holes for wiring the spinous processes should be placed as close to the base of the spinous process as possible. This reduces the risk of fracture during wire tightening.

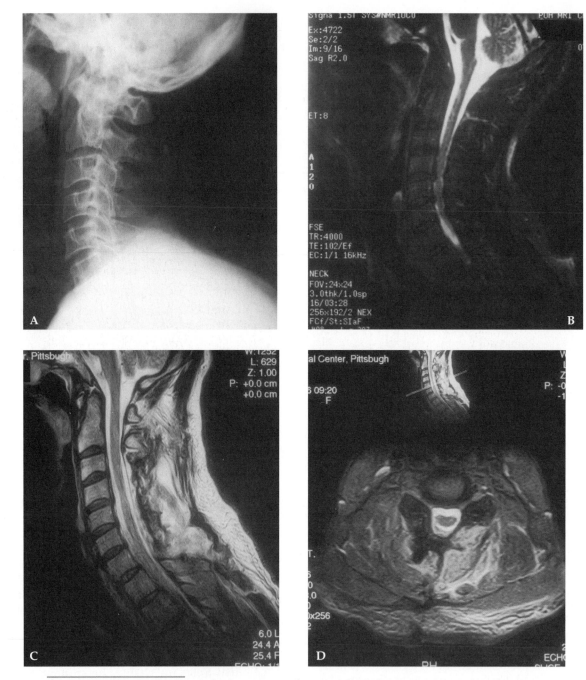

Figure 15–21   Lateral radiograph of a patient with severe cervical stenosis and myelopathy. Note the relatively normal sagittal alignment and lordosis (**A**). The MRI confirmed the severe spinal cord compression at multiple levels (**B**). The patient underwent a posterior laminoplasty with excellent clinical results. A postoperative MRI demonstrates the decompression that was achieved (**C–D**).

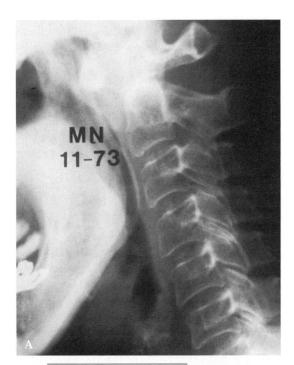 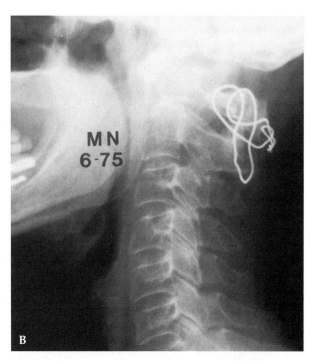

Figure 15–22 Lateral radiograph of an elderly patient with a long standing history of rheumatoid arthritis and neck pain. She has gross instability of the C1-2 segment with flexion and a posterior space available for the cord measuring 12 mm (**A**). The patient underwent a successful posterior C1-2 fusion with excellent clinical results (**B**).

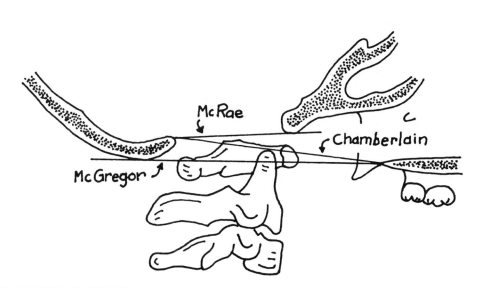

Figure 15–23 Schematic showing three techniques for assessing basilar invagination.

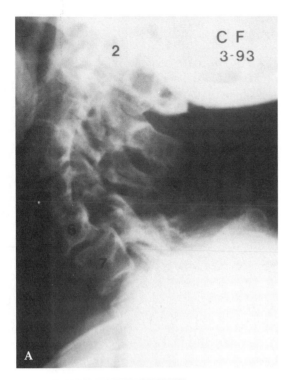

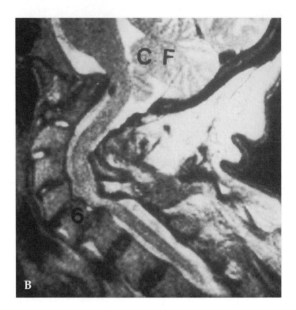

Figure 15–24 Lateral radiograph of a patient who presented with severe myelopathy and quadriparesis. Note the severe destruction of normal architecture. The patient has basilar invagination of the odontoid along with subaxial subluxations of the cervical spine (**A**). An MRI demonstrates the severity of the odontoid migration and the subaxial stenosis (**B**). The patient required a pancervical fusion from occiput to C-7 to stabilize the cervical spine.

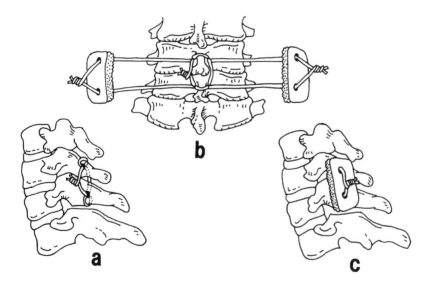

Figure 15–25 Schematic demonstrating technique of Bohlman triple wiring.

SELECTED BIBLIOGRAPHY

Biomechanics of the Cervical Spine

WHITE AA, JOHNSON RM, PANJABI MM, SOUTHWICK WO. Biomechanical analysis of clinical stability in the cervical spine. *Clin Orthop.* 1975;109:85–96.

Relevant Anatomy and Surgical Approaches

DEANDRADE JR, MCNAB I. Anterior occipito-cervical fusion using an extrapharyngeal exposure. *J Bone Jt Surg.* 1969;51:1621–1626.

RILELY LH. Surgical approaches to the anterior structures of the cervical spine. *Clin Ortho.* 1973;91:16–20.

WHITESIDES TE Jr, KELLY RP. Lateral approaches to the upper cervical spine for anterior fusions. *Southern Med. J.* 1966;59:879–883.

Biochemistry

COVENTRY MB, GHORMLEY RK, KERNOHAN JW. The intervertebral disc: its microscopic anatomy and pathology; II: changes in the intervertebral disc concomitant with age. *J Bone Jt Surg.* 1945;27:233–247.

KANG JD, GEORGESCU HI, LARKIN L, STEFANOVIC-RACIC M, EVANS CH. Herniated lumbar intervertebral discs spontaneously produce matrix metalloproteinases, nitric oxide, interlukin-6, and PGE_2. *Spine.* 1996;21:271–277.

KANG JD, GEORGESCU HI, LARKIN L, STEFANOVIC-RACIC M, EVANS CH. Towards a biochemical understanding of human intervertebral disc degeneration and herniation: the contributions of nitric oxide, interleukins, PGE_2, and matrix metalloprteinases. *Spine.* 1997;22:1065–1073.

Upper Cervical Spine Trauma

ANDERSON LD, D'ALONZO RT. Fractures of the odontoid process of the axis. *J Bone Jt Surg.* 1974;56A:1663–1674.

BROOKS AL, JENKINS EB. Atlanto-axial arthrodesis by wedge compression method. *J Bone Jt Surg.* 1978;60A:279–284.

CLARK CR, WHITE AA. Fractures of the dens: a multicenter study. *J Bone Jt Surg.* 1985;67A:1340–1348.

LEVINE AM, EDWARDS CC. The management of traumatic spondylolisthesis of the axis. *J Bone Jt Surg.* 1985;67: 217–226.

LEVINE AM, EDWARDS CC. Traumatic lesions of the occipito-atlantal complex. *Clin Orthop.* 1989;239:53–67.

Lower Cervical Spine Trauma

ALLEN BL, FERGUSON RL, LEHMANN TR, O'BRIEN RP. A mechanistic classification of closed, indirect fractures and dislocations of the lower cervical spine. *Spine.* 1982;7:1–27.

ANDERSON PA, BOHLMAN HH. Anterior decompression and arthrodesis of the cervical spine; I: long-term motor improvement. *J Bone Jt Surg.* 1992;74A:671–682.

ANDERSON PA, BOHLMAN HH. Anterior decompression and arthrodesis of the cervical spine; I: long-term motor improvement. *J Bone Jt Surg.* 1992;74A:683–692.

BOHLMAN HH. Acute fractures and dislocations of the cervical spine: an analysis of 300 hospitalized patients and review of the literature. *J Bone Jt Surg.* 1979;61A:1119–1142.

BRACKEN MB, SHEPARD MJ, COLLINS WF, et al. A randomized, controlled trial of methlyprednisolone or naloxone in the treatment of acute spinal cord injury: results of the second national acute spinal cord injury study. *New Eng J Med.* 1990;322:1405–1411.

EISMONT FJ, ARENA MJ, GREEN BA. Extrusion of an intervertebral disc associated with traumatic subluxation or dislocation of facets. *J Bone Jt Surg.* 1991;73A:1555–1560.

GARFIN SR, BOTTE MJ, WATERS RL, NICKEL VL. Complications in the use of the halo fixation device. *J Bone Jt Surg.* 1986;68A:320–325.

KANG JD, FIGGIE MP, BOHLMAN HH. Sagittal measurements of the surgical spine in subaxial fractures and dislocations: an analysis of 288 patients with and without neurological deficits. *J Bone Jt Surg.* 1994;76A:1617–1628.

Cervical Radiculopathy and Myelopathy

BOHLMAN HH. Cervical spondylosis with moderate to severe myelopathy: a report of 7 cases treated by Robinson anterior cervical disectomy and fusion. *Spine.* 1977;2:151–161.

BOHLMAN HH, EMERY SE, GOODFELLOW DB, JONES PA. Robinson anterior cervical disectomy and arthrodesis for cervical radiculopathy: a long-term follow-up of 122 patients. *J Bone Jt Surg.* 1993;75A:1298–1307.

CRANDALL PH, GREGORIUS FK. Long-term follow-up of surgical treatment of cervical spondylotic myelopathy. *Spine.* 1977;2:139–146.

HERKOWITZ HN, KURZ LT, OVERHOLT DP. The surgical management of cervical soft disc herniation: a comparison between the anterior and posterior approach. *Spine.* 1990;15:1026–1031.

HIRABAYASHI K, WATANABE K, WAKANO K, SUZUKI N, SATOMI K, ISHII Y. Expansive open-door laminoplasty for cervical spinal stenotic myelopathy. *Spine.* 1983;8:693–699.

KANG JD, BOHLMAN HH. Cervical spondylotic myelopathy. *Curr Opin Orthop.* 1996;7:13–21.

ROBINSON R, WALKER A, FERLIC D. The results of anterior interbody fusion of the cervical spine. *J Bone Jt Surg.* 1962;44A:1569–1587.

ZDEBLICK TA, BOHLMAN HH. Cervical kyphosis and myelopathy: treatment by anterior corpectomy and bone grafting. *J Bone Jt Surgery.* 1989;71A:170–182.

Rheumatoid Arthritis

BODEN SD, DODGE LD, BOHLMAN HH, RECHTINE GR. Rheumatoid arthritis of the cervical spine. *J Bone Jt Surg.* 1993;75A:1282–1297.

KRAUS DR, PEPPELMAN WC, AGARWAL AK, DE LEEUW HW, DONALDSON WF III. Incidence of subaxial subluxation in patients with generalized rheumatoid arthritis who have had previous occipital cervical fusions. *Spine.* 1991;16S: 486–489.

LIPSON SJ. Cervical myelopathy and posterior atlanto-axial subluxation in patients with rheumatoid arthritis. *J Bone Jt Surg.* 1985;67A:593–597.

MCAFEE PC, BOHLMAN HH, WILSON WL. The triple wire fixation technique for stabilization. *Orthop Trans.* 1985; 9(1):142.

PEPPELMAN WC, KRAUS DR, DONALDSON WF, AGARWAL A. Cervical spine surgery in rheumatoid arthritis: improve-ment of neurologic deficit after cervical spine fusion. *Spine.* 1993;18:2375–2379.

RANAWAT CS, O'LEARY P, PELLICCI P, TSAIRIS P, MARCHISELLO P, DORR L. Cervical fusion in rheumatoid arthritis. *J Bone Jt Surg.* 1979;61A:1003–1010.

WERTHEIM SB, BOHLMAN HH. Occipitocervical fusion: indications, technique, and long-term results in 13 patients. *J Bone Jt Surg.* 1987;69A:833–836.

SAMPLE QUESTIONS

1. Which statement is false regarding rheumatoid arthritis of the cervial spine:

   (a) The most common radiographic lesion is atlanto-axial instability.

   (b) Basilar invagination occurs due to destruction of the C-1 lateral articular masses.

   (c) The surgical treatment for patients with basilar invagination is posterior C1-2 fusion.

   (d) Posterior stabilization should be performed in those patients with a posterior atlanto-dental interval of less than 14 mm.

   (e) Significant basilar invagination has occured if the tip of the odontoid has migrated more than 4.5 mm above McGregor's line.

2. Which statement is true about upper cervical spine fractures:

   (a) Fractures of the C1-2 complex often involve severe neurologic deficits.

   (b) Type III odontoid fractures are associated with a high incidence of nonunions.

   (c) Hangman's fractures of C-2 will often require posterior surgical fusion.

   (d) The best indication for an odontoid screw is for patients with concomitant odontoid and atlas fractures.

   (e) Occipital-C1 dislocations can be effectively treated in a halo orthosis.

3. Which statement is false about subaxial fractures and dislocations:

   (a) Unilateral facet dislocations are easily reduced with tong traction.

   (b) Patients with unilateral and bilateral facet dislocations and a normal neurological examination should all undergo MRI scan prior to reduction to look for traumatic disc herniations.

   (c) Bilateral facet dislocations are highly associated with spinal cord injury and require surgical stabilization.

   (d) Teardrop fracture/dislocations are relatively stable injuries, which can be treated in a halo orthosis as the definitive treatment.

   (e) Burst fractures of the cervical spine involve axial loading as the predominant mechanism of injury.

4. Which statement is false regarding cervical radiculopathy and myelopathy:

   (a) The pathophysiology of cervical myelopathy includes chronic cord compression from spondylotic bars in patients with congenitally narrow spinal canals.

   (b) Patients with a C-7 radiculopathy will predictably have a herniated disc at the C7-T1 level.

   (c) Patients with myelopathy may present with gait disturbance, spasticity, hyper-flexia, and a Babinski's sign.

   (d) Patients with cervical stenosis and mild kyphosis should be treated with anterior cervical decompression and fusion.

   (e) Congenital stenosis of the cervical spine can be diagnosed on a plain lateral radiograph if the space availble for the cord is less than 13 mm.

5. Which statement is true about the vertebral artery in the cervical spine:

   (a) The vertebral artery enters the transverse foramen at the C-7 level.

   (b) Dissection can be safely carried out up to 3 cm lateral to the midline during posterior C1-2 fusions.

   (c) Injury to the vertebral artery can result in a cerebellar infarct in patients with a dominant vertebral artery.

   (d) The vertebral artery enters the carotid tubercle near the C4-5 level.

   (e) The vertebral artery is positioned posterior to the exiting cervical nerve root.

Answers: 1) c; 2) d; 3) d; 4) b; 5) c;

Chapter 16

Traumatic and Degenerative Conditions of the Lumbosacral Spine

Mark A. Fye, MD

Low back pain represents the second most common reason for patients to seek medical advice. Degenerative conditions of the lumbar spine are a common cause of low back or leg pain. Injuries to the lumbar spine must be diagnosed and appropriately managed to prevent long-term disability. This chapter provides an overview of the evaluation and management of common problems of the lumbar spine.

BASIC SCIENCE

Biomechanics of the Lumbar Spine

The lumbar spine is straight in the frontal plain and lordotic in the sagittal plain. The lordosis provides mobility and shock-absorbing properties. The functional unit of the lumbar spine is the motion segment, which consists of two vertebral bodies and the intervening soft tissue structures. Biomechanical studies of the motion segment have provided important clinical information on degenerative and traumatic conditions affecting the lumbar spine. The lumbar vertebral bodies and intervening discs provide support to the spine for withstanding compressive loads from the cervical and thoracic spine. The disc acts as a shock absorber, distributing loads

and preventing excessive motion. The disc contains an inner portion, the nucleus pulposus, which is surrounded by a tough outer structure, the anulus fibrosus. Studies on the physiology and mechanical behavior of an intervertebral disc have improved understanding of the degenerative processes that take place with aging. The collagen fibers of the anulus provide the necessary strength to resist the inner pressures of the nucleus and maintain the stability of the motion segment. The nucleus consists of collagen and hydrated proteoglycan, which provides the motion segment the capacity to distribute compressive loads.

Spinal stability is poorly understood. Lumbar stability can be defined using Denis's three-column fracture model of the spine (Fig. 16–1). In this model, the anterior column is composed of the anterior longitudinal ligament (ALL), the anterior half of the anulus fibrosus, and the anterior vertebral body. The middle column consists of the posterior half of the anulus fibrosus and the vertebral body and the posterior longitudinal ligament (PLL). The posterior column includes the spinous process, lamina, facets, and pedicles, as well as the supra- and interspinous ligaments and ligamentum flavum. Using this model, injuries to the lumbar spine are classified as stable or unstable. Stable injuries occur when only one column is disrupted, usually the anterior column as in compression fractures. The middle and posterior columns remain intact. Unstable injuries are further classified as mechanical or neurologic spinal instability. Mechanical instability occurs when two of the three columns are disrupted, allowing the development of abnormal motion of the spine. Neurologic instability develops when the middle column is disrupted causing compression of the neural structures.

Lumbar spine instability may be caused not only from trauma but from degeneration of the spine. Degenerative instability may be present preoperatively or may occur intraoperatively if excessive bone from the facets (> 50% of each facet or one whole facet) or pars is removed during a surgical procedure. White and Panjabi (1990) define clinical instability of the spine as "loss of the ability of the spine under physiologic loads to maintain its pattern of displacement so that there is no initial or additional neurological deficit, no major deformity, and no incapacitating pain." Lumbar instability is defined as greater than 4 mm of anterior or posterior translation or 10 degrees of angular motion between vertebral end plates on the lateral flexion-extension radiographs. The unstable level must be compared with the angular motion of the level above and below.

Orthopaedic Surgery: The Essentials. Edited by M.E. Baratz, A.D. Watson, and J.E. Imbriglia. Thieme Medical Publishers, Inc., New York © 1999

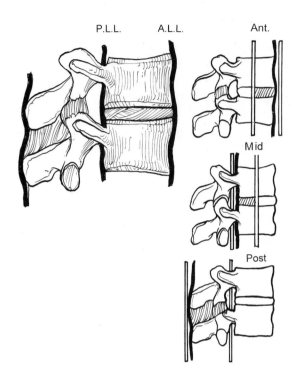

Figure 16–1 Denis's three-column model of the spine. The middle column is made up of the posterior longitudinal ligament (PLL), the posterior anulus fibrosus, and the posterior aspect of the vertebral body and disc. Reprinted with permission from Eismont FJ, Garfin SR, Abitbol JJ. Thoracic and upper lumbar spine injuries. In: Browner BD, Jupiter JB, Levine AM Trafton PG, eds *Skeletal Trauma: Fractures, Dislocations, Ligamentous Injuries*. Vol. 1. Philadelphia, PA: WB Saunders; 1992:744.

Mechanism of Low Back Pain

The lumbar spine consists of bones, joints, ligaments, muscles, and tendons. All of these structures are innervated and may cause pain in the unstable spine. The facet joints, composed of articular cartilage, absorb and distribute loads across the lumbar spine. The facet joint is innervated by afferent nerve endings from the articular and accessory articular nerves. Abnormal facet joint motion from degeneration may produce a stimulus from the nociceptive or mechanocoreceptors in the synovium or facet capsule causing localized low back pain.

Several chemical stimuli may produce pain through these nerve fibers. The neuropeptides, Substance P and calcitonin gene-related peptide (CGRP), have been implicated as mediators in pain associated with degeneration of the facet joints.

The vertebral body or posterior bony arch can cause pain through periosteal injury from tumor or infection, mechanical bony disruption secondary to trauma, and bone marrow congestion from metabolic or vascular injury. With distortion of the bone or periosteum, neuropeptides are released that activate pain receptors. Vasoactive intestinal peptide (VIP), Substance P, and CGRP are found in nerve fibers located in the cancellous bone and periosteum.

Low back pain from paraspinal muscle injury results from disruption of the nerve fibers innervating the damaged muscle tissue as well as the inflammation and distention causing stimulation of the mechanocoreceptors and chemonociceptor nerve endings. Neuropeptides also play a role in muscle pain from trauma or exercise. Low back pain from degeneration of the intervertebral disc has been the topic of much debate. The outer one third of the anulus is innervated by nerve endings that are sensitive to the pain-related neuropeptides: Substance P, VIP, and CGRP. With disc degeneration or herniation, these nerves may produce pain localized to the low back. The sinuvertebral nerve innervates the PLL, as well as the ventral dura, posterior anulus, and lateral anulus. Of all the ligaments of the lumbar spine, the PLL is the most richly innervated. The PLL and posterior outer anulus are tightly connected causing localized back pain from not only disc herniation itself but from distortion of the PLL. Nociceptive nerve endings are also present in the PLL and are stimulated by the various pain-related neuropeptides.

The dorsal root ganglion (DRG) has been implicated as a source of low back pain. Pressure from herniation of disc material, as well as chemical stimulation from neuropeptides released from damaged tissue, sensitize the DRG and cause low back pain though neural discharges.

Pathophysiology of Sciatica

Sciatica is pain radiating down the leg from irritated nerve roots in the lumbar spine. The nerve roots that make up the sciatic nerve include L4, L5, S1, S2, and S3. The lifetime prevalence of sciatica ranges from 2 to 40% of the population. Sciatica may be caused by root compression or chemical irritation. The anterior vertebral body, pedicles, and the posterior bony arch (which includes the lamina and spinous process) protect the spinal cord and nerve roots from injury. The nerve roots are anatomically, biomechanically, and physiologically different from peripheral nerves. Mechanical compression and deformation of nerve roots is different from compression and deformation of peripheral nerves. An important anatomic part of the nerve root is the DRG. Irritation of this structure may cause localized low back pain or pain radiating into the leg. The DRG can induce electrical impulses that are similar to ones seen with mechanical compression. The much talked about pain-related neuropeptides (CGRP, VIP, Substance P) are all synthesized in the DRG and are important in the transmission of pain centrally and peripherally.

Nerve root deformation occurs with spine degeneration and trauma. The nerve root is able to sustain a certain amount of deformation. After excessive compression or stretching, changes take place that alter the physiology of the nerve root thereby causing sciatica. Constriction of the dural sac to 45% or less of normal can cause nerve root injury resulting in motor and sensory deficits. Some people have sciatica without mechanical compression of the nerve roots. Cells of the nucleus pulposus may produce certain substances (interleukins, prostaglandins, phospholipase A2, nitrous oxide) that cause nerve root injury.

ANATOMY AND SURGICAL APPROACHES

Anatomy

The lumbar spine has five vertebrae, each composed of an anterior body and posterior neural arch (pedicles, lamina, and spinous processes). The conus medullaris (inferior aspect of the spinal cord) usually ends at the L1-2 disc. The rest of the lumbar spinal canal protects the cauda equina, which is composed of the spinal nerve roots enclosed by the dural sac. With the introduction of pedicle screw instrumentation for the lumbar spine, understanding the morphometry of the pedicle is required. The position of the pedicles in the lumbar spine varies depending on the level. In the lumbar spine, the angle of the pedicle at L1 inclines medially at 11 degrees compared with 30 degrees at L5. The pedicle can be found for screw insertion at the junction of the transverse process and inferior point of the superior articular facet. Between each pedicle is the neural foramen through which the nerve root exits the spinal canal. In the lumbar spine, the nerve root is numbered according to the pedicle that it passes beneath. Therefore, a disc herniation at the L4-5 disc causes compression of the L5 nerve root, which passes around the L5 pedicle below the L4-5 disc space.

PEARL

A far lateral L4-5 herniated disc causes compression of the L4 nerve root in the L4-5 foramen.

The lumbar segmental arteries arise from the abdominal aorta to supply the muscles, bones, and nerves of the lumbar spine. Each segmental branch is located at the midpoint of each vertebral body. The posterior branch is always located along the lateral border of the pars interarticularis. It is important to identify the lateral pars during surgical exposure and to cauterize this vessel to prevent excessive bleeding. It is important to understand the venous system of the lumbar spine (Batson's plexus) to keep blood loss to a minimum during lumbar surgery. This valveless system has a rich interconnecting network surrounding the spinal canal and bony elements of the spine and drains into the inferior vena cava. If the intra-abdominal pressure is increased for any reason causing decreased flow to the inferior vena cava, venous drainage from the spinal canal will be impaired, increasing blood loss during surgery.

The ligaments of the lumbar spine include the ALL, PLL, ligamentum flavum, and interspinous and supraspinous ligaments. The yellow ligament, or ligamentum flavum, originates on the superior edge of the caudal lamina and inserts on the midpoint of the ventral surface of the cephalad lamina. This ligament is generally removed for standard laminotomy and discectomy. With aging, the ligamentum flavum hypertrophies and compresses the dural sac causing spinal stenosis. The PLL becomes thin in the lower lumbar spine contributing to the fact that most disc herniations occur at the L4-5 and L5-S1 disc.

Posterior Approach to the Lumbar Spine

The posterior approach is the most common operative approach to the lumbar spine. The patient is positioned prone with the abdomen free to reduce the intra-abdominal pressure and allow drainage of the lumbar venous plexus. For noninstrumented posterior procedures, an Andrews (OSI; California) table is used to allow the abdomen to hang free. For instrumented cases requiring pedicle screws, a Jackson table (OSI; California) is used to produce a more anatomic lordosis of the lumbar spine. A standard incision using the midline spinous processes as landmarks is used for the majority of posterior lumbar surgery. The top of the iliac crest helps localize the L4-5 disc space (Fig. 16–2). A preoperative anteroposterior (AP) lumbar radiograph will confirm this. Identifying both posterior superior iliac spines and joining a line between them identifies the S-2 part of the sacrum. A finger breadth above this line generally reveals the L5-S1 interspace. Placing a Kocher (OSI; California) on the spinous process and taking an intraoperative cross-table lateral radiograph helps confirm the vertebral level. For a standard laminotomy and discectomy, dissection is carried down one side of the spinous process at the appropriate level elevating the muscles laterally and identifying the ligamentum flavum between the lamina. A laminotomy is required with removal of the ligamentum flavum folbwed by retraction of the dural sac medially to identify the disc space (Figs. 16–3 and Fig. 16–4). For decompressive surgery requiring laminectomy, as in spinal stenosis, a bilateral dissection is required with removal of the spinous process, lamina, and ligamentum flavum. The lateral border of the pars must be visualized and no more than one-half the pars resected during decompression to prevent postoperative instability. Identify

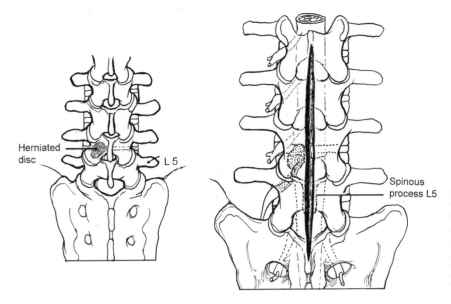

Figure 16–2 Make a longitudinal incision over the spinous process extending from the spinous process above to the spinous process below the level of pathology. A line drawn across the highest point of the iliac crest is in the L4-5 interspace.

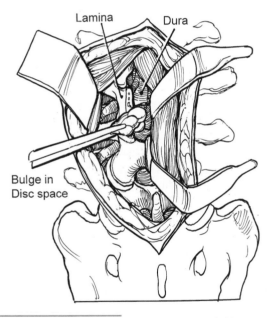

Figure 16–3 Using blunt dissection, carefully continue down the lateral side of the dura to the floor of the spinal canal; retract the dura and its nerve root medially. Reveal the posterior aspect of the disc space.

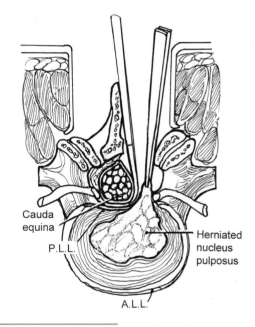

Figure 16–4 Cross section revealing the retraction of the dural tube and a herniated nucleus pulposus impinging on a nerve root.

the pedicle first, find the corresponding nerve root and protect it while decompressing each foramen. The aorta and iliac vessels lie anterior to the vertebral bodies and discs. Be careful not to penetrate the anterior anulus during a discectomy. Generally, 20 to 25 mm is the maximum depth when using a pituitary rongeur for disc removal.

Anatomy: Transperitoneal and Retroperitoneal Approaches to the Lumbar Spine

The skin of the anterior abdominal wall is supplied by segmental nerves (T7–T12), and these nerves do not cross the midline. The anterior abdominal muscles consist of the midline rectus abdominus, the external and internal obliques, and the transversus abdominus muscles. The umbilicus usually lies over the L3-4 disc space. Lying anterior to the vertebral bodies of the upper lumbar spine is the aorta. The aorta divides into the common iliac arteries over the L4 body. The common iliac vessels divide into the external and internal vessels at the S1 level. The aorta lies to the left and inferior vena cava to the right of the vertebral bodies. Both structures are held on the anterior vertebral bodies by the segmental vessels. The left iliac vein lies medial to the iliac artery, an important fact with transabdominal or retroperitoneal approaches.

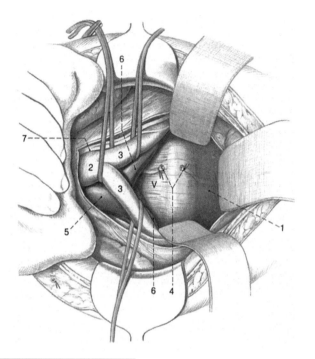

Figure 16–5 Exposure of promontory and caudal half of the fifth lumbar vertebra and upper half of the first sacral vertebra following transection of median sacral artery, snaring of aorta and left and right common iliac artery, and retraction of left and right common iliac vein. 1 = sacrum; 2 = abdominal aorta; 3 = common iliac artery; 4 = median sacral artery; 5 = inferior vena cava; 6 = common iliac vein; 7 = superior hypogastric plexus; V = lumbar vertebra.

The parasympathetic plexus lies on the anterior surface of the sacrum between the bifurcation of the aorta. This plexus is important for sexual function and preservation is impor-

tant for male ejaculation. The psoas muscle lies lateral to the vertebral bodies. The sympathetic chain lies over the medial part of the psoas, whereas the genitofemoral nerve lies on the anterior medial surface of the psoas.

Transperitoneal Approach

This approach is generally used for anterior fusion of the L5-S1 disc space. The patient is placed supine on a standard operating room table. The incision runs in the midline from the umbilicus to just above the pubic symphysis. This midline incision does not cut any nerves because of segmental innervation. Once through the anterior abdominal wall, the peritoneal contents are retracted superiorly. Ligation of the middle sacral artery is necessary to approach the L5-S1 disc space. Careful attention must be paid to preserve the anterior sacral parasympathetic plexus (Fig. 16–5). A needle may be inserted into the disc space and a cross-table lateral radiograph taken to identify the disc space.

Retroperitoneal Approach

This approach is generally utilized for access to the entire lumbar spine for infection, tumor, or trauma. The patient is placed in a semilateral position (45 degrees to horizontal) on the operating room table. A standard approach is an oblique flank incision, usually on the left side, because the aorta is on the left side and the approach allows for easier mobilization of the vessels. The incision is made between the pelvic crest and the 12th rib, extending from the posterior half of the 12th rib to the lateral border of the rectus abdominus muscle. The external and internal obliques and transverse abdominus muscle are transected in line with the incision. The peritoneal contents are mobilized to the right along with the ureter. The psoas muscle is identified, protecting the sympathetic chain and genitofemoral nerves (Fig. 16–6). The aorta is mobilized

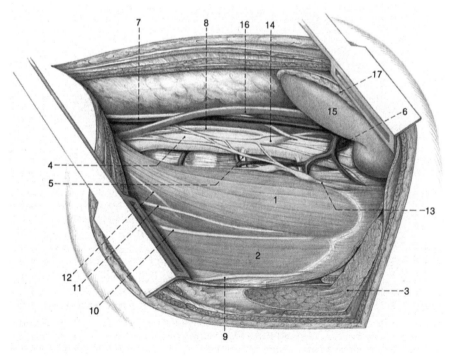

Figure 16–6 Anatomic site in retroperitoneal approach to lumbar spine. 1 = greater psoas muscle; 2 = quadratus lumborum muscle; 3 = iliocostal muscle; 4 = abdominal aorta; 5 = lumbar artery and vein; 6 = renal vein; 7 = spermatic vessels; 8 = inferior meserteric artery; 9 = subcostal nerve; 10 = iliohypogastric nerve; 11 = ilioinguinal nerve; 12 = lateral cutaneous nerve of the thish; 13 = sympathetic trunk; 14 = inferior mesenteric ganglion; 15 = left kidney; 16 = ureter; 17 = adipose capsule of the kidney.

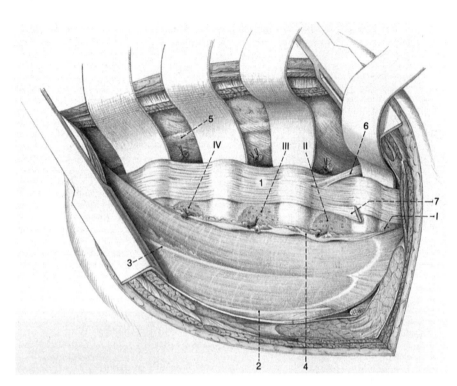

Figure 16–7 Operative site after transection of segmental vessels. 1 = anterior longitudinal ligament; 2 = subcostal nerve; 3 = ilioinguinal nerve; 4 = sympathetic trunk; 5 = ureter; 6 = right medial crus; 7 = left medial crus; I-IV = vertebrae.

along with the iliac vessels by tying off the appropriate segmental vessels (Fig. 16–7). The appropriate disc level is identified with a needle and a lateral cross-table radiograph to confirm the position.

EXAMINATION

A careful history must be obtained with details relating to the location, quality, and chronicity. Details about buttock, thigh, or leg pain must be obtained. It is important to determine if the back pain is worse than the leg pain or vice versa. Have the patient point a finger to outline where the pain begins and radiates. Determine what factors or positions aggravate or improve the pain. Determine if bowel or bladder dysfunction is present. Bowel or bladder dysfunction with buttock numbness and motor and sensory changes in the lower extremity could represent a cauda equina syndrome. This requires immediate diagnosis with magnetic resonance imaging (MRI) to rule out a large central disc herniation or tumor.

PEARL

A magnetic resonance imaging (MRI) scan or computed tomography (CT) myelogram should be ordered urgently if cauda equina syndrome is in your differential diagnosis.

Tumor, infection, and inflammatory arthritides are important conditions to rule out when evaluating patients with low back pain. "Red flags" associated with tumor or infection include back pain unrelieved with rest, night pain, unexplained weight loss, fever, malaise, and history of cancer or immunological compromise. Morning stiffness that improves through the day or after exercise is typical for inflammatory spondyloarthropathies. Visceral sources of referred pain to the back, including abdominal aortic aneurysm, pancreatitis, cholecystitis, ulcers, prostate disease in men, and genitourinary problems in females need to be excluded. Two of the most commonly encountered degenerative conditions of the lumbar spine deserve further elaboration: herniated disc and spinal stenosis. Both of these conditions may be diagnosed by history alone in most cases.

Disc herniation most often occurs between the ages of 30 and 55, whereas spinal stenosis is seen in patients over 60. The pain associated with a disc herniation increases with sitting and is relieved by lying supine with the knees and hips flexed. Symptoms start gradually in the low back and eventually radiate into the buttocks to the thigh and calf. Paresthesias, including numbness and tingling, are common and follow the dermatomes of the lower extremity (Fig. 16–8).

Lumbar spinal stenosis with neurogenic claudication can be differentiated on history from vascular claudication (Table 16–1). Palliative factors, such as sitting and bending forward (increased room in the spinal canal) after prolonged walking will decrease the pain associated with stenosis. The patient with vascular pain will only need to stop walking to have the calf pain improve. Walking uphill is painless and walking downhill is painful (increased lordosis with extension, which decreases room in the spinal canal) for the patient with neurogenic claudication. The distance the patient is able to walk is generally constant if related to vascular insufficiency. Patients with spinal stenosis will walk less overtime secondary to the progression of disease.

It is important to obtain a good history after trauma to the lumbar spine to determine the mechanism of injury and elucidate the fracture pattern. Loss of consciousness and history of movement of the extremities is important to note.

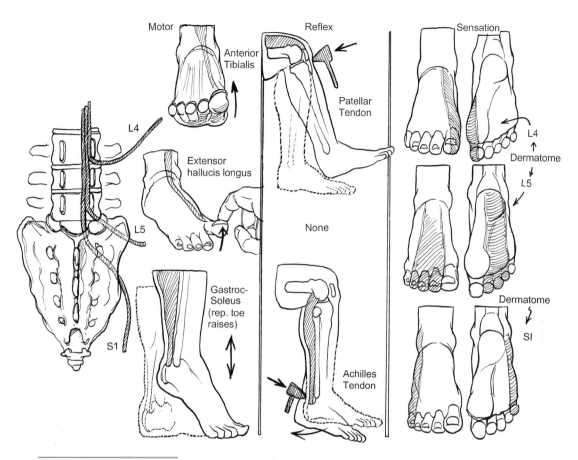

Figure 16–8 Lower extremity findings with lumbar radicular syndrome. Reproduced with permission from Kasser JR. *Orthopaedic Knowledge Update 5*. Rosemont, IL: American Academy of Orthopaedic Surgeons; 1996:609–623.

Physical examination includes gait analysis and evaluation of general movements of the patient as he or she disrobes. The patient's posture as well as any deformities should be noted. The patient should heel and toe walk to evaluate the dorsiflexors (L4, L5) and plantar flexors (S1), respectively. The patient should squat to elicit a mechanical cause of low back pain. Active motion of the lumbar spine should be assessed to identify pain with flexion as seen in herniated nucleus pulposus or extension as seen in spinal stenosis or spondylolisthesis. Inspect the skin for abnormalities for clues of underlying congenital abnormalities. Palpating the midline structures for step-offs or defects as well as for lateral muscle tenderness will help with the diagnosis of spondylolisthesis or muscle spasm, respectively.

A careful neurologic examination is necessary, especially following spine trauma. Motor, sensation, and deep tendon reflexes should be assessed for each root level (Fig. 16–8). Nerve root tension signs, the straight leg raise (SLR), contralateral SLR Lasègue's sign, "bowstring test", and femoral stretch test are used to evaluate nerve root compression from a suspected disc herniation. Active motion of the hips is performed to rule out referred pain from osteoarthritis of the hips. Examination of the sacroiliac joints using the Faber (flexion, abduction, external rotation) or Patrick's test will help rule out sacroiliitis as the cause of low back pain.

Nonorganic physical signs (Waddell's signs) are used in patients with a history of psychiatric disorders, workers'

PEARL

A positive contralateral straight leg raise (SLR) is the most sensitive test for a disc herniation in the axilla of the nerve root.

compensation, or a motor vehicle crash that has legal implications. These five signs include (1) superficial or nonanatomic tenderness, (2) simulation test that is performed by axial loading of the spine through the skull causing low back pain, (3) distraction test that attempts to reproduce exam findings while distracting the patient, (4) regional disturbances such as "give-way" weakness or stocking-glove sensory loss rather than dermatomal distribution, and, finally, the most common nonorganic finding on exam, (5) overreaction with disproportionate pain and exaggerated facial expressions.

PITFALL

If a patient has a negative straight leg raise (SLR) in the seated position and a positive SLR in the supine position, disc herniation as the cause of the patient's low back pain or leg pain is unlikely.

TABLE 16-1   Differential diagnosis of claudicant leg pain.

Findings	Vascular Claudication	Neurogenic Claudication (SCS)
Back pain	Rare	Always in the past or present history
Leg pain		
Type	Sharp, cramping	Vague and variously described as radicular, heaviness, cramping
Location	Exercised muscles (often calf, but may be buttock and thigh), may be one leg	Either typical radicular or extremely diffuse and almost always buttock, thigh, and calf in location. Always both legs in canal stenosis
Radiation	Rare after onset, but may be distal to proximal	Common after onset, usually proximal to distal
Aggravation	Walking, not standing	Usually aggravated by walking, but can be aggravated by standing
Walking uphill	Worse	Better (because back is flexed)
Walking downhill	Better (less muscular energy needed)	Worse (because back is extended)
Relief	Stopping muscular activity even in the standing position	Walking in forward, flexed position more comfortable; once pain occurs, relief comes only with lying down or sitting down
Time to relief	Quick (minutes)	Slow (many minutes)
Neurological symptoms	Not present	Commonly present
Straight leg raising tests	Negative	Mildly positive or negative
Neurological examination	Negative	Mildly positive or negative
Vascular examination	Absent pulses	Pulses present
Skin appearance	Atrophic changes	No changes

Reproduced with permission from McCulloch JA, Transfeldt EE. Disc degeneration with root irritation: spinal canal stenosis. In: Macnab I, ed. *Backache*. 3rd ed. Baltimore, MD: Williams and Wilkins; 1997: 629.

During examination for traumatic lumbar spine injuries, a rectal examination must be performed to document sphincter tone and anal sensation. Spinal shock along with sacral sparing should also be evaluated if a neurologic injury is present.

IMAGING

In patients 20 to 50 years of age with a nontraumatic history of low back pain, plain radiographs yield very little information. In patients older than 50 years of age with gradual or acute onset of low back pain, plain radiographs may provide useful information.

PEARL

No correlation exists between the radiologic findings of a narrowed disc space and low back pain in the adult.

A lumbar radiographic series includes an AP and lateral of the lumbar spine with a cone-down view of the L5 to S1 vertebral bodies. If there is any question of degenerative segmental instability on the initial lateral x-ray, then dynamic flexion-extension lateral radiographs should be obtained. Generally, 4 mm of translation or greater than 10 degrees angulation is considered an unstable lumbar spine. The amount of vertebral height loss, kyphosis, and angulation should be assessed to determine instability in a trauma patient.

Magnetic resonance imaging provides excellent visualization of the entire lumbar spine. If there is any question regarding spinal stenosis or disc herniation that has not improved with 4 to 6 weeks of nonoperative measures, an MRI should be obtained for preoperative evaluation. The physician must remember that abnormal findings on MRI are common in up to 30% of asymptomatic patients. Any findings on diagnostic imaging studies must be correlated to the patient's examination. An MRI is also the study of choice for suspected tumors or infection.

Computed tomography (CT) scans are important in evaluating patients with suspected fractures of the lumbar spine. A CT scan allows improved visualization of the bony elements over MRI but does not accurately define neural compression from disc, infection, or tumor. As with MRI, there is a 36% incidence of abnormalities on CT in asymptomatic volunteers. With the addition of myelography prior to a CT scan, visualization of the neural elements is improved. A CT myelogram is useful for evaluation of lateral recess stenosis of the lumbar spine or in patients who are unable to undergo an MRI. Electromyographic and nerve conduction velocity tests are generally not recommended in the evaluation of degenerative or traumatic conditions unless diabetic neuropathy is suspected as the cause of lower extremity motor or sensory changes.

SPECIFIC CONDITIONS, TREATMENT, AND OUTCOME

Degenerative Conditions

Low Back Pain

An estimated $50 to $100 billion a year is spent on treatment of low back pain in the United States. Acute low back pain spontaneously resolves in 4 to 6 weeks, regardless of treatment. Disc degeneration as a cause of low back pain remains controversial. Many studies have attempted to demonstrate that incompetence of the disc secondary to disc dehydration and chemical alteration causes low back pain. Low back pain should be treated nonoperatively. Table 16–2 outlines the management of low back pain.

Disc Herniation with Radiculopathy

Approximately 2% of the adult population develops symptomatic lumbar disc herniation with sciatica. Symptoms from

TABLE 16–2 Elements that may be included in the nonsurgical treatment program of low back pain.

1. Anti-inflammatory medications
2. Pain modulating medications
3. Physical modalities for pain control
4. Detoxification from addictive and psychotropic medications
5. The use of braces and orthoses
6. Ergonomic evaluation and workplace modification
7. Body mechanics instruction
8. Psychosocial evaluation and intervention
9. Psychiatric intervention (when necessary and appropriate)
10. Family counseling
11. Vocational counseling
12. Nutritional counseling and weight reduction
13. Smoking cessation
14. Establishing a successful doctor-patient relationship
15. Therapeutic exercises for pain control, flexibility, range of motion, muscular strength, muscular endurance, balance, proprioception and coordination, cardiorespiratory aerobic and anaerobic capacity, "work-hardening," and training for a particular sport, job, or activity

Reproduced with permission from Garfin SR, Vaccaro AR, eds. *Orthopaedic Knowledge Update: Spine.* 1st ed. Rosemont, IL; American Academy of Orthopaedic Surgeons; 1997: 114.

> ### PITFALL
> **More than 4 days of bed rest after an acute low back pain episode is not helpful and may prolong a patient's debilitation.**

a disc herniation are thought to result from mechanical compression of the disc on the nerve root as well as biochemical and vascular factors. Treatment options include bed rest for 2 to 3 days, anti-inflammatories, patient education, and therapy. Epidural steroids have limited benefit in patients with herniated discs. Surgery is indicated if nonoperative methods have failed after 6 to 8 weeks. Motor weakness is a relative indication for discectomy.

Prior to surgery, the neurodiagnostic studies must correlate to the history and physical examination (Fig. 16–9). The standard surgical options include a laminotomy and discectomy to relieve the compression on the nerve root. Similar results have been obtained using no magnification, loupe magnification, or a microscope. Relief of sciatica with surgery is more than 90% in properly selected patients. Relief of low back pain is not as predictable. Up to 10 to 15% of patients may have low back discomfort after a discectomy procedure.

Spinal Stenosis

Lumbar spinal stenosis is defined as a narrowing of the spinal canal. The stenosis is caused by degeneration of the disc with a resultant decrease in disc space. This results in narrowing of the neural foramen and buckling inward of the ligamentum flavum. These changes along with facet hypertrophy cause compression of the neural elements of the spinal canal (Fig. 16–10). Depending on the amount of facet changes, secondary spinal instability may occur adding to the nerve compression. The body's attempt to control the instability produces more osteophytes and facet hypertrophy.

Compression of the nerve roots in the cauda equina or the neural foramen decreases the flow of cerebrospinal fluid and vascularity around the nerve root. This chronic process eventually causes irreversible changes in the nerve root. The increased demands of the nerve root with ambulation along with the baseline compression will cause a relative ischemia of the nerve root. These events produce ectopic impulses of the spinal nerves that may contribute to the symptoms of neurogenic claudication.

Most patients present in their 50s or 60s with a 10- to 15-year history of low back pain. This is accompanied by progressive radiation of pain into their buttocks and thighs, either posteriorly or anterior laterally. Patients seek help when they develop radicular pain of claudication. Complaints include a limp with ambulation, weakness of the lower extremities, and fatigue after prolonged walking or standing. Most of the leg symptoms resolve with sitting or squatting because of the increased area of the spinal canal with these positions. This is in direct contrast to vascular claudication (Table 16–1). On examination, only 40% of patients

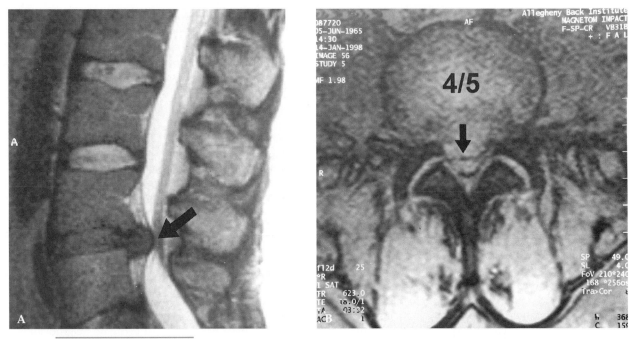

Figure 16–9   Central disc herniation of the lumbar spine. (**A**) A 36-year-old male with a large central disc herniation at L4-5. Sagittal magnetic resonance imaging (MRI) reveals the disc herniation is contained within the PLL. (**B**) Axial MRI demonstrating the central disc herniation at L4-5.

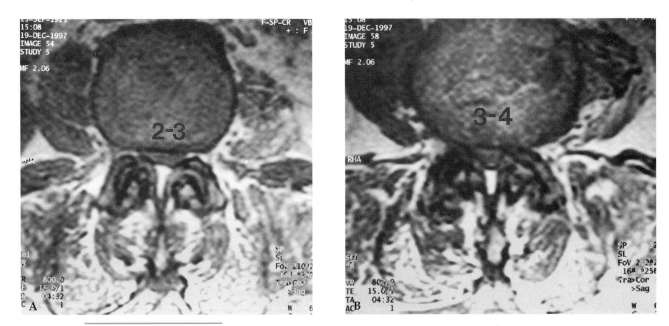

Figure 16–10   Spinal stenosis of the lumbar spine in a 68-year-old female with chronic low back pain and bilateral lower extremity neurogenic claudication. (**A**) Level 2-3 shows severe spinal stenosis centrally and mild to moderate forammal stenosis. (**B**) Level 3-4 shows moderate central stenosis and severe forammal stenosis.

present with a neurologic deficit. If degenerative spondylolisthesis or scoliosis is present along with the stenosis, patients may have increased nerve root compression with subsequent weakness on examination. Often lumbar lordosis is decreased to help prevent further nerve compression.

Tension signs are usually absent. A thorough examination must be obtained even if the history suggests degenerative spinal stenosis to rule out peripheral neuropathy, vascular disease, or an occult neoplasm. Motion of both hips must be evaluated to rule out hip pathology. One sixth of all patients with spinal stenosis will have osteoarthritis of the hips. The difficulty comes with determining which degenerative process is causing the patient's symptoms.

Laboratory studies exclude other causes of low back pain and leg pain in the patient over 50 years of age. These would include metastatic disease, multiple myeloma, infection, or inflammatory arthritis. If the diagnosis is in question, a complete blood count, sedimentation rate, serum protein electrophoresis, and a prostatic specific antigen should be obtained.

Initial radiologic studies for degenerative spinal stenosis include an AP and lateral of the lumbar spine. These studies will hopefully exclude infection and tumor as a cause of low back pain.

PEARL

It takes approximately 50% of bone loss to be able to identify any pathologic process on plain radiographs. If any degree of instability is present on the lateral radiograph of the lumbar spine, dynamic flexion-extension lateral radiographs should be obtained to further delineate the instability.

Magnetic resonance imaging is the study of choice to evaluate spinal stenosis. Myelography followed by CT is used if the patient demonstrates significant instability on flexion-extension radiographs, or if the MRI does not adequately delineate the stenosis. The CT scan will evaluate lateral recess stenosis better than the MRI. Electromyography / nerve conduction studies are helpful only if peripheral neuropathy is in the differential diagnosis.

Nonoperative treatment consists of activity restriction, weight loss, use of a cane, nonsteroidal anti-inflammatory drugs (NSAIDs), and a lumbosacral corset. A flexion exercise program, including an aerobic program such as stationary bicycle, may help reduce the low back pain and leg symptoms in spinal stenosis. Epidural steroid injections for stenosis generally are not helpful long term and remain controversial. Operative treatment includes decompression of the involved segments with or without fusion, depending on preoperative assessment of stability. Decompression involves the central spinal canal as well as the lateral recess and neural-foramen.

PITFALL

If greater than 50% of each facet or one whole facet is removed at a single level during decompression, postoperative instability may occur.

Degenerative spondylolisthesis or scoliosis with associated spinal stenosis often requires fusion of the involved motion segments to prevent further instability after decompression of the neural structures. Degenerative spondylolisthesis with stenosis is generally seen at the L4-5 level and is caused by chronic disc degeneration and facet instability (Fig. 16–11). The problem occurs in females more than 60 years of age. The translation progresses to approximately 30% of the vertebral body. Treatment for degenerative spondylolisthesis includes decompression and posterolateral fusion with or without instrumentation. Instrumentation should be used only if gross instability is documented by flexion-extension radiographs.

PEARL

Instability of the lumbar spine is defined by greater than 4 mm of translation or greater than 10 degrees angulation on flexion-extension lateral radiographs.

Degenerative scoliosis and stenosis are seen in patients greater than 60 years of age. Lumbar spine scoliosis results from disc degeneration and facet degeneration and instability. Lumbar scoliotic curves generally stay under 40 degrees. In patients with persistent symptoms of low back and leg pain, decompression and fusion are recommended. Segmental instrumentation has been advocated to restore lordosis and correct the scoliosis. Pedicle screw instrumentation also has the advantage of improving neural foraminal compression through distraction thereby decreasing the compression on the nerve root and decreasing the amount of bony decompression required.

Lumbar Trauma

Traumatic injury to the lumbar spine generally produces one of four fracture patterns (Table 16–3). The mechanism of injury must be identified to properly understand the fracture pattern and direct treatment. There are six forces that account for the majority of injuries. These include axial compression, flexion, lateral compression, flexion rotation, flexion distraction, and extension. These forces acting alone or in conjunction will produce four common injury patterns seen in traumatic conditions of the lumbar spine. To properly treat these injuries, the three-column concept of the lumbar spine by Denis must be understood (Fig. 16–1).

Compression fractures are by definition an anterior column injury with the middle column intact. If the anterior column is compressed to 40% or less of the total vertebral height and the kyphosis is greater than 30 degrees, a posterior column distraction injury is likely. For simple compression fractures, a thoracolumbar sacral orthosis (TLSO) to prevent motion and enhance healing is used for 3 months. If a posterior ligamentous distraction injury is diagnosed, a posterior fusion and instrumentation should be undertaken.

Burst fractures have disruption of the anterior and middle column. The posterior column may have compression or no injury. Anterior compression, angulation, spinal canal compromise, and neurologic deficits must be evaluated to determine whether surgical intervention is warranted. Treatment with a TLSO is indicated if anterior height loss is less than 40 to 50%, kyphotic angulation is less than 25 to 30 degrees, spinal canal compression is less than 40 to 50%, and

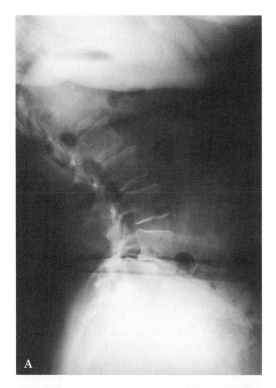

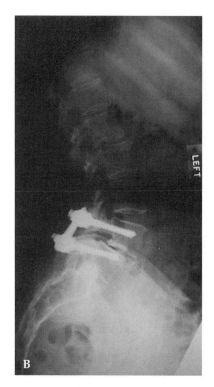

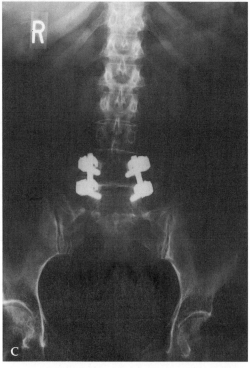

Figure 16–11 Lumbar spinal stenosis with spondylolisthesis. A 62-year-old female with chronic low back pain and bilateral leg pain. (**A**) Preoperative lateral radiograph of the lumbar spine shows grade II spondylolisthesis at L4-5. (**B**) Post-operative lateral radiograph of the lumbar spine shows partial reduction of spondylolisthesis (from positioning, no active reduction) with fusion and pedicle instrumentation at L4-5. (**C**) Postoperative anteroposterior view of the lumbar spine demonstrates wide decompression lammectomy at L4-5 with transverse process fusion and instrumentation at L4-5.

there is no neurologic deficit. Patients with greater than 50% canal compromise with and without neurologic deficit may be treated with posterior decompression and fusion with instrumentation. The posterior instrumented construct relies on distraction and "ligamentotaxis" of the PLL and the anulus of the disc. These structures allow restoration of lordosis and reduction of retropulsed fracture fragments of the middle column (Fig. 16–12).

If canal compromise with a neurologic deficit occurs, anterior decompression and fusion with instrumentation may be appropriate. If a posterior approach is initially chosen, a

---

PEARL

Laminar fractures occurring with a burst fracture are associated with a 50% chance of a posterior dural laceration with entrapment of neural elements at the fracture site.

repeat CT scan after the initial procedure should be done to evaluate the decompression if a continued neurologic deficit

TABLE 16–3   The four major types of spinal injuries.

Fracture Type	Mechanism of Injury		
	Anterior Column	**Middle Column**	**Posterior Column**
Compression	Compression	None	None; distraction
Burst	Compression	Compression	None; compression
Seatbelt	None; compression	Distraction	Distraction
Fracture-dislocation	Compression; rotation; shear	Distraction; rotation; shear	Distraction; rotation; shear

Reproduced with permission from Dennis F. The three column spine and its significance in the classification of acute thoracolumbar spinal injuries. *Spine.* 1993;8:818.

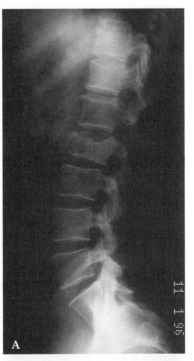

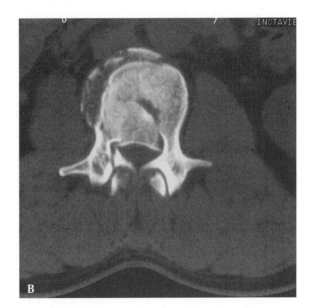

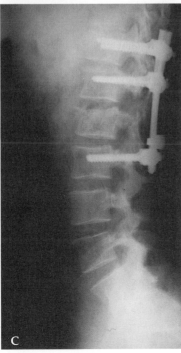

Figure 16–12   L2 burst fracture. A 24-year-old male sustained an L-2 burst fracture with neurologic deficit S/P (status post) MVA (Motor Vehicle Accident). (**A**) Preoperative lateral radiograph showing loss of height, relative kyphosis, and retropulsion of bony fragments. (**B**) Preoperative axial computed tomography scan of L2 burst demonstrating 60% canal compression. (**C**) Postoperative lateral radiograph of the lumbar spine demonstrating restoration of normal alignment with pedicle instrumentation at T12, L1, and L3.

is present. An anterior decompression and fusion may follow a posterior procedure if continued compression and neurologic deficit continues after the posterior procedure.

Flexion-distraction or seatbelt, injuries are by definition disruption of the middle and posterior columns by distraction with possible compression of the anterior column. These injuries can occur through bone or soft tissue. The Chance fracture was originally described for a flexion-distraction injury through bone. These injuries have the best potential for healing and may be treated with a TLSO for 3 to 4 months. Injuries with ligamentous or disc disruption usually require surgical stabilization with a posterior compression instrumentation construct.

PITFALL

A flexion-distraction injury (Chance) may contain an intra-abdominal injury that is commonly overlooked secondary to the fracture of the spine.

PEARL

Magnetic resonance imaging (MRI) will help determine if any soft tissue injury is present with edema of the disc or posterior ligamentous structures.

Fracture dislocation injuries involve all three columns: compression of the anterior column and distraction and rotation or shear of the middle and posterior columns. These injuries have a high rate of neurologic deficit. The majority of these injuries require posterior fusion and instrumentation. If any neurologic injury is present, a posterior decompression should be done.

SUMMARY

The lumbar spine is an important link in the human body between the upper torso and lower extremities. Degenerative conditions of the lumbar spine are a consequence of the aging process. Traumatic conditions of the lumbar spine are relatively infrequent. To treat these problems, the surgeon must understand the biomechanics, physiology, and anatomy of the lumbar spine. In recent years, the pathophysiology of degenerative conditions has been studied extensively. This new information will allow better treatment options in the future for low back pain, disc herniations, and spinal stenosis.

Evaluation of the patient with degenerative or traumatic conditions of the lumbar spine begins with a thorough history and examination. Further diagnostic workup is based on the differential diagnosis. The surgeon must use imaging studies in a cost-effective manner to define the problem when surgical intervention is necessary. Most problems encountered in the lumbar spine are dealt with nonoperatively. When the indication arises to intervene surgically, the surgeon must understand the goals, techniques, and limitations of surgery.

SELECTED BIBLIOGRAPHY

Biomechanics

WHITE AA III, PANJABI MM. *Clinical Biomechanics of the Spine.* 2nd ed. Philadelphia, PA Lippincott: 1990.

Low Back Pain

BOGDUK N. The innervation of the lumbar spine. *Spine.* 1983;8:286–293.

BOGDUK N, TYNAN W, WILSON AS. The nerve supply to the human lumbar intervertebral discs. *J Anatomy.* 1981;132:39–56.

Sciatica

CORNEFJORD M, OLMARKER K, FARLEY DB, WEINSTEIN JN, RYDE-VIK B. Neruopeptide changes in compressed spinal nerve roots. *Spine.* 1995;20:670–673.

DELAMARTER RB, BOHLMAN HH, DODGE LD, BIRO C. Experimental lumbar spinal stenosis: analysis of the cortical evoked potentials, microvasculature, and histopathology. *J Bone Jt Surg.* 1990;72A:110–120.

OLMARKER K, RYDEVIK B, NORDBORG C. Autologous nucleus pulposus induces neurophysiologic and histologic changes in porcine cauda equina nerve roots. *Spine.* 1993;18:1425–1432.

Degenerative Conditions: Low Back Pain

BIGOS S, BOYER O, BRAEN G. Acute low back pain problems in adults: clinical practice guideline No 14. Rockville, MD: Agency for Health Care Policy and Research; 1994. US Department of Health and Human Services publication 95–0642.

DEYO RA, DIEHL AK, ROSENTHAL M. How many days of bed rest for acute low back pain? a randomized clinical trial. *N Eng J Med.* 1986;315:1064–1070.

MALMIVAARA A, HAKKINEN U, ARO T et al. The treatment of acute low back pain: bed rest, exercises, or ordinary activity? *N Eng J Med.* 1995;332:351–355.

VON KORFF M. Studying the natural history of back pain. *Spine.* 1994;19 (suppl 18):2041S–2046S.

Herniated Disc

SAAL JA, SAAL JS, HERZOG RJ. The natural history of lumbar intervertebral disc extrusions treated nonoperatively. *Spine.* 1990;15:683–686.

TULLBERG T, ISACSON J, WEIDENHEILM L. Does microscopic removal of lumbar disc herniation lead to better results than the standard procedure? results of a 1-year randomized study. *Spine.* 1993;18:24–27.

Spinal Stenosis

Johnsson KE, Rosen I, Uden A. The natural course of lumbar spinal stenosis. *Clin Orthop.* 1992;270:82–86.

Katz JN, Lipson SJ, Larson MG, McInnes JM, Fossel AH, Liang MH. The outcome of decompressive laminectomy for degenerative lumbar stenosis. *J Bone Jt Surg.* 1991; 73A:809–816.

Simpson JM, Silveri CP, Balderston RA, Simeone FA, An HS. The results of operations on the lumbar spine in patients who have diabetes mellitus. *J Bone Jt Surg.* 1993;75A:1823-1829.

Imaging

Boden SD, Davis DO, Dina TS, Patronas N, Wiesel SW. Abnormal magnetic-resonance scans of the lumbar spine in asymptomatic subjects: a prospective investigation. *J Bone Jt Surg.* 1990;72A:403–408.

Boden SD, Wiesel SW. Lumbosacral segmental motion in normal individuals: have we been measuring instability properly? *Spine.* 1990;15:571–576.

Wiesel SW, Tsourmas N, Feffer HL, Citrin CM, Patronas N. A study of computer-assisted tomography; I: The incidence of positive CAT scans in an asymptomatic group of patients. *Spine.* 1984;9:549–551.

Clinical Evaluation

Keenen TL, Benson DR. Initial evaluation chapter of the spine-injured patient. In: Browner BD, Jupiter JB, Levine AM, eds. *Ligamentous Injuries.* Vol 1. Philadelphia, PA: WB Saunders; 1992;585–603.

Macnab I, ed. *Backache.* 3rd ed. Baltimore, MD: Williams and Wilkins; 1997.

Scham SM, Taylor TKF. Tension signs in lumbar disc prolapse. *Clin Orthop.* 1971;75:195–204.

Waddell G, McCullough JA, Kummel E, Venner RM. Nonorganic physical sign in low back pain. *Spine.* 1980; 5:117–125.

Lumbar Fusion

Zdeblick TA. A prospective, randomized study of lumbar fusion: preliminary results. *Spine.* 1993;18:983–991.

Trauma

Bohlman HH. Treatment of fractures and dislocations of the thoracic and lumbar spine. *J Bone Jt Surg.* 1985;67A: 165–169.

Cammisa FP Jr, Eismont FJ, Green BA. Dural laceration occurring with burst fractures and associated laminar fractures. *J Bone Jt Surg.* 1989;71A:1044–1052.

Denis F. The three column spine and its significance in the classification of acute thoracolumbar spinal injuries. *Spine.* 1983;8:817–831.

Fredrickson BE, Mann KA, Yuan HA, Lubicky JP. Reduction of the intracanal fragment in experimental burst fractures. *Spine.* 1988;13:267–271.

McAfee PC, Bohlman HH, Yuan HA. Anterior decompression of traumatic thoracolumbar fractures with incomplete neurological deficit using a retroperitoneal approach. *J Bone Jt Surg.* 1985;67A:89–104.

Degenerative Spondylolisthesis

Bridwell KH, Sedgewick TA, O'Brien MF, Lenke LG, Baldus C. The role of fusion and instrumentation in the treatment of degenerative spondylolisthesis with spinal stenosis. *J Spinal Disord.* 1993;6:461–472.

Herkowitz HN, Kurz LT. Degenerative lumbar spondylolisthesis with spinal stenosis: a prospective study comparing decompression with decompression and intertransverse process arthrodesis. *J Bone Jt Surg.* 1991;73A:802–808.

Degenerative Scoliosis

Marchesi DG, Aebi M. Pedicle fixation devices in the treatment of adult lumbar scoliosis. *Spine.* 1992;17(suppl 8):S304–S309.

Simmons ED Jr, Simmons EH. Spinal stenosis with scoliosis. *Spine.* 1992;17(suppl 6):S117–S120.

SAMPLE QUESTIONS

1. A 35-year-old male complains of pain in his back and left lower extremity. The pain radiates to the outside of his calf and top of his foot to the big toe. The pain has persisted for 3 months. Examination reveals diminished sensation over the dorsum of his foot and weakness of his (extensor hallucis longus) on the left. An MRI reveals a herniated disc that correlates to his examination. The best treatment option is:

   (a) bed rest for 2 weeks then progressive ambulation

   (b) laminotomy L5 and L5-S1 discectomy

   (c) laminectomy L4 and L4-5 microdiscectomy

   (d) lammectomy L4 and L4-5 discectomy

   (e) L4-5 micro-discectomy and fusion

2. A 65-year-old female with a 10-year history of low back pain and 8-month history of bilateral lower extremity pain with ambulation is referred to you for evaluation. On examination, she has no neurologic deficits of her lower extremities. She has pain with extension of the lumbar spine. Her pulses of the lower extremities are normal. The next step in management would be to:

   (a) obtain an MRI scan of the lumbar spine

   (b) order an arteriogram of the lower extremities

   (c) order an AP and lateral plain radiograph of the lumbar spine

   (d) start a physical therapy program and see her back in 6 months

(e) order electromyography and nerve conduction velocity tests of the lower extremities

3. A 44-year-old male is involved in a motor vehicle crash and sustains an injury to his lumbar spine. He has a neurologic deficit in his left lower extremity. Plain radiographs reveal an L1 burst fracture with 40% loss of height and 40 degrees of kyphosis. Computed tomography scan reveals 60% canal compromise. Treatment would be:
   (a) thoracolumbosacral orthosis for 3 months
   (b) posterior fusion and instrumentation
   (c) posterior laminectomy at L1
   (d) anterior L1 corpectomy with fusion and instrumentation
   (e) bed rest for 3 months then ambulation as tolerated

4. True or false:
   (a) If a patient has motor weakness from a disc herniation, surgical intervention is mandatory.
   (b) The neuropeptides substance P, VIP, and CGRP are important mediators for the production of pain in the low back and legs.
   (c) Bed rest for more than 3 to 4 days is not beneficial for the treatment of low back pain.

5. Which of the following are correct statements:
   (a) The majority of patients (90%) with a disc herniattion do not require surgery.
   (b) Most patients with low back pain will need a lumbar fusion.
   (c) Leg pain is generally improved after discectomy, whereas low back pain may persist.
   (d) The anterior tibialis muscle is innervated by the L4 nerve root.
   (e) The reflex for the L5 nerve root is checked by tapping on the Achilles' tendon.

Answers: 1) d; 2) c; 3) d; 4) a: false, b: true, c: true, 5) a, c, d

Shoulder

Chapter 17

Evaluation of Shoulder Pain

Joseph P. Iannotti, MD, PhD and Abraham Shurland, MD

The shoulder girdle is a complex anatomical structure consisting of three diarthrodial joints, two bursal articulations, four muscle groups, and four sets of ligaments. The evaluation of shoulder pain requires knowledge of the pathology of each of these components and an understanding of how these components can interact with each other.

The causes of shoulder pain can be divided into four main categories; disorders of the rotator cuff and associated structures, disorders of the glenohumeral joint, scapulothoracic disorders, and distant pathology associated with referred pain. It is not within the scope of this chapter to attempt an exhaustive discussion of the evaluation of all of the causes of shoulder pain. We have chosen to select the most common causes for discussion. Rotator cuff disease is discussed both as a primary disorder and secondary to other disorders of the shoulder girdle. The glenohumeral joint disorders discussed are glenohumeral instability, arthritis, and adhesive capsulitis. Finally, we will discuss general characteristics of cervical spine disease, thoracic outlet syndrome, and brachial plexitis. Some of the common clinical features and techniques to evaluate these disorders will be reviewed. A more complete list of the causes of shoulder pain is presented in Table 17–1.

The diagnosis of shoulder pain relies heavily on the history, physical exam, and radiographic studies. In gathering the history, it is important for the clinician to assess the patient's general state of health in addition to the chief complaint. The characterization of the patients pain should be done in a thorough manner, taking care to document its location, severity, character, time course, associated symptoms, radiation, and aggravating and relieving factors. The physical exam should include an evaluation of the joints proximal and distal to the shoulder and always involve a comparative assessment of the other shoulder. Radiographic tests should

TABLE 17–1   Common causes of shoulder pain

Rotator Cuff and Associated Structures

Tendonitis: partial and complete tears
Calcific tendonopathies
Disorders of the acromioclavicular joint
   Dislocations: distal clavicle fractures and nonunion
   Degenerative joint disease
   Os-acrominale
Disorders of the sternoclavicular joint
   Instability
   Degenerative joint disease
Disorders of the scapula
   Fractures: nonunion, malunion
   Osteochondroma
   Snapping scapula syndrome

Glenohumeral Joint

Recurrent Instability
   Voluntary
   Involuntary traumatic/atraumatic
Articular cartilage degeneration
   Rheumatoid arthritis
   Osteoarthritis
   Post-traumatic
   Recurrent instability
   Crystal induced arthropathy
   Neuropathic
   Septic
Osteonecrosis
Adhesive capsulitis and frozen shoulder syndromes
Proximal humeral fractures

Referred Sources of Pain

Cervical degenerative disc disease
Thoracic outlet syndrome
Traumatic and viral brachial plexus injuries
Isolated entrapment neuropathies
Neoplasm

be limited to plain film studies for most common shoulder disorders. Magnetic resonance imaging (MRI) has been found to be an extremely helpful tool when used judiciously but

Orthopaedic Surgery: The Essentials. Edited by M.E. Baratz, A.D. Watson, and J.E. Imbriglia. Thieme Medical Publishers, Inc., New York © 1999

should not be an initial imaging study in most cases. An MRI has been found to be most indicated when a diagnosis of soft tissue injury is suspected. It is not particularly useful in most cases of suspected adhesive capsulitis, advanced acromioclavicular and glenohumeral osteoarthritis, brachial plexus stretch injury, and cervical spondylosis.

SPECIFIC CONDITIONS

Rotator Cuff Disease

Clinical Presentation

Factors that contribute to the development of rotator cuff disease are: age related changes of the rotator cuff (intrinsic cuff disease), degenerative spur formation of the coracoacromial arch and the acromioclavicular joint (extrinsic cuff disease), and overuse microtrauma or a single event of macrotrauma. These factors can work independently or in association with each other.

Disorders of the rotator cuff are generally associated with pain localized to the region of the coracoacromial arch and the anterior and middle deltoid. Mild pain may be present at rest but is always exacerbated by reaching, pushing, and pulling activities involving the use of the hand above shoulder level. The pain may radiate to the deltoid tuberosity and occasionally to the level of the elbow. It is uncommon for patients with rotator cuff disease to have pain below the level of the elbow. Rotator cuff disease is often associated with pain at night, which can awaken the patient from sleep, particularly when laying on the affected shoulder.

PEARL

Patients with impingement syndrome frequently complain of pain on the lateral aspect of the arm near the deltoid insertion.

The physical findings associated with rotator cuff disease are quite variable and reflect the wide spectrum of clinical symptoms and disease severity. Mild tenderness can sometimes be elicited over the anterolateral aspect of the shoulder in the region of the anterior acromion, greater tuberosity, biceps tendon, and acromioclavicular joint. Severe tender-

ness can be found in acute inflammatory bursitis with calcific tendonopathy.

With chronic rotator cuff disease, contracture of the posterior capsule can result in a mild to moderate limitation of passive forward flexion, cross-body adduction, and internal rotation. Limitations in passive range of motion are often mild and will not exceed 10 or 15 degrees as compared with the opposite shoulder. If greater limitation of passive range of motion is noted, the diagnosis of frozen shoulder, either as a primary (adhesive capsulitis) or secondary problem, should be considered.

The impingement signs are useful tools for confirming that shoulder pain is associated with the rotator cuff and when positive suggest clinically significant pathology. The Neer impingement sign is performed by passive forward flexion above 130 degrees. The abduction internal rotation (ABIR) impingement sign is performed with the arm held at 90 degree elevation in the plane of the scapula while the forearm is internally rotated. Pain associated with the rotator cuff when performing the impingement signs is often localized to the anterolateral and superior aspects of the shoulder. The impingement test is one of the most useful clinical tests to help localize the shoulder pain to the subacromial space. Five to ten mL of local anesthetic is injected into the subacromial space and the impingement signs are performed 10 minutes after injection. A positive test is achieved if the anesthetic relieves at least 50% of the patient's shoulder symptoms. If there is no other pathology, subacromial injection of local anesthetic will result in temporary relief of 75 to 100% of the patient's shoulder pain. If pain persists following subacromial injection of local anesthetic and is localized to the acromioclavicular joint, then a second injection of the acromioclavicular joint with 2 or 3 mL of local anesthetic is indicated. A significant further improvement of the shoulder pain indicates clinically significant and concomitant acromioclavicular joint pathology. Local corticosteroid injection may be used in conjunction with the lidocaine injection for therapeutic purpose.

Weakness of the shoulder is a common finding in patients with shoulder pain and may be caused by disuse atrophy or full-thickness rotator cuff tears. It is important to determine whether the patient has true weakness or whether the symptom is due to avoidance of pain. True weakness of abduction of the arm will often be accompanied by abnormal scapular elevation (the shrug sign) as the patient tries to compensate by using their trapezius (Fig. 17–1). Strength assessment of

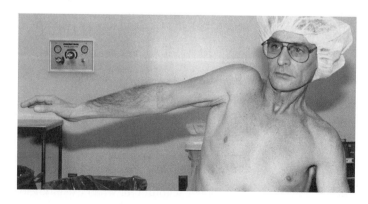

Figure 17–1   Shrug sign. With abduction there is elevation of the scapula with inability to fully elevate the arm.

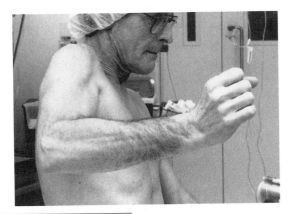

Figure 17–2 Hornblower's sign. With the arm in the abducted position the patient is unable to externally rotate the arm indicating a massive superior and posterior cuff tear.

external rotation can be performed both before and after subacromial injection of lidocaine. Significant weakness after temporary relief of pain with local anesthetic indicates true muscle weakness as opposed to antalgic-related weakness.

External rotation strength measured with the elbow at the side of the body is indicative of infraspinatus and teres minor function. The inability to actively maintain the position obtained by passive external rotation indicates a tear involving the supraspinatus and a portion of the infraspinatus tendon. Inability to maintain external rotation in the midrange of motion against minimal resistance indicates a larger tear of the infraspinatus tendon. Inability to externally rotate the

passively abducted shoulder (hornblower's sign) is indicative of a large superior-posterior cuff tear (Fig. 17–2). Weakness of the subscapularis is indicated by the lift off test (Fig. 17–3) and abdominal compression test.

Clinical Conditions Associated with Rotator Cuff Disease

It is important to remember that rotator cuff disease can be associated with other pathology or be secondary to other shoulder disorders. Most notable among these are glenohumeral joint instability, acromioclavicular joint, biceps pathology, and abnormalities of scapulo-thoracic kinematics. The clinician must determine whether observed rotator cuff abnormalities are due to a primary rotator cuff disorder or manifestations of other pathology.

A common extrinsic cause for chronic rotator cuff tendonitis is scapular dysfunction that results from weakness of the periscapular muscles. This can be an acute process secondary to trauma or chronic resulting from cervical spondylosis. Clinical evaluation of scapular rotation with active elevation of the arm is the most reliable diagnostic tool to evaluate scapula dysfunction. Scapula winging can be due to pain, generalized scapula disuse weakness, and specific neuromuscular injury. Pain-related weakness and generalized weakness is characterized by mild scapula winging with active elevation of the arm that is decreased when the muscle groups are tested by specific manual muscle resistive tests. Neuromuscular injury is characterized by more severe winging with active elevation of the arm that is excentuated by manual muscle testing. Trapezius paresis (spinal accessory

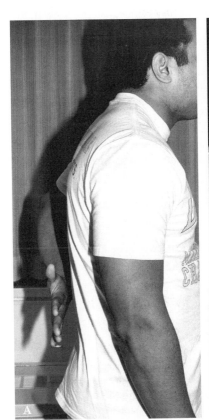

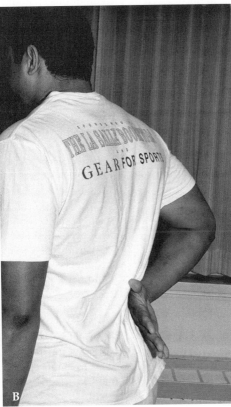

Figure 17–3 A negative lift off test is shown (**A**); the patient is able to actively bring the arm away from the lumbar spine. A positive lift off test is shown (**B**) by the patients inability to do this.

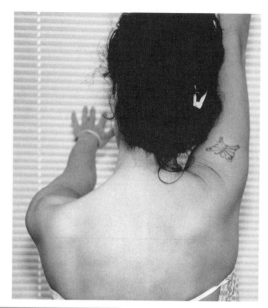

Figure 17–4 Trapezius palsy demonstrated by the drooped scapula and inability to elevate the arm above the horizontal.

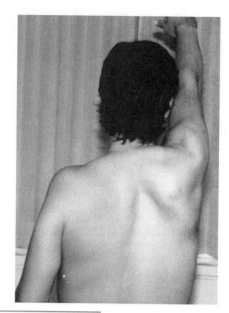

Figure 17–5 Serratus anterior palsy demonstrating inferior scapula winging.

nerve) results in upper scapula winging and abnormal clockwise rotation of the scapula (Fig. 17–4). Serratus anterior paresis (long thoracic nerve) results in lower scapula winging and counter-clockwise rotation (Fig. 17–5). Abnormal scapula function can result in secondary pathology to the rotator cuff. The cuff pathology is usually overuse-type tendonitis rather than a cuff tear.

Acromioclavicular (AC) joint arthritis is associated with pain over the superior aspect of the shoulder that is exacerbated by cross body adduction of the arm. Tenderness localized to the AC joint and its improvement with local anesthetic injection to the joint can confirm that the AC joint is the source of pain in a patient whose radiograph shows AC joint arthritis. Acromioclavicular joint arthropathy can cause subacromial impingement resulting in rotator cuff disease.

Biceps tendon rupture, which in the older individual is often associated with chronic impingement lesions and rotator cuff tears, is apparent on clinical examination by asymmetric prominence of the muscle belly. Provocative tests such as Yergason's sign and Speed's test may indicate inflammation associated with the biceps tendon. The tests may be helpful in the overall impression of rotator cuff problems but are not entirely specific or highly sensitive for biceps tendon pathology.

In the young athletic population, particularly those individuals participating in overhead sports, chronic rotator cuff tendonitis is often associated with glenohumeral instability. This instability can be so subtle that the patient does not have a sense of instability. Primary rotator cuff disease in this patient population is unusual and underlying glenohumeral instability should always be considered as a possible cause for chronic rotator cuff pain.

Imaging Studies

Plain radiographs remain the most important imaging study for evaluation of the painful shoulder. In patients suspected

of having pain associated with rotator cuff disease, plain radiographs should include an anteriorposterior view in the plane of the scapula with the arm in slight external rotation. This view is useful for evaluating the glenohumeral joint for degenerative changes, the acromiohumeral distance, and calcifications in the subacromial space. An axillary view is obtained to evaluate the anterior and posterior glenoid margin for calcification or bony lesions consistent with glenohumeral instability. It can also be used to rule out os-acromiale and glenohumeral arthritis. A 30 degree anteriorposterior caudad tilt view taken in the coronal plane is used to assess the amount of bone that extends anterior to the anterior border of the clavicle. This is necessary to rule out an anterior acromial spur. A supraspinatus outlet view is obtained as a lateral view in the plane of the scapula with a 10 to 15 degree caudad tilt. This radiograph is best used to evaluate the acromial morphology and undersurface of the coracoacromial arch. A 10 to 20 degree anteriorposterior cephalic tilt view in the coronal plane is taken to evaluate the acromioclavicular joint. These x-rays should be considered standard x-ray views for patients with the diagnosis of impingement syndrome.

Magnetic resonance imaging is now considered the most accurate imaging study for evaluation of partial- and full-thickness rotator cuff tears, rotator cuff tendon degeneration, AC joint arthritis, subacromial outlet narrowing, supraspinatus muscle atrophy, and a variety of glenohumeral abnormalities. Magnetic resonance imaging is 95 to 100% accurate in the diagnosis of full-thickness rotator cuff tear and is highly accurate for evaluating the size of the cuff tear, degree of muscle atrophy, degree of tendon retraction, and associated coracoacromial arch and AC joint pathology. Routine MRI is noninvasive and does not use ionizing radiation. The disadvantages of MRI are its cost (400–600 per study) and the technical requirements to obtain and interpret the studies accurately. Magnetic resonance imaging should not be used as a standard diagnostic test but is indicated when data from the history, physical exam, and plain films is insufficient to make appropriate management decisions.

Arthrography is the most accurate imaging study for the diagnosis of a full-thickness rotator cuff tear. It is performed by injecting contrast material into the glenohumeral joint. Plain radiographs are obtained following a brief period of shoulder exercise. If contrast material extends into the rotator cuff, a partial tear of the cuff exists. If contrast is found in the subacromial space, a full-thickness tear is diagnosed. Arthrography is nearly 100% accurate in the diagnosis of full-thickness cuff tears but less so for partial-thickness rotator cuff tears. Arthrography is easy to perform and to interpret. Its disadvantages relate to the invasive nature of the procedure and its limited diagnostic usefulness when compared with MRI.

High resolution dynamic diagnostic ultrasonography is also used for the diagnosis of full-thickness rotator cuff tears with 90 to 95% accuracy. Ultrasonography is noninvasive and will allow imaging of both shoulders at a cost of approximately 250 to $300. The disadvantages are the technical difficulty in both performing and interpreting the study. It is also much less useful for diagnosing partial rotator cuff tears and subacromial impingement.

Glenohumeral Instability

Clinical Presentation

Glenohumeral instability includes a spectrum of disorders the extremes of which include traumatic and atraumatic causes. Atraumatic instability is often associated with generalized ligamentous laxity and significant translational motion of both shoulders. There is usually no injury to the labrum, capsule, or bony structures of the joint. The instability is most often bi- or multi directional in nature with a predominant anterior-inferior or posterior-inferior component. In contrast, traumatic instability is due to either a single macrotraumatic event that causes dislocation of the glenohumeral joint or to microtrauma caused by repetitive overhead shoulder activity that results in recurrent anterior-inferior subluxation without dislocation. Traumatic instability is associated with labral tearing, capsular avulsion, and bony erosions or fractures of the glenoid and humeral head. The instability is often unidirectional in an anterior-inferior direction.

Evaluation of the patient with glenohumeral instability should include a careful history to allow accurate characterization of the type of instability. This is necessary for the formulation of an appropriate treatment plan. The history should include the mechanism of injury; the arm position in which instability occurs; activities associated with instability; and the character, severity, and duration of pain associated with both the initial and recurrent episodes of instability. It is also important to know what treatment the patient has received for both the initial episode and subsequent episodes of instability and the response to that treatment.

As described previously, patients with glenohumeral instability can often have associated rotator cuff tendonitis and biceps tendinitis as secondary factors to the underlying instability pattern. In throwing athletes, the rotator cuff disease can be severe, involving small full-thickness tears. It is important to treat the underlying glenohumeral instability to effect a cure. In addition, it is often necessary to manage the patient's rotator cuff pain to allow the patient to engage in an exercise program to improve the glenohumeral instability.

Anterior-inferior glenohumeral subluxation can be associated with the "deadarm syndrome" that often occurs with overhead throwing activities. It is characterized by a sudden sensation of shoulder pain and radicular arm pain that causes a transient sense of paralysis of the arm.

Physical Examination of the Unstable Shoulder

Evaluation of the patient with glenohumeral instability should always include testing for generalized ligamentous laxity. This includes an evaluation of elbow, knee, wrist, and metacarpal hyperextension. Because of wide variation in the amount of glenohumeral translation from one individual to another, it is important to examine the asymptomatic shoulder. In some patients, posterior translation of as much as 50% of the humeral head diameter is normal.

Provocative stress testing is a useful technique for detecting shoulder instability. It involves positioning the affected arm so that the patient feels that the shoulder is about to dislocate. This causes apprehension, guarding, and sometimes pain in a diseased shoulder. The presence of pain without apprehension is less specific for glenohumeral instability.

Testing for anterior-inferior instability requires positioning the arm in abduction and external rotation while the examiner applies an anteriorly directed force to the posterior aspect of the humeral head. Pain is often present in the posterior aspect of the glenohumeral joint. Relief of the apprehension and posterior glenohumeral pain associated with the test can be achieved with either a posteriorly directed force over the humeral head or by placing the arm anterior to the coronal plane; the positive relocation test (Fig. 17–6).

A provocative test for posterior instability is performed with the arm in 90 degrees of elevation, adduction, and internal rotation with a posteriorly directed axial load on the humerus. In this position, the humeral head is translated posteriorly over the glenoid rim (Fig. 17–7). When the arm is then brought into horizontal extension there is a palpable and occasionally audible relocation of the humeral head in the glenoid fossa. This is often associated with pain and reproduction of the patient's symptoms.

Pain or palpable grinding present with humeral translation during either provocative stress testing or with passive translation of the humeral head is seen with labral tears.

Imaging Studies

Plain radiographs for evaluating glenohumeral instability should include axillary, West Point axillary, apical oblique, and Stryker-Notch views. These are obtained to look for the presence of glenoid hypoplasia, glenoid version, glenoid fracture, or soft tissue calcification along the anterior or posterior

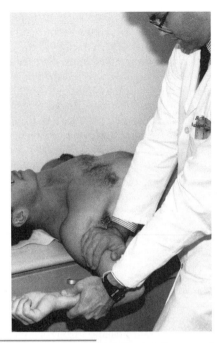

Figure 17–6   Relocation test. Relieving the apprehension by a posteriorly directed force placed at the proximal humerus.

glenoid rim, as well as humeral head defects (Hill-Sach's lesion). In patients with traumatic instability, these radiographs often may reveal evidence of glenoid fracture, capsular calcification, or humeral head defects. In the setting of unequivocal anterior-inferior instability by history and physical examination, plain radiographs are the only imaging study necessary to make a definitive diagnosis and plan appropriate treatment.

If the diagnosis of glenohumeral instability can not be made on exam alone, CT arthrography, MRI, and diagnostic arthroscopy with examination under anesthesia may be required for definitive diagnosis. Both CT arthrography and MRI have been considered useful for the diagnosis of labral

and capsular abnormalities associated with glenohumeral instability. It should be remembered that many patients with atraumatic instability will not have radiographically apparent lesions. The diagnosis in this patient population is largely based upon a careful history and physical examination.

The examination of shoulder translation under anesthesia is similar to that of an awake patient. The results must be correlated closely with the history and prior physical exam. The clinician must keep in mind that the amount of translation in any specific direction within a given shoulder cannot be used as an absolute criteria for diagnosis of pathologic instability. Arthroscopic shoulder examination is a useful clinical tool for the evaluation of the patient with suspected instability but without a definitive diagnosis. Abnormalities in the labrum, capsule, or bony structures of the shoulder must be compared with known anatomic variants before a diagnosis can be made.

Glenohumeral Arthritis

Glenohumeral arthritis occurs in a variety of disorders, the most common of which are rheumatoid arthritis, osteoarthritis, post traumatic arthritis, and osteonecrosis. Less common causes include crystalline arthropathy, cuff tear arthropathy, degenerative arthropathy secondary to glenohumeral instability and instability surgery, pyogenic and tuberculosis arthropathy, Paget's disease, glenohumeral dysplasia, and neuropathic arthropathy. In cases of osteoarthitis and rheumatoid arthritis multiple joints are usually involved. In most cases of glenohumeral arthritis the patient's chief complaints will be severe pain and range of motion limitations.

End stage glenohumeral arthritis of causes other than infection or neuropathy can be successfully managed with prosthetic joint replacement. Preoperative clinical evaluation of patients with end-stage glenohumeral arthropathy includes assessing the degree of functional limitations secondary to pain, loss of motion, and weakness, as separate but interdependent variables. The patient's overall health, especially as regards the other joints of the body and the ability to

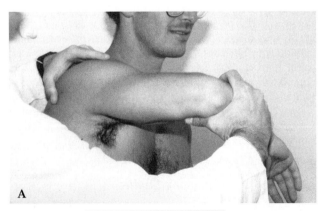

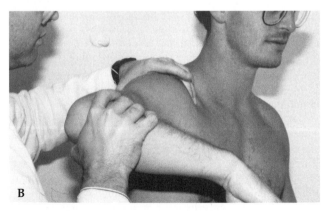

Figure 17–7   (**A**) Posterior provocative stress test. The arm is placed in 90-degree elevation in the saggital plane with a posteriorly directed axial load which will subluxate the humeral head posterior to the glenoid rim. (**B**) When the arm is placed into horizontal adduction the humeral head can be reduced back into the glenoid fossa. Reduction is felt as clucking sensation.

undertake the tasks of daily living, should be included in the evaluation. Significant disease of the opposite shoulder, elbows, hands, and lower extremities may interfere with normal postoperative rehabilitation following shoulder joint replacement. If the patient currently ambulates with crutches, the temporary use of a wheelchair will have to be considered.

The clinical factors that most significantly influence the success of shoulder arthroplasty include the degree of preoperative capsular contracture, the degree of rotator cuff insufficiency, the presence of subacromial outlet narrowing and AC joint arthropathy, and the severity of humeral and glenoid bone loss. In the case of prior humeral fractures, the degree and extent of tuberosity deformity and malunion will impact on outcome. These factors must be evaluated during the physical examination and by plain radiographs. The evaluation of the rotator cuff, biceps tendon, and AC joint are necessary for the patient with glenohumeral arthritis. The degree of capsular contracture must be measured as it relates to each position of the shoulder. Rotator cuff strength can be measured by manual muscle testing as described above, but may be unreliable in patients with advanced glenohumeral stiffness.

Imaging Studies

Anteriorposterior and lateral radiographs in the plane of the scapula and axillary views are also quite useful in the evaluation of glenohumeral arthritis, tuberosity malunion, and glenoid and humeral bone loss. In patients in which axillary radiographs are inadequate due to severe pain and stiffness of the shoulder, CT arthrography may be helpful in evaluating the severity of glenoid bone loss.

Frozen Shoulder

Frozen shoulder encompasses a large group of disorders characterized by varying degrees of pain and decreased range of motion. The classification of frozen shoulder includes primary or idiopathic disorders (adhesive capsulitis) and secondary disorders including local and systemic causes. Local causes include post-traumatic and postsurgical arthritis and rotator cuff tears. Systemic causes include diabetes and hypothyroidism. The history taken for patients with frozen shoulder should consider these classifications. The etiology of primary frozen shoulder or adhesive capsulitis is unknown. Women are more often affected than men and patients tend to be between 50 and 70 years of age.

Evaluation of the patient in the early stages of adhesive capsulitis is often quite difficult due to the vague nature of the symptoms. Patients will initially tend to have a mild loss of passive motion and diffuse shoulder pain. Tenderness may be elicited over the anterior joint line, biceps tendon, and rotator cuff. As the disease progresses, pain usually continues, and there is a gradual loss of passive motion. In the later stages of the disease, patients develop significant restrictions of internal and external rotation as well as forward flexion. In later stages pain is minimal at rest, but the patient may experience discomfort at the extremes of motion. The finding of a significant loss of humeral rotation is essential to the diagnosis of adhesive capsulitis. Shoulder muscle atrophy

may be observed due to disuse of the joint. Loss of elevation of the arm may be masked by scapulothoracic motion, which needs to be minimized to obtain meaningful data about the glenohumeral joint. If the patient presents with significant pain, injection of local anesthetic to the glenohumeral joint may assist in the diagnosis by allowing range of motion testing to be done unimpeded by shoulder pain. Corticosteroid injections may be used to reduce inflammation in the acute phase of the disorder and to allow the patient to engage fully in physical therapy.

Imaging Studies

Plain radiographs generally demonstrate normal osseous anatomy but may show bone demineralization from disuse. Routine use of arthrography for the evaluation of adhesive capsulitis is not indicated, but when performed, will show obliteration of the inferior axillary pouch and a small capsular volume. The vast majority of patients with adhesive capsulitis will have an intact rotator cuff.

Magnetic resonance imaging of patients with adhesive capsulitis may show a variety of changes within the rotator cuff that may be consistent with age-related and clinically insignificant degenerative changes of the rotator cuff, coracoacromial arch, and AC joint. An MRI may also demonstrate fluid in the biceps tendon sheath, glenohumeral joint, or subacromial bursitis. These latter findings may be consistent with but nonspecific for adhesive capsulitis and are not always present. The routine use of MRI in the diagnosis of adhesive capsulitis cannot be justified as the diagnosis is made via clinical criteria.

Referred Pain

Referred pain can be caused by any disorder that affects nerves that innervate the shoulder. Nerve impingement occurs in cervical disc disease, thoracic outlet syndrome, and by traumatic injury or viral infection of the brachial plexus. Neoplastic disease can involve the nerves at any point in their course. Pancoast's tumor is a primary lung tumor that can migrate by direct extension from the apex of the lung into the thoracic wall and brachial plexus.

Referred sources of pain should be suspected whenever a patient has radicular pain proximal or distal to the shoulder girdle. Patients with cervical spine disorders may complain of neck pain in association with their shoulder pain. Often the symptoms intensify during daytime activities and abate at night. They may also have symptoms of weakness or paresthesia below the level of the elbow, which is uncommon in rotator cuff disease. Physical exam may reveal tenderness of the paraspinal muscles and decreased range of motion of the neck. A positive Spurling test may be elicited. This involves flexion of the neck toward the side of the shoulder pain while the clinician applies axial pressure to the top of the head. A positive test results in worsening of the pain or may cause pain where it was not present immediately prior to the examination. Nerve root blocks can be used to confirm the diagnosis of cervical spine disease.

Thoracic outlet syndrome is a collection of disorders that involve compression of the brachial plexus as it passes

---

PEARL

Shoulder pain that is exacerbated by neck motion may be due to a cervical disc.

between the scalene muscles and between the clavicle and first rib. Patients complain of radicular pain associated with movements of the head. They may also have symptoms of vascular compromise in the affected arm. Several provocative tests have been developed such as Adson's maneuver, in which the patient extends the neck while turning the chin to the affected side and taking a deep breath. Plain films are usually unremarkable but may reveal the existence of a cervical rib as the causative agent.

SUMMARY

This chapter has reviewed some of the most common causes of shoulder pain and the important diagnostic principles. The history and physical exam remain the most important tools at the disposal of the clinician. Plain films are high-yield, inexpensive studies that are almost always indicated for the diagnosis of shoulder pain. Magnetic resonance imaging is a powerful imaging tool at the disposal of the clinician. It is not effective for certain disorders, such as adhesive capsulitis, and it is relatively expensive so it should be used judiciously. The appropriate use of the history, physical exam, and radiographic studies will result in a complete and accurate diagnosis for most patients with shoulder pain.

SELECTED BIBLIOGRAPHY

ANDREWS JR, CARSON WG, ORTEGA K. Arthroscopy of the shoulder: techniques and normal anatomy. *Am J Sports Med.* 1984;12:1–7.

SINGSON RD, FELDMAN F. BIGLIANI LU. CT arthrographic patterns in recurrent glenohumeral instability. *Am J. Rad* 1987;149:749–753.

BRETZKE CA. CRASS JR. CRAIG EV. FEINBERG SB. Ultrasonography of the rotator cuff. Normal and pathologic anatomy. [Journal Article] *Investigative Radiology.* 1985;20: 311–315.

BURK DL Jr. KARASICK D. KURTZ AB. MITCHELL DG. RIFKIN MD. MILLER CL. LEVY DW. FENLIN JM. BARTOLOZZI AR. Rotator cuff tears: prospective comparison of MR imaging with arthrography, sonography, and surgery. AJR. *American Journal of Roentgenology.* 1989;153(1):87–92.

CARSON WG. Arthroscopy of the shoulder: anatomy and technique. *Orthop Rev.* 1992;21:143–153.

CHANDNANI VP. YEAGER TD. DEBERARDINO T. CHRISTENSEN K. GAGLIARDI JA. HEITZ DR. BAIRD DE. HANSEN MF. Glenoid lateral tears: prospective evaluation with MRI imaging, MR arthrography, and CT arthrography. AJR. *American Journal of Roentgenology.* 1993;161:1229–1235.

CRASS JR. CRAIG EV. THOMPSON RC. FEINBERG SB. Ultrasonography of the rotator cuff: surgical correlation. *Journal of Clinical Ultrasound.* 1984;12:487–491.

CRASS JR. et al. Ultrasonography of the rotator cuff: surgical correlation. *J Clin Ultrasound.* 1984;12:487–493.

DRAKEFORD MK. QUINN MJ. SIMPSON SL. PETTINE KA. A comparative study of ultrasonography and arthrography in evaluation of the rotator cuff. *Clinical Orthopaedics & Related Research.* 1990;253:118–122.

ELLMAN H. Shoulder arthroscopy: current indications and techniques. *Orthopedics.* 1988;11:45–52.

GARTH WP, ALLMAN FL. Jr, ARMSTRONG WS. Occult anterior subluxations of the shoulder in noncontact sports. *Am J Sports Med.* 1987;15:579–585.

GARTH WP, SLAPPEY CE, OCHS CW. Roentgenographic demonstration of instability of the shoulder: the apical oblique projection. *J Bone Jt Surg.* 1984;66A:1450–1453.

COFIELD RH, BERQUIST TH, McGROUGH PF, MOFFMAYER PJ. Shoulder arthrography for determination of size of rotator cuff tears. *J Shoulder Elbow Surg.* 1992;1:98–105.

HAWKINS RJ. ABRAMS JS. Impingement syndrome in the absence of rotator cuff tear (Stages 1 and 2). *Orthop Clin North Am.* 1987;18:373–382.

HAWKINS RJ. HOBEIKA P. Physical examination of the shoulder. *Orthopedics.* 1983;6:1270–1278.

HERTEL R, HERTEL R, BALLMER FT, LAMBER SM. Lag signs in the diagnosis of roator cuff rupture. *J Shoulder Elbow Surg.* 1996;5:307–313.

HULSTYN MJ. WEISS AC. Adhesive capsulitis of the shoulder. *Orthop Rev.* 1993;22:425–433.

HURLEY J. BRONSTEIN R. Shoulder arthroscopy in the athlete. Practical applications. *Sports Medicine.* 1993;15:133–138.

HURLEY J, BRONSTEIN R. Shoulder arthroscopy in the athlete. practical applications. *Sports Med.* 1993;15:133–138.

IANNOTTI JP. ZLATKIN MB. ESTERHAI JL. KRESSEL HY. DALINKA MK. SPINDLER KP. Magnetic resonance imaging of the shoulder. Sensitivity, specificity, and predictive value. *J Bone Jt Surg.* 1991;73A:17–29.

MCNIESH LM, CALLAGHAN JJ. CT arthrography of the shoulder: variations of the glenoid labrum. *AJR.* 1987;149: 963–966.

MINK JH, HARRIS E, RAPPAPORT M. Rotator cuff tears: evaluation using double-contrast shoulder arthrography. *Radiology.* 1985;153:621–623.

MOK DW. FOGG AJ. HOKAN R. BAYLEY JI. The diagnostic value of arthroscopy in glenohumeral instability. *J Bone Jt Surg.* 1990;72B:698–700.

MURNAGHAN JP. Adhesive capsulitis of the shoulder: Current concepts and treatment. *Orthopedics.* 1988;11:153–158.

NEER CSI. Anterior acromioplasty for the chronic impingement syndrome in the shoulder: a preliminary report. *J Bone Jt Surg.* 1972;54A:41–50.

NEER CSI. Impingement lesion. *Clin Orthop.* 1983;173:70–77.

NEVIASER JS. Adhesive capsulitis of the shoulder. A study of the pathological findings in periarthritis of the shoulder. *J Bone Jt Surg.* 1945;27:211–222.

ROCKWOOD CA, LYONS FR. Shoulder impingement syndrome: diagnosis, radiographic evaluation, and treatment with a modified Neer acromioplasty. *J Bone Jt Surg.* 1993;75A:409–424.

ZANCA P. Shoulder pain: involvement of the acromioclavicular joint: analysis of 1000 cases. *AJR.* 1971;112:493–506.

ZLATKIN MB, IANNOTTI JP, ROBERTS MC. Rotator cuff tears: diagnostic performance of MR imaging. *Radiology.* 1989;172:223–229.

SAMPLE QUESTIONS

1. Shoulder pain from rotator cuff disease may:
   (a) occur at rest
   (b) increase with overhead activities
   (c) awaken the patient at night, especially if the patient rolls onto the affected shoulder
   (d) radiate to the midlateral aspect of the arm (deltoid insertion)
   (e) all of the above

2. A 22-year-old swimmer has anterior shoulder pain when doing the butterfly stroke. His initial evaluation should include all of the following *Except*:
   (a) impingement sign
   (b) subacromial injection of lidocaine, followed by impingement sign
   (c) assessment of passive shoulder range of motion
   (d) provocative tests for shoulder instability
   (e) CT arthrogram

3. The swimmer's most likely diagnosis is:
   (a) impingement syndrome
   (b) shoulder instability with secondary impingement
   (c) early post-traumatic arthritis
   (d) adhesive capsulitis
   (e) cervical radiculopathy

4. A weight lifter has pain while performing overhead lifting. You suspect he has pain in his AC joint due to osteolysis of the distal clavicle. Which of the following supports your diagnosis:
   (a) pain elicited by the apprehension maneuver
   (b) pain with adduction of the affected arm across the chest
   (c) positive push-off test
   (d) positive impingement test
   (e) pain with resisted external rotation of the arm

5. Shoulder pain from adhesive capsulitis is characterized by all of the following *EXCEPT*:
   (a) pain at rest
   (b) pain with loss of active forward flexion
   (c) lancinating pain that radiates from the neck to the fingers
   (d) pain with loss of passive external rotation
   (e) diffuse pain and tenderness about the shoulder girdle

Answers: 1) e; 2) e; 3) b; 4) b; 5) c

Chapter 18

Fractures of the Shoulder

Suzanne E. Hall, MD and Joseph D. Zuckerman MD

The shoulder is the most mobile joint in the body. The fine balance between stability and mobility is maintained predominantly by the soft tissues: the capsule, ligaments, and muscles about the shoulder joint. Restoration of function following a fracture must focus not only on union but also on reestablishment of the proper relationship of muscle length. Maintenance of mobility during recovery is desirable when treating any fracture. In the shoulder, maintenance of mobility is critical. Long periods of immobilization may create loss of motion, which may never be regained. The problem of maintaining mobility is made more complex when the fracture occurs in osteoporotic bone, in which loss of fixation occurs more easily. The responsibility of the orthopaedic surgeon is to weigh the conflicting demands for mobility of the soft tissues and stability of the fracture and to design a treatment that is appropriate for the individual and the fracture.

BASIC SCIENCE

Restoration of function of the shoulder following fracture depends on an understanding of the anatomy of this complex joint. The shoulder consists of three bones: the humerus, scapula, and clavicle; and four joints: the glenohumeral joint,

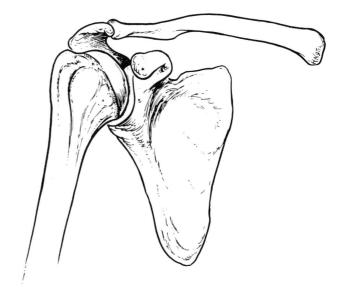

Figure 18–1   The shoulder girdle: the humerus, scapula, and clavicle.

acromioclavicular joint, sternoclavicular joint, and the scapulothoracic articulation (Fig. 18–1). The first three joints have capsules and ligaments that provide static stability. Control, movement, and dynamic stability of this complex is provided by several sets of muscles that must all work synchronously for proper shoulder function.

The shoulder is suspended from the axial skeleton via the clavicle by the ligaments and capsule of the sternoclavicular joint. The clavicle is an S-shaped bone that is tubular medially, becoming flattened laterally. The scapula is suspended from the clavicle via the coracoclavicular and acromioclavicular ligaments. The scapula has a very complex shape. The body is flat and triangularly shaped. When viewed laterally, the scapula looks like the letter Y with the small shallow glenoid sitting in its center. The Y is formed by the body of the scapula inferiorly, the coracoid anteriorly, and the scapular spine posteriorly arching superiorly to form the acromion (Fig. 18–2). The proximal humerus consists of a rounded articular surface, the greater and lesser tuberosities, and the shaft. The greater tuberosity has three facets corresponding to the attachment sites of the supraspinatus, infraspinatus, and teres minor. The biceps groove lies between the

243

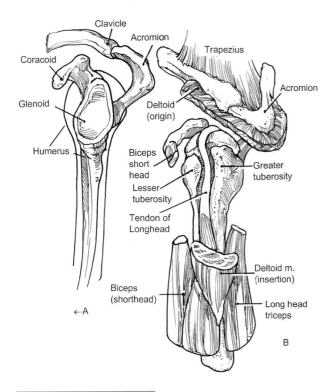

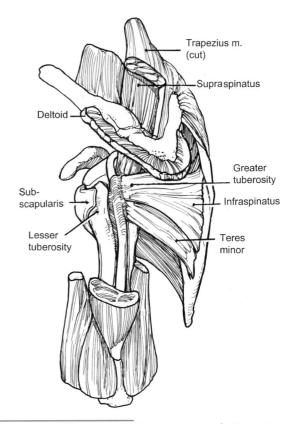

Figure 18–2 (**A**) The lateral scapula or Y view. The Y is formed by the body of the scapula inferiorly, the coracoid anteriorly, and the scapular spine posteriorly arching superiorly to form the acromion. The humeral head should be centered on the glenoid. (**B**) Schematic illustrating lateral view of humerus and musculature.

Figure 18–3 The rotator cuff as seen from the lateral scapular view: supraspinatus, infraspinatus, teres minor, and subscapularis.

tuberosities and provides a valuable guide to rotation following fracture.

ANATOMY AND SURGICAL APPROACHES

The Muscles of the Shoulder

The outer layer of muscles covering the shoulder consists of the trapezius and the deltoid. The trapezius covers the superomedial portion of the shoulder inserting on the clavicle superiorly, the medial border of the acromion, and the scapular spine posteriorly. The deltoid envelopes the shoulder anteriorly, laterally, and posteriorly. Its broad origin continues the downward path of the trapezius, originating where the trapezius inserts and ending with its own insertion midway down the lateral humerus.

The next layer of shoulder musculature includes the rotator cuff; supraspinatus, infraspinatus, teres minor, and subscapularis (remember the acronym SITS) (Fig. 18–3). The subscapularis is the only attachment to the lesser tuberosity and is an internal rotator. The other three muscles of the rotator cuff attach to the facets of the greater tuberosity. The supraspinatus passes through the top of the scapular Y. Its superior position makes it an abductor of the glenohumeral joint. The infraspinatus and teres minor are external rotators.

There are several other muscles that also cross the glenohumeral joint. They are the biceps, coracobrachialis, pectoralis major, teres major, latissimus dorsi, and triceps. Of these, the long heads of the biceps and triceps and the pectoralis major are most commonly involved as deforming forces or as interposed soft tissue in fractures of the shoulder.

Both heads of the biceps cross the shoulder. The long head of the biceps traverses a groove between the greater and lesser tuberosities, travels intra-articularly, and inserts at the supraglenoid tubercle. It acts as a secondary depressor of the humeral head. The long head of the biceps can be a key landmark for locating the interval between fractured greater and lesser tuberosities.

The pectoralis major crosses the shoulder joint inserting just inferior to the subscapularis but lateral to the bicipital-intertubercular groove. In fractures of the surgical neck, the pectoralis major is a strong deforming force that displaces the humeral shaft medially.

PEARL
Muscle pull may displace the humeral head superiorly, inferiorly, or medially, but acute *lateral* displacement of the humeral head is either blood, pus, or soft tissue interposed in the joint.

The long head of the triceps attaches to a tubercle just inferior to the glenoid rim. It can cause displacement of intra-articular glenoid fractures.

The muscles that position the scapula are the serratus anterior, the rhomboids, the levator scapula, and the trapezius. Paralysis of the serratus anterior, secondary to trauma to the long thoracic nerve, can cause winging of the scapula.

Neurovascular Anatomy of the Shoulder

The axillary artery and the brachial plexus traverse the infra-clavicular region together, passing inferior to the coracoid as they enter the arm (Fig. 18–4). The branches of the axillary artery in the shoulder include the thoracoacromial artery, the anterior and posterior humeral circumflex arteries, and the suprascapular artery. The major blood supply to the head of the humerus is from the anterior humeral circumflex artery through an ascending branch that travels along the bicipital groove and enters the greater tuberosity to become the intraosseous arcuate artery. There is some anastomosis with the posterior humeral circumflex, but it is insufficient to supply the head, thus predisposing the humeral head to osteonecrosis with comminuted fractures.

The brachial plexus gives rise to the nerves that innervate the muscles that cross the shoulder and position the scapula. The most commonly injured nerves in shoulder trauma and

> ### PEARL
> The major blood supply to the humeral head is the anterior humeral circumflex artery, a vessel that enters the greater tuberosity.

surgery are the axillary nerve, the suprascapular nerve, and the long thoracic nerve.

Surgical Approaches to the Proximal Humerus

The two approaches most commonly used for fractures of the proximal humerus are the deltopectoral approach and the deltoid splitting approach. The anterior axillary incision can be used for a deltopectoral approach but the incision is directed from the lateral edge of the coracoid inferiorly to the axilla rather than laterally along the arm (Fig. 18–5).

For all of these approaches, the patient is positioned in a semireclining or "beach chair" position. The head and back are elevated 30 degrees for the deltopectoral approach and up to 70 or 80 degrees for the superior or deltoid splitting approach. The head is supported and secured to prevent hyperextension of the cervical spine. The patient is placed

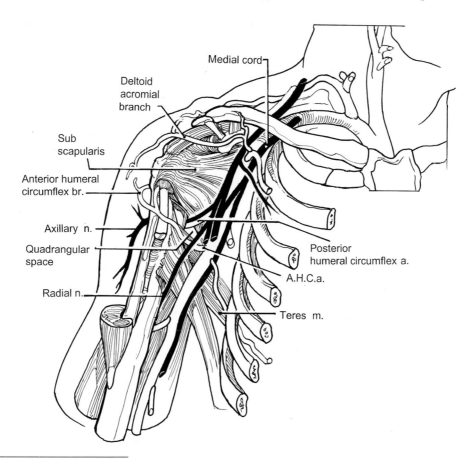

Figure 18–4 The axillary artery and the brachial plexus pass medially and inferiorly to the cora-coid process. The axillary nerve is at risk of injury in a proximal humerus fracture as it passes from anterior to posterior under the glenoid. The nerve then winds anteriorly along the surgical neck of the humerus on the undersurface of the deltoid.

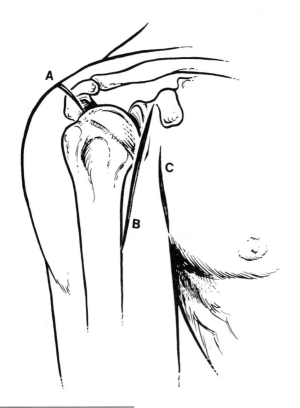

Figure 18–5 Incisions for open treatment of fractures of the proximal humerus. (**A**) Deltoid splitting approach via a strap incision that is placed over the lateral third of the acromion in Langer's lines. The deltoid is split in line with its fibers, perpendicular to the skin incision. (**B**) Deltopectoral approach. This extensile approach allows maximum access to the proximal humerus. (**C**) Anterior axillary incision, which also utilizes the deltopectoral interval, is used mainly for instability repairs. In the context of fractures, this incision is suitable for isolated lesser tuberosity fractures.

close enough to the edge of the table to allow extension of the shoulder, a requirement for insertion of an intramedullary rod or humeral prosthesis. The entire upper extremity from neck to finger tips is draped free. Excessive abduction of the shoulder is avoided to prevent injury to neurovascular structures by the fracture fragments.

Deltoid Splitting Approach

The deltoid splitting approach may be used for fixation of the greater tuberosity, repair of the rotator cuff, and intramedullary fixation of surgical neck fractures that can be close-reduced but are unstable. It is limited distally by the axillary nerve and should not be used in fractures that might require a more distal or medial exposure to accomplish an adequate reduction.

The deltoid splitting approach is performed through a skin incision that extends obliquely for 5 cm from the acromioclavicular joint in an inferolateral direction. The skin incision may also be made in Langer's lines as a strap or "saber" incision just lateral to the edge of the acromion. The deltoid is split between the anterior and middle thirds, exposing the subdeltoid bursa overlying the greater tuberosity. The

deltoid cannot be split more than 5 cm, roughly 3 finger breadths, distal to the acromion without endangering the axillary nerve. Injury to the axillary nerve at this location would denervate the anterior deltoid, seriously compromising forward flexion. A stay suture is placed at the distal end of the deltoid incision to prevent extension of the split.

The advantage of the deltoid splitting approach is that it lies directly over the fracture site. The deltopectoral approach is more anterior and requires retraction of the anterior deltoid to visualize the greater tuberosity. Avulsion of the most medial attachment of the deltoid is at risk with the deltopectoral approach if the incision is not distal enough to allow gentle retraction.

Deltopectoral Approach

The deltopectoral approach gives a broader exposure to the proximal humerus. It is used for complex, displaced fractures and for arthroplasty. A skin incision is made from lateral edge of the coracoid and extends distally and laterally along the anterior border of the deltoid. With the arm in neutral, the incision usually ends at the level of the axilla, at the junction of the proximal and middle third of the arm. The actual length of the incision is determined by the location of the fracture and the musculature of the patient. If necessary, the incision can be carried all the way to the insertion of the deltoid to allow gentle retraction of the deltoid. Subcutaneous flaps are raised up to the clavicle and medially and laterally for several centimeters. The cephalic vein is identified. Most of its branches are found laterally making lateral mobilization easiest. However, the vein crosses the top of the incision and may be injured by retraction or during insertion of an intramedullary rod or prosthesis. Medial mobilization of the vein provides the best exposure.

The split between the deltoid and the pectoralis is deepened until the clavipectoral fascia is visible. The fascia is incised along the lateral border of the conjoint tendon, exposing the subscapularis. The biceps tendon is then sought and, if present and intact, acts as a guide to the location of the fractured tuberosities. Heavy stay sutures are placed through the cuff at its insertion on each tuberosity, facilitating reduction. Fixation with the selected device may then be accomplished.

EXAMINATION

History

Specifics of the injury may help understand the force imparted as well as the chance of associated injuries. Patients should be questioned about shortness of breath (pneumothorax) or numbness (brachial plexus injury).

Exam

The shoulder should be inspected for open wounds. A complete and thorough neurovascular exam should be performed. Although movement of the injured shoulder should be minimized, the stability of the fracture should be assessed. Gentle rotation of the humerus will allow assessment of whether the proximal and distal portions move as a unit. This information may be important in determining a treatment plan.

Radiographs

Anteroposterior, scapular Y, axillary lateral, and a chest x-ray is usually sufficient to evaluate fractures involving the shoulder girdle. An apical lordotic view of the clavicle is often helpful.

AIDS TO DIAGNOSIS

Computed tomography helps evaluate intra-articular extension and displacement in fractures of the humeral head and glenoid.

A magnetic resonance image may help in the diagnosis of an associated rotator cuff tear, particularly following a fracture of the greater tuberosity.

SPECIFIC CONDITIONS, TREATMENT, AND OUTCOME

Clavicle Fractures

The clavicle is the most commonly fractured bone in the skeleton. Fortunately, the vast majority of clavicle fractures can be treated nonoperatively with a high rate of union and good functional outcome.

Classification

Clavicle fractures are classified by their location dividing the clavicle into thirds; proximal, middle, and distal. Group I fractures—fractures of the middle third—are the most common, accounting for 80% of all clavicle fractures. They are usually minimally displaced and heal uneventfully. When they are displaced, the proximal segment is pulled superiorly and posteriorly by the sternocleidomastoid muscle and the distal segment is pulled inferiorly and anteriorly due to the weight of the shoulder and the pull of the pectoralis major muscle (Fig. 18–6).

Group II fractures—fractures of the distal third of the clavicle—are subclassified according to the location of the fracture in relation to the coracoclavicular ligaments. Type 1 fractures, in which the fracture occurs between intact coracoclavicular ligaments, are the most common within group II. These fractures are stable, minimally displaced and are expected to heal with standard nonoperative treatment.

Group II, type 2 fractures occur just medial to the coracoclavicular ligaments or between the conoid and the trapezoid with the conoid torn and the trapezoid attached to the distal fragment. The resulting displacement in either situation is the same. The distal fragment is firmly attached to the coracoid and is pulled down by the weight of the shoulder, resulting in relative superior displacement of the proximal fragment. This displacement pattern results in a higher incidence of nonunion than other clavicle fractures, leading some to recommend operative management.

Type 3 fractures are intra-articular *without* ligamentous injury. A type 2 fracture may have intra-articular extension, but it is distinguished from a type 3 by the presence of ligamentous disruption. Type 3 fractures may be difficult to visualize radiographically and can be mistaken for an acromioclavicular sprain. The intra-articular location of the fracture may result in acromioclavicular joint arthritis.

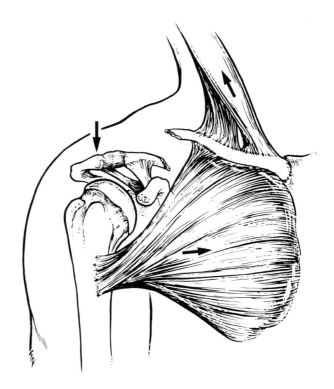

Figure 18–6 The proximal segment of a fractured clavicle is pulled superiorly and posteriorly by the sternocleidomastoid muscle. The weight of the shoulder pulls the distal fragment inferiorly while the pectoralis major pulls it medially.

Type 4 clavicle fractures occur in children. The proximal fragment displaces superiorly, tearing through the periosteum. The coracoclavicular ligaments remain attached to the periosteal sleeve. As in nearly all fractures of the clavicle in children, this injury can be treated closed due to the significant potential for remodelling in spite of the initial displacement.

Type 5 clavicle fractures are comminuted fractures in which the coracoclavicular ligaments are attached to an inferior butterfly fragment. Therefore, neither the proximal nor distal fragments have any attachment to the coracoid. The result is a fracture that is even more unstable than the type 2 pattern.

Group III fractures are fractures of the medial third of the clavicle. They account for 5% of all clavicle fractures. If the costoclavicular ligament is intact and remains attached to the lateral fragment, then little displacement occurs. If this ligament is disrupted, the lateral fragment may be pulled superiorly by the sternocleidomastoid muscle. Intra-articular fractures may lead to degenerative arthritis of the sternoclavicular joint.

Nonoperative Treatment

The majority of clavicle fractures should be treated closed. Open treatment of clavicle fractures is associated with a higher incidence of nonunion than closed treatment. Nonoperative treatment of clavicle fractures usually consists of treatment with either a "figure-of-eight" splint or sling. Studies have not shown a consistent advantage of one method over the other. The figure-of-eight sling has the potential advantage of retracting the scapulas and promoting healing of the clavicle in a position closest to its full length. The figure-of-eight may also allow more use of the ipsilateral hand. However, the figure of eight is more difficult to apply properly and is less well tolerated by patients because of associated irritation of the axilla and anterior shoulder. It requires more frequent inspection and adjustment. These issues have generally made the sling the preferred method of closed treatment.

A variety of casting techniques have been described in an attempt to reduce displaced clavicle fractures. These techniques are rarely used and have not been shown to be advantageous over a figure-of-eight or simple sling.

Operative Management

The following is a list of some of the indications for operative management of clavicle fractures.

1. Open fractures. Disruption of the soft tissue envelope may impair both the blood supply and stability of the fracture, increasing the chance of nonunion. Surgical extension of the wound, necessary for irrigation and debridement, may be used to provide access for internal fixation as well.

2. Fractures with neurovascular injury requiring repair. Fixation prevents disruption of the repair.

3. Group II fractures. Types 2 and 5 are associated with higher rates of nonunion because of the degree of displacement and comminution respectively.

4. Fractures of both the scapula and clavicle. Fixation of the clavicle aids in reduction of the scapula fracture.

5. Symptomatic nonunion after 4 to 6 months. Not all nonunions are symptomatic. Asymptomatic nonunions do not require surgery.

6. Group III, medial third, fractures with posterior displacement compressing mediastinal structures in which a stable reduction cannot be maintained with closed methods.

7. Group I fractures that are so displaced that skin integrity is compromised; or rarely, when the cosmetic deformity caused by the bony prominence is less desirable than a scar produced by surgical correction of the deformity.

Operative Treatment: Fractures of the Middle Third of the Clavicle
Fixation of a clavicle fracture may be accomplished several ways. One method of fixation of middle third fractures is intramedullary fixation. This has the advantage of minimal soft tissue stripping of the fracture site, ease of removal of hardware, and little risk of refracture after removal of hardware. Bone graft may be added when treating nonunions. Hardware crossing the acromioclavicular joint is avoided, both to preserve the integrity of the joint as well as to minimize the forces exerted across the implant. The most serious complication of this type of fixation is failure of the hardware with migration to various sites including the mediastinum, the ascending aorta, and the liver. Using threaded hardware or bending the protruding end decreases the risk of migration. Knowles or Hagie pins are much larger than Steinman pins, and therefore, decrease the risk of breakage (Fig. 18–7). The Hagie pin is a large caliber bolt on which a nut can be placed, thus decreasing the risk of migration in both directions. It requires only a strap incision in Langer's lines over

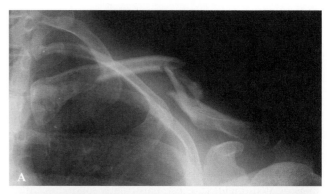
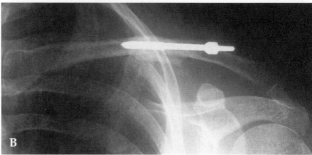

Figure 18–7   (**A**) A modified Hagie pin was used in this comminuted, midshaft clavicle fracture. (**B**) This large caliber pin adequately fills the medullary canal and maintains overall alignment, minimizing the tendency for this fracture to shorten.

the fracture and a puncture posteriorly for placement of the nut and cutting the bolt to length. Prominence of the bolt posteriorly can necessitate early removal, but union rates of more than 90% have been documented.

Plating of the fracture is another option. Plating is particularly useful in comminuted fractures and in nonunions where loss of clavicular length is an issue. Bone graft may be useful in these cases as well. If plating is chosen, 6 cortices should be engaged on each side of the fracture or, if the fragments are of insufficient length, the fixation should be supplemented with external immobilization. The plate is usually placed on the anterior or superior surface of the clavicle. The skin incision may be placed either parallel to the clavicle or obliquely along Langer's lines. Use of a plate involves greater periosteal stripping than does intramedullary fixation and, depending on placement, the hardware can be prominent and palpable. There is also a risk of refracture through screw holes if the plate is removed.

Operative Treatment: Fractures of the Distal Third of the Clavicle
Fractures of the distal third of the clavicle are challenging because of the difficulty of obtaining adequate fixation of the distal piece, which may be quite small. Fixation of a very distal fracture site may necessitate crossing the acromioclavicular joint. Kirschner wires alone placed across that joint have a high rate of failure. Coracoclavicular fixation may be used to reduce and stabilize type 2 fractures, or as a supplement to plating or intramedullary fixation.

Operative Treatment: Fractures of the Proximal Third of the Clavicle

The largest proportion of mortalities reported from pin migration have occurred with pin fixation through the sternoclavicular joint. Fixation with a heavy suture material (#5) and meticulous patient follow-up, and early removal of hardware is recommended.

Fractures of the Proximal Humerus

The proximal humerus may be fractured by a direct blow to the shoulder or by force transmitted via a fall on the elbow or outstretched hand. When fractured, the proximal humerus tends to split along the epiphyseal lines. Understanding the relationship of these fragments to their muscular attachments and blood supply is the key to recognizing fracture patterns and planning treatment.

In 1934, Codman described the proximal humerus as consisting of four parts. These parts are divided along the epiphyseal lines and consist of the greater tuberosity, the lesser tuberosity, the articular segment, and the shaft. The four parts described by Codman serve as the basis for Neer's classification system, which is the most widely used system today (Fig. 18–8). In Neer's system, to be considered a separate part, the fragment must be angulated 45 degrees or displaced 1 cm. A fracture that is minimally displaced would then be a one-part fracture no matter how many fracture lines were visible. A fracture in which only one part was displaced would then be a two-part fracture. There are, therefore, four possible types of two-part fractures; surgical neck, greater tuberosity, lesser tuberosity, and anatomic neck. Three-part fractures consist of a shaft fragment, an articular segment still attached

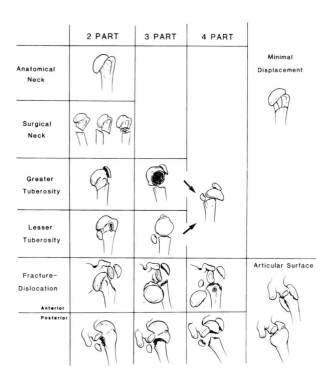

Figure 18–8   The four-part classification system for fractures of the proximal humerus. Redrawn with permission from Neer, CS II. *J Bone Jt Surg.* 1970;52A:1077.

to one tuberosity, and a separately displaced tuberosity. The head internally or externally rotates depending on which tuberosity is still attached. A four-part fracture has displacement of all four parts and the direction of dislocation. Fracture dislocations are also enumerated by parts. Impression or head-splitting fractures in which the head is crushed are yet another category.

Examination

Inspection of the patient with a proximal humerus fracture may reveal a change in the contour of the shoulder. Swelling is common. Prominence of the acromion may be seen if the humeral head is dislocated. Ecchymosis from the lateral shoulder and axilla to the elbow may become apparent over several days. Crepitus may be palpable with gentle movement. The neurovascular status should be assessed with particular attention to sensory and motor function of the axillary and musculocutaneous nerves.

Radiographs

A trauma series for proximal humerus fractures should include at least three views; a scapular anterioposterior, an axillary view, and a scapular lateral also known as the Y view.

Treatment of One-part Fractures of the Proximal Humerus

One-part fractures are by definition minimally displaced (Fig. 18–9). Treatment consists of immobilization in a Velpeau's sling until the fracture moves as a unit, usually in 3 to 4 weeks. At that time, gentle passive range of motion exercises may be started. Hand and wrist motion is begun immediately. The amount of elbow motion that is allowable is determined by whether the fracture extends into the biceps groove and lesser tuberosity.

If the greater tuberosity is fractured, the patient is advised to wear oversized shirts that drape over the affected shoulder, leaving the hand tucked inside. It is very difficult to pass the arm through a sleeve without actively abducting the shoulder and risking displacement of the greater tuberosity.

For stable, impacted fractures of the surgical neck of the humerus, gentle passive range of motion exercises may be started early, even within the first few weeks, as soon as comfort permits and the fracture fragments are palpated moving as a unit without crepitus. Pendulums are avoided initially due to the risk of disimpaction of the fracture. Usually by 6 to 8 weeks, active motion exercises are begun. Serial radiographs are essential to ensure that the fracture reduction is maintained.

Treatment of Two-part Fractures

Two-part fractures may consist of a displaced fracture of the surgical neck, the greater tuberosity, the lesser tuberosity, or the anatomic neck; fractures of the neck and greater tuberosity are by far the most common.

Surgical Neck Fractures

When the humerus is fractured at the surgical neck, the shaft fragment is pulled medially by the pectoralis major, teres major, and latissimus dorsi. Attempts at matching the angulation of an abducted proximal fragment by corresponding

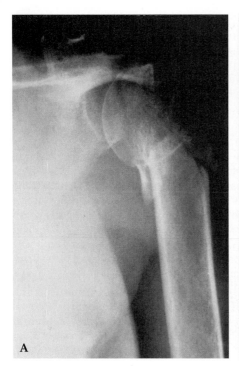
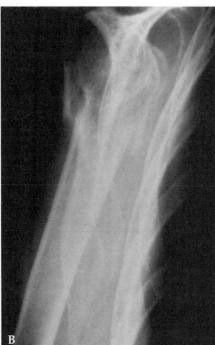

Figure 18–9 This proximal humerus has multiple fracture lines, but none of the fragments is angulated more than 45 degrees or displaced by 1 cm. This, is therefore, a one-part fracture. (**A**) Scapular anteroposterior view (**B**) Scapular lateral view.

abduction of the arm are often foiled by these powerful deforming forces. Abduction exacerbates their medial pull and may cause further displacement. Some medial translation can be accepted with little functional impairment.

If closed manipulation does not yield a stable reduction, open reduction and internal fixation is advisable. Intramedullary rods, figure-of-eight tension bands, or both may be used. If the fracture can be reduced but is unstable, a superior or deltoid splitting approach may be used (see Fig. 18–5). This approach provides good exposure of the greater tuberosity for purposes of insertion of an intramedullary device. However, if the reduction is difficult to achieve, the deltopectoral approach is recommended. This approach has several advantages. It provides access to the fracture enabling the removal of entrapped soft tissue such as the tendon of the long head of the biceps. It exposes the sternal head of the pectoralis major, the superior portion of which may be released after placement of stay sutures to facilitate a gentle reduction. This decreases the chance of brachial plexus and axillary artery injury. Lastly, impaction of the shaft into osteopenic bone in the humeral head may result in relative shortening of the muscle and, therefore, weakening of the deltoid. Through a deltopectoral approach, autologous or allograft bone may be placed into the defect in the center of the humeral head, decreasing impaction and preserving length to the deltoid insertion.

Tension banding across the fracture site ensures impaction and provides rotational stability (Fig. 18–10). Several strands of no. 5 nonabsorbable suture may be passed through drill holes in the shaft, crossed, then passed under the rotator cuff just medial to its insertion. A tension band may also incorporate fixation of an intramedullary rod depending on the device used. The tension band may pass under the hooks of Rush rods or through additional holes placed near the end of Ender's rods (see Fig. 18–10). It is critical that the proximal

end of any intramedullary device be sufficiently below the rotator cuff so that it does not cause impingement with normal shoulder motion.

Greater Tuberosity

Displaced fractures of the greater tuberosity are significant for two reasons. First, the greater tuberosity is the insertion site of the supraspinatus, infraspinatus, and teres minor. Therefore, a two-part greater tuberosity fracture fragment displaces superiorly and posteriorly (Fig. 18–11). If allowed to unite in this position, the greater tuberosity can impinge on the undersurface of the acromion with abduction and forward flexion. It can also limit external rotation. Second, significant displacement of the greater tuberosity indicates a rotator cuff tear. Reduction of the tuberosity, repair of the rotator cuff, and compliance with a postoperative rehabilitation program are all essential for optimal results.

A deltoid splitting approach is usually used for such fractures. A large, greater tuberosity fragment in good bone may be reduced and internally fixed with a screw, along with repair of the rotator cuff. However, because these fractures often occur in the elderly, the bone of this metaphyseal region is frequently poor quality. Tension banding using the stronger bone-tendon interface of the rotator cuff and drill holes in the shaft provides a more secure fixation (Fig. 18–12). In order to completely reduce the greater tuberosity, it is important to place sutures at the level of the superior, middle, and inferior facets to counteract the displacing forces of the supraspinatus, infraspinatus, and teres minor respectively.

Isolated Lesser Tuberosity Fracture

The lesser tuberosity can be avulsed from the proximal humerus when the abducted arm is resisting a posteriorly directed force. It is also associated with seizures and posterior dislocation. The lesser tuberosity is the site of insertion of the

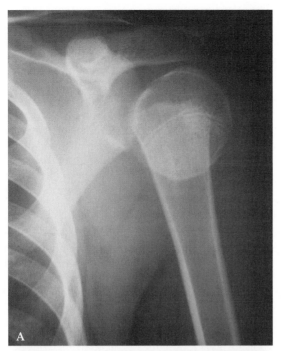

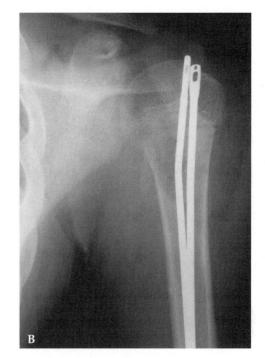

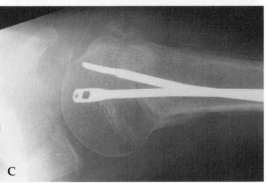

Figure 18–10   (**A**) This Salter II fracture occurred in an adolescent male nearing maturity. It was 100% displaced and could not be reduced by closed manipulation. (**B**) An open reduction was performed via a deltopectoral approach. (**C**) The reduction was maintained using modified Ender's nails and a tension band of heavy, nonabsorbable no. 5 sutures. Radiographs reproduced with permission of Frances Cuomo, MD.

subscapularis. Therefore, a two-part lesser tuberosity fracture is displaced medially and slightly inferiorly and can block internal rotation (see Fig. 18–11). Due to overlap with the humeral head and glenoid, displacement of this fracture is difficult to appreciate radiographically. It is best seen on an axillary radiograph.

Open reduction may be performed through the deltopectoral interval using an anterior axillary incision. Internal fixation can be accomplished with either a screw or heavy sutures through the bone-tendon interface to bone, similar to the technique for the greater tuberosity.

Treatment of Three-part Fractures

Three-part fractures consist of an isolated tuberosity, the other tuberosity still attached to the articular segment, and the humeral shaft. In the most common type of three-part fracture, in which the greater tuberosity is displaced and lesser tuberosity is attached to the humeral head, the pull of the subscapularis causes internal rotation so that the articular surface faces posteriorly. This is best appreciated on an axillary view.

Open reduction and internal fixation that is secure enough to allow early range of motion is the goal in treatment of these fractures. However, several factors may combine that prevent attainment of this goal. The surgeon embarking on an open reduction should always be prepared to do a hemiarthroplasty if it becomes necessary. This possibility should be discussed with the patient preoperatively.

Open reduction is accomplished through a deltopectoral approach. The tendon of the long head of the biceps, when it is intact, is a useful guide to the interval between the tuberosities.

PEARL

The tendon of the long head of the biceps is easiest to locate as it emerges from under the insertion of the pectoralis major.

The biceps groove is opened. The rotator cuff interval, which is usually partially torn, is opened to the glenoid. Heavy sutures are placed at the bone-tendon junction of each fragment to facilitate reduction. It is especially important to secure the inferior portion of the greater tuberosity

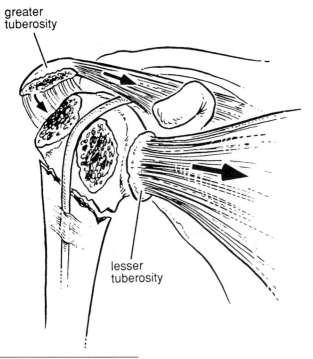

greater
tuberosity

lesser
tuberosity

Figure 18–11   The greater tuberosity is pulled superiorly by the supraspinatus and posteriorly by the infraspinatus and teres minor. The lesser tuberosity is pulled medially and inferiorly by the subscapularis.

posteriorly enough to correct the displacement that commonly occurs.

In the past, plate fixation was commonly used for three-part fractures. Problems with nonunion and loss of fixation have led to the increasing popularity of minimal fixation techniques. Minimal fixation requires less periosteal stripping and provides a better hold on the osteopenic bone frequently encountered in these fractures.

One example of minimal fixation involves using nonabsorbable no. 5 suture to tension band the tuberosities to each other and to the shaft. Two drill holes are placed in the shaft through which 3 or 4 no. 5 sutures are placed (Fig. 18–12). These sutures are then placed through the bone-tendon junction of each of the tuberosities. After all the sutures have been placed, they are tied. The shoulder is put through a range of motion to check the security of the fixation and to determine the safe range of motion that can be begun postoperatively. The wound is closed over a drain.

Following fixation, a sling and swath are applied. Active motion of the elbow, wrist, and hand are begun immediately in addition to passive motion of the shoulder. Forcible or painful passive motion is forbidden because this can lead to loss of fixation and nonunion. Active motion is begun when the pain has subsided and there is radiographic evidence of union, usually at around 6 weeks.

Treatment of Four-part Fractures

The treatment of four-part fractures is usually hemiarthroplasty. The rationale for this approach is based on the assumption that circulation to the articular portion is disrupted, creating a high risk of avascular necrosis. However, the consequences of avascular necrosis of the humeral head can vary from collapse with loss of fixation to uneventful revascularization. The results of treatment of three- and four-part fractures with hemiarthroplasty is generally a pain-free shoulder, but functionally, patients frequently have difficulty

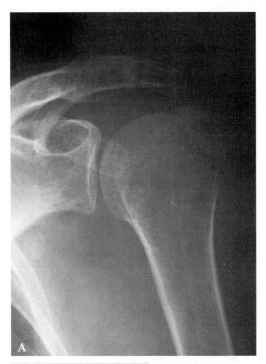
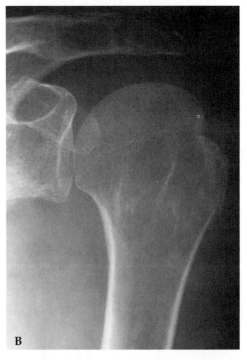

Figure 18–12   (**A**) This displaced greater tuberosity fracture signifies a rotator cuff tear. The fragment lies above the articular surface and would have caused impingement if treated nonoperatively. (**B**) It was reduced via a deltoid splitting incision. The reduction was maintained using several no. 5 nonabsorbable sutures as tension bands.

with activities above the level of the shoulder and with lifting and carrying objects. In the younger adult patient, open reduction and internal fixation is an option if the fragments can be anatomically reduced with fixation secure enough to permit early motion. Results of hemiarthroplasty done after failed attempts at open reduction internal fixation were significantly worse than for hemiarthroplasty performed as the primary treatment. If adequate fixation to permit early mobilization cannot be achieved, hemiarthroplasty is an acceptable treatment for the younger adult as well as the elderly.

A deltopectoral approach is used. The tuberosity fragments are isolated and tagged as for a three-part fracture. If hemiarthroplasty has been selected, the humeral head is removed along with any articular remnants still attached to the tuberosities. The humeral shaft is reamed to the appropriate size. Two drill holes are placed on either side of the biceps groove. Four no. 5 nonabsorbable sutures are passed in one hole and out the other. These are used to secure the tuberosities once the prosthesis has been cemented in place (Fig. 18–13).

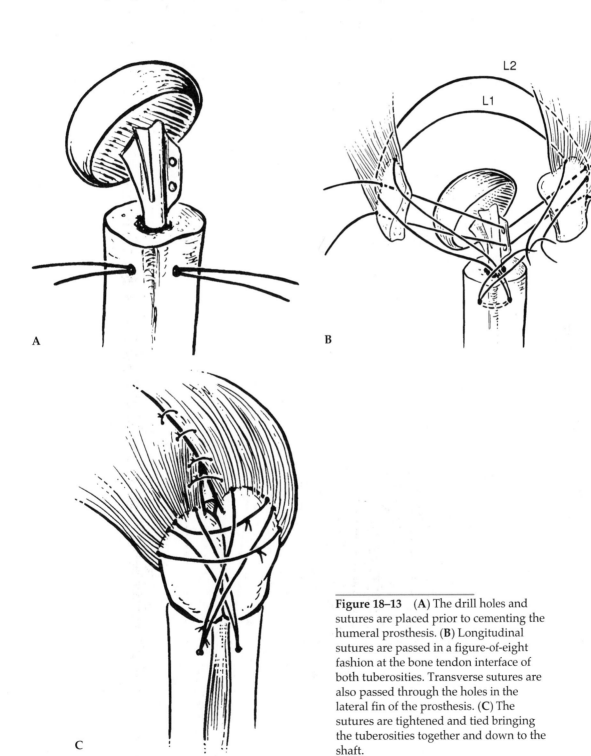

Figure 18–13 (**A**) The drill holes and sutures are placed prior to cementing the humeral prosthesis. (**B**) Longitudinal sutures are passed in a figure-of-eight fashion at the bone tendon interface of both tuberosities. Transverse sutures are also passed through the holes in the lateral fin of the prosthesis. (**C**) The sutures are tightened and tied bringing the tuberosities together and down to the shaft.

A trial prosthesis is then placed. The rotation and depth of placement and the size of the prosthesis must be determined. If the prosthesis is allowed to sink too far into the shaft, the tuberosities may sit superior to the articular surface causing impingement. It is very common for the lateral fin to be completely exposed when the prosthesis is properly positioned. The prosthesis is generally placed in 30 degrees of retroversion. Retroversion is estimated by flexing the elbow to 90 degrees and externally rotating the forearm. When the prosthesis is pointing directly toward the glenoid, the desired degree of retroversion has been achieved. The location of the anterior fin is marked on the shaft, and the depth of the implant is noted. When conducting a trial placement of the prosthesis, a prosthesis the same size as the last reamer may be used. Usually, a prosthesis one size down from the last reamer will actually be implanted to allow for an adequate cement mantle. A surgical sponge may be temporarily wrapped around the trial stem to further enhance an interference fit. Gentle longitudinal traction on the arm should elicit downward displacement of the humeral head. If there is a question about the placement, intra-operative radiographs may be obtained.

If a modular system is being used, after the stem is cemented in place the head size may be determined. With the tuberosities brought into apposition, the humeral head should be able to be posteriorly displaced of 50% the width of the humeral head. After the head has been selected and placed, sutures are passed through the bone-tendon interface of both the tuberosities in figure-of-eight patterns. The superior portion of the lesser tuberosity and the superior facet of the greater tuberosity are approximated first, then the repair moves inferiorly with subsequent figure-of-eight sutures. In addition, sutures are passed transversely from one tuberosity to another, passing through the holes in the lateral fin (see Fig. 18–13b). After all the sutures have been placed, each is securely tied (Fig. 18–13c). The tuberosities should be in direct contact with each other and with the shaft to allow union of all fragments. If there is a gap due to comminution, it should be filled with bone graft from the humeral head. The shoulder is then put through a range of motion to determine the "safe range" for postoperative therapy. The deltopectoral fascia is closed over a drain. Subcutaneous tissue and skin is closed and a sling and swath are applied. Active motion of the elbow, wrist, and hand are begun immediately.

Fractures of the Scapula

Fractures of the scapula are unusual probably due to the mobility of the scapula and to the thick layer of musculature investing it. They are frequently the result of high-energy trauma and have many associated injuries including rib fractures, hemopneumothorax and pulmonary contusion, head injuries, clavicle fractures, cervical spine injuries, and brachial plexus injuries. Anteroposterior and lateral scapular views and a chest x-ray are usually sufficient to characterize the fracture.

Classification may be made on the basis of anatomic region (Fig. 18–14). Type I is fracture of either the acromion or coracoid. Type II is fracture of the neck of the scapula. Type III is an intra-articular fracture of the glenoid (Fig. 18–15). Type IV is a fracture of the body. A computed tomographic scan may help assess intra-articular fractures or fractures with a complex configuration. Fractures of the body, even when displaced, do well with closed treatment; nonunion has not been documented in this region. Displaced fractures of the scapular neck and spine frequently cause abduction weakness and subacromial pain. Miller and Ada (1992) published the results of their large series of scapula fractures. They proposed the following indications for surgical management of the fractured scapula: displaced glenoid fractures, scapular neck fractures with more than 40-degree angulation in either the transverse or coronal plane, and fractures of the scapular neck with 1 cm or more displacement. Scapular spine fractures at the base of the acromion and those with more than 5 mm of displacement may be at risk for the development of nonunion and should also be considered for surgical treatment.

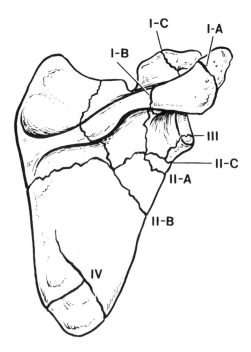

Figure 18–14 Classification of scapula fractures: I-A: acromion; I-B: spine through base of acromion; I-C: coracoid; II-A: neck lateral to base of acromion; II-B: neck extending to base of acromion; II-C: neck, transverse type; III: glenoid intra-articular; IV: body.

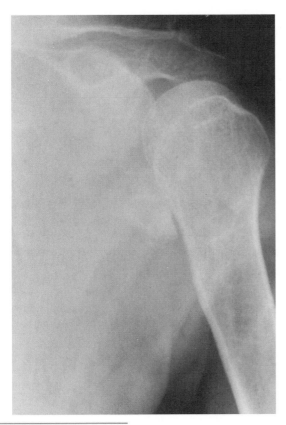

Figure 18–15   This is a displaced intra-articular glenoid fracture with inferior subluxation of the humeral head.

Surgical approaches to the scapula may be made anteriorly or posteriorly. The approach to fractures of the coracoid or anterior glenoid may be made through the deltopectoral interval in a manner similar to that for a Bankhart repair. Approaches to the scapular spine or body may be made via the Judet incision, which follows the line of the scapular spine and then curves inferiorly following the medial border of the scapula. When exposing the scapular spine, the infraspinatus must be retracted from medial to lateral to avoid traction injury to the suprascapular nerve as it rounds the base of the acromion.

Rigid fixation of scapular fractures with plates and interfragmentary screws is recommended if surgical treatment is chosen.

SUMMARY

Fractures of the shoulder girdle are common injuries that may be disabling if not judiciously managed. Most fractures of the clavicle are treated without surgery unless the fracture is open or the overlying skin is compromised by marked displacement of the fracture fragments. The treatment of proximal humerus fractures is dictated by the degree of displacement and the risk that the fracture pattern will result in avascular necrosis of the humeral head. Scapular fractures are treated nonoperatively except for those in which there is marked incongruity of the surface of the glenoid or a "floating shoulder": a displaced scapular neck fracture combined with a displaced fracture of the clavicle.

SELECTED BIBLIOGRAPHY

BIGLIANI LU. Fractures of the proximal humerus. In: Rockwood CA Jr, Matsen FA, eds. *The Shoulder.* Philadelphia, PA: WB Saunders; 1990:278.

BOEHME D, CURTIS RJ Jr, DE HAAN JT, KAY SP, YOUNG DC, ROCKWOOD CA Jr. The treatment of nonunion fractures of the midshaft of the clavicle with an intramedullary Hagie pin and autogenous bone graft. *Instr Course Lect.* 1993; 42:283–290.

ESSER RD. Open reduction and internal fixation of three- and four-part fractures of the proximal humerus. *Clin Orthop.* 1994;299:244–251.

GERBER C, SCHNEEBERGER AG, VINH TS. The arterial vascularization of the humeral head: an anatomic study. *J Bone Jt Surg Am.* 1990;72A:1486–1494.

KOFOED H: Revascularization of the humeral head: a report of two cases of fracture-dislocation of the shoulder. *Clin Orthop.* 1983;179:175–178.

KONA J, BOSSE MJ, STAEHELI JW, ROSSEAU RL. Type II distal clavicle fractures: a retrospective review of surgical treatment. *J Orthop Trauma.* 1990;4:115–120.

LEE CK, HANSEN HR. Post-traumatic avascular necrosis of the humeral head in displaced proximal humeral fractures. *J Trauma.* 1981;21:788–791.

LODMAN EA. *The Shoulder.* Boston: Thomas Todd Company; 1934.

LYONS FA, ROCKWOOD CA Jr. Migration of pins used in the shoulder. *J Bone Jt Surg.* 1990;72A:1262–1267.

MILLER ME, ADA JR. Injuries to the shoulder girdle. In: Browner BD, Jupiter JB, Levine AM, Trafton PG, eds. *Skeletal Trauma.* Philadelphia, PA: WB Saunders; 1992: 1291–1301.

NEER CS: *Shoulder Reconstruction.* Philadelphia, PA: WB Saunders; 1990:367.

SIDOR ML, ZUCKERMAN JD, LYON T et al. The Neer classification system for proximal humeral fractures: an assessment of interobserver reliability and intraobserver reproducibility. *J Bone Jt Surg.* 1993;75A:1745–1750.

STROMQVIST B, LIDGREN L, NORGREN L, ODENBRING S. Neurovascular injury complicating displaced proximal fractures of the humerus. *Injury.* 1987;18:423–425.

ZUCKERMAN JD, FLUGSTAD DL, TEITZ CC, KING HA. Axillary artery injury as a complication of proximal humerus fractures: two case reports and a review of the literature. *Clin Orthop.* 1984;189:234–237.

SAMPLE QUESTIONS

1. Which is the main blood supply to the humeral head:
   (a) the anterior humeral circumflex artery
   (b) the posterior humeral circumflex artery
   (c) the thoracoacromial artery
   (d) the suprascapular artery
   (e) the axillary artery

2. On which view is displacement of the lesser tuberosity best seen:
   (a) anteroposterior
   (b) scapular Y
   (c) axillary lateral
   (d) West Point
   (e) Naval Academy

3. True or false: Hemiarthroplasty for four-part fractures of the proximal humerus may be done without cement.
   (a) true
   (b) false

4. Name two problems commonly associated with greater tuberosity fractures.
   (a) loss of internal rotation
   (b) injury to the musculocutaneous nerve
   (c) subacromial impingement
   (d) rotator cuff tear
   (e) injury to the axillary nerve

5. List two indications for open reduction and internal fixation of the clavicle.
   (a) group I (middle third) fracture with 75% displacement
   (b) open fracture
   (c) nonunion, asymptomatic
   (d) fracture associated with a subclavian artery laceration
   (e) group I fracture with 100% displacement and overiding of the fracture ends

Answers: 1) a; 2) c; 3) b; 4) c, d; 5) b, d

Chapter 19

Shoulder Instability

Robin R. Richards, MD, FRCSC

The shoulder provides the foundation for upper extremity function. The articular surface of the glenoid is shallow. Therefore, stability of the shoulder is dependent on the integrity of the surrounding soft tissue structures and, to a lesser extent, on the underlying bony anatomy. An element of laxity is normal in the human shoulder. The shoulder is the most mobile joint in the human body. Normal shoulder function is dependent on a delicate balance between mobility and stability. The patient with shoulder instability is significantly disabled and often wishes to have surgical treatment even though the shoulder functions well between episodes of instability.

The shoulder has the highest incidence of instability of any joint. In Cave's series of 394 shoulder dislocations, 84% were anterior glenohumeral dislocations, 12% involved the acromioclavicular joint, 2.5% involved the sternoclavicular joint, and 1.5% were posterior dislocations. It is likely that acute posterior dislocations are more common than generally recognized because the diagnosis is frequently missed. It is the author's experience that patients with posterior glenohumeral dislocations may attend an emergency department, get radiographs, and be sent home with an incorrect diagnosis. Physicians and radiologists treating acutely injured patients must take great care to be certain that a good lateral radiograph (either trans-scapular or transaxillary) is obtained in every patient with an acute shoulder injury (Fig. 19–1).

ETIOLOGY

Shoulder instability most frequently develops in relation to acute trauma. Disruption of the static constraints can occur alone or in association with avulsion of a portion of the bony glenoid rim. Once dislocation has occurred, pain-induced muscle spasm locks the humeral head out of joint. Some patients are capable of sufficient muscle relaxation such that they can relocate their shoulders. However, most patients with acute dislocations will require medical assistance. A subgroup of patients with shoulder instability have generalized ligamentous laxity. These patients are usually teenagers or in

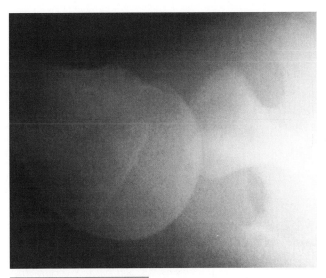

Figure 19–1 Transaxillary radiograph showing posterior dislocation of the humeral head.

Orthopaedic Surgery: The Essentials. Edited by M.E. Baratz, A.D. Watson, and J.E. Imbriglia. Thieme Medical Publishers, Inc., New York © 1999

their 20s and are more commonly female than male. Instability in these patients can develop in combination with acute injury. However, their instability can also develop as a result of repetitive forceful use of the shoulder in sports such as swimming, baseball, or volleyball. Instability can even develop without any history of trauma. Shoulder instability presents a spectrum of etiologies. Some patients have traumatic instability and others give no history of trauma at all. Many patients fall in between these two categories and each case must be assessed on an individual basis.

The incidence of recurrent dislocation following traumatic dislocation is age-dependent. Recurrent dislocation is extremely common in individuals who sustain their initial dislocation during the second decade of life. In contrast, recurrent dislocation occurs in less that 20% of individuals who sustain their initial dislocation past age 40. Recurrence is more common in athletes than in nonathletes and in males more than in females. The presence of a large Hill-Sach's lesion is correlated with a higher incidence of recurrent instability. In contrast, the presence of a greater tuberosity fracture in association with the initial dislocation is associated with a lower incidence of recurrent instability. The role of immobilization is controversial following the initial dislocation. Some studies have indicated that immobilization can reduce the incidence of recurrent dislocation. This finding has not been confirmed by all investigators. It is the author's practice to immobilize first time dislocators under age 30 with a Velpeau sling for 3 to 4 weeks. Patients under age 20 are immobilized for 4 to 5 weeks in an effort to allow healing of the soft tissues, reattachment of the labrum (if a Bankart lesion is present), and, hopefully, for an element of scar contraction to occur.

Multidirectional instability usually occurs in the context of a patient with generally more than the normal amount of ligamentous laxity (Fig. 19–2). Demonstrable inferior instability is required to make the diagnosis of inferior shoulder instability. These patients have a combination of either anterior and inferior instability, posterior and inferior instability, or instability in all three directions. The diagnosis is made by

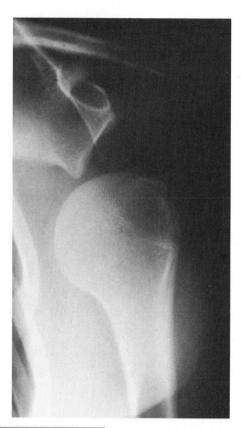

Figure 19–3 Anteroposterior radiograph showing inferior subluxation of the glenohumeral joint in a patient with multidirectional shoulder instability. Reproduced with permission from Richards, RR. *Soft Tissue Reconstruction in the Upper Extremity.* New York, NY: Churchill Livingstone; 1995.

the combination of history and physical examination. Inferior traction on the arm can produce a sulcus sign, which indicates inferior subluxation of the humeral head. This can be confirmed by a plain radiograph (Fig. 19–3). In its most severe form, patients with multidirectional instability can have anterior, posterior, and inferior instability combined.

BASIC SCIENCE

The normal shoulder has a combination of bony, cartilaginous, labral, capsular, ligamentous, and muscular constraints. Conceptually the stabilizers of the shoulder can be subclassified according to whether they have a static or dynamic function. It is felt that there is a hierarchy of constraints to shoulder motion with minimal loads resisted by the passive mechanisms, intermediate loads resisted by the action of the periarticular musculature, and extreme loads resisted by the static restraints. The role of static stabilizers varies significantly according to the position of the shoulder.

In addition to the static and dynamic stabilizers of the shoulder several phenomenon exist that are operational both at rest and with motion. Normally, the shoulder is hermetically sealed. The amount of joint fluid within the normal shoulder is less than 1 mL. Distraction of the normal joint surfaces is resisted by the normally negative intra-articular pressure. Indeed, distraction of the joint surface requires contraction of the surrounding capsule. The closely congruent chondral sur-

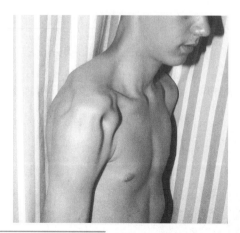

Figure 19–2 Multidirectional shoulder instability in a teenager with generalized ligamentous laxity. Reproduced with permission from Richards, RR. *Soft Tissue Reconstruction in the Upper Extremity.* New York, NY: Churchill Livingstone; 1995.

faces of the glenoid and humerus, when coapted with a small amount of intervening joint fluid, are difficult to separate. This phenomenon can be termed adhesion-cohesion or "stiction-friction." The viscous forces provide stability by this mechanism, although this phenomenon can be eliminated by the addition of excess fluid in the form of either gas or liquid to the joint. Indeed, the atmospheric pressure may contribute to shoulder stability, as it has been observed that perforation of the joint capsule will allow the humeral head to fall slightly away from the scapula. This normal passive mechanism providing stability to the shoulder can be eliminated by many mechanisms including intra-articular incongruity, joint effusion, and/or hemarthrosis.

Static Stabilizers

One of the static stabilizers of the shoulder is the geometry of the joint surface. The glenoid is very shallow and presents a small surface to the humeral head, offering little intrinsic stability. The glenoid is shaped more like a saucer than a socket. The glenoid labrum is a fibrocartilaginous structure attaching to the glenoid, which deepens and expands the glenoid, thus contributing to its stabilizing function. Detachment of the glenoid labrum is common in patients with anterior instability. However, the amount of attachment is so variable and the frequency of patients having anterior instability without detachment of their glenoid labrum is so high, that it is probably fallacious to consider the Bankart lesion to be "essential" for anterior dislocation to occur. The acromion and coracoid provide bony limits to superior and anterosuperior motion. They cannot, however, be considered primary shoulder stabilizers.

To allow motion, the capsule of the glenohumeral joint is, of necessity, loose and redundant. Portions of the capsule tighten at the extremes of motion in order to provide restraint to the joint. The important anterior glenohumeral ligaments are capsular condensations which, when placed under tension, constrain anterior translation of the humerus in relation to the scapula (Table 19–1).

The inferior glenohumeral ligament is felt to be a major anterior stabilizer of the glenohumeral joint. The posterior capsule of the shoulder is also recognized to play an important role in stabilizing the glenohumeral joint. Indeed Schwartz's work indicates that clinical instability is usually

accompanied by both anterior and posterior ligamentous lesions. The coracohumeral ligament extends from the lateral border of the coracoid process to the area of the transverse humeral ligament. This structure should also be considered to be a static stabilizer of the shoulder when the arm is abducted.

Extensive radiographic study has not demonstrated any convincing evidence that glenoid version plays a role in shoulder instability. The humeral head is normally retroverted 30 to 40 degrees in relation to the transverse axis of the elbow joint. Glenoid version is extraordinarily difficult to measure accurately on plain radiographs. Recent computed tomography studies have failed to demonstrate consistent alterations in glenoid anatomy in patients with shoulder instability.

Dynamic Constraints

With complete muscular relaxation, many patients demonstrate astounding amounts of glenohumeral laxity. Because they are asymptomatic and fully active they do not have "unstable" shoulders. The periarticular musculature is of great importance in stabilizing the shoulder. Indeed, some patients have voluntary shoulder instability and can actually dislocate the glenohumeral joint by contraction of specific periarticular muscles. Conversely, normal muscle function tends to stabilize the shoulder by centering the humeral head in the glenoid. This is particularly true of the rotator cuff musculature. A portion of the rotator cuff musculature inserts into the capsule of the shoulder and is thought to play a role in "tensioning" the capsule.

There is a subset of patients whose primary source of instability may very well be dyskinetic motion about the shoulder. This is the case in patients with multidirectional instability, where in spite of normal deltoid strength, the shoulder can subluxate inferiorly to a extraordinary extent.

ANATOMY AND SURGICAL APPROACHES

In contemplating surgery for recurrent anterior glenohumeral instability, the surgeon must consider the pathoanatomy in each patient. Many, but not all, patients with this condition have a Bankart lesion. The portion of the glenoid involved in the Bankart lesion is quite variable, ranging from huge to minuscule. Some patients do not have a Bankart lesion in the usual sense but rather a Bankart "phenomenon," with scuffing of the anterior labrum but no detachment (Fig. 19–4). Most patients have laxity of their anterior capsule and attenuation of the anterior glenohumeral ligaments. Some patients have Hill-Sach's lesions; an impaction fracture of the posterolateral portion of the humeral head. If present, this lesion may be of widely varying size. Large lesions can contribute to shoulder instability.

Surgical repair seeks to restore toward normal the pathologic anatomy present in each individual patient. Thus, a "cookbook" approach must be avoided. The surgeon must also seek to avoid overtightening of the shoulder, which can lead to arthrosis. Furthermore, an inordinate restriction of motion will prevent the patient from returning to normal activities of daily living or a desired sports activity. It is generally agreed that the use of metallic fixation devices near the

TABLE 19–1 Glenohumeral ligaments.

Ligament	Origin	Insertion
Superior	Anterosuperior glenoid	Top of lesser tuberosity
Middle (absent in 30%)	Supraglenoid tubercle, superior labrum, scapular neck	Lesser tuberosity
Inferior	Anteroinferior labrum and glenoid lip	Lesser tuberosity (beneath middle ligament)

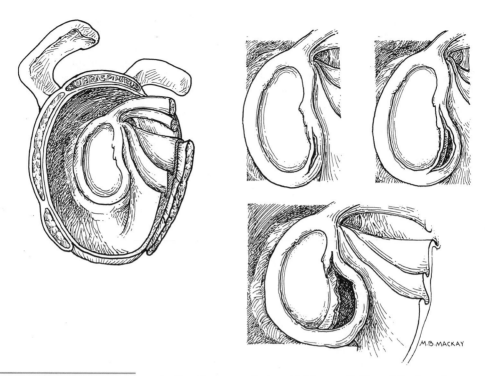

Figure 19–4   Diagram demonstrating the normal glenoid labrum (left) and Bankart lesions of varying size and significance (right). Reproduced with permission from Richards, RR. *Soft Tissue Reconstruction in the Upper Extremity.* New York, NY: Churchill Livingstone; 1995.

glenoid rim is to be avoided. Use of staples and other devices exposes the patient to the risk of the metal penetrating the joint. Even if the metallic device does not enter the joint, the head of the device can scuff or irritate the humeral head as it rotates about the glenoid. Similarly, because no abnormality of glenoid shape or version has been consistently identified, operative procedures that alter the architecture of the glenoid are best avoided. Recurrent shoulder instability is primarily a soft tissue problem, and the surgical reconstruction is directed toward balancing the soft tissues and restoring their structure towards normalcy.

PEARL

It is generally agreed that the use of metallic fixation devices near the glenoid rim is to be avoided.

Anterior Approach

Anterior shoulder repair is performed through an anterior approach. The patient is positioned semi-sitting on the operating room table and the involved extremity is draped free. A sterile, covered Mayo stand is used to support the arm during certain portions of the procedure. The author prefers a deltopectoral approach. The incision is extensile and provides superb visualization without undue traction on the soft tissues. The deltopectoral incision does leave a visible scar about which the patient should be informed preoperatively. Although axillary incisions are more cosmetic, it is the

author's opinion that it does not provide optimal exposure. If the patient has had previous surgery through a transaxillary incision, the previous incision is ignored. It is virtually impossible to incorporate an axillary incision into a deltopectoral incision and the author, in many revision cases, has not had a problem with skin healing in this situation. After incision, the deltopectoral interval is developed (Fig. 19–5). Care is taken to identify the coracoid process, the "signpost" of the shoulder. Shoulder reconstruction can be performed safely, providing dissection is kept lateral to the edge of the conjoined tendon of the coracobrachialis and the short head of the biceps. The coracobrachial fascia is incised and the coracohumeral ligament is divided. The author routinely divides the coracoacromial ligament when performing anterior shoulder surgery. The proximal portion of the conjoined tendon is partially released transversely and the areolar plane beneath the conjoined tendon anterior to the subscapularis muscle is developed. With the arm externally rotated, abducted 30 degrees, and resting on the Mayo stand, the anterior humeral circumflex artery and its vena commitantes are identified. The artery and its vena commitantes are elevated and coagulated over a broad distance. The author routinely coagulates this vessel and has never observed a case of osteonecrosis postoperatively as a result of this maneuver.

Identification and Protection of the Axillary Nerve

The axillary nerve lies in intimate relationship to the anterior and inferior aspect of the shoulder as it passes from the posterior cord into the quadrangular space. Because the

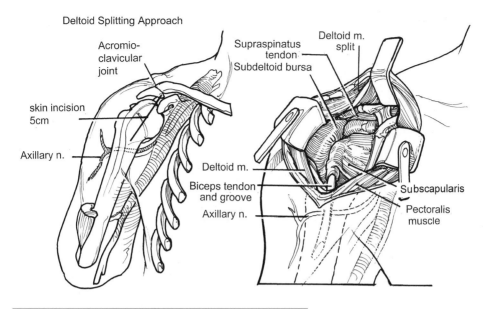

Figure 19–5 Deltopectoral incision and development of the deltopectoral interval.

pathoanatomy of anterior instability involves stretching and redundancy of the anteroinferior capsule, dissection must be performed in close vicinity to the axillary nerve. Accordingly, it is the author's preference to routinely identify, mobilize, and protect the axillary nerve when performing a repair for anterior instability. Although there is some risk of traumatizing the nerve by identifying it, this has not occurred in the author's experience in more than 300 cases. Having protected the nerve intraoperatively, if weakness of the deltoid is noted postoperatively, the surgeon and patient can take comfort in knowing that the nerve was stretched or contused but not lacerated or inadvertantly sutured or cauterized. Accordingly, recovery almost certainly will occur.

The axillary nerve can be identified by placing a finger beneath the coracoid process and gently palpating distally and medially. The nerve is felt as it arises from the posterior cord laterally and inferiorly. Careful placement of deep, right angle retractors on the subscapularis and on the conjoined tendon will identify the nerve, and the fascia overlying it can be divided. A cystic duct clamp is then gently passed around the nerve, a 1/4-inch Penrose drain is grasped with the cystic duct clamp, and the drain pulled around the nerve to protect it (Fig. 19–6). With gentle traction on the nerve, the overlying fascial fibers and areolar tissue is divided up to the origin of the axillary nerve from the posterior cord proximally to at least the midpoint of the quadrangular space distally. With the nerve identified, dissection can proceed inferiorly in a safe and uninhibited fashion.

PEARL

The axillary nerve can be identified by placing a finger beneath the coracoid process and gently palpating distally and medially.

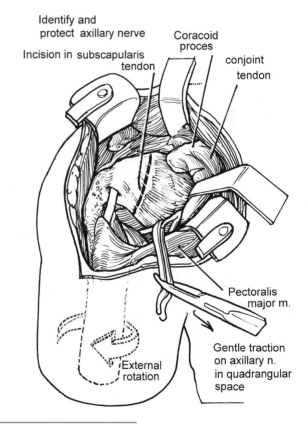

Figure 19–6 Anterior approach with identification and protection of axillary nerve.

Posterior Approach

Recurrent posterior instability is treated with the patient in the lateral position. The patient's position on the operating table is secured with a beanbag, folded sheets, and tape. The extremity is draped free, and an incision is marked out along the spine of the scapula turning distally in line with the deltoid fibers for a distance of 6 to 8 cm, depending on the size of the patient. Prior to making the incision, the skin is infiltrated with dilute saline and epinephrine (1:500,000). The subcutaneous tissues are incised in line with the skin incision. Dissection is carried down to the deltotrapezial fascia. The origin of the deltoid is detached from the angle of the acromion and the scapular spine for 7 to 8 cm (Fig. 19–7). The deltoid is detached with electrocautery and is split distally at the junction of the unipennate (posterior) and multipennate (middle) fibres. The fascial plane immediately beneath the deltoid but superficial to the supraspinatus is identified. Dissection can be performed easily in this plane. The subdeltoid fascia is divided 5 cm distal to the angle of the acromion.

After deepening the self-retaining retractors, the axillary nerve is identified as it exits from the quadrangular space (Fig. 19–8). A cystic duct clamp is used to encircle the axillary nerve and a 1/4-inch Penrose drain is placed around it. The nerve is mobilized to the extent that it can be safely retracted. Homan retractors are placed beneath the acromion superiorly and beneath the deltoid laterally to improve the exposure.

EXAMINATION

Each patient with shoulder instability must be assessed on an individual basis. In most patients, the diagnosis of shoulder instability can be made by a careful history noting:

1. the usual position of the arm when episodes of instability occur
2. the degree of activity and trauma required to produce the instability
3. the length of time required for reduction and whether or not medical attention was needed to obtain a reduction
4. the length of time after an episode of instability that the shoulder remains symptomatic

Patients should be carefully examined for translational motion and for a sulcus sign.

Plain radiographs must be carefully reviewed even though they are normal in the vast majority of patients. There may be new bone formation demonstrable on the anteroinferior aspect of the shoulder indicative of anterior instability.

If the examination and plain radiographs are not sufficient

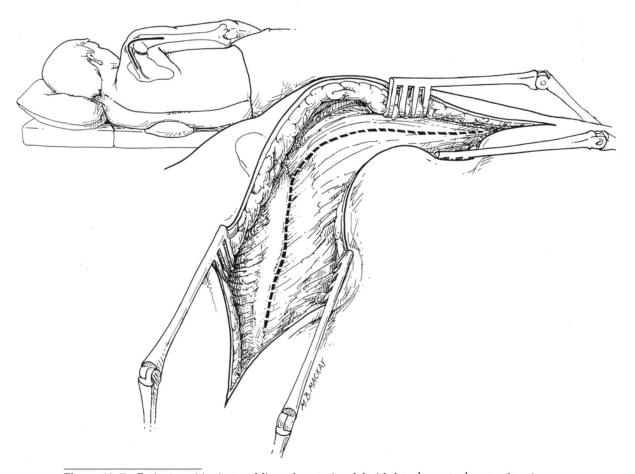

Figure 19–7 Patient positioning and line of posterior deltoid detachment when performing a posterior approach to the glenohumeral joint. Reproduced with permission from Richards, RR. *Soft Tissue Reconstruction in the Upper Extremity.* New York, NY: Churchill Livingstone; 1995.

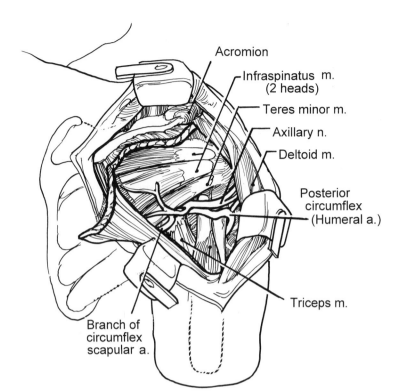

Acromion
Infraspinatus m.
(2 heads)
Teres minor m.
Axillary n.
Deltoid m.
Posterior
circumflex
(Humeral a.)
Triceps m.
Branch of
circumflex
scapular a.

Figure 19–8 Schematic illustrating posterior approach with identification of rotator cuff musculature and axillary nerve.

to make a definitive diagnosis, consideration should be given to examination of the shoulder under anesthesia with or without an arthroscopic assessment. Examination of the shoulder under anesthesia must be performed with axial compression of the joint surfaces. Such a maneuver tends to exaggerate the instability. This point deserves emphasis because it can be exceedingly difficult to demonstrate shoulder instability in the anesthetized patient. This is particularly true if the patient's arm is larger than that of the examiner. The arm is grasped with one hand while an assistant stabilizes the shoulder girdle. The examiner's second hand is placed over the shoulder, and the thumb and index finger are used to displace the humeral head.

Anterior Instability

The arm is abducted and externally rotated. The thumb is used to displace the humeral head anteriorly. With axial compression applied to the arm, the shoulder is adducted and flexed. The shoulder is observed and palpated for relocation of the humeral head. The findings can be subtle, particularly in an obese patient or in a patient whose periarticular musculature is well developed.

Posterior Instability

The arm is adducted and internally rotated. An assistant stabilizes the shoulder girdle. Axial pressure is applied to the upper extremity in line with the humerus with the arm abducted. The shoulder is observed and the second hand palpates whether or not relocation occurs.

Associated Injuries

Shoulder instability can occur in association with fracture of the proximal humerus or of the glenoid rim. In this situation, open reduction is usually indicated if the fracture is displaced. Glenoid rim fractures involving more than one third of the joint surface that do not anatomically reduce after relocation of the shoulder often require surgical treatment.

Vascular injuries can occur in association with shoulder instability, most frequently in elderly patients.

Injury to the axillary nerve is common with anterior dislocations. The incidence of axillary nerve injury in association with anterior shoulder dislocations is variable. It appears that nerve injury is more common than is generally recognized. If electromyograms are performed (as by Blom and Dahlback, 1970) the incidence is as high as 35%. Axillary nerve injury is associated with increasing age. Nerve injury following anterior dislocation can involve the axillary nerve, the posterior cord, or other neural elements including, in some cases, the entire brachial plexus. The majority of axillary nerve injuries recover following closed reduction of the humeral head. If neurologic recovery is not progressing, or has not occurred after 3 months, consideration should be given to exploration of the nerve.

In older patients, anterior shoulder dislocations are associated with a high frequency of rotator cuff tears. In patients past age 60, rotator cuff tears are the rule rather than the exception. Similarly, patients with fracture-dislocations of the shoulder involving the greater tuberosity often have significant rotator cuff pathology. Repair is not indicated providing the greater tuberosity reduces when the shoulder is reduced. If the residual displacement is greater than 1 cm, then open reduction of the tuberosity fragment is indicated to avoid malunion of the tuberosity and subsequent impingement.

CLASSIFICATION OF SHOULDER INSTABILITY

Shoulder instability can be classified by the following criteria:

1. the direction of displacement of the humeral head in relation to the glenoid
2. the acuity of the episodes of displacement
3. whether or not the patient has voluntary control over the instability

Direction of Instability

The most common direction of displacement is anterior. Anterior instability can be subclassified according to whether the humeral head resides in a subcoracoid, subglenoid, or subclavicular position. A rare variant of anterior instability is the intrathoracic dislocation, which can occur with major trauma. In posterior instability the humeral head lies behind the glenoid. Almost all posterior dislocations are subacromial, although subglenoid and subspinal dislocations have been described. Inferior instability is rare. If seen acutely, it is usually associated with severe soft tissue injury (luxatio erecta). Patients with an anterior dislocation can develop an inferior dislocation if the arm is abducted to obtain an axillary view. Inferior dislocation is most commonly seen in the context of multidirectional shoulder instability.

Timing

Shoulder instability is subclassified according to the time or chronology of the episodes of instability. Congenital instability is rare. Acute shoulder instability refers to episodes seen within the first few days of injury. If an acutely dislocated shoulder is not reduced the dislocation is considered chronic after 3 weeks. Recurrent instability refers to repeated episodes of either subluxation or dislocation. Some patients experience both subluxation and dislocation. Apprehension refers to the sensation that subluxation or dislocation may occur and is common in patients with shoulder instability.

Neuromuscular Control

Instability can be further subclassified according to the degree to which the patient has neuromuscular control of the instability. Patients who dislocate their shoulders at will are referred to as having voluntary shoulder instability. Voluntary shoulder instability is uncommon and is felt to be a relative contraindication for surgical treatment successfully stabilizing the shoulder. Voluntary instability can coexist with involuntary instability.

Habitual shoulder instability refers to episodes of instability occurring habitually in relationship to positioning of the arm. This most frequently occurs in patients with posterior instability when the patient forward flexes the shoulder in internal rotation. In this position, the humeral head subluxes or dislocates posteriorly.

AIDS TO DIAGNOSIS

If an examiner cannot be certain whether dislocation or subluxation is occurring, or if the direction of instability is in doubt, an image intensifier can be used to confirm the direction and degree of displacement as described by Norris (1985). An arthroscopic examination is not necessary for the diagnosis of shoulder instability if the instability is to be treated by open means.

SPECIFIC CONDITIONS, TREATMENT, AND OUTCOME

Indications for Surgery

Surgical stabilization of the shoulder is indicated for the patient with sufficient instability that he or she cannot enjoy the normal activities of daily living or participate in sports at the desired level. Patients need to be appraised of the success rate of the surgery, the quality of the anticipated result, the location and length of the scar that will be created, the length and intensity of the rehabilitation process, the failure rate of the procedure with the passage of time, and the possible risk of complications. Recurrent shoulder instability most commonly develops following acute dislocations in young patients. Surgical treatment is considered if symptomatic recurrent instability develops. A key consideration determining whether or not a patient will wish to have surgery is whether the patient can perform self-reduction. If a visit to the emergency department is required for every episode of shoulder instability, the patient will usually consider surgical treatment at an earlier stage. The degree of activity or trauma required to induce an episode of instability is also important in the decision-making process. Patients whose shoulders dislocate turning over in bed or while reaching into the back seat of an automobile will more commonly consider surgery.

Anterior Instability

Anterior instability that does not respond to therapy can be treated with open or arthroscopic stabilization. At present, the role of arthroscopy in the treatment of shoulder instability is evolving. There is no question that Bankart lesions can be reattached arthroscopically, although, at present, the recurrence rates following arthroscopic repair are higher than those following open surgery. The presence of anterior instability without a Bankart lesion (a relatively common circumstance) is somewhat problematic. However, there are techniques of arthroscopic capsulorrhaphy that may be considered in this situation. The author does not perform arthroscopic stabilization, and the technique will not be discussed further in this chapter. A description of the technical aspects of an open approach to shoulder stabilization follows.

Elevation of the Subscapularis

One of the most difficult aspects of anterior shoulder surgery is the dissection between the subscapularis muscle and capsule. Although the joint can be entered by directly cutting through the subscapularis muscle, the surgeon must recognize that the muscle provides a much less satisfactory material with which to accomplish a repair or closure of the joint. Furthermore, it is easy to disrupt the complex myotendinous junction, altering the normal length-tension relationship of the subscapularis myotendinous junction. The author prefers to elevate the subscapularis muscle and tendon from the capsule, preserving its integrity as a muscle-tendon unit. The insertion of the subscapularis muscle is sharply outlined on the lesser tuberosity. A no. 15 blade is used to dissect the tendon insertion from the lesser tuberosity. As soon as the tendon has been elevated from the tuberosity, dissection proceeds medially, sharply separating the fibers of the subscapularis insertion from the fibers of the anterior capsule (Fig. 19–9). Care must be taken not to make either the subscapularis flap or the capsular flap too thin. Traction is placed on the elevated tendon with Kocher clamps, and the arm is progressively externally rotated as the dissection continues medially. The rotator interval is always entered during this dissection. Visualization of the rotator interval can be used as a guide to the line of separation between the subscapularis muscle and the anterior capsule. As the dissection proceeds medially, muscle fibers are first encountered inferiorly. Once the layer between the muscle and the capsule is identified, blunt dissection with a blade can be used to elevate the muscle from the capsule. Superiorly, the dissection is more difficult. Many subscapularis fibers insert onto the anterior capsule in this area. At this level, the plane of separation must be developed more medially by sharp dissection. Blunt dissection can then proceed over the mid and superior portions of the subscapularis. Once the dissection is within a centimeter of the glenoid rim, the level of the Mayo stand is raised and the humerus is manually thrust posteriorly. This maneuver improves visualization of the capsule at the level of the joint. By blunt dissection, the subscapularis muscle is elevated from the anterior aspect of the capsule and from the

anterior aspect of the glenoid neck and body of the scapula. Once the subscapularis muscle and tendon have been elevated, an identification suture is placed in its tendinous insertion. The muscle is released and retracted medially beneath the border of the conjoined tendon.

Arthrotomy

Two clamps are placed along the superior and anterior border of the capsule at the level of the rotator interval. An arthrotomy is performed creating equal medial and lateral flaps (see Fig. 19–9). The arthrotomy is carried down to the 6-o'clock position, carefully protecting the previously identified axillary nerve. The posterior aspect of the humeral head is palpated for the presence or absence of a Hill-Sach's lesion. After the arthrotomy has been completed, a humeral head retractor is inserted, and the head is retracted posteriorly. The joint surface is carefully inspected at this point in time. Inspection of the joint surface is performed with particular attention to the status of the chondral surfaces, the presence or absence of a Hill-Sach's lesion, loose body formation, and the possible presence of pedunculated flaps of glenoid labrum. The glenoid labrum is carefully inspected for detachment and attritional change. The surgeon must determine whether a surgically significant Bankart lesion is present or whether the pathology noted represents a Bankart phenomenon, with limited functional importance. The incidence of detachment varies. Labral detachment is a common phenomenon in the athletic patient with recurrent instability following an episode of traumatic anterior instability. Bankart lesions are less common in patients whose shoulders dislocate by less traumatic mechanisms and who have a history of ligamentous laxity.

Repair of the Bankart Lesion

If a sizable Bankart lesion is present surgical repair is performed. The technique of Bankart repair is well described by Rowe and colleagues (1978). Specialized instruments are needed to perform a Bankart repair. The goal is to suture the glenoid labrum down to the anterior aspect of the glenoid neck and glenoid rim. This is accomplished by placing two or three drill holes along the anterior rim of the glenoid (Fig. 19–10). A towel clip is used to enlarge these holes so that sutures may be passed through them. The author prefers to use no. 1 braided, polyester suture, which is tied over the external surface of the reattached labrum and capsule (Fig. 19–11). Alternatively, a suture anchor can be used.

Capsulorrhaphy

The author performs anterior capsulorrhaphy in every case as part of the reconstruction for recurrent anterior glenohumeral instability. Although patients with large Bankart lesions can be treated by Bankart repair alone, it is the author's experience that almost all such patients, in addition to the Bankart lesion, have an element of stretching of the anterior capsule. This is particularly true inferiorly, where there is often gross capsular redundancy. In the author's experience, approximately 40% of patients with anterior instability have either no Bankart lesion or a trivial Bankart phenomenon. In these patients, the primary pathology of the condition seems to be

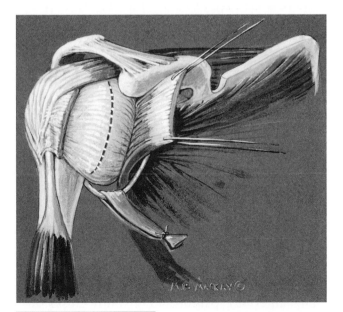

Figure 19–9   Elevation of the subscapularis muscle-tendon unit. The axillary nerve has been identified and protected by a Penrose drain.

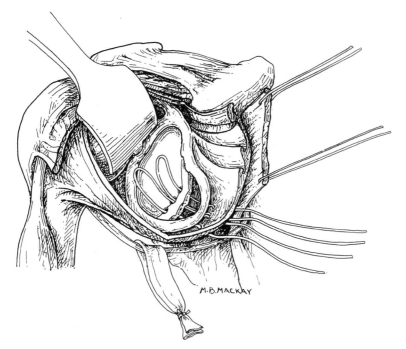

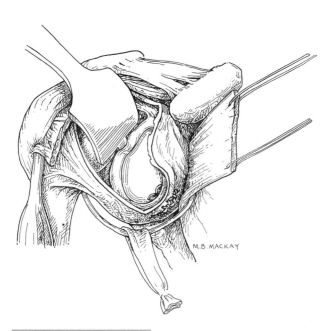

Figure 19–10   Placement of two sutures through the anterior rim of the glenoid to repair a Bankart lesion. Reproduced with permission from Richards, RR. *Soft Tissue Reconstruction in the Upper Extremity*. New York, NY: Churchill Livingstone; 1995.

Figure 19–11   The Bankart lesion has been repaired to the anterior rim of the glenoid. The sutures have been tied over the capsule and labrum. Reproduced with permission from Richards, RR. *Soft Tissue Reconstruction in the Upper Extremity*. New York, NY: Churchill Livingstone; 1995.

a stretch injury to the anterior capsule. Anterior capsulorrhaphy begins inferiorly, with placement of horizontal mattress sutures using no. 1 braided polyester suture on a tapered needle (Fig. 19–12). The author does not perform a shift procedure but rather gathers together the capsule as one would grasp two lapels of a coat to tighten it. Care must be taken to avoid overtightening of the capsule. This restricts external rotation, making the rehabilitation process more difficult. It can also lead to osteoarthritis, presumably due to an increase

in the cartilage contact forces. The first horizontal suture is placed in the inferior aspect of the capsule to reduce the size of the inferior pouch. Repositioning of the retractors is crucial when placing each of the capsulorrhaphy sutures. Care must be taken to pass the needle only through the tissue that is under direct visualization. The author uses four or five horizontal mattress sutures when performing anterior capsulorrhaphy. The amount of capsular tissue gathered together is variable depending on the size of the patient, the degree of redundancy, and the patient's anticipated demands. Care must be taken when performing capsulorrhaphy in athletes who use overhead arm movements to avoid overtightening the capsule (Fig. 19–13). It must be possible to tie the sutures with the shoulder in neutral or slight external rotation. None of the sutures are tied until all have been placed. The superior suture is very important. This is a purse-string suture, which gathers together the superomedial and superolateral corners and attaches them to the rotator cuff superiorly. The object of the most superior suture is to close the rotator interval and "suspend" the anterior capsule from the supraspinatus tendon. Care is taken to avoid catching or damaging the biceps tendon, which passes in close proximity to the superior margin of the rotator interval. The capsulorrhaphy sutures are tied with the shoulder flexed 30 to 40 degrees and resting on the sterile-covered Mayo stand. The arm should be in neutral or slight external rotation. After the sutures have been tied, the capsule is palpated for any defects. At this point the surgeon should palpate along the course of the axillary nerve to be certain that it has not been caught up in the repair.

PEARL

The superior capsulorrhaphy suture closes the rotator interval and suspends the anterior capsule from the supraspinatus tendon.

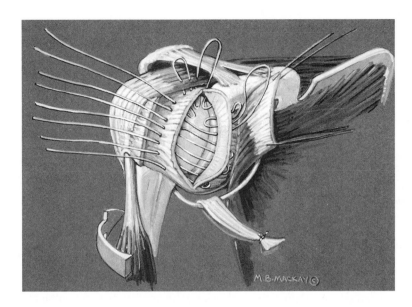

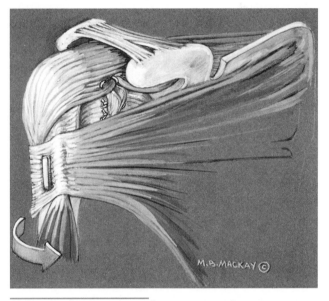

Figure 19–12 Placement of the capsulorrhaphy sutures. Care is taken to avoid injury to the axillary nerve and to close the rotator interval superiorly.

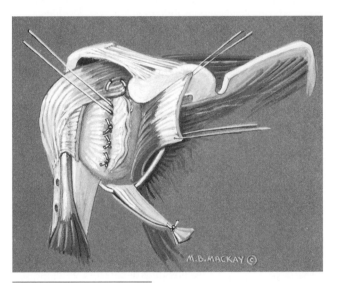

Figure 19–13 Completion of the capsular repair. The sutures are tied with the arm in neutral or slight external rotation to avoid overtightening of the capsule.

Figure 19–14 Transfer of the insertion of the subscapularis laterally and distally. The transfer is held in position with a barbed staple.

Transfer of the Subscapularis Insertion

The surgeon must choose between anatomic repair of the subscapularis insertion or transfer. The author prefers to transfer the insertion distal to the lesser tuberosity and lateral to the bicipital groove. This preserves the integrity of the subscapularis yet changes the force vector of the tendon to reduce inferior subluxation and to provide a type of dynamic "sling" for the humeral head when the arm is abducted and externally rotated (Fig. 19–14). The advantage of this transfer is that it augments the strength of the repair inferiorly and reinforces the repaired tissues when the arm is abducted and externally rotated. The disadvantage is that it restricts external rotation by tightening the subscapularis muscle-tendon unit. In the author's experience, the mean restriction of external rotation following transfer of the subscapularis insertion is approximately 15 degrees and the

mean loss of flexion is trivial. For the majority of patients, this minor loss of motion is of no functional significance (Fig. 19–15). However, for an athlete who uses overhead arm movements, maintaining the terminal range of external rotation may be of great importance.

Patients with large Hill-Sach's lesions are good candidates for tendon transfer because some loss of external rotation is desirable to avoid loads on the posterior aspect of the humeral head.

The transfer is performed by placing Homan retractors beneath the deltoid over the lateral aspect of the humerus. Electrocautery is used to divide the periosteum just lateral to the biceps tendon down to bone. A periosteal elevator is used to elevate the periosteum and the Homan retractors are repositioned beneath the periosteum. A 2-mm drill is used to

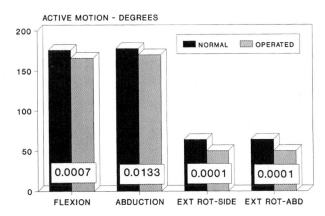

Figure 19–15 There is a small decrease in the range of external rotation, abduction, and flexion when the author's technique is used (sample of 54 patients). Patients are able to perform most activities of daily living without symptoms postoperatively. Throwing overhead may be impaired in some patients, and they are forced to use a slightly side-arm type of motion.

make 3.5 small holes in the humeral cortex on the lateral border of the bicipital groove. These holes reduce the chance of splitting the humerus and encourage healing of tendon to bone. The subscapularis insertion is retrieved from beneath the conjoined tendon. Kocher clamps are placed on the tendon, and the tendon is brought inferiorly and laterally to the area of its new insertion. The arm is internally rotated. A barbed staple is used to attach the tendon to the humerus. The point of attachment is lateral to the bicipital groove and approximately 2 cm inferior to the normal insertion on the lesser tuberosity. The surgeon must be certain not to overtighten the repair by first checking that the subscapularis has adequate excursion and has been adequately released prior to completing the transfer. Once the transfer has been stapled in place, the arm should rotate at least to neutral or slightly beyond without the transfer pulling out. The author has used this transfer in more than 100 cases, and staple fixation has been uniformly successful in maintaining the subscapularis in its transferred position. Staple pull-out has not been observed. This method of fixation is desirable because it makes early rehabilitation of the shoulder possible.

Postoperative Care

A program of physiotherapy is begun 3 weeks after anterior shoulder repair. Initially, shoulder elevation is encouraged with the arm in internal rotation. Forward elevation is not restricted, and patients receive both passive and active range of motion exercises. The patient is instructed to lie flat several times a day and, with the help of his or her normal extremity, to bring the arm overhead. External rotation past neutral is not allowed for the first 6 weeks. At 6 weeks, a radiograph is taken to check the position of the staple, if one was used. At this point, active external rotation is encouraged and nonimpact resistive exercises can begin. A program of stretching and strengthening continues until the patient's progress plateaus, which is usually 3 to 4 months postoperatively. Patients can return to noncontact sports 3 months postoperatively and to contact sports 4 months postoperatively.

In the author's experience, complications are rare following anterior shoulder repair. The most devastating complication is infection and, fortunately, the infection rate is quite low. Other complications that can occur are:

1. recurrent instability
2. neurovascular injury
3. articular damage from hardware
4. severe postoperative stiffness
5. osteoarthritis
6. scar widening

Bony Procedures

In the past, many bony procedures have been described to stabilize the shoulder (Table 19–2). The success rates following bony procedures for anterior shoulder instability are no better than the success rates using soft tissue procedures. There is no convincing evidence that there is an abnormality of bony alignment in patients with anterior instability. The reported complication rates following bone block transfer and coracoid transfer about the shoulder are higher than with soft tissue procedures. Most bone transfers require the use of internal fixation, which is not desirable in the area of the glenoid. Furthermore, revision of a failed repair following a

TABLE 19–2 Bony procedures to treat anterior shoulder instability.

Procedure	Description
Eden-Hybbinette	Augmentation of anterior glenoid with iliac crest bone graft
Lange	Osteotomy of anterior glenoid combined with bone graft
Oudard	Prolongation of coracoid process with tibial bone graft
Trillat	Coracoid osteotomy and displacement combined with subscapularis displacement
Bristow-Helfet	Transfer of tip of coracoid and conjoined tendon to anterior scapular neck (suture fixation)
McMurray	Fixation of coracoid process to anterior glenoid with screw
Latarjet	Transfer of a large portion of the coracoid process to anteroinferior glenoid neck
Meyer-Burgdorff	Posterior closing wedge osteotomy of glenoid
Saha	Anterior opening wedge osteotomy of glenoid
Weber	Proximal humeral rotational osteotomy

bony transfer is exceedingly difficult due to scarring and distorted anatomy. For these reasons, the only bony operation that the author ever considers is the rotational osteotomy of the proximal humerus.

Proximal Humeral Osteotomy

Proximal humeral osteotomy is reserved for the uncommon situation of persistent instability following a soft tissue repair together with a large Hill-Sach's lesion. The proximal humerus is exposed through a deltopectoral incision. A longitudinal mark is made on the neck of the humerus with the saw blade so that rotation can be assessed after the osteotomy. The proximal portion of a T-plate (Synthes; Paozi, PA) is attached with three screws to the head, then the plate is removed prior to creating the osteotomy. The osteotomy is performed with a sagittal saw at the level of the surgical neck. The humerus is turned externally, and the osteotomy is fixed with the plate. Postoperatively, patients are immobilized in a Velpeau sling for 7 to 10 days. On the first postoperative visit, the Velpeau sling is converted to a regular sling. As soon as the staples or sutures have been removed, the patient is allowed to bathe. Movement of the arm is allowed, although the patient is instructed to avoid externally rotating the arm.

Repair Following Previous Surgery

More than one third of the surgical repairs for anterior instability performed by the author have been revision repairs. When confronted with a patient who has had previous surgery, it is important to determine what repair had been performed. Radiographs help assess hardware position, condition of the glenoid, size of the Hill-Sach's lesion, and the glenohumeral joint space. Patients who are to undergo revision surgery should be informed that the success rate for revision repair is lower than for primary repair. Nevertheless, the majority of patients who have recurrent instability can be successfully treated.

PEARL

Identification of both the musculocutaneous and the axillary nerves is advisable in patients who have had a coracoid transfer.

The surgical approach is no different from that described above. A deltopectoral incision is used regardless of previous incisions. The amount of scarring is variable in a revision surgery. Indeed, some patients have minimal scar, suggesting that a less than extensive soft tissue repair has been performed. The pathologic anatomy is variable in these cases. The exposure can be particularly difficult in patients who have had a coracoid transfer. Such patients require a exploration of both the musculocutaneous and the axillary nerves. These nerves are often lying in an altered position and can be surrounded by dense scar tissue. Great care must be taken to identify both nerves prior to attempting to mobilize the coracoid tendon, which may not be united firmly to the glenoid neck. After the space between the conjoined tendon and the subscapularis has been defined, the condition of the anterior soft tissues is determined. It is usually possible to dissect a

good portion of the subscapularis off the capsule and then repair the capsule and transfer the subscapularis, as described above. In some cases, particularly following multiple procedures, there is a severe anterior soft tissue deficiency. In this rare instance, consideration should be given to performing an external rotation, humeral osteotomy, particularly if there is a large Hill-Sach's lesion. If a sizable Bankart lesion is identified the labrum should be reattached. The conjoined tendon is sutured to the coracoid with a single Bunnell-type suture of no. 1 polyglycolic acid using a tapered needle. The sutures should be placed only in the tendinous portion of the muscle-tendon unit, because the musculocutaneous nerve may be close to the coracoid process. The suture is tied with the elbow flexed.

Following any revision procedure, there tends to be more restriction of external rotation than is seen following a primary procedure.

Posterior Instability

Patients requiring surgery for unidirectional posterior instability fall into two groups. The most common is recurrent posterior instability. Patients with posterior instability can present with subluxation, dislocation, or both. Posterior instability is more common than is recognized in most textbooks. Patients with recurrent posterior instability frequently have an element of pain associated with forceful or overhead use of the shoulder. Patients with recurrent posterior dislocations have an increased frequency of voluntary instability, although this is not necessarily due to a pathological personality. Forward elevation of the arm past 80 degrees with internal rotation can produce an uncomfortable (yet still voluntary) posterior subluxation or dislocation.

The second category of posterior instability is the chronic (locked) posterior dislocation of the glenohumeral joint. Patients with unreduced posterior dislocations may have associated fractures involving the posterior aspect of the glenoid and anterior aspect of the humeral head (reverse Hill-Sach's lesion). The method of surgical reconstruction is different for the two groups of patients. Treatment of the patient with a recurrent dislocation is described below.

Posterior Exposure

Through a posterior, J-shaped incision (Fig. 19–7) the insertion of the infraspinatus tendon is exposed. The muscle tendon unit is brought into view by flexing the arm 15 degrees. A horizontal, mattress suture is placed in the infraspinatus insertion. The interval between infraspinatus and teres minor is developed, and the posterior capsule of the glenohumeral joint is identified (Fig. 19–16). The muscle can be easily separated from the capsule if the dissection is performed in the correct plane. Laterally, the tendon becomes contiguous with the capsule. Once the plane between the capsule and the muscle is developed, a 1/2-inch Penrose drain is passed beneath the muscle with a Kelly clamp and grasped with a snap. A similar maneuver is used to separate the muscle belly of the teres minor from the posterior capsule. Sutures are placed in the tendinous insertion of both the infraspinatus and the teres minor. Sharp dissection with a no. 15 blade is used to elevate

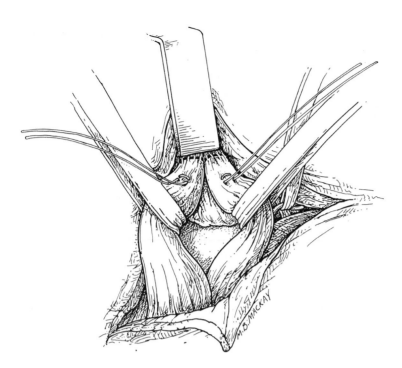

Figure 19–16 Separation of the infraspinatus and the teres minor from the posterior capsule of the glenohumeral joint. Reproduced with permission from Richards, RR. *Soft Tissue Reconstruction in the Upper Extremity.* New York, NY: Churchill Livingstone; 1995.

the infraspinatus and teres minor tendons from the posterior capsule en masse. The posterior capsule is exceedingly thin, and care must be taken not to cut into it. Elevation of the muscle from the capsule with the Penrose drain aids this dissection. Care is taken to avoid excess traction on the infraspinatus so as to avoid injuring the suprascapular nerve as it enters the muscle belly near the spinal-glenoid notch. Laterally sharp dissection must be used to define the capsular layer.

After mobilization of both the teres minor and infraspinatus insertions, the muscle tendon units are pushed medially. With the second assistant holding the arm in neutral rotation, the posterior capsule is grasped with two Kocher clamps midway between the capsular insertion on the tuberosity and the capsular origin on the glenoid. A longitudinal (vertical) arthrotomy is performed (Fig. 19–17). A humeral head retractor is used to displace the humerus anteriorly. The posterior

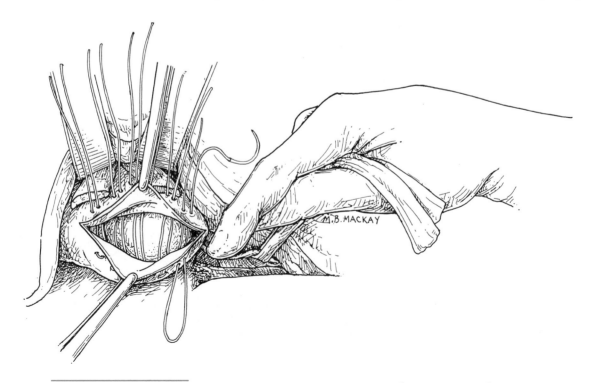

Figure 19–17 Placement of capsular sutures to repair posterior arthrotomy and tighten posterior capsule. Reproduced with permission from Richards, RR. *Soft Tissue Reconstruction in the Upper Extremity.* New York, NY: Churchill Livingstone; 1995.

labrum is carefully inspected. Loose bodies or cartilage fragments within the joint are debrided. The anterior aspect of the humeral head is palpated for the presence of a reverse Hill-Sach's defect. The pathology in patients with recurrent posterior instability is variable. A Bankart lesion is distinctly uncommon. The Bankart phenomenon with scuffing of the capsule posteriorly is seen frequently. If detachment of the labrum has occurred, the labrum should be reattached with sutures. The primary pathology in most patients is laxity of the posterior and inferior capsule.

PITFALL

During the posterior exposure, care must be taken to avoid excess traction on the infraspinatus so as to avoid injuring the suprascapular nerve as it enters the muscle belly near the spinal-glenoid notch.

Posterior Capsulorrhaphy

Retractors are positioned to protect the axillary nerve. Horizontal, mattress sutures of no. 1 nonabsorbable braided polyester suture are placed to reduce the volume of the inferior and posterior capsule (Fig. 19–18). All four sutures are placed prior to tying any single suture. The amount of tissue gathered together should be such that the arm can internally rotate to just past neutral after placement of these sutures.

Although this may seem to be an inordinate amount of capsule to imbricate, the posterior capsule is thin and flimsy. The repair usually stretches in the postoperative period. It is better to have it tight rather than loose at the conclusion of the procedure. The sutures are tied with the arm in neutral rotation. The posterior capsule is palpated to be certain that the closure is water tight.

Transfer of Teres Minor and Infraspinatus Insertions

With the arm held in external rotation, a Homan retractor is placed beneath the deltoid. The teres minor and infraspinatus insertions are transferred 2.5 cm laterally. Two horizontal sutures are placed in each tendon, and the tendon is sutured to the soft tissues overlying the humeral head in the new position. The knot in the horizontal mattress suture should lie on top of the tendon insertion in its new location. Because the arm is held in external rotation, these sutures should be placed as deeply as possible to provide secure fixation. The muscle tendon units are usually quite pliable, and transfer laterally is not met with significant resistance. Once completed, the arm usually cannot be passively internally rotated past the neutral position. This is not a concern because the repair will stretch out with the passage of time.

The axillary nerve is again palpated making certain that no suture material has penetrated the nerve. The Penrose drain on the axillary nerve is removed, and the wound is irrigated. The deltoid is reattached to the spine of the scapula (Fig. 19–19). Three or four drill holes are made in the spine of

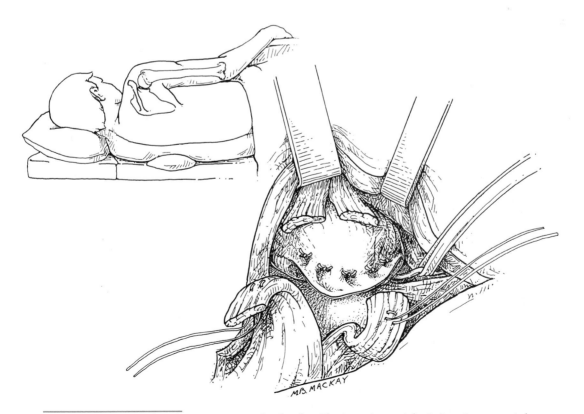

Figure 19–18   Completed posterior capsulorrhaphy. The insertions of the infraspinatus and the teres minor are about to be transferred laterally. Reproduced with permission from Richards, RR. *Soft Tissue Reconstruction in the Upper Extremity.* New York, NY: Churchill Livingstone; 1995.

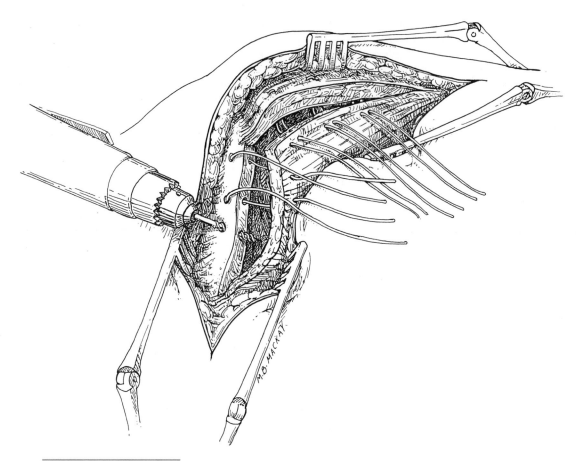

Figure 19–19 Reattachment of the deltoid to the spine of the scapula through drill holes. Reproduced with permission from Richards, RR. *Soft Tissue Reconstruction in the Upper Extremity.* New York, NY: Churchill Livingstone; 1995.

the scapula. To provide secure fixation, the reattachment is performed with interrupted horizontal sutures with no. 1 polyglycolic acid. The fascia overlying the deltoid is closed with no. 2-0 polyglycolic acid sutures on a tapered needle. The subcutaneous tissues and skin are closed in a routine fashion. In the operating room, a padded dressing is applied to the wound. The arm is held in external rotation, and a pillow is placed between the arm and the chest. A swath is applied to immobilize the upper extremity in neutral rotation with the elbow flexed 90 degrees. It is necessary to sit the patient up with the endotracheal tube in place while the pillow and swath is applied.

Postoperative Care

On the first postoperative day a thermoplastic splint is constructed. This splint rests on the iliac crest and is suspended by a padded strap from the opposite shoulder. A gutter-type attachment is constructed for the arm with the shoulder in adduction, slight extension, and neutral rotation. Velcro straps are used to secure the arm to the gutter portion of the splint. Care is taken to pad the elbow in the vicinity of the ulnar nerve to avoid a compressive neuropathy.

The splint is worn full-time for 1 month. It can be removed to bathe once the skin sutures or staples have been removed. After 1 month, a program of active and passive assisted exercises begins. The assistance of a physiotherapist is required to supervise the rehabilitation program. Patients exercise their shoulders several times per day and at least 3 times per week under supervision. Nonimpact strengthening is begun 6 weeks after surgery, and a program of stretching and strengthening continues until the patient's progress plateaus; usually 3 or 4 months after surgery. It is expected that patients will regain full forward elevation with some restriction of internal rotation. Some surgeons prefer a less extensive soft tissue repair for recurrent posterior instability. It has been the author's practice to tighten virtually all of the posterior soft tissues. Further comparative studies are needed to determine whether this is necessary. Certainly, patients with posterior instability fall into different demographic subgroups according to age, sex, and activity level. As experience with posterior repair develops, it is possible that subgroups of patients may be defined that require less repair than those described here. However, the author has not had cause to regret the extent of the repair described above because the recurrence rate following surgery is low. The author has not found it necessary to perform glenoid osteotomy or a bone block procedure when reconstructing shoulders for recurrent posterior instability.

Multidirectional Instability

The capsular shift procedure has been advocated for patients with multidirectional instability. Patients with multidirectional instability have, in addition to anterior or posterior instability (or both), inferior subluxation of the humeral head. The capsular shift procedure seeks to tighten the inferior capsule to "suspend" the capsule from the superior structures. The capsular shift can be performed either anteriorly or posteriorly, depending on the primary direction of instability. Because the capsular tissue is much thicker anteriorly, the procedure is more easily performed anteriorly. Key components of the capsular shift procedure include rotation of the capsule to reduce the size of the inferior capsular pouch. In addition the rotator interval must be carefully closed. The reader is referred to the paper by Neer and Foster (1980) for the details of the operative technique.

It is not certain that the capsular shift procedure is superior to other forms of capsulorrhaphy. The author uses one of the repairs described above for patients with multidirectional instability. The choice of which repair to use is dependant on the primary (most symptomatic) direction of instability. If the primary direction of instability is uncertain after history, physical examination, review of the radiographs, and examination of the shoulder under anesthesia, the repair is done anteriorly. The reason for this is that the capsule is much thicker anteriorly and postoperative treatment does not require the use of a brace.

SUMMARY

Reconstructive procedures are indicated for recurrent episodes of shoulder instability. At present, there is no role recognized for early surgery apart from inability to reduce the shoulder due to soft tissue interposition or the presence of a displaced fracture of the glenoid rim as described above. The role of early surgery for patients who have had a single dislocation is quite controversial and needs further scientific study before a definitive statement can be made in this regard.

Shoulder instability is primarily a soft tissue problem. The bony changes that occur in patients with shoulder instability are usually secondary. An accurate diagnosis is required to direct surgical treatment appropriately. Surgical rebalancing of the soft tissues necessitates an accurate diagnosis, good exposure, and an understanding of the periarticular anatomy. Surgery is combined with a comprehensive rehabilitation program so that a functional range of motion is obtained postoperatively. Recurrence rates following surgery should be low if the pathology observed in any single patient is addressed at the time of surgery. Revision surgery is required for patients with recurrent instability after a previous repair or unrecognized or untreated chronic dislocations that are symptomatic. Only a minority of patients with shoulder instability require bony procedures to restore stability to the shoulder.

ACKNOWLEDGMENT

The author wishes to thank Margot MacKay, ANSCA, BSc AAM, Division of Biomedical Communication, Department of Surgery, University of Toronto, for creating some of the illustrations.

SELECTED BIBLIOGRAPHY

BANKART ASB. Recurrent or habitual dislocation of the shoulder joint. *Br Med J.* 1923;2:1132.

BANKART ASB. The pathology and treatment of recurrent dislocation of the shoulder joint. *Br J Surg.* 1939;26:23.

BLOM S, DAHLBACK LO. Nerve injuries in dislocations of the shoulder joint and fractures of the neck of the humerus. *Acta Chir Scand.* 1970;136:461–466.

BROSTROM LA, KRONBERG M, SODERLUND V. Surgical and methodologic aspects of proximal humeral osteotomy for stabilization of the shoulder joint. *J Shoulder Elbow Surg.* 1993;2:93–98.

BURKHEAD WZ, SCHEINBERG RR, BOX G. Surgical anatomy of the axillary nerve. *J Shoulder Elbow Surg.* 1992;1:31–36.

CAVE EF, BURK JF, BOYD RJ: *Trauma Management.* Chicago, IL: Year Book Medical Publishers; 1974.

COOPER DE, ARNOCZKY SP, O'BRIEN SJ, WARREN RF, DICARLO E et al. Anatomy, histology, and vascularity of the glenoid labrum; an anatomical study. *J Bone Jt Surg.* 1992;74A:46–52.

COOPER RA, BREMS JJ. The inferior capsular shift procedure for multidirectional instability of the shoulder. *J Bone Jt Surg.* 1992;74A:1516–1521.

FLATOW EL, MILLER SR, NEER CS. Chronic anterior dislocation of the shoulder. *J Shoulder Elbow Surg.* 1993;2:2–10.

HARRYMAN DT, SIDLES JA, HARRIS SL, MATSEN FA. Laxity of the normal glenohumeral joint: a quantitative in vivo assessment. *J Shoulder Elbow Surg.* 1992;1:66–76.

HARRYMAN DT, SIDLES JA, HARRIS SL, MATSEN FA. The role of the rotator interval capsule in passive motion and stability of the shoulder. *J Bone Jt Surg.* 1992;74A:53–66.

HAWKINS RJ, ANGELO RL. Glenohumeral osteoarthrosis: a late complication of the Putti-Platt repair. *J Bone Jt Surg.* 1990;72A:1193–1197.

HAWKINS RJ, KOPPERT G, JOHNSTON G. Recurrent posterior instability (subluxation) of the shoulder. *J Bone Jt Surg.* 1984;66A:169–174.

HOVELIUS L. Anterior dislocation of the shoulder in teenagers and young adults: five year prognosis. *J Bone Jt Surg.* 1987;69A:393–399.

LIPPIT SB, VANDERHOFFT JE, HARRIS SL, SIDLES JA, HARRYMAN DT, MATSEN FA. Glenohumeral stability from concavity-compression: a quantitative analysis. *J Shoulder Elbow Surg.* 1993;2:27.

LUSARDI DA, WIRTH MA, WURTZ D, ROCKWOOD CA. Loss of external rotation following anterior capsulorraphy of the shoulder. *J Bone Jt Surg.* 1993;75A:1185–1192.

JOBE FW, GIANGARRA CE, KVITNE RS et al. Anterior capsulolabral reconstruction of the athlete in overhand sports. *Am J Sports Med.* 1991;19:429–434.

MATSEN FA III, THOMAS SC, ROCKWOOD CA JR. Anterior glenohumeral instability. In: ROCKWOOD CA JR, MATSEN FA III, eds. *The Shoulder.* Philadelphia, PA: WB Saunders; 1990;526–622.

NEER CS II, FOSTER CR. Inferior capsular shift for involuntary inferior and multidirectional instability of the shoulder: a preliminary report. *J Bone Jt Surg.* 1980;62A:897–908.

NORRIS TR. Diagnostic techniques for shoulder instability. *Instr Course Lect.* 1985;34:239–257.

O'DRISCOLL SW, EVANS DC. Long-term results of staple capsulorraphy for anterior instability of the shoulder. *J Bone Jt Surg.* 1993;75A:249–258.

POLLOCK RG, BIGLIANI LU. Glenohumeral instability: evaluation and treatment. *J Am Acad Orthop Surg.* 1993;1:24.

RICHARDS RR, DELANY J. Syringomyelia presenting as shoulder instability. *J Shoulder Elbow Surg.* 1992;1:151–161.

RICHARDS RR, HUDSON AR, BERTOIA JT, URBANIAK JR, WADDELL JP. Injury to the brachial plexus during anterior shoulder repair: a report of eight cases. *Am J Sports Med.* 1987;15:374–380.

ROWE CR, PATEL D, SOUTHMAYD WW. The Bankart procedure: a long-term end-result study. *J Bone Jt Surg.* 1978;60A:1–16.

SCHWARTZ RE, TORZIN PA, WARREN RE. Capsular restraints to antero-posterior shoulder motion of 5 Trans. *Orth. Ros. Soc.* 1987;12, 78.

TAMAI K, SAWAZAKI Y, HARA I. Efficacy and pitfalls of the STATAK soft-tissue attachment device for the Bankart repair. *J Shoulder Elbow Surg.* 1993;2:216–220.

WEBER BG, SIMPSON LA, HARDEGGER F, CALLEN S. Rotational humeral osteotomy for recurrent anterior dislocation of the shoulder associated with a large Hill-Sach's lesion. *J Bone Jt Surg.* 1984;66A:1443–1450.

YONEDA B, WELSH RP, MACINTOSH DL. Conservative treatment of shoulder dislocations in young males. *J Bone Jt Surg.* 1982;64B:254.

YOUNG DC, ROCKWOOD CA JR. Complications of a failed Bristow procedure and their management. *J Bone Jt Surg.* 1991;73A:969–981.

ZUCKERMAN JD, MATSEN FA III. Complications about the glenohumeral joint related to the use of screws and staples. *J Bone Jt Surg.* 1984;66A:175–180.

SAMPLE QUESTIONS

1. The most common type of shoulder instability is:
   (a) sternoclavicular
   (b) acromioclavicular
   (c) posterior glenohumeral
   (d) anterior glenohumeral
   (e) multidirectional

2. When intermediate loads are applied to the shoulder it is stabilized by:
   (a) "stiction-friction"
   (b) periarticular muscle action
   (c) passive mechanisms
   (d) static constraints
   (e) all of the above

3. Bankart lesions are _____ present in cases of anterior shoulder instability.
   (a) always
   (b) never
   (c) often
   (d) sometimes
   (e) rarely

4. Patients over age ____ usually tear their rotator cuff when they sustain an anterior shoulder dislocation.
   (a) 25
   (b) 30
   (c) 40
   (d) 50
   (e) 60

5. Bony procedures are _____ indicated for the surgical treatment of anterior shoulder instability.
   (a) never
   (b) often
   (c) frequently
   (d) almost never
   (e) usually

Answers: 1 (d); 2 (b); 3 (c); 4 (e); 5 (d)

Chapter 20

Rotator Cuff Disease

Julian S. Arroyo, MD, Evan L. Flatow, MD, and Louis U. Bigliani, MD

Shoulder disorders, in particular disorders of the rotator cuff, are one of the most common pathologies encountered by orthopaedists today. In 1972, Charles Neer, MD, revolutionized the understanding of rotator cuff problems by demonstrating that impingement is a common cause of rotator cuff pathology. Treatment of rotator cuff disorders has been directed by Neer's principles. Recently, with the increasing use of arthroscopy, more information is becoming available for rotator cuff pathology and new methods are being successfully developed to treat these disorders.

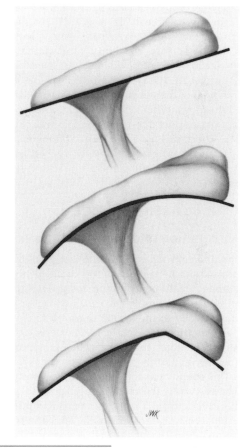

Figure 20–1 Acromion morphology. When seen on the supraspinatus outlet view, the acromion has one of three shapes. Type I is flat, type II is curved, and type III is hooked.

ETIOLOGY

More than 60 years ago, Meyer (1937) implicated mechanical attrition under the acromion in the pathogenesis of rotator cuff tendon defects. In 1972, Neer described the impingement syndrome, in which the supraspinatus tendon is compressed at its insertion on the greater tuberosity as it passes underneath the coracoacromial arch when the arm is used in the overhead position. Neer hypothesized that variation in acromial shape and morphology is clinically relevant and suggested that 95% of cuff tears are caused by subacromial impingement. Bigliani and coworkers (1986) demonstrated a

relationship between acromial morphology and the incidence of rotator cuff tears in cadavers. They described three acromial shapes: type I, flat, with a low incidence of rotator cuff tears; type II, curved; and type III, hooked, with a high incidence of tears (Fig. 20–1).

More recently, it has been suggested that impingement may not be the initiating event but may occur secondary to upward subluxation of the head in the absence of structural abnormalities in the coracoacromial arch. Another hypothesis is that tendon degeneration occurs first, causing kinematic

Orthopaedic Surgery: The Essentials. Edited by M.E. Baratz, A.D. Watson, and J.E. Imbriglia. Thieme Medical Publishers, Inc., New York © 1999

abnormalities and secondary impingement. However, theories of intrinsic tendon degeneration do not explain why the supraspinatus is almost always the site of initial tendon failure, or why all shoulders do not develop rotator cuff tears.

Rathbun and Macnab (1970) looked at the vascularity of the rotator cuff through injection studies. They found that when the arm is at the side there is a relatively avascular area at the insertion of the supraspinatus, correlating with the most frequent site of cuff tears. They have proposed that this relative avascularity may play a role in the origin of rotator cuff tears. Other investigators have failed to find an avascular zone. There is still debate in the literature regarding the vascularity of the rotator cuff tendons and its role in tendon failure.

Other proposed mechanisms for tendon failure include varying material properties leading to shear between fiber bundles, repetitive overhead arm use, acute trauma, glenohumeral dislocations, tensile overload, aging, altered glenohumeral kinematics (i.e., instability), and matrix changes induced by the loading environment. A consensus is emerging that rotator cuff disease has a multifactorial etiology. However, not all of these factors are amenable to treatment (e.g., tendon aging). Whether subacromial impingement is the primary cause rather than one among several, or even just a secondary effect, it is usually a source of ongoing tendon damage. For this reason, acromioplasty has become a standard part of most rotator cuff surgery.

BASIC SCIENCE

Function and Biomechanics

The primary function of the rotator cuff is to act as a humeral head depressor and dynamic stabilizer of the glenohumeral joint. Its other functions include forming a fulcrum from which the deltoid can elevate the arm. The rotator cuff also contributes directly to the torque required to elevate the shoulder and contributes to internal and external rotation of the humerus. The supraspinatus lies across the top of the glenohumeral joint and its contraction provides joint compression. This counteracts the shear force generated by the deltoid while elevating the arm. The supraspinatus also aids the deltoid in abduction. The infraspinatus and teres minor both function as external rotators of the arm. The subscapularis acts as an internal rotator as well as a powerful dynamic barrier to anterior displacement of the humeral head. The long head of the biceps tendon is thought to contribute to the dynamic superior stability of the humeral head, however, electromyographic studies show the biceps to be electrically silent during shoulder elevation.

Elevation of the arm is produced by a combination of the deltoid and rotator cuff acting through the glenohumeral joint and scapulothoracic articulation. The overall contribution of the glenohumeral-scapulothoracic motion is 2:1.

Rotation of the scapula is important in overhead arm activity. Through the scapulothoracic articulation, the trapezius and serratus anterior act on the scapula to rotate it during abduction. The glenoid is therefore rotated with the humerus, maintaining stable contact with the humeral head. Rotation of the scapula also results in elevation of the acromion, consequently reducing impingement.

Remarkable function can be present in some patients despite massive rotator cuff tears, while in others loss of active elevation and/or external rotation can be extreme. Many biomechanical theories have been proposed to explain such findings, but confusion still exists. It has been shown that experimental tendon defects will permit superior humeral subluxation, but usually only when the edge of the tear approaches the humeral equator. In smaller tears, the remaining tendon transmits the force of the uninvolved muscles, and the thickness of the remaining tendon can have a "spacer effect," stuffing the subacromial space. In massive tears, the head can protrude through the defect, resulting in loss of active shoulder elevation.

PEARL

Rotator cuff repair appears to restore normal kinematics.

Recent interest has focused on the coracoacromial (CA) arch. In the past, it had been believed that all contact of the arch on the rotator cuff was potentially deleterious, encouraging a "more is better" approach to bone removal at acromioplasty. However, it has been shown that contact of the acromion and CA ligament on the underlying rotator cuff tendons and the greater tuberosity occurs in normal shoulders. This may have an important passive, stabilizing role against superior humeral subluxation, especially when a large rotator cuff tear has compromised the dynamic stabilizers.

ANATOMY AND SURGICAL APPROACHES

Anatomy

The shoulder girdle is made up by the humerus, scapula, and clavicle. The true diarthrodial joints include the glenohumeral, acromioclavicular, and sternoclavicular joints. There is also articulation between the humeral head and the CA arch as well as the scapula and thorax.

The CA arch includes the acromion, acromioclavicular (AC) joint, distal clavicle, and CA ligament. Between the CA arch and the head of the humerus lies the subacromial space with bursa and rotator cuff tendon.

There are 26 muscles controlling the shoulder girdle, 4 of which constitute the rotator cuff. The subscapularis arises from the anterior surface of the scapula and inserts onto the lesser tuberosity. It is innervated by the upper and lower subscapular nerves. The supraspinatus arises from the supraspinatus fossa of the scapula and attaches to the upper aspect of the greater tuberosity after passing beneath the acromion and AC joint. It is innervated by the suprascapular nerve. The infraspinatus originates from the infraspinatus fossa of the scapula and inserts onto the posterolateral aspect of the greater tuberosity. It is innervated by the suprascapular nerve as well. The fourth muscle making up the rotator cuff is the teres minor, arising from the lateral border of the scapula and inserting on the lower aspect of the greater tuberosity. It is innervated by a branch of the axillary nerve. The primary vascular supply to the rotator cuff arises from the anterior humeral circumflex, the subscapular, and the suprascapular arteries. There is a definable separation between the subscapularis and the supraspinatus termed the rotator cuff interval.

PEARL

A consistent landmark for the interval is the long head of the biceps tendon, which travels in the interval, separating the supraspinatus and subscapularis tendons.

Surgical Approaches

Proper patient positioning greatly enhances the exposure to the rotator cuff, whether an open or arthroscopic procedure is planned. We perform all our surgeries in a modified "beach chair" position with the torso angled approximately 60 degrees from the horizontal plane (Fig. 20–2). A head rest is used which allows access to the superior and posterior aspects of the shoulder. The arm is draped free allowing shoulder rotation, extension, and elevation. Two small towels are placed under the scapula to elevate the shoulder off the table. Typically, a regional anesthesia is given (i.e., interscalene block) with intravenous sedation.

Standard Superior Approach

Many skin incisions can be used to gain access to the rotator cuff, but in our experience the most versatile and cosmetic

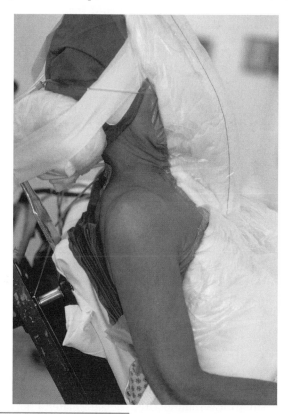

Figure 20–2 "Beach chair" position with the torso angled approximately 60 degrees from the horizontal plane.

incision is one extending from the middle of the acromion anteriorly to approximately 2 cm lateral to the coracoid in the lines of Langer (Fig. 20–3). This incision can be moved medially if access to the AC joint is necessary, or laterally if a large tear is anticipated, and the AC joint does not need to be addressed. We use this approach for all large and massive tears.

Following the skin incision, flaps are created at the level of the deltoid fascia extending from the AC joint to 6 cm lateral from the tip of the acromion. Great care needs to be taken not to injure the deltoid. The anterior deltoid is detached from the acromion. We prefer to use needle tip electrocautery and incise the deltoid approximately 5 mm anterior to the acromial edge. Electrocautery helps maintain hemostasis, particularly over the coracoacromial ligament, where the acromial branch of the thoracoacromial artery is frequently encountered. Incising the deltoid at this level leaves a stout remnant of deltoid fascia attached to the acromion for closure. The deltoid is incised from the AC joint to the anterolateral edge of the acromion and then split in line with its muscle fibers 3 to 5 cm laterally (Fig. 20–4). If the posterior portion of the cuff is thought to be intact, then the lateral split can be placed along the anterolateral raphe of the deltoid. However, by moving the split more posteriorly, greater exposure of the back of the cuff is possible. A stay suture is placed at the end of the split to avoid extension of the split and possible damage to the axillary nerve, which generally lies 5 to 6 cm from the tip of the lateral acromion. The split is deepened through the deltoid until the subacromial bursa is encountered. Medially, the deltoid is carefully incised to expose the CA ligament. The ligament is then detached subperiosteally.

Following a subacromial decompression (see Specific Conditions, Treatment, and Outcome), and mobilization and repair of the rotator cuff, the deltoid is repaired. A perfect repair of the deltoid is as important as the rotator cuff repair

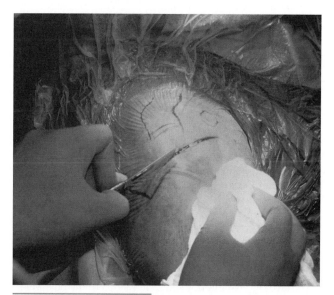

Figure 20–3 Skin incision in Langer's lines at the superoanterior aspect of the shoulder extending from the lateral aspect of the anterior third of the acromion inferiorly to the lateral aspect of the coracoid.

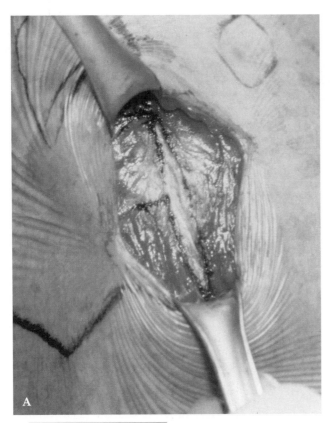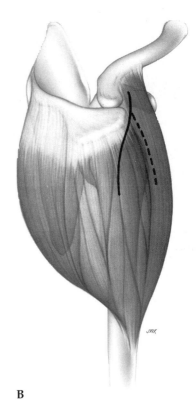

Figure 20–4   (**A**) Deltoid incision starting just anterior to the acromioclavicular joint and extending laterally to the lateral edge of the acromion, where it curves slightly posteriorly ending approximately 3 to 4 cm lateral to the lateral acromial edge. (**B**) The posterior curve of the deltoid incision allows the exposure to be centered over the greater tuberosity for better access to the cuff. The dotted line demonstrates the less desirable anterior exposure provided by the older and more anterior type of deltoid incision.

itself. Heavy No. 1 or No. 2 nonabsorbable suture is used to reattach the deltoid back to the remnant of tissue left on the anterior acromion. On occasion, sutures through the acromion itself will be necessary if the fascia on the deltoid does not provide a secure closure. The deltoid split is closed in a side-to-side fashion.

Arthroscopy

As previously mentioned, we perform all arthroscopies in the beach chair position with regional interscalene anesthesia. Prior to starting the arthroscopy, 10 to 15 mL of 0.25% bupivacaine with epinephrine is injected into the subacromial space. This distends the subacromial bursa, provides hemostasis, and also helps provide anesthesia for an extended period of time. The glenohumeral joint is accessed through a posterior portal located in the "soft spot" made up of the interval between the infraspinatus and the teres minor. The location of the soft spot varies from patient to patient, but typically it is 2 cm inferior and 2 cm medial to the posterolateral corner of the acromion. Care must be taken not to go below the teres minor because this is the quadrangular space that transmits the axillary nerve and posterior humeral circumflex artery. The glenohumeral joint is inspected with par-

ticular attention to the long head of the biceps tendon and the rotator cuff. The insertion of the rotator cuff is best visualized with the arm abducted 90 degrees and externally rotated. If a working portal is needed, it is placed anteriorly 1 cm lateral to the coracoid and brought in at the rotator cuff interval (between the biceps tendon and the subscapularis) under direct visualization from within the joint (Fig. 20–5). This is a dangerous portal in that if it is placed medial to the coracoid, the brachial plexus or brachial artery could be injured. If the portal is placed inferior to the coracoid, the axillary or musculocutaneous nerves may be injured.

Once the glenohumeral joint arthroscopy is completed, the subacromial space is entered through posterolateral and anterolateral portals. An arthroscopic bursectomy, anterior acromioplasty, and CA ligament resection is performed (see Specific Conditions, Treatment, and Outcome).

Mini-open Approach

All small or medium cuff tears are approached through a mini-open portal-extending incision following an arthroscopic anterior acromioplasty. The anterolateral portal is extended to a length of 3 cm, anterior to posterior, in the lines of Langer (Fig. 20–6). Once again, skin flaps are elevated at

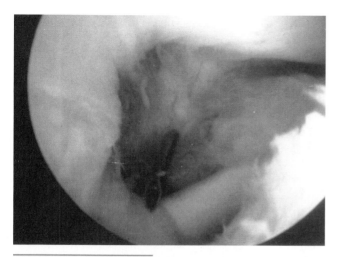

Figure 20–5 Creating an anterior portal under direct visualization. A 18-gauge spinal needle is introduced into the joint in the interval between the biceps tendon (top) and the tendon of the subscapularis (bottom).

the level of the deltoid myofascia to the lateral edge of the acromion. The deltoid is then split in line with its fibers to the lateral edge of the acromion and 3 to 5 cm laterally. The deltoid split should incorporate the small defect caused by the introduction of arthroscopic instruments. None of the deltoid is detached from the acromion. A stay suture is then placed in the deltoid to prevent propagation of the split and possible damage to the axillary nerve. By maneuvering the arm, the entire extent of the tear can be seen.

The mini-open approach provides good exposure of the supraspinatus and infraspinatus tendons, but access to the subscapularis and teres minor is difficult. For this reason, we use this approach only for small and medium cuff tears.

EXAMINATION

Patients with rotator cuff problems will typically complain of pain in their shoulder, especially with overhead arm activities. Their pain may be localized around the acromion or may be felt down the arm due to the extensive bursa extending under the deltoid. Patients will frequently have pain at night.

Visual inspection for shoulder symmetry will often reveal atrophy of the supraspinatus or infraspinatus. Range of motion of the shoulder should be performed actively and passively and compared with the asymptomatic side. Patients will often have decreased active range of motion with full passive motion. This deficit can be caused by weakness or pain. Subacromial injections with 1% lidocaine (Xylocaine) can be used to help distinguish between the two. If there is limited range of motion but no difference between active and passive, then adhesive capsulitis should be suspected.

Strength of the shoulder should be examined in forward elevation, abduction, and external rotation. For large or massive tears, strength may be reduced when compared with the contralateral side. The long head of the biceps tendon is frequently involved in large rotator cuff tears, and biceps symmetry and strength should be evaluated.

Provocative tests are used to elicit symptoms of impingement by maneuvering the biceps and rotator cuff under the CA arch. The Neer impingement test entails forward elevation with the arm internally rotated, while Hawkin's test for impingement is forward elevation to 90 degrees, adduction across the chest, and internal rotation. Both of these tests bring the biceps, rotator cuff, and greater tuberosity directly under the CA arch. However, these maneuvers may also cause pain in other shoulder conditions such as instability, stiffness, calcium deposits, arthritis, and bone lesions. In patients with classic impingement syndrome, pain will not only be produced by these impingement maneuvers but should be nearly completely eliminated following a subacromial injection of 10 mL of 1% Xylocaine.

AIDS TO DIAGNOSIS

Radiographs

Patients with rotator cuff pathology are evaluated with five views of the shoulder. Neutral, internal, and external rotation views are obtained to visualize the glenohumeral joint and greater and lesser tuberosities, and to bring small calcium deposits into relief. An axillary view is also obtained, again to visualize the glenohumeral joint, especially the glenoid and humeral tuberosities. This is the view used to see if there are any defects in the anterior or posterior aspects of the humeral head or glenoid. Finally, a supraspinatus outlet view will show the subacromial space and the CA arch. This view will reveal any spurs encroaching on the subacromial space and will determine the acromial shape (Fig. 20–7).

Arthrograms

Arthrograms are extremely accurate for the detection of full-thickness rotator cuff tears, but they do not give accurate information regarding tear size or the condition of the rotator cuff muscles.

PITFALL

An arthrogram is an invasive procedure.

Magnetic Resonance Imaging

As the quality improves and the price falls, magnetic resonance imaging (MRI) is rapidly replacing arthrograms as the study of choice to evaluate the rotator cuff. This noninvasive

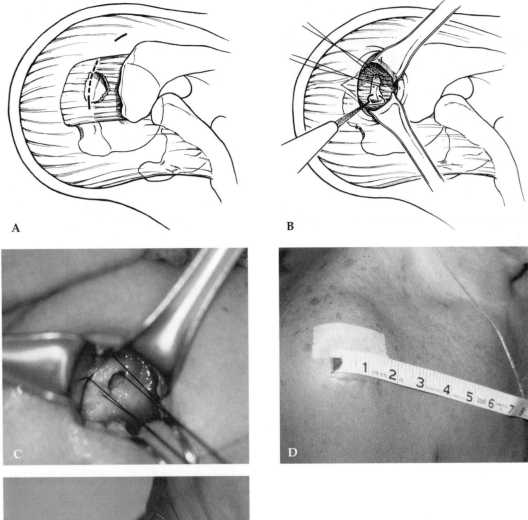

A

B

C

D

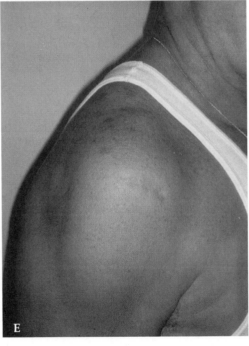

E

Figure 20–6 (**A**) The mini-open incision is placed directly over the tear as localized arthroscopically. Usually, the tear can be rotated to be under the anterolateral portal. The anterolateral portal is then extended to make a 3 cm-long incision in line with the skin creases. The deltoid is then split (but not detached) for 3 or 4 cm in line with fibers. (**B**) Rotator cuff repair is then performed as in a standard open procedure. (**C**) Stay sutures have been placed to mobilize a small supraspinatus tear. (**D**) The incision at 1-week follow-up. (**E**) Same incision at 1-year follow-up showing the cosmetic healing obtained with transverse incisions.

test provides much more information than an arthrogram. The quality of the rotator cuff muscles, the size of the tear, involvement of the biceps tendon, and partial cuff tears can clearly be determined. The accuracy in detecting full-thickness cuff tears has been reported to be between 93 and 100%. Partial-thickness tears are less accurately detected (Fig. 20–8).

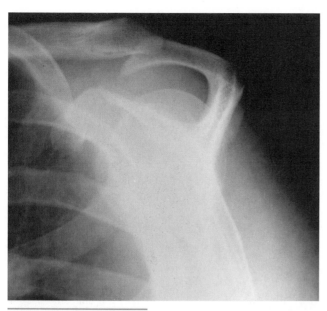

Figure 20–7 Supraspinatus outlet view showing a type III acromion.

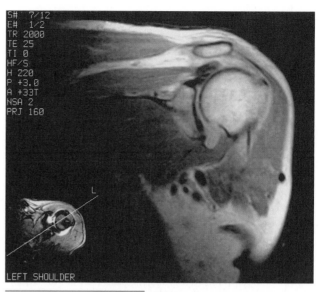

Figure 20–8 T1-weighted magnetic resonance image of a left shoulder with a large full-thickness rotator cuff tear. The supraspinatus tendon is retracted to the middle of the humeral head.

Not all patients with rotator cuff tears are symptomatic. Sher and associates (1995) looked at asymptomatic shoulders by MRI and found that 34% of patients had a rotator cuff tear. Of the patients past the age of 60, 54% had a rotator cuff tear, which was significantly higher than those patients between the ages of 40 and 60 (28%). The older patient group had significantly more full-thickness tears whereas the younger group had more partial-thickness tears. Based on these findings, caution must be used when interpreting MRI without clinical correlation.

SPECIFIC CONDITIONS, TREATMENT AND OUTCOME

Subacromial Impingement

Subacromial impingement results from contact between the rotator cuff and biceps tendon against the CA arch. This contact can cause an inflammatory response resulting in a subacromial bursitis, reducing the space for the rotator cuff tendons to glide beneath the acromion. Frequently, a spur will form from the anterior acromion in the CA ligament. This is best seen radiographically on the supraspinatus outlet view (Fig. 20–7). Neer (1972) demonstrated that this encroachment on the subacromial space by spurs and bursa leads to rotator cuff irritation. He described three phases of impingement based on the severity of disease. Phase I is acute inflammation with edema and hemorrhage in the rotator cuff tendon. Phase II involves fibrosis and tendonitis. In phase III, there is bone spur formation and a full-thickness cuff tear.

For phase I and II stages of impingement, patients will frequently respond to conservative therapy including rest, anti-inflammatories, subacromial injections of corticosteroids, and rotator cuff strengthening exercises. For resistant impingement and impingement associated with cuff tears, subacromial decompression is effective. A decompression can be performed through an open incision or arthroscopically. When there is no cuff tear or a small or medium tear, the authors prefer to perform the decompression arthroscopically.

Arthrsoscopic acromioplasties begin with glenohumeral joint inspection. Inflamed synovium is debrided, and glenohumeral pathology is addressed as indicated. Attention is then focused on the undersurface of the rotator cuff, evaluating for any irritation or tears (see Partial-thickness Rotator Cuff Tears). Once the glenohumeral joint has been examined, the subacromial space is entered with the arthroscope. Typically, a thick bursitis is encountered. This is removed with a 5.5-mm full-radius resector. Once there is good visualization of the subacromial space, the undersurface of the acromion and CA ligament are inspected. Often there is deep hemorrhage in the ligament and anterior aspect of the acromion from chronic impingement. The CA ligament often extends to the lateral aspect of the acromion and is frequently the primary source of subacromial impingement. Adequate removal of the CA ligament is an important step in an arthroscopic acromioplasty. Using electrocautery, the CA ligament is sequentially removed from the undersurface of the acromion and then at the CA ligament's margins laterally and medially. At this point, a full-radius resector will remove the ligament, or it can be removed in one piece with a grasper. The undersurface of the acromion, and frequently a spur, are now exposed with the ligament resection. A 6-mm tapered burr is used to perform the bony acromioplasty. The thickness and shape of the acromion, as well as the size of any bone spur, will dictate the amount of bone removed. On the average, only a small amount of bone is removed from the undersurface of the anteroinferior acromion. A smooth acromial undersurface should be achieved while establishing a smooth transition to the deltoid insertion. After decompression, the instruments are removed and portals are closed with absorbable suture. Postoperative exercises are started immediately and progressed as tolerated.

For open subacromial decompressions, see Rotator Cuff Repair.

There are a number of advantages of performing arthroscopic rather than open decompressions. The deltoid is damaged less because it does not have to be detached from the acromion as is necessary with an open decompression. Use of the arthroscope allows inspection of the glenohumeral joint as well as the undersurface of the rotator cuff. Any pathology encountered can then be addressed.

The results of arthroscopic subacromial decompressions are comparable with open decompressions. In a prospective, randomized study, Sachs and associates (1994) found that patients having an arthroscopic acromioplasty did better in the first 3 months following surgery than did patients undergoing an open procedure. After 3 months the two groups were equal. Long-term follow-up showed no difference between the two procedures, with an overall success rate of 90%. These findings are consistent with other reports in the literature.

Partial-thickness Rotator Cuff Tears

The literature remains unclear on treatment of partial-thickness rotator cuff tears. Recommendations range from conservative therapy to open rotator cuff debridement and repair. Our philosophy is to treat partial cuff tears the same as phase I and II impingement. We begin with conservative measures as outlined above. If conservative therapy fails, we will perform a shoulder arthroscopy to determine the depth and size of the tear. If the tear is less than 50% in thickness, then we will perform an arthroscopic cuff debridement followed by an anterior acromioplasty with CA ligament excision (Fig. 20–9). If the tear is greater than 50% in thickness in an active patient, we will perform the arthroscopic anterior acromioplasty and proceed to a portal extending mini-open rotator cuff debridement and repair. This will typically include an elliptical excision of the degenerative portion of the cuff tissue followed by a side-to-side repair. Occasionally, a tendon to bone repair will be required. For patients with partial tears of less than 50%, rehabilitation is the same as for patients undergoing arthroscopic anterior acromioplasty for chronic impingement. Those patients with tears greater than 50% having a mini-open procedure receive the same rehabilitation as patients with small full-thickness tears.

Snyder and coworkers (1991) reported their results for arthroscopic cuff debridement with or without subacromial decompression. They had 85% satisfactory results, with similar results between those patients having a decompression and those not having a decompression. The literature is still unclear whether an open debridement should be performed on tears less than 50% thick.

Weber (1994) reported on patients undergoing debridement of cuff tears that were greater than 50% both arthroscopically and through a mini-open approach. A higher percentage of the arthroscopic group had less than excellent

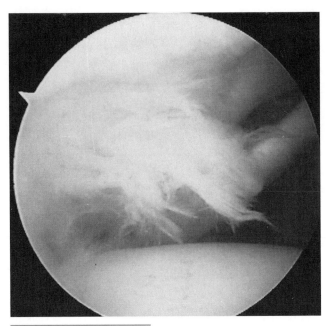

Figure 20–9 Arthroscopic view of a partial-thickness rotator cuff tear on the undersurface of the tendon. This tear involves less than 50% of the tendon and will be treated with debridement followed by an anterior acromioplasty.

results. These results are consistent with the literature supporting open debridement and tendon repair when there is greater than 50% thickness involved.

Full-thickness Rotator Cuff Tears

As previously mentioned, not all patients with rotator cuff tears are symptomatic. The indication for rotator cuff repair includes patients that are having pain and are limited in activities of daily living. Patients that are not having much pain but are weak should undergo a complete evaluation to ensure there is not an underlying neurological problem. Patients that are having pain with limited passive range of motion are initially placed on a physical therapy program to regain motion prior to any surgical intervention.

Prior to 1972, the results of rotator cuff repairs were less than acceptable. The failure rate was reported as high as 50%. In 1972, Neer described the association of subacromial impingement of the CA arch and rotator cuff tears. He recommended a subacromial decompression at the time of all rotator cuff repairs. Since that time, results have been consistently higher with predictable satisfactory results in both pain relief and function with the use of this approach.

As previously mentioned, for small and medium cuff tears we perform an arthroscopic anterior acromioplasty and a portal extending mini-open repair of the rotator cuff (Fig. 20–6). For large and massive tears, an open procedure is performed. (for approach see Anatomy and Surgical Approaches). For the large and massive tears, preservation and medialization of the CA ligament is routinely performed. The reason for this is to preserve the static superior stabilization for the humeral head and prevent any anterosuperior instability should the humeral head migrate superiorly. Preliminary results have been favorable. The ligament is separated from the deltoid prior to detachment from the acromion

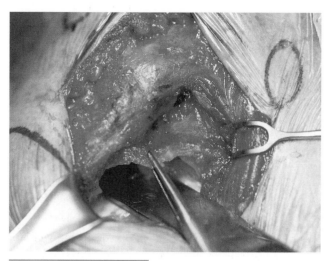

Figure 20–10 The coracoacromial (CA) ligament is identified as it inserts into the undersurface of the anterolateral aspect of the acromion.

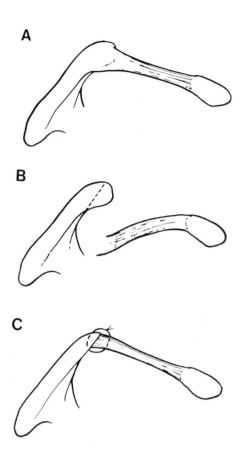

Figure 20–11 (**A**) An acromial spur will originate within the CA ligament. (**B**) Detachment of the ligament exposes the acromial spur. Depicted is the removal of the spur. This is routinely performed with a sharp osteotome and then smoothed with burr or rasp. (**C**) Reattachment of the CA ligament in its new position. After removal of the spur, the ligament is able to be reattached in a more superior position, thus preventing recurrence of any impingement.

(Fig. 20–10). The ligament is then detached with electrocautery from its insertion on the acromion, preserving as much length as possible. Removal of the acromial spur will also create length in the ligament (Fig. 20–11). The ligament is kept intact throughout the entire case and then reattached in a more medial position with heavy nonabsorbable suture. After removing the acromial spur, the ligament attachment is now superior to its previous position, reducing the chance of recurrent impingement.

Once the CA ligament is detached, there is excellent exposure of the anterior acromion and any spurs that may have developed (Fig. 20–12). An acromioplasty is performed. A wide osteotome is used to remove the anterior aspect of the acromion from the AC joint to the lateral edge of the acromion (Fig. 20–13). Depending on the thickness of the acromion and the size of any spurs, from 3 to 5 mm of bone is removed. The emphasis should be on contouring a smooth undersurface of the acromion. The wedge of bone excised should include the full width of the acromion from the medial to the lateral border (Fig. 20–14). If the AC joint is tender preoperatively, a distal clavicle excision is performed. This is done from the undersurface using either a rongeur or a burr. The superior AC ligaments are left intact for distal clavicle stability.

Once the acromioplasty is performed, the rotator cuff is more easily visualized. A bursectomy is performed for better visualization as well as to free the rotator cuff from any adhesions. Mobilization of the rotator cuff is the first step in repairing the tendon. Stay sutures are placed in the retracted rotator cuff tendon beginning anteriorly and working posteriorly. These can be used for traction while mobilizing the tendon. To mobilize the tendon, all adhesions are freed beginning on the superior, or bursal side. A periosteal elevator or scissors can be used to mobilize the cuff and its associated bursa from the undersurface of the acromion and deltoid. After the bursal surface is released and exposed, the posterior tissues are assessed to determine the full extent of the cuff tear. Usually, a portion of the posterior cuff remains attached to the humeral head.

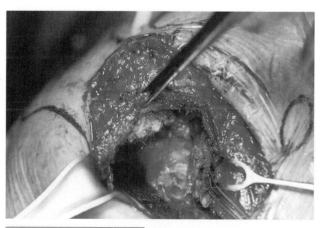

Figure 20–12 The cuff of strong, deltoid insertion tissue is meticulously elevated in a superior direction from the anterior part of the acromion allowing access for the anterior acromioplasty.

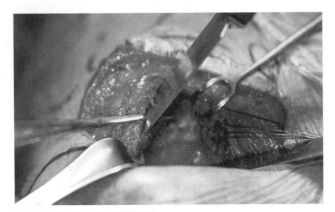

Figure 20–13 A thin and sharp beveled osteotome is used to perform the anterior acromioplasty. The osteotome is oriented in such a way as to remove a wedge of bone approximately 7 to 8 mm thick at the undersurface of the anterior one third to one half of the acromion.

Next the articular surface of the tendon is mobilized. This is typically done by spreading scissors or by blunt dissection because injury to the suprascapular nerve at the base of the scapular spine can occur as well as injury to the biceps tendon insertion (Fig. 20–15). Once the undersurface is freed, the excursion of the tendons is assessed (Fig. 20–16). For healing of the tendons to occur, there should be minimal tension with the tendons reaching the anatomic neck of the humerus while the arm is in 10 to 15 degrees of forward elevation and 10 degrees of abduction. If there is insufficient tendon to create a tension free repair, then an "interval slide" can be performed. This entails opening the rotator cuff interval between the supraspinatus and subscapularis to the base of the coracoid (Fig. 20–17). This will allow the supraspinatus to be mobilized 1 to 1.5 cm. The coracohumeral ligament is often contracted and can also be released to the base of the coracoid. If there is still tension posteriorly, a posterior release may be necessary. This is done by incising the tendon from the apex of the tear to the base of the scapular spine, which is the interval between the supraspinatus and infraspinatus. In

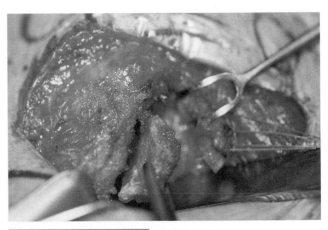

Figure 20–14 The piece should consist of the full width of the acromion from the medial to the lateral border as shown.

the majority of cases, these maneuvers will provide sufficient cuff mobilization to obtain a tension-free repair.

The greater tuberosity is prepared for tendon repair by freshening or "scarifying" the anatomical neck area with a rongeur or curette. A deep trough is not used as it requires more tendon mobilization and is not necessary to promote tendon-to-bone healing. Multiple drill holes are placed through the anatomic neck and lateral cortex at the greater tuberosity. No. 0 or No. 1 braided, nonabsorbable sutures are passed through the tunnels with a curved needle. The tendon is repaired to the greater tuberosity with the arm held in 10 to 15 degrees of flexion and 10 degrees of abduction (Fig. 20–18).

As previously discussed, if there is a large or massive tear, the CA ligament is repaired in a medial position. This provides a superomedial buttress, which may provide restraint from superior migration or anterosuperior instability of the humeral head. The deltoid is meticulously repaired as outlined in Surgical Approaches.

Depending on the quality of tissue and repair, postoperative rehabilitation follows the Neer protocol or a modification of this protocol to protect the repair. In all cases, a physician-directed rehabilitation program is begun on the first

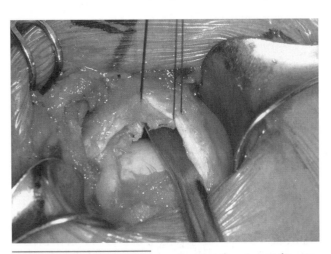

Figure 20–15 Stay sutures are placed at the edge of the rotator cuff tear and mobilization is begun with an elevator, which is used to free bursal adhesions and also to bluntly mobilize the cuff at the glenoid rim.

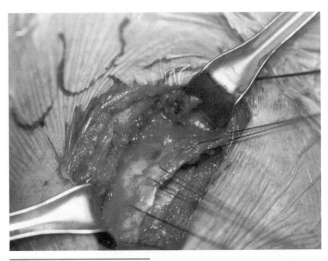

Figure 20–16 With mobilization completed in a sequential fashion, the cuff is able to be brought over the anatomical neck for repair.

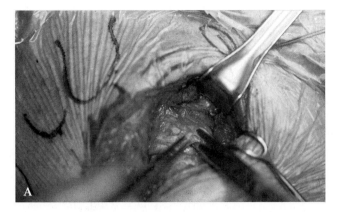

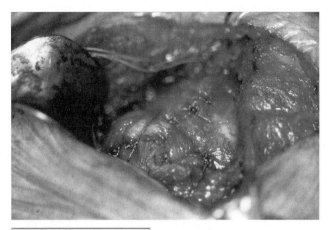

Figure 20–18 The sutures are tied over the bony bridges formed by the bone tunnels and excellent apposition of the bone and healing cuff edge is obtained.

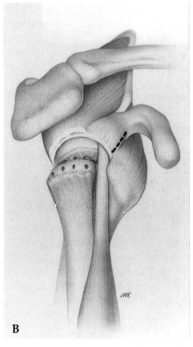

Figure 20–17 **(A)** To release scarring of the coracohumeral ligament at the base of the coracoid, an interval release is sharply performed with scissors, beginning laterally and incising directly to the coracoid base. **(B)** The complete release of the rotator interval and coracohumeral ligament is termed the "interval slide" as the tissues, once incised, are slid along the dotted line, thus mobilizing the retracted tissue in a lateral direction. Sliding the tissues in a lateral direction at the interval allows for 1 to 1.5 cm of new length for repair.

postoperative day. Passive motion is maintained for the first 6 weeks, and then active assisted and active exercises are added between 6 and 8 weeks postoperatively.

Using these principles for rotator cuff repair, Cofield (1985), in a review of the literature, found an average of 85% of patients having satisfactory results. Bigliani et al (1994) recently reported the results of rotator cuff repair in 486 patients and found 96% had satisfactory pain relief and 80% had substantial functional improvement. Functional outcome has been less predictable. Reports in the literature range from 75% to 95% of patients achieving significant improvement in shoulder function following rotator cuff repair. The literature

supports the premise that pain remains the primary indication for rotator cuff repair.

The results of arthroscopic acromioplasty with a mini-open rotator cuff repair are promising. Levy and coworkers (1991) reported 80% satisfactory results overall, while all patients with small or medium size cuff tears had a satisfactory result. Of the patients in the study, 96% were satisfied with the procedure. O'Boyle et al (1997) have recently reported their experience with mini-open rotator cuff repairs following an arthroscopic acromioplasty. All 30 of the patients had an excellent result at an average of 25 months of follow-up. The average hospital stay was only 1 day. All the tears in this study group were either small or medium.

Factors that influence the outcome of rotator cuff repair are the size of the tear, patient age, and preoperative function. Hattrup (1995) evaluated patient age with regard to outcome following rotator cuff repair. He was able to show that patients past the age of 65 tended to have poorer results as well as larger cuff tears. Cofield and coworkers (1995) found that tear size is the single most important factor influencing long-term results. Ellman and co-workers (1986) were able to show a correlation between a poor result and preoperative strength and active range of motion. If patients had grade 3/5 strength or less or were unable to abduct their shoulders beyond 100 degrees, there was an increased risk of a poor result. When patients have unsatisfactory results, it is usually associated with poor function and not pain relief. This is supported by Bigliani (1992) and Hawkins (1985), who found that there is good pain relief for repairs of massive tears, but functional improvement was less predictable.

Cuff Tear Arthropathy

Superior migration of the humeral head is frequently seen in rotator cuff deficient shoulders. The pull of the deltoid without the rotator cuff results in the humeral head translating superiorly and articulating with the undersurface of the acromion and CA arch.

The combination of a nonfunctioning rotator cuff, inactivity of the shoulder, leaking of synovial fluid, and instability of the humeral head results in both nutritional and mechanical factors that cause atrophy of the glenohumeral articular cartilage and osteoporosis of the subchondral bone of the humeral head. Eventually, radiographic evidence of degenerative changes becomes apparent. It is this combination of degenerative changes with a superiorly migrated humeral head that Neer in 1977 termed cuff-tear arthropathy. Patients will have pain associated with the degenerative changes and poor function due to the nonfunctioning rotator cuff.

Treatment of cuff-tear arthropathy begins with nonoperative measures including anti-inflammatories, physical therapy, and corticosteroid injections. If patients have continued pain despite a long course of conservative therapy, then surgery may be indicated. We prefer humeral head replacement both to avoid glenoid loosening (more likely due to eccentric superior loading in a cuff-deficient shoulder) and to maintain the new fulcrum the head has usually gained under the CA arch.

An extended deltopectoral approach is used, preserving the deltoid origin and insertion. The incision starts inferior to the clavicle and proceeds over the coracoid and obliquely toward the deltoid insertion. The interval between the deltoid and the pectoralis major is identified and developed, retracting the cephalic vein either medially or laterally. Slight abduction of the arm will release tension on the deltoid and facilitate this dissection. The clavipectoral fascia is incised, starting lateral to the coracoid and strap muscles. The subacromial space is cleared of bursal adhesions or scar. It is important to avoid damaging or resecting the CA ligament. Preserving the CA arch provides a buffer and superior stabilizer in such shoulders. The long head of the biceps also functions as a humeral depressor and superior stabilizer and should also be preserved, if it is intact.

The subscapularis tendon is often inferiorly retracted and the head protrudes superiorly, creating a boutonnière deformity. The subscapularis is incised at its bony insertion to maintain maximum length. The underlying capsule is often thin and attenuated, and it is usually incised together with the subscapularis. Traction sutures are placed in the cut edge of the subscapularis to allow gentle mobilization while minimizing tissue trauma.

The humeral head is dislocated by gentle external rotation and extension. If the biceps tendon is intact, care is taken to preserve it. It is helpful to fully visualize the posterior cuff insertion on the greater tuberosity to avoid damage during humeral head resection. The humeral head is resected with an oscillating saw. Osteophytes are removed to prevent impingement of the humerus on the glenoid and to allow maximal capsular mobility.

Attention is now turned to the rotator cuff. The posterior cuff is mobilized using traction sutures and both blunt and sharp dissection. The rotator cuff insertion is never detached posteriorly, as this can lead to further weakness of external rotation. The humeral head replacement is placed as described by Pollock et al (1992). The mobilized rotator cuff is repaired.

The wounds are irrigated. Suction drains are placed between the deltoid and rotator cuff and are brought through the deltoid and the skin through separate stab incisions. The deltopectoral interval is closed and, finally, the skin is closed with a subcuticular suture. The patient's arm is placed in a sling and swathe in the operating room.

On the first postoperative day, the swathe is removed, and the arm is maintained in a sling. Suction drains are likewise removed. Administration of perioperative antibiotics is continued for 24 to 48 hours. Passive range of motion exercises are begun on the first or second postoperative day, consisting of pendulum, elevation in the scapular plane, and external rotation exercises. These are performed with a physical therapist, under the surgeon's supervision, to stretch the tissues and maintain motion. Results with this approach have been surprisingly good.

SELECTED BIBLIOGRAPHY

ARROYO JS, HERSHON SJ, BIGLIANI LU. Special considerations in the athletic throwing shoulder. *Orthop Clin. North Am.* 1997;28:69–78.

BASMAJIAN J, DELUCA C. *Muscles Alive: Their Function Revealed by Electromyography.* Baltimore, MD: Williams and Wilkens; 1985.

BIGLIANI LU, CODD TP, FLATOW EL. Arthroscopic coracoacromial ligament resection. *Tech Orthop.* 1994;9:95–97.

BIGLIANI LU, CORDASCO FA, MCILVEEN SJ, MUSSO ES. Operative repair of massive rotator cuff tears: long-term results. *J Shoulder Elbow Surg.* 1992;1:120–130.

BIGLIANI LU, CORDASCO FA, MCILVEEN SJ, MUSSO ES. Operative treatment of failed repairs of the rotator cuff. *J Bone Jt Surg.* 1992;74A:1505–1515.

BIGLIANI LU, DURALDE XA, WEINSTEIN DM, BLACK AD, et al. Rotator Cuff Repair: Tecnhique and Long Term Results. *Orthop Trans.* 1994;18:1154–1155.

BIGLIANI LU, MORRISON DS, APRIL EW. The morphology of the acromion and its relationship to rotator cuff tears. 1986; *Orthop Trans.* 10:228.

BIGLIANI LU, RODOSKY MW. Techniques of repair of large rotator cuff tears. *Tech Orthop.* 1994;9:133–140.

BLEVINS FT, DJURASOVIC M, FLATOW EL, VOGEL KG. Biology of the rotator cuff tendon. *Orthop Clin. North Am.* 1997; 28:1–16.

COFIELD RH. Current concepts review: rotator cuff disease of the shoulder. *J Bone Jt Surg.* 1985;67A:974–979.

COFIELD RH, HOFFMEYER P, LANZAR WH. Surgical repair of chronic rotator cuff tears. *Orthop Trans.* 1990;14:251–252.

ELLMAN H. Arthroscopic subacromial decompression: analysis of one to three-year results. *Arthroscopy.* 1987;3:173–181.

ELLMAN H. HANKER G. BAYER M. Repair of the rotator cuff: end-result study of factors influencing reconstruction. *J Bone Jt Surg.* 1986;68A:1136–1144.

FLATOW EL, SOSLOWSKY LJ, TICKER JB et al. Excursion of the rotator cuff under the acromion: patterns of subacromial contact. *Am J Sports Med.* 1994;22:779–788.

FLATOW EL, WEINSTEIN DM, DURALDE XA, COMPITO CA, POLLOCK RG, BIGLIANI LU. Coracoacromial ligament preservation in rotator cuff surgery. *J Shoulder Elbow Surg.* 1994;3:S73.

FUKUDA H, HAMADA, K, NAKAJIMA T, TOMONAGA A. Pathology and pathogenesis of the intratendinous tearing of the rotator cuff viewed from en bloc histologic sections. *Clin Orthop.* 1994;304:60–67.

HATTRUP SJ. Rotator cuff repair: relevance of patient age. *J Shoulder Elbow Surg.* 1995;4:95–100.

HAWKINS RJ, ABRAMS J. Impingement syndrome in the absence of rotator cuff tear. *Orthop Clin North Am.* 1992;18:373–382.

HAWKINS RJ, MISAMORE GW, HOBEIKA PE. Surgery for full-thickness rotator-cuff tears. *J Bone Jt Surg.* 1985; 67A:1349–1355.

INMAN VT, SAUNDERS JB, ABBOTT LC. Observations on the function of the shoulder joint. *J Bone Jt Surg.* 1944;26:1–30.

LEVY HJ, GARDNER RD, LEMAK LJ. Arthroscopic subacromial decompression in the treatment of full-thickness rotator cuff tears. *Arthroscopy.* 1991;7:8–13.

LINDBLOM K. On pathogenesis of ruptures of the tendon aponeurosis of the shoulder joint. *Acta Radiol.* 1939; 20:563–577.

MEYER AW. Chronic functional lesions of the shoulder. *Arch Surg.* 1937;35:646–674.

MOSELEY HF, GOLDIE I. The arterial pattern of the rotator cuff of the shoulder. *J Bone Jt Surg.* 1963;45B:780–789.

NEER CS, II. Anterior acromioplasty for the chronic impingement syndrome in the shoulder: a preliminary report. *J Bone Jt Surg.* 1972;54A:41–50.

NEER CS, II. Impingement lesions. *Clin Orthop. North Am.* 1983;173:70–77.

O'BOYLE NT, ARROYO JS, CONNOR PM, LEVINE WN, et al. *Arthoscopically Assisted Rotator Cuff repair Through a Limited Portal-Extension.* Am Acad Orthop Surgeons, Sixty-fourth Annual Meeting, San Francisco, CA, February, 1997.

POLLOCK RG, DELIZ ED, MCILVEEN SJ, FLATOW EL, BIGLIANI LU. Prosthetic replacement in rotator cuff-deficient shoulders. *J Shoulder Elbow Surg.* 1992;1:173–186.

RATHBUN JB, MACNAB I. The microvascular pattern of the votator cuff. *J Bone Jt Surg.* 1970;52B:540–553.

SACHS RA, STONE ML, DEVINE S. Open vs. arthroscopic acromioplasty: a prospective, randomized study. *Arthroscopy.* 1994;10:248–254.

SHER JS, URIBE JW, POSADA A, MURPHY BJ, ZLATKIN MB. Abnormal findings on magnetic resonance images of asymptomatic shoulders. *J Bone Jt Surg.* 1995;77A:10–15.

SNYDER SJ, PACHELLI AF, DEL PIZZO W, FRIEDMAN MJ, FERKEL RD, PATTEE G. Partial-thickness rotator cuff tears: results of arthroscopic treatment. *Arthroscopy.* 1991;7:1–7.

SOSLOWSKY LJ, CARPENTER JE, BUCCHIERI JS, FLATOW EL. Biomechanics of the rotator cuff. *Orthop Clin North Am.* 1997;28:17–30.

SWIONTKOWSKI MF, IANNOTTI JP, BOULAS HJ, ESTERHAI JL. Intraoperative Assessment of Rotator Cuff Vascularity Using Laser Doppler Flowmetry. In: Post M, Morrey BF, Hawkins RJ, eds. *Surgery of the Shoulder.* St. Louis, MO: Mosby Year Book; 1990;202–212.

TURKEL SJ, PANIO MW, MARSHALL JL, GIRGIS FG. Stabilizing mechanisms preventing anterior dislocation of the glenohumeral joint. *J Bone Jt Surg.* 1981;63A:1208–1217.

WEBER SC. Arthroscopic vs. open treatment of significant partial-thickness rotator cuff tears. *Arthroscopy.* 1994;10: 356–366.

YAMAGUCHI K, FLATOW EL. Arthroscopic evaluation and treatment of the rotator cuff. *Orthop Clin North Am.* 1995;26: 643–659.

SAMPLE QUESTIONS

1. Which factor(s) has (have) been associated with patient outcome following rotator cuff surgery:
   (a) cuff tear size
   (b) patient age
   (c) preoperative strength
   (d) all of the above

2. Which anatomic structure is a part of the coracoacromial arch:
   (a) greater tuberosity
   (b) medial head of clavicle
   (c) acromion
   (d) coracoclavicular ligaments

3. Which tendon is most commonly involved in rotator cuff tears:
   (a) supraspinatus
   (b) infraspinatus
   (c) teres minor
   (d) subscapularis

4. Which lies in the rotator cuff interval:
   (a) infraspinatus
   (b) short head of the biceps
   (c) long head of the biceps
   (d) supraspinatus

5. Which type of acromion is associated with the highest incidence of rotator cuff tears:
   (a) type I (flat)
   (b) type II (curved)
   (c) type III (hooked)
   (d) none of the above

6. Which occupies the quadrangular space:
   (a) radial nerve
   (b) axillary nerve
   (c) anterior humeral circumflex artery
   (d) suprascapular nerve

Answers: 1) d; 2) c; 3) a; 4) c; 5) c; 6) b

Arthritis of the Shoulder

Mark W. Rodosky, MD

ETIOLOGY

Glenohumeral Arthritis

Degenerative disorders of the glenohumeral (GH) joint result in pain and dysfunction. The most prevalent of these include: primary osteoarthritis, post-traumatic osteoarthritis, rheumatoid arthritis, cuff tear arthropathy, avascular necrosis, and septic arthritis.

Osteoarthritis

Primary GH osteoarthritis is a common condition that should not be confused with the end stages of severe rotator cuff deficiency. Patients with primary GH osteoarthritis usually have an intact rotator cuff and long head of the biceps tendon. The disease is characterized by limited GH motion. The humeral head becomes enlarged by marginal osteophytes, particularly at the inferior margin of the joint (Fig. 21–1). Initially, thinning of the articular cartilage of the humeral head occurs in that area of the head that is in contact with the glenoid cavity when the humerus is in abduction. This results in greater wear on the superior part of the articular surface.

At the glenoid fossa, the wear is more pronounced posteriorly than anteriorly resulting in posterior bone loss (Fig. 21–1). Excessive posterior glenoid wear will create retroversion of the glenoid. Contractures of the anterior capsular structures and subscapularis increase the potential for posterior erosion of the glenoid.

Post-traumatic Arthritis

Post-traumatic arthritis can occur as a result of nonunion, proximal humeral fracture malunion and articular incongruency, recurrent dislocation or subluxation, and after surgical intervention for instability (Fig. 21–2). Soft tissue contractures are universally present in patients with post-traumatic arthritis. Most of the contracture involves the coracohumeral ligament and rotator interval tissue, resulting in an internal rotation contracture. Malunion of the tuberosity fragments results in an offset of the normal line of action for the rotator cuff muscles. This can lead to eccentric loading of the glenoid cavity compounded by soft tissue contracture. Tuberosity malunion can also result in subacromial impingement or coracoid impingement. Nonunion of the tuberosity fragments can cause contracture of that portion of the rotator cuff that attaches to the nonunited tuberosity. These nonunited tuberosity fragments may scar near the axillary nerve.

Rheumatoid Arthritis

Rheumatoid arthritis is a systemic disease that involves all the tissues of the GH joint including the muscles, bursa, and joint surfaces. Rheumatoid pannus will erode the joint surfaces. Erosion of the glenoid occurs in a protrusio pattern of destruction (Fig. 21–3). In some patients, the inferior aspect of the glenoid fossa remains intact, giving the glenoid surface a cephalic tilt. In others, the erosive pattern may be anterior or posterior, causing excessive anteversion or retroversion of the glenoid cavity.

Orthopaedic Surgery: The Essentials. Edited by M.E. Baratz, A.D. Watson, and J.E. Imbriglia. Thieme Medical Publishers, Inc., New York © 1999

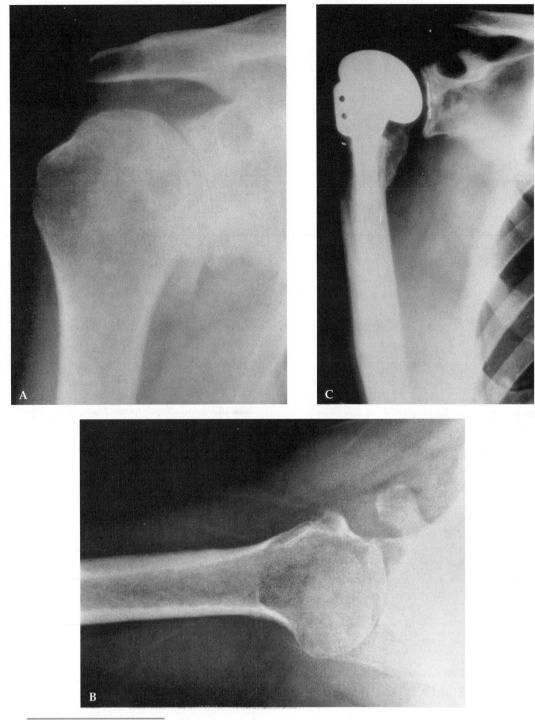

Figure 21–1 **(A)** Anteroposterior (AP) radiograph of a patient with primary glenohumeral (GH) osteoarthritis, demonstrating loss of cartilage space and large inferior humeral head osteophyte. **(B)** Axillary radiograph in the same patient demonstrating the posterior glenoid erosion that is commonly seen with primary GH osteoarthritis and results in glenoid retroversion. **(C)** AP radiograph in the same patient after a nonconstrained total shoulder replacement with a cemented metal humeral component and a cemented polyethylene glenoid component whose stem is marked by a staple.

As the disease progresses, the rotator cuff tissue is eroded by pannus, becoming thin and dysfunctional. Rotator cuff tears are present in 20 to 30% of patients with rheumatoid arthritis. With loss of the glenoid and humeral head surfaces and thinning of the rotator cuff, the humeral head migrates in a cephalad direction causing further erosion of the rotator cuff.

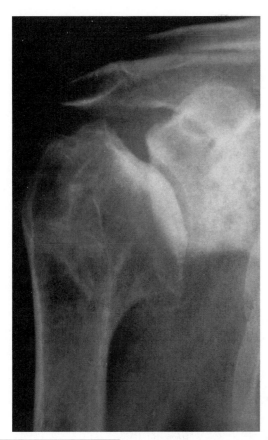

Figure 21–2   AP radiograph of a patient after a humeral head splitting fracture that resulted in a combination of post-traumatic arthritis (inferior GH incongruency) and avascular necrosis of the humeral head (superior collapse).

Cuff Tear Arthropathy

Rotator cuff tear arthropathy is related to a deficiency in rotator cuff function. This leads to an inability to keep the humeral head in contact with the glenoid fossa. The humeral head migrates proximally to abut the coaracoacromial (CA) arch, including the undersurface of the acromion and the acromioclavicular (AC) joint (Fig. 21–4). In addition, the humeral head may dislocate in an anteroinferior direction from the loss of the stabilizing effects of the posterior muscles of the rotator cuff. Abutment against the CA arch and the instability subjects the humeral head to unusual wear. The end result is cuff tear arthropathy characterized by an incongruous and distorted humeral head with superior erosion and subchondral collapse, as well as erosion of the undersurface of the acromion and AC joint. With advanced disease, the glenoid cavity can become eroded and incongruous.

Avascular Necrosis

Avascular necrosis of the humeral head is caused by a lack of blood supply to the bone. The etiology includes corticosteroid use, alcoholism, sickle cell disease, and trauma. The clinical manifestations are similar to that of primary osteoarthritis; however, motion is usually maintained even in the late phases of the disease process. The superior portion of the humeral head, which comes into contact with the glenoid at

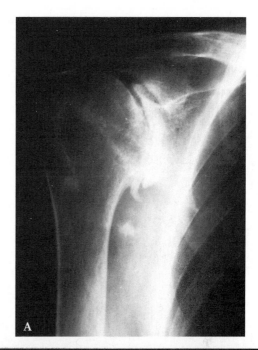

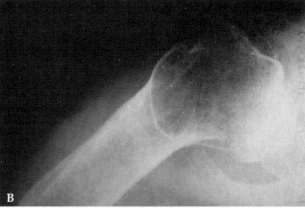

Figure 21–3   (**A**) AP radiograph of a patient with rheumatoid arthritis demonstrating osteoporosis and minimal osteophytic formation but extensive concentric erosion of the glenoid. (**B**) Axillary radiograph in same patient demonstrating extensive loss of glenoid with central erosion to the base of the coracoid process.

approximately 60 to 90 degrees of abduction, is the area prone to collapse (Fig. 21–2). The glenoid cavity is rarely affected to a degree that would necessitate glenoid resurfacing. The lesser and greater tuberosities are usually spared and the soft tissues and rotator cuff do not become significantly contracted. Shoulder arthroplasty in patients with avascular necrosis of the humeral head is usually successful. A small number of such patients present with rapid collapse of the humeral head that progresses to the point of fracturing of the greater and/or lesser tuberosities.

The pathological changes that occur in avascular necrosis are explained by the type of joint contact that occurs at the glenoid fossa. The glenoid contacts the humeral head with maximal pressure at approximately 90 degrees of elevation, which correlates to contact at 60 degrees of GH elevation. This area of contact at the humeral head is the site of collapse. Four

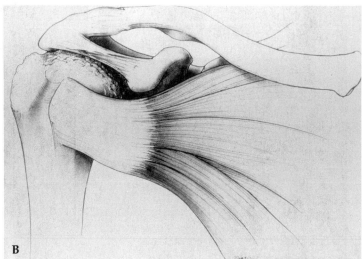

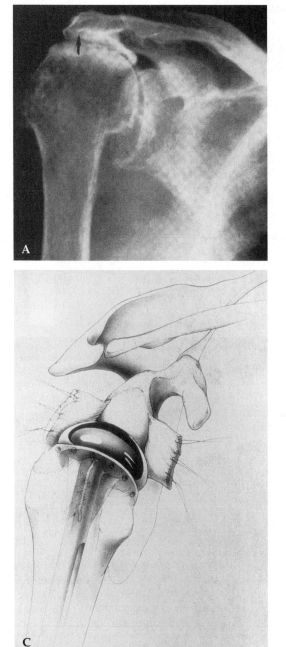

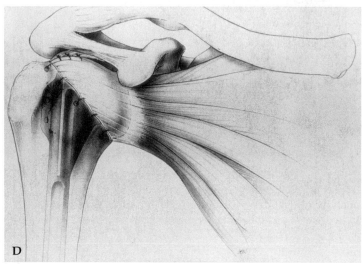

Figure 21–4 (**A**) AP radiograph of the GH joint in a patient with cuff tear arthropathy. (**B**) The rotator cuff deficiency allows proximal migration of the humeral head with erosive changes occurring at the acromion. (**C**) The rotator cuff is mobilized and the humeral head replaced. (**D**) The rotator cuff is repaired to bone around the prosthesis with an emphasis towards anteroposterior stability over complete superior coverage. Reproduced with permission from Rodosky MW, Bigliani LU. Indications for glenoid resurfacing. *J Shoulder Elbow Surg.* 1996;5:244.

stages of avascular necrosis of the humeral head have been described by Neer (1990). Stage I shows subtle sclerotic changes in the humeral head. In stage II, a "meniscal sign" is visible that represents a small area of subchondral collapse. In stage III, the disease is characterized by a "step off" sign with collapse of subchondral bone and the overlying cartilage. In stage IV, the collapse continues resulting in further incongruencies and degenerative changes in the glenoid cavity.

Acromioclavicular Arthritis

Acromioclavicular degenerative arthritis can result from trauma, such as an intra-articular distal clavicle fracture. Osteolysis of the distal clavicle may also follow trauma to the AC joint (Fig. 21–5a). This is often the result of repetitive

microtrauma such as occurs with weightlifting or gymnastics. Most of the time, the etiology of AC arthritis is idiopathic with an insidious onset (Fig. 21–5b and Fig. 21–5c). The degenerative process produces large osteophytes at the AC joint, which may protrude into the rotator cuff and contribute to symptoms of impingement.

BASIC SCIENCE

Biomechanics of Total Shoulder Replacement

Prosthetic arthroplasty of the GH joint was introduced in the early 1950s at New York Orthopaedic Hospital by Charles S.

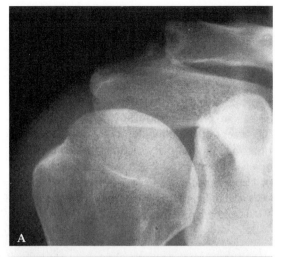

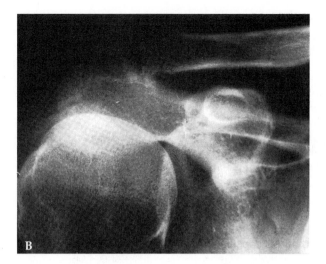

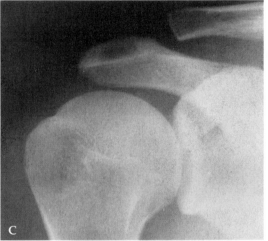

Figure 21–5   (**A**) AP radiograph with 10-degree cephalic tilt in a patient with osteolysis of the distal clavicle. The findings include loss of subchondral bone detail, cystic resorption of the distal clavicle, and a generalized osteopenia of the distal clavicle. (**B**) AP radiograph with 10-degree cephalic tilt showing osteoarthritis of the distal clavicle. The findings include cartilage space narrowing, subchondral sclerosis, and marginal osteophytes. (**C**) AP radiograph after arthroscopic acromioclavicular (AC) resection in which approximately 5 mm of bone was resected from the distal clavicle of the patient with osteolysis (**A**).

Neer II, MD. Several designs have been introduced since that time. These include totally constrained or fixed-fulcrum prosthesis that were produced in an effort to treat patients with absent or dysfunctional rotator cuffs (Fig. 21–3). The constrained designs were found to have a high failure rate and were abandoned. As with many other joints of the body, nonconstrained designs have proven to be a better choice because they reduce stress concentration at sites of component fixation (Fig. 21–1c).

Several different nonconstrained designs are currently being used, many with modular components. These designs vary as to whether the humeral head radius of curvature matches the glenoid radius of curvature. Soslowsky et al (1992) showed that the articular surfaces of the humerus and glenoid are highly congruent. For this reason, Neer (1982) advocated matching of the components. Other studies have shown an obligate translation of the humeral head on the glenoid during GH motion. This has prompted some manufacturers to produce glenoid components with a slightly larger radius of curvature than the humeral component, to allow for translation.

Humeral components are either cemented (Fig. 21–1c) or press-fit with or without the potential for biologic fixation (i.e., porous ingrowth pads). Humeral loosening has not been

a significant clinical problem. However, press-fit components without porous ingrowth capacity were shown by Pollock et al (1992) to have a nearly 100% subsidence rate. Glenoid components are either cemented or press-fit with porous ingrowth pads that are temporarily held with screws (Fig. 21–10f). The ingrowth components require a metal backing, whereas the cemented components can be constructed with polyethylene with or without a metal backing. The use of metal backing makes the component thicker, which places the glenoid surface in a more lateral position. This has been shown by Friedman et al (1992) to produce high, nonphysiologic stresses on the GH articulation. In clinical studies, metal-backed components appear to have a disproportionally high rate of failure.

Glenoid Component Failure

Glenoid component loosening is a concern in the treatment of GH arthritis with total shoulder replacement. Studies have shown a higher failure rate in certain clinical situations. Patients without adequate bone to support the glenoid component have had problems with loosening and breakage. The absence of bone support allows the component to toggle and can result in fatigue failure of the cement fixation or of the component itself. This can be avoided through precise reaming of the glenoid to allow for circumferential support of the component (Fig. 21–10f).

Glenoid components may also loosen or fail due to "edge loading." This occurs when a glenoid component is used for rotator cuff tear arthropathy. Proximal migration of the humeral head results in superior edge loading, described by Franklin et al as the "rocking horse glenoid" (Fig. 21–6). This can also occur after complex proximal humerus fractures where the tuberosities heal in a malunited position. The rotator cuff attachment sites are distorted, resulting in abnormal anterior or posterior translation of the humeral head with edge loading. For this reason, glenoid resurfacing is avoided in patients with the above described conditions.

ANATOMY AND SURGICAL APPROACHES

The shoulder consists of the bones, capsuloligamentous structures and muscles of the GH, AC, SC and scapulothoracic (ST) joints.

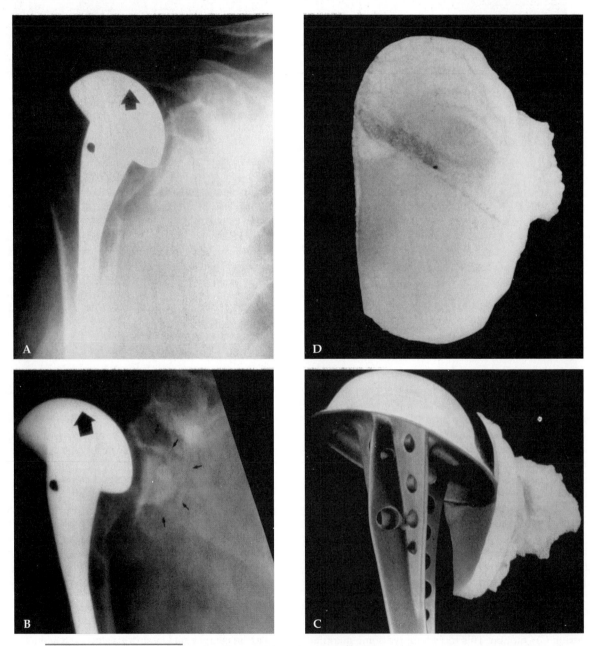

Figure 21–6 (**A**) AP radiograph of the GH joint after total shoulder replacement in a patient with a dysfunctional rotator cuff and proximal migration of the humeral component. (**B**) The dysfunctional rotator cuff resulted in superior eccentric loading of the glenoid component, which eventually caused it to loosen as demonstrated by the progression of lucencies (small arrows) seen in this radiograph. (**C**) The humeral component continually loaded the superior aspect of the glenoid resurfacing component resulting in the "rocking horse" phenomenon. (**D**) Superior eccentric wear of the glenoid component was seen at the time of revision.

Bones of the Shoulder Complex

The clavicle, scapula, and humerus form an intercalated complex that work together during shoulder motion. The clavicle serves as a strut that helps suspend the arm. It articulates with the manubrium of the sternum medially at the SC joint. The lateral aspect of the clavicle articulates with the acromion at the AC joint.

The scapula is encased in muscle and, therefore, has a pseudo-articulation with the chest wall. The scapula is tilted forward at an angle of approximately 30 degrees from the coronal plane and 3 degrees medially from the sagittal plane.

The thickened lateral aspect of the scapula forms the glenoid socket, which serves as an articular platform for the humeral head. The glenoid is separated from the body of the scapula by the scapular neck. The glenoid has an average superior tilt of 5 degrees that helps control inferior stability. It is retroverted with respect to the body of the scapula at an average of 7 degrees (Fig. 21–7).

The scapula projects two notable prominences. The coracoid process arises from the anterosuperior portion of the scapular neck and protrudes at the anterosuperior aspect of the GH joint. It serves as the attachment site for the CA, coracohumeral, and transverse scapular ligaments. The coracohumeral ligament is part of the rotator interval and can become contracted in some arthritic conditions of the GH joint. The CA ligament is part of the CA arch and can serve as a restraint to antero-superior subluxation of the humeral head in rotator cuff-deficient shoulders. This can be important in patients with rotator cuff tear arthropathy who rely on the CA arch to provide a fulcrum for motion.

The acromion projects over the humeral head as a broad, flat expansion of the scapular spine. It serves as the major site of origin for the deltoid muscle and articulates with the clavicle at the AC joint.

The proximal aspect of the humerus consists of the humeral head, anatomic neck, and metaphysis. The humeral head has an average retroversion of 30 to 40 degrees relative

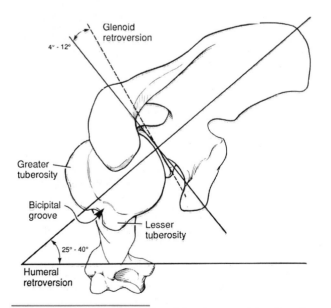

Figure 21–7   The humeral head is retroverted to allow it to "point" to the glenoid socket, which is angled forward with the scapula as it rests on the posterior chest wall.

to the transcondylar axis of the distal humerus (Fig. 21–7). The anatomic neck shaft angle of the proximal humerus averages 130 to 140 degrees. The greater and lesser tuberosities arise from the metaphyseal region and are located on opposite sides of the bicipital groove. The tuberosities play an important role in shoulder function, serving as the attachment site for the rotator cuff tendons. The subscapularis inserts on the lesser tuberosity. The supraspinatus, infraspinatus, and teres minor tendons insert on the greater tuberosity. The bicipital groove serves as a trochlea for the long head of the biceps tendon. After crossing the bicipital groove, the biceps tendon passes into the GH joint to insert at the supraglenoid tubercle. The tendon is constrained in the groove by the transverse humeral ligament as well as the rotator cuff insertions into the tuberosities. In arthritis surgery of the GH joint, the bicipital groove is used to localize the most lateral aspect of the lesser tuberosity.

Articulations of the Shoulder Complex

Glenohumeral Articulation

The GH joint is the major articulation of the shoulder complex. It is formed by the articulation between the surfaces of the hemispherical humeral head and a relatively smaller, shallow glenoid fossa (Fig. 21–7). Despite the similar radius of curvatures, a significant mismatch in size between the two surfaces leaves the articulation with little inherent stability. O'Brien et al (1990) demonstrated that the glenoid fossa is pear shaped with an average vertical and horizontal dimension of 35 mm and 25 mm, respectively. The articular surface of the larger humeral head has an average vertical dimension of 48 mm and an average transverse dimension of 45 mm. The relative area of contact between the two surfaces is analogous to that of a basketball sitting on top of a tea-cup saucer with only 25 to 30% of the humeral head articulating with the glenoid socket at any time. This geometry allows more motion than any other joint in the body at the expense of intrinsic stability. Stability of the joint is provided by surrounding soft tissue structures, which can be separated into static and dynamic restraints. The static restraints consist of the GH capsule and ligaments. The dynamic restraints consist of the rotator cuff and long head of the biceps muscles. As will be discussed later, these soft tissue restraints must be balanced to obtain stability and motion after surgery for GH arthritis.

Acromioclavicular Articulation

The AC joint is a diarthrodial joint of varying inclination between the concave surface of the anteromedial aspect of the acromion and the convex surface of the distal clavicle. This inclination is easily seen on radiographs and, when noted, can greatly improve the accuracy of needle placement during injection studies (Fig. 21–5). A fibrocartilaginous disc exists within the joint. This disc is most often incomplete, projecting downward into the joint as a rim of tissue from the superior capsule. Petersson (1983) suggested that a complete meniscal disc may protect the cartilaginous surfaces of the AC joint from arthritic degeneration.

The scapula moves in synchrony with the clavicle, therefore very little motion actually occurs at the AC joint. The main function of the AC joint is to serve as a connection between the scapula and clavicle, allowing for support of the shoulder girdle on the chest wall. The forces that are experienced by the AC joint are predominantly compressive. Because the area of the AC joint is relatively small and the forces transmitted from the chest wall to the humerus are large, the stresses at this articulation can be extremely high. For this reason, it is not surprising to see compressive failure of this joint, especially in weight lifters (Fig. 21–5a).

The stability of the AC joint is maintained by two sets of ligaments: the AC capsuloligamentous complex and the coracoclavicular ligaments (conoid and trapezoid). The AC ligaments (the inferior and the thicker superior) act as primary restraints to posterior clavicular displacement, controlling 90% of posterior motion. The coracoclavicular ligaments (the trapezoid and conoid) provide restraint to superior and anterior displacement of the clavicle. The conoid ligament seems to provide the majority of this support.

Sternoclavicular Articulation

The SC joint is formed where the inferior portion of the medial end of the clavicle articulates with the manubrial portion of the sternum. It sits directly in front of the great vessels, resulting in a dangerous situation when a posterior dislocation occurs. It is considered a gliding joint with an intervening articular disk and an extensive fibrous envelope. To permit motion at the ST articulation, the clavicle may rotate as much as 60 degrees at the SC ligament. The joint is stabilized by the costoclavicular ligament, the interclavicular ligament, and the anterior and posterior SC ligaments. When excising the medial clavicle for arthritic conditions, it is important to maintain the costoclavicular ligaments to prevent instability of the medial end of the clavicle.

Soft Tissues of the Shoulder Complex

Cooper et al (1993) showed that the shoulder can be approached as a structure consisting of four layers. The deltoid, trapezius, and pectoralis major muscles constitute the outer layer. The deltoid muscle is one of the most important muscles of the shoulder. The pennate deltoid muscle can be divided into posterior, middle and anterior portions. The anterior portion is the most important to the overall function of the arm.

Injury to the deltoid is poorly tolerated. Very little can be done to reconstruct a damaged deltoid muscle. It is important to prevent deltoid damage by making sure that its innervation, the axillary nerve, is protected from injury.

The inner three layers of the shoulder include the clavipectoral fascia, conjoined tendon, and pectoralis minor (second layer); the rotator cuff and bursae (third layer); and the GH capsule and ligaments (fourth layer).

Surgical Approaches

Extended Deltopectoral Approach

Surgical approaches are designed to provide access to pertinent pathology while minimizing the chance of morbidity from the approach. The extended deltopectoral approach provides access to the GH joint by taking advantage of the interval between the deltoid and pectoralis major muscles

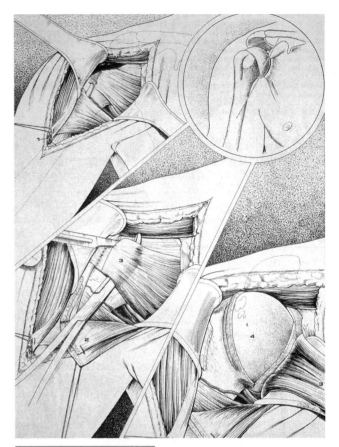

Figure 21–8 The extended deltopectoral approach for total shoulder replacement is carried out by separating the deltoid (1) and pectoralis muscles (2). The pectoralis muscle can be partially resected to aid in inferior visualization. Next, the subscapularis muscle and capsule (3) are incised to expose the humeral head (4). Reproduced with permission from Randelli M, Gambrioli PL, Minola R et al. *Surgical Techniques for the Shoulder*. Padua, Piccin; 1995; 115.

(Fig. 21–8). This approach preserves the origin and insertion of the important deltoid muscle, reducing the chance for the morbid complication of deltoid deficiency. It is a useful approach for both replacement and resection arthroplasty.

The patient is placed in a "beach chair" position with the torso 25 to 70 degrees from the horizontal. A head holder allows the shoulder to extend past the edge of the table and permits access to the superior aspect of the shoulder.

For shoulder arthroplasty an incision is made from the clavicle to the lateral edge of the coracoid down to the anterior edge of the deltoid. (Fig. 21–8). The cephalic vein is used as landmark to locate the deltopectoral interval. The vein is taken either medially or laterally as the interval between the deltoid and pectoralis major muscles is opened. The conjoined tendon (coracobrachialis and short head of biceps muscles) is identified and retracted medially. The clavipectoral fascia immediately lateral to the short head of the biceps muscle is incised, exposing the subscapularis muscle. Access to the GH joint is carried out by either splitting the subscapularis muscle along the line of its fibers or by incising the subscapularis laterally at the lesser tuberosity.

The vascular structures at greatest risk with this approach are the anterior humeral circumflex vessels, which run along the inferior border of the subscapularis tendon. These can be ligated to prevent uncontrolled bleeding. The axillary nerve is at risk as it crosses over the subscapularis and then runs beneath the anterior humeral circumflex vessels and medial aspect of the axillary pouch on its way through the quadrilateral space.

PEARL

The axillary nerve can be located during an anterior approach to the shoulder using the tug test. As described by Flatow and Bigliani (1992), the index finger is swept beneath the coracoid process, over the subscapularis, and gently hooks the axillary nerve (Fig. 21–9).

Flatow et al (1989) showed that the musculocutaneous nerve is also at risk during the anterior approach because it enters the conjoined tendon as high as 1.5 mm distal to the coracoid process. Excessive force during retraction of the conjoined tendon should be avoided. Early localization of the tip of the coracoid process is important since the brachial plexus and axillary artery are located medial to it and can be protected from harm by staying lateral to the coracoid process.

Acromioclavicular Approach

The skin incision is generally made in Langer's lines and is centered over the AC joint. The deltotrapezial fascia is incised directly over the lateral portion of the clavicle and is continued laterally across the AC joint to the medial aspect of the acromion. The periosteum is elevated to allow a 1-cm resection of the distal clavicle. The suprascapular muscle and its nerve should be protected when performing a distal clavicle excision by placing retractors under the distal aspect of the clavicle.

Sternoclavicular Approach

An oblique incision is made that runs anterior to the SC joint and perpendicular to the joint surfaces. The capsule is incised directly over the SC joint. It is important to use blunt elevators and retractors to prevent damage to the great vessels directly beneath the SC joint.

EXAMINATION

Glenohumeral Arthritis

The patient with GH arthritis presents with shoulder pain and loss of motion and strength. The pain of GH arthritis is often more intolerable than hip or knee pain because it is not alleviated by recumbency and is in most cases made worse. Recumbency eliminates the distracting force created by the weight of the arm. As GH arthritis progresses, GH motion diminishes, and the patient must compensate with increased ST motion. Because ST movement contributes little to rotation, limitation of external rotation is a more sensitive physical sign than that of loss of forward elevation. Other signs specific to GH arthritis include posterior joint line tenderness and crepitus at the GH joint.

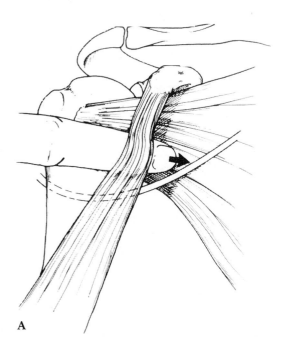
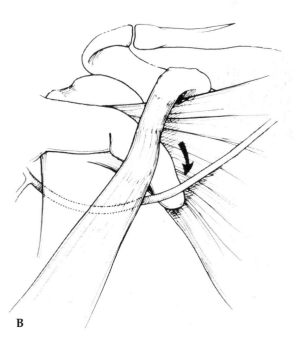

A   B

Figure 21–9 (**A**) The tug test is used to locate the axillary nerve when using the deltopectoral approach. The index finger is passed directly medially over the subscapularis and under the coracoid. (**B**) The finger is then rotated and swept down until the axillary nerve is palpated. Reproduced with permission from Flatow EL, Bigliani LU. Locating and protecting the axillary nerve in shoulder surgery: the tug test. *Orthop Rev.* 1992;21:503.

Radiographs

When the clinician suspects GH arthritis, standard radiographs should be obtained. This includes an anteroposterior (AP) view of the GH joint shot perpendicular to the plane of the scapula and an axillary view (Figs. 21–1 through 21–3).

Laboratory Studies

Laboratory studies are important in the evaluation of a patient with GH arthritis. A complete blood count with differential and an erythrocyte sedimentation rate are used to screen for infection. If these studies are positive, an aspiration arthrogram can be used to obtain a fluid specimen for culture and sensitivity. A rheumatoid factor or antinuclear antibodies can be helpful in screening for inflammatory arthritis.

Acromioclavicular Arthritis

Anterosuperior shoulder pain and difficulty sleeping on the affected side are common symptoms of AC joint arthritis. The pain often radiates to the trapezius muscle, which has fascia that is confluent with the superior capsule of the AC joint. This can lead to painful spasm of the trapezius. Tenderness to direct palpation of the joint is the most reliable physical finding on clinical examination. Osteophytic enlargement of the joint may also be appreciated.

Provocative maneuvers that compress the AC joint, such as horizontal adduction of the arm or internal rotation of the shoulder, may also elicit pain. These provocative tests are not entirely specific and may show overlap with other painful conditions such as those associated with excessive posterior capsular tightness.

Radiographs

A standard shoulder series may overpenetrate the distal clavicle. An AP radiograph with a 10 degree cephalic tilt using "soft-tissue" technique (reduced penetration) can reveal subtle changes in the distal clavicle (Fig. 21–5). Radiographic findings associated with degenerative arthritis of the AC joint include cartilage space narrowing, subchondral sclerosis, and marginal osteophytes (Fig. 21–5b). Radiographic findings indicative of osteolysis include loss of subchondral bone detail, cystic resorption of the distal clavicle, and a generalized osteopenia of the distal clavicle.

Sternoclavicular Arthritis

Pain localized to the medial aspect of the clavicle and SC joint is the most common symptom of SC arthritis. Tenderness to direct palpation of the joint is the most reliable physical finding on clinical examination. Osteophytic enlargement of the joint may also be appreciated.

Radiographs

Sternoclavicular changes are difficult to evaluate with plain radiographs and may sometimes be viewed with the help of special radiographic views such as the serendipity view. This is an oblique view used to eliminate overlap of the joint with the other structures of the thorax.

AIDS TO DIAGNOSIS

Computed Tomography

In patients with significant erosion of the humeral head or glenoid, a computed tomographic (CT) scan can help quantify the extent of bone loss. This may be important when shoulder arthroplasty is being considered. In patients with post-traumatic arthritis, the CT scan can be helpful in evaluating deformity of the greater and lesser tuberosities.

PEARL

The best study to evaluate for the presence of SC arthritis is a CT scan.

Magnetic Resonance Imaging

When a concomitant rotator cuff tear is suspected, a magnetic resonance imaging (MRI) study can verify the diagnosis. The MRI study may have the added benefit of providing information about loss of bone or bone deformity, negating the need for a CT scan. Because of the significant cost of an MRI scan, the test should be limited to those cases where the results of the test will impact the treatment.

Magnetic resonance images of the AC joint may reveal soft-tissue hypertrophy and synovitis at the AC joint.

Injections of Local Anesthetic

The most valuable diagnostic tool that can be utilized to determine whether the AC joint is contributing to a patient's shoulder pain is an AC joint lidocaine injection. It can help predict the value of surgical resection of the distal clavicle and has the added benefit of providing a therapeutic intervention if a steroid preparation is added. Multiple steroid injections should be avoided.

Lidocaine injections into the GH joint may be help determine if that joint is the source of the patient's pain. Steroid injections into the GH joint are used only in those patients with advanced degeneration.

SPECIFIC CONDITIONS, TREATMENT, AND OUTCOME

Glenohumeral Arthritis

Initial treatment consists of anti-inflammatory medications and activity modification. When these methods fail, surgical intervention is indicated.

Arthroplasty is by far the most successful type of treatment for most arthritic involvements of the GH joint. However, it is important to understand that other forms of surgical intervention are available and may be indicated in selected cases.

Debridement and Soft-tissue Balancing

Debridement and soft-tissue balancing can be useful in treating young patients with mild or moderate arthritis with a concomitant internal rotation contracture. These patients may have increased load on the posterior aspect of the glenoid as a result of the contracture. The goal of the treatment is to restore an even distribution of GH joint forces across the glenoid surface.

Arthroscopic Debridement

The use of GH arthroscopy for irrigation and debridement, combined with soft tissue release, has been successful in patients who are poor candidates for joint replacement. Weinstein et al (1993) found that arthroscopy for GH arthritis provided significant pain relief and increased motion in 78% of patients at an average of $2\frac{1}{2}$ years follow-up. This procedure was not helpful in patients with complete loss of joint space, large osteophytes, or significant posterior humeral subluxation. The long-term value of this treatment is unknown. Open debridement for synovectomy and bursectomy is rarely indicated. It may be helpful in the patient with rheumatoid arthritis who has synovitis with minimal joint destruction.

Resection Arthroplasty

Humeral head resection can be used as a salvage procedure in patients with resistant infections and failed arthroplasties with extensive bone loss. As noted by Cofield (1985), one half to two thirds of patients achieve satisfactory pain relief after humeral head excision. Motion was limited to 40 to 90 degrees of forward elevation with minimal or no active external or internal rotation. After humeral head resection, the patient's arm should be placed in a sling for 6 to 8 weeks, and the patient should be allowed pendulum range of motion exercises. The goal is to develop scar that will improve the stability of the proximal humerus and diminish the chances for abutment against surrounding structures.

Shoulder Arthrodesis

Prior to the introduction of a shoulder arthroplasty, shoulder arthrodesis was a commonly indicated procedure for GH arthritis. The fused shoulder eliminated pain at the GH joint and provided stability and durability enabling the patient to perform heavy labor activities. However, many patients with shoulder fusion developed periscapular pain and all have significantly limited rotational motion. Currently, shoulder arthrodesis is used for patients with paralysis or compromise of both the rotator cuff and deltoid muscles. The young, active laborer may be better served with a humeral head replacement.

Glenohumeral Arthroplasty

Indications

The primary indication for shoulder arthroplasty is pain that persists after nonoperative treatment. Loss of function is a secondary indication of surgery. Shoulder arthroplasty is rarely performed to improve range of motion if no concomitant pain is present. The patient should have a stable medical status and should be capable of playing an essential role in the postoperative rehabilitation. Absolute contra-indications to arthroplasty of the GH joint include the presence of an active infection and paralysis or complete functional loss of the rotator cuff and deltoid muscles.

Humeral Head versus Total Shoulder Replacement

Arthroplasty options for GH arthritis include resurfacing of the humeral side alone or resurfacing of both the humeral and glenoid articular surfaces. The advantages of total shoulder replacement include a better fulcrum for improved strength and motion, increased stability, decreased friction, and elimination of glenoid socket pain. These advantages come with a price. Inserting a glenoid component requires additional operating time and can result in additional blood loss. Over time, there may be radiographic evidence of radiolucency about the glenoid, which could suggest the eventual need for revision of the glenoid component. For these reasons, most shoulder surgeons advocate caution in considering use of a glenoid component in a younger patient. In addition, the revision rate for glenoid components increased in individuals with abnormal GH mechanics. This includes patients with rotator cuff deficiency who have an tendency towards eccentric loading (superior edge) of the glenoid socket. It may also be a problem in patients with post-traumatic arthritis who have tuberosity deformities and soft tissue contractures that may increase anterior or posterior edge loading.

Total shoulder replacement with glenoid resurfacing is advocated for patients with painful glenoid incongruity, adequate bone stock, and normal functioning rotator cuff muscles without significant tuberosity deformity (Fig. 21–1c). Fortunately, the great majority of patients with primary osteoarthritis, post-traumatic osteoarthritis, and rheumatoid arthritis have these characteristics. Patients with avascular necrosis have sparing of the glenoid cavity until the very late phases of the disease, and, therefore, glenoid resurfacing is unnecessary.

Patients with rotator cuff tears that have a smaller tear with good quality tissue are treated with total shoulder arthroplasty and cuff repair. When the cuff tissue is atrophic or the rotator cuff tear is larger, humeral hemiarthroplasty is performed, and the rotator cuff is repaired with an emphasis towards anterior-posterior stability of the implant over complete superior coverage (Fig. 21–4c and 21–4d).

Technique for Humeral Head Replacement

The extended deltopectoral approach is used and the axillary nerve is identified and protected with either a finger or retractor (Fig. 21–8). The approach allows direct access to the subscapularis and capsule. The subscapularis and capsule are released at the most lateral aspect of the lesser tuberosity to maintain maximal length. At the end of the surgery the subscapularis can be repaired to the edge of the humeral head resection, effectively lengthening the tendon. This is often necessary in patients with anterior soft tissue contracture and loss of external rotation. To maximize excursion of the subscapularis tendon, humeral and glenoid osteophytes must be excised and osteochondral loose bodies must be removed. The anterior GH capsule must be released from the glenoid margin to allow maximal excursion of the subscapularis tendon. A contracted coracohumeral ligament and rotator cuff interval tissue must be released from the base of the coracoid. If these steps are not taken, the patient will have tight anterior structures postoperatively, which can lead to posterior subluxation of the humeral component.

After release of the subscapularis and anterior capsule, the humeral head is dislocated by gently externally rotating the shoulder and extending the humerus. This step is greatly

PITFALL

Anterior soft tissue contractures are most common in patients with GH osteoarthritis or arthritis after "tight anterior" instability repairs. It may be necessary to lengthen the subscapularis to gain adequate anterior soft tissue tensioning. These patients will generally have an internal rotation contracture. The subscapularis tendon can be easily lengthened with a coronal or Z-plasty technique.

facilitated by adequate release of the inferior and posterior inferior capsule around the humeral neck. It is necessary to determine the precise location of the posterior cuff insertion into the greater tuberosity to avoid damage of the cuff tissue during humeral head resection. Osteophytes along the inferior margin of the head at the calcar area must be removed to

better delineate the true articular surface of the humerus. A guide is then used to assist in planning and performing the osteotomy for removal of the arthritic head (Fig. 21–10a). In most cases of arthritis, the inferior portion of the head becomes enlarged with osteophytes whereas the superior portion of the head is eroded. This gives the illusion that the center of the humeral head is lower than it actually is. The surgeon should recognize this fact to prevent excessive removal of the head, which may jeopardize the rotator cuff insertion (Fig. 21–10b).

The humeral cut is made orthogonal to the humeral shaft by externally rotating the humerus 30 to 40 degrees and cutting directly parallel to the torso. The same effect is achieved by using the humeral epicondyles as a landmark and making a cut approximately 30 to 40 degrees retroverted to their axis (Fig. 21–10c).

The superior aspect of the osteotomy should exit just above the insertion of the posterior cuff. By making the osteotomy in this manner, the rotator cuff insertion is preserved, and the prosthesis can be seated with the appropriate

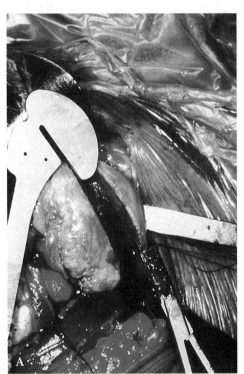

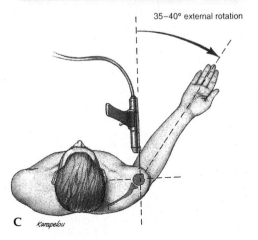

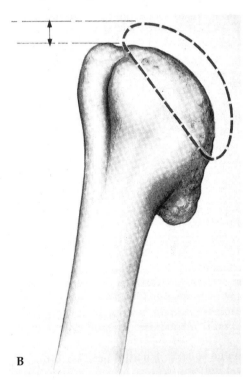

Figure 21–10 (**A**) After exposure and dislocation of the humeral head, osteophytes are removed and a template is used to determine the line of humeral resection. (**B**) The surgeon must be sure that the humeral osteotomy is above the level of the tuberosities. (**C**) The humeral cut is made orthogonal to the humeral shaft by externally rotating the humerus 30 to 40 degrees and cutting directly parallel or by using the humeral epicondyles as a landmark and making a cut approximately 30 to 40 degrees retroverted to them. Reproduced with permission from Knetsche RP, Friedman RJ. Cement versus noncement: humerus. *Op Tech Orthop.* 1994;4:213.

PEARL

When the cut is done appropriately, the lateral fin of the humeral prosthesis should lie 5 to 10 mm posterior to the posterior margin of the bicipital groove.

---

30 to 40 degrees of retroversion. In patients with arthritis after a locked humeral dislocation, the version of the humeral cut is adjusted to compensate for the instability that results from chronic expansion of the soft tissues. The retroversion is decreased for posterior instability and increased for anterior instability. In a similar fashion, the humeral retroversion can be lessened to account for excessive posterior glenoid erosion. For each degree of glenoid retroversion related to posterior bone erosion, the surgeon should subtract a degree of humeral retroversion to compensate.

The medullary canal of the humerus is prepared with manual reaming.

PEARL

A slot is made for the lateral fin of the prosthesis posterior to the bicipital groove with a small rongeur. This slot reduces the chance of a tuberosity fracture during reaming or when placing trial humeral components.

The trial implant is placed in the canal in the appropriate amount of retroversion and the GH joint is reduced.

During the trial process, component version and soft-tissue balance are assessed. The goal is to have the humeral component translate to approximately 50% of the humeral

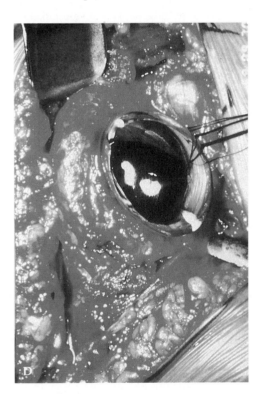

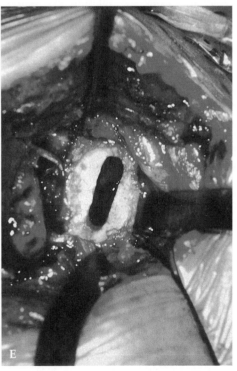

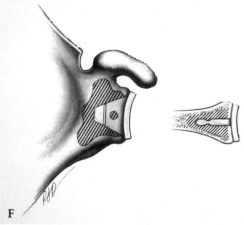

Figure 21–10 *(continued)* (**D**) Replacement of humeral head. (**E**) The glenoid bone is prepared for the glenoid component. (**F**) The glenoid bone is contoured to ensure concentric fit and support of the glenoid component.

head diameter and to allow 45 degrees of external rotation with the arm at the side.

Once appropriate humeral sizing is obtained, the humeral trial prosthesis is removed. Drill holes placed at the anterior humeral neck are filled with No. 2 nonabsorbable, braided nylon sutures. These sutures are used to repair the subscapularis tendon. Next, the surgeon verifies that a glenoid resurfacing prosthesis is not indicated, and the appropriate size humeral component is cemented or press-fit into position (Fig. 21–10d). The cement is not pressurized to avoid cement extrusion through the humeral bone.

The wound is irrigated, followed by closure of the deltopectoral interval and skin. Suction drains may be used between the deltoid and rotator cuff and should be brought out through separate stab incisions. The patient's arm is placed in a sling and swath. Physical therapy is begun on the first postoperative day.

Glenoid Replacement Technique

After the humerus has been prepared for prosthetic implantation, attention is focused on the glenoid cavity. Soft tissues at the glenoid margin, including labral tissue, are released and a blunt retractor is placed along the anterior neck of the glenoid. Any remaining labral tissue is sharply resected to allow a complete view of the entire glenoid cavity. Throughout this procedure, the axillary nerve must be carefully protected. The glenoid is evaluated to make certain that bone stock is adequate. The glenoid cavity is prepared to accept the glenoid component so that the glenoid component will have complete peripheral support (Figs. 21–10e and 21–10f).

The most common pattern of glenoid wear is posterior erosion. In this instance, the surgeon must either lower the anterior surface of the glenoid, recreating a normal glenoid tilt or lessen the amount of humeral retroversion. The combined retroversion of the two components should not be greater than 30 to 40 degrees. In certain cases, it may be necessary to bone graft the glenoid cavity to eliminate abnormal tilt and provide adequate bone stock for a glenoid replacement.

In most cases, the glenoid component is fixed with methylmethacrylate. Once the glenoid is fixed, trial components for the humerus are inserted to ensure proper humeral size and version.

Rehabilitation After Glenohumeral Arthroplasty

Rehabilitation after shoulder arthroplasty is based on Neer's three-phase shoulder rehabilitation program. Phase I emphasizes passive motion in forward elevation and external rotation. Phase II progresses to active assisted and active exercises of the shoulder, generally beginning 6 to 8 weeks after surgery. In many patients, it is safe to start gentle active forward elevation exercises within 1 to 2 weeks after surgery. In Phase III, advanced muscle stretching and progressive resistive strengthening exercises are initiated, usually at three months following surgery. The patient's specific pathology and bone and soft tissue quality direct the timing of the rehabilitation program. Premedication with oral narcotics during the early postoperative phase is necessary.

Results of Glenohumeral Arthroplasty

The overall results for both humeral head replacement and total shoulder replacement have been very satisfactory. Most series (Rodosky, 1994) show greater than 80 to 90% pain relief. The total shoulder replacement series have slightly greater relief of pain as compared with the humeral replacement series.

The postoperative results for total shoulder replacement vary depending on the type of arthritis. Patients with primary GH osteoarthritis and avascular necrosis have the best functional results. These patients are most likely to have a normal rotator cuff and deltoid muscle, which are the main determinants of active GH motion. In a recent report by Pollack et al (1995) a homogeneous group of primary osteoarthritic patients were followed prospectively for an average of 3.3 years and were found to have postoperative active elevation of 160 degrees with 97% significant pain relief. In contrast, patients with rheumatoid arthritis or post-traumatic arthritis often have more soft tissue abnormalities and, therefore, have a variable return of function postoperatively. In Neer's report (1982) of 194 patients, the gain in active elevation for the primary osteoarthritic shoulders was 77 degrees versus 57 degrees for rheumatoid shoulders and only 33 degrees for the post-traumatic shoulders.

Complications of Glenohumeral Arthroplasty

Fortunately, the incidence of complications after shoulder arthroplasty has been less than that noted for other major joint reconstructions. The incidence of infection after shoulder arthroplasty is less than 0.5%. This compares very favorably with reported infection rates following other major joint replacements. An early hematogenous infection can often be treated with irrigation, debridement, and wound closure over a closed drainage system and appropriate antibiotics. Delayed infections require removal of the prosthesis and all cement, foreign bodies, and sequestra, as well as long term antibiotic therapy. With less virulent organisms such as *Staphylococcus aureus*, the prosthesis can be replaced after adequate treatment of the infection. In cases with more virulent organisms, it may be advisable to maintain the state of resection arthroplasty and/or perform GH fusion.

Nerve injuries during shoulder arthroplasty are extremely uncommon. These injuries most often result in a neuropraxia, which can be followed. The axillary nerve is the nerve most likely to be injured, as it runs on the inferior aspect of the capsule and then curves posteriorly at the undersurface of the deltoid muscle.

Intra-operative fractures of the humerus or scapula are uncommon but can occur in osteoporotic bone. Fractures are more likely to occur when inserting a press-fit porous component rather than a cemented component. When a humeral shaft fracture occurs, a long stem prosthesis may be utilized to help stabilize the fracture. Tuberosity fragments can also fracture, especially in osteoporotic patients with rheumatoid arthritis. These fragments must be secured by heavy suture after the humeral component is cemented in position. Bone graft from the humeral head can be added to enhance healing.

Instability has been reported to occur in only 1 to 2% of shoulder arthroplasty cases. Stability of an unconstrained implant depends on preservation of humeral length, proper version of the components, and appropriate soft tissue balance. In Neer's report (1994) of 194 total shoulder replacements with an average of 37 months follow-up, there were only 4 dislocations. All were treated with closed reduction and immobilization for 3 to 6 weeks and then rehabilitation. Only 1 of the 4 had recurrent subluxations. When the instability is caused by significant abnormalities in humeral or glenoid component orientation, one or both of the components must be revised.

Postoperative tearing of the rotator cuff is one of the more frequent complications following total shoulder arthroplasty. Cofield and Edgerton (1990) reported an incidence of 3 to 4%. When the rotator cuff tear results in pain or instability, an open repair should be performed. This can be difficult, especially when little bone stock is available for transosseous sutures. Subscapularis tendon pull-off occurs when the anterior soft tissues have not been adequately released or when the size of the humeral head component is large and abuts the subscapularis repair. Failure of the subscapularis repair must be treated early to avoid retraction and scarring. If extensive scarring occurs and significant anterior instability results, Moeckel et al (1993) recommends insertion of a fascial autograft or allograft.

Prosthetic loosening is a rare complication. In a review of the current peer-reviewed literature by Rodosky and Bigliani (1996), the overall glenoid revision rate was 3.2% versus 1.8% for humeral components. When the glenoid component loosens and becomes symptomatic, it is necessary to revise or remove the glenoid component to prevent pain and dysfunction. When the glenoid bone stock is adequate and the GH mechanics are stable, the component is replaced. When bone stock is inadequate or there are concerns about the potential for abnormal GH mechanics with eccentric loading of the glenoid, it may be prudent to simply remove the glenoid component and increase the size of the humeral head component. In some cases with extensive glenoid or humeral bone loss following loosening of GH arthroplasty components, it may be necessary to use osteochondral allografts in conjunction with humeral and glenoid prostheses. In a recent report on surgical treatment of glenoid component failures, Rodosky et al (1995) found that relief of pain was successful in 79% of patients.

Acromioclavicular Arthritis

The majority of patients will respond to conservative management, which includes nonsteroidal anti-inflammatory medications, activity modifications, and a steroid injection. If the patient does not respond, operative intervention with resection of the distal clavicle should be considered.

Open resection of the distal clavicle has been a relatively successful operation for AC joint pathology. Open resection, however, requires violation of the deltoid and trapezial fascial insertions at the distal clavicle. This impacts on the time needed for postoperative rehabilitation. In addition, the superior aspect of the AC capsuloligamentous complex is also incised and stripped for visualization and access to the distal clavicle. This has the potential to interfere with its role in preventing posterior translation of the distal clavicle. In contrast, the arthroscopic approaches to distal clavicle excision limit the amount of interference with the distal clavicular insertions of the deltoid and trapezius, and active motion can begin shortly after surgery. The arthroscopic procedure can be carried out via a bursal or direct approach. It is important to remove no more than approximately 1 cm of bone.

PITFALL

In arthroscopic resections, 5 to 7 mm of bone removal is all that is necessary (see Fig. 21–5c). Loss of the insertion of the acromioclavicular (AC) capsuloligamentous complex can result in instability of the distal clavicle in an anterior-posterior direction with abutment against the base of the acromion and scapular. The success rate of distal clavicle excision is greater than 90% in most series.

Sternoclavicular Arthritis

In the individual with unremitting pain and functional deficits, surgical intervention is indicated. Surgical treatment consists of resection of the medial clavicle at the sternoclavicular joint. When the ligaments are intact and the medial clavicle is stable, a subperiosteal dissection is performed leaving the costoclavicular ligament intact. The resection is performed in an oblique fashion removing approximately 5 mm inferiorly and 10 mm superiorly. In patients with concomitant instability at the sternoclavicular joint, the medial clavicle is stabilized with autologous tendon graft (palmaris or plantaris) by passing the tendon through the first rib and medial clavicle after resection. Dead space is filled with the clavicular head of the sternocleidomastoid muscle. In the routine patient, activities are advanced as soon as wound healing allows. Patients who have undergone tendon grafting are immobilized for several weeks to allow scar formation.

SELECTED BIBLIOGRAPHY

COFIELD RH. Shoulder arthrodesis and resection arthroplasty. *Instruct Course Lect.* 1985;34:268–277.

COFIELD RH, EDGERTON BC. Total shoulder arthroplasty. complications and revision surgery. *Instruct Course Lect.* 1990;39:449–462.

COOPER DE, O'BRIEN SJ, WARREN RF. Supporting layers of the glenohumeral joint: an anatomic study. *Clin Orthop.* 1993;289:144–155.

DEPALMA AF. *Degenerative Changes of the Sternoclavicular and Acromioclavicular Joints in Various Decades.* Springfield, IL: CC Thomas; 1957.

DINES DM, WARREN RF, ALTCHECK DW, MOECKEL B. Post-traumatic changes of the proximal humerus: malunion, nonunion, and osteonecrosis: treatment with modular hemiarthroplasty or total shoulder arthroplasty. *J Shoulder Elbow Surg.* 1993;2:11–21.

FLATOW EL. The biomechanics of the acromioclavicular, sternoclavicular, and scapulothoracic joints. In: Heckman JD, ed. *Instruct Course Lect.* 1993;42:237–245.

FLATOW EL, BIGLIANI LU. Locating and protecting the axillary nerve in shoulder surgery. the tug test. *Orthop Rev.* 1992;21:503–505.

FLATOW EL, BIGLIANI LU, APRIL EW. An anatomic study of the musculocutaneous nerve and its relationship to the coracoid process. *Clin Orthop.* 1989;244:166–171.

FRANKLIN JL, BARRETT WP, JACKINS SE, MATSEN FA. Glenoid loosening in total shoulder arthroplasty: association with rotator cuff deficiency. *J Arthroplasty.* 1988;3:39–46.

FRIEDMAN RJ, LABERGE M, DOOLEY RL, O'HARA AL. Finite element modeling of the glenoid component: effect of design parameters on stress distribution. *J Shoulder Elbow Surg.* 1992;1:261–270.

KELLY IG. Surgery of the rheumatoid shoulder. *Ann Rheum Dis.* 1990;49:824–829.

MOECKEL BH, ALTCHEK DW, WARREN RF, WICKIEWICZ TL, DINES DM. Instability of the shoulder after arthroplasty. *J Bone Jt Surg.* 1993;75A:492–497.

NEER CS II. Replacement arthroplasty for glenohumeral osteoarthritis. *J Bone Jt Surg.* 1974;56A:1–13.

NEER CS II. Unconstrained shoulder arthroplasty. *AAOS Instruct Course Lect.* 1985;34:278–286.

NEER CS II, MORRISON DS. Glenoid bone-grafting in total shoulder arthroplasty. *J Bone Jt Surg.* 1988;70A:1154–1162.

NEER CS II, WATSON KC, STANTON FJ. Recent experience in total shoulder replacement *J Bone Jt Surg.* 1982;64A:319–337.

O'BRIEN SJ, ARNOCZKY SP, WARREN RF et al. Developmental anatomy of the shoulder and anatomy of the glenohumeral joint. In: Rockwood CA Jr, Matsen FA III, eds. *The Shoulder.* Vol 1. Philadelphia, PA: WB Saunders; 1990;1–33.

POLLOCK RG, DELIZ ED, MCILVEEN SJ, FLATOW EL, BIGLIANI LU. Prosthetic replacement in rotator cuff deficient shoulders. *J Shoulder Elbow Surg.* 1992;1:173–186.

POLLOCK RG, HIGGS GB, CODD TP, WEINSTEIN DM, SELF EB, FLATOW EL, BIGLIANI LU. Total shoulder replacement for the treatment of primary glenohumeral osteoarthritis. *J Shoulder Elbow Surg.* 1995;4:S12.

POST M, JABLON M. Constrained total shoulder arthroplasty. Long-term follow-up observations. *Clin Orthop.* 1983;173:109–116.

RODOSKY MW, BIGLIANI LU. Surgical treatment of nonconstrained glenoid component failure. *Oper Tech Orthop.* 1994;4:226–236.

RODOSKY MW, BIGLIANI LU. Indications for glenoid resurfacing. *J Shoulder Elbow Surg.* 1996;5:231–248.

RODOSKY MW, WEINSTEIN DM, POLLOCK RG, FLATOW EL, BIGLIANI LU, NEER CS. On the rarity of glenoid failure. *J. Shoulder Elbow Surg.* 1995;4:513.

SOSLOWSKY LJ, FLATOW EL, BIGLIANI LU, MOW VC. Articular geometry of the glenohumeral joint. *Clin Orthop.* 1992;285:181–190.

WARNER JJP. The gross anatomy of the joint surfaces, ligaments, labrum and capsule. In: Matsen FA III, Fu FH, Hawkins RJ, eds. *The Shoulder: A Balance of Mobility and Stability.* Rosemont, IL: The American Academy of Orthopaedic Surgeons; 1993;7–27.

WEINSTEIN DM, BUCCHIERI JS, POLLOCK RG, FLATOW EL, BIGLIANI LU. Arthroscopic debridement of the shoulder for osteoarthritis. *Arthroscopy.* 1993;9:366.

SAMPLE QUESTIONS

1. Primary GH osteoarthritis is a common condition that:

   (a) is often the end result of a rotator cuff tear

   (b) usually presents with anterior-inferior glenoid bone loss and resultant glenoid anteversion

   (c) result in superior humeral head bone loss with associated large superior marginal head osteophytes

   (d) usually presents with posterior glenoid bone loss and resultant glenoid retroversion

   (e) is usually associated with greater wear on the inferior part of the humeral articular surface

2. Rheumatoid arthritis of the GH joint is an inflammatory condition that:

   (a) results in destruction of the articular surfaces through pannus formation with formation of large inferior humeral head osteophytes

   (b) results in destruction of the articular surfaces through pannus formation with a protusio pattern of glenoid bone loss

   (c) results in destruction of the articular surfaces through pannus formation with associated thinning and dysfunction of the rotator cuff and proximal humeral migration

(d) a, b, and c

(e) b and c

3. In the treatment of AC arthritis it is essential to:

(a) remove at least 15 mm of bone to prevent any further contact of the resected surfaces of the joint

(b) fully release the AC capsuloligamentous complex from the distal clavicle to get an adequate resection of distal clavicle bone

(c) preserve the AC capsuloligamentous complex by resecting no more than 1 cm of distal clavicle in order that the distal clavicle remains stable in an anterior-posterior direction

(d) preserve the AC capsuloligamentous complex by resecting no more than 1 cm of distal clavicle in order that the distal clavicle remains stable in a superior-inferior direction

(e) a and b

4. Total shoulder replacement with glenoid resurfacing should be avoided in most patients with:

(a) primary GH osteoarthritis and posterior glenoid bone erosion

(b) rotator cuff tear arthropathy

(c) rheumatoid arthritis

(d) a, b and c

(e) b and c

5. Postoperative motion after arthroplasty of the GH joint is usually best in patients with:

(a) primary GH osteoarthritis

(b) post-traumatic arthritis

(c) rheumatoid arthritis

(d) rotator cuff tear arthropathy

(e) c and d

Elbow

Chapter 22

Fractures of the Humeral Shaft

Gregory G. Degnan, MD

Outline

Humeral shaft fractures are relatively common fractures, accounting for about 3% of all fractures. These injuries can be appropriately managed in a variety of ways. Satisfactory results can be achieved using both operative and nonoperative techniques. The most appropriate treatment plan is determined by the pattern of the fracture, the biology of the fracture, and the overall condition and age of the patient. The surgeon should be familiar and comfortable with a number of different treatment modalities. Treatment of these fractures should not be handled with a cookbook approach but rather should be tailored to the individual patient.

BASIC SCIENCE

Fracture Healing

To intelligently manage humeral shaft fractures it is important to understand how the fracture "personality" affects fracture healing. It is also critical to understand how the treatment will affect fracture healing.

In the mid-1970s Cruess and Dumont described three overlapping phases of fracture healing. Subsequent to this, several authors have modified and added to these phases. All agree, however, that a fracture initiates a predictable biologic cascade that begins with an inflammatory reaction and ends, potentially, with fracture healing.

The first phase is an inflammatory phase that begins immediately after injury, peaks by 48 hours, and is essentially complete by 1 week post injury. This process is identical to the inflammatory response of any tissue to trauma. Vasodilatation and hyperemia accompany invasion of the injury site by neutrophils, basophils, and phagocytic cells that clear the cellular debris. Various growth factors that regulate cell migration and differentiation are released and activated. The fracture hematoma becomes organized and provides a fibrin network pathway for cell migration. During this phase pain inhibition causes the patient to protect the extremity, and the swelling provides for hydrostatic splinting of the bone if the soft tissue envelope is intact.

The second, or reparative, phase begins shortly after injury and may persist for several months. The hallmark feature of this phase is the formation of fracture callus. This callus may consist of fibrous tissue, cartilage, osteoid, and blood vessels.

The primary callus response is not unique to fractures. It is, in fact, the direct response of bone to inflammation and may be caused by infection, foreign body, or tumor. The marrow and periosteum provide the cells from which the primary callus is derived. The osteoblasts and osteocytes present at the fracture site are inadequate to meet the demands of growing callus. The primary source, therefore, of callus cells is the pluripotential mesenchymal cells, fibroblasts, and chondroblasts that differentiate into the callus cells.

The primary callus response does not continue indefinitely. If the two ends of the fracture have not bridged within a few weeks, the provisional callus may be resorbed. This is seen in an atrophic nonunion. If bridging callus does form, the callus calcifies and becomes rigid. This leads into the final phase of bone healing, the remodeling phase.

The remodeling phase consists of the replacement by lamellar bone of the calcified cartilage and woven bone of callus. This is accomplished by osteoclastic and osteoblastic remodeling in response to physiologic stresses on the bone. Remodeling may take several years to complete.

Primary Bone Healing

When rigid fixation is applied to perfectly apposed fracture fragments, callus will not form. Healing proceeds in this case by normal osteonal bone remodeling. Osteons cross the fracture site ultimately uniting it. Radiographically, no callus

Orthopaedic Surgery: The Essentials. Edited by M.E. Baratz, A.D. Watson, and J.E. Imbriglia. Thieme Medical Publishers, Inc., New York © 1999

should be visible. This is a slow process in the adult and offers no specific advantage over callus-mediated healing.

PEARL

When callus is evident on a radiograph following open reduction and internal fixation of a fracture, it usually indicates inadequate fixation, hardware loosening, or infection.

ANATOMY AND SURGICAL APPROACHES

Anatomy

The humeral shaft is the diaphyseal portion of the humerus extending from the superior edge of the pectoralis major insertion proximally to the supracondylar ridge distally (Fig. 22–1). The shaft is cylindrical in the proximal two thirds and becomes triangular as it approaches the supracondylar ridge. The shaft is divided into three roughly equal surfaces: the anterolateral surface, the anteromedial surface, and the posterior surface. The anteromedial surface has no distinguishing bony landmarks and forms the floor of the intertubercular groove. The posterior surface contains the spiral groove, through which the radial nerve transits the posterior compartment, and also gives origin to the medial and lateral heads of the triceps. The anterolateral surface is marked by

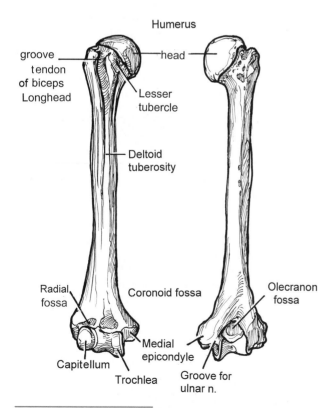

Figure 22–1 Schematic illustrating osseous anatomy of the humerus.

the deltoid tuberosity and the radial sulcus, which houses the radial nerve and the profunda brachii artery.

The humeral diaphysis receives its blood supply from segmental vessels off the brachial artery. Nutrient vessels arise off the brachial, profunda brachii, and posterior humeral circumflex arteries and provide for the intramedullary circulation. The periosteal circulation also depends on these segmental vessels, as well as small muscular branches, and the arterial anastamosis around the elbow.

The medial and lateral intermuscular septa separate the brachium into anterior (flexor) and posterior (extensor) compartments (Fig. 22–2). The posterior compartment contains the radial nerve and the triceps brachii. The anterior compartment contains the coracobrachialis, biceps brachii, and brachialis muscles. The neurovascular bundle tracks along the medial border of the biceps and includes the brachial artery and vein and the musculocutaneous, median, and ulnar nerves. The bundle may deviate from its normal course in the presence of a supracondylar process. This is a bony projection off the anteromedial humerus in the distal one third. When a supracondylar process is present the median nerve and brachial artery pass behind it and then beneath a fibrous band, which connects the process to the medial epicondyle.

An understanding of the muscular anatomy is crucial in the treatment of humerus fractures (Fig. 22–3). The location of the fracture in relation to the various origins and insertions will determine the deforming forces. Fracture above the level of the pectoralis insertion results in the proximal fragment abducting and rotating due to the forces of the rotator cuff. Fracture between the insertion of the pectoralis major and the deltoid insertion results in abduction and proximal migration of the distal fragment by the deltoid and adduction and internal rotation of the proximal fragment by the pectoralis major, latissimus dorsi, and teres major. Fracture distal to the deltoid insertion results in abduction of the proximal fragment by the deltoid and shortening of the distal fragment due to pull of the coracobrachialis and biceps brachii.

Surgical Approaches

Proximal Approach for Intramedullary Devices

The patient is placed in a "beach chair" position with the arm draped free. Care must be taken to ensure that the patient is at the edge of the table and the arm hangs freely off of the table. A 4- to 5-cm incision is made starting at the lateral border of the acromion. The deltoid is split in line with its fibers, and the greater tuberosity is exposed. The supraspinatus tendon may be split and the awl introduced directly into the tuberosity, or the awl may be placed slightly posterior to the tuberosity to avoid impingement. When interlocking nails are used, the interlocking screws are placed through limited incisions with spreading of the underlying soft tissues (Fig. 22–4).

Distal Approach for Intramedually Devices

This approach may be performed with the patient in various positions: lateral, prone, or supine. The distal approach is very useful in the multiply traumatized patient who has other injuries that are being addressed under the same anesthetic.

A posterior triceps splitting approach is used. The triceps is split just proximal to the olecranon exposing the olecranon

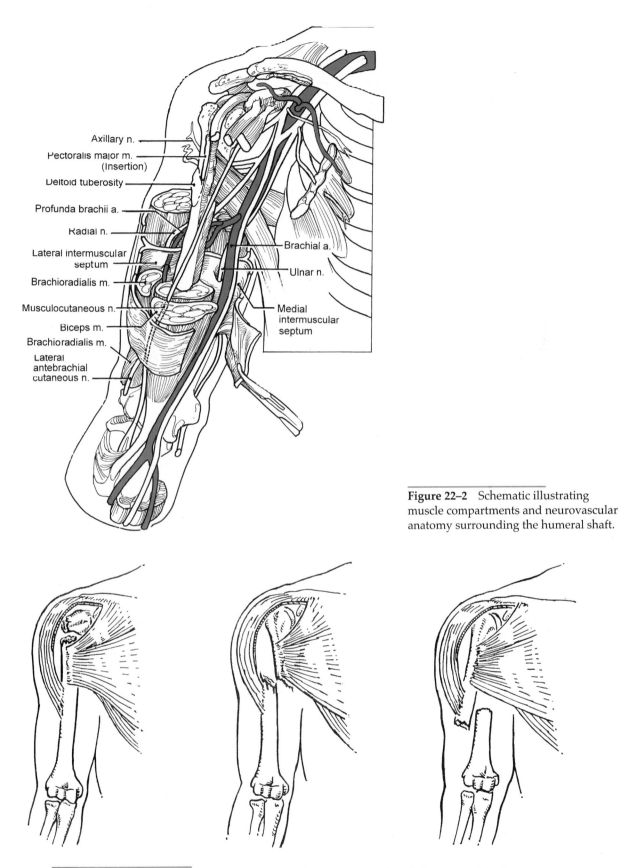

Axillary n.
Pectoralis major m.
(Insertion)
Deltoid tuberosity
Profunda brachii a.
Radial n.
Lateral intermuscular septum
Brachioradialis m.
Musculocutaneous n.
Biceps m.
Brachioradialis m.
Lateral antebrachial cutaneous n.
Brachial a.
Ulnar n.
Medial intermuscular septum

Figure 22–2 Schematic illustrating muscle compartments and neurovascular anatomy surrounding the humeral shaft.

Figure 22–3 Schematic illustrating deforming forces associated with fractures of the humeral shaft. (Reprinted with permission from Johnson ET and DeLong WG Jr. Diaphyseal fractures of the humerus. In: Dee R, Hurst LC, Gruber MA, Kottmeier SA; eds. *Principles of Orthopaedic Practice*. New York: McGraw Hill, 1997;406.)

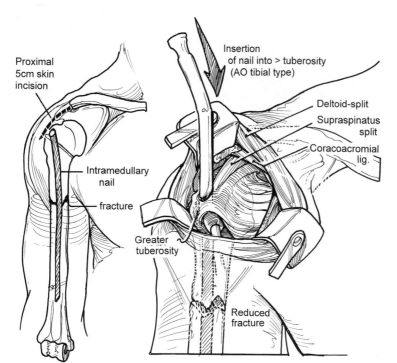

Figure labels:
Proximal 5cm skin incision

Insertion of nail into > tuberosity (AO tibial type)

Deltoid-split

Supraspinatus split

Coracoacromial lig.

Intramedullary nail

fracture

Greater tuberosity

Reduced fracture

Figure 22–4 Schematic illustrating insertion of an interlocking nail for stabilization of a humeral shaft fracture.

fossa and the posterior aspect of the distal humerus. The triceps split does not extend proximally enough to jeopardize the radial nerve in the spiral groove. The starting hole in the cortex is placed 2 cm above the olecranon fossa and is enlarged with a burr (Fig. 22–5). Care must be taken to ensure that the hardware does not impinge in the olecranon fossa.

Open Reduction and Plate Osteosynthesis

The anterolateral, anteromedial, and posterior approaches are the three approaches to the humerus. The anteromedial approach is rarely used because of the significant risk of neurovascular injury.

Anterolateral Approach

This approach is most commonly used for fractures of the proximal and middle thirds of the humerus (Fig. 22–6). This exposure is made with the patient supine and the shoulder abducted. The skin incision is an extension of an extended deltopectoral incision and begins 5 cm distal to the coracoid process. It is placed along the anterior border of the deltoid and then travels along the lateral border of the biceps to within 7 to 8 cm of the elbow joint. Proximally, the plane of dissection is between the deltoid and the pectoralis major muscles. Distally, the biceps is taken medially, and the brachialis is split in the midline. This does not denervate the muscle as the brachialis receives dual innervation. The lateral half is innervated by the radial nerve and the medial half by the musculocutaneous nerve. After splitting the brachialis

muscle, a subperiosteal dissection exposes the medial and lateral aspects of the humerus while protecting the radial nerve with the muscle belly. Retraction of the muscle is facilitated by elbow flexion. Distally the approach continues between the biceps medially and the brachioradialis laterally. At this level, care must be taken to identify and protect the lateral antebrachial cutaneous nerve.

Anteromedial Approach

This rarely used approach allows visualization of the anteromedial surface of the humeral shaft. Deep dissection is carried out posterior to the intermuscular septum and requires mobilization and retraction of the ulnar nerve. The biceps, brachial artery and vein, and the median nerve are retracted anteriorly. The triceps is elevated off the intermuscular septum and subperiosteally dissected off the humerus exposing the shaft.

Posterior Approach

The posterior approach is a triceps-splitting approach that exposes the humeral shaft from the olecranon fossa to the junction of the proximal and middle thirds (Fig. 22–7). A straight posterior incision is made in a line between the posterior edge of the acromion and the tip of the olecranon. The interval between the long and lateral heads is developed bluntly, and the medial or deep head is split in the midline. At the proximal edge of the medial head, the radial nerve and profunda brachii run across the field in the spiral groove and must be identified and protected. Proximally, the dissection is

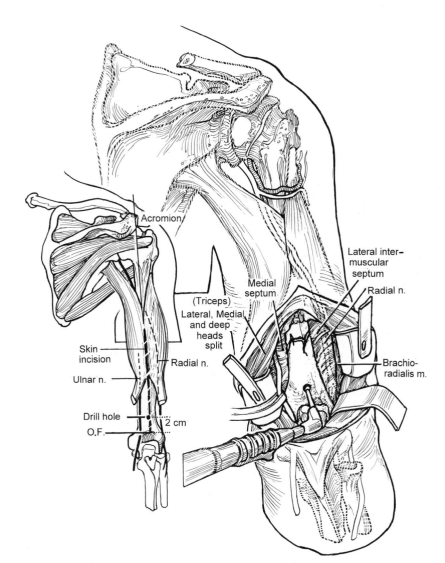

Acromion

Lateral inter-
muscular
septum

Radial n.

Medial
septum

(Triceps)

Lateral, Medial
and deep
heads
split

Skin
incision

Radial n.

Brachio-
radialis m.

Ulnar n.

Drill hole

2 cm

O.F.

Figure 22–5 Schematic illustrating distal approach for the insertion of intramedullary nails.

limited by the axillary nerve and posterior humeral circumflex artery.

AIDS TO DIAGNOSIS

History and Physical Examination

In the acutely traumatized patient, the history is unfortunately often allocated only a few seconds in the initial assessment and a single line on the chart. This is a common and unfortunate mistake. A careful history of the mechanism of the injury and a detailed history of past injury or illness can dramatically change the management of these patients (Table 22–1). In the pediatric population, for instance, it is critical to obtain a detailed history of the injury from all parties involved and then to determine whether the described mechanism matches the fracture pattern. If there is any doubt that the history matches the injury, child abuse must be considered. In this same population, it is critical to obtain past history of injuries or emergency department visits. In the young adult who describes a minor trauma resulting in fracture of the humeral shaft, a pathologic process must be considered. In any patient with a neurological deficit associated with this injury, a thorough history must be obtained with specific attention to head injury and neurological injury or disease. This simple, yet often overlooked, aspect of the workup can prevent the disaster of an unnecessary exploration of a previously injured nerve.

When performing a physical exam on a patient with a humeral shaft fracture, it is important to perform an appropriate overall assessment of the patient based on the history of the injury. The patient with a fracture secondary to a gunshot wound, for example, should be examined from head to toe for other wounds. It is not uncommon for there to be multiple unrecognized entry and exit wounds.

After the initial screening examination, attention is focused on the affected extremity. The extremity will usually be shortened, swollen, and painful. There will be crepitus and tenderness about the fracture site. The vascular status of the extremity is evaluated first. A description of capillary refill alone is insufficient. Specific documentation should be made

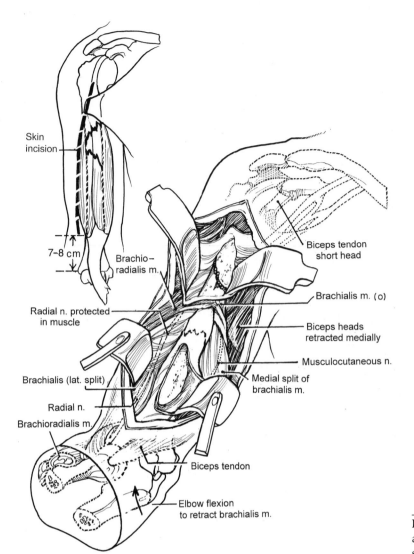

Skin incision

7-8 cm

Brachio-radialis m.

Radial n. protected in muscle

Brachialis (lat. split)

Radial n.

Brachioradialis m.

Biceps tendon short head

Brachialis m. (o)

Biceps heads retracted medially

Musculocutaneous n.

Medial split of brachialis m.

Biceps tendon

Elbow flexion to retract brachialis m.

Figure 22–6   Schematic illustrating anterolateral exposure of the humeral shaft.

of the brachial, radial, and ulnar pulses. These pulses should be compared between the two extremities. A thorough neurological examination is performed with specific documentation of each nerve's sensory and motor function. If a specific motor or sensory function cannot be appropriately assessed, then this should be clearly stated in the chart. The soft tissues are examined for abrasions, lacerations, or puncture wounds. The compartments are assessed with consideration of compartment syndrome always in mind, and finally the joints above and below are examined for point tenderness, motion, and crepitus.

PEARL

Remember that your initial evaluation establishes the baseline from which all future decisions will be made. It is critical to be thorough and specific in both your evaluation and your documentation.

Radiographs

Radiographic evaluation of humeral shaft fractures must include two views of the humerus taken at 90 degrees to one another. These views must include the shoulder and elbow joints.

In a suspected pathologic fracture, staging studies may be necessary prior to definitive treatment. These usually include, but are not limited to, bone scan, magnetic resonance imaging, and computed tomography scan.

PEARL

Remember that to obtain two views at 90 degrees, it will be necessary to turn the patient on the table. Often, the radiology technicians will rotate the arm at the elbow. This gives 90 degree views of the distal shaft but does not allow rotation of the proximal fragment and causes undue pain to the patient.

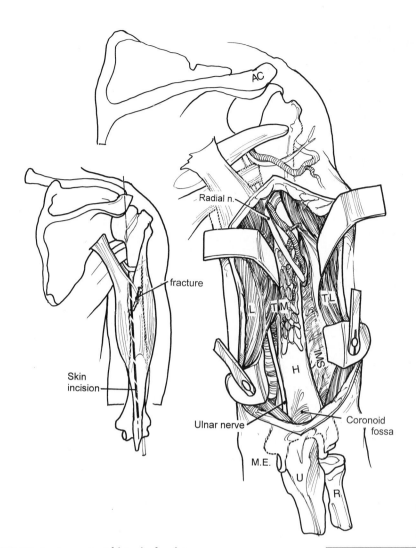

Figure 22–7 Schematic illustrating posterior approach to the humerus.

TABLE 22–1   Important historical points

Mechanism
Does it fit the fracture pattern?
Should pathologic lesion be considered?
Do other organ systems need to be further evaluated (e.g., closed head injury)?

Past History
Is there a history of medical illness which precludes surgery?
Is there a previous peripheral or central neurologic injury affecting the extremity?
Is there a history of metabolic bone disease or malignancy?
Is there a history of lower extremity injury or impairment requiring use of upper extremities for ambulation?

Classification

There is no single classification scheme for humeral shaft fractures. These injuries can be classified according to a number of factors related to the fracture. Intelligent decisions should be based on all the variables outlined in Table 22–2.

SPECIFIC CONDITIONS, TREATMENT, AND OUTCOME

General Considerations

There are a number of methods available for treatment of humeral shaft fractures. Historically, these injuries were associated with a significant incidence of delayed union or nonunion. During the last 20 years, the use of fracture bracing and improved techniques of fracture stabilization have almost eliminated these problems.

There are a number of variables that must be taken into consideration when selecting a treatment plan. The fracture level and its pattern, the soft tissue injuries, associated injuries, and the patient's age, body habitus, and ability to cooperate will influence the choice of the most appropriate treatment. When choosing a treatment, it should be remembered that the humerus can tolerate up to 20 degrees of anterior angulation, 30 degrees of varus angulation, and 1 inch of shortening without functional or cosmetic compromise.

Nonoperative Treatment

The vast majority of humeral shaft fractures can and should be treated nonoperatively, with expected union rates between

TABLE 22–2   Classification scheme for humeral fractures

I. Soft tissue injury
  A. Open fracture
    1. High energy
    2. Low energy
  B. Closed injury
    1. High energy: large zone for injury
    2. Low energy: small zone of injury

II. Fracture location
  A. Above pectoralis insertion
  B. Between pectoralis and deltoid insertions
  C. Below deltoid insertion
  D. Periprosthetic

III. Fracture pattern
  A. Tranverse
  B. Oblique
  C. Spiral
  D. Comminuted
  E. Segmental

IV. Associated injuries
  A. Nerve injury
  B. Vascular injury
  C. Bony injury
    1. Floating elbow
    2. Intra-articular extension
    3. Multiple long bone fractures
  D. Multi system/multiple trauma

V. Condition of bone
  A. Normal
  B. Pathologic
    1. Osteoporotic
    2. Neoplastic
    3. Metabolic bone disease

90 and 100%. Close supervision is essential to ensure a good result. Although there are a number of nonoperative options available, in recent years functional fracture bracing has become the treatment of choice for most of these fractures. Other options include the hanging cast; coaptation splint; Velpeau's dressing and sling and swath; abduction cast or splint; and skeletal traction. Table 22–3 lists the treatment options, their advantages and disadvantages, and the indications for their use.

Hanging Arm Casts

The hanging arm cast is still a commonly used technique for closed treatment of humeral shaft fractures. It is most useful in obtaining reduction in shortened fractures. It can, however, be used in comminuted fractures and even in fractures of the distal shaft. Appropriate use of this device requires adherence to certain treatment principles. The cast must be lightweight to prevent overdistraction and the potential for nonunion. It should extend from 1 inch proximal to the fracture to the wrist. The elbow must be at 90 degrees, and the forearm should be in neutral rotation. The cast is held in position by a sling that is attached to the wrist through loops made in the cast using plaster or wire material. Loops should be placed on the radial border, the dorsal, and the palmar aspect of the wrist (Fig. 22–8). These loops are used to control fracture angulation. Lateral angulation is corrected by placing the loop on the dorsum of the wrist. Medial angulation requires placement of the sling in the palmar loops. Posterior angulation is corrected by lengthening the sling and anterior angulation by shortening the sling. Patients must remain erect or semierect to keep the cast in a dependent position, even during sleep. They must be instructed to prevent the elbow from resting on the arm of the chair when seated. Radiographs should be obtained weekly for the first 4 weeks. Hand, wrist, and shoulder motion should be instituted immediately. Shoulder pendulum exercises are critical to prevent adhesive capsulitis.

The hanging cast requires a compliant patient and can be problematic in the obese patient. Transverse fractures with a small surface area for healing must be observed closely for overdistraction, which may lead to nonunion. If supervised carefully, in an appropriate patient union rates of 93 to 96% have been reported. At the present time, the hanging cast is used as an initial treatment to bring the fracture out to length and hold the reduction. Once the fracture pain has subsided, usually in 7 to 10 days, a functional brace is applied.

Coaptation Splint

The coaptation splint, or U-splint, applied with a collar and cuff is probably the most widely used treatment for closed humeral fractures in the acute setting. This device is very useful in the treatment of fractures that are minimally displaced, or that would be distracted by a hanging cast. This technique involves the use of a plaster slab that runs from the axilla around the elbow and over the deltoid. The cast may be applied over benzoin to prevent slippage and is held in place with elastic bandages (Fig. 22–9). This technique does allow motion of the hand, wrist, and shoulder and so offers some advantage over the hanging cast. Most commonly, it is used to stabilize the fracture in the acute setting and is then replaced with a fracture brace once the initial pain and swelling have resolved.

Velpeau's Dressing and Sling and Swath

The Velpeau's dressing and sling and swath are methods whereby the humerus and forearm are strapped to the body using either plaster or soft materials (elastic wraps, stockinette, etc.) to immobilize the fracture. The fracture angulation is controlled by the use of appropriately placed pads or bolsters between the arm and the trunk. This technique is used only rarely. It is indicated for use in unmanageable

PITFALL

When placing the coaptation splint, it is critical to pad the edge of the splint that lies in the axilla and to make sure that there is no pressure in the axilla with the arm at the patient's side. It is also crucial to ensure that the splint does not place pressure on the ulnar nerve at the elbow. Brachial plexus and ulnar nerve irritation are not uncommon when this splint is improperly applied.

pediatric or geriatric patients until healing has progressed to a point when something less restrictive can be applied.

Abduction Humeral Splint

Some authors have advocated the use of an abduction splint or cast for the treatment of humeral shaft fractures. This technique is rarely used today. It does not allow early motion of the shoulder or elbow and places pressure on the rotator cuff. If this technique is used, the splint should be replaced with a fracture brace or coaptation splint as soon as the fracture shows evidence of healing so that motion can be initiated.

Skeletal Traction

Skeletal traction is another option that is rarely indicated. It can be useful in the patient who must remain recumbent and has extensive soft tissue injuries requiring open wound care.

The traction pin is placed percutaneously through the olecranon just proximal to the level of the coronoid process. It is

TABLE 22–3   Nonoperative treatment of humeral shaft fractures

Treatment Method	Advantages	Disadvantages	Indications
Hanging arm cast	Helps restore length Can control angulation through loops at wrist	Patient must stay erect or semierect Distraction can lead to nonunion Limits range of motion of hand, wrist, elbow, and shoulder	Mostly used for initial treatment to obtain reduction in shortened fracture Usually changed to functional bracing after initial period of Rx
Coaptation splint	Inexpensive Easy to apply Allows motion of hand and wrist	May allow shortening of fracture Axillary irritation Angular union in obese patients	Initial management of nondisplaced or minimally displaced fractures Usually changed to functional bracing
Velpeau's dressing/sling and swath	Can be useful in unmanageable children or elderly who are uncooperative	Restricts motion to all joints Potential for skin maceration	Used as initial treatment in uncooperative children or elderly patients
Abduction cast/splint	No clear advantages	Poorly tolerated awkward position with rotator cuff pressure	Always listed as an option in textbooks, but no clear indication for its use
Skeletal traction	Can be used in recumbent patients Can be used with large soft tissue defects and allows access to wounds	Requires patient cooperation Risk of infection Requires close supervision Potential for ulnar nerve injury	Rarely used as there is no clear advantage over external fixation
Functional fracture bracing	Allows motion of all joints Lightweight and well tolerated Decreased nonunion rate	Is not useful for initial reduction or bringing fracture out to length	The current gold standard for most shaft fractures after an initial period in hanging cast or coaptation splint

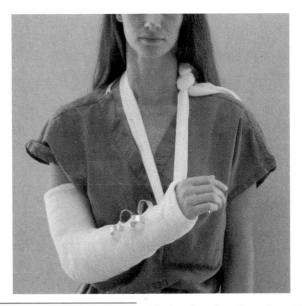

Figure 22–8 Hanging cast. Notice that the elbow is at 90 degrees and the forearm is in neutral. The loops control fracture angulation. Lateral angulation is corrected by dorsal placement. Medial angulation is corrected by palmar placement. Posterior angulation is corrected by lengthening the sling and anterior angulation is corrected by shortening the sling. The arm must remain in a dependent position for this technique to be successful.

passed from medial to lateral to avoid injury to the ulnar nerve. The traction pin is attached to a Kirschner bow, and the forearm is supported with overhead skin traction. Traction is applied in a line parallel to the floor so the elbow is flexed 90 degrees. Active excercises of the hand and wrist are begun immediately. This technique offers no real advantage over external fixation except that it can be easily applied in the intensive care unit in a patient who cannot be brought to the operating room for medical reasons.

Functional Bracing

Sarmiento popularized the use of functional bracing of humerus fractures in the late 1970s. Since that time, fracture bracing has become the treatment of choice in most closed fractures of the humeral shaft. The device is constructed of orthoplast or polypropylene material and is composed of anterior and posterior shells that encircle the arm (Fig. 22–10). The anterior shell has a contour for the biceps muscle, and the posterior shell has a similar contour for the triceps. Proximally, the brace reaches the lateral edge of the acromion laterally and the axilla medially. Distally, it extends to the epicondyles medially and laterally but is recessed in the antecubital fossa and the olecranon fossa to allow elbow flexion and extension. The anterior shell slides inside the posterior shell (or vice versa) and the two are tightened using Velcro straps. These devices may be custom molded or are available "off the shelf." For more distal injuries or fracture with concomitant forearm injuries, a hinged fracture brace with forearm extension may achieve the same goals.

Functional bracing maintains fracture alignment by utilizing the externally applied pressure of the brace to increase the hydraulic pressure of the soft tissue envelope. This pressure combined with the force of gravity acting on the dependent arm allows for the maintenance of fracture alignment while allowing early mobilization of all joints of the upper extremity.

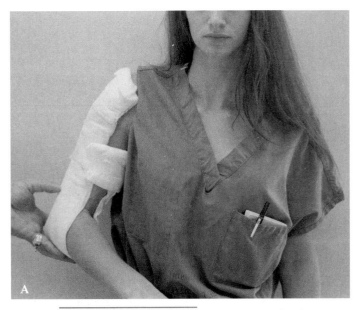
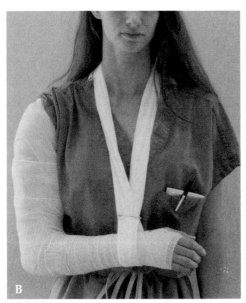

Figure 22–9 **(A)** Coaptation splint. Notice that the splint extends well into the axilla medially, and that there is padding placed over the edge of the splint in the axilla. Care must be taken not to place pressure over the ulnar nerve in the cubital tunnel. **(B)** The collar and cuff is used to prevent posterior or anterior angulation. As with the hanging cast, the arm should remain dependent.

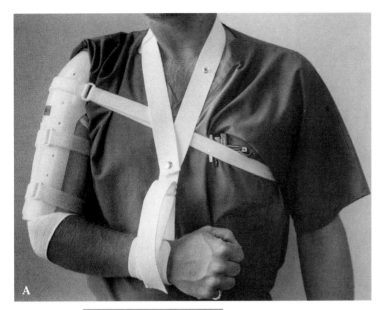 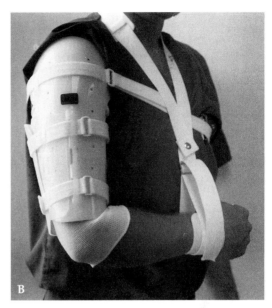

Figure 22–10 Functional fracture brace. **(A)** Anterior and **(B)** posterior shells of orthoplast or polypropylene encircle the arm. The shells are contoured to the biceps and triceps. This device allows for early motion of all joints.

The functional fracture brace is the present treatment of choice for most closed fractures of the humeral shaft. In general, the fracture is stabilized using one of the previously mentioned methods until the acute pain and swelling have resolved. At that time, usually 4 to 7 days postinjury, the patient is placed in the brace and instructed in early motion. Patients should be encouraged to use the arm as can be tolerated and to keep the arm dependent as much as possible. Additionally, they should be instructed not to abduct the arm past 60 degrees until there is radiographic evidence of healing. The patient may remove the brace for hygiene as long as the arm remains dependent. The patent remains in the brace for a minimum of 8 weeks, or until there is radiographic and clinical evidence of healing. Fracture bracing of humeral shaft fractures produces union rates of 96 to 100%.

Contraindications to this form of treatment include fractures with associated soft tissue defects, noncompliant or unreliable patients, fractures that shorten in the brace, and inability to maintain adequate alignment.

PITFALL

Gravity is an important component of fracture bracing for humeral shaft fractures. The use of a sling eliminates the force of gravity and may lead to varus or internal rotation deformities. It also can lead to elbow stiffness in the older patient. Patients should be instructed to discard the sling as soon as comfort allows.

Operative Treatment

The vast majority of humeral shaft fractures can be managed nonoperatively with a high rate of union and low complication rate. There are, however, a number of factors that may dictate operative treatment. Open fractures, failure of closed reduction, pathologic fractures, floating elbow, associated injuries to the joint, polytrauma, and associated neurovascular injuries are all possible indications for surgical intervention.

Surgical options include external fixation, open reduction and internal fixation with a plate and screws, flexible intramedullary devices, and locked intramedullary nails. Table 22–4 lists these methods and their relative advantages and disadvantages.

External Fixation

The major indication for the use of external fixation in the treatment of these fractures is the stabilization of fractures associated with large, soft tissue defects or burns that require easy, frequent access to the soft tissues. Additionally, patients with bone defects or extensively comminuted fractures who require mobilization may be candidates for external fixation.

External fixation in the humerus requires the placement of two pins above and two pins below the fracture site (Fig. 22–11). These pins should be placed under direct visualization to avoid injury to the neurovascular structures. The pins should engage both cortices and should be in the same plane. After placement of the pins the fracture is manipulated under fluoroscopic control, and the frame is applied. Compression may be placed across the fracture if the fracture pattern permits.

TABLE 22–4   Operative treatment of humeral shaft fractures

Operative Method	Advantages	Disadvantages	Specific Indications
External fixation	Allows direct access to soft tissues Allows manipulation of the fracture	Not well tolerated High complication rate	Fractures with large soft tissue defects Fractures associated with burns
Open reduction and internal fixation	Anatomic reduction Allows exploration of the nerve Allows compression of transverse fractures High rate of union Allows early motion of all joints	Potential for radial nerve injury during exposure Difficult to get adequate fixation in distal fractures Cannot use as weight-bearing extremity during early healing	Transverse fractures which are amenable to compression Fractures requiring radial nerve exploration Fractures with large butterfly fragments amenable to interfragmentary fixation
Flexible intramedullary rods	Ease of insertion Low cost of implant Can be easily placed antegrade or retrograde	Poor rotational control Can distract fracture site Potential rotator cuff problems with antegrade passage	Multitrauma patient Pathologic fractures
Rigid intramedullary nails	Can be locked for rotational control Allow early use of arm for crutch walking Allow early motion of all joints	Potential propagation of fracture with nail passage Possible distraction at fracture site Possible radial nerve injury with reaming	Indications increasing Multitrauma patient requiring crutches Segmental fractures

The major problems with external fixation include pin-tract infection, soft tissue impalement, neurovascular injury, and nonunion. These complications can be minimized by good pin-tract care, placement of pins using a limited open technique, and compression through the frame whenever possible.

Open Reduction and Internal Fixation

When plate fixation has been chosen, preoperative planning is essential for choosing the most appropriate surgical approach and method of fixation. After fracture exposure, the fracture is reduced and provisionally fixed using clamps or K-wires. Butterfly fragments should be reduced to a shaft fragment until two large reconstructed fragments remain. These are then reduced, provisionally fixed, and finally fixed definitively with a plate. Whenever possible, interfragmentary compression screws should be used. These may be placed through or outside the plate. If the size of the shaft will allow, a broad 4.5-mm dynamic compression plate should be used.

It is essential that a minimum of six, and preferably eight cortices, be obtained on both sides of the fracture (Fig. 22–12). The plate should be placed in a compression mode for transverse fractures and as a neutralization plate for all other fractures. Following plate fixation, a functional fracture brace is applied and early mobilization is started.

Complications of plate fixation include infection, radial nerve injury, and failure of fixation. Radial nerve injury can be avoided by good exposure and soft tissue technique. Fixation failure is usually avoidable by adhering to proper fixation technique.

Flexible Intramedullary Devices

Flexible intramedullary devices such as Rush rods or Enders pins are still popular for the treatment of humeral shaft fractures (Fig. 22–13). These devices can be placed antegrade or retrograde, although there have been reports of problems with the rotator cuff when placed antegrade. It is important to place multiple rods to provide stability at the fracture site.

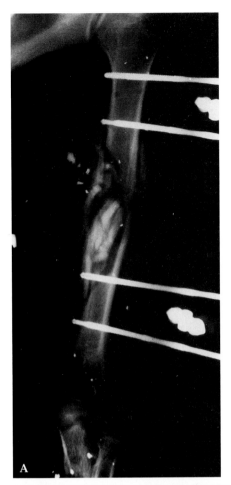

Figure 22–11 (A) Radiographs of a patient with an open humeral fracture with a large area of soft tissue loss. (B) An external fixator was placed to stabilize the fracture and allow management of the soft tissues.

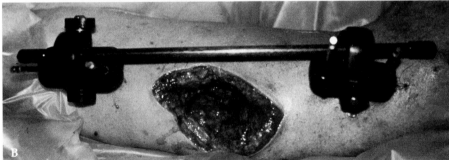

Care must also be taken to prevent distraction at the fracture site. A functional brace is used in conjunction with the rods to prevent fracture displacement

Advantages of these devices include ease of insertion, minimal morbidity, and cost of the implant. Disadvantages include poor rotational control, fracture distraction, impingement of the rotator cuff if the rods are passed antegrade, and fracture through the window used to pass the rods in a retrograde fashion.

Intramedullary Nailing

Rigid, locked intramedullary nails have been gaining popularity in recent years. This is due to the success of locked nails in the treatment of tibia and femur fractures and also to the development of several nails designed specifically for use in

PEARL
When using retrograde Enders nails, the nails have a tendency to back out. Prevent this by wiring the nails together and fixing the wire to the humerus with a unicortical 3.5-mm screw.

the humerus. Indications are similar to those for plating with the addition of segmental fractures and pathologic or impending pathologic fractures. Contraindications include fractures with associated neurologic deficit, open fractures with severe soft tissue injuries, and atrophic nonunions.

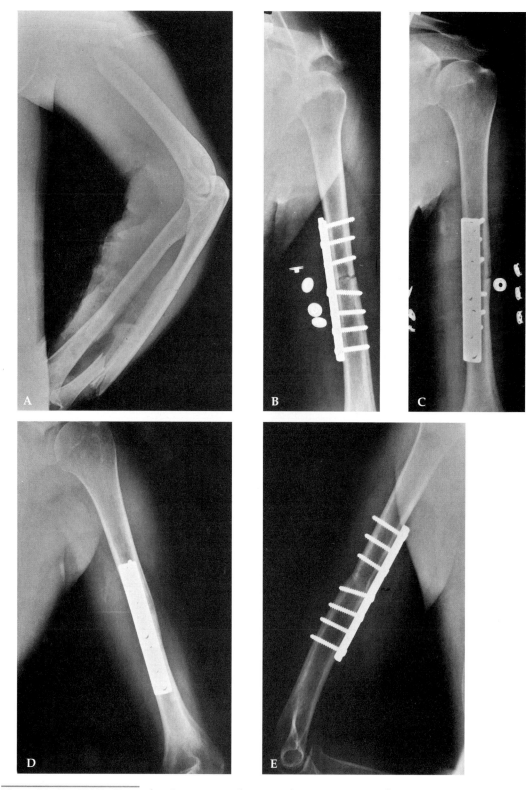

Figure 22–12 **(A)** Radiographs of a transverse humerus fracture treated with open reduction and internal fixation. **(B, C)** A broad dynamic compression plate should be used and a minimum of six (preferably eight) cortices should be obtained above and below the fracture. The plate should be placed in compression for transverse fractures and as a neutralization plate for other fracture patterns. **(D and E)** Anteroposterior and lateral radiographs of healing fractures.

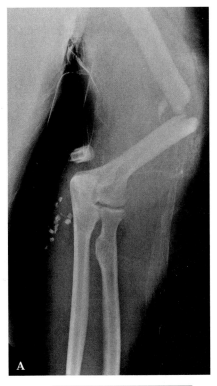
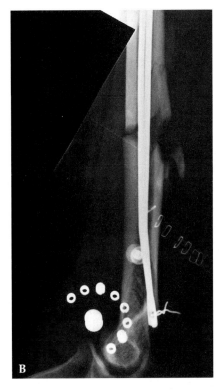
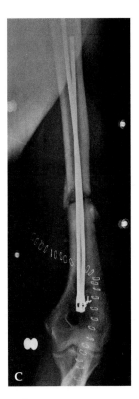

Figure 22–13   Radiographs of a patient with multiple injuries who was treated with retrograde Enders nails. **(A)** Anteroposterior projection of transverse diaphyseal fracture. This patient had contralateral lower extremity injuries. Both sides were treated simultaneously with the patient supine. Retrograde nailing with flexible devices can be performed with the patient in almost any position. **(B** and **C)** Lateral and anteroposterior of humerus with Enders nails.

These nails may be placed as unlocked or statically locked devices (Fig. 22–14). The proximal locking screws are placed using a jig attached to the nail, and the distal screws are usually placed freehand using image intensification. These nails may also be placed antegrade or retrograde.

Complications include nonunion, impingement of the nail with shoulder abduction, loss of shoulder motion, radial nerve injury due to reaming (fractures located near the radial sulcus), and propagation of fractures distally into the joint.

PEARL

Intramedullary fixation is specifically indicated in the multitrauma patient who will require crutches for weight bearing. Using the nailed extremity for weight bearing can speed the healing process. This is in contrast to the patient with a plated humerus who would require several weeks before the extremity could be bear weight.

Complications

The primary complications of this fracture include nonunion, malunion, infection, and radial nerve injury. Epps (1985) has defined a number of factors that predict the prognosis for these injuries. He noted that fractures that are in close proximity to or involving the joint carry a poorer prognosis. Associated neurovascular injury results in a worse functional outcome. Poor patient compliance will affect the outcome, particularly

in closed treatment requiring gravity dependence and early mobilization. Transverse, short oblique, and segmental fractures will heal more slowly than spiral oblique fractures.

Malunion

Because of the wide range of motion at the glenohumeral and scapulothoracic joints, the humerus can tolerate up to 20 to 30 degrees of angular malunion and up to 2 cm of shortening without loss of arm function. Additionally, rotational malunion of up to 15 degrees is well tolerated. The obese patient tends to develop angular deformity. The very body habitus that predisposes the fracture to angular malunion tends to minimize the cosmetic deformity as the deformity is masked by the soft tissue folds. Cosmesis should rarely be an indication for corrective surgery. When there is functional restriction secondary to malunion, osteotomy with rigid internal fixation is the treatment of choice.

Nonunion

Nonunion occurs in 2 to 5% of patients treated nonoperatively and has been reported in up to 25% of fractures treated by open reduction and internal fixation (Ward et al., 1992). Recent reports have demonstrated a significant incidence of nonunion with the use of unlocked intramedullary nails. There are a number of factors that will affect the incidence of nonunion. Metabolic disease, poor nutritional status, high velocity injuries, open fractures, and extensive soft tissue injuries all adversely impact the healing process. The fracture

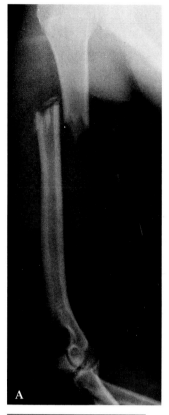 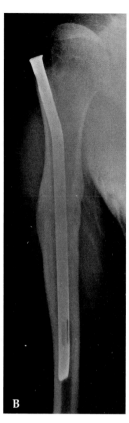

Figure 22–14 (A and B) Radiographs of a humeral shaft fracture in a multiple trauma patient treated with antegrade nailing using an AO tibial nail. Note the callus formation, which is characteristic of healing with intramedullary nailing.

personality is defined by all these variables and should be considered when selecting the appropriate treatment method.

Radial nerve injury

Radial nerve injury has been reported in up to 18% of humeral shaft fractures (Ward et al., 1992). Greater than 90% of these are neuropraxias, and 95% of these will recover spontaneously by 4 months post injury. The exceptions to this rule are the injuries associated with sharp penetrating trauma, open fractures, or nerve injuries that occur during the reduction maneuver. These all represent probable lacerations to the nerve, and primary exploration and repair in conjunction with internal fixation is indicated. The Holstein-Lewis fracture or the spiral oblique fracture at the middistal third of the shaft is commonly discussed as an indication for early exploration of the nerve. Exploration in such cases is somewhat more controversial than those discussed above, and there is literature to support either observation or early exploration.

In the face of an injury that is believed to be a neuropraxia, the patient should be followed for 6 weeks. At that time, if there is no evidence of nerve recovery on clinical exam the patient should undergo baseline electromyographic and nerve conduction velocities. If there is evidence of reinnervation (motor unit recruitment) in the wrist extensors or brachioradialis, then conservative management should be continued. If there is no electrical evidence of recovery, the nerve studies should be repeated at 12 weeks postinjury. If there is no clinical or electrical evidence of recovery after 3 months, the radial nerve should be explored.

PEARL

Low velocity gunshot wounds do not represent sharp penetrating trauma. The vast majority of these will be neuropraxias and will resolve spontaneously. Median nerve palsy can be associated with these fractures when a supracondylar process is present on the distal humerus.

SUMMARY

Satisfactory functional outcome and primary healing should be achieved in greater than 90% of humeral shaft fractures if proper treatment is applied. Functional bracing following a period of splinting or casting facilitates early rehabilitation and has an excellent rate of union. This should be considered the nonoperative treatment of choice and is the mainstay of treatment for closed humeral shaft fractures. Operative treatment of these fractures with compression plating or intramedullary nailing should produce similar results if meticulous technique and appropriate implants are used. Familiarity with the anatomy and the biology of fracture healing is critical to the development of a rational approach to these fractures.

SELECTED BIBLIOGRAPHY

Fracture Healing

BARRON SE, ROBB BA, TAYLOR WF, and KELLY PJ. Effect of fixation with intramedullary rods and plates on fracture site blood flow and bone remodeling in dogs. *J Bone Jt Surg.* 1977;59A:376–385.

CRUESS RL, DUMONT J. Healing of bone, tendon, and ligament. In: Rockwood CA, Green DP, eds. *Fractures.* Philadelphia, PA: Lippincott, 1975:147–168.

FROST HM. The biology of fracture healing. *Clin Orthop Rel Res.* 1989;248:283–293.

Nonoperative Treatment

BALFOUR GW, MOONEY V, ASHBY M. Diaphyseal fractures of the humerus treated with a ready-made fracture brace. *J Bone Jt Surg.* 1982;64A:11–13.

GILCHRIST DK. A stockinette Velpeau for immobilization of the shoulder girdle. *J Bone Jt Surg.* 1967;49A:750–751.

HOLM CL. Management of humeral shaft fractures. Fundamentals of nonoperative techniques. *Clin Orthop.* 1970; 91:132–139.

SARMIENTO A, KINMAN PB, CALVIN EG. Functional bracing of fractures of the shaft of the humerus. *J Bone Jt Surg.* 1977;59A:596–601.

Operative Treatment

BELL MJ, BEAUCHAMP CG, KELLAM JK, MCMURTRY RY. The results of plating humeral sahft fractures in patients with multiple injuries. *J Bone Jt Surg.* 1985;67B:293–296.

BRUMBECK RJ, BOSSE MJ, PKA A, BURGESS AR. Intamedullary stabilization of humeral shaft fractures in patients with multiple trauma. *J Bone Jt Surg.* 1986;68A:960–969.

CHAPMAN MW. Closed intramedullary nailing of the humerus. *Instr Course Lect.* 1982;31.

FOSTER RJ, DIXON GL, BACH AW, APPLEYARD RW, GREEN TM. Internal fixation of fractures and nonunions of the humeral shaft: Indications and results in a multi-center-study. *J Bone Jt Surg.* 1985;67A:857–864.

HALL RF, PANKOVICH AM. Ender nailing of acute fractures of the humerus. *J Bone Jt Surg.* 1987;69A:558–567.

KUNEC JR, LEWIS RJ. Closed intramedullary rodding of pathologic fractures with supplemental cement. *Clin Orthop.* 1984;188:183–186.

STERN PJ, MATTINGLY DA, POMEROY DL. Intramedullary fixation of humeral shaft fractures. *J Bone Jt Surg.* 1984;66A:639–646.

VANDER GRIEND RA, TOMASIN J, WARD EF. Open reduction and internal fixation of humeral shaft fractures. *J Bone Jt Surg.* 1986;68A:430–433.

WARD EF, WHITE J. Interlocked intramedullary nailing of the humerus. *Orthopaedics.* 1989;12:135–141.

Complications

BOSTMAN O, BAKALIM G, VAINIONPAA S, WILPPULA H, ROKKANEN P. Immediate radial nerve palsy complicating fracture of the shaft of the humerus. when is early exploration justified? *Injury.* 1985;16:499–502.

EPPS CH Jr, COTLER JM. Complications of treatment of fractures of the humeral shaft. In: Epps CH Jr ed. *Complications in orthopedic surgery.* 2nd ed. Philadelphia, PA: Lippincott; 1985;231–243.

GARCIA A, MAEK BH. Radial nerve injuries in fractures of the shaft of the humerus. *Am J Surg.* 1960;99:625–627.

HOLSTEIN A, LEWIS GB. Fractures of the humerus with radial nerve paralysis. *J Bone Jt Surg.* 1963;45A:1382–1388.

WARD EF, SAVAGE FW, HUGHES JL. Fractures of the diaphyseal humerus. In: Bronner BD, Jupiter JB, eds. *Skeletal Trauma.* Philadelphia: Saunders, 1992;1177–1200.

SAMPLE QUESTIONS

1. Which of the following statements regarding hanging casts is false:
   (a) may be used to help obtain an acceptable reduction
   (b) may be difficult to use in the obese patient
   (c) the cast should be as heavy as can be tolerated to maximize anatomical alignment.
   (d) can be used for 7 to 10 days before converting to a functional brace
   (e) Adjusting the length of the suspension straps can help correct angulation of the fracture.

2. Which of the following statements regarding fracture braces is true:
   (a) should be used with a sling to help control fracture rotation
   (b) will facilitate healing of most humeral shaft fractures
   (c) can be used for open fractures if the wound has been carefully irrigated
   (d) is particularly efficacious in the obese patient

3. A 47-year-old man falls from a ladder and sustains an open fracture of his humeral shaft. He is unable to extend his fingers, wrist, or thumb. Appropriate management includes:
   (a) wound incision and debridement with application of a fracture brace, check nerve studies in 3 weeks.
   (b) wound incision and debridement with application of an external fixator; check nerve studies in 3 weeks.
   (c) wound incision and debridement with plate fixation; check nerve studies in 3 weeks.
   (d) wound incision and debridement; explore radial nerve. Plate or rod fixation.
   (e) closed humeral rodding

4. Closed humeral rodding with a flexible intramedullary rod may be associated with all of the following except:
   (a) rapid healing
   (b) poor rotational control
   (c) impingement with rods placed in an antegrade (proximal to distal) fashion
   (d) backing of nails placed in retrograde (distal to proximal) fashion
   (e) union rates superior to functional bracing

5. A 17-year-old falls off a skateboard and sustains a closed, long oblique fracture of her humeral shaft. The fracture is angulated 30 degrees and shortened 1 cm. She has a complete radial nerve palsy. Appropriate management consists of:
   (a) Closed treatment of the fracture; follow recovery with exam. If no change at 6 weeks, check nerve study. Consider exploration at 3 to 4 months if no improvement in exam or on a nerve study repeated at 12 weeks.
   (b) Open treatment of fracture; explore the radial nerve.
   (c) Closed treatment of fracture. Check nerve study in 3 to 5 days; if it confirms complete palsy, proceed with nerve exploration.
   (d) Closed treatment of fracture; check nerve study in 6 weeks. If study shows evidence of reinnervation but exam shows no sign of recovery, explore the radial nerve.

Answers: 1) c; 2) b; 3) d; 4) e; 5) a

Chapter 23

Fractures and Dislocations of the Elbow

Peter G. Mangone, MD, Thomas T. Dovan, MD, and John G. Seiler III, MD

Outline

Elbow fractures and dislocations can result from either a direct blow or an axial load transmitted through the forearm. Most commonly, these injuries are the result of either a fall or a blunt trauma injury such as a motor vehicle accident. The type injury depends on the position of the limb and direction and magnitude of the applied force. For example, radial head fractures are often the result of either a direct blow to the proximal radius or a fall onto an outstretched hand with a valgus stress at the elbow. Each elbow injury has its own unique characteristics. Thorough examination of the patient and the radiographs help define the nature of the injury. Knowledge of the anatomy and biomechanics of the elbow combined with the clinical data about the injury is critical for successful treatment.

BASIC SCIENCE

Kinematics of the Elbow Joint

The elbow joint is composed of three separate articulations: the ulnohumeral, the radiohumeral, and the radioulnar. The ulnohumeral joint is the main site of flexion and extension. The radioulnar joint is the main site of pronation and supination. The radiohumeral joint participates in both of these motions.

Range of Motion

The normal range of motion of the elbow is from 0 to 150 degrees of flexion. Normal pronation and supination are 75 degrees and 85 degrees, respectively. Most activities of daily living can be accomplished with flexion from 30 to 130 degrees, pronation of 50 degrees, and supination of 50 degrees.

Carrying Angle

When examining the elbow joint in full extension, the forearm rests in slight valgus (10 to 15 degrees in males and 15 to 20 degrees in females) compared with the straight line axis of the brachium.

Flexion and Extension of the Elbow Joint

Elbow flexion and extension occurs at both the ulnohumeral and radiocapitellar joints of the elbow. Due to the obliquity of the trochlear groove running anterolateral to posteromedial, the ulnohumeral joint is not a true hinge joint. Instead it is a "sloppy hinge," allowing both rotation about a central axis and a sideways translation, creating a helical-type motion with flexion and extension (Fig. 23–1).

There is a cluster of points that individually acts as the axis of rotation depending on the joint load, joint position, and other factors. The average axis of rotation passes through the center region of the lateral epicondyle and the inferior border, not the center, of the medial epicondyle.

The axis of rotation of the radiocapitellar joint is the mechanical axis of the forearm rotation. This is a straight line that passes through the center of the radial head and the center of the distal head of the ulna. It is distinct from the anatomic axis of the forearm (Fig. 23–2).

Orthopaedic Surgery: The Essentials. Edited by M.E. Baratz, A.D. Watson, and J.E. Imbriglia. Thieme Medical Publishers, Inc., New York © 1999

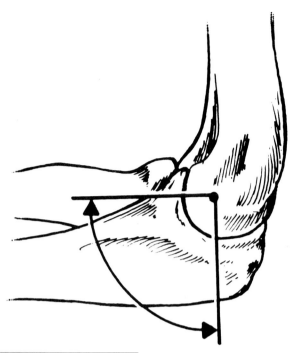

Figure 23–1   The functional axis of elbow flexion and extension.

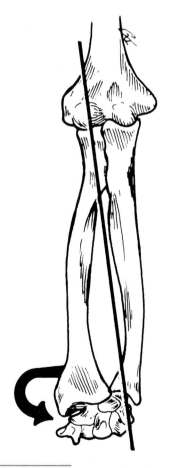

Figure 23–2   The axis of forearm rotation (drawn here) is distinctly different from the anatomic axis of the forearm. Reproduced with permission from An KN, Morrey BF. *The Elbow and its Disorders*. Philadelphia: Saunders, 1993, 54.

Biomechanics of the Elbow
Capsule and Ligaments of the Elbow Joint

The elbow capsule covers the elbow joint. The capsule's strength is derived from the cruciate arrangement of the fibers. The medial and lateral sides of the capsule are reinforced by collateral ligaments (thickened intracapsular bands). The medial collateral ligament consists of three elements: the anterior oblique band, the posterior oblique band, and the transverse band (Fig. 23–3). The anterior oblique band originates on the medial epicondyle and inserts on the anteromedial aspect of the ulna at the base of the coronoid. The posterior band originates on the medial epicondyle and inserts on the medial olecranon. The transverse band runs from the posterior olecranon to the anterior coronoid.

The major lateral structures include the radial collateral ligament, the annular ligament (LCL), the lateral collateral ligament the accessory lateral collateral ligament, and the lateral ulnar collateral ligament (LUCL). Unlike the medial collateral ligament, the LCL complex originates at the axis of rotation and is isometric during elbow flexion and extension. The thin, radial collateral ligament originates on the lateral epicondyle and inserts on the annular ligament. The annular ligament is a thick, multilayered fibrous band that attaches to the anterior and posterior edges of the lesser sigmoid notch and wraps around the radial head covering the entire surface, except that portion articulating with the ulna. The accessory LCL is a thin layer that attaches the annular ligament to the supinator tuberosity, helping to resist varus stress. The most stout and identifiable lateral capsular structure is the LUCL. This ligament originates on the the lateral epicondyle and inserts on the supinator crest of the ulna. Several studies have demonstrated both the presence of a discrete LUCL and its importance for posterolateral rotational stability of the elbow.

Elbow Stability

Valgus stability of the flexed elbow depends primarily on the medial collateral ligament and the radial head. Using a serial sectioning method it appears that the primary valgus stabilizer is the anterior oblique band of the medial collateral ligament, and that the radial head is a secondary stabilizer (Table 23–1). Valgus stability in full extension is dependent on the radial head, medial collateral ligamant, and the anterior joint capsule, each element contibuting about one third of the stability. Valgus stability should be tested in both 0 and 30

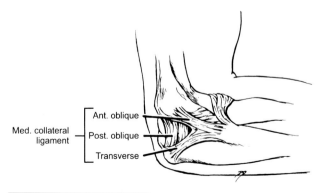

Figure 23–3   The three major elements of the medial collateral ligament.

TABLE 23–1 Valgus Elbow Stability

MCL	Radial head	Elbow stability
present	present	stable
present	absent	stable
absent	present	subluxes but stable
absent	absent	grossly unstable

MCL, medial collateral ligament.

degrees of flexion. When the elbow is extended, the olecranon tip in the olecranon fossa can theoretically stabilize the joint when a valgus stress is applied.

Varus instabilty of the elbow depends on the integrity of the ulnohumeral joint, the anterior joint capsule, and the lateral collateral ligament. Anatomic studies have reported that the ulnohumeral articulation is the primary stabilizer in both flexion and extension. With the elbow extended, the ulnohumeral joint was responsible for 55% of the resistance to varus stress; in full flexion, the percentage increases to 75%. In both positions, the anterior capsule was the secondary stabilizer and the LCL was the third most important stabilizer. Division of the LUCL band of the LCL can cause posterolateral rotational instability.

Elbow Joint Loading and Contact Forces

Joint loading and contact forces for the ulnohumeral joint depend on the resultant vector of the applied forces across the elbow. These variable forces depend on factors such as the number of muscles contracting, the position of the elbow, the total muscle force, and the forearm and hand position.

Forces at the ulnohumeral articulation are dependent on the resultant vector from muscle contraction and applied external loads. For example, flexion forces that act across an extended elbow will produce higher forces in the distal aspect of the greater sigmoid notch than in the posterior aspect. As flexion increases the resultant force vector intersects the greater sigmoid notch in the region of the bare area and distributes the force more equally across the anterior and posterior contact areas.

The loading forces across the radiocapitellar joint also depend on elbow position. The highest radiocapitellar joint forces occur between 0 to 30 degrees of flexion. Pronation results in a greater joint loading force than supination in all positions of elbow flexion and extension because the radius translates proximally (corkscrews) during forearm pronation. In the extended arm, approximately 60% of an axial load passes through the radiocapitellar joint while 40% goes through the ulnohumeral joint.

RELEVANT ANATOMY AND SURGICAL APPROACHES

Osseous Anatomy

Distal Humerus

The distal humerus consists of two separate columns, medial and lateral. Each supports a separate articulation with an articular segment, condyle, and epicondyle. The distal humerus has a fossa just above the articular surface that constrains the the bony prominences of the radius and ulna during elbow flexion and extension (Fig. 23–4).

The medial and lateral epicondyles are tuberosities that are points of muscular origin. The medial epicondyle serves

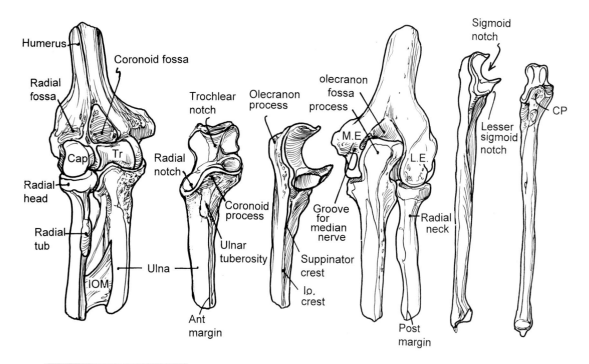

Figure 23–4 Schematic illustrating osseous anatomy of the elbow.

as the origin for the flexors of the elbow and wrist. The lateral epicondyle provides the origin for the extensors.

The trochlea and capitellum are the articulating components of the distal humerus. The trochlea consists of a larger medial and smaller lateral facet separated by a midline groove that gives the trochlea a spool-like appearance. It articulates with the greater sigmoid notch of the proximal ulna. The trochlea is internally rotated 5 to 7 degrees and is in approximately 6 degrees of valgus. The capitellum articulates with the concave surface of the radial head. The capitellum and trochlea are angled 30 degrees anterior to the long axis of the humerus.

Proximal Ulna

The proximal ulna is composed of the olecranon, greater and lesser sigmoid notch, coronoid process, crista supinatoris, supinator crest, and attachment points for several forearm muscles.

The tip of the olecranon provides the insertion point for the triceps tendon. The olecranon forms the proximal, two thirds of the greater sigmoid notch. The anterior and distal portion of the proximal ulna is composed of the coronoid. The coronoid is an attachment point for the caspsule and the anterior oblique band of the medial collateral ligament. It forms the distal, one third of the greater sigmoid notch and lies just medial to the lesser (radial) sigmoid notch (Fig. 23–5).

The greater sigmoid notch is an elliptical concavity that articulates with the trochlea of the distal humerus. The lesser sigmoid notch is a smaller concavity in the proximal ulna lateral and inferior to the coronoid that articulates with the radial head.

Inferior and superior to the lesser sigmoid notch are the attachment points for the annular ligament. The supinator crest extends laterally and distally from the lesser notch and is the origin for the supinator muscle. Slightly inferior and distal to the supinator crest is the crista supinatoris, an insertion point for the LUCL.

Proximal Radius

The proximal radius is composed of the radial head, the radial neck, and the radial tuberosity. Articular cartilage covers the concave surface of the radial head, as well as 240 degrees of the outer surface of the cylinder. The remaining anterolateral portion of the radial head's outer surface is bare. The concave surface articulates with the capitellum and allows for both rotation and translation. The outer surface of hyaline cartilage articulates with the lesser sigmoid notch as the radius rotates about the ulna during pronation and supination.

The radial head and neck lie in approximately 15 degrees of valgus relative to the shaft of the radius.

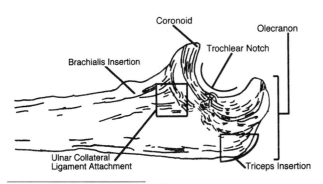

Figure 23–5 Medial view of elbow shows ligaments responsible for elbow stability. Reprinted with permission from Baratz ME, Shanan IF. Fractures of the olecranon. *J South Orthop. Assoc.* 1995;4:285.

Neurovascular Structures of the Elbow Joint

Radial Nerve

The radial nerve originates from spinal nerve roots C6, C7, and C8, with variable contributions from C5 and T1. It lies in the arm posteriorly between the long head and medial head of the triceps muscle, traveling distally to enter the spiral groove (Fig. 23–6). At the distal, one third of the humerus, it pierces the lateral intermuscular septum gaining access to the anterior compartment of the brachium. From there it descends anterior to the lateral epicondyle between the brachioradialis laterally and the brachialis medially. Just anterior to the radio-capitellar joint, it divides into the posterior interosseous nerve (PIN) and the superficial sensory branch

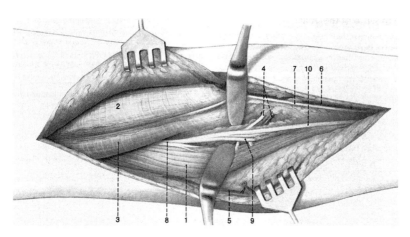

Figure 23–6 Exposure of radial nerve between brachial is and brachioradial is muscles. 1 = Brachioradialis; 2 = Biceps; 3 = Brachialis; 4 = Radial recurrent artery and vein; 5 = Cephalic vein; 6 = Basilic vein; 7 = Lateral artebrachial cutaneous nerve; 8 = Radial nerve; 9 = Deep branch of radial nerve; 10 = Superficial branch of radial nerve. Reprinted with permission from Bauer Operative Approaches in Orthopaetic Surgery and Traumatology. p. 270.

of the radial nerve. The superficial sensory branch runs distally under the brachioradialis. The posterior interosseous nerve runs laterally and posteriorly around the radius passing under the proximal edge of the supinator muscle and diving between the leading edge (the arcade of Frohse) of the superficial and deep layers of this muscle.

Median Nerve

The median nerve originates from the C5, C6, C7, C8, and T1 nerve roots. In the middle of the humerus, the nerve crosses anterior to the artery and takes a straight path to the elbow. When it reaches the antecubital fossa, medial to the biceps tendon and brachial artery, it passes under the bicipital aponeurosis and courses into the forearm between the two heads of the pronator teres muscle (Fig. 23–7).

Ulnar Nerve

The ulnar nerve originates from nerve roots C8 and T1. Descending along the medial side of the brachial artery, it pierces the medial intermuscular septum in the middle of the brachium. It runs distally in a plane that is beneath the arcade of Struthers, posterior to the medial intermuscular septum and anterior to the medial head of the triceps (Fig. 23–7). Passing posterior to the medial epicondyle, it enters the cubital tunnel and rests in a groove bordered laterally by the posterior portion of the medial collateral ligament. From here it continues distally between the humeral and ulnar heads of the flexor carpi ulnaris.

Musculocutaneous Nerve

The musculocutaneous nerve originates from nerve roots C5, C6, C7, and C8 and travels in the arm deep to the biceps muscle and superficial to the brachialis muscle. At the level of the elbow joint, it pierces the brachial fascia lateral to the biceps tendon, where it terminates as the lateral antebrachial cutaneous nerve.

Brachial Artery

The brachial artery is the continuation of the axillary artery. At the midlevel of the arm the artery runs in a plane anterior to the brachialis muscle and medial to the biceps. It enters the antecubital fossa beneath the biceps aponeurosis, medial to the biceps tendon and lateral to the median nerve, branching into the radial and ulnar arteries at the level of the radial head (Fig. 23–8).

Ulnar and Radial Arteries

From its origin, the ulnar artery travels deep to the ulnar head of the pronator teres. It then courses between the flexor carpi ulnaris and the flexor digitorum profundus (deep to the flexor digitorum superficialis) and travels distally with the ulnar nerve. The radial artery runs between the brachioradialis and the pronator teres, continuing down the forearm under the brachioradialis with the superficial sensory branch of the radial nerve (Fig. 23–8).

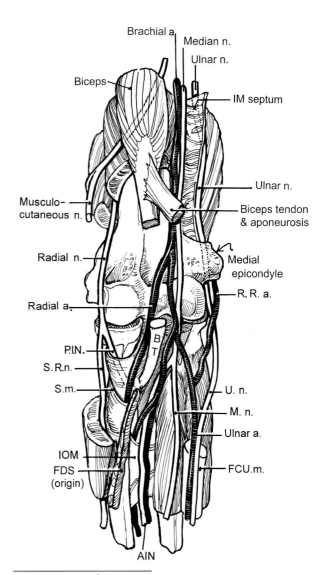

Figure 23–7 Schematic illustration neurovascular anatomy about the elbow.

Collateral Circulation

Arising from the brachial artery are the superior and inferior ulnar collateral arteries and the deep brachial artery, which gives rise to the radial and middle collateral arteries.

The profunda brachii artery travels with the radial nerve and terminates as the radial and medial recurrent arteries. The radial collateral accompanies the radial nerve through the lateral intermuscular septum to the anterior aspect of the elbow into the antecubital fossa, where it anastomoses with the radial recurrent artery at the level of the lateral epicondyle (Fig. 23–8).

Muscles of the Elbow Joints
Major Rotators of the Forearm

Understanding the function of the muscles about the elbow joint is easier once you know the origin, insertion, and innervation.

Table lists the muscles along with function, location, origin, insertion, innervation, and secondary function.

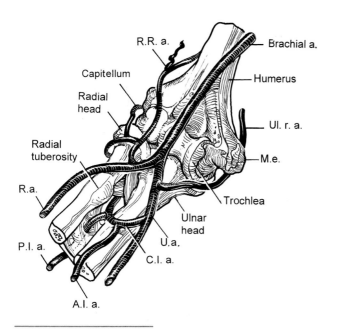

Figure 23–8 Schematic illustrating the vascular anatomy about the elbow.

Surgical Approaches
Anterior Approach (Fig. 23–9)

Uses include anterior capsular release, repair of the brachial artery, median nerve, radial nerve, and distal biceps tendon ruptures.

A curvilinear incision is made beginning on the anteromedial border of the biceps brachii. The incision curves laterally into a transverse incision across the elbow crease. The incision is carried distally along the medial border of the brachioradialis.

PITFALL

During an anterior approach to the elbow, do not cross the flexion crease at 90°.

In the proximal exposure, the internervous plane lies between the brachialis (musculocutaneous nerve) and the brachioradialis (radial nerve). Dissect between the brachialis and biceps brachii. Identify and retract the brachial artery and median nerve. The median nerve is medial to the brachial artery. Identify the biceps tendon and bicipital aponeurosis (lacertus fibrosis). The brachialis muscle overlies the anterior humerus and anterior elbow joint capsule. Identify the median nerve distally as it passes between the two heads of the pronator teres. Dissect and retract the brachialis muscle from the anterior humerus. Identify and open the elbow capsule beneath the brachialis muscle.

PITFALL

Avoid damage to the lateral antebrachial cutaneous nerve as it emerges between the brachialis and biceps brachii and crosses obliquely over the brachioradialis.

To achieve distal exposure, identify the biceps tendon, the radial nerve and its division into radial sensory branch and the posterior interosseous nerve (PIN), which runs through the supinator at 90° to the muscle fibers. Supinate the forearm to move the PIN away from the line of dissection. Identify the PIN to facilitate exposure of the radial head and neck.

PITFALL

Avoid damage to the brachial artery, radial artery, and ulnar artery, as well as the radial recurrent artery, which runs along the proximal border of the supinator.

Posterior Approach (Fig. 23–10)

The posterior surgical approach is indicated for olecranon fractures, distal humerus fractures, posterior capsular release, and total elbow arthroplasty. The patient in a prone position should have his elbow flexed 90° over a radiolucent table with the shoulder abducted. The patient in a supine position should have his elbow flexed 90° resting on a pillow across his thorax with shoulder abducted. A sterile tourniquet is useful in both instances.

For olecranon fractures, a curved incision should be made 4 cm proximal to 8 cm distal and curving around the olecranon tip. The incision may be extended proximally depending on the nature of the distal humerus fracture.

Identify the triceps and ulnar nerve from the arcade of Struthers to the cubital tunnel.

PEARL

Protect the ulnar nerve by transposing it to the anterior elbow.

Exposure for extra-articular distal humerus fractures can be performed through either a longitudinal triceps splitting approach or by using a triceps tenotomy. For the triceps splitting approach, bluntly divide the muscle fibers until the humeral shaft is reached. Periosteally dissect the triceps muscle off the posterior humeral shaft. Place retractors subperiosteally to expose the humerus and the fracture. For a triceps tenotomy, protect the ulnar nerve. Make a transverse z-cut through the middle of the triceps tendon. If access to the middle of the humeral shaft is necessary, the radial nerve must be identified. It will be coursing obliquely from medial

TABLE 23–2   Muscles of the Elbow Joint

Major Rotators of the Elbow

Muscle	Function	Location	Origin	Insertion	Innervation	Secondary functions
Biceps bracii (two heads)	supination	anterior	coracoid (short head) superior glenoid (long head)	radial tuberosity	musculocutaneous nerve	flex elbow
Supinator	supination	anterolateral	lateral epicondyle and proximal ulna	posterolateral radius	PIN	none
Pronator teres (two heads)	pronation	anteromedial	medial epicondyle and medial coronoid	lateral midshaft radius	median nerve	flex elbow (weak)
Brachioradialis	supination when elbow flexed	lateral	lateral supracondylar humerus	distal lateral radius	radial nerve	flex elbow
Flexor Carpi Radialis	pronation	medial	medial epicondyle	base of second and third metacarpal	median nerve	flex elbow when elbow flexed (weak)

Major Extensors of the Elbow

Muscle	Function	Location	Origin	Insertion	Innervation	Secondary functions
Triceps brachii (three heads)	extend elbow	posterior	inferior glenoid (long head) post/lateral humerus (lateral head) post/medial humerus (medial head)	olecranon (proximal)	radial nerve	none
Aconeus	extend elbow	posterior	lateral epicondyle	olecranon (distal)	radial nerve	none

Major Flexors of the Elbow

Muscle	Function	Location	Origin	Insertion	Innervation	Secondary functions
Brachialis	flex elbow	anterior	anterior humerus	anterior coronoid	musculocutaneous and radial nerves	none
Biceps brachii	flex elbow	anterior	coracoid (short head) superior glenoid (long head)	radial tuberosity	musculocutaneous nerve	supination
Pronator teres (two heads)	flex elbow	anteromedial	medial epicondyle and medial coronoid	lateral midshaft radus	median nerve	pronation
Brachioradialis	flex elbow	lateral	lateral supracondylar humerus	distal lateral radius	radial nerve	supination when elbow flexed

(continued)

TABLE 23–2   *(continued)*   **Muscles of the Elbow Joint**

Wrist and Digit Extensors that Cross the Elbow

Muscle	Function	Location	Origin	Insertion	Innervation	Secondary functions
Extensor carpi radialis brevis	extend wrist	lateral	lateral supracondylar humerus	base of second metacarpal	radial nerve	radial deviation of wrist
Extensor carpi radialis longus	extend wrist	lateral	lateral epicondyle	base of third metacarpal	radial nerve	elbow flexion
Extensor carpi ulnaris	extend wrist	posterior	lateral epicondyle	base of fifth metacarpal	PIN	ulnar deviation of wrist
Extensor digitorum comminis	extend fingers	posterior	lateral epicondyle	extensor apparatus of fingers	PIN	none
Extensor digitorum quinti	extend small finger	posterior	lateral epicondyle	ulnar aspect of EDC tendon to small finger	PIN	none

Wrist and Digit Flexors that Cross the Elbow

Muscle	Function	Location	Origin	Insertion	Innervation	Secondary functions
Flexor carpi radialis	flex wrist	anteromedial	medial epicondyle	base of second and third metacarpals	median nerve	radial deviation of wrist
Flexor carpi ulnaris (two heads)	flex wrist	medial	medial epicondyle and posterior ulna	pisiform	ulnar nerve	ulnar deviation of wrist
Palmaris longus	flex wrist	anteromedial	medial epicondyle	palmar aponeurosis	median nerve	none
Flexor digitorum superficialis	flex PIP joints of fingers	anteromedial	medial epicondyle anterior radius	base of middle phalanx of each finger	median nerve	none

to lateral on the posterior surface of the humerus. Elevate the triceps from the posterior shaft of the humerus. The extra-articular distal one-third of the humerus and the fracture should be visible.

PITFALL

The radial nerve is in danger if periosteal dissection is carried to the middle one-third of the humerus.

For intra-articular distal humerus fractures, dissect medial and lateral to identify the medial and lateral collateral ligaments. Dissect the FCU and aconeus from the olecranon. A transverse drill hole is made in the proximal posterior shaft of the ulna, and an 18 gauge wire is placed through the hole. This will be used for tension band wire fixation of the olecranon osteotomy. A chevron type olecranon osteotomy is made at the midpoint of the olecranon. The osteotomy is retracted proximally by releasing the capsular attachments to the proximal ulnar fragment. After fracture fixation, the olecranon osteotomy is repaired with tension band wiring.

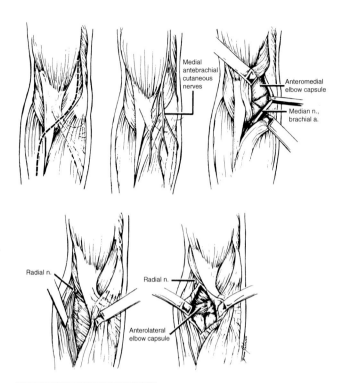

Figure 23–9 The anterior approach to the elbow.

Lateral Approach (Proximal Thompson)
(Fig. 23–11)

This approach is used for radial head excision, exploration of the proximal PIN, lateral epicondyle and capitellum fractures, anterior capsular release, anterior elbow synovectomy, distal radial tunnel exploration and release, as well as ORIF of the proximal radius.

The patient should be placed supine with the arm on a radiolucent hand table. The elbow is flexed 60° to 90° with the forearm pronated. The incision is made from the lateral epicondyle to 8 cm proximal to Lister's tubercle.

Identify the EDC and ECRB. The division is easier to discern more distally in the incision. Retract the EDC and ECRB, exposing the supinator muscle.

Palpate the cordlike PIN as it runs perpendicular to the fibers of the supinator. Supinate the forearm, retract the PIN,

and subperiosteally dissect the supinator from the proximal radius. Identify and open the anterior/lateral capsule to expose the radial head, proximal radial neck, and the capitellum.

Lateral Approach (Kocher)
(Fig. 23–12)

This approach can be used for radial head fractures, radial head excision, lateral epicondyle fractures and release. Place the patient supine, arm on a radiolucent hand table, elbow flexed 60° to 90°, and the forearm pronated. A curvilinear incision is made from the lateral epicondyle to the posterior aspect of the ulna, approximately 6 cm distal to the olecranon tip. The incision should lie just posterior to the radial head.

Identify the aconeus and ECU. This division is easier to appreciate distally. Dissect proximally to the common origin of the lateral epicondyle. Reflect the anconeus and ECU, exposing the elbow capsule. Pronate the forearm to protect the PIN. This approach may be extended proximally with an incision along the lateral supracondylar ridge of the humerus.

Incise the capsule in line with the radius but not beyond the annular ligament. Identify the capitellum, radial head, and annular ligament. If the approach is extended proximally, elevate the triceps from the lateral condyle exposing the posterolateral corner of the distal humerus.

PITFALL

Dissection to the annular ligament places the PIN in danger. The radial nerve is anterior to the lateral epicondyle and is in danger if dissection is carried anteriorly.

Medial Approach (Fig. 23–13)

This approach is useful for anterior and posterior capsular release, ulnar nerve exploration and anterior transposition, medial epicondylar release, medial epicondyle fractures, coronoid process fractures and exploration of the brachial artery and proximal median nerve.

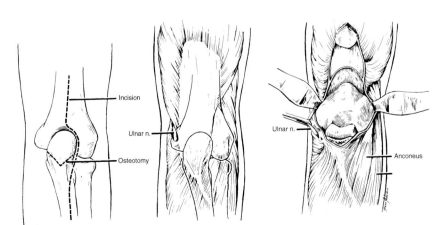

Figure 23–10 The posterior approach to the elbow.

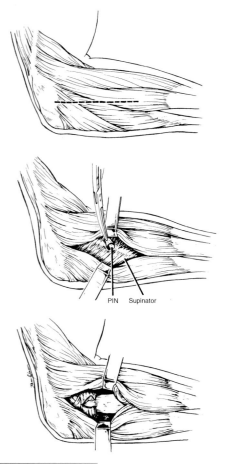

Figure 23–11   The proximal Thompson lateral approach to the elbow.

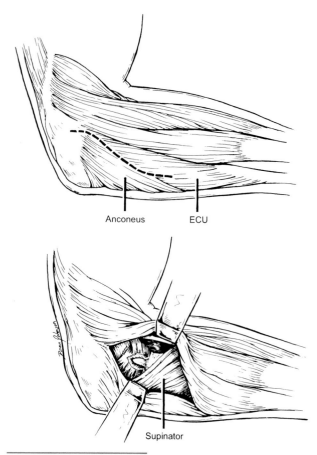

Figure 23–12   The Kocher lateral approach to the elbow.

A curvilinear incision is made with its apex over the medial epicondyle.

In the proximal half of the dissection, identify the ulnar nerve behind the medial intermuscular septum and dissect distally to the cubital groove and into the FCU on the posterior aspect of the medial epicondyle.

Identify and retract the medial antebrachial cutaneous nerves as it courses obliquely across the distal portion of the incision. Trace the ulnar nerve from the posterior aspect of the medial epicondyle into the FCU. Identify the first motor branch of the FCU. Identify and retract the median nerve as it runs between the two heads of the pronator teres. Retract the pronator teres medially by partial release from its origin to gain access to the brachialis and anterior elbow capsule.

Identify the medial collateral ligament, especially the anterior oblique band at the anterior and inferior edge of the medial epicondyle. Incise the capsule to access the medial elbow joint. Elevate the triceps to access the posterior elbow capsule.

EXAMINATION

Always carefully document physical findings on the chart. Examine the skin and perform a complete neurovascular examination. Assess compartments of the forearm and hand.

Palpate bony prominences, check motion, and assess stability of both the elbow and distal radioulnar joint of the wrist.

Radiographs

Anteroposterior (AP), lateral, and radiocapitellar views of the elbow—*true* AP and lateral views are critical. If wrist pain and tenderness are present, obtain posteroanterior and lateral views of the wrist.

AIDS TO DIAGNOSIS

Stress Views

Radiographs taken while a varus or valgus stress is applied to the elbow can help document laxity of the elbow joint.

Traction Radiographs

Traction radiographs performed intra-operatively are an inexpensive method of obtaining better vizualization of comminuted fracture of the distal humerus.

Tomography

Trispiral or computed tomography (CT) may provide superior images of comminuted fractures and intra-articular fragments.

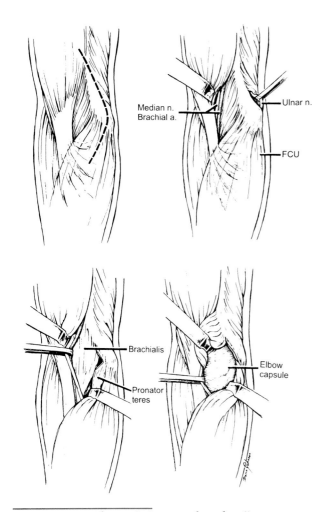

Radial Head and Neck Fractures

Classification and Treatment

Radial head and neck fractures have been classifild by a system described by Mason (1954) and later modified by Johnston (1962) (Fig. 23–14). Type I fractures are minimally displaced. Type II fractures are "marginal sector fractures with displacement." Johnston further defined them as having "widening of the head and depression or tilting of the segment". Type III fractures are comminuted. Type IV fractures are associated with an elbow dislocation.

Although the classification system developed by Mason and Johnston has been useful for common fracture patterns of injury, it does not incorporate clinical information that often guides treatment. For example, elbow motion is an important variable. A classification system is proposed that not only describes the injury but guides treatment (Table 23–3).

Type I fractures are nondisplaced or minimally displaced. Type IA fractures have unimpeded elbow motion. Type IB fractures have a mechanical block or click. Patients will benefit from either a CT arthrogram to look for an osteochondral fragment or surgery to assess the joint. Examination for mechanical block is done by aspiration of the hematoma and injection of a local anesthetic.

Type IIA fractures are displaced, segmental, and noncomminuted or minimally comminuted fractures without mechanical block or click. These fractures are treated nonoperatively with early motion. Type IIB are similar radiographically but have a mechanical block or click on exam. For these fractures, we recommend operative treatment (Fig. 23–15). There are several options for internal fixation including mini-compression plate, Herbert screw, and polyglycolide pins. Smith and Hotchkiss (1996) helped to define the safest area on the radial head for hardware placement. The forearm is placed in full supination, full pronation, and neutral rotation. In each of these positions, a longitudinal line is drawn on the lateral surface of the radius that bisects the AP width of the radial head and neck. Both the posterior and anterior borders of the hardware "safe zone" can be determined from these three lines. The posterior border is defined by a line that bisects the lines made in full pronation and neutral rotation (45 degrees from the most posterior mark). The anterior border is defined by moving 2 to 3 mm anterior to the line that bisects the lines made in full supination and neutral rotation

.**Figure 23–13** The medial approach to the elbow.

SPECIFIC CONDITIONS TREATMENT, AND OUTCOME

Initial Treatment

Uncomplicated injuries can be treated with a well-padded, posterior splint with the elbow in 60 degrees of flexion with neutral rotation of the forearm.

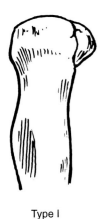
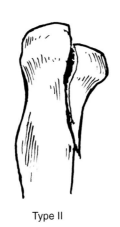
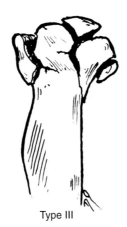

Type I
Type II
Type III

Figure 23–14 The Mason classification of radial head fractures

TABLE 23–3 Modification of the Mason-Johnston classification of radial head and neck fractures

	Radiologic Description	Clinical Exam	Treatment
Type IA	Nondisplaced *or* minimally displaced	No mechanical block No click	Conservative Sling or posterior splint Early motion
Type IB	Nondisplaced *or* minimally displaced	Mechanical block present *or* Click present	Arthroscopy *or* Open exploration and osteochondral fragment excision Early motion
Type IIA	Displaced, segmental, noncomminuted *or* minimal comminution	No mechanical block No click	Conservative Sling or posterior splint Early motion
Type IIB	Displaced, segmental, noncomminuted *or* minimally comminuted DRUJ subluxation/dislocation	Mechanical block present *or* Click present *or* DRUJ injury/tender IOM	Fragment excision if < 30% radial head AP width ORIF Radial head excision and placement of prosthetic spacer if unable to ORIF* Possible pinning DRUJ (if injured)
Type III	Comminuted	Mechanical block present or absent	Radial head excision and placement of prosthetic spacer* ORIF
Type IVA	Elbow dislocation Radial head fracture of Type IA or Type IIA variant	*After reduction* No mechanical block No click No instability	Sling or posterior splint Early motion (initially limit extension to 45 degrees)
Type IVB	Elbow dislocation Radial head fracture of Type IB, Type IIB, or Type III variant	*After reduction* Mechanical block present Click present Instability present	Type-IB open excision of fragment Type-IIB ORIF Type-III radial head excision and placement of prosthetic spacer*

* If silastic radial head prosthesis used, plan for removal eight weeks after insertion. IOM, interosseous membrane; ORIF, open reduction internal fixation.

(about 35 degrees from the most anterior mark). With these fixation techniques, authors report good results. Although these fracture can be treated with radial head excision, late proximal radius migration, wrist pain, and loss of strength can develop. In the isolated case of a small fragment that involves 30% or less of the articular surface, excision has been reported to be a successful alternative.

Type III fractures are comminuted. Treatment options include early excision of the fractured radial head with or without a prosthetic spacer or open reduction and internal fixation (ORIF). The results following open reduction and internal fixation have not been as good as excision. The use of a prosthetic radial head depends on the injury and the clinician's judgment. Coleman et al (1987) reported virtually no complications in the 17 patients they reviewed who had been treated with radial head excision alone. When interosseous membrane injury or elbow instability is suspected, excision without prosthetic replacement can lead to a valgus deformity, proximal migration of the radius and distal radioulnar joint subluxation.

For these cases, the use of a prosthetic radial head spacer is recommended until the soft tissues heal. If a silastic implant is used, it should be removed after 8 weeks to prevent prosthesis fracture and silicone synovitis.

Type IV fractures are associated with elbow dislocation (Fig. 23–16). Treatment consists of elbow reduction and treatment of the fracture according to the algorithm described above.

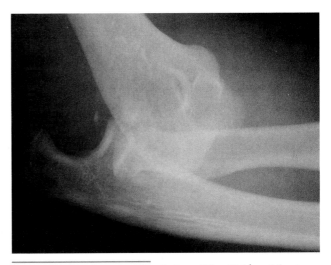

Figure 23–16 An example of a type IV radial head fracture.

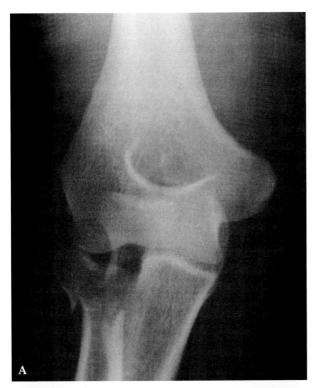

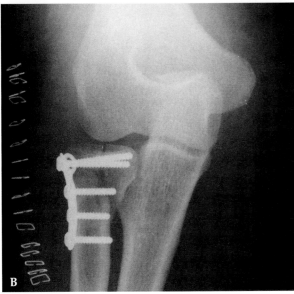

Figure 23–15 (**A**) This patient sustained a type IIB radial head fracture. (**B**) She subsequently underwent open reduction and internal fixation.

Essex-Lopresti Fractures

A rare but clinically important variant of radial head and neck fractures are those associated with distal radioulnar joint (DRUJ) subluxation or dislocation.

The force that fractures the proximal radius can disruption of the interosseous membrane and the restraining ligaments of the distal radioulnar joint. When this occurs, the radius migrates proximally resulting in a shortened radius and subluxated ulnar head at the wrist. If overlooked, it is associated with wrist and elbow dysfunction. Patients pre-

sent with wrist pain and tenderness. The diagnosis can be confirmed by comparing radiographs of the injured wrist with radiographs from the uninjured wrist.

Treatment consists of either open reduction and internal fixation of the radial head or excision and placement of a prosthesis. This decision depends on the severity of the radial head fracture. Either percutaneous pinning or splinting the forearm in supination may be used to keep the DRUJ reduced. The prosthetic implant is removed after the interosseous membrane has healed, about 8 weeks after insertion.

Olecranon Fractures

Classification and Treatment

Many classification systems have been developed for the olecranon fracture. Our preferred system is a combination of Colton's, Schatzker's, and Wolfgang's systems and is based on both injury pattern and treatment options (Table 23–4 and Fig. 23–17).

Type I fractures are nondisplaced and can be treated with immobilization for 4–6 weeks. Close followup is necessary as these fractures may displace.

Type II fractures include displaced avulsion (extra- and intra-articular) and transverse fractures. These fractures can be treated with either open reduction and internal fixation or fracture fragment excision with triceps advancement. The treatment depends on the age and demands of the patient, the quality of the bone, and the size of the fractured fragment. Many methods of fixation of transverse fractures have been described, including tension-band wire alone, K-wires and tension band, large compression screw, and large compression screw with tension band. We recommend that two-part transverse fractures be fixed with a tension band wire combined with two longitudinal K-wires. Prominent hardware has been reported with this method and is often attributed to inadequate seating of the K-wires at the time of surgery.

There are reports in the literature of large, fracture fragments (even greater than 50% of the greater sigmoid notch) being excised without untoward effect on strength, stability, and range of motion. However, biomechanical studies by An et al (1986) have suggested increasing elbow instabilty that is linearly proportional to the amount of proximal ulna excised.

TABLE 23–4   Classification of olecranon fractures

Type	Radiographic Description	Treatment
Type I	Nondisplaced (< 2mm displacement or articular incongruity)	Splint/cast in slight extension (45 to 60 degrees) until healing seen
Type II	*Displaced and noncomminuted* Avulsion (extra/intra-articular) Transverse without comminution	Tension-band wire* Fragment excision
Type III	*Displaced and noncomminuted* Oblique (either direction)	Compression plate with interfragmentary lag screw
Type IV	Comminuted	Compression plate Supplemental interfragmentary lag screw if possible ICBG (if needed) Fragment excision if fracture beyond repair
Type V	Fracture of any type with associated elbow dislocation	*After reduction* Treat olecranon fracture based on its type

*We recommend 2 K-wires with tension band wiring. ICBG, Iliac crest bone graft.

We discourage excision of the fracture fragment as the primary operative treatment for the typical two-part transverse olecranon fracture. Fragment excision is indicated for severely comminuted fractures that cannot be adequately reconstructed with internal fixation.

The noncomminuted oblique olecranon fracture should be treated differently than the transverse fracture. Tension-band wiring creates unequal compressive forces across the fracture site. We prefer fixing these fractures with an interfragmentary lag screw perpendicular to the fracture line and a compression plate on the posterior olecranon (Fig. 23–18).

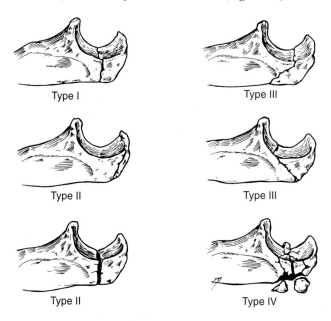

Figure 23–17   Modified classification of olecranon fractures (type V not shown).

Type IV fractures (comminuted), are best treated with a compression plate and interfragmentary lag screws. These fractures may require bone grafting. Highly comminuted fractures may not be amenable to plate fixation. In this event, K-wires with tension-band wiring and bone graft can be used (Fig. 23–19). If the fracture is comminuted beyond repair, excision and triceps advancement is recommended.

Monteggia Fractures

The Monteggia fracture is a fracture of the proximal, one-third of the ulna, with a concommitant radial head dislocation. This injury occurs in 1 to 2% of forearm fractures. Radiographs must focus on the radiocapitellar joint as the radial head dislocation can be subtle. A line drawn through the radial head and shaft should intersect with the capitellum on any view of the elbow.

Four types of Monteggia fractures have been described. The first three types (I, II, and III) are classified according to the direction of the fracture apex and radial head dislocation. Type I is an anterior radial head dislocation, type II a posterior radial head dislocation, and type III lateral. The type IV Monteggia fracture is a type I injury with a concommitant fracture of the proximal one third of the radius.

Monteggia fractures require open reduction and internal fixation of the ulna fracture and reduction of the radial head. If reduction of the ulna fracture restores ulnar length, the radial head will often reduce in a stable position. Intra-operatively, the stability of the radial head can be assessed by moving the elbow under fluoroscopy. If the ulna is accurately reduced and the radial head remains unstable, the radial head must be exposed and reduced. Reduction may require removal of interposed soft tissue from the joint capsule such as a portion of the annular ligament.

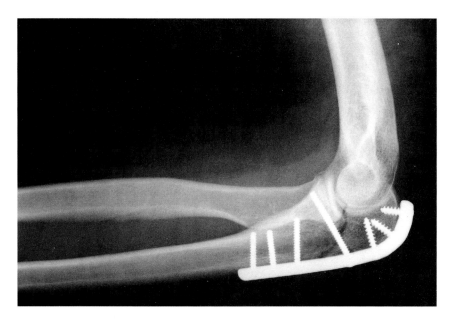

Figure 23–18 An example of a type III (oblique) olecranon fracture treated with open reduction and internal fixation using a compression plate and interfragmentary screw.

Fractures of the Coronoid Process

Classification and Treatment

The beak-shaped coronoid process is the insertion point for the anterior bundle of the medial collateral ligament and middle half of the anterior portion of the capsule. It forms the anterior buttress of the greater sigmoid notch, contributing to elbow stability.

Isolated fractures of the coronoid process are rare. They are typically associated with significant elbow trauma and occur in 2 to 10% of elbow dislocations. The mechanism of injury is usually elbow hyperextension or forced posterior displacement of the proximal ulna.

Radiographic assessment of coronoid fractures requires oblique views because visualization on lateral projections is difficult due to superimposition of the radial head.

Regan and Morrey (1992) classified coronoid process frac-

tures into three types. A type I fracture is an avulsion of the tip of the coronoid process. Type II is a single or comminuted fragment involving 50% or less of the coronoid process. A type III injury is a single or comminuted fragment involving greater than 50% of the coronoid process.

For type I fractures, the elbow joint should be immobilized for 3 weeks or less (at 45 to 60 degrees of flexion) followed by active motion. Associated osseous injuries should be treated by standard methods but avoiding an immobilization period of more than 3 weeks. Treatment is the same for type II injuries unless the elbow is unstable. For type II coronoid fractures with associated ulnohumeral instability, consideration should be given to reduction and stabilization of the coronoid fragment. Occasionally, the fragments are not amenable to direct stabilization techniques. In these cases, the patient may benefit from application of an external fixator. Type III fractures are almost always associated with signifi-

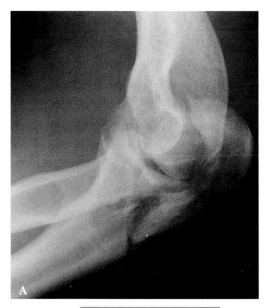
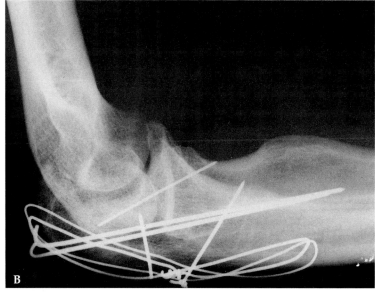

Figure 23–19 (**A**) An example of a type V (comminuted) olecranon fracture (**B**) reconstructed using K-wire fixation, tension band wiring and bone grafting.

cant elbow instability and are a challenging clinical problem. If there is a single coronoid fragment, then open reduction and internal fixation is recommended. Occasionally, an external fixator is necessary to stabilize the fracture and allow protected motion while the bone and soft tissues repair. If there is severe comminution, the fragments should be stabilized with No. 5 braided, Dacron sutures placed through the ulna. Fragment resection is usually not recommended. The treatment methods described by Regan and Morrey yield satisfactory results in 90% of type I, 67% of Type II, and 20% of type III coronoid process fractures.

Distal Humerus Fractures

Classification and Treatment

Distal humerus fractures are currently classified using either the AO system or the Mehne and Matta system. The AO classification is based on the fracture's location, comminution, and involvement of the articular surface. Mehne and Matta's classification divides fractures into intra-articular, extra-articular/intracapsular, and extra-articular and extracapsular variants (Jupiter and Mehne, 1992). The fractures are subdivided by individual anatomic pattern (Table 23–5).

Distal humerus fractures are a challenge to the orthopaedic surgeon. Over the last 30 years, techniques of internal fixation have improved giving surgeons the ability to stabilize most distal humerus fractures. Improvements in outcome from the use of open reduction and internal fixation techniques have three goals in common: accurate intra-articular reconstruction, stable fixation, and early active motion.

The distal humerus is exposed through an olecranon osteotomy or triceps-sparing approach. The ulnar nerve is exposed and transposed anteriorly. Fracture fragments are reassembled, usually starting with the articular surface (see Tools of the Trade). If the joint is comminuted, start rebuild-

ing the column that has the least comminution. Provisional pin fixation is helpful. A fully threaded 3.5-mm screw is used to fix the articular surface. Two 3.5-mm reconstruction plates are used to fix the two columns. One is placed on the medial aspect of the medial column. The second is placed on the posterior aspect of the lateral column. Areas of cortical discontinuity are filled with corticocancellous graft. Cancellous defects are filled with cancellous bone. The olecranon osteotomy is rigidly fixed with a screw or pins supplemented with tension-band wiring. If a triceps-sparing approach is used, the reflected triceps is sutured to the olecranon tuberosity with No. 2 nonabsorbable suture. Before closure, motion is checked and intra-operative radiographs are obtained. The elbow is splinted until the wound is sealed, usually within 3 to 5 days. Gentle active-assisted motion is then begun.

Stiffness remains a common complication of distal humerus fractures. In a study of 29 patients, Aitken and Rorabeck (1986) report that "the most important indicator of end result was the starting time of physiotherapy." Those patients starting therapy before 6 weeks had a significantly better outcome than those immobilized longer. Other complications include nonunion, malunion, infection, neuritis, heterotopic bone formation, and arthrosis.

Capitellum Fractures

This injury is usually the result of a fall onto an outstretched hand with the elbow in slight flexion. These fractures have been divided into three types. Type I is a large fragment with both cartilage and bone (an osteochondral fragment). Type II is a fragment involving just the articular surface. Type III fractures are comminuted. Type I fractures have been treated with excision in the past, but several authors now report good success using countersunk screw fixation to obtain accurate reduction and stable fixation. Another option is fixation by placement of two 3.5-mm screws from the "bare spot" on the

TABLE 23–5   Mehne and Matta classification of distal humerus fractures

Intra-articular fractures	Extra-articular/ intracapsular fractures	Extra-articular/ extracapsular fractures
Single column	Transcolumn fractures	Medial epicondyle
Medial	High	Lateral epicondyle
High	Extension	
Low	Flexion	
Lateral	Abduction	
High	Adduction	
Low	Low	
	Extension	
	Flexion	
Bicolumn		
T pattern		
High		
Low		
H pattern		
Lamda pattern		
Medial		
Lateral		
Capitellum fractures		
Trochlea fractures		

posterior aspect of the humerus into the capitellar fragment. This spot can be exposed through an extended Kocher approach. The triceps is elevated. The ulnohumeral ligaments are preserved. Type II and III fractures are often treated by excision of the fracture fragments. Active elbow motion should be started soon after surgery.

Elbow Dislocations

Classification and Treatment

Elbow dislocations can be divided into two categories: simple (without fracture) or complex (with fracture). Each is then divided based on the direction of the dislocation: anterior, posterior, lateral, and medial, the most common type being posterior. In rare circumstances, the radius and ulna will be displaced in opposite directions. This is a divergent dislocation. Isolated, radial head dislocation has also been reported.

Neurovascular injuries with elbow dislocations are common and include entrapment or injury to the brachial artery, median nerve, and ulnar nerve. The forearm should also be assessed for compartment syndrome.

The direction of the dislocation determines the technique used for reduction. For posterior dislocations, the patient is placed prone on the stretcher or bed, and the affected arm is allowed to dangle over the side of the bed. Conscious sedation is administered. Traction is applied by pulling down on the arm with one hand while the other hand gently guides the olecranon in a distal direction. When the elbow reduces, a palpable "clunk" will often occur. The elbow is then placed through a full range of motion. Varus and valgus stability are tested in full extension and 30 degrees of flexion. Examination of the neurovascular status and forearm compartments should be repeated. The elbow is placed in a well-padded posterior splint (with about 90 degrees of flexion). Passive motion should be avoided, as it has been reported to increase the occurrence of myositis ossificans. Instead, early, active motion appears to be the key to better outcome. Mehlhoff et al (1988) examined the results of 52 patients who had sustained a simple elbow dislocation. They found that patients who were immobilized longer than 4 weeks had more pain and significantly less motion than those who began motion early. They recommended "that gentle active flexion be started as soon as pain will allow and that unprotected flexion and extension should be initiated before 2 weeks." Mehlhoff et al and Protzman reported no long-term instability in patients with stable reductions who were treated with early, active motion. Operative treatment of simple dislocations is not necessary and offers no advantage to closed reduction and early motion. The long-term outcome for patients who sustain a simple elbow dislocation is generally good, with the most common sequelae being loss of full elbow extension.

Complex Elbow Dislocations

Complex elbow dislocations are common injuries occurring in up to 49% of all elbow dislocations. The radial head, coronoid, and medial and lateral epicondyles are the most frequent areas of fracture. Early reduction of the elbow joint, and splint stabilization should be accomplished. After imaging studies have been completed, the operative plan must be tailored to the injury. If the radial head is comminuted, valgus stability of the elbow must be assessed. If the anterior oblique band of

medial collateral ligament is also injured, the elbow may be unstable to valgus stress. In this case, the medial collateral ligament is repaired or a prosthetic radial head spacer placed to prevent chronic valgus instability.

Outcome from complex elbow dislocations is generally worse than simple dislocations and often results in decreased motion with increased pain after the injury. Thompson and Garcia (1967) reported myositis ossificans in 24 of 136 (18%) patients with complex dislocations compared to only 11 of 311 (4%) patients with simple dislocations (Fig. 23–20).

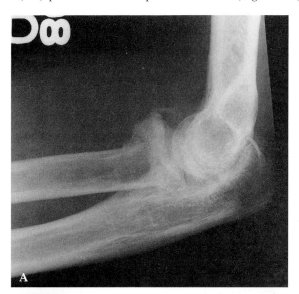

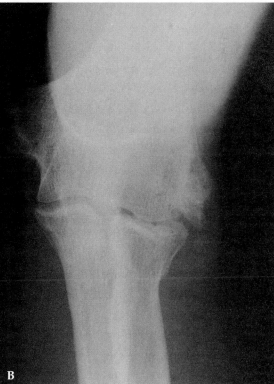

Figure 23–20 (**A** and **B**) These radiographs demonstrate myositis ossificans at the elbow. This patient had sustained a type IV radial head fracture/dislocation approximately 1 year prior to these radiographs. His range of motion was severely limited.

Like simple dislocations, early, active motion is the goal of treatment. Broberg and Morrey (1987) reviewed the results of 24 patients with Type IV radial head fractures (ulnohumeral dislocation with a radial head fracture) and reported that immobilization greater than 4 weeks compromised outcome.

While uncommon, chronic, recurrent elbow dislocation may result from insufficiency of LCL complex. Several operative procedures have been developed to reconstruct the LCL.

Tools of the Trade

Open Reduction Internal Fixation Distal Humerus	• Patient prone • AP and lateral radiographs • Tomograms of the elbow (1-mm cuts) • Sterile touniquet • 3.5-mm pelvic reconstruction plates • 3.5-mm limited contact dynamic compression plates may be necessary • Large and small fragment sets • Bone graft set • Bone graft site prepped/draped • Extra Hohman retractors • C-arm
Open Reduction Internal Fixation Proximal Ulna	• Patient prone or lateral decubitis • AP and lateral radiographs • Possibly tomograms of the elbow (1-mm cuts) • Sterile tourniquet • 3.5-mm pelvic reconstruction plates • 3.5-mm limited contact dynamic compression plates • Kirshner wires • 18- and 20-gauge wires • Large and small fragment sets • Bone graft set • Bone graft site prepped/draped • Extra Hohman retractors • C-arm
Open Reduction Internal Fixation Proximal Radius	• Patient supine • AP, lateral, and radiocapitellar view radiographs • Tourniquet • Small and mini-fragment sets • Specialized instrumentation (i.e., Herbert screw) • Prosthetic radial head (if excision is a possibility) • Extra Hohman retractors • C-arm

SELECTED BIBLIOGRAPHY

Elbow Fractures and Dislocations: General

JUPITER JB, MEHNE DK. Trauma to the adult elbow and fractures of the distal humerus. In: Browner BD, Jupiter JB, Levine AM, et al, eds. *Skeletal Trauma*. Vol. 2. 1st ed. Philadelphia, PA: WB Saunders Co; 1992.

MORREY BF. Current concepts in the treatment of fractures of the radial head, the olecranon, and the coronoid. *Instruct Course Lect*. 1995;44:175–185.

Anatomy and Biomechanics

AMIS AA, DOWSON D, WRIGHT V. Elbow joint force predictors for some strenuous isometric actions. *J Biomech*. 1980;13:765–775.

AN KN, HUI FC, MORREY BF, LINSCHEID RL, CHAO EY. Muscles across the elbow joint: a biomechanical analysis. *J Biomech*. 1981;14:659–669.

AN KN, MORREY BF. Biomechanics of the elbow. In: Mow VC, Ratcliffe, A, Woo SLY, eds. *Biomechanics of Diarthrodial Joints*. Vol 2. 1st ed. New York, NY: Springer-Verlag; 1990; 441–464.

AN KN, MORREY BF. Biomechanics of the elbow. In: Morrey BF, ed. *The Elbow and Its Disorders*. 2nd ed. Philadelphia, PA: WB Saunders; 1993;53–72.

BASS RL, STERN PJ. Elbow and forearm anatomy and surgical approaches. *Hand Clin*. 1994;10:343–356.

KOLB LW, MOORE RD. Fractures of the supracondylar process of the humerus: Report of two cases. *J Bone Jt Surg*. 1967;49A:532–534.

LONDON JT. Kinematics of the elbow. *J Bone Jt Surg.* 1981; 63A:529–535.

MORREY BF. Applied anatomy and biomechanics of the elbow joint. *Instruct Course Lect.* 1986;35:59–68.

MORREY BF. Anatomy of the elbow joint. In: Morrey BF, ed. *The Elbow and Its Disorders.* 2nd ed. Philadelphia, PA: WB Saunders;1993.

MORREY BF. Acute and chronic instability of the elbow joint. *J Am Acad Orthop Surg.* 1996;4:117–128.

MORREY BF, AN KN. Articular and ligamentous contributions to the stability of the elbow joint. *Am J Sports Med.* 1983; 11:315–319.

MORREY BF, TANAKA S, AN KN. Valgus stability of the elbow. *Clin Orthop.* 1991;265:187–195.

O'DRISCOLL SW, MORREY BF, KORINEK S, AN KN. Elbow subluxation and dislocation: a spectrum of instability. *Clin Orthop.* 1992;280:186–197.

OLSEN BS, VAESEL MT, SOJBJERG JO, HELMIG P, SNEPPEN O. Lateral collateral ligament of the elbow joint: anatomy and kinematics. *J Shoulder Elbow Surg.* 1996;5:103–112.

SCHWAB GH, BENNETT JB, WOODS GW, TULLOS HS. Biomechanics of elbow instability: the role of the medial collateral ligament. *Clin Orthop* 1980;146:42–52.

TULLOS HS, SCHWAB G, BENNETT JB, WOODS GW. Factors influencing elbow instability. *Instruct Course Lect.* 1981; 30:185–199.

WERNER FW, AN KN. Biomechanics of the elbow and forearm. *Hand Clin.* 1994;10:357–373.

Radial Head Fractures

ADLER JB, SHAFTAN GW. Radial head fractures, is excision necessary? *J Trauma.* 1964;4:115–136.

BAKALIM G. Fractures of the radial head and their treatment. *Acta Orthop Scand.* 1970;41:320–331.

BROBERG MA, MORREY BF. Results of delayed excision of the radial head after fracture. *J Bone Jt Surg.* 1986;68A:669–674.

BROBERG MA, MORREY BF. Results of treatment of fracture-dislocations of the elbow. *Clin Orthop.* 1987;216:109–119.

BUNKER TD, NEWMAN JH. The Herbert differential pitch bone screw in displaced radial head fractures. *Br J Accident Surg* 1985;16:621–624.

CARN RM, MEDIGE J, CURTAIN D, et al. Silicone rubber replacement of the severely fractured radial head. *Clin Orthop.* 1986;209:259–269.

COLEMAN DA, BLAIR WF, SHURR D. Resection of the radial head for fracture of the radial head: long-term follow-up of seventeen cases. *J Bone Jt Surg.* 1987;69A:385–392.

EDWARDS Jr GS, JUPITER JB. Radial head fractures with acute distal radioulnar dislocation: Essex-Lopresti revisited. *Clin Orthop.* 1988;234:61–69.

GEEL CW, Palmer AK. Radial head fractures and their effect on the distal radioulnar joint. *Clin Orthop.* 1992;275:79–84.

HOLDSWORTH BJ, CLEMENT DA, ROTHWELL PNR. Fractures of the radial head; the benefit of aspiration: a prospective controlled trial. *Injury.* 1987;18:44–47.

JOHNSTON GW. A follow-up of one nundred cases of the head of the radius with a review of the literature. *Ulster Med J.* 1962;31:51–56.

KHALFAYAN EE, CULP RW, ALEXANDER AH. Mason type II radial head fractures: operative versus nonoperative treatment. *J Orthop Trauma.* 1992;6:283–289.

KING GJW, EVANS DC, KELLAM JF: Open reduction and internal fixation of radial head fractures. *J Orthop Trauma.* 1991;5:21–28.

KNIGHT DJ, RYMASZEWSKI LA, AMIS AA, MILLER JH. Primary replacement of the fractures radial head with a metal prosthesis. *J Bone Jt Surg.* 1993;75B:572–576.

MASON ML. Fractures of the head of the radius: some observations on fractures of the head of the radius with a review of 100 cases. *Br J Surg.* 1954;42:123–132.

MCARTHUR RA. Herbert screw fixation of fracture of the head of the radius. *Clin Orthop.* 1987;224:80–87.

MIKIC ZD, VUKADINOVIC SM. Late results in fractures of the radial head treated by excision. *Clin Orthop.* 1983; 181:220–228.

Orthopaedic Trauma Association Committee for Coding and Classification. Fracture and dislocation copendium. *J Orthop Trauma.* 1996;10(suppl 1):16–20.

PELTO K, HIRVENSALO E, BOSTMAN O, ROKKANEN P. Treatment of radial head fractures with absorbable polyglycolide pins: a study on the security of the fixation in 38 cases. *J Orthop Trauma.* 1994;8:94–98.

SMITH GR, HOTCHKISS RN. Radial head and neck fractures: anatomic guidelines for proper placement of internal fixation. *J Shoulder Elbow Surg.* 1996;5:113–117.

VANDERWILDE RS, MORREY BF, MELBERG MW, et al. Inflammatory arthritis after failure of silicone rubber replacement of the radial head. *J Bone Jt Surg.* 1994;76B:78–81.

WEXNER SD, GOODWIN C, PARKES JC II Webber BR, Patterson AH. Treatment of fractures of the radial head by partial excision. *Orthop Rev.* 1985;14:83–86.

Olecranon Fractures

AN KN, MORREY BF, CHAO EYS. The effect of partial removal of proximal ulna on elbow constraint. *Clin Orthop.* 1986;209:270–279.

BADO JL. The Monteggia lesion. *Clin Orthop.* 1967;50:71–86.

GORDON ML. Monteggia fracture: a combined surgical approach employing a single lateral incision. *Clin Orthop.* 1967;50:87–93.

GARTSMAN GM, SCULCO TP, OTIS JC. Operative treatment of olecranon fractures: excision or open reduction with internal fixation. *J Bone Jt Surg.* 1981;63A,5:718–721.

HUME MC, WISS DA. Olecranon fractures: a clinical and radiographic comparison of tension band wiring and plate fixation. *Clin Orthop.* 1992;285:229–235.

INHOFE PD, HOWARD TC. The Treatment of olecranon fractures by excision of fragments and repair of the extensor mechanism: historical review and report of 12 fractures. *Orthopedics.* 1993;16:1313–1317.

JOHNSON RP, ROETKER A, SCHWAB JP. Olecranon fractures treated with AO Screw and tension bands. *Orthopedics.* 1986;9:66–68.

MACKO D, SZABO RM. Complications of tension-band wiring of olecranon fractures. *J Bone Jt Surg.* 1985;67A:1396–1401.

MURPHY DF, GREENE WB, DAMERON TB. Displaced olecranon fractures in adults: clinical evaluation. *Clin Orthop* 1987; 224:215–223.

MURPHY DF, GREENE WB, GILBERT JA, et al. Displaced olecranon fractures in adults: biomechanical analysis of fixation methods. *Clin Orthop.* 1987;224:210–214.

TOMPKINS DG. The anterior Monteggia fracture. *J Bone Jt Surg.* 1971;53A:1109–1114.

WADSWORTH TG. Screw fixation of the olecranon after fracture osteotomy. *Clin Orthop.* 1976;119:197–201.

WOLFGANG G, BURKE F, BUSH D, et al. Surgical treatment of displaced olecranon fractures by tension band wiring technique. *Clin Orthop.* 1987;224:192–204.

Coronoid Fractures

CABANELA ME, MORREY BF. Fractures of the proximal ulna and olecranon. In: Morrey BF ed. *The Elbow and Its Disorders.* 2nd ed. Philadelphia, PA: WB Saunders; 1993;405–428

HANKS GA, KOTTMEIER SA. Isolated fracture of the coronoid process of the ulna: a case report and review of the literature. *J Orthop Trauma.* 1990;4:193–196.

REGAN W, MORREY BF. Fractures of the coronoid process of the ulna. *J Bone Jt Surg.* 1989;71A:1348–1354.

REGAN W, MORREY BF. Elbow trauma: classification and treatment of coronoid process fractures. *Orthopaedics.* 1992; 15:845–848.

SCHARPLATZ D, ALLGOWER M. Fracture dislocations of the elbow. *Injury.* 1975;7:143–159.

SELESNICK FH, DOLITSKY B, HASKELL SS. Fracture of the coronoid process requiring open reduction and internal fixation: a case report. *J Bone Jt Surg.* 1984;66A:1304–1305.

Distal Humerus Fractures

AITKEN GK, RORABECK CH. Distal humeral fractures in the adult. *Clin Orthop.* 1986;207:191–197.

GABEL GT, HANSON G, BENNETT JB, NOBLE PC, TULLOS HS. Intra-articular fractures of the distal humerus in the adult. *Clin Orthop.* 1987;216:99–108.

GRANTHAM SA, NORRIS TR, BUSH DC. Isolated fracture of the humeral capitellum. *Clin Orthop.* 1981;161:262–269.

HELFET DL, SCHMELING GJ. Bicondylar intra-articular fractures of the distal humerus in adults. *Clin Orthop.* 1993;292: 26–36.

JOHANSSON H, OLERUD S. Operative treatment of intercondylar fractures of the humerus. *J Trauma.* 1971;11:836–843.

JUPITER JB, NEFF U, HOLZACH P, ALLGOWER M. Intercondylar fractures of the humerus: an operative approach. *J Bone Jt Surg.* 1985;67A:226–239.

JUPITER JB, MEHNE DK. Elbow trauma: fractures of the distal humerus. *Orthopaedics.* 1992;15:825–833.

JUPITER JB, MORREY BF. Fractures of the distal humerus in the adult. In: Morrey BF, ed. *The Elbow and Its Disorders.* 2nd ed. Philadelphia, PA: WB Saunders; 1993;328–366.

MCKEE MD, JUPITER JB. A contempory approoch to the management of complex fractures of the distal humerus and their sequelae. *Hand Clin.* 1994;10:479–494.

RISEBOROUGH EJ, RADIN EL. Intercondylar T-fractures of the humerus in the adult. *J Bone Jt Surg.* 1969;51A:130–141.

SILVERI CP, CORSO SJ, ROOFEH J. Herbert screw fixation of a capitellum fracture: a case report and review. *Clin Orthop.* 1994;300:123–126.

Elbow dislocations

HASSMANN GC, BRUNN F, NEER CS. Recurrent dislocations of the elbow. *J Bone Jt Surg.* 1975;57A:1080–1084.

HEIDT RS, STERN PJ. Isolated posterior dislocation of the radial head. *Clin Orthop.* 1982;168:136–138.

JOSEFSSON PO, GENTZ CF, JOHNELL O, et al. Surgical versus nonsurgical treatment of ligamentous injuries following dislocation of the elbow joint: a prospective randomized study. *J Bone Jt Surg.* 1987;69A:605–608.

JOSEFSSON PO, JOHNELL O, GENTZ CF. Long-term sequelae of simple dislocation of the elbow. *J Bone Jt Surg.* 1984; 66A:927–930.

LOUIS DS, RICCIARDI JE, SPENGLER DM. Arterial injury; a complication of posterior elbow dislocation: a clinical and anatomical study. *J Bone Jt Surg.* 1974;56A:1631–1636.

MATEV I. A radiological sign of entrapment of the median nerve in the elbow joint after posterior dislocation: a report of two cases. *J Bone Jt Surg.* 1976;58B:353–355.

MEHLHOFF TL, NOBLE PC, BENNETT JB, et al. Simple dislocation of the elbow in the adult. *J Bone Jt Surg.* 1988; 70A:244–249.

MEYN MA, QUIGLEY TB. Reduction of posterior dislocation of the elbow by traction on the dangling arm. *Clin Orthop.* 1974;103:106–108.

O'HARA JP, MORREY BF, JOHNSON EW, JOHNSON DA. Dislocations and fracture-dislocations of the elbow. *Minn Med.* 1975;58:697–700.

PROTZMAN RR. Dislocation of the elbow. *J Bone Jt Surg.* 1978;60A:539–541.

ST. CLAIR STRANGE FG. Entrapment of the median nerve after dislocation of the elbow. *J Bone Jt Surg.* 1982;64B:224–225.

SYMEONIDES PP, PASCHALOGLOU C, STAVROU Z, PANGALIDES T. Recurrent dislocation of the elbow: report of three cases. *J Bone Jt Surg.* 1975;57A:1084–1086.

THOMPSON HC, GARCIA A. Myositis ossificans: aftermath of elbow injuries. *Clin Orthop.* 1967;50:129–134.

SAMPLE QUESTIONS

1. Motion after an elbow fracture or dislocations should:

(a) begin 6 weeks after the injury to allow the fracture and soft tissues adequate healing time

(b) consist of early, active and passive motion within 3 weeks of the injury

(c) only occur after the patient is pain free from the injury

(d) start within 3 weeks and include active motion exercises

(e) include only passive motion exercises

2. The decision to operate on a radial head fracture depends mainly on what information:

(a) the amount of pain the patient is experiencing

(b) the range of motion after intra-articular anesthetic injection

(c) the patient's age

(d) the number of fracture fragments

(e) the patient's hand dominance

3. The major reason the lateral Kocher approach cannot be extended distally is:

   (a) The radial nerve lies just anterior to the radial head.

   (b) The radial artery crosses too close to the field of dissection.

   (c) The posterior interosseous nerve cannot be adequately protected from injury.

   (d) The anterior interosseous nerve cannot be adequately protected from injury.

   (e) The annular ligament prevents distal dissection.

4. A patient with a radial head fracture complains of distal forearm pain. The forearm and wrist films show no fracture. Which would be the next appropriate test to order:

(a) AP lateral of the opposite (uninjured) wrist

(b) CT scan of the elbow

(c) compartment pressures in the forearm

(d) AP grip view of the carpus

(e) electromyogram of the PIN to rule out a compression neuropathy

5. The amount of elbow motion considered to be adequate for activities of daily living is:

   (a) 75 degrees pronation, 50 degrees supination, 130 degrees flexion, and 30 degrees extension

   (b) 50 degrees pronation, 50 degrees supination, 150 degrees flexion, and 30 degrees extension

   (c) 75 degrees pronation, 85 degrees supination, 150 degrees flexion, and 0 degrees extension

   (d) 75 degrees pronation, 50 degrees supination, 130 degrees flexion, and 0 degrees extension

   (e) 50 degrees pronation, 50 degrees supination, 130 degrees flexion, and 30 degrees extension

Answers: 1) d; 2) b; 3) c; 4) a; 5) e

Chapter 24

Overuse Syndromes of the Elbow

Neal S. ElAttrache, MD and Arthur L. Valadie, III, MD

Outline

ETIOLOGY

- Lateral epicondylitis
- Medial epicondylitis
- Medial ligamentous insufficiency
- Osteochondritis dissecans
- Valgus extension overload
- Little league elbow

BASIC SCIENCE

Elbow Biomechanics

The elbow is a complex joint that permits flexion and extension as well as pronation and supination. The humeroulnar joint is a hinge joint with a constant center of rotation allowing stable flexion and extension. The humeroradial joint permits pronation and supination via rotation through this articulation. These articulations and the associated ligamentous structures experience tremendous forces during sports. The humeroulnar articulation provides a significant amount of intrinsic stability to the elbow joint by virtue of its bony congruence. Resection of increasing amounts of the proximal ulna results in a proportional decrease in elbow stability.

The radiocapitellar joint is a significant contributor to valgus stability of the elbow. The radial head is responsible for approximately 25% of valgus stability at 0 degrees of flexion, 30% at 45 degrees of flexion, and up to 45% at 90 degrees of flexion. This contribution may be clinically important when treating radial head fractures with associated elbow ligamentous injuries. The potential for instability determines the need to salvage the radial head or use a prosthetic replacement.

The medial collateral ligament (MCL) is the primary medial stabilizer of the elbow (Fig. 24–1). The MCL consists of anterior, posterior, and transverse bands, with the anterior band being functionally the most significant. The most anterior fibers of the anterior band are tense in elbow extension, and the posterior fibers are most tense in elbow flexion. In 0 to 20 degrees of elbow flexion the MCL plays a limited role in valgus stability. Stability in this range is predominantly due to skeletal constraints. At 20 to 120 degrees of flexion the MCL is the predominant valgus stabilizer.

Orthopaedic Surgery: The Essentials. Edited by M.E. Baratz, A.D. Watson, and J.E. Imbriglia. Thieme Medical Publishers, Inc., New York © 1999

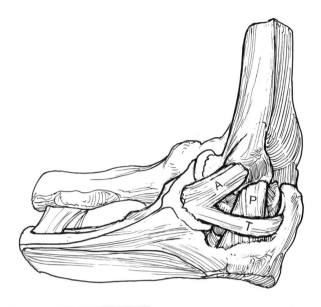

Figure 24–1 Medial collateral ligament (MCL) consisting of anterior band, posterior band, and transverse band.

PEARL

The medial collateral ligament (MCL) is the primary restraint to a valgus stress when the elbow is positioned between 20 and 120 degrees of flexion.

Lateral ligamentous stability is provided by the radial collateral ligament, annular ligament, accessory collateral ligament, and lateral ulnar collateral ligament. Lateral ligamentous deficiency results in posterolateral instability. The lateral ulnar collateral ligament is the primary restraint against this instability pattern.

The Elbow in Throwing

The elbow is subject to extreme mechanical demands during the throwing motion. The phases of the throwing motion have been well described and are helpful for analyzing the dynamics of the elbow during this activity (Fig. 24–2). Late

cocking, acceleration, and deceleration are the most demanding phases of throwing for the elbow. During late cocking, the radial wrist extensors have the greatest muscle action about the elbow while the humerus rapidly externally rotates. During the acceleration phase, the elbow extends at a rate of approximately 2200 degrees per second and a significant valgus moment is experienced. The MCL is the primary restraint to this valgus force. The medial epicondylar muscles become very active during this phase. Deceleration then occurs and involves a complex interplay of elbow flexors and extensors resulting in a significant deceleration rate at the elbow.

ANATOMY AND SURGICAL APPROACHES

Medial

Anatomy

The flexor-pronator muscle group originates on or near the medial epicondyle. The musculature can be divided into superficial and deep layers. The superficial layer includes the pronator teres, flexor carpi radialis (FCR), palmaris longus (PL), flexor carpi ulnaris (FCU), and flexor digitorum superficialis (FDS). The pronator teres has a humeral head and an ulnar head, between which passes the median nerve. The common flexor origin is a blend of fibers from the FCR, PL, and FCU. The FDS has a broad origin under which pass the median and anterior interosseous nerves. The deep layer includes the flexor digitorum profundus and flexor pollicis longus. The flexor-pronator group is supplied by the median nerve except for the FCU, which is ulnar nerve innervated.

The MCL lies just deep to the muscle mass and has three bands: anterior, posterior, and transverse. The functionally important anterior band arises from the medial epicondyle and inserts onto a small tubercle on the medial ulna.

Surgical Approaches

A gently curved incision is made based over the medial epicondyle. Care is taken to avoid branches of the medial antebrachial cutaneous nerve (Fig. 24–3). The medial epicondyle and flexor-pronator muscles are then exposed. Examination

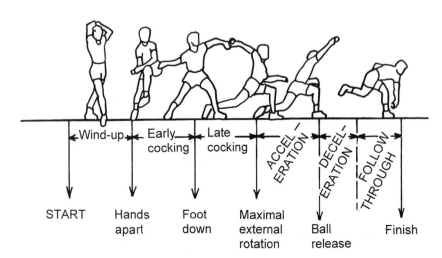

Figure 24–2 Six phases of pitching. Reproduced with permission from DiGiovine NM, Jobe FW, Pink M et al. An electromyographic analysis of the upper extremity in pitching. *J Shoulder Elbow Surg.* 1992;1:15–25.

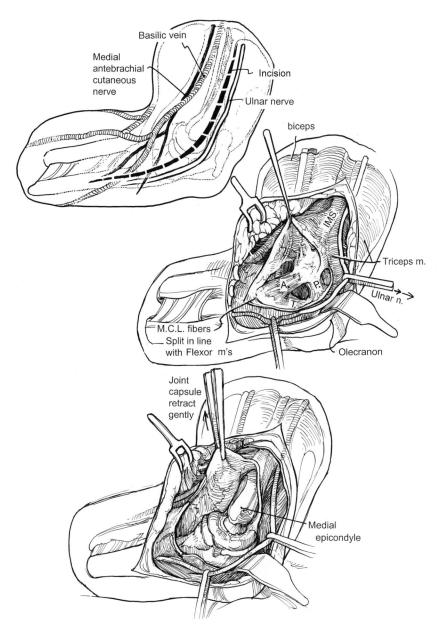

Figure 24–3 Incision for medial approach to the elbow.

of the MCL can be done by splitting the muscle in line with its fibers. The common flexor origin can be released from the epicondyle, leaving a small cuff of tissue for later repair, for the purpose of submuscular ulnar nerve transposition. The ulnar nerve lies just posterior to the medial epicondyle in the cubital tunnel and passes under the cubital tunnel retinaculum.

PITFALL

Transection of branches of the medial antebrachial cutaneous nerve during a medial approach to the elbow often results in formation of painful neuromas.

Lateral

Anatomy

The extensor-supinator muscles originate from the lateral epicondylar region. These can be divided into superficial and deep groups. The superficial group includes, in order from radial to ulnar, the brachioradialis, extensor carpi radialis longus (ECRL), extensor carpi radialis brevis (ECRB), extensor digitorum communis, extensor digiti minimi, extensor carpi ulnaris, and anconeus (Fig. 24–4a). The ECRL originates from the distal supracondylar ridge, whereas the ECRB originates from the lateral epicondyle via the common extensor tendon. The ECRB is most commonly implicated in lateral epicondylitis. The deep layer includes the supinator, abductor pollicis longus, extensor pollicis brevis, extensor pollicis

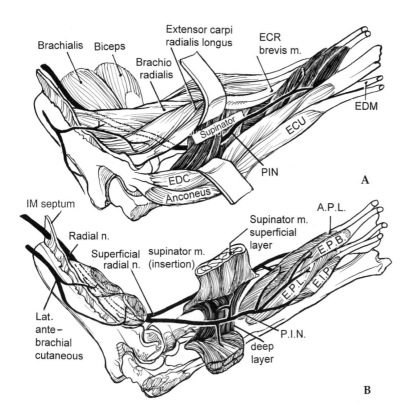

Figure 24–4 (**A**) Schematic illustrating superficial layer of forearm extensors. (**B**) Schematic illustrating deep layer of forearm extensors.

longus, and extensor indicis proprius (Fig. 24–4b). The supinator is divided into superficial and deep lamina by the posterior interosseous nerve, which passes directly through the substance of the muscle. The extensor-supinator muscles are innervated by the posterior interousseous nerve except for the brachioradialis and ECRL, which are innervated by the radial nerve before it braches into the superficial radial nerve and posterior interosseous nerves.

The lateral ligamentous complex comprises the radial collateral ligament, lateral ulnar collateral ligament, annular ligament, and accessory lateral collateral ligament. The lateral ulnar collateral ligament is believed to contribute most to lateral stability. The annular ligament encircles 4/5 of the radial head and stabilizes it within the ulnar notch (Fig. 24–5).

Surgical Approaches

The lateral approach of Kocher is the preferred lateral approach to the elbow joint. A curvilinear incision is made centered over the lateral epicondyle. The interval between the anconeus and ECU is developed. The lateral capsule can be incised to access the radiocapitellar joint.

Posterior
Anatomy

The triceps muscle inserts onto the olecranon posteriorly and is the only muscle in the posterior compartment. The ulnar nerve lies medially in the cubital tunnel.

Surgical Approaches

The preferred approach posteriorly depends on the type of access required. A triceps-splitting approach via a posterior

incision can be used for limited exposure to the posterior compartment. The incision should be kept off the tip of the olecranon to prevent a tender weight-bearing surface (Fig. 24–6). An olecranon osteotomy can be done through a posterior incision for wide exposure of the joint surfaces. The posterior compartment can also be reached via medial and lateral incisions by reflecting the triceps tendon. The entire aspect of the distal humerus can be exposed with a triceps-sparing approach (Fig. 24–6).

PEARL

A posterior incision made off the tip of the olecranon will prevent a painful scar from forming on the point of the elbow.

Anterior
Anatomy

The antecubital fossa covers the anterior aspect of the elbow joint. The brachialis passes in front of the joint to insert on the coranoid process of the proximal ulna. The biceps inserts via the distal biceps tendon and the broad lacertus fibrosis. The median nerve and brachial artery pass in front of the elbow joint, the artery being more medial than the nerve.

Surgical Approaches

The anterolateral approach to the elbow utilizes the plane between the brachioradialis and brachialis. A curved incision is made along the anterior aspect of the elbow joint (Fig. 24–7). Proximally, the brachioradialis is retracted laterally, and the brachialis and biceps are retracted medially. More distally, the brachioradialis is retracted laterally, and the

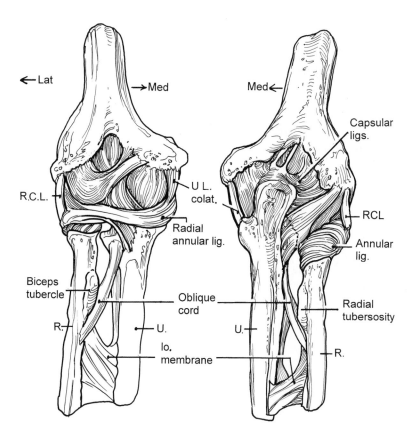

Figure 24–5 Schematic illustrating ligamentous support of the elbow.

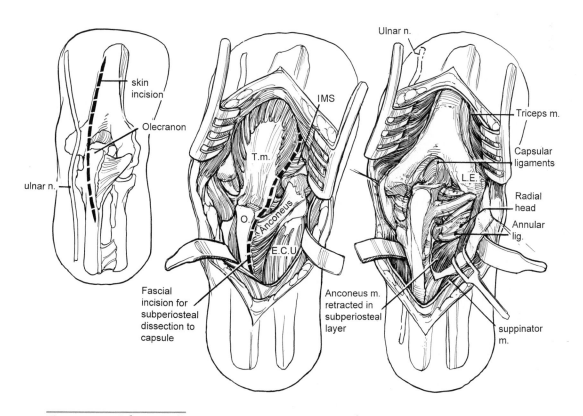

Figure 24–6   Schematic illustrating triceps-sparing approach.

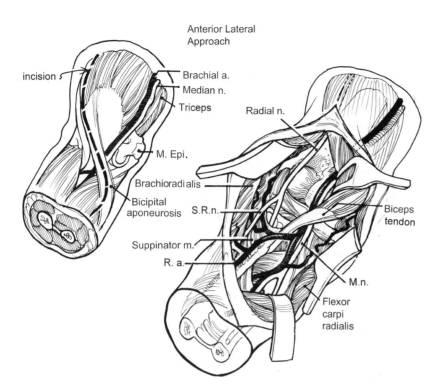

Figure 24–7   Schematic illustrating anterolateral approach to the elbow joint.

pronator teres is retracted medially. This provides good exposure of the lateral half of the elbow joint and proximal radius. The direct anterior approach to the cubital fossa is uncommonly used, but can be used to provide good access to the neurovascular structures of the elbow.

Arthroscopic Anatomy

A thorough knowledge of the neurovascular anatomy of the elbow is vital when performing elbow arthroscopy. Three standard portals are used routinely, with a fourth portal available to improve posterior access (Fig. 24–8). The proximal-medial portal lies 2 cm proximal to the medial epicondyle and just anterior to the intermuscular septum. This

portal is useful for visualization of the radial head, capitellum, trochlea, coranoid process, and anterior joint capsule. The mid-lateral portal is located in the anconeus triangle, which is formed by the lateral epicondyle, radial head, and olecranon. This can be used for outflow, instrumentation, and for a view of the posterior aspect of the radiocapitellar joint. The anterolateral portal is created directly anterior and lateral to the radiocapitellar joint. This portal is excellent for instrumentation and can be used to visualize the distal humerus, coranoid process, and radial head. The direct posterior portal is located 2 cm proximal to the tip of the olecranon and passes through the triceps tendon. The posterolateral portal lies just lateral to the triceps tendon. These portals permit visualization and instrumentation of the posterior

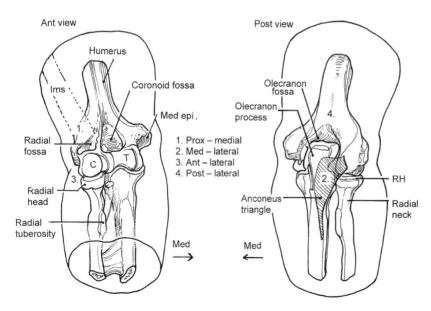

Figure 24–8   Schematic illustrating arthroscopic portals of the elbow.

aspect of the joint. The portals to be used depend on the pathology present, patient position, and surgeon preference.

EXAMINATION

History

A careful history is essential for all patients presenting with elbow pain. The type and location of pain should be noted, as well as details about provocative activities. The history of sports and occupational activities should be carefully noted, as well as any significant change in the patient's usual level of activity. One should question the patient about the presence of neurologic symptoms more distally in the arm.

Physical Examination

Inspection

Inspect the elbow carefully for atrophy, swelling, and deformity.

Palpation

Palpation of the medial epicondyle and flexor-pronator muscle mass and the lateral epicondyle and extensor-supinator muscle mass should be performed. Palpate the antecubital fossa, olecranon, and olecranon fossa, as well as the ulnar nerve.

Range of Motion

Active and passive ranges of motion should be noted. Normal maximal range of motion is approximately 0 to 140 degrees of flexion and 75 degrees of pronation to 85 degrees of supination. The range of motion necessary for most activities of daily living is 30 to 130 degrees of flexion along with 50 degrees of pronation to 50 degrees of supination. Athletes usually need a range of motion closer to normal to perform sporting activities.

Provocative Maneuvers

Stability tests include tests for medial and lateral ligamentous insufficiency. Valgus stress on the elbow in 30 degrees of flexion best tests the MCL. Reproduction of pain or palpable instability is diagnostic for MCL pathology. Patients with chronic medial ligamentous insufficiency may experience only pain over the anterior band of the MCL with valgus stress rather than obvious instability. Lateral ligamentous deficiency, or posterolateral instability, is best tested by the posterolateral rotatory instability test described by O'Driscoll (1991) (Fig. 24–9). The test involves placing an axial load and valgus stress on the supinated elbow while moving it from extension to flexion. This test is positive if it causes a sense of apprehension, pain, or true subluxation of the elbow joint.

Resisted wrist flexion and and forearm pronation may be provocative for medial epicondylitis. Resisted wrist extension with an extended elbow may be provocative for lateral epicondylitis. A complete neurovascular examination should be performed to elucidate nerve entrapment lesions about the elbow. Percussion of the ulnar nerve behind the medial epicondyle or sustained elbow flexion may produce dyesthesias diagnostic of cubital tunnel syndrome.

AIDS TO DIAGNOSIS

Radiographs

Look for signs of degenerative arthritis, calcification in the soft tissue, or osteochondritis, typically in the capitellum of adolescents.

Magnetic Resonance Imaging

Magnetic resonance imaging can be used to evaluate the integrity of the MCL and to evaluate lesions of the capitellum suggestive of osteochondritis dissecans (OCD).

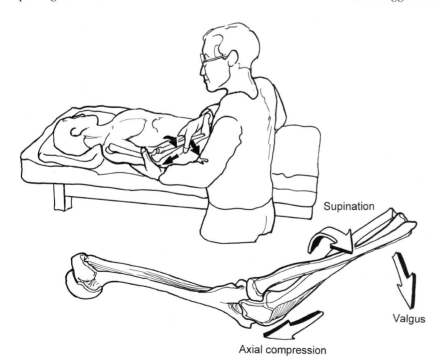

Supination

Valgus

Axial compression

Figure 24–9 Stability test for posterolateral rotatory instability. Flexion of the supinated, valgus-stressed elbow reduces the radial head.

Bone Scan

A bone scan is a good screening tool for early arthritis and chronic ligament tears.

Electrodiagnostic Studies

Such studies may help with the diagnosis of cubital tunnel syndrome or cervical radiculopathy presenting as elbow/arm discomfort.

SPECIFIC CONDITIONS, TREATMENT, AND OUTCOME

Lateral Epicondylitis

The lateral aspect of the elbow is the most common site of elbow pain in athletes. Initially described as lawn tennis elbow, lateral epicondylitis, or tennis elbow, may occur from a variety of sports, occupational, and daily activities. Lateral epicondylitis likely results from the cumulative affect of microtrauma to the common extensor origin, paticularly the ECRB. This repetitive trauma likely results in mucoid degeneration and reactive granulation within the tendinous origin of the ECRB. This leads to pain, swelling, and decreased performance. Clinical diagnosis is made by the presence of a consistent history, tenderness over the ECRB origin, and pain with resisted wrist extension.

PEARL

Lateral epicondylitis is characterized by pain and weakness that occurs with resisted wrist extension, particularly during elbow extension.

Nonoperative treatment of lateral epicondylitis yields successful results in the vast majority of cases. Nonoperative measures include rest from the offending activity, anti-inflammatory medications, physical therapy, and steroid injections. Operative treatment is reserved for failure of a thorough trial of nonoperative methods. The authors utilize an extra-articular technique of debridement of the pathologic tendon tissue, followed by reattachment of the tendon.

A lateral incision is made centered over the lateral epicondyle. The common extensor origin is identified, sharply detached subperiosteally from the lateral epicondyle, and reflected distally. The undersurface of the extensor mechanism is inspected for granulation tissue or tears. The radiocapitellar joint is also inspected through an incision in the lateral capsule. Any abnormal portions of the tendon are sharply excised (Fig. 24–10). This abnormal tissue usually occurs on the undersurface of the ECRB but may extend to the other tendinous origins. The lateral epicondyle is then debrided to a bleeding surface for tendon reattachment, which is done using braided nonabsorbable sutures through drill holes (Fig. 24–11). Postoperative care involves use of a posterior splint on the elbow for approximately 7 days. The splint and sutures are then removed, and the patient is started on a program of progressive mobilization. Passive motion is encouraged, but resisted wrist and finger extension are avoided. Strengthening can be started at 4 to 6 weeks. Return to normal activities is encouraged by the third to fourth month.

This technique results in an 85% rate of return to full activities without pain. Persistant strength deficits without significant functional consequences may occur.

Medial Epicondylitis

Medial epicondylitis, sometimes known as golfer's elbow, occurs less commonly than lateral epicondylitis. Valgus forces at the elbow and contraction of the flexor pronator muscle group creates stress at the medial epicondylar muscle mass, leading to microtrauma and inflammation. The pronator teres and FCR have been most commonly implicated as the focus of the inflammatory changes. Ulnar neuritis is a commonly associated condition.

The diagnosis of medial epicondylitis is made clinically by the presence of tenderness over the flexor-pronator origin. Resisted wrist flexion and forearm pronation usually exacerbate the pain. One should be sure to examine the patient for medial ligamentous instability and for ulnar neuritis. Nonoperative treatment principles for lateral epicondylitis apply to medial epicondylitis as well and are successful in the majority of cases. If nonoperative treatment fails, the authors again utilize the principle of resection of pathologic tissue and reattachment of the flexor-pronator origin. An incision is made centered over the medial epicondyle, protecting the cutaneous nerves. Care is taken to confirm the position of the ulnar nerve posterior to the epicondyle. The common flexor orgin is sharply incised and reflected distally, taking care not to violate the MCL and joint capsule. The pathologic tissue is resected from the undersurface of the tendinous origin. The medial epicondyle is debrided down to bleeding bone, and the tendon is reattached using heavy braided nonabsorbable suture. The postoperative regimen includes splinting of the elbow for approximatly 7 days. Gentle motion is then initiated. Resisted wrist flexion and pronation exercises are avoided for 4 to 6 weeks postoperatively. This is then followed by a progressive strengthening program. Return to normal activities is usually encouraged by the third to fourth postoperative month.

For properly selected patients, a high rate of return to normal elbow function can be anticipated. Vangsness and Jobe (1991) reported good to excellent results in 97% of their patients treated operatively for medial epicondylitis using the above-described technique.

Medial Collateral Ligament Insufficiency

Chronic repetitive valgus stress to the elbow, as in throwing, may lead to medial ligamentous insufficiency. The patient may not complain of frank instability but may describe pain and decreased performance with throwing activities. Repetitive stress with microtrauma to the MCL likely causes tissue attenuation and degeneration leading to functional laxity. Occasionally, the patient may present after an acute injury to the MCL, during which he or she experienced a pop or sharp pain in the medial aspect of the elbow.

Physical examination includes stability testing as previously described. The patient should be carefully inspected for associated ulnar neuritis as well. Stress radiographs may demonstrate medial joint opening with valgus stress (Fig. 24–12).

Figure 24–10 (**A**) Skin incision overlying the lateral epicondyle. (**B**) Reflection of the extensor mechanism, exposing the captillum and radial head. (**C**) Debridement of pathological tissue from the undersurface of the extensor mechanism. (**D**) Decortication of the lateral epicondyle.

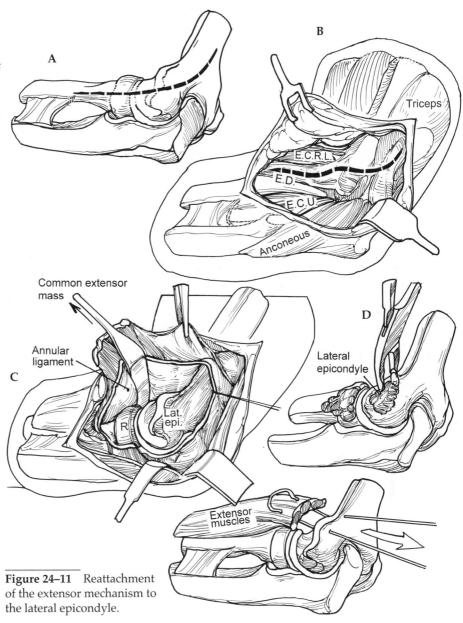

Figure 24–11 Reattachment of the extensor mechanism to the lateral epicondyle.

In patients with symptomatic medial ligamentous insufficiency, reconstruction as described by Jobe (1996) is recommended. An incision is made over the medial epicondyle. Care is taken to avoid the branches of the medial antebrachial cutaneous nerve. The flexor-pronator muscle orgin is split in line with its fibers. The MCL is exposed and is incised in line with its fibers. This permits inspection of the joint and evaluation of the degree of valgus laxity that is present. If the injury is acute and sufficient tissue is present, a direct repair may be performed. If the local tissue is not suitable for repair, or if it is a chronic injury, reconstruction with a graft is done. A 3.2-mm drill bit is used to make bone tunnels for the ligamentous reconstruction. Two drill holes are made in the medial epicondyle with a single entrance hole anteriorly that diverges

anterosuperiorly and posterosuperiorly, avoiding the ulnar nerve posteriorly. These drill holes are made midway between the base and tip of the medial epicondylar prominence at the anatomic origin of the anterior bundle of the MCL. A drill hole is also placed in the proximal ulna at the level of the coronoid tubercle. A PL graft or other suitable tendon graft 15 to 17 in length is harvested. The tendon is then passed through the drill holes in a figure-of-eight fashion with the elbow held in 45 degrees of flexion, making sure to avoid valgus stress (Fig. 24–13). The tendon is then tightened and sutured to itself and to the native MCL. Isometry and stability of the ligament reconstruction is manually tested.

Postoperatively, the patient is placed in a long-arm posterior splint in 90 degrees of elbow flexion and neutral forearm

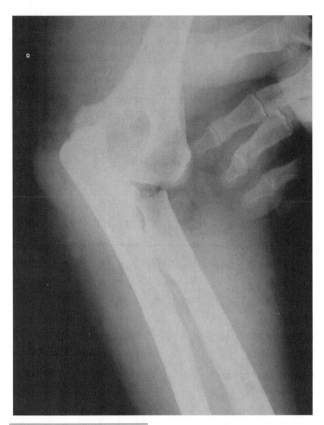

Figure 24–12 Stress radiograph of MCL-deficient elbow.

rotation. Gentle hand squeezing is initiated immediately. At 7 to 10 days, the splint is removed and active elbow and shoulder range of motion is started. At four weeks postoperatively, strengthening exercises of the elbow are initiated while avoiding valgus stress. At approximately 4 months postoperatively, if elbow range of motion and strength are normal, a progressive throwing program can be started. Performance should return to normal within 12 to 18 months after surgery. Conway and associates (1992) examined the results of medial elbow reconstruction with this technique. If no previous surgery had been performed, 74% of patients had an excellent result, and 85% considered the result satisfactory. The results were less favorable for revision surgery.

PITFALL

Medial ligamentous insufficiency is often confused clinically with medial epicondylitis and ulnar neuritis. Stress radiographs with comparison views may be helpful.

Osteochondritis Dissecans

Osteochondritis dissecans is an injury to the articular surface of a joint involving separation of a segment of articular cartilage and subchondral bone and is commonly the result of an overuse injury. In throwing athletes and gymnasts, the capitellum is most commonly affected. Panner's disease, an osteochondrosis of the entire ossific nucleus of the capitellum, may be a related entity. Patients with OCD of the elbow usually present with gradual onset of dull, lateral elbow pain, which is aggravated by activity. A flexion contracture may be present. If loose bodies have formed, locking and catching may occur. Radiographs reveal lucency and irregularity of the capitellum. Magnetic resonance imaging is very useful in evaluating these lesions.

In the early stages of disease when the fragment has not separated from the capitellum, avoidance of the offending activity may relieve symptoms and permit the fragment to heal. Operative treatment is indicated for lesions that fail to resolve with nonoperative care and for partial or complete separation of the fragment. The presence of loose bodies with locking or catching also warrants surgery. Arthroscopic treatment is preferred. Any fragmented pieces are removed, and the base of the lesion is debrided with a curette or motorized bur. It is important to thoroughly examine the joint for the presence of loose bodies. Stabilization of large fragments has been described. Postoperative care for arthroscopically treated OCD includes early range of motion followed by progressive strengthening exercises.

McManama et al (1985) evaluated the results of surgical treatment of OCD of the capitellum. Patient results were: 8 excellent, 5 good, and 1 fair. There were no poor results. Of 14 patients, 12 returned to organized competitive activity without restrictions.

PEARL

Early recognition of osteochondritis dessicans (OCD) of the capitellum and immediate rest from the offending activity are the keys to successful nonoperative treatment.

Valgus Extension Overload

Repetitive throwing and its associated valgus and extension forces may result in valgus extension overload syndrome. If repetitive throwing results in attenuation of the MCL, the olecranon will impinge on the olecranon fossa during the throwing motion. This may result in local inflammation, synovitis, ostyeophyte formation, and loose body formation. Patients with valgus extension overload syndrome usually complain of elbow pain during the acceleration phase of throwing. Physical examination reveals posterior pain with full extension and valgus stress. Locking and catching can occur if loose bodies are present.

Nonoperative treatment aims to relieve pain, decrease inflammation, and increase functional strength through the use of anti-inflammatory medications and strengthening exercises. Operative indications include failure of nonoperative treatment and the presence of loose bodies. Arthroscopic treatment of valgus extension overload is preferred. Posterior elbow portals are utilized. Osteophytes are removed from the olecranon and olecranon fossa using a motorized

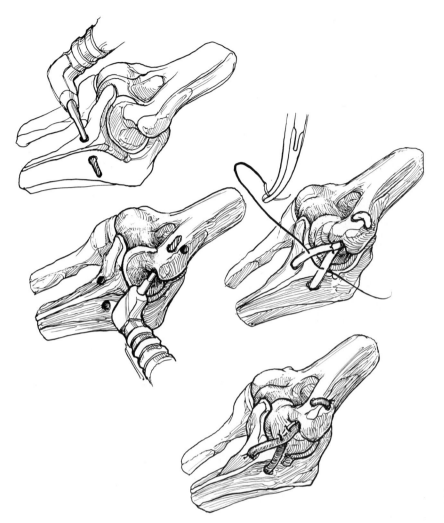

Figure 24–13   Suture fixation of autogenous tendon graft.

burr (Fig. 24–14). Loose bodies are removed if present. The joint is thoroughly irrigated. The postoperative regimen includes progressive range-of-motion exercises within 7 days. Strengthening exercises are initiated as tolerated. A progressive throwing program is started at 8 to 12 weeks postoperatively.

Excellent results have been obtained for properly selected patients. At the Kerlan-Jobe clinic, 115 professional baseball players were treated with arthroscopic removal of loose bodies and proximal olecranon resection. At a minimum 2-year followup, 74% excellent results were achieved. Of the patients treated, 17% had poor results, but most of these had symptomatic medial elbow instability and/or radiocapitellar chondrosis. If significant MCL laxity appears to be present, this should be addressed with medial ligamentous reconstruction.

Little League Elbow

Little League elbow is probably best thought of as a combination of clinical entities that occur as a result of repetitive valgus stress to the skeletally immature elbow. The most common injury is to the medial epicondylar apophysis. There is repetitive microinjury secondary to tensile forces causing fragmentation of the apophysis. There is resultant pain, swelling, and difficulty throwing. The lateral elbow is subject to compressive forces with throwing, and in the immature athlete this may result in OCD of the capitellum, which has been previously discussed. Osteochondritis dissecans of the trochlea may also occur. The immature olecranon experiences tensile forces during throwing and traction apophysitis of the olecranon may occur as well.

Medial epicondylar apophysitis is diagnosed by pain medially with valgus stress and localized tenderness of the epicondyle. Radiographs demonstrate fragmentation of the apophysis. Acute avulsion of the apophysis is a separate entity but is often described as Little League elbow.

Skeletally immature patients with OCD of the capitellum usually present with chronic, dull, lateral elbow pain. Radiographs may demonstrate a discreet OCD lesion or diffuse changes in the capitellum (Panner's disease).

The treatment for these conditions is almost always rest from the offending activity. Indications for surgical intervention include gross displacement of the medial epicondyle or

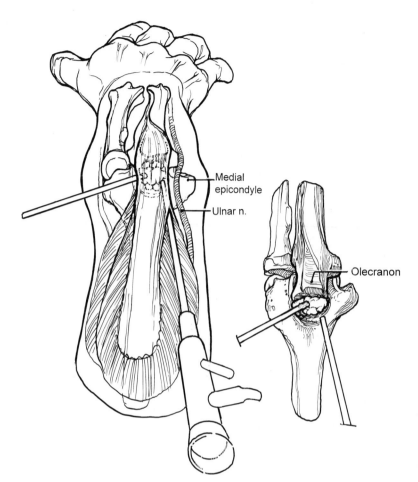

Medial
epicondyle

Ulnar n.

Olecranon

Figure 24–14 Resection of hypertrophic olecranon spurs. The shaded area represents posteromedial bony impingement that is to be arthroscopically resected.

olecranon as well as a displaced OCD lesion. If acute displacement of an apophysis occurs, surgical fixation is indicated. The surgical technique involves open reduction of the displaced apophysis to the anatomic position. Internal fixation can be accomplished with a variety of fixation devices.

SELECTED BIBLIOGRAPHY

Biomechanics

JOBE FW. *Operative Techniques in Upper Extremity Sports Injuries*. St. Louis, MO: Mosby; 1996.

MORREY BF. *The Elbow and Its Disorders*. Philadelphia, PA: WB Saunders; 1985.

SISTO DJ, JOBE FW, MOYNES DR, ANTONELLI DJ. An electromyographic analysis of the elbow in pitching. *Am J Sports Med*. 1987;15:260–263.

Surgical Approaches

JOBE FW. *Operative Techniques in Upper Extremity Sports Injuries*. St. Louis, MO: Mosby; 1996.

Physical Examination

O'DRISCOLL SW, BELL DF, MORREY BF. Posterolateral rotary instability of the elbow. *J Bone Jt Surg*. 1991;73A:440–446.

Arthroscopy of the Elbow

LYNCH GJ, MEYERS JF, WHIPPLE TL, CASPARI RB. Neurovascular anatomy and elbow arthroscopy: inherent risks. *Arthroscopy*. 1986;2:1911–197.

POEHLING GG, EKMAN EF. Arthroscopy of the elbow. *AAOS Instruct Course Lect*. 1995;44:217–223.

Lateral Epicondylitis

LEACH RE, MILLER JK. Lateral and medial epicondylitis of the elbow. *Clin Sports Med*. 1987;6:259–272.

NIRSCHL RP, PETTRONE FA. Tennis elbow: the surgical treatment of lateral epicondylitis. *J Bone Jt Surg*. 1979;61A:832–839.

Medial Epicondylitis

VANGSNESS CT, JOBE FW. Surgical treatment of medial epicondylitis. *J Bone Jt Surg*. 1991;73B:409–411.

Medial Ligamentous Insufficiency

CONWAY JE, JOBE FW, GLOUSMAN RE, PINK M. Medial instability of the elbow in throwing athletes. *J Bone Jt Surg*. 1992;74A:67–83.

MORREY Bf, TANAKA S. AN K. Valgus stability of the elbow. *Clin Orthop*. 1991;265:187–195.

Osteochondritis Dissecans

McMANAMA GB Jr, MICHELI LJ, BERRY MV, SOHN RS. The surgical treatment of osteochondritis of the capitellum. *Am J Sports Med*. 1985;13:11–21.

Valgus Extension Overload

MILLER CD, SAVOIE FH III. Valgus extension injuries of the elbow in the throwing athlete. *JAAOS*. 1994;2:261–269.

WILSON FD, ANDREWS JR, BLACKBURN TA, McCLUSKEY G. Valgus extension overload in the pitching elbow. *Am J Sports Med*. 1983;11:83–88.

Little League Elbow

GRANA WA, RASHKIN A. Pitcher's elbow in adolescents. *Am J Sports Med*. 1980;8:333–336.

PAPPAS AM. Elbow problems associated with baseball during childhood and adolescence. *Clin Orthop*. 1982;164:30–41.

SAMPLE QUESTIONS

1. The portion of the MCL that confers stability to a valgus stress is the:
   (a) anterior band
   (b) oblique band
   (c) posterior band
   (d) transverse band
   (e) b and d

2. Maximal medial tensile forces at the elbow occur during which phase of the throwing motion:
   (a) early cocking
   (b) late cocking
   (c) acceleration
   (d) deceleration
   (e) follow-through

3. Which tendinous origin is most commonly implicated in lateral epicondylitis:
   (a) ECRL
   (b) ECRB
   (c) ECU
   (d) supinator
   (e) EDC

4. Chronic medial ligamentous laxity at the elbow may result in:
   (a) ulnar neuritis
   (b) valgus extension overload
   (c) decreased pitching performance
   (d) all of the above
   (e) b and c

5. Repetitive throwing by the immature athlete may result in:
   (a) OCD of the trochlea
   (b) OCD of the capitellum
   (c) fragmentation of the medial epicondylar apophysis
   (d) radiocapitellar chondrosis
   (e) all of the above

Chapter 25

Arthritis of the Elbow

Heather Brien, MD, FRCSC and Graham J. W. King, MD, FRCSC

Outline

Arthritis of the elbow is commonly seen as a result of joint injuries and rheumatoid arthritis. The stiffness and pain which occur can be helped using appropriate non-operative and operative treatments. This chapter will outline the etiology, anatomy, and biomechanics of elbow arthritis. Treatment options and outcomes for the management of elbow osteoarthritis and rheumatoid arthritis will be reviewed.

ETIOLOGY

Inflammatory Arthritis

Inflammatory arthritis of the elbow includes rheumatoid arthritis, juvenile rheumatoid arthritis, lupus, psoriatic arthritis, crystalline arthropathies, and enteropathic arthritis. Rheumatoid arthritis is the most frequent of the inflammatory arthropathies, and elbow involvement is seen in 20 to 50% of afflicted patients.

The etiology of rheumatoid arthritis is poorly defined. Recent investigations suggest environmental factors or infection may be the cause, similar to the mechanism of arthritis in infections such as Lyme disease. Both mycobacterium and

an unidentified retrovirus have been implicated. (Paliard et al, 1991).

The extent of joint destruction in rheumatoid arthritis has been classified and is useful in deciding the appropriate surgical management. We have found the Mayo classification system to be most helpful in clinical practice (Morrey, 1992). It describes four stages of joint destruction, which are summarized below:

I.   Normal joint space with periarticular osteoporosis
II.   Narrowed joint space with joint contour maintained
IIIA. Moderate architectural changes
IIIB. Severe architectural changes
IV.   Gross joint destruction

Osteoarthritis

Osteoarthritis can be classified as primary or secondary. Primary osteoarthritis occurs spontaneously, and its etiology is unknown. Secondary osteoarthritis refers to that associated with trauma, avascular necrosis, and metabolic abnormalities such as haemochromatosis and crystal deposition disease.

The etiology of primary osteoarthritis remains elusive in spite of considerable research efforts. Imeokparia et al (1994) showed that in a mechanically sound joint, exercise has no correlation with the onset of osteoarthritis. Genetic factors have been implicated through the studies of familial patterns of osteoarthritis. The pathophysiology of osteoarthritis shows change in both the cartilage and in subchondral bone, where there is early formation of new bone. Smith et al (1992) felt that new bone formation changes the subchondral bone stiffness and may lead to secondary cartilaginous change. Other researchers, including Brand et al (1991) have suggested that the primary pathology is in the chondrocytes. There is an increase in the formation of type II collagen, the primary component of cartilage, which is responsible for tensile strength. Type II collagen is encoded on a chromosome 12 gene called COL2A1. Eyre showed an association between an abnormal promoter region (arginine to cysteine base substitution) and hereditary forms of osteoarthritis. There are also other areas of the COL2A1 gene that are susceptible to mutation. Hulth (1993) postulated that growth factors released into the joint cause the changes seen in osteoarthritis.

Orthopaedic Surgery: The Essentials. Edited by M.E. Baratz, A.D. Watson, and J.E. Imbriglia. Thieme Medical Publishers, Inc., New York © 1999

Increased age has been a constant determinant associated with increased rates of osteoarthritis in epidemiological studies. Obesity has also been demonstrated to be a risk factor for osteoarthritis of the knee.

BASIC SCIENCE

Relevant Anatomy and Biomechanics of The Elbow

An understanding of the treatment options for elbow arthritis cannot be adequately discussed without reference to the relevant anatomy and biomechanics of the elbow joint.

The important anatomical considerations about the elbow can be divided according to (1) osseous anatomy, (2) capsuloligamentous structures, and (3) biomechanics.

The osseous anatomy has important significance for both elbow stability and mechanical function. The distal humerus has two articular portions: the trochlea and the capitellum. The articular portion is flexed 40 degrees relative to the long axis of the humerus. The anterior position of the articular surface is important in allowing a full range of motion of the joint. The ulna articulates with the humerus at the greater sigmoid notch and with the radial head at the lesser sigmoid notch. The coronoid process anteriorly and the olecranon process posteriorly both contribute to the stability of the joint by locking into their respective fossae on the humerus in flexion and extension, respectively. The proximal radius articulation is an elliptically shaped, concave dish that articulates with the capitellum and proximal ulna.

Capsuloligamentous structures play an important role in stabilization of the elbow. The anterior joint capsule and olecranon provide significant stability in full extension, whereas the posterior capsule and coronoid are important stabilizers in flexion. Varus and valgus stability in the midrange of elbow motion is primarily provided by the collateral ligaments. The medial and lateral collateral ligaments have been well described in the literature and are critical in the maintenance of a stable, functional range of motion. The medial collateral ligament has an anterior bundle, posterior bundle, and transverse portion all arising from the undersurface of the

medial epicondyle (Fig. 25–1). This origin is posterior to the flexion axis of the humerus. The anterior bundle is the strongest portion; inserting into the anteromedial coronoid and greater sigmoid notch, it provides significant resistance to valgus forces in flexion. The posterior bundle inserts into the posteromedial margin of the greater sigmoid notch and is even more posterior to the axis of rotation. As a consequence of its anisometry, this bundle may need to be divided to improve flexion range in an elbow with restricted motion. The posterior bundle provides little contribution to valgus stability of the elbow.

The lateral collateral ligament complex has three components: annular, radial, and ulnar (lateral ulnar collateral ligament) portions. They all originate on the lateral epicondyle near the axis of rotation, an important landmark for arthroplasty (Fig. 25–2). The ulnar portion, inserting on the cristae supinatoris of the ulna, provides the strongest resistance to rotational forces. Because the lateral collateral ligament is isometric through the range of motion, release is usually not required to improve motion of a stiff elbow. The radial portion of the ligament stabilizes the proximal radius as it inserts in to the annular ligament. Finally, the funnel-shaped annular ligament attaches to both the anterior and posterior sigmoid notch, where it stabilizes the radial head through pronation and supination.

The biomechanics of the elbow in relation to reconstructive procedures have been well described in the recent literature. The most important aspects include definition and reconstruction of the axis of rotation, as well as maintenance of varus-valgus and anterior-posterior stability. It is important to remember that the function of the elbow is to position and stabilize the hand in space for bimanual activity. The elbow acts as a "sloppy-hinge" joint with the majority of

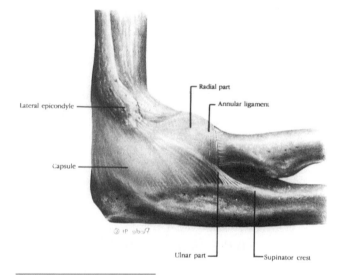

Figure 25–2 The anatomy of the lateral collateral ligament. The three parts of the lateral collateral complex include the ulnar part, annular ligament, and radial part. The ulnar portion is most important as a varus and posterolateral rotatory stabilizer, originating from the lateral epicondyle to the supinator crest. The lateral collateral ligament is isometric. Reproduced with permission from O'Driscoll SW, Horii E, Morrey BF, Carmichael SW. Anatomy of the ulnar part of the lateral collateral ligament of the elbow. *Clin Anat.* 1992;5:298.

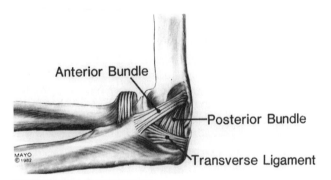

Figure 25–1 The anatomy of the medial collateral ligament. Anterior and posterior bundles are identified based on their site of attachment on the ulna. The anterior bundle is most important structurally. Reproduced with permission from Morrey BF. Anatomy of the elbow joint. In: Morrey BF, ed. *The Elbow and Its Disorders.* Philadelphia, PA: WB Saunders; 1993:29.

motion in the flexion-extension plane (0 to 140 degrees). Pro-supination of the proximal radius and ulna traverses approximately 170 degrees.

The axis of motion through the predominant flexion-extension movement is located along a line joining the center of the capitellum and the center of curvature through the trochlear groove (Fig. 25–3). The external landmarks used to define this axis are the center of the arc of curvature of the capitellum laterally and the anteroinferior aspect of the medial epicondyle medially. These landmarks are critical in allowing an anatomical reconstruction of the joint axis in reconstructive procedures. The axis does not correspond to the carrying angle of the elbow, which is defined as the angle between the long axis of the humerus and the long axis of the ulna in full extension. In contrast, the axis of rotation is 3 to 5 degrees internally rotated with respect to the epicondylar plane and 4 to 8 degrees valgus with respect to the humerus.

Joint stability following elbow arthroplasty can be maintained either through appropriate ligamentous balancing or intrinsic prosthetic constraint. Both the medial and lateral collateral ligaments are essential in maintaining varus-valgus stability and must be preserved or reconstructed in unconstrained (unlinked) prosthetic implants. The medial collateral ligament (anterior bundle) is the primary restraint to valgus stability of the elbow. It works in combination with the osseous stability provided by the radial head along with the musculotendonous structures in the common flexor origin.

The lateral collateral ligament is the primary structure resisting varus and rotation at the elbow. This works as well with the osseous stability provided by the greater sigmoid notch of the ulna.

SURGICAL APPROACHES

In the treatment of arthritis around the elbow, standard approaches used for joint debridement and arthroplasty

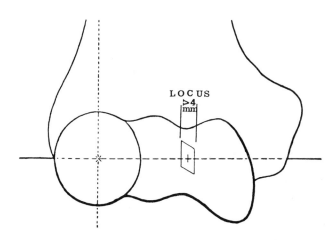

LOCUS
>4 mm

Figure 25–3 Locus of instant centers of rotation of the elbow. The axis of rotation runs through the center of curvature of the capitellum and the trochlea. Reproduced with permission from Morrey BF. Post traumatic stiffness: distraction arthroplasty. In: Morrey BF, ed. *The Elbow and Its Disorders*. Philadelphia, PA: WB Saunders; 1993:484.

include lateral and posterolateral approaches (Kocher, Kaplan) and posterior approaches (Bryan-Morrey, triceps-splitting).

Lateral and Posterolateral Approaches

Indications: joint debridement, radial head excision, removal of loose bodies, interpositional arthroplasty, and unconstrained total elbow arthroplasty.

Kocher Approach

Advantages: protects the radial nerve and lateral ulnar collateral ligament (Fig. 25–4). It may also be extended to approach the distal humerus.

The skin is incised proximal to the lateral epicondyle of the humerus and taken distally and posteriorly over the fascia of the anconeus and extensor carpi ulnaris (ECU). The interval between the anconeus and the ECU is identified once the fascia of the forearm is exposed. Dissection through this interval is taken down to the joint capsule. The origin of the anconeus is dissected posteriorly to expose the full extent of the posterior joint capsule, which may then be excised posterior to the lateral ulnar collateral ligament. Elevation of the ECU anteriorly off the radial collateral ligament allows division of the capsule anterior to this structure for exposure of the anterior portion of the elbow. The radial nerve remains protected throughout this approach by the muscle belly of the ECU.

Extended Kocher Approach

Advantages: wide exposure of posterolateral aspect of the elbow. This is an extension of the Kocher approach in which the anconeus is reflected with the triceps tendon off its insertion onto the olecranon using sharp dissection. The triceps is then taken medially to expose the whole posterior aspect of the elbow. A modification of this technique has been described where a wafer of bone off the olecranon is taken with the triceps tendon (Wolfe and Ranawat, 1990). This can be useful in the patient with a thin/attenuated triceps insertion.

Kaplan Approach

Advantages: useful to expose the anterior aspect of the elbow joint, radial nerve, and/or posterior interosseous nerve for surgical decompression. Requires pronation of the forearm to protect the nerve. Incision of the skin begins just proximal to the lateral epicondyle and extends distally over the radiohumeral joint. The interval between the extensor carpi radialis longus muscle anteriorly (radial nerve) and the extensor carpi radialis brevis posteriorly (posterior interosseous nerve) is identified and carefully dissected to expose the belly of the supinator muscle deep to the extensor muscles. The incision is extended along the lateral supracondylar ridge elevating the origin of the brachioradialis and the extensor carpi radialis longus to expose the anterior aspect of the elbow joint (Fig. 25–5).

Posterior Approaches
Bryan-Morrey Triceps-sparing Approach

Indications: elbow arthroplasty, release of ankylosis, and interposition arthroplasty. *Advantages*: triceps preserved in continuity.

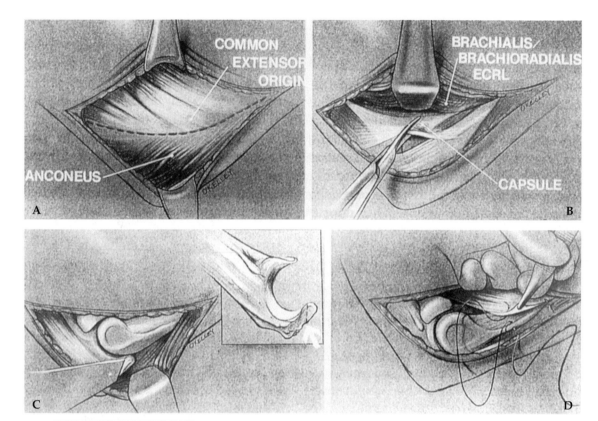

Figure 25–4   The Kocher approach to the elbow. (**A**) The deep fascia is incised laterally in a plane between extensor carpi ulnaris and anconeus. (**B**) Proximally, the fascia is taken off the lateral condyle. (**C**) The lateral margin of the triceps may be elevated and the posterior joint exposed by partially releasing triceps from the ulna. The common extensor origin is taken off the lateral collateral ligament. (**D**) The anterior joint capsule is then exposed. The joint may be entered through a longitudinal capsulotomy or the lateral collateral is taken off its origin for later repair to bone. Reproduced from Morrey BF. Post traumatic stiffness: distraction arthroplasty. In: Morrey BF, ed. *The Elbow and Its Disorders*. Philadelphia, PA: WB Saunders;1993:482.

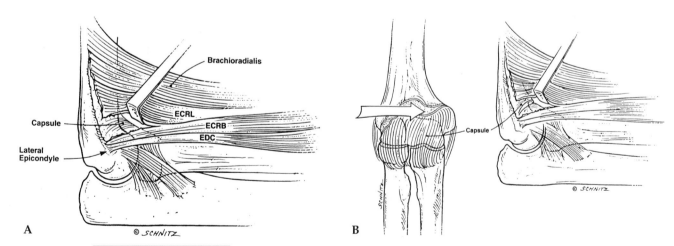

Figure 25–5   The Kaplan approach to the elbow. This is a direct lateral approach. The interval between extensor digitorum communis (EDC) and the extensor carpi radialis longus (ERCL) and brevis (ERCB) is entered, and these structures are retracted away from the capsule (**A**). The supinator muscle and posterior interosseous branch of the radial nerve along with the radial head are then exposed if neccessary (**B**). Reproduced with permission from Hastings H. Elbow contractures and ossification. In: Peimer CA, ed. *Surgery of the Hand and Upper Extremity*. Vol 1. McGraw-Hill; 1996:516.

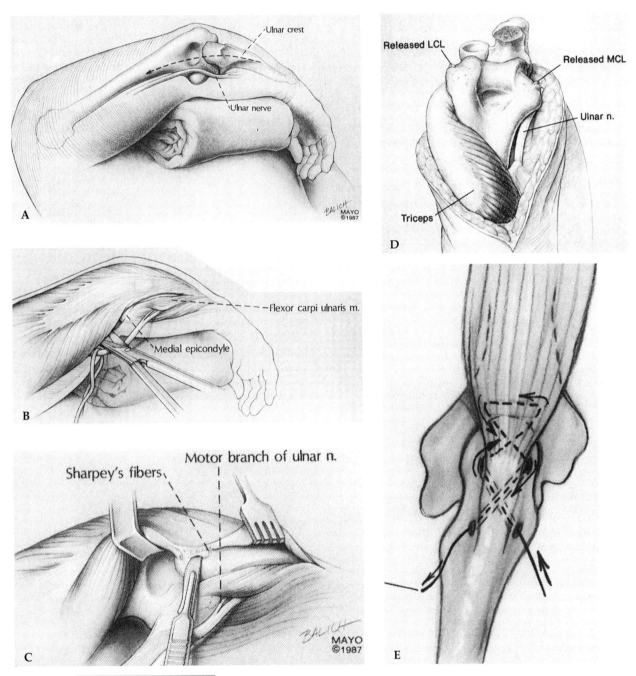

Figure 25–6   The Bryan-Morrey approach. (**A**) Straight posterior incision exposed the triceps and superficial forearm fascia. The distal incision line between the fascia and periosteum is shown. (**B**) The ulnar nerve is anteriorly translocated, and the interval between the medial border of the triceps and ulna is created. (**C**) The triceps is further reflected off the ulna, exposing joint capsule and the flexor group taken medially. (**D**) With the extensor mechanism laterally displaced, the joint is exposed. The proximal olecranon is osteotomized to improve exposure. (**E**) The triceps must be carefully repaired to bone to ensure a functional extensor mechanism. Reproduced with permission from Morrey BF and Adams RA. Semiconstrained Elbow Replacement Arthroplasty: rationale, technique, and results. In: Morrey BF, ed. *The Elbow and Its Disorders*. Philadelphia, PA: WB Saunders; 1993:652–653.

A posteromedial, extensile triceps-sparing approach (Bryan and Morrey, 1982) is commonly used when exposure of the ulnar collateral ligament or ulnar nerve is required (Fig. 25–6). In this approach, the interval begins by elevation of the medial aspect of the triceps tendon after the ulnar nerve has been anteriorly transposed. The interval is carried distally on to the medial subcutaneous border of the ulna, elevating the triceps subperiosteally off the olecranon in continuity with the anconeus fascia. In both the Bryan Morrey and extended Kocher approaches, the triceps is reattached onto the olecranon using a heavy, nonabsorbable suture through drill holes in the bone.

Triceps-splitting Approach

Indications: Debridement and ulnohumeral arthroplasty. *Advantages*: triceps attachment in continuity and excellent visualization of the olecranon fossa.

Using a straight, posterior midline incision, care is taken to identify and protect the ulnar nerve or to transpose it if indicated. The triceps tendon is split longitudinally down to its insertion on the olecranon. This allows the surgeon direct visualization of the olecranon fossa and permits anterior debridement after fenestration of the distal humerus when performing the Outerbridge-Kashiwagi procedure.

Universal Skin Incision

In our institution, we use a posterior, midline skin incision for almost all elbow surgery. This incision has been shown to have the least effect on the cutaneous nerves surrounding the elbow, limiting the incidence of neuromas. Elevation of the fasciocutaneous flaps allows global approach to the elbow through medial, lateral, or posterior internervous planes.

PEARL

Skin incisions should not cross the tip of olecranon. Place the incision slightly medially or laterally. Posterior approach is optimal.

PEARL

Identify and protect the ulnar nerve. Subcutaneous or submuscular anterior transposition may be required.

EXAMINATION

History

Pattern of Symptoms

1. Pain: onset, duration, progression, radiation, night symptoms
2. Stiffness: onset, progression, location in arc of motion
3. Stability: provocative maneuvers
4. Function: activities of daily living, vocation
5. Treatment: types and response

Physical Examination

1. Inspection: skin, scars, atrophy, discoloration, alignment, joint effusion (over radial head)
2. Palpation: skin, tendon, muscle, bone, nerves
3. Range of motion: flexion-extension, pronation-supination, active and passive
4. Strength: flexion-extension, prosupination, grip strength

5. Neurovascular: sensation, reflexes, note posterior interosseous and ulnar nerve function
6. Special Tests: varus-valgus stability, posterolateral rotatory instability of radial head, Tinel test of ulnar nerve

---

PEARL

Always rule out infection before considering total elbow arthroplasty.

AIDS TO DIAGNOSIS

Radiographs

Anteroposterior, lateral, oblique, and stress views with fluoroscopy. Radiographs should include anteroposterior, lateral, oblique, and stress views with fluoroscopy. Computed tomography, with or without contrast, and arthrography are useful for evaluating periarticular deformity or loose bodies. A technetium bone scan may be useful for detecting occult fractures of early degenerative changes. Soft tissue lesions and ligamentous injuries are most clearly seen by magnetic resonance imaging.

SPECIFIC CONDITIONS, TREATMENT, AND OUTCOME

Rheumatoid Arthritis

Treatment of the rheumatoid elbow in a surgical manner begins after appropriate medical treatment has failed. Medical management includes pharmacological intervention and steroid injection in combination with physical therapy and splinting. Prior to any surgical treatment, it is important to check for involvement in the cervical spine, as well as to assess other joints, particularly the shoulder, wrist, and hand to decide on a coordinated approach to treatment.

Surgical Techniques

Synovectomy

Synovectomy and radial head excision with or without radial head replacement has been reported to have good results in those patients with stage II and, occasionally, stage III disease. Timing of the synovectomy is critical. Gross ligamentous instability, severe stiffness secondary to fibroarthrosis, and advanced articular cartilage destruction are the main contraindications to synovectomy. Excision of the radial head at the time of surgery is performed to improve the surgical exposure, increase forearm rotation, and decrease impingement at the radiocapitellar joint.

This procedure is done through the posterolateral Kocher approach. The radial head is identified and excised in a manner so as to maintain ligamentous support at the proximal radialulnar joint. Once the head has been removed, synovectomy of the anterior portion of the joint can be completed with good visualization. The posterior aspect of the joint can be addressed by elevating the anconeus and opening up the interval bordering the lateral aspect of the triceps tendon. Using this approach, the medial joint is difficult to visualize and clear entirely, but the approach is usually adequate for a successful synovectomy. If further medial visualization is required, the triceps may be taken off the olecranon, or a supplementary medial incision may be used.

Postoperatively, we recommend immediate motion, preferably using a continuous passive motion machine and continuous axillary block for the first 48 hours. This is followed by outpatient active physiotherapy and a resting extension splint at night.

Arthroscopic synovectomy has been performed with success. There may be an increased risk of neurovascular injury due to the reduced capsular volume as a consequence of capsular contracture, decreasing displacement of the neurovascular structures from the arthroscopic portals. In addition, the anterior capsule is often attenuated in rheumatoid arthritis, further increasing the risk of nerve injury. Additional experience with this technique is needed.

The results of open synovectomy have shown (1) pain relief in more than 90% of patients for 3 years postoperatively and 75 to 80% of patients at 5 years and (2) maintenance of range of motion in 45% and improvement in 40% of patients, respectively.

Patient satisfaction with the procedure is high, although recurrent synovitis is common after 5 years postoperatively. Most importantly, synovectomy and repeat synovectomy does not compromise later arthroplasty of the joint.

PITFALL

Beware of the anterior capsule: The neurovascular structures are very close (within 2 mm) and easily injured when the capsule is attenuated by rheumatoid synovitis.

Arthroplasty
Elbow arthroplasty has the best outcome in advanced rheumatoid arthritis of the elbow. Indications include painful stage III and IV joint disease and disabling ankylosis. Many advances have been made in elbow arthroplasty over the past decade. There are currently two popular types of prostheses: unconstrained and semiconstrained. Unconstrained devices are joint resurfacing prostheses that require intact muscles and ligaments of the joint, (e.g., Capitellocondylar, Souter and Pritchard). The semiconstrained device is used most frequently when there is more severe joint and ligamentous erosion, as the implant has inherent stability due to its linked design as a sloppy hinge (e.g., Coonrad-Morrey, Triaxial).

Surgical technique is dependent on the type of implant selected for the individual patient, but certain generalities apply. In our institution, we use the Bryan-Morrey posteromedial triceps reflecting approach for the Coonrad-Morrey implant and routinely anteriorly transpose the ulnar nerve. The extended Kocher approach is preferred for resurfacing

devices. Meticulous care of the skin edges and soft tissues is critical to decrease wound infection and skin slough, common in the rheumatoid patient. The collateral ligaments are released for the semiconstrained device but preserved or repaired for resurfacing designs. The radial head is excised and the humeral and ulnar surfaces are prepared for trial implantation. Full extension with the trial in place is essential as is adequate tracking of the implant surfaces and tension in the triceps. We favor the use of intramedullary cement restrictors to aid cement fixation in both the humeral and ulnar canals. The bone is often very fragile in the rheumatoid patient, and the cortex can easily be penetrated with the rasp. This is of particular concern in the humerus, where cement extrusion from the canal can cause radial nerve injury.

Postoperatively, the patient is splinted in extension for the Coonrad-Morrey and to 60 degrees of flexion for resurfacing devices. Active, assisted flexion exercises are started under the supervision of a physiotherapist beginning on the second day postoperatively. Passive extension is performed for 6 weeks to avoid avulsion of the triceps tendon repair. Resting flexion and extension splints are fabricated. The patient should be at a functional range of motion (30 to 130 degrees) prior to discharge.

Results of elbow arthroplasty in the rheumatoid patient have been very encouraging. Range of motion averages 35 to 125 degrees of flexion with 40 degrees pronation-supination, in most cases. Satisfactory pain relief along with a functional range can be expected in 90% of cases. Patients who undergo arthroplasty with semiconstrained devices often have greater postoperative motion due to the extensive release required for insertion and the ability to permit full extension in the early postoperative period (Fig. 25–7).

Complications of elbow arthroplasty include wound healing complications (2%); nerve injury, usually transient ulnar parasthesias (2–26%); instability (5–10%); perioperative fracture (5%); infection (1–5%), and loosening (1–2%). Instability is seen exclusively in the resurfacing type of arthroplasty (Fig. 25–8).

Arthrodesis and Interpositional Arthroplasty
Elbow arthrodesis is relatively contraindicated in the rheumatoid patient due to the stresses that it places on the adjacent joints. Interpositional arthroplasty is indicated for young patients with painful, stiff joints who are too young to be considered for total elbow arthroplasty. While this procedure is usually helpful, the results are far inferior to that of total elbow arthroplasty.

Osteoarthritis

The majority of patients with primary osteoarthritis of the elbow are male and present at the age of 40 or older. Pain at the limits of extension or flexion is a common initial symptom, which later progresses to pain throughout the arc of motion. Flexion contracture occurs with increasing severity of the disease. Rotation of the forearm is maintained in the majority of cases, as the disease primarily affects the ulnohumeral joint. Ulnar nerve symptoms are frequently present. Nonoperative treatment, rest and activity modification,

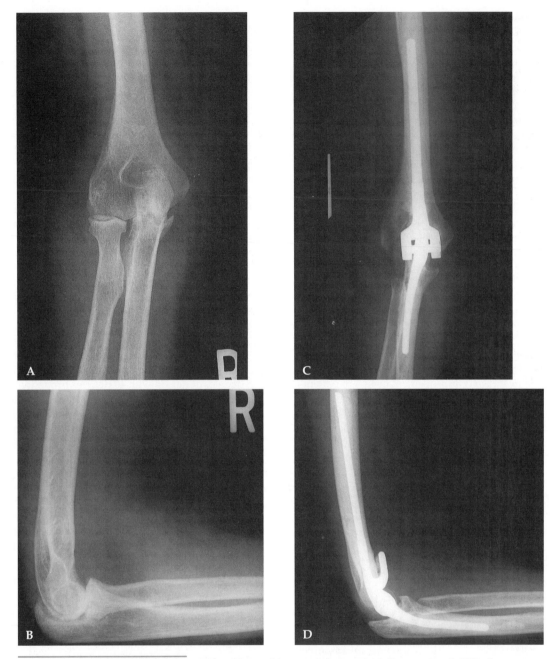

Figure 25–7   A 65-year-old patient with a 20-year history of rheumatoid disease. Grade IIIA changes are seen on the anterior-posterior (AP) (**A**), and lateral (**B**) radiographs. This was treated with a Coonrad-Morrey arthroplasty, seen in the AP (**C**) and lateral (**D**) postoperative radiographs.

splinting, and anti-inflammatory medications are helpful in relieving symptoms in the early stages of the disease, but surgical treatment is required if symptoms are progressive and debilitating.

Surgical Management

Arthroscopy
The most promising indication for arthroscopy in osteoarthritis of the elbow is for mild disease with removal of a loose body. Excision of loose bodies causing impingement symptoms is usually successful (89%) at relieving the patient's symptoms. Arthroscopic debridement of osteoarthritic

elbows has a lower success rate when loose bodies are not found at the time of surgery. As further experience is gained with these techniques, the indications for arthroscopic debridement may increase in the future.

Joint Debridement
Debridement of the joint has been shown to provide pain relief and an improved range of motion. The most common procedure is the Outerbridge-Kashiwagi procedure. The Tsuge procedure is also used for a more extensive debridement (Tsuge, 1994).

The Outerbridge-Kashiwagi procedure was initially described in 1978 and has been modified by Morrey, (1992,

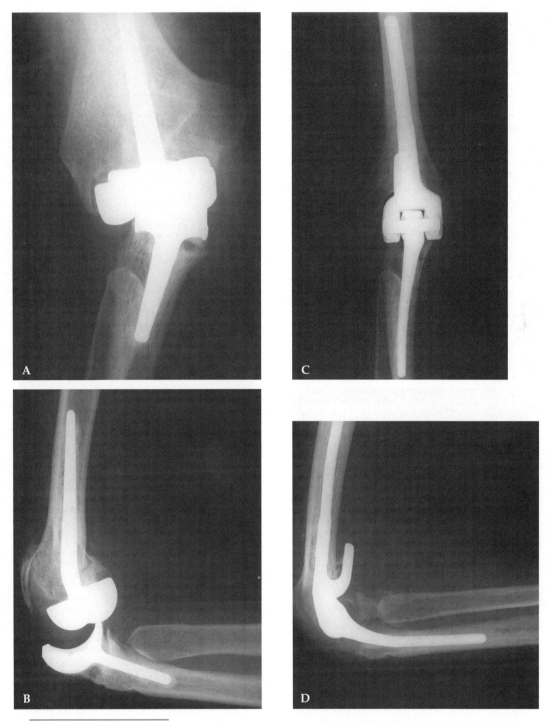

Figure 25–8   This patient presented with severe pain and instability three years after a capitellocondylar arthroplasty. Radiographs taken at that time show valgus instability in the AP view (**A**), and subluxation in the lateral view (**B**). The joint was revised to a semiconstrained Coonrad Morrey device (**C and D**) after which the patient was left with a pain-free, stable, and functional joint.

described as the ulnohumeral arthroplasty). The patient is positioned for a posterior approach to the elbow, either prone, or supine with the arm across the chest. A straight posterior incision is made and subcutaneous dissection is made to expose triceps fascia. Transposition of the ulnar nerve is performed if necessary. The triceps is split in the midline and

the tip of the olecranon is removed to assist exposure, as well as to improve extension. The olecranon fossa is cleared of osteophytes and opened with a Cloward trephine. Care must be taken to position the fenestration correctly so as not to compromise the medial or lateral columns, capitellum, and trochlea. The coronoid tip can be visualized and removed by

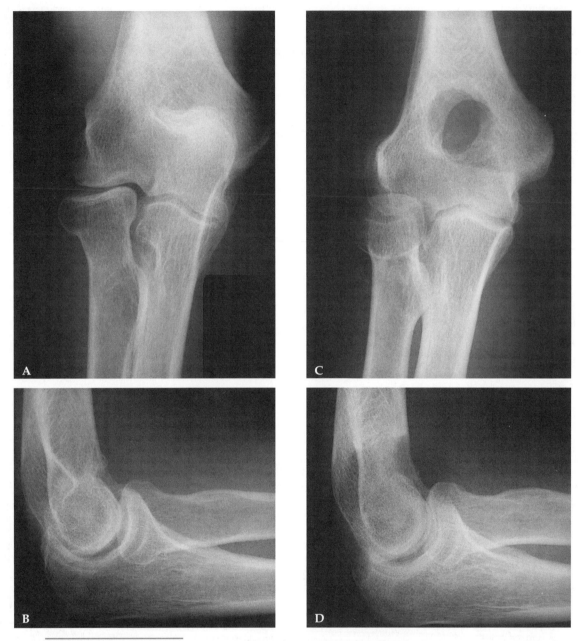

Figure 25–9   A 40-year-old male presented with impingement pain and a flexion-extension range of 45 to 120 degrees. The anterior (**A**) and lateral (**B**) radiographs show a roof osteophyte in the coronoid fossa. Post operative views following treatment with an Outerbridge-Kashiwagi procedure show the characteristic fenestration in the olecraneon fossa in the AP view (**C**) and removal of osteophytes in the lateral view (**D**). Functionally, the patient had decreased pain and range of motion from 20 to 145 degrees of flexion.

flexion of the elbow. Partial release of the anterior capsule may be done at the same time if needed. (Fig. 25–9).

The ulnohumeral arthroplasty has been shown to reliably relieve pain symptoms and improve range of motion. In one series, improvement in pain occured in all cases; 39% complete relief, 91% improved extension, and 76% improved flexion (Morrey, 1992). The results appear to be of limited duration, and symptoms often gradually recur as the disease continues to progress. Complications include ulnar neuropathy, periop-erative fracture, and recurrence of osteophyte formation along with haematoma, infection, and ectopic ossification.

Interposition Arthroplasty

Interposition arthroplasty has been used successfully for many years as a treatment for elbow arthritis. It originally developed from resection arthroplasty, which was used in

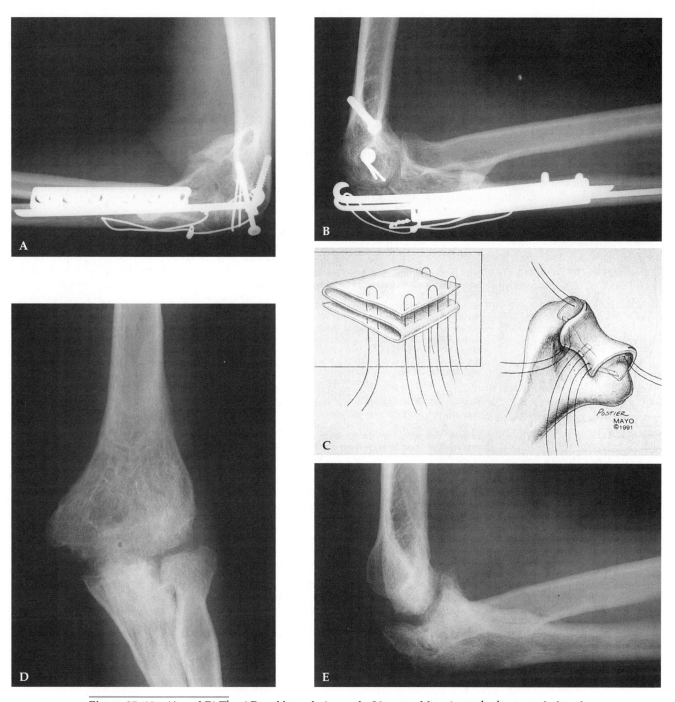

Figure 25–10   (**A** and **B**) The AP and lateral views of a 21-year-old patient who has an ankylosed elbow 1 year following surgery for a fracture caused by a motor vehicle accident. Note the synostoses between the radius and ulna, as well as the decreased joint space and ossification of the medial collateral ligament. The patient went on to operative management with interposition arthroplasty (**C**) using a fascial interposition technique. At 18 months postoperatively, the patient has a range of 20 to 140 degrees flexion and minimal discomfort. (**D** and **E**) The AP and lateral radiographs at that time.

cases of late untreated dislocations, arthrodeses in nonfunctional positions, and other conditions of unremitting joint pain. A variety of substances, both biological and man-made, have been used as interposition substances to provide a painless but stable joint. Fascial interposition arthroplasty has proved one of the most reliable for this procedure (Fig. 25–10).

The indications for interposition arthroplasty include treatment of the post-traumatic, painful, stiff joint for which other options have been exhausted and for which total elbow arthroplasty is contraindicated due to age or history of previous sepsis. For this procedure to be successful, there must be pre-existing ligamentous stability. Contraindications include active sepsis, open physes, a patient who is a heavy laborer or who is required to use crutches, and multiple ankylosed joints.

The procedure is done through an extended posterolateral Kocher approach. The patient is positioned supine, with the extremity draped free and positioned across the chest. Once the posterior midline incision has been made, the interval between the anconeus and ECU is identified, and the plane of dissection through this interval is created. The insertion of the triceps is reflected from the posterior ulna using sharp dissection and retracted medially while keeping the extensor mechanism in continuity. The tip of the olecranon is then removed with a rongeur or oscillating saw, and the joint is fully exposed. The radial head is preserved, if possible. If there is bony ankylosis of the joint, this is osteotomized to allow the full exposure and dislocation of the elbow. As always, care is taken to identify and protect the ulnar nerve throughout the procedure. The trochlea is deepened, removing all osteophytes and releasing contracted capsule anteriorly and posteriorly. The proximal ulna is then smoothed, and the sigmoid notch is contoured to allow the fascial interposition. Tensor fascia latae is harvested from the ipsilateral thigh. A sheet of fascia 4- to 5-cm $\times$ 15-cm is harvested for this purpose. The graft is folded (smooth surface inside) three times and attached to the distal humerus using drill holes through bone. The joint is then reduced with the graft in place. Range of motion and stability are checked and closure proceeds with lateral collateral ligament repair and closure of the fascial plane, as previously described for this surgical approach. An articulated elbow distraction device is used for 4 to 6 weeks postoperatively. One pin is placed through the distal humerus axis of rotation, and two pins are placed into the ulna. All pin placement is done under fluro-

scopic control to correctly place the axial pin and to position the joint in 3 to 5 mm of distraction. Particular care is taken to protect the ulnar nerve during insertion of the distal humerus axial pin.

Results of this procedure have been successful with reports of 75% good pain relief and somewhat lesser results for increasing range of motion. The best results are seen in younger patients and those with intact periarticular structures. However, total elbow arthroplasty has shown superior results and does not compromise bone stock as much as this procedure.

Total Elbow Arthroplasty

Arthroplasty for osteoarthritis of the elbow is less successful than that for rheumatoid disease. Indications include osteoarthritis with pain and limited motion in an elderly, low-demand patient, preferably past age 60. Elderly patients with a chronic nonunion of a supracondylar humerus fracture are also considered good candidates for total elbow arthroplasty. Absolute contraindications are the same as for any elbow arthroplasty and include sepsis, triceps/biceps insufficiency, and some neurological disorders. Arthroplasty should be contemplated only after options such as capsular release and debridement/ distraction arthroplasty have been exhausted, particularly in the younger patient.

The technique is the same as that previously described for rheumatoid arthroplasty, and the risks and complications are similar. Morrey (1990) described a series of elbow arthroplasty for post-traumatic arthritis with a satisfactory outcome in 86% of cases, including 100% stable joints and an 18% complication rate. The concern is a higher loosening rate with total elbow arthroplasty for osteoarthritis versus rheumatoid arthritis.

SELECTED BIBLIOGRAPHY

Rheumatoid Arthritis: Etiology and Basic Science

PALIARD X, WEST SG, LAFFERTY JA et al. Evidence for the effects of a superantigen in rheumatoid arthritis. *Science.* 1991;253:325–29.

MORREY BF, ADAMS RA. Semi-constrained total elbow arthoplasty for rheumatoid arthritis. *J Bone Jt Surg.* 1992;74A: 479–490.

Osteoarthritis: Etiology and Epidemiology

BRAND HS, DEKOENING MH, VAN KAMPEN GP, VANDER KORST JK. Age related changes in the turnover of proteoglycans from explants of bovine articular cartilage. *J Rheum.* 1991;18:599–605.

EYRE DR, WEIS MA, MOSKOWITZ RW. Cartilage expression of a type II collagen mutation in an inherited form of osteoporosis with a mild chondrodysplasia. *J Clin Invest.* 1991;357–61.

FELSON DT. The epidemiology of knee osteoarthritis. Results of the Framingham osteoarthritis study. *Sem Arthritis Rheum.* 1990;20(suppl 1):42–50.

HULTH A. Does osteoarthritis depend on growth of the mineralized layer of cartilage? *Clin Orthop,* 287;1993:19–24.

IMEOKPARIA RL, BARRETT JP, ARRIETA MI, et al. Physical activity as a risk factor for osteoarthritis of the knee. *Ann Epidemiol.* 1994;4:221–230.

SMITH RL, THOMAS KD, SCHURMAN DJ, CARTER DR, WONG M, VANDER MERLEN MC. Rabbit knee immobilization: bone remodelling preceeds cartilage degeneration. *J Orthop Res.* 1992;10:88–95.

WILLIAMS CJ, CONSIDINE EL, KNOWLTON RG, et al. Spondyloepiphyseal dysplasia and precocious arthritis in a family with Arg 75- Cys mutation in the procollagen type II gene (COL2A1). *Human Genet*. 1993;92:499–505.

Elbow Biomechanics

KING GJW, ITOI E, NIEB UR, MORREY B, AN K. Motion and laxity of the capitellocondylar total elbow prosthesis. *J Bone Jt Surg*. 1994;76A:1000–1007.

KING GJW, MORREY BF, AN K. Stabilizers of the elbow. *Shoulder Elbow Surg*. 1993;2:165–174.

O'DRISCOLL SW, AN KN, KORINEK S, MORREY BF. Kinematics of semiconstrained total elbow arthroplasty. *J Bone Jt Surg*. 1992;74B:297–299.

SOJBJERG JO, OVESEN J, NIELSEN S. Experimental elbow instability after transection of the medial collateral ligament. *Cinical Orthop Rel Res*. 1987;218:186–190.

Surgical Approaches

BRYAN RS, MORREY BF. Extensive posterior exposure of the elbow. A triceps-sparing approach. *Cinical Orthop*. 1982;166:188–192.

DOWDY PA, BAIN GI, KING GJW, PATTERSON SD. The midline posterior elbow incision. *J Bone Jt Surg*. 1995;77B:696–698.

WOLFE SW, RANAWAT CS. The osteoanconeus flap: an approach for total elbow arthroplasty. *J Bone Jt Surg*. 1990;72A:684–688.

Arthroscopic Synovectomy

O'DRISCOLL S, MORREY BF. Arthroscopy of the elbow: Diagnostic and therapeutic benefits and hazards. *J Bone Jt Surg*. 1992;72A:84–94.

OGILVIE-HARRIS DJ, SCHEMITSCH E. Arthroscopy of the elbow for removal of loose bodies. *Arthroscopy*. 1993;9:5–8.

Elbow Arthroplasty

KNIGHT RA, VAN ZANDT IL. Arthroplasty of the elbow: an end result study. *J Bone Jt Surg*. 1952;34A:610–618.

LJUNG P, JONSSON K, LARSSON K, RYDHOLM U. Interpositional arthroplasty of the elbow with rheumatoid arthritis. *J Shoulder Elbow Surg*. 1996;5:81–85.

MORREY BF. Post-traumatic contracture of the elbow, *J Bone Jt Surg*. 1990;72A:601–618.

O'DRISCOLL SW, AN K, KORINICK S, MORREY BF: Kinematics of semiconstrained total elbow arthroplasty. *J Bone Jt Surg*. 1992;74B:297–9.

Osteoarthritis: Debridement and Ulnohumeral Arthroplasty

KASHIWAGI D. Intra-articular changes of the osteoarthritic elbow especially about the fossa olecrani. *J Japanese Orthop Assoc*. 1978;52:1367.

MINAMI NM, ISHII S. Outerbridge-Kashiwagi arthroplasty for osteoarthritis of the elbow joint. In: Kashiwagi D, ed. *Proceedings of the International Congress*, Kobi, Japan. Amsterdam, The Netherlands: Excerpta medica; 1986.

MORREY BF. Primary degenerative arthritis of the elbow: treatment by ulnohumeral arthroplasty. *J Bone Jt Surg*. 1992;74B:409–413.

TSUGE K, MIZUESKI T. Debridement arthroplasty for advanced primary osteoarthritis of the elbow: results of a new technique used for 29 elbows. *J Bone Jt Surg*. 1994;76B:641–646.

SAMPLE QUESTIONS

1. Early symptoms of primary osteoarthritis of the elbow include:
   (a) a hot, reddened, swollen joint
   (b) pain at rest
   (c) pain at the end of flexion and extension
   (d) morning stiffness
   (e) restriction of pronation and supination

2. Advantages to excision of the radial head during synovectomy for rheumatoid arthritis include:
   (a) greater exposure to the posterior joint
   (b) improved range of motion and stability postoperatively
   (c) greater exposure to the anterior joint
   (d) ease of later arthroplasty

3. Joint aspiration in the rheumatoid elbow typically reveals:
   (a) white blood cells greater than 50×10^9/liter
   (b) decreased glucose relative to serum
   (c) increased polymorphs

   (d) hemarthrosis
   (e) gram negative rods

4. Absolute contraindications to total elbow arthroplasty include:
   (a) ankylosis of the joint
   (b) total shoulder arthroplasty
   (c) triceps paralysis
   (d) aseptic loosening of a previous total joint

5. The most frequent complication of open debridement of the elbow for osteoarthritis is:
   (a) infection
   (b) perioperative fracture
   (c) heterotopic ossification
   (d) paraesthesia of the ulnar nerve

Answers: 1) c; 2) c; 3) b; 4) c; 5) d

Chapter 26

Diaphyseal Forearm Fractures

T. Michael Dye, MD and John Clifford, MD

Outline

The bones of the forearm rotate in a precise manner during forearm pronation and supination. To maintain this relationship, anatomic alignment of the radius and ulna is necessary. Restoration of this alignment is a priority in treating fractures of the diaphyseal forearm.

ETIOLOGY

The mechanism of injury in adult diaphyseal forearm fractures is often high-energy trauma such as a motor vehicle accident, fall from a height, or gunshot wound. Pathological fractures are rarely seen in this area.

BASIC SCIENCE

Stress Shielding

Most fractures of the forearm are treated with plate fixation. Following surgery, the bone is subject to two undesirable conditions: stress shielding and the development of stress risers. Stress shielding occurs when a decrease in stress develops around bone due to the sharing of stresses by a stiffer structure, such as a plate, nail, or screw. Stress shielding can cause loss of bone beneath the plate. This has been attributed to unloading of bone and structural adaptation according to Wolff's law; remodeling of bone in response to the stress. There are other factors that may contribute to loss of cortical bone under an implant. It has been shown that compression under a plate leads to loss of blood flow in periosteal vessels.

This compounds the avascularity resulting from the fracture and the stripping that occurs during the surgical exposure.

With rigid plate fixation, bone healing occurs primarily. Vascular ingrowth of secondary osteons and cutting cones leads to the development of porous cortical bone beneath the implant. The thinned cortex combined with the stress risers resulting from screw holes results in a high incidence of refracture if the plates are removed. Several studies have shown refracture rates higher when plates are removed than when they are left in place. The recommendation has been that plates placed on the diaphysis of the radius and ulna should not be removed.

The use of 1/3 tubular steel plates for fixation of diaphyseal forearm fractures has proven inadequate. The plate frequently breaks at the screw holes; a stress riser in the plate that is often too weak to withstand forces seen in the forearm. Refracture of the radius and ulna has also been associated with the use of 4.5-mm plates.

PEARL

Optimal open reduction and fixation of forearm fractures is achieved with the use of 3.5-mm compression plating. In most instances, the plate should not be removed after the fracture has healed.

ANATOMY AND SURGICAL APPROACHES

Restoration of proper bony alignment is essential in preserving normal motion of the forearm. The shaft of the ulna is relatively straight and serves as a fixed point about which the radius rotates. The radius, on the other hand, has a more complex shape, with a bow that creates an arc of rotation. Restoration of this bow in fracture care is important in maintaining proper forearm rotation.

Restoration of proper radial bow will also restore the interosseous space. This space is occupied by the interosseous membrane (IOM), an important structure in maintaining longitudinal stability of the forearm. The central portion of the IOM has been found to be most important in maintaining this

377

stability. The function of the IOM becomes especially important in injuries that compromise the stability and function of the radiocapitellar joint.

Deforming forces in forearm fractures are related to muscular attachments along the bones. The primary deforming forces result from contraction of the biceps, brachialis, supinator, pronator teres, and pronator quadratus. A fracture of the radius distal to the supinator insertion and proximal to the pronator insertion results in supination of the proximal fragment and pronation of the distal fragment. If the fracture is distal to the pronator teres attachment, the proximal fragment assumes a neutral position. Understanding the anatomy and deforming forces is useful when performing open reductions.

The distal radioulnar joint (DRUJ) is stabilized by the triangular fibrocartilage complex (TFCC) and the distal aspect of the IOM. Injuries that propagate along the IOM can disrupt the TFCC leading to instability of the DRUJ. This will be discussed in the section on Galeazzi fractures.

Surgical Approaches

There are three surgical approaches to the forearm that are commonly used: anterior (Henry), posterior (Thompson), and the subcutaneous approach to the ulna.

We prefer the anterior approach for most fractures of the radial diaphysis. The ulna is approached along its subcutaneous border.

Anterior Approach

The anterior approach is made along a line between the radial styloid and a point just lateral to the biceps tendon. All or part of the incision can be used. It can also be extended proximally and distally to expose the wrist, elbow, or humerus (Fig. 26–1).

The approach follows the interval between the brachioradialis and flexor carpi radialis in the distal half of the wound. The superficial radial nerve is taken with the brachioradialis radially. The radial artery is taken either radially or ulnarly, depending on the need for proximal or distal exposure. Proximally, the plane of dissection is between the brachioradialis and the pronator teres.

Deep dissection proximally should be radial to the biceps tendon and the radial artery. To avoid the posterior interosseous nerve (PIN), the forearm should be supinated. The supinator attachment can be elevated off the ulnar aspect of the radius. Care should be taken to avoid excessive lateral traction on the supinator and the placement of retractors posterior to the radius to avoid injury to the PIN.

In the middle third of the forearm, the pronator teres and superficial flexor muscles are elevated off bone by pronating the forearm and elevating muscle from its lateral attachment. In the distal third, the pronator quadratus and flexor pollicis longus are elevated from the radial aspect of the radius.

Posterior Approach

The skin incision for the posterior approach is made on a line connecting a point just anterior to the lateral epicondyle to a point just ulnar to Lister's tubercle. Normally, only part of this incision is needed.

Proximally, the plane is between the extensor carpi radialis brevis (ECRB) and extensor digitorum communis (EDC). This plane is easier to find distal to their common origin and in the middle third of the forearm, where the abductor pollicis longus (APL) and extensor pollicis brevis (EPB) emerge between the two muscles (Fig. 26–2).

In the interval between the ECRB and the EDC, the supinator is found draped over the radius. The PIN emerges from this muscle 1 cm proximal to its distal edge. The nerve must be identified and isolated, either by tracing it from proximal to distal or distal to proximal. Following isolation of the nerve, the supinator is elevated off the radius along its anterior margin.

In the middle third of the exposure, the APL and the EPB are elevated off the radius. Distally, the exposure of the radius is made either between the EPB and the EDC, or between the extensor pollicis longus and the ECRB.

Exposure of the Shaft of the Ulna

The skin incision is made along the subcutaneous border of the ulna. The shaft is exposed by incising deep fascia and elevating muscle in the plane between the extensor carpi ulnaris and the flexor carpi ulnaris. Subperiosteal exposure of the ulna is then performed.

EXAMINATION

Forearm fractures are often high energy injuries. Attention should be paid to assessing the patient for concommitant injuries. Thoracic, abdominal, cranial, and other musculoskeletal injuries should be ruled out.

The status of the soft tissues of the injured extremity should be assessed. Evidence of an open injury must be ruled out. A thorough neurovascular exam should be performed. Usually, the surrounding soft tissue envelope will protect vessels and nerves, but in severe trauma there may be a deficit. Although rare, compartment syndromes of the forearm do occur, and the examiner should be alert to this. Tense swelling, pain with passive motion, and paresthesias are important diagnostic clues. Pulselessness is a very late finding.

Measurement of compartment pressures may be necessary to establish the diagnosis, especially in obtunded or comatose patients. Compartment pressures may be measured by a variety of techniques, including infusion techniques, wick catheter, or continuous monitoring. The absolute pressure measurement indicating need for fasciotomy is debatable. Various numbers have been used, including a pressure within 10 to 30 mm of diastolic pressure or an absolute pressure of 30 mm Hg. It should always be remembered, however, that a strong clinical suspicion is more important than pressure measurements.

The status of the entire upper extremity should be examined, checking for evidence of trauma to the shoulder, humerus, elbow, wrist and hand.

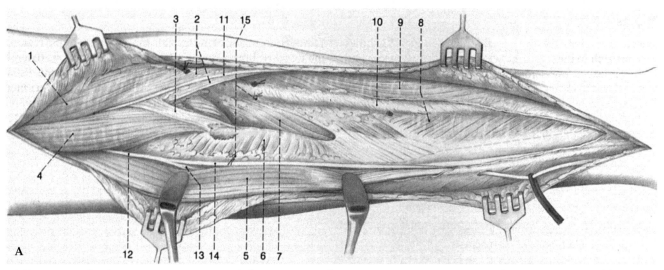

A

1 Biceps muscle of arm	6 Supinator muscle	11 Lateral cutaneous nerve of foream
2 Aponeurosis of biceps muscle of arm	7 Pronator teres muscle	12 Radial nerve
3 Tendon of biceps muscle of arm	8 Long flexor muscle of thumb	13 Deep branch of radial nerve
4 Brachial muscle	9 Radial flexor muscle of wrist	14 Superficial branch of radial nerve
5 Brachioradial muscle	10 Radial vessels	15 Radial recurrent artery

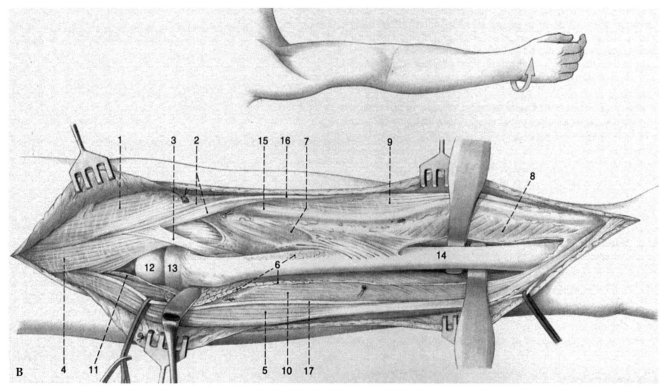

B

1 Biceps muscle of arm	7 Pronator teres muscle	13 Head of radius
2 Aponeurosis of biceps muscle of arm	8 Long flexor muscle of thumb	14 Body of radius
3 Tendon of biceps muscle of arm	9 Radial flexor muscle of wrist	15 Radial vessels
4 Brachial muscle	10 Long radial extensor muscle of wrist	16 Lateral antebrachial cutaneous
5 Brachioradial muscle	11 Cubital joint capsule	nerve
6 Supinator muscle	12 Capitellum of humerus	17 Superficial branch of radial nerve

Figure 26–1 Anterior approach (Henry) to the radius. **(A)** Superficial dissection. **(B)** Deep dissection. Reproduced with permission from Bauer R, Kerschbaumer F, Poisel S. Operative approaches in Orthopaedic Surgery and Traumatology. New York: Thieme Medical Publishers. 1987;276.

AIDS TO DIAGNOSIS

Radiographs should include standard anteroposterior (AP) and lateral views. Positioning of the injured arm may preclude good orthogonal views, and oblique views may be necessary to properly visualize the extent of injury. It is important to get good views of the wrist and elbow with any forearm fracture, with special attention to the DRUJ and the radiocaptellar joint.

SPECIFIC CONDITIONS, TREATMENT, AND OUTCOME

Diaphyseal Fractures of the Radius and Ulna

Most displaced, both-bone forearm fractures in adults will require open reduction with internal fixation. Nondisplaced both-bone fractures may be amenable to closed treament but must be followed closely because of a tendency to angulate in the cast. The forearm should be placed in a long-arm cast at 90 degrees elbow flexion and neutral forearm rotation.

Isolated fractures of the ulna (nightstick fractures) with minimal or no displacement can also be treated closed (Fig. 26–3). Generally, some form of cast immobilization is used, but functional bracing and no immobilization have also been reported with good results. If there is angulation greater than 10 degrees, displacement greater than 50%, or comminution, open reduction and plate fixation is recommended.

Plate fixation of both-bone forearm fractures

As mentioned above, operative fixation will be the treatment choice for most forearm fractures. Compression plate fixation is the preferred method (Fig. 26–4). Numerous studies have shown a 95 to 98% rate of union, with good restoration of anatomy and a functional range of motion.

Most authors advocate fixation within 48 hours. This makes for easier fracture reduction and reduces recovery time.

The surgical approaches have been previously described. We prefer the anterior approach for fractures of the radial shaft and an incision along the subcutaneous border of the ulna for fractures of the ulnar shaft. Exposure at the fracture site should be subperiosteal. The periosteum should be stripped just enough to allow reduction and plate application.

Reduction techniques vary according to fracture configuration. A bone-holding forceps can be used to hold the plate to the reduced fracture. Lag screws can be placed in oblique or spiral fractures outside or within the plate. This significantly improves the strength of the reconstruction. With comminuted or unstable fractures, it is sometimes easier to fix one side of the fracture to the plate with one or two screws, and then reduce the rest of the fracture to the plate-bone construct. Occasionally, reduction of very comminuted fractures will be facilitated with the use of a mini-distractor. The distracter provides initial alignment and length, comminuted fragments are teased into place, and a plate is applied.

The optimal plate to use for fixation is a 3.5 mm dynamic compression (DC) plate. These plates provide the strength necessary to ensure healing of the fracture.

The length of plate used depends on fracture configuration. For transverse fractures, six cortices on each side of the fracture should be engaged. For oblique or comminuted fractures, eight cortices on each side of the fracture should be engaged (Fig. 26–5).

Segmental fractures can be fixed either with one long plate, or with two plates at 90 degrees to each other. Plates in all fractures should be contoured to reproduce normal anatomy. This is especially important for the radius, and care should be taken to reproduce the normal bow of the radius by proper contouring of the plate.

Intramedullary Rodding of Both-bone Diaphyseal Fractures

Due to the superior results obtained with plate fixation, intramedullary rod fixation is very seldom used. Rod fixation presents problems with fracture stability, restoration of proper alignment, and has a lower union rate than plating. Error in selection of the size of the rod can lead to side-to-side and rotatory movement with resultant malunion or nonunion. Too large a rod can split the cortex. Use of square or diamond shaped rods helps rotation, but maintenance of the proper radial bow is a problem. There are occasions when an isolated ulna fracture can be supported with the use of rods, but plate fixation is the standard by which all other forms of management should be judged.

Galleazzi Fractures

In any isolated fracture of the radius, disruption of the DRUJ should be suspected. This combination of injuries, the Galleazi fracture, has been dubbed the "fracture of necessity" due to the poor outcome with nonoperative treatment. The typical pattern of injury consists of fracture at the junction of the middle and distal thirds of the radius, with disruption of the interosseous membrane from that level through the DRUJ. The radius fracture is usually apex dorsal, and the distal ulna is usually prominent dorsally.

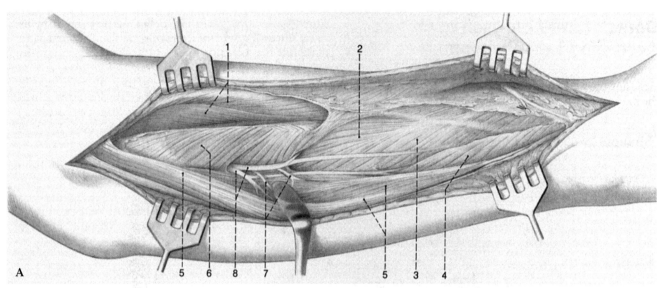

1 Short radial extensor muscle of the wrist
2 Long abductor muscle of the thumb
3 Short extensor muscle of the thumb
4 Long extensor muscle of the thumb
5 Extensor muscle of fingers
6 Supinator muscle
7 Posterior interosseus artery (muscular branches)
8 Deep branch of radial nerve

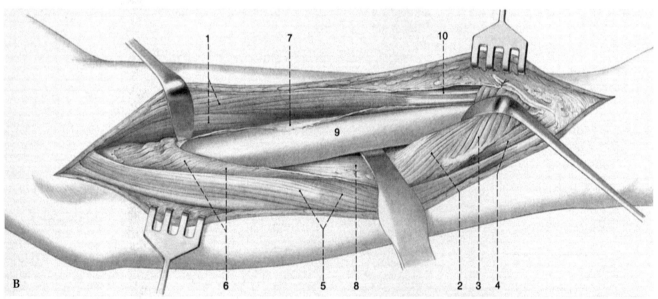

1 Short radial extensor muscle of wrist
2 Long abductor muscle of thumb
3 Short extensor muscle of thumb
4 Long extensor muscle of thumb
5 Extensor muscle of fingers
6 Supinator muscle
7 Pronator tares muscle (insertion)
8 Periosteum
9 Body of radius
10 Tendon of long radial extensor muscle of wrist

Figure 26–2 Posterior approach (Thompson) to the radius. **(A)** Superficial dissection. **(B)** Deep dissection, mid-radius. Reproduced with permission from Bauer R, Kerschbaumer F, Poisel S. Operative approaches in Orthopaedic Surgery and Traumatology. New York: Thieme Medical Publishers. 1987;279, 284.

Diagnosis of Galleazzi fracture can be made clinically and on radiographs. Key features are isolated distal radius fracture with:

1. ulnar styloid fracture
2. widened DRUJ on AP radiograph of wrist
3. apex dorsal fracture and subluxation/dislocation of radius on ulna seen on lateral radiograph
4. shortened radius greater than 5 mm relative to the ulna

This fracture pattern is inherently unstable and requires open reduction and internal fixation. The radius is plated through an anterior approach. The forearm is supinated and the stability of the DRUJ is assessed. If the ulnar head is stable, the arm is held in full supination for 4 weeks. If the head remains unstable, it is pinned to the radius for 4 weeks. If the DRUJ is unreducible, then the joint should be opened dorsally, inspected for interposed tendon (usually the extensor carpi ulnaruis) or loose bodies, and reduced. The capsule should

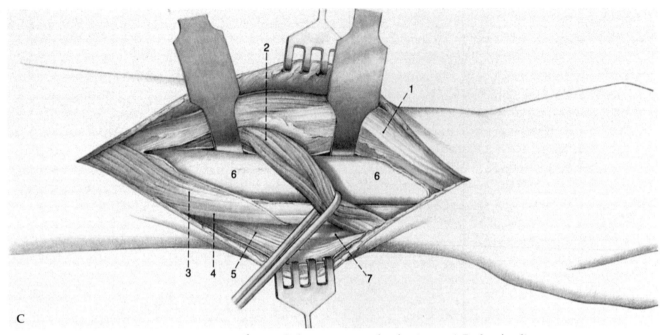

C

1 Extensor muscle of fingers
2 Short extensor and long abductor
   muscle of thumb

3 Short radial extensor muscle of wrist
4 Long radial extensor muscle of wrist
5 Brachioradial muscle

6 Body of radius
7 Superficial branch of radial nerve

Figure 26–2 *(continued)*   Posterior approach (Thompson) to the radius. **(C)** Deep dissection, distal radius.

be repaired in the closure, and the joint should then be pinned and splinted as above.

Management of Open Fractures

The management of open fractures of the forearm is different from that of the lower extremity. Open fractures of the forearm have been successfully treated with immediate (within 24 hours) open reduction and internal fixation. The

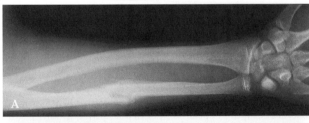
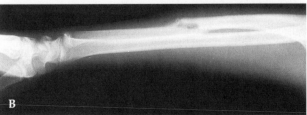

Figure 26–3 Anteroposterior (**A**) and lateral (**B**) radiograph of the forearm in a 17-year-old girl.

key to good results is meticulous debridement, adequate irrigation, and rigid internal fixation. In the emergency department, and the patient should be given tetanus prophylaxis and started on intravenous cefazolin. For grossly contaminated wounds, an aminoglycoside and penicillin should be added. A careful neurovascular exam should be performed. Open fractures, in general, are associated with a higher incidence of nerve laceration (Fig. 26–6).

At operation, the wound should be meticulously debrided of devitalized, contaminated tissue and then copiously irrigated with saline irrigation to which an antibiotic has been added. Fracture fixation should proceed as has been described. After fixation of the fracture, the wound should again be irrigated. Wounds are packed open and secondarily closed. If the wound requires soft tissue coverage, a flap should be performed within 7 to 10 days for good results. It is usually best to delay bone grafting until the final operation, just before closure.

This approach has yielded very good results. Good to excellent results have been achieved for Gustilo and Anderson type I, II, and IIIA fractures. The results have not been as good for type IIIB and IIIC fractures. This may be related more to the severity of the injury than the fact that the fracture was open versus closed. It may be prudent to consider other management techniques such as external fixation in these injuries.

External fixation is reserved for open fractures that cannot be managed easily with internal plate fixation such as Gustilo type IIIB and IIIC fractures with soft tissue and bone loss. Half pins with a rigid frame in two planes will help avoid neurovascular injury and provide stable fixation.

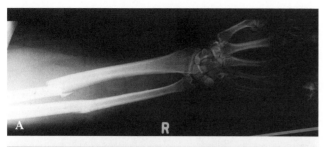

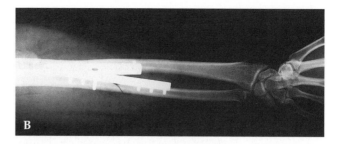

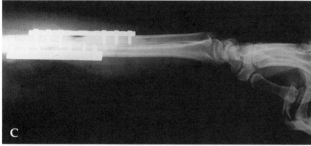

Figure 26–4 Both-bone forearm fracture in a 41-year-old female treated with 3.5-mm AO dynamic compression plating. (**A**) AP radiograph demonstrates mid-diaphyseal fracture of the radius and ulna. (**B**) AP and (**C**) lateral radiographs of same fracture after open reduction and internal fixation.

Meticulous debridement is imperative intraoperatively. External fixation is usually converted to internal fixation when soft tissue coverage permits.

Comminuted Fractures

Most fractures with comminution can be managed with standard plating techniques. If the fracture fragments are large, the pieces should be anatomically reduced. Lag-screw fixation of the pieces should result in good alignment of the fracture. The construct can then be stabilized using normal plating, either in compression or neutralization as appropriate. Fragments of bone that are stripped of their soft tissue attachments should be removed and discarded, especially in open fractures. The resultant defects can be bone grafted immediately in closed fractures and in 3–5 days in open fractures.

If the fragments are small or do not lend themselves to lag-screw fixation, then the comminuted area may be spanned with a plate and the fragments teased into position after the reduction and fixation of the major sections of bone have been accomplished. It is often helpful in this instance to use ligomentotaxis to aid in reduction. A distraction device can be used to distract and reduce the fracture site. This is accomplished through the use of two 4.5-mm Shantz pins placed away from the proposed area of internal fixation. The distracter helps to hold the reduction while the neutralization plate is applied. Another helpful technique is to attach the plate to one of the fracture ends with a single screw. Reduction of the major fragments is performed, then the plate is clamped to the other end while the comminuted fragments are reduced. Do not attach the plate with more than a single screw initially, or you may not be able to achieve proper alignment of the plate in the final reduction.

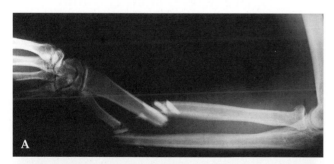

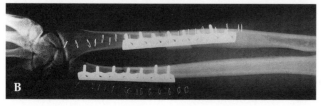

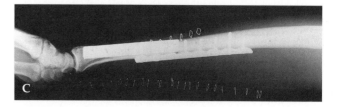

Figure 26–5 Both-bone forearm fracture in a 35-year-old male treated with 3.5-mm AO low-contact dynamic compression plating. Note the notched undersurface of the plate on the lateral view. (**A**) AP radiograph of forearm demonstrates comminuted mid-diaphyseal radius and ulna fracture. (**B**) AP and (**C**) lateral radiographs after open reduction and internal fixation.

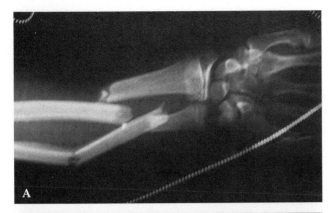
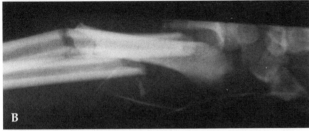

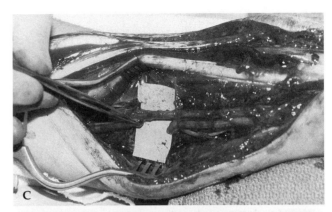
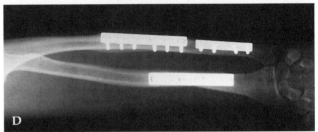
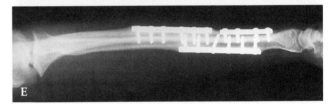

Figure 26–6   Open fracture of both bones of the forearm in a 17-year-old patient. Note the segmental fracture of the ulna. This patient had complete loss of median nerve function below the level of injury. (**A**) AP and (**B**) lateral radiographs demonstrate a segmental fracture of the ulna and diaphyseal fracture of the radius. (**C**) At operation the median nerve was found to be transected and was repaired primarily. (**D**) AP and (**E**) lateral radiographs of the forearm after repair with dynamic compression plating. Ideally, the ulna should have been fixed with either one long plate or two plates oriented at 90 degrees to each other.

SELECTED BIBLIOGRAPHY

Anatomy

RABINOWITZ RS, LIGHT TR, HAVEY BS, GOURINENI P, PATWARD-HAN AG, SARTORI MJ, VRBOS L, MAYWOOD IL. The role of the interosseous membrane and triangular fibrocartilage complex in forearm stability. *J Hand Surg.* 1994;19A: 385–393.

Surgical Approaches to the Forearm

HOPPENFELD S. DEBOER P. *Surgical Exposures in Orthopaedics: The Anatomic Approach.* 2nd ed. Philadelphia, PA: Lippincott; 1994:118–146.

Closed Treatment of Forearm Fractures

KNIGHT RA, PURVIS GD. Fractures of both bones of the forearm in adults. *J Bone Jt Surg.* 1949;31A:755–764.

Internal Fixation of Both Bone Forearm Fractures

ANDERSON LD, SISK TD, TOOMS RE, PARK WI. Compression plate fixation in acute diaphyseal fractures of the radius and ulna. *J Bone Jt Surg.* 1975;57A:287–297.

CHAPMAN MW, GORDON JE, ZISSIMOS AG. Compression plate fixation of acute fractures of the diaphysis of the radius and ulna. *J Bone Jt Surg.* 1989;71A:159–169.

Open Fractures of the Forearm

DUNCAN R, GEISSLER W, FREELAND AE, SAVOIE FH. *J Orthop Trauma.* 1992;6:125–131.

MOED BR, KELLAM JF, FOSTER RJ, TILE M, HANSEN ST. Immediate internal fixation of open fractures of the diaphysis of the forearm. *J Bone Jt Surg.* 1986;68A:1008–1017.

External Fixation

DELEE JC. External fixation of the forearm and wrist. *Orthop Rev.* 1981;6:43–48.

Galeazzi Fractures

BENEYTO ME, ARANDES RENU JM, FERRERES CLARAMUNT A, RAMON SOLER R. Treatment of Galeazzi fracture-dislocations. *J Trauma.* 1994;36:352–355.

MIKIC ZD. Galeazzi fracture-dislocations. *J Bone Jt Surg.* 1975;57A:1071–1080.

Complications

DELUCA PA, LINDSEY RW, ROWE PA. Refracture of bones of the forearm after removal of compression plates. *J Bone Jt Surg.* 1988;70A:1372–1376.

SAMPLE QUESTIONS

1. All of the following may be found in a forearm with a compartment syndrome of the anterior compartment except:
   (a) pain in excess of that expected, given the injury
   (b) tense swelling along the entire length of the compartment
   (c) a compartment pressure of 40 mm Hg
   (d) pain with passive finger flexion
   (e) a compartment pressure of 20 mm Hg in a patient with a blood reading of 95/40

2. The optimal surgical approach to a mid-diaphyseal both-bone forearm fracture is:
   (a) a single volar approach
   (b) a single dorsal approach
   (c) volar approach to the ulna, dorsal approach to the radius
   (d) volar approach to the radius, lateral approach to the ulna
   (e) lateral approach to the radius, dorsal approach to the ulna

3. A 48-year-old woman falls onto her outstretched arm and presents to the emergency department complaining of pain and deformity in her right arm. Radiographs reveal a dorsally angulated fracture of the radius at the junction of the middle and distal thirds. The distal ulna is subluxated dorsally on the radius, but reduces with manual pressure. Proper management of this fracture entails:
   (a) closed reduction and splinting in pronation
   (b) closed reduction and splinting in supination
   (c) open reduction, internal fixation of the radius, and splinting in pronation
   (d) open reduction, internal fixation of the radius, and splinting in supination
   (e) open reduction, internal fixation of the radius, and open reduction and pinning of the DRUJ

4. A 28-year-old construction worker sustains an open, comminuted both-bone forearm fracture after being struck by a backhoe. The wound is 7 cm long with bone stripped of soft tissue and dirt ground into the bone ends. The patient is neurovascularly intact. Proper management of this fracture includes meticulous debridement and irrigation, and:
   (a) reduction and splinting with wounds treated open, then open reduction and internal fixation with primary closure 3 to 10 days after injury
   (b) open reduction and internal fixation with wounds closed over a drain
   (c) external fixation with wound loosely approximated, then redebridement with plate fixation in 5 to 7 days
   (d) open reduction and internal fixation with bone graft and wound closed at a second procedure
   (e) open reduction and internal fixation with bone graft and primary closure

5. Which of the following statements concerning fixation of both-bone forearm fractures is incorrect:
   (a) Optimal fixation of the radius and ulna are acheived with 4.5-mm dynamic compression plating.
   (b) Low-contact dynamic compression plating may decrease stress shielding by allowing greater periosteal blood flow than dynamic compression plates.
   (c) One-third tubular plates are inadequate fixation for most forearm fractures due to their relative weakness.
   (d) The use of 3.5-mm dynamic compression plates is associated with decreased incidence of fracture after plate removal.
   (e) The use of titanium low-contact dynamic compression plates may decrease stress shielding because titanium's modulus of elasticity is closer to that of bone than stainless steel.

Wrist/Hand

Chapter 27

Fractures and Dislocations of the Wrist and Hand

Stanley Marczyk, MD, Adrienne J. Towsen, MD, Bruce Jacobs, OT, and Mark E. Baratz, MD

Outline

Fractures and dislocations of the wrist and hand occur frequently with varying degrees of severity. The intricate anatomy of the wrist and hand makes complications such as nerve and tendon damage a serious consideration when managing these types of injuries. Numerous classification systems and eponyms exist to describe these injuries which often require surgical management. Accurate diagnosis, proper treatment and supervised rehabilitation are the keys to recovery of strength, range of motion, and function. This chapter will cover many of the major fractures and dislocations of the wrist and hand with emphasis on basic science, anatomy, surgical approaches, diagnostics, treatment and outcome.

ETIOLOGY

To better understand the etiology of fractures and dislocations of the hand and wrist, it is important to elicit the mechanism of injury. A direct blow or crush will more frequently result in a transverse or comminuted fracture pattern, whereas a twisting injury will often result in a spiral or oblique pattern. The position of the hand or wrist when it is injured will frequently determine the fracture pattern or ligament injury.

BASIC SCIENCE

Blood Supply of the Scaphoid

The blood supply of the scaphoid accounts for its susceptibility, following a fracture, to delayed union, nonunion, and avascular necrosis (Fig. 27–1). The radial artery sends branches to the dorsal ridge of the scaphoid, which supplies the proximal 70 to 80% of the bone. A second branch of the

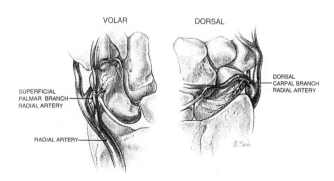

Figure 27–1 Blood supply of the scaphoid, dorsal, and volar views. Reproduced with permission from Amadio, Taleisnik. Fractures of the carpal bones. In: DP Green, ed. *Operative Hand Surgery.* 3rd ed. New York, NY: Churchill Livingstone; 1993:80.

Orthopaedic Surgery: The Essentials. Edited by M.E. Baratz, A.D. Watson, and J.E. Imbriglia. Thieme Medical Publishers, Inc., New York © 1999

radial artery enters the distal palmar aspect of the scaphoid to supply the tuberosity. There is no interosseous anastamosis between these two branches. Fractures through the waist and proximal pole of the scaphoid can interrupt the blood supply to the proximal fragment, reducing the chance that the fracture will heal.

Keinbock's Disease

Another entity in which there is compromise in the vascularity of a carpal bone is Keinbock's disease. This involves avascular necrosis of the lunate. The most consistent blood supply to the lunate enters palmarly and arises from both the radial and ulnar arteries through an intercarpal arch.

The cause of Keinbock's is unknown. Possible etiologies include previous fracture, repeated minor wrist trauma, and a wrist in which the radius is longer than the ulna (ulnar minus variance). Treatment of Keinbock's includes procedures designed to reduce the forces crossing the lunate by shortening the radius or capitate and procedures designed to restore blood supply to the lunate via a vascularized bone graft. A commonly used classification for the stages of Keinbock's disease is shown in Fig. 27–2.

Progressive Perilunar Instability

Dislocations and fracture-dislocations of the wrist can be severely disabling injuries. Pure lunate and perilunate dislocations involve only ligamentous damage but can lead to long term instability and wrist arthritis. The concept of progressive perilunar instability describes the progressive disruption of ligaments attached to the lunate as the wrist is hyperextended. This type of injury can result in a spectrum of injuries ranging from a simple scapholunate ligament tear to a lunate dislocation.

Mayfield 1980 described four stages of progressive perilunar instability (Fig. 27–3). Stage I involves tearing of the scapholunate interosseous as well as palmar radio-scaphoid ligaments, resulting in a scapholunate dissociation. This may be misdiagnosed as a "wrist sprain" in the acute setting. Stage II involves a dissociation of the capitolunate joint. The radiotriquetral and lunotriquetral ligaments are torn in stage III, resulting in a separation of the lunate and triquetrum.

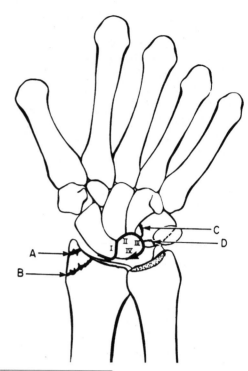

Figure 27–3   Mayfield's classification of progressive perilunar instability. Reproduced with permission Mayfield JL, *J Hand Surg*. 1980;5A:239.

Finally, stage IV involves a dorsal radiocarpal tear allowing the lunate to dislocate palmarly.

ANATOMY AND SURGICAL APPROACHES

Interphalangeal Joints

The proximal interphalangeal (PIP) joints and the distal interphalangeal (DIP) joint structures are very similar. Each interphalangeal joint in the hand is a hinge joint with motion limited to flexion and extension. Stability is derived from the articular contours of the bones as well as the surrounding ligaments. Secondary reinforcement is supplied by adjacent tendons and the retinacular system. The joint capsules are composed of strong radial and ulnar collateral ligaments and the stout palmar plate. Each of these three structures insert into bone as well as into each other. The DIP joint gains additional support from the proximity of insertion of the flexor and extensor tendons. This anatomic difference, and a shorter lever arm, makes the DIP joint less susceptible to dislocation.

Metacarpophalangeal Joints

The metacarpophalangeal joints are multiaxial, condyloid joints that allow flexion, extension, lateral motion, and a small amount of circumduction. The metacarpal heads have an irregular spheroidal shape, and the bases of the phalanges are broad and concave. The articulation of these reciprocally shaped bones is stabilized by the collateral ligaments, the volar plate, and the accessory collateral ligaments. The sagit-

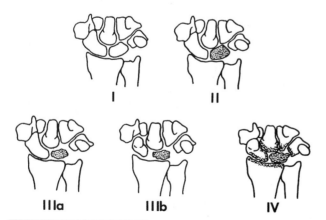

Figure 27–2   The staging of Keinbock's disease. Reproduced with permission Weiss from APC. *J Bone Jt Surg*. 1991; 73A:388.

tal bands and the tendons of the intrinsic musculature also play a reinforcing role.

The collateral and accessory collateral ligaments originate from the metacarpal metaphysis. The collateral ligaments insert onto the palmar aspects of the proximal phalanges. The eccentric origin of these ligaments produces a camlike effect, which causes them to be lax in extension and and maximally taut in flexion (Fig. 27–4). Therefore, with the joint in extension there is little ligamentous support against lateral motion; but in full flexion, the joint is extremely stable laterally. The accessory ligaments insert on the lateral aspect of the palmar plate. This fibrocartilaginous structure forms the anterior wall of the joint and is responsible for resisting excessive hyperextension.

Carpometacarpal joints

The carpometacarpal (CMC) joints (fingers) of the hand can be broken down into three separate functional and anatomic units. The most mobile and most susceptible to injury is the thumb CMC joint. The first metacarpal articulates with the trapezium, an articulation frequently described as two perpendicular "saddles." This joint possesses some inherent stability, but the joint capsule and palmar ligaments are the primary stabilizers.

The CMC joints of the index and long fingers are the central, fixed portion of the hand. There is essentially no motion at these joints. The index articulates primarily with the trapezoid, and the long metacarpal articulates with the capitate. Strong palmar, dorsal, and interosseus ligaments, as well as wrist flexor and extensor insertions, serve to make these two joints very immobile and stable.

The ring and small metacarpals share an articulation with the hamate. These two, ulnar CMC joints have 10 to 20 degrees of flexion and extension as well as some supination.

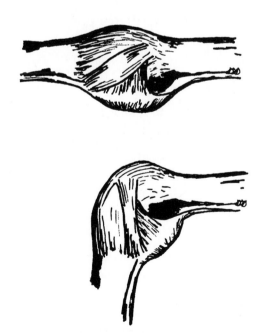

Figure 27–4   Metacarpophalangeal joint in extension and flexion, demonstrating the collateral ligaments.

The mobility of these two digits allows them to enhance the gripping strength of the hand.

Intercarpal and Radiocarpal Joints

The wrist joint is composed of not only the radiocarpal and distal radioulnar joints but also the intercarpal articulations. The radiocarpal joint is made up of articulations between the radius and lunate and the radius and scaphoid. These articulations are supported by strong palmar ligaments including the radiolunate, radioscaphocapitate, and radial collateral complex. Ulnar-sided wrist ligaments include the ulnolunate, ulnar collateral, and the triangular fibrocartilage complex, which helps to stabilize the distal radioulnar joint. Dorsal and palmar views of these ligamentous structures are seen in Fig. 27–5. Intercarpal ligaments include the lunotriquetral and scapholunate ligaments which aid in stabilizing the proximal carpal row. The scapholunate ligament is composed of strong dorsal and palmar connections with a weak membranous portion between them. The physician must maintain a high index of suspicion for a scapholunate ligament tear in what is thought to be a wrist sprain. The ligamentous connections between the proximal and distal rows include the arcuate or deltoid ligament, which runs from the scaphoid and triquetrum to the capitate, and the previously mentioned radioscaphocapitate. An area void of any ligament support is the palmar capitolunate joint, referred to as the space of Poirier.

Scaphoid Surgical Exposure: Palmar and Dorsal

The scaphoid can be approached through either a palmar or dorsal approach. More commonly, the palmar approach is used to protect the dorsal blood supply. The dorsal approach is sometimes utilized for proximal pole fractures, scaphoid excisions, or scaphoid fractures associated with other injuries (perilunate dislocations).

The palmar approach (Fig. 27–6) involves a longitudinal incision in the interval between the flexor carpi radialis (FCR) and radial artery beginning approximately 3 cm proximal to the wrist crease and continuing distally over the base of the thenar eminence. The FCR is mobilized and retracted ulnarly. The radial artery is mobilized radially. The wrist capsule is then exposed by opening the floor of the FCR sheath longitudinally. The exposed section of the wrist capsule can then be entered through a longitudinal incision. It is important to repair this section of capsule during closure due to the strong palmar radiocarpal ligaments traversing it. The capsule is split to the base of the trapezium. The superficial palmar branch of the radial artery may need to be ligated as it crosses the distal aspect of the wound. Dorsiflexion of the wrist will allow better visualization of the proximal pole.

Distal Radius Exposure: Palmar and Dorsal

Like the scaphoid, the distal radius may be exposed through either a palmar or dorsal approach.

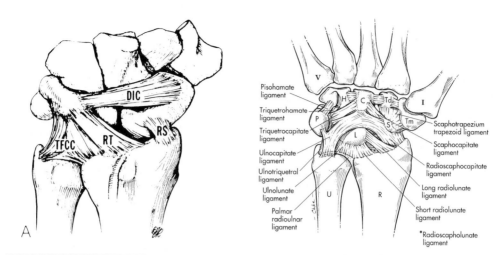

Figure 27–5 (A) Dorsal view of ligaments of the wrist. RS, radioscaphoid; RT, radiotriquetral; TFCC, triangular fibrocartilage complex; DIC, dorsal intercarpal ligaments. Reproduced with permission from AK Palmer. Fractures of the distal radius. In: DP Green, ed *Operative Hand Surgery*. 3rd ed. New York, NY: Churchill Livingstone; 1993:933–934. **(B)** Carpal ligaments from a palmar perspective. (*) denotes the space through which the radioscapholunate ligament pierces the palmar radiocarpal joint capsule. C, capitate; H, hamate; L, lunate; P, pisiform; R, radius; S, distal pole of scaphoid; Td, trapezoid; Tm, trapezium; U, ulna; I, first metacarpal; V, fifth metacarpal. Reproduced with permission from Berger RA. Ligament anatomy. In Cooney WP, Linscheid RL, Dobyns JH, eds *The wrist – diagnosis and operative treatment*. St. Louis: Mosby; 1998:79.

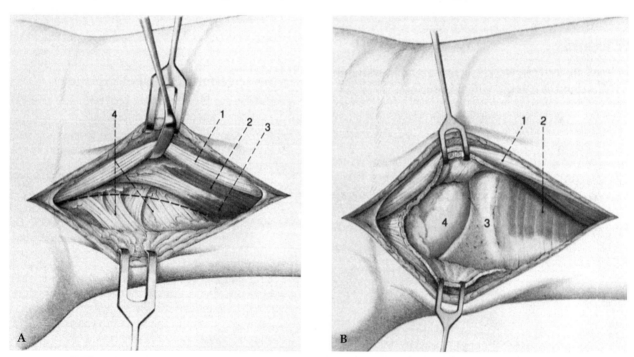

Figure 27–6 Palmar approach to the scaphoid. **(A)** The FCR is retracted ulnarly. 1. Tendon of FCR. 2. Flexor digitorum superficialis (FDS). 3. Flexor pollicus longus. 4. Palmar intercarpal ligaments. **(B)** The joint capsule is opened to expose the scaphoid and distal radius. 1. Tendon of FCR. 2. Pronator teres. 3. Distal radius. 4. Scaphoid. Reproduced with permission from Bauer R, Kerschbaumer F, Poisel S. *Operative Approaches in Orthopedic Surgery and Traumatology*. New York, NY: Thieme; 1987:304.

The incision for a dorsal approach (Fig. 27–7) runs longitudinally along the dorsal aspect of the wrist to the midforearm. The dissection is carried through the subcutaneous tissues, which are then elevated off the extensor retinaculum.

Next, the extensor retinaculum is divided between the tendons of the third and fourth extensor compartments. The extensor pollicis longus is released from its compartment and retracted toward the radial aspect of the wrist. The fourth

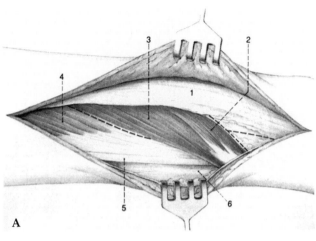

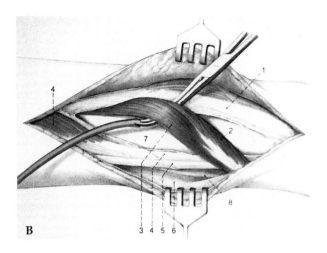

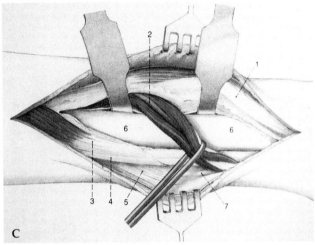

Figure 27–7 Dorsal approach to the distal radius. **(A)** Status after incision of fascia. 1. Extensor digitorum. 2. Extensor pollicus brevis. 3. Abductor pollicus longus. 4. Extensor carpi radialis brevis. 5. Extensor carpi radialis longus. 6. Superficial branch of the radial nerve. **(B)** 1. Extensor digitorum. 2. Extensor pollicus brevis. 3. Abductor pollicus longus. 4. Extensor carpi radialis brevis. 5. Extensor carpi radialis longus. 6. Brachioradialis. 7. Radius. 8. Superficial branch of radial nerve. **(C)** Subperiosteal exposure of the distal radius. 1. Extensor digitorum. 2. Extensor pollicus brevis and abductor pollicus longus. 3. Extensor carpi radialis brevis. 4. Extensor carpi radialis longus. 5. Brachioradialis. 6. Radius. 7. Superficial branch of radial nerve. Reprinted with permission from Bauer R, Kerschbaumer F, Poisel S. *Operative Approaches in Orthopedic Surgery and Traumatology.* New York, NY: Thieme; 1987:283–284.

extensor compartment can be elevated subperiosteally from the dorsal cortex. Alternatively, the retinaculum can be open with a Z-cut lengthening and the tendons retracted ulnarly.

The palmar approach (Fig. 27–8) begins with a longitudinal or Bruner incision across the wrist just superficial to the FCR tendon. The tendon sheath of the FCR is opened, and the tendon is retracted toward the ulnar side of the wrist. An incision through the floor of the FCR sheath will expose the radial aspect of the pronator quadratus. The pronator quadratus is stripped off the radius and retracted ulnarly to expose the palmar cortex of the distal radius.

EXAMINATION

History

Key points to elicit are how the injury occurred, when it occurred, and prior treatment. It is important to find out about previous injuries, which may have left the patient with residual deformity or limitations.

Wounds

The history of how and where the injury occurred can help determine the extent of wound contamination. Note the presence of exposed bone or tendon. Wounds should be covered with an antiseptic-soaked gauze until a formal exploration with debridement can be performed.

Swelling

The local swelling that often accompanies a fracture or dislocation makes the site of injury readily apparent. A hand that has suffered a crush injury is at risk of compartment syndrome of the thenar, hypothenar, or interosseous muscles. Clinical assessment with pressure monitoring and a low threshold for fasciotomies can prevent irreversible damage to the hand.

Neurovascular Examination

Thorough assessement of the neurovascular status of the affected extremity is critical, particularly distal to the injury. One must note both motor and sensory function of the radial, median, and ulnar nerves. A radial pulse should be palpated if possible. If not, an attempt to find the pulse with a Doppler device should be made. Capillary refill can also be used as a measure of vascular status.

Adjacent Joints

The exam of any injured extremity is not complete without evaluating the joints adjacent to the injury. These joints should be assesed in a similar manner to the affected area, with attention to wounds, swelling, range of motion, and tenderness. It is also standard practice to image these joints in the trauma patient.

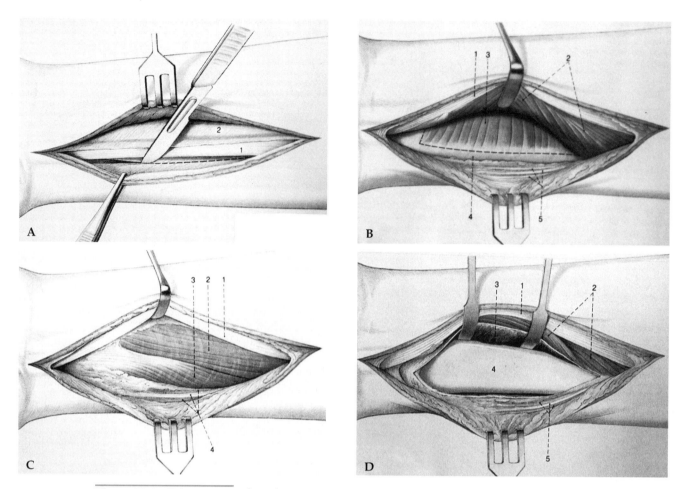

Figure 27–8 Palmar approach to the distal radius. **(A)** Splitting of the tendon sheath of FCR. 1. FCR. 2. FDS. **(B)** Exposure of FDS. 1. FCR. 2. FDS. 3. Flexor pollicus longus. 4. Radial artery and accompanying veins. **(C)** Detachment of pronator quadratus along dashed line. 1. FCR. 2. FDS and flexor pollicus longus. 3. Pronator quadratus. 4. Radius. 5. Radial artery and accompanying veins. **(D)** Subperiosteal exposure of the distal radius. 1. FCR 2. FDS and flexor pollicus longus. 3. Pronator quadratus. 4. Radius. 5. Radial artery and accompanying veins. Reproduced with permission from Bauer R, Kerschbaumer F, Poisel S. *Operative Approaches in Orthopedic Surgery and Traumatology.* New York, NY: Thieme; 1987:288–289.

AIDS TO DIAGNOSIS

Plain Radiographs

Plain radiographs are often the first and only imaging modality needed when treating fractures and dislocations. A standard series includes an anteroposterior (AP), lateral, and oblique views of the injured area and its adjacent joints. A nondisplaced scaphoid fracture will not infrequently be missed on routine AP, lateral, and oblique wrist radiographs. When one has a high suspicion for a scaphoid fracture an additional view, termed the scaphoid oblique, will show an elongated view of the scaphoid (Fig. 27–9).

Tomograms

Tomograms are an excellent means to define complex fractures, especially intra-articular distal radius fractures.

PEARL

A scaphoid oblique radiograph is performed by placing the wrist in ulnar deviation and directing the radiographic beam 30 degrees proximal to distal. This is an excellent technique to identify occult scaphoid fractures.

Magnetic Resonance Imaging

The use of magnetic resonance imaging (MRI) in the acute setting of fractures or dislocations of the hand and wrist is limited. It may be useful as an aid to diagnosis of ligamentous injuries about the wrist, particularly those to the triangular fibrocartilage complex (TFCC). Magnetic resonance

Computed Tomography Scan

Computed tomography (CT) scan may be useful in evaluating intra-articular distal radius fractures, injuries to the distal radioulnar joint, and fractures through the hook of the hamate.

SPECIFIC CONDITIONS, TREATMENT, AND DIAGNOSIS

Distal Phalanx Fractures

Fractures of the distal phalanx are common. They include extra-articular tuft fractures as well as intra-articular flexor or extensor tendon avulsion injuries.

Tuft fractures are commonly associated with nail-bed injuries. Technically an open fracture, treatment consists of nail-bed repair and splinting of the fracture. It is important to start early motion, to prevent DIP joint stiffness.

Flexor digitorum profundus (FDP) avulsions often involve a small piece of palmar bone fracturing from the distal phalanx. They can be classified as types I through IV. All FDP avulsions require operative treatment.

A mallet finger involves avulsion of the extensor tendon, with or without a bony fragment, at its attachment to the distal phalanx (Fig. 27–10). Most mallet fingers are treated with full-time splinting in extension for 6 weeks, followed by night splinting for 6 to 8 weeks. Even fractures with palmar subluxation can be managed in this fashion. Operative treatment has been associated with a higher complication rate than closed treatment. The outcome does not seem to be significantly different.

Dislocations of the DIP joint are less common than PIP joint dislocations. These injuries are frequently open. They are treated with closed reduction and splinting for 2 to 3 weeks. It is important to check stability as well as flexor and extensor function following reduction. If the joint is irreducible due to volar plate, sesamoid, or tendon interposition, open reduction will be required.

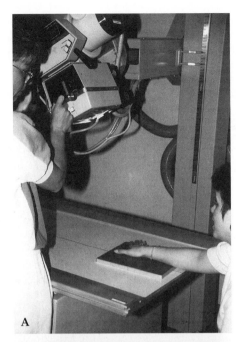
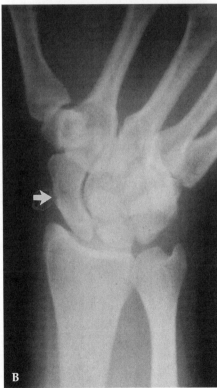

Figure 27–9 **(A)** Technique for taking a scaphoid oblique radiograph; note the ulnar deviation of the patient's wrist. **(B)** A scaphoid oblique radiograph demonstrating a fracture of the scaphoid.

imaging is also used as a diagnostic tool to define the vascularity of the scaphoid and lunate in cases of suspected Keinbock's disease or avascular necrosis of the scaphoid.

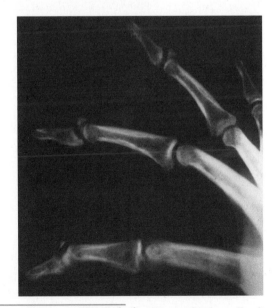

Figure 27–10 Radiograph showing multiple mallet fingers; distal phalanx fractures with avulsion of the extensor tendon.

Middle Phalanx Fractures

The key deforming forces in fractures of the middle phalanx are the flexor digitorum superficialis (FDS) tendon on the palmar surface and the central slip of the extensor tendon on the dorsal surface. Fractures distal to the FDS insertion angulate apex palmarly. Fractures proximal to the insertion angulate apex dorsal. Intra-articular fractures of the middle phalanx are treated with open reduction and internal fixation (ORIF) if there is greater than 2 mm of displacement or a deformity due to malrotation.

Proximal Phalanx Fractures

Proximal phalanx fractures may lead to finger stiffness if the flexor or extensor tendons adhere to the healing bone. Stable, nondisplaced fractures can be treated by splinting, followed by "buddy" taping and early motion. Displaced fractures of the shaft invariably angulate with the apex palmar. This is due to the central slip extending the distal fragment and the interossei or lateral bands flexing the proximal fragment.

Displaced extra-articular fractures that cannot be adequately managed with a splint can be treated with closed reduction and percutaneous pinning. Displaced intra-articular fractures of the base or condyles are best treated with percutaneous reduction and pin or screw fixation (Fig. 27–11).

Fractures that cannot be treated with percutaneous reduction may require ORIF. We prefer the use of lag screws, when the fracture pattern permits. We reserve the use of plates for combined injuries: comminuted fractures with skin or extensor tendon injuries. A dorsal approach is used working on either side of the extensor or splitting the extensor, as the fracture dictates. Proximal phalanx fractures with bone loss (e.g., gun shot wounds) may require external fixation to promote soft tissue healing and preserve length.

Common complications of proximal phalanx fractures include loss of PIP joint motion and malunion, especially malrotation, which creates "cross-over" of the injured finger with normal grip (Fig. 27–12).

Proximal Interphalangeal Joint Fracture-Dislocations

Proximal interphalangeal joint fracture-dislocations (Fig. 27–13) are common and can cause significant disability if not managed appropriately. Most occur as a result of an axial load, that is, a "jammed" finger. The palmar articular surface of the base of the middle phalanx fractures, and the remaining portion of the bone subluxates dorsally on the head of the proximal phalanx. The degree of damage to the base of the middle phalanx is a key factor in treating this injury.

The goal of treatment is a concentric reduction on a lateral radiograph. Fractures that involve one third of the base of the middle phalanx may be amenable to closed treatment. The finger is flexed approximately 45 degrees, a dorsal splint is applied, and a lateral radiograph is taken. If the flexion succeeds in eliminating the dorsal subluxation of the middle phalanx, then the static splint is kept in place for 2 weeks. Protected motion is begun at the end of the second week in a figure-of-eight splint and continued for 2 weeks.

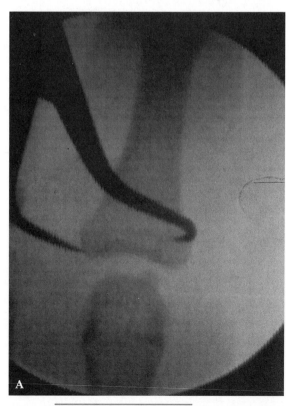 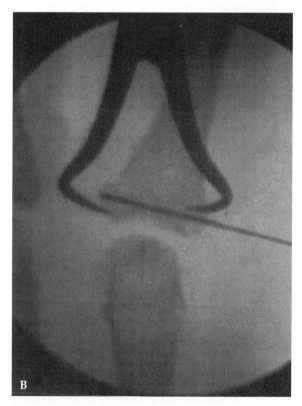

Figure 27–11   (A) Image of the reduction of a proximal phalanx fracture. (B) Image demonstrating placement of the pin, postreduction.

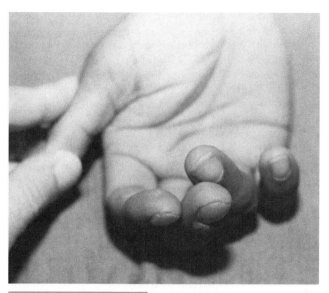

Figure 27–12 Cross-over of the fourth digit as a result of malrotation of a proximal phalanx fracture.

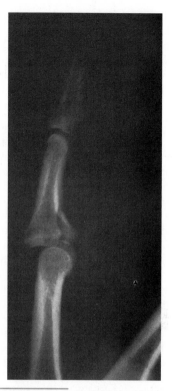

Figure 27–13 Radiograph depicting a proximal interphalangeal (PIP) joint fracture-dislocation.

PEARL

If you choose to plate a fractured finger phalanx remember:

1. The drill bits must be sharp, straight, and centered in the drill chuck. A dull or off-centered bit will split the fracture fragment you have reduced.

2. Avoid the apex of the fracture. Phalangeal cortex is brittle in the diaphysis; you may break the spike.

3. Use a counter sink. It will place the screw head flush with the bone.

4. Pay attention to where the tips of the screws exit. The cross-section of the phalanx is shaped like a kidney bean. Flexor tendons don't like to share their space with a screw.

5. If despite your efforts you create a fracture pattern worse than the one you started with, use one or two pins to fix the major fragments. The fracture will heal if you align the fracture and splint the hand. Not every fracture is amenable to rigid fixation with early range-of-motion exercises.

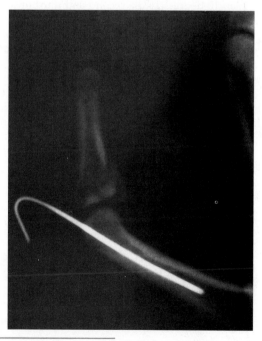

Figure 27–14 Radiograph showing placement of a pin to treat a PIP joint fracture-dislocation.

If the fracture involves more than 30% of the middle phalanx, closed treatment is usually unsuccessful. We use closed reduction and percutaneous pin fixation for PIP joint fracture-dislocations that cannot be managed with a splint. Using a digital block for anesthesia, the finger is flexed approximately 45 degrees. A single 0.045-inch pin is placed in the head of the proximal phalanx, just dorsal to the base of the middle phalanx (Fig. 27–14). A lateral radiograph of the PIP joint should be taken intra-operatively to confirm concentric reduction of the joint. The pin is kept in place for 2 to 3 weeks, after which active motion is begun. Most patients will achieve close to 80% of PIP joint motion.

Fractures involving greater than 50% of the base of the middle phalanx are best managed with dynamic traction. Our personal preference is Schneck traction. The reader is referred to his article (Schenck, 1986) for a description of this technique.

Metacarpal Fractures

The metacarpal is the second most commonly fractured bone in the hand after the distal phalanges. Fractures of the metacarpal can be classified according to anatomic region: head, neck, shaft, and base. Fractures of the metacarpal head are commonly associated with collateral ligament injuries. Those involving more than 20 to 30% of the articular surface and displaced greater than 2 mm may require surgical treatment.

Metacarpal neck fractures are more common injuries, generally resulting from a direct blow. The fifth metacarpal is most frequently involved, and commonly is referred to as a boxer's fracture. Palmar angulation greater than 15 degrees warrants an attempt at closed reduction. Residual angulation of up to 40 degrees can be accepted in the fourth and fifth digits. Due to the lack of mobility at the second and third CMC joints, residual angulation of 15 degrees or less is acceptable with the index and long metacarpals.

Fractures of the metacarpal shaft often result in shortening and malrotation. Indications for surgery after an attempt at closed reduction include shortening greater than 2 to 3 mm, malrotation, multiple metacarpal fractures, and angulation greater than 10 degrees in the second and third or greater than 20 degrees in the fourth and fifth metacarpals. Fractures of the base of the metacarpals can occur with or without dislocation. Several of theses fractures are more commonly known by their eponyms.

Intra-articular fractures of the base of the fifth finger are referred to as reverse Bennett's fractures. A radial fragment remains in place due to the strong intermetacarpal ligaments. The shaft is displaced by the pull of the extensor carpi ulnaris.

These generally require closed reduction and pinning or ORIF, if irreducible.

Fractures of the base of the thumb are commonly referred to as Bennett's or Rolando's fractures. Bennett's fractures are unstable fractures that leave a single fragment from the palmar-ulnar base of the thumb metacarpal. The normal metacarpal-trapezial articulation creates a "V" along the radial aspect (Fig. 27–15a). When the metacarpal fractures and subluxates, due to the pull of the abductor pollicis longus, it creates the "broken V sign" (Fig. 27–15b). Due to their instability, they are usually treated by closed reduction and pinning (Fig. 27–15c). A Rolando fracture is described as a fracture of the base of the thumb metacarpal with a "Y" or "T" configuration. Treatment involves the restoration of the articular surface by closed reduction and pinning, ORIF, or external fixation.

Carpal Fractures

The scaphoid is the most commonly fractured of the eight carpal bones (Fig. 27–16). It is imperative when treating fractures of the scaphoid to understand its blood supply, as previously discussed in this chapter. The scaphoid can be divided into proximal, middle, and distal segments with approximately 70% of fractures occurring through the middle or waist segment. Another 20% occur in the proximal pole, with the remaining 10% occurring distally. A high index of suspicion is essential in diagnosing a nondisplaced scaphoid fracture that is not apparent on routine radiographs. A scaphoid oblique radiograph may be helpful. Rarely, a bone scan or MRI may aid in the diagnosis of an occult scaphoid fracture. Nondisplaced fractures should be immobilized based on the location and pattern of the fracture. Stable, transverse fractures can be treated with a short, arm-thumb spica cast. Oblique fractures may be unstable and are usually held for the first 3 to 4 weeks in a long-arm cast. Distal fractures can generally be immobilized for 4 to 8 weeks. Waist fractures will require longer periods of immobilization, often

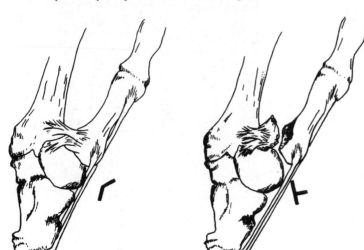
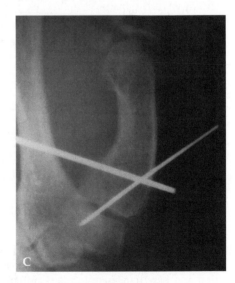

Figure 27–15   **(A)** The first metacarpal-trapezium articulation creates a "V" along the radial aspect. **(B)** The abductor pollicis longus tendon causes the metacarpal to subluxate following a Bennett's fracture. This creates the "broken V" sign. **(C)** Radiograph demonstrating pinning of a base of the thumb metacarpal fracture-subluxation with restoration of the V.

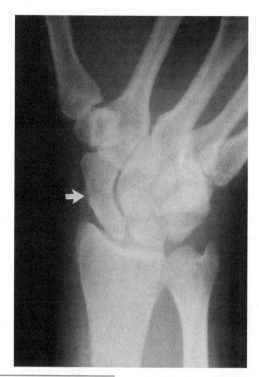

Figure 27–16 Radiograph of a nondisplaced fracture through the "waist" of the scaphoid.

12 weeks or greater. Proximal pole fractures treated with immobilization may require casting of 3 to 5 months before

union (although many authors recommend immediate ORIF due to the high risk of avascular necrosis and nonunion).

Displaced fractures of the scaphoid and those associated with complex injuries (perilunate dislocations) require early ORIF. Nonunions of the scaphoid may remain asymptomatic for years and become clinically troublesome after minor trauma. Late surgical reconstruction depends on the amount of arthritis associated with the nonunion. Surgical options include open reduction with bone grafting, radial styloidectomy, proximal row carpectomy, intercarpal fusion, or wrist arthrodesis.

The lunate is the carpal bone most likely to dislocate; however, fractures are rare. The anatomy of the lunate, particularly its vascular supply, makes this bone vulnerable to long-term sequelae following fracture. The blood supply of the lunate is limited to small areas of dorsal and palmar periosteum with an anastomosis in the center. Fractures of the palmar and dorsal poles can disrupt this vascular pattern, which may lead to Keinbock's disease, avascular necrosis of the lunate.

Fractures of the hamate are uncommon injuries. They can occur through an articular surface, the proximal pole or the body; but the most common hamate fracture is through the hook. The mechanism of injury in this instance is usually the swing of a golf club, tennis raquet, or baseball bat that comes to an abrupt stop as it hits a firm surface. Fractures of the body are often associated with CMC dislocations of the fourth and fifth joints (Fig. 27–17).

Patients with hamate fractures experience ulnar-sided hand pain. They have localized tenderness over the hamate

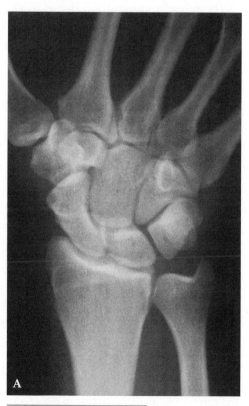

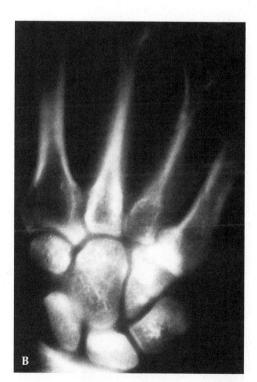

Figure 27–17 **(A)** Radiograph showing normal alignment of the carpometacarpal (CMC) joints. Note the "sawtooth" image of the CMC. **(B)** Tomogram showing the loss of the saw tooth, which results after a CMC dislocation of the fourth and fifth joints.

hook, which can be palpated approximately 2 cm proximal to the palmar wrist crease in a line drawn between the fourth and fifth finger rays. They can also have ulnar nerve or fifth-digit flexor tendon symptoms, as these structures are both in close proximity to the hamate. Hook of the hamate fractures may be apparent on a carpal tunnel view or on a 45-degree oblique. If suspected but not visualized on plain radiographs, a CT scan will confirm the diagnosis.

It is generally believed that fractures of the hook are best treated with excision of the fragment. The hamate hook is exposed through a longitudinal incision placed 5 to 10 mm ulnar to that used for a carpal tunnel release. The ulnar nerve and artery are dissected from proximal to distal and retracted ulnarly as the hamate hook is exposed. The fracture fragment is removed and any remaining portion of the hook rongeured flush with the body of the hamate. After suture removal, full activities may be resumed.

Carpal Dislocations

Perilunate and lunate dislocations may be isolated injuries or found in association with carpal fractures (Fig. 27–18). Two categories of injuries have been described based on the presence or absence of fracture. Pure ligamentous injuries are referred to as lesser arc injuries, while those with fracture are termed greater arc injuries.

The dorsal perilunate dislocation and the transscaphoid perilunate dislocation are the two most common types of dislocations. Open reduction with internal fixation is recommended for any carpal dislocation or fracture-dislocation.

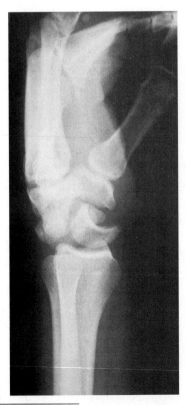

Figure 27–18 Lateral view of a perilunate dislocation.

There is some controversy as to whether to use a dorsal approach alone or a combined dorsal-palmar approach. We favor the combined approach.

The palmar aspect of the wrist is exposed through an extended carpal tunnel approach. In a lunate dislocation, the lunate will be resting in the carpal canal. After the lunate is reduced, the transverse rent in the palmar capsule is repaired with interrupted sutures. With perilunate dislocations, the same rent is present and can be similarly repaired. Assessment of carpal fractures and ligament injuries is performed through a dorsal approach. In a transscaphoid perilunar fracture-dislocation, the arc of injury runs through the scaphoid and around the lunate. The scaphoid is reduced and held with a Herbert screw. The capitolunate joint is reduced and pinned with 0.062 inch wire, as is the lunotriquetral joint if the lunotriquetral ligament is torn. In pure perilunate or lunate dislocations, the arc of injury passes through the scapholunate joint, requiring that this joint be pinned as well.

PEARL

An adequate reduction is achieved following carpal dislocation when there is a colinear alignment of the metacarpal, capitate, lunate, and radius on a lateral radiograph. This can be assessed clinically during the dorsal exposure. Due to disruption of the scapholunate ligament, the lunate sits in a dorsiflexed position. This leaves the capitate head exposed: the "naked-capitate" sign. With palmar-directed pressure on the neck of the capitate, the lunate will cover the capitate head. In this position the carpal alignment should be near-anatomic.

Distal Radius Fractures

Distal radius fractures are the most common fracture of the upper extremity. They usually occur as a result of a fall on an outstretched hand. These fractures can be broadly classified as either extra-articular or intra-articular, but numerous patterns exist within these categories. We prefer the "universal" classification system described by Cooney et al. (1993). This system emphasizes the stability of the fracture, which is helpful in directing treatment. The important issues to consider when planning treatment and predicting outcome include bone quality, degree of comminution and displacement, associated injuries, energy of the injury, and function of the patient prior to the fracture.

In addition to the classification system, there are several eponyms which are used to describe distal radius fractures. A Colles' fracture is a fracture of the distal metaphysis with dorsal angulation, dorsal displacement, and radial shortening. A Smith's fracture is sometimes referred to as a reverse Colles' because it involves palmar angulation of the distal fragment. A Barton's fracture is a fracture-dislocation or subluxation of the carpus on the distal radius in either a palmar or dorsal direction. The Chauffeur's fracture is an oblique fracture through the radial styloid.

When evaluating a patient with a distal radius fracture, it is important to identify associated injuries. Acute carpal tunnel syndrome is common with high-energy fractures and those fractures with palmar displacement of the proximal fragment. Hematoma formation may contribute to carpal canal compression, but direct pressure on the nerve from a fracture fragment is often sited as the primary source of injury. Immediate reduction is warranted, followed by close observation. The patient's symptoms should begin to resolve within a couple of days. If the symptoms linger on or worsen, the carpal tunnel should be decompressed.

Another associated injury in the setting of distal radius fractures is ligamentous damage. The soft tissues found in this region that tend to be most at risk are the scapholunate ligament and the TFCC. The more complex fractures with significant displacement, comminution, or associated subluxation of the carpus allow for greater disruption of the surrounding soft tissues. Injuries of the TFCC come in several forms including avulsion from the ulnar styloid, tears of the rim, and displacement with the lunate fossa. Treatment of this injury is suggested only if there is considerable instability of the distal ulna.

Treatment of Distal Radius Fractures

Principles of Treatment

The objective of treatment for any fracture of the distal radius is to maximize wrist and hand function. Toward that end the priorities in order of importance are:

1. Preserve median nerve function.
2. Preserve finger motion.
3. Restore the shape of the distal radius.

In restoring the shape of the distal radius, the most important parameters are:

1. radial length
2. articular congruity
3. palmar tilt

PEARL

There are many ways to restore wrist function following malunion of a distal radius fracture. It is far more difficult to recover feeling and motion to fingers that have become stiff or numb in the course of treatment. Hence, the first goal of treatment is to preserve median nerve function and finger motion.

Methods of Treatment
Casting

Casting is used for all minimally displaced and stable fracture patterns. It must be nonconstrictive. The distal edge should end at the distal palmar crease to allow full flexion at the metacarpophangeal joints.

Closed Reduction and Pinning

This method is used for unstable, reducible fractures. It is best for extra-articular fractures but is also useful for unstable fracture with acute carpal tunnel syndrome. If carpal tunnel release is necessary, don't use a constrictive cast. The surgeon can pin the radius and apply a splint without fear of loss of reduction.

Make a small incision over the radial styloid. Spread through the subcutaneous tissues to the tip of styloid. Insert two 0.062-inch pins from styloid to ulnar cortex, proximal to the fracture. Leave the pins outside of the skin. Splint for 2 weeks and cast for an additional 2 to 4 weeks.

PEARL

Consider immediate carpal tunnel release in patients who have numbness and abnormal 2-point discrimination (compare with contralateral hand).

External Fixation

Use this method for unstable, intra-articular fractures of the distal radius. Percutaneous pins can be used for reducible fractures. Combine this method with open reduction and pin fixation through a dorsal approach for irreducible fractures. If the fracture has metaphyseal comminution, consider bone grafting. Use a corticocancellous graft for metaphyseal comminution with cortical defect; we refer to this as a structural defect. External fixation can be used with a cancellous graft if there is cortical continuity.

We recommend placing external fixation pins in the metacarpal and radius under direct visualization to avoid injury to the radial sensory nerve or tendons. The surgeon can use distraction to help effect reduction. Once the reduction is achieved, it should be held with internal fixation. The distraction should then be released to the point that the carpus is barely elevated off the distal radius. Excessive distraction will place traction on the nerves and tendons crossing the wrist. This may lead to compromised nerve function or finger stiffness.

PITFALL

The external fixator should be used to neutralize forces across the wrist to protect fracture reduction. Excessive distraction may contribute to finger stiffness.

Open Reduction, Plate Fixation

Use a dorsal plate for displaced fractures with dorsal comminution. Use a palmar plate for palmarly angulated fractures and intra-articular fractures with palmar subluxation of the carpus.

Expose the dorsal aspect of the radius with longitudinal incision centered over Lister's tubercle. Release the extensor pollicus longus and retract radially. Elevate entire fourth compartment subperiosteally. Release the brachioradialis from the radial styloid. If the fracture is extra-articular, the distal fragment can be stabilized with one or two screws through the plate and into the distal fragment.

If the fracture is intra-articular, the radial styloid is usually the least comminuted fragment. Re-establish length by fixing the styloid to the proximal fragment. Reduce the lunate fossa to the styloid fragment. If the fragment is large, it may be fixed with a screw. If the lunate fossa fragment is small, its position may be maintained with a Kirschner wire inserted from the styloid to the lunate fossa fragment. If there is a metaphyseal defect from comminution and the fracture fixation is stable, the defect can be filled with cancellous bone. If the fixation is not stable, the fracture is at risk of shortening. Corticocancellous bone from the iliac crest should be used to help maintain fracture stability and to fill the defect.

Fractures with palmar displacement can be stabilized with a palmar buttress plate. The palmar aspect of the radius is approached via a longitudinal incision over the FCR. The FCR sheath is opened, and the FCR is retracted radially. The finger flexors and median nerve are retracted ulnarly. The pronator quadratus is elevated off the radius exposing the fracture. A T-plate placed on the palmar aspect of the radius will buttress the fracture without the need for screws in the distal fragment.

Guidelines for Treatment
Extra-articular Fractures
Fractures that are nondisplaced and nonangulated can be treated with cast immobilization.

For fractures that are displaced or angulated, a closed reduction can be attempted. If reducible, the fracture can be stabilized with percutaneous Kirshner wires. If an adequate reduction cannot be achieved, open reduction and plate fixation should be considered.

Intra-articular Fractures
Nondisplaced fractures without cortical comminution can be considered stable. A trial of cast immobilization is warranted. Displaced, unstable fractures without metaphyseal comminution can be managed in several ways: closed reduction with percutaneous pin fixation, closed reduction with external fixation and percutaneous pin fixation, open reduction with percutaneous pin fixation, and open reduction with plate fixation. Any of these methods may be effective in restoring joint congruity and radial length. We do not recommend the use of external fixation alone. Treatment with pins alone usually requires immobilization in a splint followed by a cast for 6 weeks. If an external fixator is used, it remains in place for 6 weeks. Four weeks of immobilization is usually sufficient after plate fixation of a displaced distal radius fracture.

Displaced unstable fractures with metaphyseal comminution are at risk of shortening after treatment. To maintain length and congruity, we prefer to use either external fixation, percutaneous pin fixation and corticocancellous graft, or plate fixation with cancellous graft. External fixation with pin fixation may be the only option when there is severe comminution of the articular surface. The fragments can be reassembled and pinned. The external fixator may be used with distraction to help effect reduction. After the reduction

is achieved and stabilized with pins, the distraction should be released until the carpus is barely elevated off the radius. Excessive distraction is to be avoided, as it may cause pain and finger stiffness.

PEARL

Pay careful attention to the alignment of the carpus and radius on the lateral radiograph when treating an intra-articular fracture of the distal radius. Fractures with a displaced palmar cortex may have associated palmar subluxation of the carpus. This is best treated with a palmar buttress plate.

Complications of Distal Radius Fractures

There are several complications associated with fracture of the distal radius. Despite adequate treatment, the more complex fractures may go on to have suboptimal outcomes due to the severity of the initial injury. However, in some cases, the treatment is the culprit.

Perhaps the most important factor in avoiding complications is maintenance of a good reduction. Unfortunately, loss of reduction with a secondary malunion is not uncommon. Malunited fractures may cause a host of problems including nerve compression, wrist pain, and midcarpal instability. Surgery is indicated to correct a malunion, as it is not a benign complication.

Conversely, nonunions of distal radius fractures are quite rare. However, when they do occur, the patients are usually symptomatic. Factors that contribute to nonunion include severe comminution, osteoporotic bone, overdistraction, and lack of bone grafting during ORIF. The ultimate goal when this problem arises is to achieve a union with internal fixation and bone grafting. If the radiocarpal joint is also involved, most authors advocate wrist arthrodesis.

Factors related to the onset of the post-traumatic arthritis include articular incongruity of 1 mm or more, radial shortening of 5 mm or more and dorsal angulation of 20 degrees or more.

Another complication, which is typically iatrogenic, is stiff fingers. Cooney et al. (1980) found this to be a severe, debilitating complication of distal radius fractures in only 2% of the patients in their study; however, this is generally thought of as a common occurrence. The hallmark of this syndrome is swelling in the hand with loss of finger motion. There can be contracture of the joints of the fingers along with the intrinsic muscles. Fibrosis of the joint surfaces is also seen. This complication is usually the result of improper application of a cast, causing significant distal edema. Therefore, it is crucial to make patients aware of certain warning signs after they are casted. If the hand becomes increasingly swollen despite elevation, if there is any numbness or tingling, and most importantly, if it becomes painful to extend the fingers, the patient should be instructed to return to the emergency department to be evaluated and to have the cast split. Even if this results in loss of reduction, the outcome will be superior because the patient will have full function of the digits.

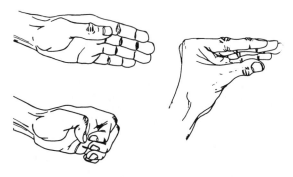
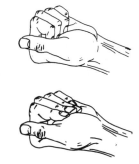

Figure 27–19 The five common exercises used to achieve finger motion after a distal radius fracture.

The final significant complication of distal radius fractures is reflex sympathetic dystrophy (RSD). This complication is included in every review of radius fracture outcomes as a potential cause of major disability. Knirk (1986) reported on several studies that looked at the incidence of RSD. There was a range from 2.1% to 10.3% in four studies. The literature consistently sites median nerve compression as a common precursor to RSD in the setting of a distal radius fracture. The characteristics of this disease include pain, swelling, and finger stiffness. These symptoms are best recognized and addressed early. Interventions such as splitting a cast, aggressive hand therapy, and treatment of median nerve compression can all lead to significant improvement. In patients who are refractory to such treatments, other options include sympathetic blockade or steroid therapy.

Hand Therapy for Patients with Fractures of the Distal Radius

Finger motion is a major concern in the treatment of distal radius fractures. A stiff wrist does not compromise the function of the hand to nearly the extent of stiff fingers. Efforts to control edema and encourage finger motion will maximize hand function.

Edema Control

Elevation of the limb will minimize edema in the first several days following fracture of the distal radius. Constrictive dressings and casts can be devastating. Patients should be specifically asked if their dressing is too tight before leaving the hospital or office. Finger motion will help reduce edema as will compressive wraps and gloves. Wraps and gloves must be used judiciously as they will limit joint mobility.

Range of Motion Excercises

Active range of motion excercises preserve neuromotor function, facilitate tendon gliding, promote blood flow, reduce edema, and help maintain the integrity of articular cartilage, ligaments, and bone. Blocking excercises facilitate full excursion of the tendons and the finger joints. Active assistive range of motion and passive range of motion can help achieve maximum finger motion. These techniques should be used cautiously to avoid pain and increased edema. Five commonly used excercises are illustrated in Fig. 27–19.

SELECTED BIBLIOGRAPHY

Scaphoid Blood Supply

GELBERMAN RH, PANAGRIS JS, TALEISNIK J, BAUMGAERTNER M. The arterial anatomy of the human carpus; Part I: the extraosseous vascularity. *J Hand Surg.* 1983;8:367–375.

LESLIE IJ, DICKSON RA. The fractured carpal scaphoid: natural history and factors influencing outcome. *J Bone Jt Surg.* 1981;63B:225–230.

RUBY LK, STINSON J, BELSKY MR. The natural history of scaphoid nonunion: a review of 55 cases. *J Bone Jt Surg.* 1985;67A:428–432.

Keinbock's Disease

BECKENBAUGH RD, SHIVES TC, DOBYNS JH, LINSCHEID RL. Kienbock's disease: the natural history of Kienbock's disease and consideration of the lunate fractures. *Clin Orthop.* 1980;149:98–106.

WEISS APC, WEILAND AJ, MOORE R, WILGIS EF. Radial shortening for Kienbock's disease. *J Bone Jt Surg.* 1991;73A: 384–391.

WERNER FW, MURPHY DJ, PALMER AK. Pressures in the distal radioulnar joint: effect of surgical procedures use for Kienbock's disease. *J Orthop Res.* 1989;7:445–450.

Progressive Perilinear Instability

MAYFIELD JK, JOHNSON RP, KILCOYNE RK. Carpal dislocations: pathomechanics and progressive perilinear instability. *J Hand Surg.* 1980;5:226–241.

Finger Fractures and Dislocations

BELSKY, MR, EATON, RG, LANE, LB. Closed reduction and internal fixation of proximal phalangeal fractures. *J Hand Surg.* 1984;9A:725–729.

HAGBERG W, SCHILKEN R, BARATZ M, IMBRIGLIA J. *Percutaneous Pin Fixation of Dorsal Fracture: Subluxation of the Proximal Interphalangeal Joint.* Kansas City, MO: American Society for Surgery of the Hand; 1993.

LEDDY JP, PACKER JW. Avulsion of the profundus tendon insertion in athletes. *J Hand Surg.* 1977;2:66–69.

LUBAHN JD, HOOD JM. Fractures of the distal interphalangeal joint. *Clin Orthop.* 1996;327:12–20.

MALERICH MM, EATON RG. The volar plate reconstruction for fracture-dislocation of the proximal interphalangeal joint. *Hand Clin.* 1994;10:251–260.

OUELLETTE EA, FREELAND AE. Use of the minicondylar plate in metacarpal and phalangeal fractures. *Clin Orthop.* 1996;327:38–46.

ROBINS PR, DOBYNS JH. Avulsion of the insertion of the flexor digitorum profundus tendon associated with fracture of the distal phalanx. In: *AAOS Symposium on Tendon Surgery in the Hand.* St Louis, MO: CV Mosby; 1975.

SCHENCK RR. Dynamic traction and early passive movement for fractures of the proximal interphalangeal joint. *J Hand Surg.* 1986;11A:850–858.

STERN PJ, ROMAN RJ, KEIFHABER TR, MCDONOUGH JJ. Pilon fractures of the proximal interphalangeal joint. *J Hand Surg.* 1991;16A:844–850.

WEHBE MA, SCHNEIDER LH. Mallet fractures. *J Bone Jt Surg.* 1984;66A:658–669.

WEISS AC, HASTINGS H. Distal unicondylar fractures of the proximal phalanx. *J Hand Surg.* 1993;18A:594–599.

Carpal Fractures and Fracture-Dislocations

MAYFIELD, JK, JOHNSON, RP, KILCOYNE, RK. Carpal dislocations: pathomechanics and progressive perilunar instability. *J Hand Surg.* 1980;5A:226–241.

RUBY, LK, STINSON, J, BELSKY, MR. The natural history of scaphoid nonunion: a review of 55 cases. *J Bone Jt Surg.* 1985;67A:428–432.

Fractures of the Distal Radius

BRADWAY JK, AMADIO PC, COONEY WP. Open reduction and internal fixation of displaced, comminuted intra-articular fractures of the distal end of the radius. *J Bone Jt Surg.* 1989;71A:839–847.

COONEY WP. Fractures of the distal radius. A modern treatment-based classification. *Orthop. Clin. of North America.* 1993;24(2):211–216.

COONEY WP, DOBYNS JH, LINSCHEID RL. Complications of Colles' fractures. *J Bone Jt Surg.* 1980;62A:613–619.

FERNANDEZ DL, GEISSLER WB. Treatment of displaced articular fractures of the radius. *J Hand Surg.* 1991;16A:375–384.

KNIRK JL, JUPITER JB. Intra-articular fractures of the distal end of the radius in young adults. *J Bone Jt Surg.* 1986;68A:647–659.

TRUMBLE TE, SCHMITT SR, VEDDER NB. Factors affecting functional outcome of displaced intra-articular distal radius fractures. *J Hand Surg.* 1994;19A:325–340.

SHORT WH, PALMER AK, WERNER FW, MURPHY DJ. A biomechanical study of distal radial fractures. *J Hand Surg.* 1987;12A:529–534.

SAMPLE QUESTIONS

1. Which of the following statements regarding evaluation of wrist injuries is incorrect:

   (a) An MRI is a highly sensitive tool for the diagnosis of intercarpal ligament injuries.

   (b) A scaphoid oblique projection is a good screening tool for an occult scaphoid fracture.

   (c) A bone scan is a test with high sensitivity and low specificity for occult wrist fractures.

   (d) A CT scan is the definitive test for diagnosing a hook of the hamate fracture.

   (e) Trispiral tomograms can help characterize the fracture pattern in a comminuted intra-articular distal radius fracture.

2. Finger stiffness following a proximal phalanx fracture can be the result of:

   (a) flexor tendon adhesions

   (b) extensor tendon adhesions

   (c) metacarpophalangeal joint stiffness

   (d) proximal interphalangeal joint stiffness

   (e) all of the above

3. Which of the following types of scaphoid fracture are at greatest risk of nonunion:

   (a) proximal pole fractures

   (b) fractures with 2 mm or more of displacement

   (c) distal pole fractures

   (d) a and b

   (e) all of the above

4. Parameters that should be corrected in displaced distal radius fractures include:

   (a) radial length

   (b) palmar tilt

   (c) articular congruity

   (d) a and c

   (e) all of the above

5. Reflex sympathetic dystrophy is a complication of distal radius fractures characterized by pain, stiffness, and swelling. Early treatment consists of:

   (a) finger range-of-motion excercises

   (b) mild analgesics

   (c) psychoactive agents (e.g., amitriptyline hydrochloride [Elavil]

   (d) stress loading

   (e) all of the above

Answers: 1) a; 2) e; 3) d; 4) e; 5) e

Chapter 28

Tendon Injuries of the Wrist and Hand

Joseph M. Failla, MD

This chapter deals with acute and chronic problems involving flexor and extensor tendons. Traumatic injuries such as tendon transection, avulsion, or subluxation make up the bulk of the acute flexor and extensor tendon injuries, but acute inflammatory conditions are also common. The chronic tendon conditions include the various forms of tenosynovitis, and their accompanying differential diagnoses, with which they can be confused. A detailed physical examination is the key to preventing an acute tendon problem from becoming chronic and often more difficult to treat.

Acute and chronic flexor and extensor tendon problems of the hand and wrist fill primarily two large categories; these are traumatic tendon injuries and inflammatory conditions affecting tendon. Tendons can also be involved in acute and chronic infections, such as purulent tenosynovitis or granulomatous tenosynovitis, neoplasia, such as giant cell tumor of the flexor sheath and ganglia, or acute and chronic presentation of metabolic disease, such as crystal deposition or diabetes. However, the focus of this chapter will be on the traumatic and inflammatory etiologies. The traumatic tendon problems include acute injuries such as flexor and extensor tendon laceration, flexor digitorum profundus avulsion, wrist extensor avulsion, extensor pollicis longus (EPL) rupture, extensor carpi ulnaris (ECU) subluxation, extensor digitorum communis (EDC) subluxation, boutonniere injury, and mallet

finger. Chronic traumatic conditions include extensor or flexor tendon adherence after fracture, chronic laceration, the quadriga effect, lumbrical plus finger, and intrinsic tightness. Inflammatory conditions involving tendon include DeQuervain tendinitis, extensor intersection syndrome, tenosynovitis of the extensor pollicis longus, extensor digiti quinti, extensor carpi ulnaris, and flexor carpi radialis, rheumatoid tenosynovitis, trigger finger, acute calcific tendinitis and capsulitis, and conditions that can mimic inflammation such as the Linburg connection, extensor indicis proprius (EIP) syndrome, and Secretan's disease.

SELECTED BASIC SCIENCE

Flexor Tendon Healing

Flexor tendons receive nutrition through the vincular blood supply and also through synovial fluid of the flexor sheath. The vessels enter the tendon in a relatively dorsal position. During tendon repair, sutures are placed in the palmar aspect of the tendon to avoid injuring the circulation. Tendons heal by making scar internally with participating cells coming from the tendon itself. This was shown in experiments using isolated flexor tendon segments that were repaired and replaced in the synovial environment of a rabbit knee joint. Tendons can also heal by external scar between the flexor sheath and the tendon surface. Repair techniques are aimed at minimizing this external scar to prevent adherence to the sheath. This includes atraumatic grasping of the tendon within its substance at either stump, gently passing tendon ends through the sheath for repair in the cruciate synovial zones to avoid damaging the sheath's inner surface, and early postoperative motion. It has also been suggested that the use of nonsteroidal anti-inflammatory agents may limit formation of external scar. The strength of the tendon repair with time depends on the patient's intrinsic ability to make scar. Future research centers on the possibility of allowing early active motion after tendon repair.

Histopathology of Trigger Finger

The tissue changes that occur in chronic trigger finger have been described as fibrocartilaginous metaplasia of the A1 pulley and thickening with fibrous tissue that includes chondro-

Orthopaedic Surgery: The Essentials. Edited by M.E. Baratz, A.D. Watson, and J.E. Imbriglia. Thieme Medical Publishers, Inc., New York © 1999

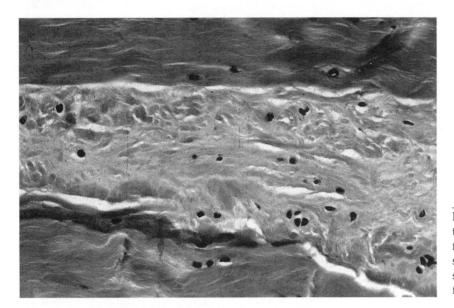

Figure 28–1 Histology of tendon in trigger finger. The palmar surface of the flexor digitorum superficialis FDS (left) shows fibrocartilaginous tissue (lightly stained) between and disrupting tendon fascicles (darkly stained).

cyte-like cells. It is theorized that increased pressure between the tendon and pulley causes the soft tissue to respond with a fibrocartilaginous change. Tension placed on tendons will cause the tendon microstructure to show longitudinally oriented collagen fibers rather than fibrocartilage. The histological changes in the tendon in trigger finger have not been extensively investigated. It has been showed that there can be areas of calcification within the flexor tendon, and that the fibrocartilaginous changes may also occur within the flexor tendon (Fig. 28–1). The ability of corticosteroid injection to eliminate symptoms of trigger finger suggests that there is an inflammatory component. The cases in which steroid injection into the flexor sheath is ineffective, however, suggest permanent thickening of the tendon and pulley rather than a true synovitis.

Overuse Syndrome

Patients who complain of pain and swelling in the hand related to repetitive use can be difficult to manage, particularly when examination of the hand is normal. Physicians tend to attach the diagnosis of "tendinitis," or nerve entrapment, even without evidence of inflammation or neuritis on exam. Overuse syndrome may present as poorly localized pain and swelling that can not be demonstrated on exam. Tendinitis, on the other hand, shows some swelling and tenderness over the musculotendinous units with direct palpation and with resisted tendon excursion. The exact tissue microscopic changes, if any, in overuse syndrome are not known. They may relate to microdamage to collagen fascicles of tendon, tendon insertion, or musculotendinous junction, but this remains to be demonstrated.

ANATOMY AND SURGICAL APPROACHES

Extensor Mechanism Anatomy

The extensor tendons at the wrist are in six dorsal compartments, defined at the level of the extensor retinaculum (Fig. 28–2). The first compartment contains the abductor pollicis longus (APL) and extensor pollicis brevis (EPB) tendons.

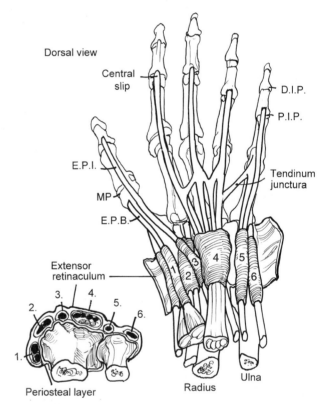

Figure 28–2 Extensor apparatus. Note the six extensor compartments.

Inflammation of these two tendons within their compartment at the wrist causes the condition known as DeQuervain tendinitis. Enroute to the wrist, the APL and EPB pass from ulnar to radial in the distal third of the forearm, dorsal to the radial wrist extensors in the second compartment. The crossover point is called the extensor intersection and can be a site of tenosynovial inflammation called the "intersection syndrome."

The third dorsal extensor compartment contains the EPL, which runs around the ulnar side of Lister's tubercle and then crosses from ulnar to radial over the second compartment tendons. The fourth compartment contains the EIP, and EDC tendons. The fifth compartment contains the EDQ. The sixth compartment contains the ECU tendon. The ECU tendon passes along a groove on the dorsal distal ulna, independent of the overlying extensor retinaculum.

Distal to the extensor compartments at the wrist, both proprius tendons run ulnar to the corresponding communis tendons and can be found ulnar at the metacarpophalangeal (MP) joint level. The junctura tendinum is a connection from the ring finger EDC to the little and middle finger EDC just proximal to the MP joint. These connections are significant because they can mask a complete adjacent extensor tendon laceration proximal to their insertion on the middle finger, for example.

The EDC tendons do not insert directly on the dorsal base of the proximal phalanx. They are stabilized centrally over the MP joint by the sagittal bands, or dorsal hood. The dorsal hood overlies the MP joint capsule, attaches radially and ulnarly to the EDC tendon, courses circumferentially around the MP joint, and inserts into the palmar plate. The function of the saggital band is to maintain the EDC in the midline and to extend the proximal phalanx by lifting it dorsally as a sling from below (Fig. 28–3). A closed, crush injury of the radial saggital band can cause ulnar subluxation of the tendon and an underlying MP joint capsule tear, which may require repair.

The extensor tendon continues distally over the proximal phalanx and is known at this level as the central tendon, as it inserts on the dorsal middle phalanx base; it is the primary extensor of the proximal interphalangeal (PIP) joint. Rupture of the extensor at this level can lead to a "boutonniere" deformity. The extensor tendon distal to the PIP joint is a confluence of the radial and ulnar lateral bands dorsal to the middle phalanx that insert on the base of the distal phalanx. Rupture of the extensor at the base of the distal phalanx leads to a "mallet" deformity.

The EPL tendon exits the third compartment and continues distally dorsal to and on the ulnar side of the thumb MP joint. The adductor pollicis aponeurosis ulnarly and abductor pollicis aponeurosis radially attach to the EPL. The EPL in some cases is joined by the EPB tendon to form a distal insertion on the base of the distal phalanx. More commonly, the EPB inserts on the base of the proximal phalanx or directly into the MP joint dorsal capsule. Rupture of the EPB at this level, when associated with thumb radial collateral ligament tear, leads to MP joint extensor lag and palmar subluxation. The APL tendon attaches to the thumb metacarpal base and proximal thenar muscle fascia.

The intrinsic tendon system flexes the MP joints and extends the PIP and distal interphalangeal (DIP) joints. The four dorsal interosseous muscles continue as tendons palmar to the transverse intermetacarpal ligaments to flex the MP joint. They then run dorsally to continue as the lateral bands that extend the PIP and DIP joints (Fig. 28–4). The first, second, and fourth interossei also have a separate head that inserts on the base of the proximal phalanx. The three palmar interossei also course palmar to the MP joint, then continue as the lateral band to insert dorsal to the PIP and DIP joints, radially for the ring and little finger and ulnarly for the index finger. The lumbrical muscles originate on the FDP tendons, course palmar to the MP joint, and continue as the lateral band on the radial side of each finger (Fig. 28–5). Contraction of the lumbrical will pull the FDP tendon distally, facilitating PIP and DIP extension. The interosseous muscles form an aponeurotic expansion dorsally over the proximal phalanx and central tendon. It courses dorsally from the lateral band to converge in the midline over the central tendon. The proximal portion of the aponeurosis is made of transversely oriented fibers and pulls the proximal portion of the proximal phalanx into flexion. The distal portion is made of oblique fibers, which insert onto the middle phalanx dorsal base radially and ulnarly. These oblique fibers are transected when performing an "intrinsic release."

Retinacular ligaments link the extrinsic and intrinsic portions of the extensor mechanism. The transverse retinacular ligament (TRL) courses lateral to the PIP joint from the flexor sheath to the lateral band, preventing the lateral band from traveling dorsal to the PIP joint. Some patients have enough laxity at this level to allow the lateral bands to shift dorsal to the PIP joint, causing PIP hyperextension. In the boutonniere injury, with loss of central tendon insertion the lateral bands displace palmarly and with time, the TRL will fibrose and maintain the lateral band palmar to the PIP joint where it will act as a PIP flexor, and via attachment to the terminal extensor tendon, a DIP extensor.

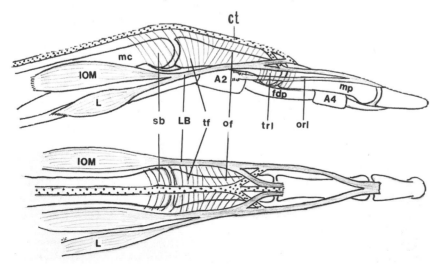

Figure 28–3 The extrinsic (*dotted*) and intrinsic (*shaded*) components of the extensor mechanism of the finger. mc, metacarpal; mp, middle phalanx; IOM, interosseous muscle; L, lumbrical muscle; LB, lateral band; ct, central tendon; sb, sagittal band; tf, transverse fibers; of, oblique fibers; trl, transverse retinacular ligament; orl, oblique retinacular ligament.

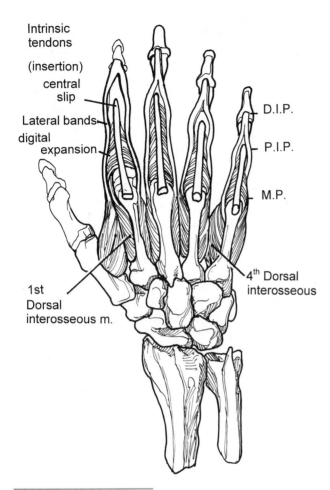

Figure 28–4 Schematic illustration of dorsal interosseous muscles.

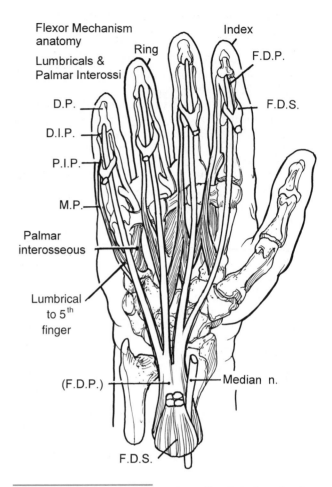

Figure 28–5 Schematic illustration of lumbricals and palmar interossei.

The oblique retinacular ligament (ORL) courses from the palmar and lateral aspect of the proximal phalanx shaft, palmar to the PIP joint, and then dorsal the DIP joint to insert into the terminal extensor tendon. It is thought that normal PIP extension will cause tension in the ORL and facilitate DIP extension. With a chronic boutonniere deformity, an ORL contracture will maintain PIP flexion and DIP extension, thus adding to the deformity. Leaving the DIP joint free for flexion while splinting the PIP joint in extension allows passive stretch of the ORL by flexing the DIP joint.

Flexor Mechanism Anatomy

In the forearm, the FDS muscle divides into four separate tendons, one for each finger. The ring and middle finger tendons enter the carpal canal superficial to the index and little finger tendons. The median nerve travels with the FDS muscle belly. The FDP muscle is linked to all four tendons deep to the FDS. The FPL (Flexor Pollicis Longus) takes origin off the radius in the distal forearm and travels radial to the index FDP. Occasionally the FDP to the index and FPL are linked by a tendon slip known as Linburg's connection. This connection may cause tenosynovial inflammation and limit thumb and index independent flexion. In the carpal tunnel, the median nerve lies palmar to the FDS tendons. The FPL is deep and radial to

the median nerve. The FDS tendons for the ring and little finger contact the radial surface of the hamate hook as a pulley. The lumbricals take origin off the FDP tendons distal to the carpal canal. Distal to the carpal tunnel, the FDS is superficial to the FDP as both enter the palmar aponeurosis pulley. Both tendons enter the flexor sheath at the A1 pulley at the MP joint level. The A2 pulley is attached to the proximal phalanx shaft and often blends with the A1 pulley. The C1 pulley connects the A2 pulley to the A3 pulley at PIP level. The C2 pulley connects the A3 to the A4 pulley, which is attached to the middle phalanx shaft. The C3 pulley connects the A4 to the A5 pulley, which is at DIP joint level. Thus, there are two types of annular pulleys, namely joint pulleys (A1, A3, A5) and bone pulleys (A2, A4) (Fig. 28–6). The A2 and A4 pulleys are the most important in preventing bowstringing of the tendons. The three cruciate synovial pulleys (C1, C2, C3) allow the flexor sheath to fold upon itself to occupy less space with digital flexion.

The FDS divides into two slips that decussate to form the chiasma of Camper dorsal to the FDP tendon at proximal phalanx level. The FDS slips insert on the proximal half of the middle phalanx palmar shaft, and the FDP tendon inserts on the distal phalanx base.

The FPL tendon enters the A1 pulley of the thumb at the MP joint level, with the pulley anchored to the sesmoids and

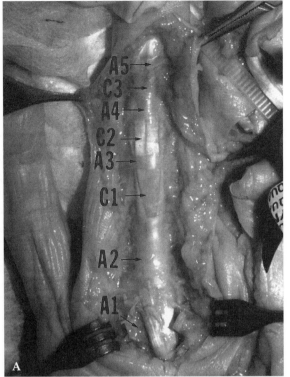

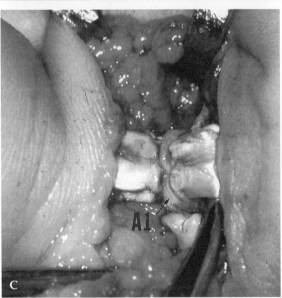

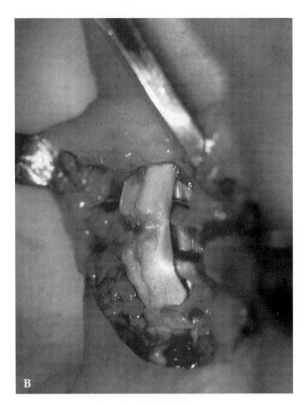

Figure 28–6 The flexor sheath annular (A1-5) and cruciate pulleys (C1-C3. A1 has been cut **(A)**. A partial FDS laceration **(B)** caught on the Al pulley **(C)**.

palmar plate. The oblique pulley of the thumb is analogous to the A2 pulley of the finger because it prevents bowstringing of the FPL tendon. The A2 pulley is the final pulley of the thumb sheath and is attached to the interphalangeal joint palmar plate.

Surgical Approach to the Extensor Mechanism

For a laceration on the dorsal aspect of the wrist a zigzag or curvilinear incision is used. Full-thickness skin and subcutaneous flaps are elevated off the extensor retinaculum. Dissection proceeds from radial to ulnar, using the EPL as a guide, first removing the EPL from the third compartment, then the ECRL-ECRB tendons radial to the EPL, then the APL and EPB in the first compartment, taking care to identify the radial sensory nerve. The fourth compartment is dissected ulnar to the EPL, leaving some retinaculum intact, if possible, followed by the fifth compartment ulnarly, then the ECU tendon, leaving the tunnel intact, if possible, to prevent subluxation.

For release of the first compartment, a transverse incision is placed in a skin crease, with careful subcutaneous spreading to avoid radial sensory nerve injury.

For exposure of extensor tendons over the fingers, a direct dorsal linear or curvilinear incision is used over metacarpals;

transverse, curvilinear, or longitudinal approaches over the MP joint; curvilinear incisions over the PIP joint, and transverse, linear, H-shaped, or S-shaped incisions over the DIP joint.

Surgical Approach to the Flexor Mechanism

A palmar wrist laceration can be explored through a zigzag incision, dissecting skin and full-thickness subcutaneous flaps off the fascia. An organized plan of dissection decreases surgical time. For example, dissection is done radial to ulnar, superficial to deep, first finding the radial artery, thenar cutaneous nerve branch, median nerve within the FDS, individual FDS tendons, the FPL, FDP tendons, and the plane between the FDP and the ulnar neurovascular bundle. Opening the carpal tunnel may be necessary, with a zigzag incision across the wrist flexion crease, ulnar to the palmaris longus and median nerve (Fig. 28–7).

For single tendon exposure, for example, tenosynovectomy of the FCR or digital flexors, a linear or zigzag incision is used, only opening the carpal canal if necessary. For lacerated digital flexor tendons, a modified Bruner zigzag or midlateral incision is used, elevating skin and subcutaneous tissue full thickness off the flexor sheath and identifying the neurovascular bundles palmar to Grayson's ligament.

EXAMINATION

The physical examination for each tendon injury will be discussed separately. In general, the extremity is inspected, palpated, and put through a range of motion. Inspection will show scars; color changes suggesting circulation disturbance or inflammation; abnormal shapes such as swelling, masses, or muscle wasting; and unusual posture such as flexion or extension contracture, rotation or deviation deformity, clawing, or isolated loss of finger extension or flexion. Palpation will reveal skin quality, hidden soft tissue or bony masses, and joint contour. Active motion will demonstrate the rhythm of motion, tenderness with motion, triggering, or crepitus. Passive motion will show joint contracture and extrinsic and intrinsic tightness, and the tenodesis effect. Resisted motion can allow localization of painful musculotendinous units and assessment of muscle strength.

AIDS TO DIAGNOSIS

Most abnormalities involving tendons will be evident after careful history and physical examination. An x-ray should be done to rule out arthrosis, which could contribute to finger stiffness being attributed to loss of tendon excursion or to rule out a painful joint near a region of tendon inflammation. An example would be thumb carpometacarpal arthrosis adjacent to FCR tenosynovitis. Occasionally, ultrasound will help to precisely visualize a subluxating tendon, the ends of a ruptured tendon, or a mass within a tendon.

SPECIFIC CONDITIONS, TREATMENT, AND OUTCOME

Traumatic Conditions

Extensor Tendon Laceration

The level of extensor tendon injuries is separated into five zones. Zone 5 is at the level of the tendons exiting the muscle bellies, zone 4 is beneath the extensor retinaculum, zone 3 is from the extensor retinaculum to the metacarpal neck level, zone 2 is from the metacarpal neck to the PIP joint, and zone 1 is from the central slip insertion to the distal phalanx. Repair in each zone is achieved with nonabsorbable monofiliment or braided synthetic suture. Sutures are either core or mattress, depending on the tendon shape at each level. Zone 5 repairs may be difficult and require tendon suture to fascial elements of the muscle belly. Zone 4 injuries may require that a portion of the retinaculum over a repair be judiciously excised to prevent adherence. Distally in the finger, a colorless suture with a few knots should be used where skin is thin to prevent prominence or ability to see the colored suture through thin, scarred skin and subcutaneous tissue. Central tendon lacerations that enter the PIP joint capsule often lead to PIP joint stiffness due to tendon adherence or joint damage. A zone 3 injury can be masked by a junctura tendinum. A central tendon laceration can be masked by intact lateral bands. Postoperative care is zone dependent. Zone 3, 4, or 5 repairs can be treated with immobilization for 3 to 4 weeks with wrist extension, MP relaxed extension, and interphalanged joints free, followed by active and gentle passive motion out of a protective orthoplast splint. An alternative method is a dynamic extension splint with gentle active flexion of the MP joints analogous to the Kleinert technique for flexor tendons (Fig. 28–8). Repairs of the central tendon in zone 2 are protected with the MP joint in mild flexion and the PIP joint extended for 3 to 4 weeks. Zone 1 repair is protected with the DIP joint extended for 4 weeks.

Reconstruction of a chronic extensor tendon injury in zone 3, 4, or 5 is either by tendon graft or tendon transfer because in old injuries approximation of the retracted tendon stumps is often not possible. If there is a scarred subcutaneous bed with tendon loss, then flap coverage and silastic rods, followed by a second stage tendon graft or tendon transfer, may be needed.

Extensor Pollicis Longus Rupture

Zone 5 extensor tendon rupture is rare and could occur with direct blunt trauma or by attrition over a prominent fixation screw. Zone 4 rupture occurs with chronic tenosynovial swelling of the wrist often involving the EPL tendon at Lister's tubercle. This condition was common in military drummers due to the adducted thumb position when holding the drumstick with the left hand. Extensor pollicis longus rupture can also occur with nondisplaced Colles' fracture in which the third compartment is filled to tension with hematoma, which disturbs the circulation to the tendon (Fig. 28–9). Late rupture may also be due to rubbing of the tendon on bony callus. Repair of the ruptured EPL depends on whether the stumps are retracted and the time between injury

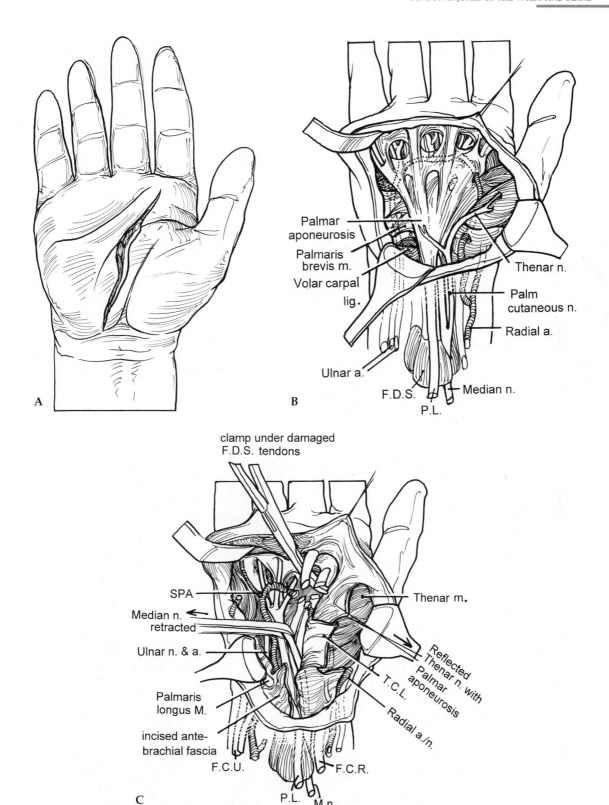

Figure 28–7 **(A)** Palmar laceration **(B)** Exposure of palmar fascia **(C)** Exposure of injured tendons with carpal tunnel depression.

and diagnosis. Direct suture may be possible occasionally, but more often a tendon graft, tendon transfer with the EIP, or proximal advancement and distal lengthening may be necessary.

Extensor Carpi Ulnaris Tendon Subluxation

The ECU tendon can be torn from its sheath on the dorsal aspect of the distal radioulnar joint with a hypersupination

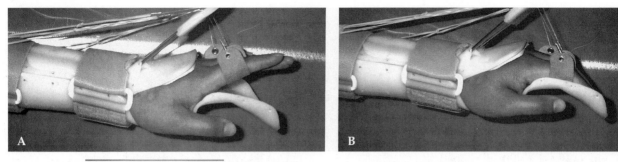

Figure 28–8 Dynamic extension splint for postoperative controlled motion of a zone 5 extensor tendon repair. Passive extension **(A)** and active flexion **(B)**.

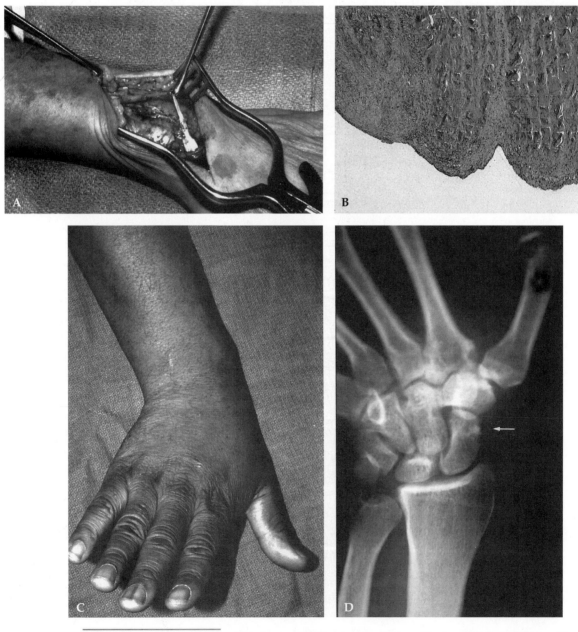

Figure 28–9 **(A)** Extensor pollicis longus (EPL) rupture after nondisplaced Colles' fracture. The tendon stumps are connected by tenosynovium. **(B)** Histology shows necrotic tendon fascicles and inflammation. **(C)** Extensor carpi radialis longus-brevis (ECRL-B) avulsion shows wrist ulnar deviation. **(D)** X-ray shows a small ossicle adjacent to the scaphoid tubercle.

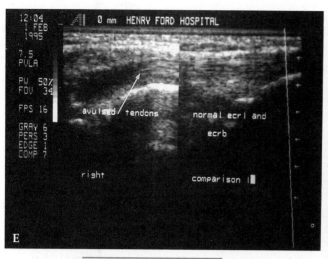
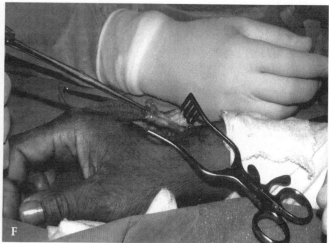

Figure 28–9 *(continued)* **(E)** Ultrasound shows the retracted stump. **(F)** The avulsed ends at surgery.

injury, either during a fall on the outstretched hand or with sports such as hockey or golf. The patient usually presents late with swelling over the ECU tunnel in the ulnar styloid area and a history of palpable and sometimes audible snapping of the dorsal ulnar wrist. Physical exam shows palpable subluxation of the ECU tendon in an ulnar palmar direction with supination and ulnar deviation of the wrist. In some cases, the tendon can also be manually pushed out of its groove at the ulnar head level. The acute injury can theoretically be treated with splinting of the forearm in pronation, with the wrist in neutral. In a patient with chronic ECU subluxation, tendon reconstruction can be performed with a flap of extensor retinaculum. The flap is passed beneath the tendon, then brought over on top of the tendon and sutured to itself proximal to the ECU tunnel. The patient is treated with a long arm cast in pronation for 4 weeks, followed by an orthoplast splint in the same position for an additional 4 weeks. At 8 weeks, rehabilitation begins with gradual grip strengthening and gentle active supination of the forearm. Resubluxation is rare, and symptoms are generally resolved with normal activity.

Extensor Carpi Radialis Longus and Brevis Rupture

The ECRL and ECRB tendons can be avulsed from their insertions on the index and middle metacarpal bases respectively (Figs. 28–9c through 28–9f). This occurs with forceful, resisted wrist extension. If the tendon is avulsed with a bone fragment, it may heal with the wrist immobilized in extension. If there is no bone fragment, the tendon can be sutured into a trough created at the base of the metacarpal. The wrist is immobilized in extension for 4 weeks followed by protected, gentle active motion for an additional 2 weeks.

Extensor Digitorum Communis Subluxation

The EDC can subluxate to the ulnar side of the metacarpal head following a tear to the sagittal band. This can occur with a closed crush injury of the MP joint, most often involving the middle finger. On physical exam, the tendon subluxation

is either visible or palpable and can often be manually reduced with finger extension. If the injury is diagnosed acutely, it can be treated by splinting with the MP joint extended. If repair becomes necessary, the ruptured saggital band is sutured along with the rent in the joint capsule (Fig. 28–10). It is essential that the extensor tendon tracks directly over the MP joint with finger flexion and extension. Postoperatively, the MP joint is splinted in extension for 3 to 4 weeks, followed by gentle active motion.

In the chronic tear, the ulnar sagittal band may be extremely contracted and may need to be released to bring the tendon to the midline. Also, the radial saggital band tissue may be very friable and unsuitable for repair. In this case, the EDC is sutured to the dorsal capsule using a distally based strip of the EDC tendon from the radial side.

Boutonniere Injury

The boutonniere injury is a form of zone 2 extensor tendon rupture. In this injury, the central slip tendon is avulsed from the base of the middle phalanx. The acute injury is often difficult to diagnose because PIP extension may be preserved through the action of the uninjured lateral bands. Initially, only dorsal PIP joint swelling and tenderness may be present. The Boyes test may help with the diagnosis of a suspected boutonniere deformity. The patient will have difficulty flexing the DIP joint when the PIP joint is held extended. This is because the extensor mechanism, disrupted at the PIP joint, has retracted proximally and is pulling on the lateral bands, making DIP flexion difficult. Central tendon disruption is also suggested by the lack of passive PIP joint extension when the MP joint and wrist are in flexion.

Acute boutonniere injuries are treated with the PIP joint splinted in extension for 4 to 6 weeks. The DIP joint is left free for active and passive flexion. This helps prevent extension contracture of the DIP joint and encourages distal pull on the ruptured central tendon via distal excursion of the lateral bands. Distal interphalangeal joint flexion also prevents oblique retinacular ligament contracture. An additional 2

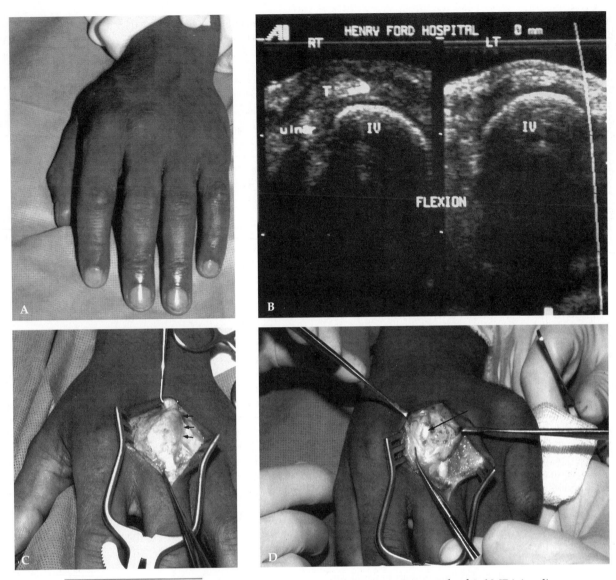

Figure 28–10   Extensor digitorum communis (EDC) subluxation ulnary at the third MP joint clinically **(A)**. An example of subluxation ulnar to the fourth metacarpal by ultrasound **(B)**. The case in A at surgery **(C)** shows the ulnar position of the EDC (arrows), and the underlying MP joint capsular tear **(D)** and exposed metacarpal head (arrow).

weeks of PIP extension splinting is carried out allowing flexion to 40 degrees. At 6 weeks, attempts at full flexion of the PIP joint are begun. With further use of the hand, some elongation of the healed central tendon can be expected with a mild PIP joint extensor lag.

If the boutonniere injury goes untreated, the unopposed PIP flexion becomes evident as the lateral bands subluxate palmar to the axis of the PIP joint. With time, the lateral bands are held in a subluxated position due to contracture of the TRL. Contracture of the palmar plate and collateral ligaments of the PIP joint will create a static, flexion deformity. The ORL

fibroses in a shortened position maintaining the DIP joint extended via attachments to the terminal extensor tendon. Loss of insertion of the extensor mechanism on the middle phalanx base also allows the proximal stump of the central tendon to retract proximally. This exerts a pull on the lateral bands, further increasing DIP joint extension.

If the chronic boutonniere injury remains supple, or if the flexed PIP joint can be straightened by serial finger casting, nonoperative treatment may be successful. However, stretching of the chronically healed extensor tendon is very likely to result in some extensor loss at the PIP joint. If splinting fails in the supple case, a surgical release of the terminal tendon at the level of the middle phalanx (Dolphin tenotomy), taking care to preserve the ORLs laterally, can improve PIP extension and decrease DIP hyperextension. This occurs because the lateral bands retract proximally and exert a proximal pull on the elongated central tendon.

The PIP joint with degenerative changes is not reconstructable. Full passive PIP motion is necessary for a successful boutonniere reconstruction. This can be obtained by preoperative hand therapy or by surgical release of the flexion contracture as needed. Anatomic repositioning of the extensor mechanism includes release of the contracted TRLs, dorsal mobilization of the subluxated lateral bands and suture to the central tendon, which is shortened and repaired. Loss of central tendon substance is replaced by either lateral band transfer or tendon graft. The PIP joint is pinned in extension to protect the repair for 3 to 4 weeks, followed by gentle, protected active flexion supervised by a hand therapist.

PITFALL

Boutonniere reconstruction may improve finger extension at the expense of finger flexion. The patient's expectations must be clearly defined.

Acute boutonniere injury also occurs with palmar PIP joint dislocation. In this setting, it is associated with rupture of a collateral ligament and the palmar plate. Exam can show rotary subluxation of the PIP joint. One condyle of the proximal phalanx may become interposed between the ruptured central tendon and the lateral band. Closed reduction and PIP extension splinting is the preferred treatment. PIP extension pinning or direct repair may be necessary.

Mallet Finger

Rupture of the extensor in zone 1 is known as a mallet finger. The terminal tendon is avulsed from the base of the distal phalanx with or without a fracture fragment. The diagnosis on exam is evident by swelling and tenderness on the dorsal aspect of the DIP joint and an inability to extend the distal phalanx. The mallet finger is treated with 8 weeks of continuous splinting with the DIP joint in extension. The splint must be changed carefully to avoid DIP joint droop and often to avoid skin maceration.

In the chronic, supple mallet injury, increased extensor force is directed at the PIP joint. The patient with relative laxity of the palmar plate of the PIP joint will develop a hyperextension deformity. The combination of a flexed DIP and hyperextended PIP joint is referred to as the swan neck deformity. The chronic injury can still be treated closed but is more likely to result in some DIP joint extensor lag. If closed treatment of a supple mallet finger fails, the central slip tenotomy

(Fowler tenotomy) can be used to decrease PIP hyperextension and increase DIP extension. This occurs as the extensor mechanism is allowed to retract proximal to the PIP joint, exerting a proximal pull on the lateral bands via their connection to the central tendon. This will extend the DIP joint through the elongated terminal extensor tendon.

Extensor or Flexor Tendon Adherence After Fracture

Extensor or flexor tendon adherence to a healing proximal phalanx fracture is possible especially after a dorsal approach for open reduction internal fixation. Bleeding from the fracture into the flexor sheath can lead to flexor tendon adherence. A tenolysis of the central tendon dorsal to the proximal phalanx shaft or the FDS and FDP tendons beneath the A2 pulley may be necessary (Fig. 28–11). Active and passive motion begins immediately postoperatively to prevent readherence.

Flexor Tendon Laceration

If both the FDS and FDP tendon are lacerated, the injured finger remains extended at the PIP and DIP joints. The fingers will not flex when the wrist is extended (tenodesis effect) or when pressure is applied to the muscles and tendons of the finger flexors in the forearm. These two tests help in the diagnosis of flexor tendon lacerations in the unconscious patient and in children.

Function of the FDP tendon is tested by extending the PIP joint and asking the patient to flex DIP joint. The FDS is tested by holding all but the injured finger in extension and checking for PIP flexion. The little finger FDS may be absent or linked to the ring finger FDS. It can be tested by allowing the ring finger to flex with the small finger or by passively flexing the MP joint to relax the FDP tendon and then testing PIP flexion. Two-point discrimination is checked to rule out digital nerve injury. The digital vessel is usually lacerated with the corresponding digital nerve, so care is taken not to injure the intact neurovascular bundle. Bleeding from a tendon wound should never be treated by blunt clamping. Instead, pressure should be applied until operative exploration under loupe magnification can be performed.

Flexor tendon laceration is classified according to the zone of injury. Zone 5 is the area of the forearm proximal to the carpal tunnel. Zone 4 is within the carpal tunnel. Zone 3 is from the lumbrical origin to the A1 pulley. Zone 2 is within the flexor sheath from the A1 pulley to the FDS insertion. Zone 1 is FDP tendon laceration distal to the FDS insertion.

Zone 5 tendon injuries are associated with nerve and vessel damage, the extent of which depends on the depth and width of the laceration. All injured structures are repaired, with the possible exception of a single vessel injury if circulation is intact and the vessel is too damaged to be repaired without a vein graft. The zone 5 tendons are oval and accept core sutures well. Postoperatively, the wrist is held in 30-degree flexion and the fingers in 80-degree flexion at the MP

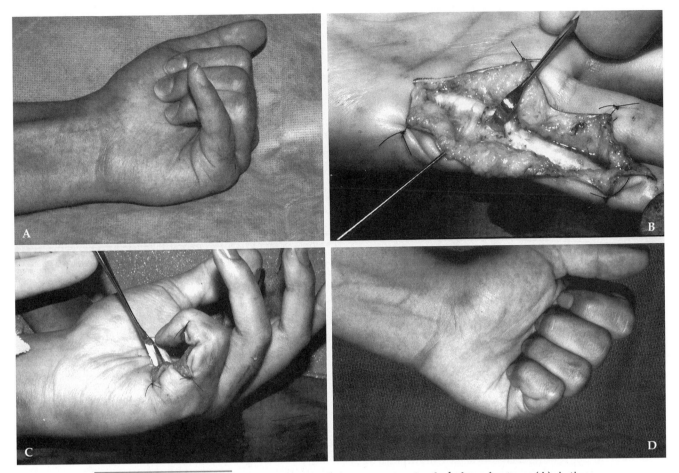

Figure 28–11 Tenolysis of flexor tendons adherent to a proximal phalanx fracture. **(A)** Active flexion. **(B)** Exposure of flexor sheath, with tendons adherent beneath A2 pulley. **(C)** Passive flexion and **(D)** active flexion after tenolysis.

joints with relaxed PIP and DIP flexion. Dynamic splinting can also be used.

Zone 4 injuries require release of the transverse carpal ligament to define the injury and to repair it. Zone 3 injuries often include digital nerve injury and retraction of the FDP stumps to a hidden position within the lumbrical muscles.

Zone 2 injuries often involve both the FDS and FDP tendons and the digital neurovascular bundles. Extensile exposure of the flexor sheath is performed through a Bruner incision; a zigzag incision with the apices at the flexion creases. Loupe magnification facilitates safe dissection, protecting the neurovascular bundles. It is essential to preserve the A2 and A4 pulleys and to open the sheath for tendon repair in the cruciate area. The inner surface of the flexor sheath and tendon are handled with care to limit scar formation. Once the proximal end of the tendon is delivered into an open window in the sheath, it can be held in place by placing a 21-gauge needle through the sheath, and tendon. A standard core suture technique is used with braided, polyester No. 4-0 suture. Either 2-, 4-, or 6-strand techniques are used. The 2-strand technique is the classic and the easiest. The 4-strand technique can be done without difficulty and adds to the strength of the repair. The 6-strand technique is very difficult to perform because of small tendon width. Strength of repair

is dependent on both the number of strands and on the knot strength. Strength is increased by an epitendinous No. 6-0 nylon suture in addition to the core suture. Partial lacerations that create a flap of tendon could catch on a pulley edge and should be trimmed if less than 60% of tendon diameter or repaired otherwise (Fig. 28–6).

Finger motion begins immediately postoperatively using the Kleinert protocol with a dynamic flexion splint and protected, active extension or the Duran passive motion technique.

Complications include flexor tendon adherence, rupture of the repair, or PIP and DIP joint flexion contracture. Adherence is treated by tenolysis after a minimum of 6 months of excercises to gain flexion by active and gentle passive motion. Rupture should be diagnosed quickly and treated by a second attempt at repair.

In the thumb, zone 5 and zone 4 FPL injuries are similar to that for the FDP and FDS tendons. Zone 3 FPL injuries are defined from the MP joint level to the carpal tunnel. Zone 2 injury is at the A1 pulley at the MP joint, and zone 1 injury is distal to the MP joint. Direct repair is often possible. If the proximal stump is retracted, shortened, and must be advanced more than 1 cm, it can be Z-lengthened in the forearm. A chronic FPL laceration for which primary repair and immobilization of the stumps is not possible may be treated by a tendon graft, a transfer of the FDS tendon of the ring finger, or an interphalangeal joint fusion.

Chronic Flexor Tendon Laceration

A tendon graft may be used for flexor tendon laceration in zone 2 that is not repaired within 3 weeks, provided the pulley system is intact and not scarred. After excision of the FDS and FDP, the palmaris longus is used if the graft is inserted from fingertip to palm; the plantaris tendon is used if the graft is placed from fingertip to the forearm. Postoperatively the wrist is splinted in 20 degrees of flexion and the MP joints in 80 degrees of flexion. Motion is begun in the splint immediately with passive finger flexion and active finger extension.

Complications of tendon grafting include tendon adherence, rupture of a graft junction, hyperextension of the PIP joint due to loss of the FDS tendon, or the lumbrical plus finger with paradoxical extension due to flexor profundus pull on the lumbrical originating from it.

Late reconstruction for zone 4 and 5 can be by direct repair, tendon graft, tendon transfer, or side-to-side suture to intact tendons.

Two-stage flexor tendon reconstruction is used if there is severe crush, fracture, infection, tendon or pulley avulsion, failed tenolysis, or dense scarring of the tendon and sheath. It is used when a standard tendon graft would not be feasible due to scar or pulley loss. In stage 1, the scarred tendons are excised and the A2 and A4 pulleys are reconstructed using palmaris tendon. A silastic tendon rod is sutured to the base of the distal phalanx, passes through the reconstructed sheath, through the carpal canal, and ends in the distal forearm. Passive motion is begun immediately to establish a gliding surface between the reconstructed sheath and the implant. The rod is left in place for 3 months.

In stage 2, a tendon graft is sutured to the end of the tendon rod in the forearm. The silicone rod is detached from the distal phalanx. As the rod is withdrawn from the tip of the finger, the graft is pulled into place. The graft is attached to the base of the distal phalanx with a pull-out suture. It is placed under tension in the forearm and sutured to the FDP stump with a Pulvertaft weave. Postoperatively, the hand is placed in a dorsal block splint. Passive motion is allowed for 4 weeks, followed by active motion in a dorsal block splint for 2 additional weeks.

Complications of the two-stage procedure include synovitis and infection in stage 1. Synovitis is treated by temporary immobilization and continuing with stage 2 when possible. A superficial infection can be treated with antibiotics. If the rod is infected is should be removed. Stage 2 complications include pulley stretching with bowstringing and loss of motion, scarring, or graft junction rupture.

Flexor Digitorum Profundis Rupture

The FDP tendon can rupture off its insertion on the base of the distal phalanx. The ring finger is commonly injured in football and rugby. The mechanism of injury is forced extension of a flexed finger, as happens when trying to tackle an opponent by grabbing his jersey. A mass in the palm signals a type 1 injury. In this case, the tendon rup-

tures and retracts out of the flexor sheath and into the palm. The vinculae rupture, creating relative ischemia in the tendon. Repair must be performed within 10 days. In the type 2 injury, a fleck of bone is avulsed with the tendon. The bone becomes trapped in the tendon sheath beneath the PIP joint. The vinculae remain intact. Successful repair has been accomplished up to 1 month following injury. The type 3 injury is rupture of the FDP with a large avulsion fragment that gets caught at the A4 pulley. Repair should be performed as soon as possible, but may be successful up to 1 month after the initial injury.

Quadriga Effect

The term quadriga refers to an analogy between the four horses attached by reins to a Roman chariot and the four FDP tendons attached to a common muscle belly. The quadriga effect is the limitation of proximal excursion of the noninjured FDP tendons when one FDP tendon is scarred to an amputation stump or advanced too far distally after DIP joint amputation. Quadriga is also physiologic in that with one finger held in full extension, the other digits can not fully flex. It also occurs with the EDC tendons because with one finger held in flexion the other fingers can not fully extend, despite the proprius tendons. Another example of quadriga effect is limitation of DIP flexion with mallet-finger hyperextension DIP splinting of an adjacent finger (Fig. 28–12).

PEARL

A patient who has trouble flexing all fingers following injury to one flexor tendon may be a victim of the quadriga effect. The common muscle belly of the profundus tendons means that all four tendons must contract in concert. If one FDP tendon is tethered distally, the excursion of the other three will be limited.

Lumbrical Plus Finger

With loss of the insertion of the FDP tendon after distal phalanx amputation, the FDP tendon will retract toward the palm. Active contraction of the FDP muscle will then pull on the unanchored FDP tendon. With the DIP joint lost, active FDP excursion places tension on the corresponding lumbrical muscle causing the PIP joint to paradoxically extend via the radial lateral band. This is treated by release of the radial lateral band.

PEARL

A patient who has suffered an amputation at the level of the DIP joint may find that the finger actually extends when the patient tries to make a fist. This "paradoxical extension" may be the result of a "lumbrical plus" finger.

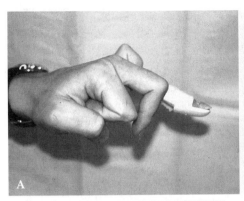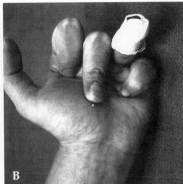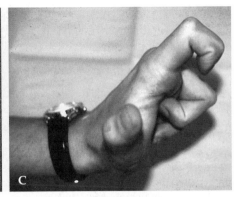

Figure 28–12 The quadriga effect that occurs when a ring mallet finger is placed in a hyperextension splint, advancing the flexor digitorum profundis (FDP) distally, and preventing FDP proximal excursion, and thus distal interphalangeal (DIP) flexion of the adjacent middle finger **(A,B)**. With removal of the mallet splint, DIP flexion of the middle finger is possible **(C)**.

Intrinsic Tightness

Fibrosis and shortening of the intrinsic muscles and tendons result in decreased PIP joint flexion and the intrinsic plus deformity. The MP joint is held tightly in flexion while the PIP joint is held tightly in extension. This can be due to swelling and fibrosis of the interosseous muscles after a crush injury, scarring after a burn, or simply due to swelling and lack of finger motion after any hand fracture, but commonly after Colles' fracture. The intrinsic tightness test places the MP joint in passive extension to use up all available excursion of the tight intrinsics; simultaneous PIP passive flexion will be very limited but will increase when the MP joint is passively flexed. The extrinsic tightness test shows the opposite; more PIP joint passive flexion with MP joint passive extension. Treatment is by hand therapy with passive intrinsic stretching and active stretching by PIP flexion over a Bunnell block. If therapy fails and only the PIP joint is affected, then a distal intrinsic release of the lateral band and oblique fibers of the interosseous hood is done. If the MP joint is also involved, then a more proximal release of the interosseous muscle origin on the metarcarpals may be necessary.

PEARL

A weak grip with limited finger flexion following blunt hand trauma may be the result of intrinsic tightness. Passive flexion of the PIP joint will be limited when the MP joint is hyperextended and will improve when the MP joint is flexed. This is Bunnell's intrinsic tightness test.

Inflammatory Conditions

DeQuervain's Tendinitis

DeQuervain's tendinitis is inflammation of the APL and EPB tendons. This condition occurs randomly, but it is very common in mothers taking care of newborn infants. The patient presents with swelling dorsally over the first extensor tendon compartment. Thumb and wrist motion are painful. There also may be triggering of the thumb as the EPB tendon catches at the edge of the first compartment retinaculum. This can be mistaken for a trigger thumb. The Finkelstein test helps make the diagnosis. The patient flexes the thumb into the palm and the wrist is ulnarly deviated passively. A patient with DeQuervain's tendinitis will experience pain over the first compartment at the radial styloid. Initial treatment is by immobilization with a thumb spica splint or injection of steroid and lidocaine into the first dorsal compartment. More than one injection may be necessary for relief. Patients who fail conservative treatment often have the anatomic variation of having multiple tendon slips of the APL and a separate compartment for the EPB (Fig. 28–13).

Surgical release of the compartment is done under local anesthetic with a transverse incision over the first dorsal compartment at the level of the radial styloid. Careful dissection is necessary to prevent injury to the radial sensory nerve, which often overlies the compartment. Division of the first compartment retinaculum is done in the midline. If there are separate compartments for the EPB and APL tendons, these are both released throughout their length, and the septum between the two is excised to create one compartment. Complications include radial sensory neuritis and, occasionally, radial tendon subluxation out of the first compartment. Postoperative care includes gentle motion of the wrist with a bulky soft dressing and the thumb free for motion. Most patients can expect resolution of symptoms within 2 to 4 weeks and may resume full activity after this time.

Extensor Intersection Syndrome

The extensor intersection syndrome is inflammation of tenosynovial tissue between the first and second compartment tendons. The first compartment tendons cross obliquely over the second compartment tendons. At this intersection tenosynovial connections between the tendons can become inflamed. On exam, this presents as pain and swelling proximal to the radial styloid area. This condition is often mistaken for DeQuervain tendinitis (Fig. 28–13). One distinguishing feature is that the inflammation in this area can cause loud crepitation with wrist and thumb motion, which is also palpable on exam. Treatment can be rest with immobilization in a thumb spica splint, injection of corticosteroid, or tenosynovectomy of the affected area if conservative treatment fails.

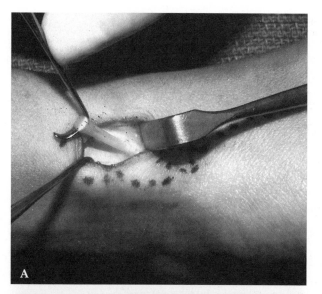

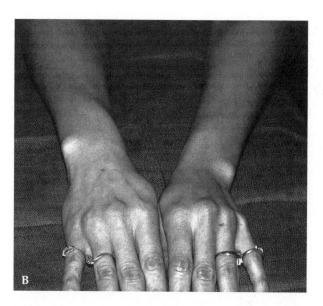

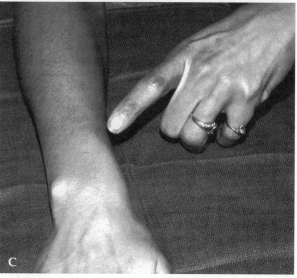

Figure 28–13 Separate extensor pollicis brevis (EPB) tendon compartment in DeQuervain tendinitis **(A)**. Extensor intersection syndrome of the right forearm with swelling proximal to the first dorsal compartment **(B,C)**.

Extensor Pollicis Longus Tenosynovitis

Tenosynovitis of the EPL tendon has been called drummer's palsy. Military drummers who held the left drumstick tightly between the thumb and index finger would develop synovitis and even tendon rupture. On exam, there is pain and swelling over the third extensor compartment (Fig. 28–14). The inflammation may respond to rest, splints, or a cortisone injection. Refractory cases should be treated with release of the third compartment, synovectomy, and transposition of the tendon into the subcutaneous tissues.

Extensor Digiti Quinti Tenosynovitis

Extensor tenosynovitis of the fifth dorsal compartment causes swelling just radial to the ulnar head and pain with little finger motion. Triggering is possible due to catching of the EDQ tendon at the edge of the fifth compartment retinaculum. This will respond to immobilization, steroid injection, or release of the fifth compartment. Surgical findings include tenosynovial thickening requiring tenosynovectomy of the fifth compartment, or duplication of the extensor tendon as in DeQuervain tendinitis. Anomalous muscles intruding into the fifth

compartment, such as the muscle belly of an EDQ tendon coursing distally over the hand, have been reported (Figs. 28–14e and 28–14f).

Extensor Carpi Ulnaris Tenosynovitis

The ECU tendon can become inflamed within the sixth extensor compartment of the wrist. This can occur spontaneously or after injury and must be distinguished from an ECU tendon subluxation. Exam shows isolated swelling over the compartment with tenderness to palpation of the ECU tendon within its groove, without subluxation with forearm supination and wrist ulnar deviation.

Treatment can be by either immobilization of wrist in extension, injection of the sixth compartment with steroid, or by surgical release and tenosynovectomy.

Rheumatoid Tenosynovitis

Rheumatoid extensor tenosynovitis is easily diagnosed by the large tenosynovial mass over the fourth compartment. The other extensor compartments of the wrist can be involved as well. Dorsal subluxation of the distal ulna combined with extensor tenosynovitis can lead to sequential rupture of the

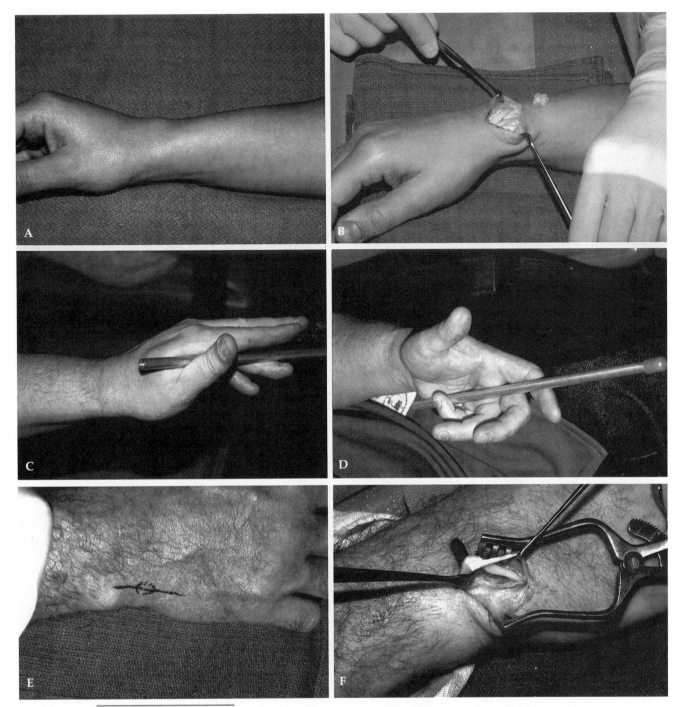

Figure 28–14   Extensor pollicis longus (EPL) tenosynovial swelling treated by tenosynovectomy
(A,B). Position of risk for EPL rupture in nineteenth-century military drummers **(C)** and the safe
position **(D)**. Duplicated extensor digiti quinti (EDQ) tendon and tenosynovitis causing little-finger triggering. The site of triggering and pain marked before surgery **(E)**. The duplicated EDQ
tendon after synovectomy **(F)**.

extensors of the fifth, fourth, and third fingers. This is called
the Vaughn-Jackson syndrome. Tenosynovectomy is recommended after 6 months failed medical management. When
combined with distal ulna resection (if dorsally subluxated),
tendon rupture can be prevented.

Rheumatoid flexor tenosynovitis that persists in spite of 6
months of anti-inflammatory medications is treated by

tenosynovectomy to prevent flexor tendon rupture. The FPL
is at risk due to tenosynovitis and prominent osteophytes on
the palmar aspect of the scaphoid (the Mannerfelt lesion). The
digital flexors are treated by synovectomy of the flexor
sheath, with preservation of the A1 pulley to prevent ulnar
migration of the flexor tendons and worsening of MP joint
ulnar drift.

Secretan's Disease

Secretan's disease is a dorsal, hard, subcutaneous thickening over the extensor tendons at metacarpal shaft level after direct injury.

There is dense fibrosis, which surrounds the extensor tendons and limits motion. A factitious injury is often suspected in these patients. It is possible that the condition is a variant of sympathetic dystrophic phenomenon. Surgical excision results in recurrent fibrosis and does not guarantee success. Symptoms are often chronic and debilitating.

Extensor Indicis Proprius Syndrome

Extensor indicis proprius (EIP) syndrome is due to pain on the dorsum of the wrist after strenuous use of the hand. The cause is an anomalous muscle belly of the EIP, which continues distally into the fourth compartment and is constricted by the extensor retinaculum. Treatment is by release of the extensor retinaculum to free the muscle belly and prevent swelling and pain due to entrapment.

The extensor digitorum brevis manus is another anomalous muscle that presents as dorsal hand swelling. It is often bilateral and suspected of being a ganglion or vascular tumor. Treatment is by excision if the EDC is normal. Other muscle anomalies that can cause similar pain in the dorsum of the wrist include duplicated extensor tendons of the fifth compartment and extensor medius proprius, which attaches to the middle finger proximal phalanx.

Flexor Carpi Radialis Tenosynovitis

Flexor carpi radialis tenosynovitis presents as swelling directly over the region of the scaphoid tubercle and the trapezial ridge where the FCR tendon enters its tunnel. Swollen synovium will bulge in a palmar direction proximally along the FCR sheath. There is pain with resisted wrist flexion and direct palpation of the FCR tendon on exam. Treatment is by either immobilization, steroid injection into the FCR tendon sheath, or release of the FCR tendon sheath and synovectomy.

Linburg Syndrome

The Linburg connection is a tendon slip between the FPL and index FDP. Tenosynovium connecting the two tendons can become inflamed and limit thumb and index finger flexion. This presents as pain directly over the palmar radial wrist and can be mistaken for FCR tenosynovitis or trigger finger. It can be diagnosed by resisting thumb flexion and palpating the index pulp to detect simultaneous index DIP flexion, with pain at the wrist flexion crease. Treatment is by tenosynovectomy and release of the tendinous connection between the FPL and the FDP of the index finger if symptoms are severe.

Flexor Tendinitis

The most common form of flexor tendinitis is the trigger finger due to thickening of the tendon and the tendon sheath.

Triggering is experienced when the flexor tendon catches on the proximal edge of the A1 pulley. Triggering is most common in the middle and ring fingers. It occurs spontaneously and very seldom after an injury. Tenderness is elicited directly over the A1 pulley of the affected finger. Palpable triggering can be felt with attempted extension or flexion. In some cases the finger becomes "stuck" in a flexed or extended position.

Trigger finger is treated with corticosteroid injection, with approximately two thirds of patients having relief from a single injection. Operative treatment involves dividing the A1 pulley through a transverse incision protecting the neurovascular bundles. Complications are rare but include bowstringing of the flexor tendon if the A2 pulley is released, local wound maceration if the hand is used too quickly or moistened after surgery, or residual triggering due to another cause of triggering that is missed. In the typical case with triggering at the A1 pulley, relief of symptoms is excellent with surgery. A recent method of surgical release is closed, A1 pulley release with an 18-gauge needle. This is a demanding procedure and requires expertise so as not to injure neurovascular bundles, completely release the A1 pulley, or lacerate the tendon. It is usually reserved for people with visible and palpable locking of the PIP joint, which can noticeably be decreased after percutaneous release. It is a dangerous procedure in the thumb because of oblique crossing of the radial digital nerve proximal to the A1 pulley.

The differential diagnosis of triggering is important because there are many conditions that can mimic trigger finger. The most common cause of failure of release of triggering after A1 pulley release is triggering in another anatomic location. Flexor tendinitis more distally than the A1 pulley in the flexor sheath, such as at the A3 pulley, can cause the flexor profundus tendon to catch if it is swollen and nodular. Triggering at the wrist is possible because of masses within the flexor tendons in the carpal canal catching on the edge of the transverse carpal ligament. Another cause at the wrist is extensor tendinitis where one of the extensor tendons is swollen and thickened or duplicated causing impingement within the extensor compartment. Examples are triggering of the EPB tendon in DeQuervain tendinitis, which mimics trigger thumb, and triggering of the EDQ tendon within the fifth compartment, which could mimic little-finger triggering. The extensor mechanism on the dorsum of the finger can also mimic trigger finger if the lateral bands snap dorsally as the PIP joint moves from a slightly flexed position to an extended position and then snap palmarly as the PIP joint moves from hyperextension into slight flexion. The EDC tendon can subluxate in an ulnar direction off the dorsum of the MP joint with a sagittal band tear or with chronic stretching of the extensor mechanism in rheumatoid arthritis. Locking of the MP joint is an arthritic condition where an osteophyte on the radial aspect of the metacarpal head can catch on a collateral ligament as the MP joint is moving from extension to flexion. It is most common in the index finger and often involves a sesmoid or palmar plate that gets caught in the palmar aspect of the joint.

The physical exam of patients with trigger finger should include examination of the area of the carpal canal, the thumb CMC joint, and the distal forearm to rule out proximal triggering and to rule out carpal tunnel syndrome and thumb arthrosis. A radiograph of the wrist and thumb should be done to rule out an arthritic cause of loss of normal excursion of the finger or thumb.

Acute Calcific Tendinitis

Acute calcifying disease involving the joint capsules of flexor tendons presents as diffuse swelling, pain, and redness over the affected area and is often suspected of being infection. The condition occurs spontaneously with few patients having a history of trauma. The etiology is not known, but the pathology involves calcification of either an injured or degenerated area of joint capsule or tendon. The differential diagnosis includes infection. Many of these patients are taken for incision and drainage at which time a white toothpaste-like material is found. Differential diagnosis also includes gout or pseudogout. The clinical course is gradual, spontaneous resolution with symptoms decreased by anti-inflammatory agents. Knowledge of the classic picture of an area of calcification of the soft tissues around a joint or tendon on radiograph associated with these symptoms can lead to the diagnosis and prevent unnecessary surgery.

SELECTED BIBLIOGRAPHY

CURTISS RM, REID RL, PROVOST JM. A staged technique for the repair of the traumatic boutonniere deformity. *J Hand Surg.* 1983;8:167–171.

DOYLE JR. Anatomy of the finger flexor sheath and pulley system. *J Hand Surg.* 1988;13A:473–484.

KONIUCH MP, PEIMER CA, VANGORDER T, MONCADA A. Closed crush injury of the metacarpophalangeal joint. *J Hand Surg.* 1987;12A:750–757.

LOMBARDI RM, WOOD MB, LINSCHEID RL. Symptomatic restrictive thumb-index flexor tenosynovitis: incidence of musculoskeletal anomalies and results of treatment. *J Hand Surg.* 1988;13A:325–328.

MURPHY D, FAILLA JM, KONIUCH MP. Steroid versus placebo injection for trigger finger. *J Hand Surg.* 1995;20A:628–631.

POSNER MA, LANGA V, GREEN SM. The locked metacarpophalangeal joint: diagnosis and treatment. *J Hand Surg.* 1986;11A:249–253.

RITTER MA, INGLIS AE. The extensor indicis proprius syndrome. *J Bone Jt Surg.* 1969;51A:1645–1648.

SAMPSON SP, BADALAMENTE MA, HURST LJ, SEIDMAN J. Pathobiology of the human A1 pulley in trigger finger. *J Hand Surg.* 1991;16A:714–721.

SELBY CL. Acute calcific tendinitis of the hand: an infrequently recognized and frequently misdiagnosed form of periarthritis. *Arthrithis Rheum.* 1986;27:337–440.

SMITH RJ. Intrinsic muscles of the fingers: function, dysfunction, and surgical reconstruction. *Instruct Course Lect.* 1975; 21:200–220.

STERN PJ. Tendinitis, overuse syndromes, and tendon injuries. *Hand Clin.* 1990;6:467–476.

STRICKLAND JW. Flexor tendon injuries, I: foundations of treatment. *J Am Acad Orthop Surg.* 1995;3:44–54.

SAMPLE QUESTIONS

1. The lumbrical plus finger involves all structures except the:
   (a) PIP joint
   (b) FDP
   (c) ulnar lateral band
   (d) radial lateral band
   (e) lumbrical origin

2. Which condition is not included in the differential diagnosis of trigger finger:
   (a) locking MP joint
   (b) EDC subluxation
   (c) snapping lateral bands
   (d) extensor intersection syndrome
   (e) EDQ tenosynovitis

3. Surgical release of intrinsic tightness includes release of which structure:
   (a) sagittal band
   (b) transverse fibers
   (c) TRL
   (d) ORL
   (e) oblique fibers

4. Partial flexor tendon lacerations should be:
   (a) repaired primarily in all cases
   (b) completed and repaired primarily
   (c) treated by early motion if > 60%
   (d) trimmed if < 60% and with a flap that catches on the flexor sheath
   (e) repaired only if the tendon ruptures

5. Traumatic boutonniere deformity of the PIP joint involves all the following except:
   (a) lateral band
   (b) sagittal band
   (c) TRL
   (d) ORL
   (e) central extensor tendon

Answers: 1) c; 2) d; 3) e; 4) d; 5) b

Chapter 29

Ligament Injuries
of the Wrist and Hand

John M. Bednar, MD

Ligament injuries involving the hand and wrist are a common cause of pain and disability. These injuries are frequently misdiagnosed in the immediate post injury period, a time when they are most amenable to closed treatment. Accurate early diagnosis requires a high index of suspicion, a knowledge of anatomy, and common injury pattern as well as pertinent physical findings. This chapter reviews the common ligament injuries which occur in the wrist and hand. Relevant anatomy and surgical approaches are discussed highlighting important technical points and pitfalls. Physical examination and relevant diagnostic studies are discussed as they relate to specific conditions. Surgical treatment options are reviewed for the commonly seen ligament injuries of the wrist and hand.

WRIST

Basic Science

Carpal Anatomy and Kinematics

The carpus is composed of eight bones arranged in two rows that articulate with the distal radius and triangular fibrocartilage complex (TFCC) (Fig. 29–1). The proximal row consists of the scaphoid, lunate, and triquetrum. The distal row consists of the trapezium, trapezoid, capitate, and hamate. The pisiform is a sesamoid bone in the tendon of the flexor carpi

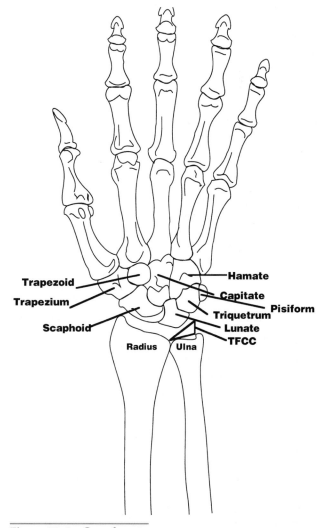

Figure 29–1 Carpal anatomy.

ulnaris. The scaphoid is the link between the proximal and distal row. There are no muscle or tendon attachments to the carpus. The stability of the carpal bones is therefore dependent on bone surface anatomy and ligament attachments.

Two major ligament groups are present in the wrist: extrinsic and intrinsic. The extrinsic ligaments are extracapsular and pass from radius or metacarpal to carpus. The

423

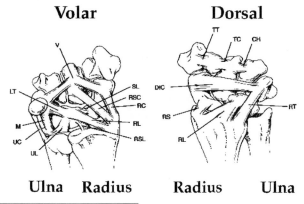

Volar   **Dorsal**

Ulna Radius   **Radius Ulna**

Figure 29–2 Wrist ligaments. Volar: RSL, radioscapholunate; RL, radiolunate; RSC, radioscaphocapitate; RC, radiocarpal; UL, ulnolunate; UC, ulnotriquetral; M, meniscal homologue; SL, scapholunate; LT, lunotriquetral; V, deltoid. Dorsal: RS, radioscaphoid; RL, radiolunate; RT, radiotriquetral; DIC, dorsal intercarpal; TT, trapezialtrapezoid; TC, trapezoid capitate; CH, capitohamate.

intrinsic ligaments are intracapsular and originate from and insert on adjacent carpal bones (Fig. 29–2).

The extrinsic ligaments have dorsal and volar components. The volar system is composed of the radial collateral ligament, the volar radiocarpal ligament complex, and the ulnocarpal ligament complex. The volar radiocarpal complex is made up of the radioscaphocapitate ligament, radiolunate ligament, and radioscapholunate ligament (ligament of Testut). The radioscaphocapitate ligament crosses the waist of the scaphoid as it passes from radius to capitate. It may be a factor in scaphoid waist fractures. The radiolunate ligament passes from radius to triquetrum with an insertion on the lunate. The radioscapholunate ligament passes from radius to lunate and the proximal pole of scaphoid. It provides a check to motion of the scaphoid proximal pole. The ulnocarpal complex consists of the ulnolunate ligament, ulnotriquetral ligament, ulnar collateral ligament, the dorsal and volar radioulnar ligaments, and the TFCC. These ligaments function as a unit rather than individual ligaments to support the ulnar carpus and stabilize the distal radioulnar joint. The dorsal system is composed of the radiotriquetral ligament, the radiolunate ligament, and the dorsal radioscaphoid ligament. All of these ligaments originate on the radius and insert distally onto the carpus.

The intrinsic ligaments are thicker and stronger volarly than dorsally and are grouped according to length. The short intrinsic ligaments connect the bones of the distal row. These ligaments seldom fail with injury. The intermediate intrinsic ligaments include the scapholunate ligament, lunatotriquetral ligament, and the ligaments connecting the scaphotrapezial joint. The long intrinsic ligaments include the dorsal intrinsic ligament, which passes from scaphoid to capitate and triquetrum, and the volar V, or deltoid, ligament, which originates from the scaphoid and triquetrum and inserts on the capitate in a V-shaped pattern. This ligament provides stability to the midcarpal joint.

The articulations of the carpus allow motion in two planes: flexion-extension and radial-ulnar deviation. Half of flexion-extension motion occurs at the radiocarpal joint and half at

the midcarpal joint. About 60% of radial-ulnar deviation occurs at the midcarpal joint and 40% at the radiocarpal joint. The center of rotation of the wrist is the head of the capitate. As the wrist moves from radial to ulnar deviation, the proximal carpal row rotates from a position of volar flexion to extension. Linscheid and colleagues (1972) believe that this rotation occurs through pressure on the distal pole of the scaphoid. The scaphoid is forced into flexion with radial deviation. This causes flexion of the lunate and triquetrum through the interosseous ligament connections of the proximal row. Weber (1984) believes that the helicoid shape of the triquetralhamate joint causes the distal carpal row to translate volarly with radial deviation. This puts pressure on the volar aspect of the proximal carpal row causing it to rotate into flexion. Both of these theories emphasize the concept of the proximal row as the intercalated segment that is controlled by both ligamentous and surface contact restraints.

Mechanism of Injury

Mayfield and associates (1980) studied carpal injury patterns in cadaver wrists. The wrists were loaded in extension, ulnar deviation, and carpal supination. A pattern of progressive perilunar instability was observed and divided into four stages (Fig. 29–3). Stage I was a scapholunate diastasis. As loading progressed, a dorsal dislocation of the capitate occured at stage II. Lunatotriquetral dissociation occured at stage III and lunate dislocation at stage IV. This experimental work correlates well with the pattern of injury with a fall on to an outstretched arm. The wrist usually assumes a position of extension, ulnar deviation, and carpal supination. The direction, point and magnitude of the force on impact determines whether there will be a fracture or ligament injury, as well as the type of ligament injury.

Traumatic injuries of the TFCC also occur by application of an extension, pronation force to the axially loaded wrist or by a distraction force to the ulnar aspect of the forearm or wrist. Tears of the TFCC are commonly associated with distal radial fractures, as well as scapholunate ligament injuries.

Classification
Carpal Instability

Carpal instability has been divided into two groups by Dobyns and his colleagues (1975): carpal instability dissociative (CID) and carpal instability nondissociative (CIND). Dissociative carpal instability results from a tear of an intrinsic ligament. Nondissociative instability results from a tear of an extrinsic ligament.

Four major types of carpal instability are seen: dorsiflexion instability, volar flexion instability, ulnar translocation, and midcarpal instability. Dorsiflexion instability occurs from a disruption of the scapholunate ligament. This allows the scaphoid to rotate into volar flexion. The lunate and triquetrum rotate into extension. The capitate migrates proximally with shortening of the carpus. This produces a zigzag collapse deformity with a dorsally rotated lunate referred to as dorsal intercalated segment instability (DISI) (Fig. 29–4). This is the most common pattern of carpal instability. It is classified as a carpal instability dissociative, dorsal intercalary segment type.

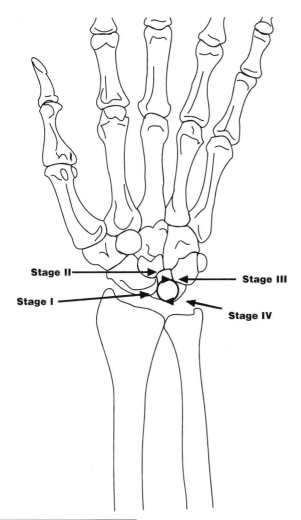

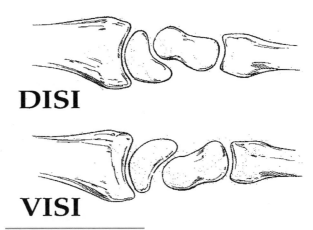

DISI

VISI

Figure 29–4 Carpal collapse patterns. DISI: dorsal intercalary segment instability, VISI: volar intercalary segment instability.

Figure 29–3 Stages of perilunar instability Stage I: scapholunate instability, Stage II: midcarpal instability, Stage III: lunatotriquetral dissociation, Stage IV: lunate or perilunate dislocation.

Volar flexion instability occurs from disruption of the lunatotriquetral ligament. This results in volar rotation of the lunate and extension of the triquetrum producing a volar intercalated segment instability (VISI) (see Fig. 29–4). Ulnar translocation occurs from a disruption of the ulnocarpal ligament complex. This pattern rarely occurs with trauma but is frequently seen in rheumatoid wrists. Midcarpal instability is commonly seen after a malunited fracture of the distal radius with reversal of the normal palmar tilt of the articular surface. This causes subluxation of the carpus and instability. Midcarpal instability can also occur with ligamentous injury to the midcarpal joint.

Carpal instabilities are also classified as static or dynamic. Static instability exists when routine x-rays clearly demonstrate the loss of normal carpal alignment. Dynamic instability exists when routine x-rays are normal, but instability is demonstrated by active motion or manipulation on fluoroscopy.

Triangular Fibrocartilage Complex Injuries

The classification system described by Palmer (1989) is the most useful for TFCC injuries. Traumatic injuries are classi-

fied according to the location of the tear within the TFCC (Fig. 29–5). A Class 1A lesion is a tear in the central portion, class 1B is a tear of the peripheral aspect of the TFCC from its insertion on the distal ulna, class 1C is a tear at the TFCC attachment to the ulnocarpal ligaments, and class 1D is a tear at the radial attachment of the TFCC. Class 1B lesions frequently result in instability of the distal radial ulnar joint. Class 1C lesions result in ulnar carpal instability with volar translocation of the carpus.

Anatomy and Surgical Approaches
Arthroscopic

Arthroscopic evaluation of the wrist is an excellent method for defining pathology. In acute injuries, arthroscopy allows surgical treatment to be performed without significant disruption of uninjured tissue. The relevant anatomy for an arthroscopic approach to the wrist relates to the extensor tendons and dorsal sensory nerves. The surgeon must be able to visualize the location of these structures to properly place arthroscopic portals without injury. The arthroscopic portals are named according to their relation to the extensor compartments of the wrist (Fig. 29–6). The main working portal is the 3–4 portal. To create this portal, a 5-mm longitudinal incision is made dorsally over the radial carpal joint at the interval between the third and fourth extensor compartments. This location is a soft spot just distal to Lister's tubercle. The incision should be made only through skin to avoid injury to extensor tendons or branches of the radial sensory nerve. Blunt dissection is made to the level of the extensor retinaculum. The arthroscopic sleeve is then introduced using a blunt obturator.

PEARL

The surgeon must consider the normal volar tilt of the radial articular surface at the time of obturator insertion and hold the obturator at an equivalent angle to enter the joint without causing damage to the articular surface of the carpus.

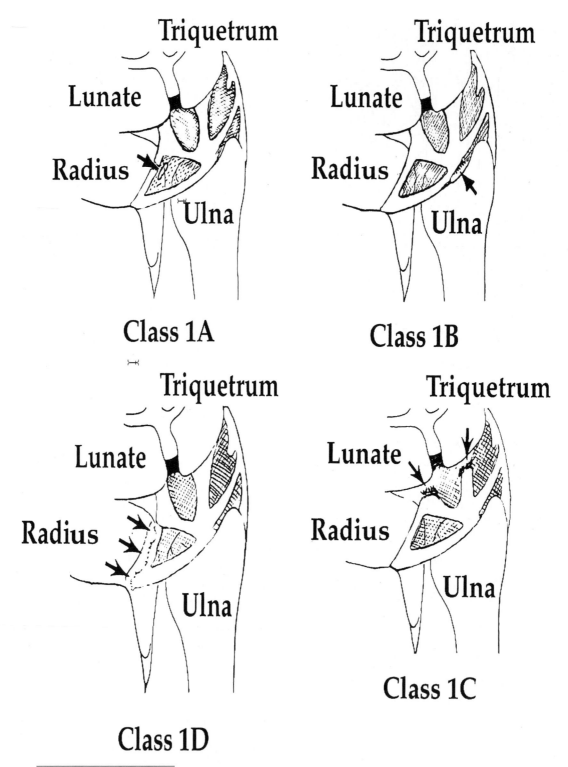

Figure 29–5 Triangular fibrocartilage complex (TFCC) traumatic injury classification. **(A)** Class 1A, central tear. **(B)** Class 1B, peripheral tear. **(C)** Class 1C, ulnocarpal ligament tear. **(D)** Class 1D, radial detachment.

The arthroscope is introduced and the prestyloid recess of the TFCC visualized. Under direct visualization, a drainage portal is then established through the 6U portal. This portal is ulnar to the flexor carpi ulnaris tendon at the level of the radial carpal joint.

The working portals for the radial carpal joint are now made at the 4–5 portal between the fourth and fifth extensor compartments or radial to the tendon of the flexor carpi ulnaris tendon, the 6R portal (Fig. 29–7). The midcarpal joint is visualized through either the midcarpal ulnar or midcarpal

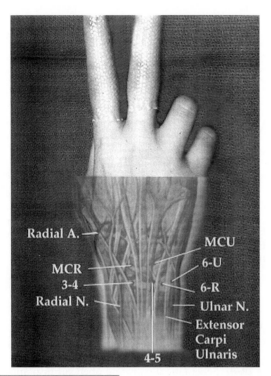

Figure 29–6   Arthroscopic portals with their relationship to important tendons and nerves.

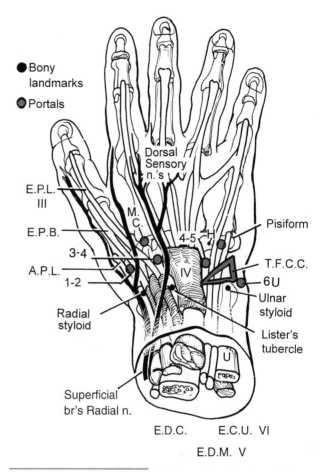

Figure 29–7   Schematic illustrating arthroscopic portals.

PITFALL

Blind insertion of this drainage portal can result in a significant disruption of the periphery of the TFCC and secondary instability from the operative approach.

---

radial portals. These portals are in line longitudinally with, and 1 cm distal to, the 3–4 and 4–5 portals.

Open

The open surgical approach to the wrist involves a longitudinal incision centered over the radiocarpal joint in line with the long finger metacarpal. Skin flaps should be raised as full-thickness flaps at the level of the extensor retinaculum. Preserve as many dorsal veins as possible to minimize postoperative venous congestion and swelling in the hand. Branches of the radial sensory nerve and dorsal ulnar sensory nerve should be identified and protected. The retinaculum of the fourth extensor compartment is divided longitudinally, and the extensor tendons are retracted. The terminal branch of the posterior interosseous nerve is identified. It lies on the dorsal radius at the radial aspect of the fourth extensor compartment along with the posterior interosseous artery. The artery is coagulated. The nerve is crushed and transected (Fig. 29–8). This neurectomy may help alleviate a portion of the wrist pain experienced by the patient. The posterior interosseous nerve enters the dorsal wrist capsule at the scapholunate interval. This anatomic fact allows the surgeon to precisely

place the arthrotomy to minimize injury to normal capsular structures.

The open surgical approach to the TFCC consists of a longitudinal incision over the distal ulna at the dorsal aspect of the extensor carpi ulnaris tendon (Fig. 29–9). Skin flaps are raised at the level of extensor retinaculum taking care to protect branches of the dorsal ulnar sensory nerve. The retinaculum of the sixth extensor compartment is longitudinally divided and the extensor carpi ulnaris tendon retracted. Dissection through the floor of the sixth extensor compartment will expose the TFCC. The proximal and distal edge of the TFCC must be identified. A transverse arthrotomy is made at the proximal edge of the TFCC, if the surgeon is planning to repair a peripheral detachment. If the arthrotomy is to repair a lunatotriquetral ligament tear or perform a lunatotriquetral fusion, a longitundinal arthrotomy is made distal to the TFCC to expose the lunatotriquetral joint. Care must be taken to avoid TFCC injury with this arthrotomy or distal radioulnar instability will occur postoperatively.

Examination

Examination of the wrist in a patient with a carpal ligament injury will demonstrate tenderness over the injured structure. Pain may be present with extremes of motion as well as a click. Decreased wrist motion is measured as well as weakness of grip on dynamometer grip strength testing.

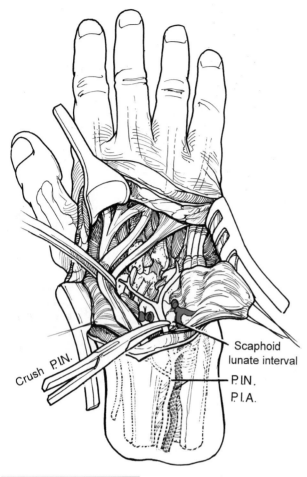

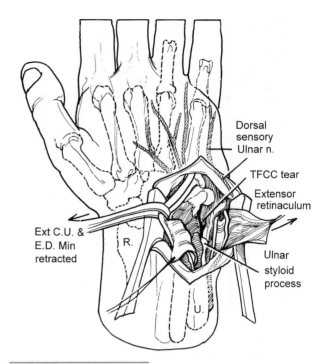

Figure 29–8   Schematic illustrating open surgical approach and identification of the posterior interosseous nerve.

Specific dynamic maneuvers have been described to diagnose specific instabilities. Watson's test for scapholunate instability involves pressure by the examiner's thumb on the scaphoid tubercle, the palmar aspect of the distal pole of the scaphoid. As the wrist is moved from ulnar to radial deviation the distal pole of the scaphoid normally volar flexes. If a scapholunate ligament tear is present, this volar flexion is blocked by the pressure of the examiner's thumb. The proximal pole of the scaphoid subluxes dorsally on the rim of the radius, causing pain and possibly a click.

PEARL

If the Watson's test is performed with the wrist in extension, the subluxation may be blocked giving a false negative result.

Kleinman has described the "shear" test for lunatotriquetral instability. The examiner's contralateral thumb is placed over the dorsal aspect of the lunate. With the lunate supported, the examiner's ipsilateral index finger pushes the pisiform dorsally. This drives the triquetrum dorsally, creating a shear force across the lunatotriquetral joint. Pain or a click will ocurr if instability is present.

Figure 29–9   Schematic illustrating open surgical approach to the TFCC.

Triangular fibrocartilage complex instability is differentiated from lunatotriquetral instability by the point of maximal tenderness and wrist motion that causes pain. A TFCC tear will be tender at its insertion on the distal ulna. There is often pain with forearm rotation, especially if the wrist is forced into ulnar deviation.

Aids to Diagnosis

Radiographic evaluation of a patient with carpal instability should consist of a posteroanterior (PA) view of the wrist in neutral rotation and a lateral view. If scapholunate instability is suspected, a PA clenched-fist view in ulnar deviation is helpful to accentuate widening at the scapholunate interval.

Typical radiographic findings in a patient with a scapholunate instability include a scapholunate space greater than 3 mm, a cortical ring sign produced by the volar flexed scaphoid distal pole viewed in cross section, and a volar flexed scaphoid seen on lateral with a dorsally rotated lunate. Measurement of the scapholunate angle on lateral x-ray is used to define this instability. The normal scapholunate angle is 47 degrees with a range of 30 to 60 degrees. Patients with a scapholunate instability will have a scapholunate angle greater than 70 degrees. This is the classic DISI pattern.

Lunatotriquetral dissociation will also show a cortical ring sign on a PA view of the wrist but without widening at the scapholunate interval. The lunate is volar flexed and triangular in appearance. Widening is not seen at the lunatotriquetral joint. On the lateral view, the lunate is volar flexed and the scapholunate angle is less than 30 degrees. This is the classic VISI pattern.

In patients with dynamic instability, routine x-rays will be normal. Cineradiography will be required to document instability, as it occurs with motion and manipulation of the wrist.

Arthrography is useful in defining tears in the interosseous ligaments and the TFCC. If the radiocarpal injection is negative, then both a midcarpal and distal radioulnar injection should be performed. The arthrogram is most useful if positive in defining the pathology. It evaluates the membranous interosseous portion of the intercarpal ligaments and not the dorsal or volar ligamentous portions, which are responsible for stability. Likewise, a tear can be filled with scar tissue, which will prevent dye flow, but is still mechanically inadequate as a stabilizing ligament. A negative arthrogram is therefore not useful in the patient with abnormal physical exam.

Magnetic resonance imaging (MRI) is a noninvasive method of evaluating the TFCC and intercarpal ligaments. Its role in treatment is evolving as the technology improves to create better images. A study looking for ligament pathology must be performed using a wrist coil to obtain resolution sufficient to visualize these structures. The MRI, like the arthrogram, is most helpful if it is positive. It is not helpful if it is negative in a patient with a clinical exam that suggests instability.

Specific Conditions, Treatment, and Outcome

The treatment of carpal instability is based on the time of presentation after injury, the degree of ligamentous injury, and the presence of degenerative arthritis in the wrist. Acute injuries should have routine x-rays in all cases. If the x-rays are negative, but point tenderness is present on clinical exam and aspiration of the joint produces a bloody aspirate, an injury should be presumed and immobilization instituted for 6 weeks. If tenderness or clinical exam for instability remain positive after immobilization, additional study is advised either as an arthrogram, MRI, or arthroscopic evaluation.

All acute tears with abnormal initial radiographs should be treated by arthroscopic evaluation and either arthroscopically guided reduction and pinning or open reduction and repair.

Open repair of subacute tears diagnosed from 4 weeks to 6 months gives excellent results if the collapse deformity can

be reduced to restore normal intercarpal alignment and ligament repair is performed.

Chronic tears, defined as those present for more than 1 year, are usually not amenable to repair. The carpal collapse has become rigid and irreducible. Any attempt at ligament repair or reconstruction will fail if proper reduction does not restore normal carpal alignment. If a rigid carpal collapse is present with secondary arthritic changes, then a salvage procedure should be considered. Salvage procedures include limited intercarpal fusions, proximal row carpectomy, and total wrist arthrodesis.

Scapholunate Ligament Injury

An acute or subacute scapholunate tear should be treated by arthoscopic evaluation. The evaluation from the radiocarpal joint will demonstrate a tear of the membranous portion of the scapholunate ligament. The volar radiocarpal ligaments must also be assessed for integrity. The midcarpal, ulnar portal will give the best view of the dorsal scapholunate ligament, as well as an appreciation of the scaphoid collapse. A probe through the midcarpal radial portal will allow the examiner to determine if a partial or complete detachment of the scapholunate ligament has occurred. The relation of the articular surfaces of the scaphoid and lunate at the midcarpal joint should be congruous. If a scapholunate tear produces instability, there will be a step-off between the midcarpal articular surfaces of the scaphoid and lunate as the scaphoid rotates into volar flexion and the lunate rotates dorsally (Fig. 29–10). In an acute or subacute injury, the insertion site for the ligament can be debrided and the bone roughened to a bleeding base. A Kirschner wire placed into the scaphoid is used as a joystick to reduce the collapse and realign the articular surfaces at the midcarpal joint. The pressure from the arthroscope on the volar aspect of the lunate aids in reduction. Two pins can then be placed across the scapholunate joint to maintain this reduction. The correct alignment is achieved when a congruous scapholunate articular surface is created as viewed from the midcarpal joint (Fig. 29–11).

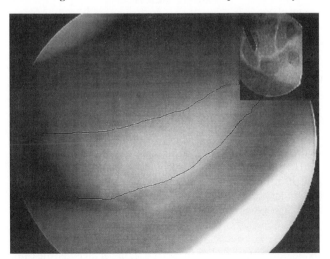

Figure 29–10 Arthroscopic view of scapholunate instability. Seen from the midcarpal ulnar portal, the articular surfaces of the scaphoid and lunate are incongruous (edges are oulined by black line).

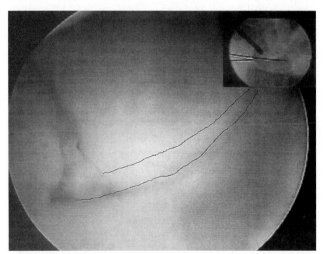

Figure 29–11 Arthroscopic view of reduced scapholunate ligament tear. The scaphoid and lunate surfaces are now congruent (black lines). The radiograph inset shows corresponding radiographic appearance.

Anatomic alignment of the bones allows the torn ligament to return to its proper insertion position at the area of bone previously roughened to provide a good bed for reattachment.

Chronic scapholunate instability can be treated by ligament reconstruction and capsulodesis using the method described by Blatt (1987) if the carpal collapse deformity is reducible. Blatt uses a proximally based flap of dorsal capsule as a tether (Fig. 29–12). It is inserted into the dorsal aspect of the distal pole of the scaphoid to hold it in a reduced position. This prevents volar flexion of the scaphoid and shortening of the carpus due to capitate migration. If the carpal collapsed is fixed, intercarpal arthrodesis is recommended either as a scaphocapitate fusion or a scapho-trapeziotrapezoid fusion.

Lunatotriquetral Ligament Injury

Treatment of tears of the lunatotriquetral ligament follows an algorithm similar to that for the scapholunate ligament. Acute tears are treated by repair either arthroscopically or open. Chronic tears that are reducible require lunatotriquetral ligament reconstruction. Unreducible tears are treated by lunatotriquetral arthrodesis.

Triangular Fibrocartilage Complex Tears

The majority of TFCC tears can be treated arthroscopically. Class 1A tears are treated by debridement of the central tear until a stable rim is present. The central one third of the TFCC can be debrided without affecting its function and ability to transfer load. In a patient whose ulna is longer than the radius (ulnar positive), ulnar shortening must also be performed to prevent persistent symptoms. Shortening is either performed arthroscopically by wafer resection of the distal ulna using a bur or by open ulnar shortening osteotomy with plate fixation. This procedure requires the removal of a piece of ulna large enough to create an ulnar neutral or slight ulnar negative alignment.

Class 1B tears result in instability of the distal ulna. They can be treated by open repair approaching the tear through the floor of the sixth extensor compartment, as previously described. These tears are also ammenable to arthroscopic repair with results comparable to those obtained by open

repair. The arthroscopic technique utilizes the arthroscope in the 3–4 portal. A shaver is placed through the 4–5 and 6R portals to debride the synovitic reaction that occurs around a peripheral tear and to trim the edges to create a vascular bed. Percutaneously, two 18-guage spinal needles are passed across the tear (Fig. 29–13). A small, wire loop is passed into the joint through one of the spinal needles. A No. 2-0 suture is passed through the other needle and through the wire loop. The loop is then pulled out of the joint pulling the suture externally, where it is tied over a button and foam bolster. This technique places a horizontal, mattress-type suture through the TFCC, reattaching it peripherally. The patient is immobilized in a long, arm cast for 6 weeks until the suture is removed and therapy is started. Results of this type of repair have produced excellent and good results in 83% of our patients.

Class 1C tears result in ulnocarpal instability. The arthroscope is useful in defining the extent of the tear. A shaver is used to debride scar and to establish healthy ligament edges. Due to the overlying ulnar artery and nerve, arthroscopic repair is not feasible. An open approach on the volar ulnar aspect of the wrist is required. The flexor carpi ulnaris tendon and ulnar neurovascular bundle must be retracted to place sutures in the ulnocarpal ligament tear. Arthroscopic confirmation of suture placement aids in peforming a precise repair.

Class 1D repairs of a radial detachment can be performed either by open or arthroscopic methods. The primary portion of the TFCC that must be reattached is the dorsal thickening, which forms the radioulnar ligament. This portion must be reattached to radius either by suture anchor or by passing suture through radius and tying over the radial aspect of the wrist. Jantea et al. (1995) have developed a jig to allow this procedure to be performed arthroscopically, with good success in 92% of patients.

HAND

Basic Science

Ligamentous injuries of the small joints of the hand are common injuries. Inadequate treatment can result in significant morbidity affecting the entire hand. The carpometacarpal (MC) joints are tethered by six volar and six dorsal ligaments. The dorsal ligaments are stronger than the volar ones. The index and long (CMC) joints are stable and permit only a few degrees of flexion and extension. These form the fixed unit of the hand. The ring and little finger metacarpals articulate with a shallow saddle-shaped articular surface of the hamate and are mobile, allowing 30 degrees of motion.

The metacarpal phalangeal (MP) joints of the fingers are diarthrodial with the primary motion in the sagittal plane. The collateral ligaments originate from the dorsal sides of the metacarpal head and insert into tubercles on the sides of the proximal phalanx. The metacarpal head is trapezoidal, being more narrow dorsal than volar. In addition, in the sagittal plane, the metacarpal head has the shape of an eccentric cam. The distance from the axis of motion to the volar surface is greater than to the dorsal surface. These anatomic facts result in the collateral ligaments at the MP joint being loose when

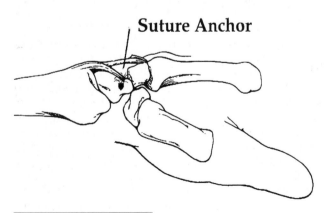

Suture Anchor

Figure 29–12 Capsulodesis using dorsal capsule to stabilize the scaphoid in chronic scapholunate instability.

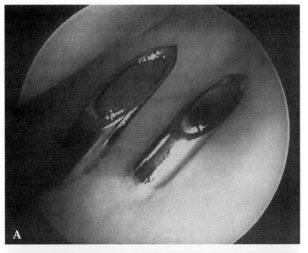

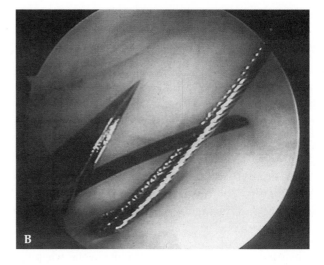

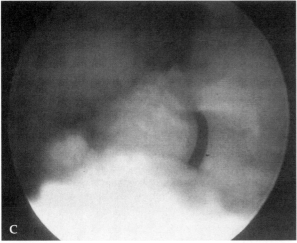

Figure 29–13 Arthroscopic TFCC repair technique. **(A)** Needle placement. **(B)** Wire loop to pass suture. **(C)** Horizontal, mattress-type suture secures TFCC.

the joint is in extension and tight when in flexion. This point is important to remember when the joint is to be immobilized or pinned.

PITFALL

If the metacarpophalangeal (MP) joint is immobilized in an extended position, the ligaments will become contracted in a shortened position and prevent MP joint flexion.

The proximal interphalangeal joints (PIP) of the fingers are bicondylar hinge joints. They achieve their stability by articular contour, the collateral ligaments, accessory collateral ligaments, and the volar plate. The collateral ligaments originate from wide, shallow fossae on either side of the neck of the proximal phalanx and insert on the sides of the middle phalanx. The accessory collateral ligaments are the volar obliquely oriented fibers of the collateral ligaments, which insert on to the volar plate. They function to maintain the

shortest possible moment arm for the flexor tendon. The volar plate is a rectangular fibrocartilagenous structure that inserts across the base of the middle phalanx with its strongest attachments at the lateral margins.

Anatomy and Surgical Approaches

The surgical approach to the CMC joint is dorsal either through a longitudinal or transverse incision. The extensor tendons and branches of the radial sensory and ulnar sensory nerves must be identified and preserved. Carpometacarpal dislocations that are not able to be reduced closed will have either a small articular avulsion fragment blocking reduction or soft tissue in the joint in the form of capsule or ligament. These structures must be cleared from the joint to allow symmetric reduction. Pin fixation will support the reduction during the healing phase. Suture repair of the disrupted dorsal ligament should be performed with nonabsorable suture.

The surgical approach for a complex MP dislocation of a finger can be either volar or dorsal. The volar approach will require identification of the digital nerves and arteries. Note that they are stretched over the volarly dislocated metacarpal head and can easily be transected with an overly aggressive skin incision. The A1 pulley is released, and the volar plate removed from the joint.

PEARL

If the dorsal approach is used to reduce a dislocated MP joint, the ulnar sagittal bands should be divided rather than the radial bands to prevent extensor subluxation of the extensor tendon with MP flexion. The joint capsule is then opened to visualize and disengage the volar plate.

The surgical approach to the PIP joint is volar when the primary pathology is the volar plate, dorsal for the central slip, and midlateral for collateral ligament reconstruction. The volar approach utilizes a Brunner, zigzag incision. The neurovascular bundles are identified, and the flexor retinaculum opened between the A2 and A4 pulleys. The flexor tendons are retracted to visualize the volar plate and accessory collateral ligaments. The dorsal approach is a longitudinal incision centered over the PIP joint. Full-thickness skin flaps are raised at the level of the extensor mechanism. The collateral ligaments can be approached by mobilizing the lateral bands. The central slip attachment to the base of the middle phalanx is easily visualized and may be repaired.

The midlateral approach is through an incision at the apex of the flexion creases of the finger. Cleland's ligaments are opened to identify the neurovascular bundle. Retraction of the nerve and artery will give direct access to the collateral ligament.

The thumb ulnar collateral ligament is approached through a curvilinear incision on the dorsal ulnar aspect of the thumb at the MP joint. The skin flaps are raised at the level of retinaculum after identifying branches of the radial sensory nerve. The adductor aponeurosis is divided longitudinally and reflected in a dorsal and volar direction. The dorsal capsule is frequently torn, allowing visualization of the joint and the ulnar collateral ligament avulsion. If the capsule is not torn, a longitudinal arthrotomy should be made dorsal to the ulnar collateral ligament.

Examination

Physical examination will reveal soft tissue swelling with ecchymosis and tenderness at the affected joint. Carpometacarpal dislocations are usually dorsal. This will clinically be seen as tenderness and swelling at the dorsal aspect of the CMC joint. Pain is present with motion at the CMC joint. The examiner can elicit this by grabbing the metacarpal head and moving in a flexion-extension motion.

Metacarpophalangeal joint ligament injury will cause swelling and tenderness along the injured collateral ligament. Stability of the joint is tested with the MP joint in full flexion.

Dislocations of the MP most frequently occur in a dorsal direction. The MP joint is held in a hyperextended position.

Passive flexion is painful. With local anesthesia, a simple dislocation is easily reducible. If one or two attempts at traction and flexion do not reduce the joint, assume that a complex dislocation is present and that open reduction will be required. Further attempts to perform a closed reduction on a complex dislocation will not be successful and will risk damage to the articular surface.

Thumb MP joint ulnar collateral ligament injuries are very common, especially in sports injuries. The examiner will find tenderness and swelling at the ulnar collateral ligament insertion at the base of the proximal phalanx. The examiner must determine if the tear is partial or complete and if the distal end of the ligament is superficial to the adductor aponeurosis (Stener lesion). Instability is best determined by stressing the joint in 30 degrees of MP flexion. If stress produces 15 degrees of deviation more than seen on the uninjured side, there is a complete rupture. A Stener lesion is suggested if a fullness or mass is noted on the ulnar aspect of the metacarpal head. Proximal interphalageal ligament injuries occur with a PIP joint dislocation. The direction of the dislocation will determine the major structures injured. A dorsal dislocation will injure volar plate and collateral ligament. This injury is immobilized with the PIP joint in 10 to 15 degrees of flexion. A volar dislocation of the PIP joint will result in injury to the central slip and collateral ligament. This injury must be immobilized with the PIP joint in full extension to prevent a late Boutonniere deformity. If the direction of dislocation is not obvious to the examiner, the point of maximal tenderness must be determined to identify the injured structures. This is best evaluated by pressing over each collateral ligament, volar plate, and central slip with the eraser of a pencil or blunt end of a pen.

Aids to Diagnosis

Radiographic evaluation of the CMC joint requires two oblique views each rotated 30 degrees with one in pronation and the other in supination. This will allow adequate visualization of each CMC joint. Tomography and computed tomography scans are also helpful to assess CMC dislocations and to evaluate reduction, especially when articular fractures are present.

Metacarpophalangeal and PIP joint injuries are adequately seen on routine PA and lateral radiographs. Stress PA views for the thumb MP joint are helpful in assessing the degrees of instability. The stress maneuver must be performed by the examining physician. Magnetic resonance imaging may become more useful as finger coils are perfected. Some authors have reported being able to identify a collateral ligament rupture and Stener lesion by MRI.

Specific Conditions, Treatment, and Outcome

Ulnar Collateral Ligament Injury Thumb Metacarpophalangeal Joint

Injury to the ulnar collateral ligament of the thumb is treated based on the clinical examination. If a partial tear is present without instability, a short, arm-thumb spica cast is worn for

3 weeks followed by a removable splint for an additional 3 weeks. If instability is present, operative repair is recommended. The approach described previously is recommended. The ligament is reattached to the proximal phalanx by either a suture anchor placed into bone or by passing the sutures through the proximal phalanx using a straight Keith needle and tying directly over bone on the radial side of the phalanx. Cast immobilization is recommended for 3 weeks followed by a splint for an additional 3 weeks.

If the injury is approached after 3 weeks, the surgeon should prepare the patient for the possible need to reconstruct the ligament with tendon graft. The ligament quickly becomes stiff and shortened and is not able to be reattached at its proper insertion point.

PITFALL

Attempts to "stretch" contracted ulnar collateral ligament of the metacarpophalangeal (MP) joint may cause ulnar subluxation of the joint.

Late reconstruction of the ulnar collateral ligament is performed by creating bony tunnels at the origin and insertion sites of the collateral ligament. A tendon graft, such as the palmaris longus, is passed through the tunnels to form a rectangular ligamentous structure. Crossing the tendon graft in a figure-of-eight fashion will result in less MP motion and is not advisable.

Complex Metacarpophalangeal Dislocation

A complex dislocation of the MP joint occurs when the volar plate becomes interposed in the joint, and the metacarpal head "buttonholes" between the lumbrical muscle and flexor tendons. This author's preferred approach is volar. An oblique incision is made in the palm from the distal palmar crease to the base of the finger. Care must be made not to lacerate the digital nerve with the skin incision. The A1 pulley is released, and the volar plate is disengaged from the joint. Frequently, the volar plate must be released at its attachment to the deep, transverse metacarpal ligament to achieve reduction. After reduction, the volar plate is repaired with nonabsorbable suture. The joint is supported by a dorsal splint with the MP joint in flexion, and range of motion exercises are started early to prevent stiffness.

Proximal Interphalangeal Joint Dislocations

Dislocations of the PIP joint are major injuries to the ligamentous structures of the joint. Insufficient treatment causes a significant amount of morbidity and functional deficit. All PIP dislocations must be carefully examined to determine the injured structures and splinted accordingly. The finger is immobilized in a splint for 3 to 6 weeks. If the joint can not be maintained in a reduced position by closed means, then open reduction is utilized. The approach is dictated by the injured structures. A volar approach is used if volar plate injury is present and a dorsal approach if the central slip is involved. The repair must provide sufficient stability to allow early motion or PIP stiffness and contracture will result.

SELECTED BIBLIOGRAPHY

Anatomy

BERGER RA, LANDSMEER JM. The palmar radiocarpal ligaments: a study of adult and fetal human wrist joints. *J Hand Surg.* 1990;15A:847–854.

PALMER AK, WERNER FW. The triangular fibrocartilage complex of the wrist: anatomy and function. *J Hand Surg.* 1981;6A:153–162.

TALEISNIK J. The ligaments of the wrist. *J Hand Surg.* 1976;1A:110–118.

Kinematics

LINSCHEID RL, DOBYNS JH, BEABOUT JW, BRYANS RS. Traumatic instability of the wrist: diagnosis, classification, and pathomechanics. *J Bone Jt Surg.* American Volume 1972; 54(8):1612–1632.

RUBY LK, COONEY WP III, AN KN, LINSCHEID RL, CHAO EY. Relative motion of selected carpal bones: a kinematic analysis of the normal wrist. *J Hand Surg.* 1988; 13A:1–10.

COONEY WP III, LINSCHEID RL, DOBYNS JH. Carpal instability: treatment of ligament injuries of the wrist. *Instruct Course Lect.* 41:33–44, 1992.

COONEY WP III, LINSCHEID RL, DOBYNS JH. Triangular fibrocartilage tears. *J Hand Surg.* 1994;19A:143–154.

MINAMI A, AN KN, COONEY WP III, LINSCHEID RL, CHAO EY. Ligament stability of the metacarpophalangeal joint: a biomechanical study. *J Hand Surg.* 1985;10A;255–260.

SARRAFIAN SK, MELAMED JL, GOSHGARIAN GM. Study of wrist motion in flexion and extension. *Clin Orthop* 1977;126: 153–159.

SPAETH HJ, ABRAMS RA, BOCK GW, TRUDELL D, HODLER J, BOTTE MJ, PETERSEN M, RESNICK D. Gamekeeper thumb: differentiation of nondisplaced and displaced tears of the ulnar collateral ligament with MR imaging. Work in progress. *Radiology.* 1993;188:553–556.

WEBER ER. Concepts governing the rotational shift of the intercalated segment of the carpus. *Orthop Clin North Am.* 1984;15(2):193–207.

Classification of Wrist Injuries

DOBYNS JH, LINSCHEID RL, CHAO EY, WEBER ER, SWANSON GE. Traumatic instability of the wrist. *Instruct Course Lect.* 1975;24:182–199.

MAYFIELD JK, JOHNSON RP, KILCOYNE RK. Carpal dislocations: pathomechanics and progressive perilunar instability. *J Hand Surg.* 1980;5A:226–241.

PALMER AK. Triangular fibrocartilage complex lesions: a classification. *J Hand Surg.* 1989;14A:594–606.

Treatment of Wrist Ligament Injuries

BLATT G. Capsulodesis in reconstructive hand surgery: dorsal capsulodesis for the unstable scaphoid and volar capsulodesis following excision of the distal ulna. *Hand Clin.* 1987;3:81–102.

COONEY WP III, LINSCHEID RL, DOBYNS JH. Carpal instability: treatment of ligament injuries of the wrist. *Instruct Course Lect.* 1992;41:33–44.

COONEY WP III, LINSCHEID RL, DOBYNS JH. Triangular fibrocartolage tears. *J Hand Surg.* 1994;19A:143–154.

JANTEA CL, BALTZER A, RUTH W. Arthroscopic repair of radial-sided lesions of the fibrocartilage complex. *Hand Clin.* 1995;11:31–36.

PALMER AK, DOBYNS JH, LINSCHEID RL. Management of posttraumatic instability of the wrist secondary to ligament rupture. *J Hand Surg.* 1978;3A:507–532.

WHIPPLE TL. The role of arthroscopy in the treatment of scapholunate instability. *Hand Clin.* 1995;11:37–40.

Carpometacarpal and Finger Joint Anatomy

BOWERS WH, WOLF JW, NEHIL JL et al. The proximal interphalangeal volar plate; I: an anatomical and biomechanical study. *J Hand Surg.* 1980;5A:79–88.

GUNTHER SF. The carpometacarpal joints. *Orthop Clin North Am.* 1984;15:259–277.

MINAMI A, AN KA, COONEY WP III et al. Ligament stability of the metacarpophalangeal joint: a biomechanical study. *J Hand Surg.* 1985;10A:255.

SPAETH HJ, ABRAMS RA, BOCK GW et al. Gamekeeper's thumb: differentiation of nondisplaced and displaced tears of the ulnar collateral ligament with MR imaging. *Radiology.* 1993;188:553.

SAMPLE QUESTIONS

1. The mechanism of injury for most wrist ligament injuries requires application of force with the wrist in the following position:
   (a) neutral, radial deviation, and carpal supination
   (b) extension, ulnar deviation, and carpal pronation
   (c) flexion, ulnar deviation, and carpal supination
   (d) extension, ulnar deviation, and carpal supination
   (e) extension, radial deviation, and carpal supination

2. Scapholunate instability is classified as:
   (a) carpal instability dissociative, dorsal intercalary segment type
   (b) carpal instability dissociative, volar intercalary segment type
   (c) carpal instability nondissociative, dorsal intercalary segment type
   (d) carpal instability nondissociative, volar intercalary segment type
   (e) carpal instability dissociative, midcarpal type

3. A 30-year-old laborer with a scapholunate collapse deformity that is 12 months old has radiographic evidence of collapse and arthritic changes at the midcarpal joint. The recommended treatment is:
   (a) arthroscopic repair of the scapholunate ligament
   (b) open scapholunate ligament reconstruction
   (c) intercarpal arthrodesis
   (d) dorsal capsulodesis
   (e) TFCC repair

4. A patient with a ski-pole injury to the thumb should have surgical repair if:
   (a) The ski glove can not be removed.
   (b) The MP joint stressed in 30 degrees of flexion deviates 10 degrees.
   (c) Tenderness is present at the insertion of the ulnar collateral ligament.
   (d) A masslike fullness is palpable at the ulnar aspect of the thumb MP joint.
   (e) Tenderness is present at the radial collateral insertion on the proximal phalanx.

5. Volar dislocation of the PIP joint will result in injury of the following structures:
   (a) central slip and collateral ligaments
   (b) volar plate and collateral ligaments
   (c) central slip and sublimus insertion
   (d) terminal extensor
   (e) flexor digitorum profundus tendon

Answers: 1) d; 2) a; 3) c; 4) d; 5) a

Chapter 30

Vascular Injuries of the Wrist and Hand

L. Scott Levin, MD, Richard S. Moore, Jr., MD, and Rey Aponte, PA-C

Patients with vascular disorders of the upper extremity may present with symptoms ranging from acute limb-threatening ischemia to chronic insufficiency. This spectrum of clinical manifestations makes the evaluation of vascular disorders in the upper extremity exceptionally challenging to the clinician. The potentially devastating consequences of these disorders necessitate a timely, thoughtful, and thorough approach to assessment, diagnosis, and management. The purpose of this chapter is to provide a review of the etiology, evaluation, and treatment of selected acute and chronic vascular injuries and disorders of the wrist and hand.

ETIOLOGY

Vascular disorders of the wrist and hand can be associated with multiple etiologies including acute trauma, cumulative trauma, and vasospastic disorders. Injuries attributed to acute trauma result from a single insult such as a laceration, pene-trating trauma, or crush unjury. Disorders attributed to cumulative trauma result from a series of minor insults that alone would not result in significant injury but when combined over a period of time lead to pathologic changes. Finally, vasospastic disorders are the result of elevated tone in the sympathetic nerves supplying the small arteries and arterioles of the wrist and hand. The elevated sympathetic tone results in symptomatic decreases in blood flow and symptoms of ischemia. Each of these etiologies will be further discussed in the following text.

BASIC SCIENCE

Histologic Anatomy

The arterial wall is made up of three distinct layers. The innermost, or intima, consists of the luminal lining of endothelial cells, their basement membrane, and the underlying subendothelial connective tissue. The outermost layer is formed by connective tissue and transitional fibroblasts, which gradually merge with the surrounding connective tissue. This layer is referred to as the adventitial layer and contains the sympathetic innervation of the vessel. The media lies between these two layers and consists of connective tissue and smooth muscle cells. An internal and external elastic lamina separate the media from the intimal and adventitial layers. The lamina are well developed in larger arterial vessels, such as the aorta, where the vessel wall must withstand relatively high pressures. This elastic layer acts to maintain blood pressure during diastole.

The smaller, more peripheral vessels have a less prominent elastic layer, and the walls has more smooth muscle. These vessels are more vasoactive, or capable of changes in vessel diameter. This activity is regulated by the sympathetic nerve fibers of the adventitial layer and helps to regulate blood flow in response to injury, activity, and temperature.

The veins also have an intimal, medial, and adventitial layer; however, these layers are much less easily distinguished. In larger veins, the connective tissue of the intima is prominent and the media is poorly developed. The adventitial layer makes up the largest portion of the vessel wall and contains elastin fibers, collagen fibers, and prominent smooth muscle cells. The lumen contains fine leaflets, which function as valves and prevent backflow in this low pressure system. Although the changes in vessel diameter are not as significant in the venous system, the sympathetic innervation allows alterations in vessel tone and pliability, which play a major role in hemodynamics.

435

Intimal Injury

The delicate balance between the thrombogenic and thrombolytic pathways depends on the precise interaction of many factors. The endothelial cells that line the vascular lumen play an active role in the regulation of this system. The cells themselves form an antithrombogenic surface by presenting molecules with antithrombin III binding activity on their luminal sides. Additionally, the endothelial cells actively bind and remove thrombin from forming clots and secrete factors that inhibit platelet aggregation.

The endothelial cells also provide coverage for the underlying basement membrane, connective tissue, and vascular collagen. These substances are highly thrombogenic. When the endothelial layer is disrupted platelet aggregation is rapidly initiated, and the extrinsic clotting cascade is activated. This results in an intravascular thrombus and partial or complete vessel occlusion. Once an intravascular thrombus has formed, it has the potential to serve as a nidus for local propagation or embolization to smaller vessels.

Disruption of the intima is a common mechanism of vascular injury in blunt trauma. Often, the injury is unrecognized on initial evaluation. Thrombosis ensues and the insult is discovered after the onset of ischemia. A high index of suspicion is necessary to detect intimal injury in patients with an appropriate mechanism of injury.

Tissue Perfusion and Ischemia

Tissue perfusion is based on adequate pressure to deliver oxygen and nutrient-rich blood to the capillary bed. Perfusion pressure is a function of blood pressure and tissue resistance and is tightly regulated by multiple mechanisms. Inflammatory changes occurring in the capillary beds due to injury or systemic disease can have a profound effect on tissue perfusion.

In instances of hypoperfusion tissues become ischemic. If tissue ischemia persists for prolonged periods of time irreversible changes in cellular architecture occur. The anoxic insult leads to alterations in the cellular membrane, which progress to cell lysis and tissue necrosis. Prevention of hypoperfusion and restoration of flow are the main treatments for ischemia.

Revascularization of ischemic tissues can lead to severe physiologic changes. Toxic metabolites produced during the period of hypoperfusion can produce electrolyte imbalances, and myoglobin released from necrotic muscle cells cause renal injury. The ischemic alterations in cell membrane function can lead to reactive hyperemia and extravasation of fluid into the tissues with reperfusion. This can result in profound increases in intracompartmental pressures and a reperfusion compartment syndrome. With limb revascularization following extended ischemia, faciotomies should be performed and patients monitored for the clinical manifestations of these problems.

ANATOMY AND SURGICAL APPROACHES

Vascular Anatomy

The brachial artery crosses the elbow superficial to the brachialis muscle belly. It is accompanied by the median nerve medially and the biceps tendon laterally. In the cubital fossa it divides into its terminal branches, the radial and ulnar arteries.

The ulnar artery descends into the forearm deep to the flexor carpi ulnaris and is accompanied by the ulnar nerve on its medial side. At the wrist, these structures enter Guyon's canal between the pisiform and hook of the hamate and pass into the palm. The ulnar artery continues as the superficial palmar arch, which courses radially (Fig. 30–1). In the palm, the arch lies superficial to the branches of the median nerve; however, this relationship is reversed in the digits.

The first constant branch of the superficial arch is the proper digital artery to the ulnar side of the small finger. This is usually followed by three common digital arteries to the adjacent sides of the four fingers. The proper digital arteries arise from the common digital arteries and form the major supply to the fingers. These travel distally adjacent to the flexor tendons and dorsal to the digital nerves. The radial and ulnar digital arteries form an arch across the distal phalanx. After giving origin to the common digital arteries, the arch continues radially into the thenar muscles where it normally forms an anastomosis with the superficial branch of the radial artery.

The radial artery descends toward the wrist under the flexor carpi radialis. The artery is palpable just proximal to the wrist, where it overlies the pronator quadratus. At this level it gives off the superficial palmar branch, which courses into the palm to join the terminal superficial arch. The radial artery proper then turns dorsally and radially to enter the anatomic "snuffbox," which is defined by the tendons of the first and third extensor compartments. Here it gives off branches that form the dorsal radiocarpal, intercarpal, and metacarpal arches. The artery then dives between the two heads of the first dorsal interosseous muscle, where it divides to form the princeps pollicis and the deep palmar arch. The deep branch passes ulnarly, where it usually anastomoses with a deep branch of the ulnar artery (Fig. 30–1b). The princeps pollicis artery runs between the first dorsal interosseous and adductor pollicis before dividing into the radial and ulnar digital arteries of the thumb.

There are multiple perforating arteries between the deep and superficial arches. These collaterals allow the hand to survive following division of the radial or ulnar arteries. However, incomplete arches have been noted in up to 20% of hands. In these individuals, loss of flow from one artery can leave some or all of the hand ischemic (Fig. 30–1c). In a small percentage of individuals, a persistent median artery, which enters the palm through the carpal tunnel, will make a significant contribution to distal perfusion.

The venous drainage of the hand consists of superficial and deep systems. The superficial system is the dominant source of drainage and is formed by longitudinal trunks, which join to form a dorsal network ultimately emptying into the basilic and cephalic veins. The deep system is of much smaller caliber and accompanies the arterial arches.

Surgical Approaches

In the forearm, the radial and ulnar arteries are approached through longitudinal palmar incisions over the flexor carpi radialis and flexor carpi ulnaris tendons, respectively. If both arteries must be exposed, an extended midline incision is rec-

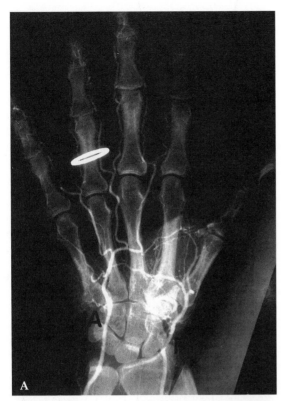

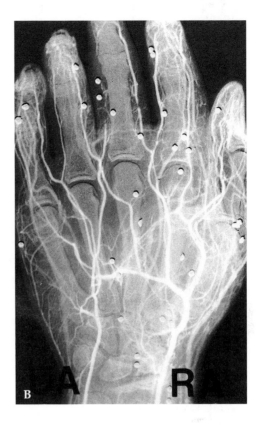

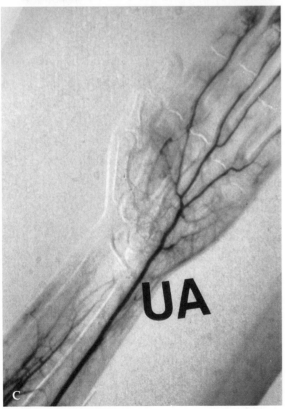

Figure 30–1 **(A)** Arteriogram of the wrist and hand in a 59-year-old female who complained of index-finger cold intolerance. The ulnar artery (UA) crosses the wrist and turns radially forming the superficial arch, which gives origin to the common digital vessels. Note the occlusion of the terminal portion of the superficial arch and the digital vessels to the index finger: the pathology underlying her cold intolerance. The radial artery (RA) passes ulnarly as the deep arch. Note the collaterals between the two arches. **(B)** Arteriogram of the wrist and hand in an 18-year-old male who sustained a shotgun blast to the upper extremity. The RA traverses the anatomic "snuffbox" to emerge between the first and second metacarpals and turns ulnarly to continue as the deep palmar arch. The UA forms an anastomosis with the terminal segment of the deep arch. The superficial palmar arch is not visualized, and the common digital vessels appear to take origin directly from the deep arch. Note the injury to the ulnar digital vessel of the long finger. **(C)** Arteriogram of the wrist and hand in a 28-year-old female who developed ischemia of the thumb following blunt trauma to the wrist. The study reveals an incomplete arch and thrombosis of the radial artery. The thrombosed segment of the RA was resected, and a reverse interpositional vein graft was placed with complete resolution of symptoms.

ommended (Fig. 30–2 and Fig. 30–3). This allows access to both the radial and ulnar arteries, a complete fascial release, and can be extended across the wrist to release Guyon's canal and the transverse carpal ligament. Care should be taken to preserve a flap to cover the median nerve and tendons at the wrist. A Bruner, zigzag incision across the wrist with the apex pointing radially will help in avoiding the palmar cutaneous branch of the median nerve (Fig. 30–4).

The radial artery in the anatomic snuffbox is accessible through a dorsal-radial incision (Fig. 30–5). In this area, the

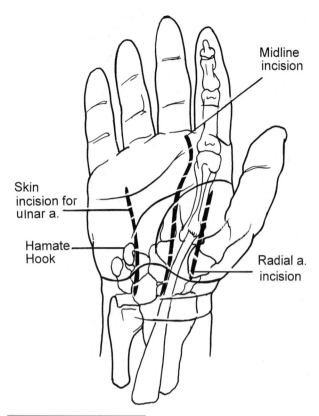

Figure 30–2 Schematic illustrating longitudinal palmar incisions.

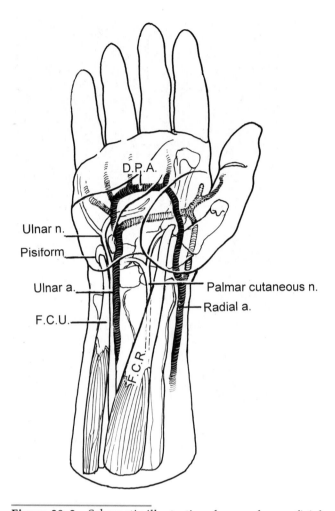

Figure 30–3 Schematic illustrating deep and superficial arch.

branches of the superficial radial nerve should be identified and carefully preserved.

The approach to Guyon's canal classically follows the hypothenar skin crease at the base of the ring finger. The incision is extended across the wrist flexion crease in an oblique fashion and then can be carried up the forearm in a gentle curve or Bruner fashion. The incision is extended distally into the palm using a Bruner incision. The ulnar nerve and artery should be identified beneath the flexor carpi ulnaris and followed into Guyon's canal. The nerve is located ulnar to the artery at this level. The roof of the canal, formed by the volar carpal ligament, is divided. The dissection can be carried into the palm to expose the entire superficial arch.

The level of the superficial palmar arch is defined by a line drawn from the radial side of the proximal palmar flexion crease to the ulnar side of the distal palmar flexion crease (Fig. 30–6). It is at this level that the common digital arteries take their origin. An oblique incision is recommended for their exposure, as it can easily be extended into the digit in either a standard palmar zigzag or midlateral approach. In the digits, the neurovascular bundles are suspended between Grayson's ligament palmarly and Cleland's ligament dorsally. The artery lies dorsal to the nerve at this level.

EXAMINATION

History

Perhaps the most crucial component in the evaluation of vascular disorders is the history. A tremendous amount of information is available if carefully obtained. In the setting of

acute injury, the mechanism should always be identified. This provides the physician with an idea regarding the nature of the vascular injury and allows thorough preoperative planning. Difficulties with repair, such as the need for vein grafting due to segmental loss with blast or avulsion injuries, can be anticipated. It is also helpful to determine the position of the extremity at the time of injury to identify what structures were within the zone of injury. This is especially important in the upper extremity due to the gliding nature of tendons and their significant excursions. Furthermore, the volume and character of bleeding at the time of injury should be confirmed.

Although arterial lacerations in the setting of acute trauma may present very dramatically, occult injuries associated with penetrating trauma are not uncommon. These injuries must be rapidly and accurately diagnosed to prevent limb-threatening ischemia. Perry, Thal, and Shires (1971) conducted an extensive review of civilian arterial injuries and set forth seven criteria to alert the treating physician to the possibility of underlying arterial injury. Surgical exploration is indicated if any of the following criteria are met:

1. decreased or absent distal pulse
2. history of persistent arterial bleeding

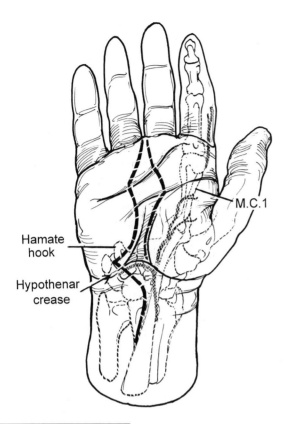

Figure 30–4 Schematic illustrating a Bruner zigzag incision across the wrist.

3. large or expanding hematoma
4. major hemorrhage with hypotension
5. bruit
6. injury to an anatomically related nerve
7. anatomic proximity to a major artery.

Additionally, the authors reported an associated major venous or nerve injury in nearly 40% of cases.

Outside the setting of acute trauma, a complete medical history should be obtained to identify factors that can contribute to vascular disorders. The patient should be questioned with regards to systemic disorders such as scleroderma, atherosclerosis, or abnormalities in coagulation. Any history of injury or surgery in the extremity should be identified, as well as any extrinsic causes of vascular insufficiency such as tobacco use, caffeine, or vasoconstrictive drugs.

The characteristics of the symptoms can provide insight into the etiology. Vasospastic disease is characterized by episodes of pallor, which can be triggered by cold temperatures and are followed by periods of hyperemia. Thrombotic and embolic events are associated with an acute onset and progressive, typically unrelenting, symptoms.

Physical Exam

The physical examination should always begin with inspection of the extremity. Note should be made of skin color, including areas of pallor, hyperemia, cyanosis, and mottling. Scars and ulcerations should be documented, as well as a description of the healing process.

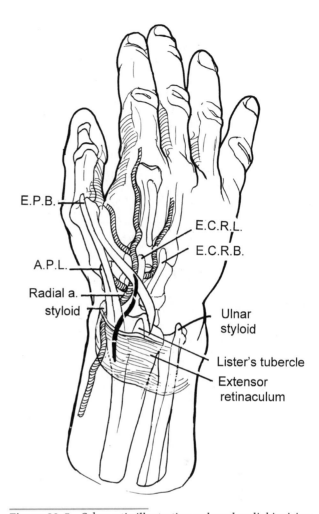

Figure 30–5 Schematic illustrating a dorsal-radial incision.

The heart should be ascultated for irregularity and murmurs. Cardiac dysfunction, such as valve incompetence and muscular dysmotility, can lead to thrombus formation and embolic events. Similarly, the subclavian system should be auscultated to assess for the presence of a bruit, which would indicate a large proximal lesion. Such lesions can have a profound effect on the distal extremity by acting as an embolic source or an obstruction to adequate flow.

Pulses should be palpated beginning with the subclavian and proceeding to the axillary, brachial, ulnar, radial at the wrist and in the anatomic snuffbox, and the digital arteries. Bilateral blood pressures should be recorded for the brachial artery. Digital pressures can be obtained to calculate a digital brachial index (DBI). This is calculated by dividing the digital pressure by the brachial pressure with values < 0.70 considered abnormal. An obstruction between the brachial and digital vessels will cause the DBI to fall; however, vasospastic disease may not affect the value. Provocative testing may be beneficial in patients with vasospastic syndromes.

The relative contributions of the radial and ulnar arteries to the hand can be assessed by the Allen test. The test is conducted by compression of both the radial and ulnar arteries. The patient helps exsanguinate the hand by repetitively clenching the fingers into a fist. The hand is relaxed and the

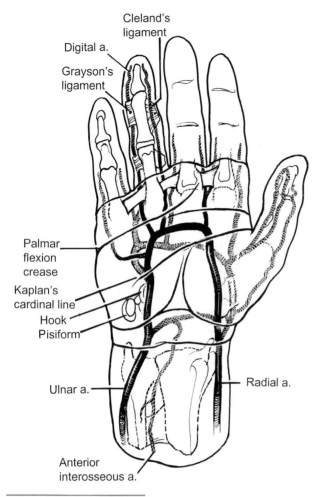

Cleland's ligament

Digital a.

Grayson's ligament

Palmar flexion crease

Kaplan's cardinal line

Hook
Pisiform

Ulnar a.

Radial a.

Anterior interosseous a.

Figure 30–6   Schematic illustrating level of superficial palmar arch.

radial artery is released. Both the time until refill and the distribution of refill in the hand is recorded. This process is then repeated for the ulnar artery and in the other hand. Gelberman has reported that the average time to refill in the radial artery is 2.4 + 1.2 seconds and in the ulnar 2.3 + 1.0 seconds. He reported that 7% of ulnar and 2% of radial arteries failed to fill the hand in 6 seconds. A delay in filling indicates an incomplete arch. Loss of either artery may place a portion of the hand at risk of ischemia. The Allen test can be performed on the digits to assess the patency of the radial and ulnar digital vessels.

AIDS TO DIAGNOSIS

Doppler Studies

Dopplers provide a simple, accurate, and noninvasive method of evaluating vascular flow. These units function by emitting a low frequency, ultrasonic wave that passes through the soft tissues. When the beam encounters a vessel, the frequency is altered by the blood flow and is reflected back to the device. The unit gathers the reflected beam converting it into an audible signal. The amount of alteration in the beam's

frequency is proportional to the velocity of blood flow. Therefore, the quality of the flow within the vessel can be assessed by the quality of the signal. These devices are relatively inexpensive and available in most clinics and hospitals.

Ultrasound Imaging

Diagnostic ultrasound units use high-frequency sound waves to produce real-time images of vascular structures. High-frequency sound waves are transmitted into and reflected by the soft tissues. Differences in tissue density result in alterations in the reflected signal, which are electronically converted into images. Vascular structures can be readily visualized. These systems can be utilized in conjunction with doppler technology to image flow within the vessels.

Digital Plethysmography

The volume of blood within an appendage can be assessed by measuring changes in the circumference of the appendage. This is carried out by the use of a device called a plethysmograph. The device consists of a cuff placed around the digit that measures changes in circumference and converts them into a wave pattern. This pattern can, in turn, be used to measure the volume and quality of flow to the digit. Differences in pressure of 15 mm Hg between adjacent digits or 30 mm Hg between a digit and the radial or ulnar artery are considered abnormal. This technique provides a quantitative assessment of digital flow and is useful in the evaluation of replants, vasospastic disease, and thrombosis.

Radiographic Studies

Plain x-rays are of limited value in assessing vascular disorders. However, associated soft tissue masses, intraosseous lesions, and vascular calcifications can often be visualized. Advances in magnetic resonance imaging has led to the development of magnetic resonance angiography. This technology is expensive and is not universally available. However, it is noninvasive and produces high-resolution images of the vascular structures and surrounding soft tissues. It is likely that over the next several years this technique will come to play a much larger role in the evaluation of vascular problems in the upper extremity.

Cold-stress Testing

Controlled cooling of the hands with monitoring of finger pulp pressures and temperature is a valuable technique in the assessment of circulatory disorders in the upper extremity (Fig. 30–7). Responses have been classified into three types by Koman et al (1993). Type I patients have baseline pulp temperatures of 30 degrees Celsius or greater that fall only 3 to 4 degrees with cooling. During the rewarming period, these patients rapidly return to baseline with no pain or discomfort during testing. Type II patients are characterized by baseline temperatures below 30 degrees Celsius that fall 8 to 10 degrees during cooling. These patients take significantly longer to rewarm and experience moderate pain with testing. This response indicates an isolated nerve injury or collateralization following vascular injury. Type III patients have baseline temperatures of 28.5 degrees Celsius or less

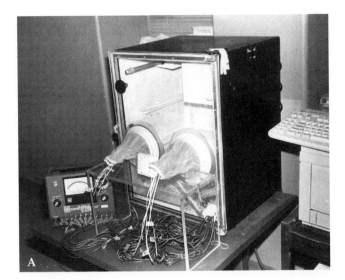

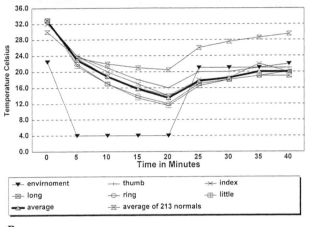

Figure 30–7 **(A)** Cold-stress testing apparatus. **(B)** Cold-stress test in patient with abnormal response. Note the significant decrease in temperature and delayed return to baseline when compared with the normal curve.

that drop 8 to 13 degrees with cooling. These patients rewarm extremely slowly and experience severe pain with testing. The type III pattern is indicative of arterial injury or severe vasospastic disease.

This technique has been combined with other technologies, such as plethysmography, to provide a more detailed evaluation of vascular disorders. Cold-stress testing is also a valuable tool in evaluating recovery and response to treatment.

Arteriography

Arteriography is the gold standard in the evaluation of vascular disorders. The intravascular injection of radiographic contrast agents allows visualization of the vascular structures and assessment of their quality and integrity. Although invasive, the technique plays a prominent diagnostic and therapeutic role.

Historically, angiography was fraught with complications. Early contrast agents were highly charged, requiring administration in hypertonic solutions, and were associated with a high incidence of systemic reactions. Modern contrast agents

are more isotonic and less prone to elicit a systemic response. Advances in radiographic technology have led to higher resolution images with lower dye loads. Current complication rates are less than 1%.

Although the vascular tree of the upper extremity can be accessed through the axillary or brachial arteries, cannulation at this level does not allow visualization of the subclavian system. Proximal lesions can lead to profound vascular changes in the upper extremity and will be missed if not studied. The authors recommend that all upper extremity arteriograms be performed through a femoral puncture to allow visualization of the proximal vessels. With this technique, the surgeon can determine the location and size of a lesion, as well as the involvement and condition of the other vessels. This additional information allows a complete assessment and accurate preoperative planning.

Perhaps the most important advancement in arteriography has been the development of digital subtraction technology. This technique utilizes computer technology to remove bone and soft tissue shadows, allowing unobstructed visualization of the vascular structures. In modern angiographic suites, procedures producing high-resolution images can be carried out more quickly and with less radiation.

Over the past decade, vascular radiologists have developed interventional techniques that play a vital role in the treatment of vascular disorders. Intra-arterial access allows precise catheter placement. Diagnosis of a lesion can be rapidly followed by local administration of vasodilators or thrombolytic agents. Thrombectomy and atherectomy have also become commonplace, and in many centers interventional radiologic procedures are the first line in the management of vascular lesions. These techniques are available for intra-operative imaging and are valuable for assessing clinical response to therapy.

SPECIFIC CONDITIONS, TREATMENT, AND OUTCOME

Acute Injuries

Intimal Injuries

As previously noted, intimal integrity is essential for the maintenance of vessel competence. The intimal lining is susceptible to injury via chemicals and blunt or penetrating trauma. With invasive monitoring techniques, intimal injuries caused by cannulation are relatively common. Intimal trauma from cannulation and indwelling devices can lead to thrombosis of the vessel and ischemia or embolization to the distal vasculature.

At the wrist, this problem is seen with radial artery cannulation for intra-arterial pressure monitoring. Patients with complete arches usually have sufficient flow through the ulnar system to supply the digits. However, in the 20% of patients with an incomplete arch some or all of the digits may be threatened. Additionally, the thrombosis may act as an embolic source or may increase sympathetic tone leading to severe vasospasm. An Allen test is mandatory prior to cannulation of either artery at the wrist.

Some authors recommend treating these lesions with thrombolytics and have reported acceptable results. Others have not been as successful with this approach and have recommended surgical management. The authors recommend prompt surgical exploration and resection of the thrombosed segment to normal intima followed by reconstruction. A preoperative arteriogram is recommended to evaluate the location and extent of injury as well as the arterial anatomy. Primary repair is optimal; however, the resected segment often leaves a gap and reverse interpositional vein grafting is preferable to inadequate resection of injured intima.

Lacerations

In the past, arterial lacerations of any type were potentially limb threatening. Over the past two decades, advances in microsurgical techniques have led to a dramatic change in the treatment and prognosis of these injuries.

In the setting of acute trauma, a high index of suspicion for arterial injury should be maintained. Intimal injuries may have subtle presentations with devastating outcomes. Severed arterial stumps will often retract and go into spasm resulting in surprisingly little bleeding. However, this can lead to late bleeding if not recognized. Partial arterial lacerations are unable to adequately contract with spasm and will often result in profuse bleeding. This can be difficult to control with pressure and elevation and usually requires surgical treatment.

Laceration of both the radial and ulnar arteries in the forearm is associated with significant distal ischemia. Immediate repair by a skilled surgeon is recommended. The management of an injury to a single vessel with no evidence of ischemia in the hand is controversial. Isolated, unrepaired arterial lacerations in the forearm have been shown by Gelberman et al (1979) to result in diminished distal perfusion. However, these changes rarely result in cold intolerance or clinically significant ischemia. Long-term patency rates for repair of single arteries has been reported to be as low as 50%. Some authors suggest better regeneration of ulnar nerve function following repair at the wrist if the ulnar artery is also repaired; however, others have reported no significant difference.

Despite the controversy, the authors recommend exploration of all major arteries near the zone of injury. If ischemia is present, repair of the injured vessel is mandatory. If the hand is well perfused, ligation of the arterial stumps is acceptable. Care should be taken to identify and ligate both the proximal and distal stump to prevent late complications such as bleeding or aneurysm formation.

When complete, the superficial arch in the palm receives contributions from both the radial and ulnar arteries. Therefore, laceration of a complete arch in the palm should not significantly compromise flow to the digits, as each stump will be supplied by its contributing artery. Upon exploration, if active bleeding is encountered from both ends of the severed arch, then ligation of the stumps should not place the digits at risk. However, if there is evidence of inadequate flow from one segment, the arch must be repaired or reconstructed.

A significant number of collaterals exist between the radial and ulnar digital vessels in the fingers; therefore, laceration of a single digital vessel is well tolerated and rarely results in symptoms of ischemia. It should be noted that digital artery laceration by a palmar wound is almost always associated with laceration of the accompanying digital nerve due to the palmar position of the nerve relative to the artery in the finger.

PEARL

Disruption of a digital artery due to a palmar laceration is almost always associated with a digital nerve laceration due to the proximity of the nerve and vessel in the finger.

Amputations

Recent advances in the field of microsurgery now allow replantation of amputated parts with a high probability of survival. The decision of whether to replant an amputated appendage must be made on an individual basis. Experience with replants has resulted in the following indications for replantation. Patients with amputations through the thumb, palm, wrist or distal forearm, multiple digits, or a single digit distal to the insertion of the flexor digitorum superficialis (FDS) are believed to be good candidates for replantation. Additionally, elbow and above-elbow amputations with minimal avulsion injuries and nearly any part in a child, are generally felt to be appropriate indications.

Amputations due to crush or severe avulsion injuries, amputations at multiple levels, and amputations with greater than 6 hours warm ischemia time or 12 hours cool ischemia time should not be replanted. Replantation of a single digit proximal to the insertion of the FDS is generally not recommended as useful range of motion is unlikely and the patient will tend to bypass the digit. An associated serious injury or disease is an absolute contraindication. Relative contraindications include advanced age, cigarette smoking, and mental illness. Preparation of the amputated part for transport to the microsurgical team is crucial. The authors recommend wrapping the amputated part in a gauze soaked in saline or Ringer's lactate. This should then be placed in a plastic bag, which is immersed in a container of iced saline. This ensures that the part remains cool while preventing frostbite. The patient should be transported as quickly as possible, provided that his or her medical condition is stable. If appropriately cooled, a part should survive for at least 12 hours. Digits can often be replanted at up to 24 hours due to the absence of muscle tissue.

Replantation is accomplished most efficiently by two teams working simultaneously to prepare the amputated part and amputation site. The surgery should proceed in a systematic fashion beginning with skeletal stabilization followed by tendon repair, arterial repair, venous repair, and finally nerve repair. As a general rule, two veins should be repaired for every artery. The artery should be stripped back to healthy intima and often cannot be repaired primarily. The artery can be mobilized by division of tethering branches, but will often require vein grafting. The bony elements should be shortened to allow easier approximation of the neurovascular structures, often obviating the need for grafting (Fig. 30–8).

Dressings should be nonconstrictive and the digit should be monitored for capillary refill and temperature. Postoperative venous congestion is often a more significant threat to

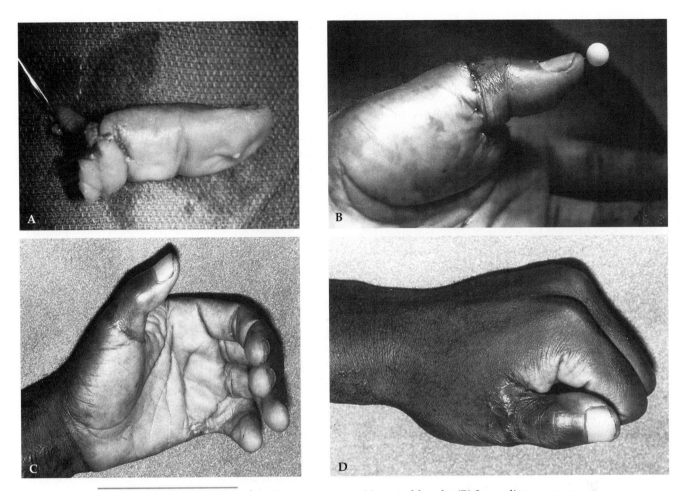

Figure 30–8   **(A)** Complete thumb amputation in 30-year-old male. **(B)** Immediate post operative. **(C, D)** One-year follow-up with excellent functional result.

viability than inadequate arterial inflow and requires aggressive action. Options to supplement venous outflow include removal of the nail and placement of heparin-soaked gauze on the nail bed, construction of an arterial venous shunt, or medicinal leeches. Leeches reduce congestion by direct removal of blood from the tissue and by secretion of a natural anticoagulant, hirudin. Judicious use of leeches can be a critical factor in saving a threatened replant.

With modern microsurgical techniques one can expect a viability rate of nearly 80%; however, functional results vary. Young patients with sharp amputations at the wrist or distal to the FDS insertion tend to have the best results. This is related to the regenerative potential of the tissues, the lack of crush or avulsion injury to the neurovascular structures, and the fact that the tendon injury occurs at a level where gliding is not crucial. Amputations proximal to the FDS insertion rarely regain a functional range of motion and the patients tend to bypass these digits in everyday activities. Multiple-level crush and avulsion injuries tend to have poor return of function due to the higher degree of soft tissue injury.

The decision of whether to replant an amputated body part can be difficult and is best left to the experienced microsurgeon. Many factors such as expectations of the patient and

the patient's family, the cost and time commitment of replantation, and the significant period of rehabilitation can all place pressure on the physician. It is crucial that the surgeon consider each patient individually and opt for the course of treatment that will result in the most functional limb possible.

Ring Avulsion Injuries

Digital injuries caused by traction on a ring can produce a spectrum of injury ranging from a simple abrasion to a complex degloving or amputation. These injuries present a difficult management problem to the physician and deserve special mention.

Urbaniak et al (1981) reviewed a large series of these injuries and stratified them into three classes. Class I injuries have adequate distal circulation. Class II have inadequate distal circulation but have preservation of the majority of the soft tissues. Class III have complete degloving or amputation of the digit. This method of classification has subsequently been subclassified by other authors; however, a reasonable treatment plan can be formulated from this simple system.

Class I injuries require only standard bone and soft tissue treatment adhering to established orthopaedic principles. An excellent outcome can be expected, with the majority of patients having no long-term disability. Class II injuries are more complex and require restoration of vascular flow by microsurgical techniques. A subgroup of these injuries, classified as IIA by Nissenbaum (1989), are characterized by arterial injury only with no significant bony, tendonous, or nerve injuries. Due to the relatively benign initial presentation, these significant vascular injuries are often missed, with dire consequences. These digits can be salvaged with relatively simple microvascular techniques. It is, therefore, imperative that a thorough vascular exam be conducted on any patient who presents with a ring-avulsion-type injury.

PITFALL

Ring avulsion injuries require a careful vascular evaluation as profound vascular injuries can occur in the absence of significant soft tissue injury and can lead to digit threatening ischemia (Class IIA injuries).

Class III injuries present the greatest challenge to the treating surgeon and require the most astute judgment. The avulsion mechanism results in severe, soft tissue injuries that make attempts at replantation difficult if not impossible (Fig. 30–9). A successful replantation is often a functional failure, leaving the patient less functional than if a primary amputation had been performed. As with replantation from other

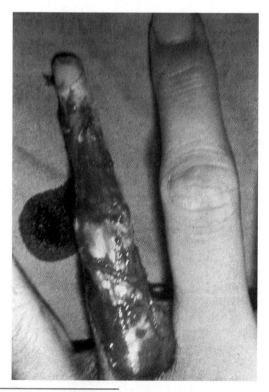

Figure 30–9 Class III ring avulsion injury. Note the complete degloving of soft tissues. This patient was treated with primary amputation.

mechanisms, the surgeon must consider the functional, economic, and cosmetic demands of each patient.

Chronic Conditions
Ulnar Artery Thrombosis

The superficial position of the ulnar artery at the wrist, combined with its confinement within the unforgiving boundaries of Guyon's canal, leave it subject to injury. Since its initial description by Van Rosen (1934), thrombosis of the ulnar artery at the wrist due to trauma, the "hypothenar hammer syndrome," has been widely reported. Despite its presence in the medical literature, it often remains unrecognized or misdiagnosed.

Ulnar artery thrombosis most often occurs in males of working age and is associated with activities that involve repetitive, blunt trauma to the hands. The disorder primarily affects the dominant hand and has been related to hammering with the heel of the palm, use of pneumatic devices, and prolonged pressure over the hypothenar eminence. An association with cigarette smoking has also been suggested.

The pathogenesis of the disease is felt to stem from intimal damage. The artery is fixed within Guyon's canal and is susceptible to trauma. The intimal disruption leads to activation of the clotting cascades and subsequent thrombus formation. This assumption is supported by histologic studies of resected specimens that reveal organized thrombus within the lumen in association with intimal hyperplasia and inflammatory infiltration of the vessel wall. Ishemic effects of the disruption in flow may be magnified by embolization to the distal vasculature or vasospasm related to an increase in sympathetic tone.

Patients with ulnar artery thrombosis present with complaints of pain, cold intolerance, and numbness. They will almost always have a history of repetitive or isolated blunt trauma to the hand. Pain is localized to the ulnar aspect of the hand and may be associated with a tender mass. Pain may be exacerbated by repetitive activity. Night pain and pain at rest can occur; however, this is unusual in the absence of significant ischemia, and these findings are often associated with ulcerations.

The ulnar artery is intimately associated with the ulnar nerve in Guyon's canal. It is not surprising that a significant number of patients will present with complaints of numbness in the ulnar nerve distribution. Objective testing may be normal; however, subjective decreases in sensation and alteration in sweating in the ulnar nerve distribution have been reported in as many as 30% of patients.

Discomfort associated with exposure to cold is quite common. Symptoms usually involve the ulnar two or three digits and often follow a classic Raynaud's pattern. In patients with unilateral symptoms of Raynaud's, ulnar artery thrombosis should be considered. Cold-stress testing has confirmed alterations in blood flow, and a characteristic, digital temperature response has been described.

The physical exam of the patient with ulnar artery thrombosis is definitive. A careful evaluation of the ulnar artery should be conducted to evaluate its patency. The ulnar palm should be carefully inspected for any masses or tenderness overlying Guyon's canal, and a careful examination of the sensory and motor components of the ulnar nerve should be conducted. The digits should be evaluated for ulcerations and trophic changes associated with chronic ischemia, and the nail beds should be inspected for subungal splinter hemorrhages.

The definitive diagnosis of ulnar artery thrombosis is made by the Allen test (Fig. 30–10). Failure of the hand to reperfuse or absence of a dopplerable ulnar pulse during radial artery occlusion is diagnostic of ulnar artery occlusion. The exact location and extent of the thrombosis can be determined by Doppler evaluation of the radial and ulnar arteries and the superficial arch. Digital plethysmography has also been found to be useful in the evaluation of these patients. By recording the flow response to sequential radial and ulnar artery occlusion, a digital plethysmograph provides a quantitative digital Allen's test.

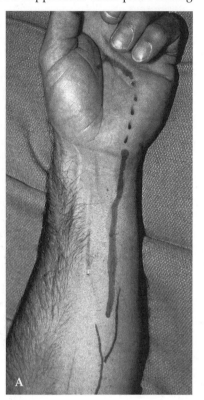

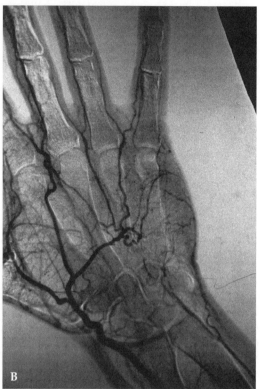

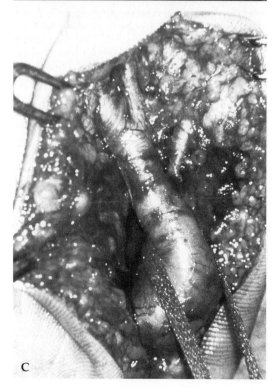

Figure 30–10 Ulnar artery occlusion in 32-year-old laborer. **(A)** Physical exam reveals arterial segment with absence of flow indicated by broken line. **(B)** Digital subtraction arteriogram demonstrates occluded ulnar artery. **(C)** Intraoperative photograph of occluded segment.

Arteriography, although not necessary for the diagnosis of ulnar artery thrombosis, provides invaluable information for formulating a course of treatment (Fig. 30–10b). The exact location and extent of the lesion, as well as the general health of the vessels and the amount of collateralization, can be accurately determined by arteriography. Although it is invasive, the authors feel that the value of the information it provides far outweighs the risk. In patients undergoing surgical intervention, it should be considered mandatory. Additionally, arteriography can provide a potent therapeutic tool by delivering intra-arterial thrombolytics and vasodilators.

The management of ulnar artery thrombosis has been controversial. Treatments have included pharmacologic management, sympathectomy, thrombectomy, and arterial reconstruction. Recently, there has been a trend toward surgical management. If the thrombus is acute or the patient is a poor surgical candidate, an attempt can be made to treat with intra-arterial thrombolytics. However, if the lesion is chronic or there is significant intimal injury, it is unlikely that this will be of significant long-term benefit.

The artery is approached in Guyon's canal through a zigzag palmar incision (Fig. 30–5c). The ulnar nerve is decompressed and protected, and the thrombosed segment of artery is identified and resected to normal intima. In a hand with a complete arch and strong bleeding from the distal aspect of the ulnar artery, simple ligation of the stumps has been recommended. This removes the thrombus as a source of sympathetic irritation and emboli. This treatment does not create a significant risk of ischemia. However, recent reports have indicated better results with arterial reconstruction, and this is the preference of the authors. If the patient had clinical signs of significant ischemia preoperatively or there is inadequate backflow through the arch, arterial reconstruction is mandatory. This is best accomplished with the use of a reverse interposition vein graft harvested from the forearm.

Postoperatively, the patient's digit should be placed in a bulky dressing, and a short term course of an antithrombotic agent should be administered. A high incidence of recurrent thrombosis has been reported; however, if this occurs there is no need for reoperation unless there is clinical evidence of significant ischemia. Results are usually very good with the majority of patients noting a significant improvement in symptoms. Residual cold intolerance is common following either vessel reconstruction or resection. These symptoms are best managed by cessation of smoking, biofeedback and relaxation techniques, environmental modifications, and sympathetic blocks or sympathectomy.

Vasospastic Disease

Episodic vasospasm of the digital arteries was described by Maurice Raynaud in 1862 and is referred to as Raynaud's phenomenon. The disorder is characterized by a progression of symptoms initiated by stress or cold exposure. An initial period of blanching due to vasospasm is followed by a period of cyanosis. With rewarming, a reactive hyperemia leads to flushing in the digits and is often accompanied by pain and dysesthesias. Although the "white, blue, and red" is considered to be the classic presentation, patients with this disorder may experience a spectrum of symptoms with or without color change.

Episodic digital ischemia has been associated with a number of underlying organic disorders and environmental factors. When an associated disorder or factor is identified, the condition is referred to as Raynaud's syndrome. When there is no identifiable underlying disorder, the condition is referred to as Raynaud's disease. In 1932, Allen and Brown published the criteria that must be met to establish the diagnosis of Raynaud's disease. These include (1) intermittent attacks of discoloration of the acral parts, (2) symmetrical or bilateral involvement, (3) absence of occlusion of peripheral arteries, (4) gangrene or atrophic changes, which when present, are limited to the distal digital skin, (5) symptoms present for a minimum of 2 years, (6) absence of previous disease to which the abnormal vascular reactivity may be attributed, and (7) a predominance in women.

The etiology of Raynaud's syndrome is unclear. It is associated with a number of disorders and factors including collagen vascular diseases, autoimmune disorders, hematologic and occlusive diseases, and occupational exposure to cold and vibration. This association would seem to be related to the fact that the vast majority of these conditions produce a spastic or obstructive arterial phenomenon. The pathophysiology of the disorder is felt to be secondary to several mechanisms. Pathological changes within the vasculature can lead to narrowing of the vessel lumens. These structural changes can also act to diminish the vessel's intrinsic ability to remain patent. Abnormalities in vasomotor tone can result in vasospasm and interruption of flow, and alterations in blood viscosity can lead to diminished flow. These mechanisms, occurring alone or in combination, result in the characteristic pattern of ischemia.

The diagnosis of Raynaud's is usually suggested by the history. Patients typically present with the classical pattern of symptoms preceded by stress or cold exposure. Noninvasive studies such as Dopplers, plethysmography, and temperature monitoring are valuable tools in the evaluation of these patients, especially when combined with cold-stress testing. Patients with Raynaud's have been shown to exhibit lower than normal resting temperatures and digital flow. They experience more significant decreases in temperature with cooling and take significantly longer to return to baseline with rewarming.

Arteriography plays a less prominent role in the evaluation of a patient with Raynaud's. It is useful in delineating proximal vascular lesions when suspected and should be obtained in cases of unilateral disease. Arteriography is also indicated in cases with progression of ischemic changes despite maximal medical management and in evaluating the response to vasodilators in vasospastic disease.

The diagnosis of Raynaud's phenomenon is less important than the differentiation between the disease and the syndrome. Every effort must be made to exclude an underlying disorder, the treatment of which may take precedence over the Raynaud's. Late presentation such as the fifth decade, male sex, unilateral disease, and systemic symptoms should alert the physician to the probability of an associated disorder. Additionally, patients should be carefully followed for several years as the Raynaud's may be the presenting symptom of a subclinical disorder. Differentiation of these groups also has prognostic significance. Patients with underlying disorders tend to follow a more progressive course and are less responsive to therapy.

The initial treatment of patients with Raynaud's is nonoperative. Efforts should be directed at limiting environmental factors that may contribute to the symptoms. Patients should be instructed to avoid cold exposure, dress warmly, and keep the hands protected. They should be urged to stop smoking and to limit their intake of caffeine. Some authors have advocated the use of biofeedback. This technique allows patients to gain voluntary control over the autonomic mechanisms that contribute to vasospasm by monitoring digital bloodflow and temperature.

Pharmacologic therapy is directed at the suspected underlying disorder. Significant attention has been directed at blocking the sympathetic nerves that are believed to be responsible for the increase in vasomotor tone. Intra-arterial reserpine, which acts by depleting catecholamines, has been trialed with some success; however, it has been abandoned due to the deleterious effects of repeated injections. Oral administration of sympatholytic agents has been unsuccessful due to the unpleasant side effects of therapeutic doses. Calcium, channel blockers such as nifedipine and angiotensin converting enzyme (ACE) inhibitors such as captopril have been utilized in an attempt to inhibit the smooth muscle of the vessel walls and thereby limit vasospasm. These agents may currently offer the most promise in the pharmacological management of this disorder. Anticoagulants have been advocated to prevent small vessel thrombosis, and aspirin and persantine have been utilized to inhibit platelet aggregation.

Great care should be taken in the management of skin lesions. Established principles of wound care should be strictly followed and aggravating environments and agents avoided. Some studies have reported healing of ulcers with topical wound care and antibiotics. With progressive necrosis, amputation is often necessary. Attempts should be made to preserve as much length as possible; however, wound complications are common, and the surgeon must resect to a level of viable tissue.

In some patients with progressive pain and ischemia that is unresponsive to medical therapy, surgical intervention may be indicated (Fig. 30–11). Historically, efforts had been directed at removing the sympathetic input to the extremity by cervicothoracic sympathectomy. This approach met with only temporary success due to the fact that the brachial plexus receives additional sympathetic input through other sources and has been abandoned.

The technique of distal digital sympathectomy entails separating the proper digital artery from the common digital nerve and stripping the adventitia of the artery for a distance of 2 cm. This technique has met with some success in carefully selected patients. Only patients who demonstrate improvement in pulse volume recording and cold-stress testing after local anesthetic block are candidates.

As with other treatment modalities, patients with underlying collagen vascular disorders do not have as favorable a response. Jones felt that this may be related to periarterial fibrosis causing extrinsic compression of the vessels and contributing to vasospasm. He recommended a more extensive approach to expose the entire superficial arch and release fibrous septa. Segmental occlusions could be bypassed and an aggressive adventitial stripping conducted distally to the digital vessels.

With careful patient selection, these techniques have met with good short-term results; however, it must be remembered that the majority of these patients have underlying disorders. It is likely that with time the progression of these diseases will lead to further small vessel disease and a recurrence of symptoms. These patients must be followed over an extended period of time. Regular examinations are necessary to identify changes early, maximize therapy, and prevent complications.

Thromboangitis Obliterans

Thromboangitis obliterans is a rare syndrome of migratory superficial phlebitis and severe ischemia of the extremities. This disease occurs almost exclusively in young adult males with a strong history of cigarette smoking. The presentation is characterized by severe pain, cold intolerance, Raynaud's phenomenon, and digital ischemia manifested as well-demarcated areas of necrosis. In contrast to atheromatous lesions, which primarily involve the larger vessels in a segmental pattern, thromboangitis obliterans primarily affects the small vessels of the hands and feet. Histologically, these lesions are found to contain arterial and venous thrombosis in association with a significant inflammatory reaction.

The etiology of thromboangitis obliterans is unclear and likely multifactorial. Family studies and racial prevalence indicate a heritable factor predisposing an individual to the disease. A hypercoagulable state has been postulated and recent studies seem to implicate an autoimmune response. The presence of this genetic predisposition combined with environmental factors leads to the development of the disease. The strong association with cigarette smoking implies an etiological role.

The management of patients with this disorder is difficult. The associated pain is often excruciating and commonly requires narcotics for adequate control. There is no single, accepted pharmocological management, although anticoagulants, vasodilators, and prostaglandin inhibitors have been advocated. There may be a role for sympathetic blockade in the treatment of the vasospastic component. By far, the primary objective in the treatment of these patients is to stop the use of tobacco products. Abstinence from smoking is often associated with indefinite remissions; however, these patients are often unwilling or unable to overcome their addictions.

The chronic course of this disease is painful and protracted, and patients often require multiple amputations. These patients tend to heal distal wounds better than those with diffuse intravascular disease; therefore, more distal and functional amputations are possible without fear of wound complications. Life-threatening complications are uncommon, and life expectancy is only slightly lower than that of the general population.

SUMMARY

Vascular disorders of the upper extremity present a complex and challenging problem to the treating physician. The presentation is often subtle, and the consequences of misdiagno-

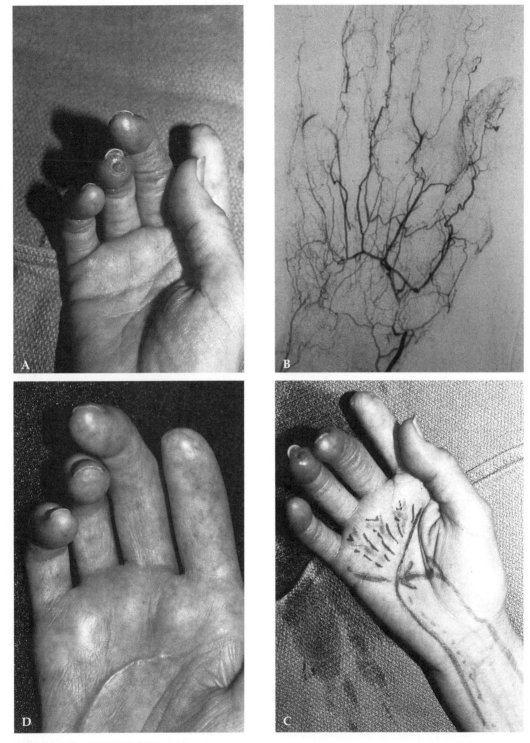

Figure 30–11 (**A**) 55-year-old female with scleroderma and Raynaud's syndrome. Note the hyperemia and ulceration of the ring finger and previous amputation of the distal portion of the index finger. (**B**) Digital subtraction arteriogram of the patient reveals ulnar artery occlusion at the wrist and absence of the superficial palmar arch. The deep palmar arch fills centrally via collaterals. (**C**) Preoperative planning for sympathectomy and reconstruction of the superficial palmar arch. The digital vessels are outlined in the distal palm, and the planned vein graft for reconstruction of the arch is indicated by the arrow. (**D**) One-year postoperative followup. The ring finger ulceration has healed. Note the J-shaped palmar incision.

sis or mistreatment severe. A thoughtful and thorough approach combining the history, physical exam, and appropriate diagnostic aids will provide the physician and patient with the greatest opportunity for a satisfactory outcome.

SELECTED BIBLIOGRAPHY

Selected Basic Science

OEGEMO T, AN K-N, WEILAND A, FURCH L. Peripheral blood vessels. In: Woo SL-Y, Buckwalter JA, eds. *Injury and Repair of the Musculoskeletal Soft Tissues.* Rosemont Illinois: American Academy of Orthopaedic Surgeons; 1988: 353–400.

Relevant Anatomy and Surgical Approaches

COLEMAN SS, ANSON BJ. Arterial patterns in the hand based upon a study of 650 specimens. *Surg Gynecol Obstet.* 1961;113:409–424.

KLEINERT JM, FLEMING SG, ABEL CS, FIRRELL J. Radial and ulnar artery dominance in normal digits. *J Hand Surg.* 1989;14A:504–507.

Examination

ALLEN EV. Thromboangitis obliterans: methods of diagnosis of chronic occlusive arterial lesions distal to the wrist with illustrative cases. *Am J Med Sci.* 1929;178:237–244.

BUEHNER JW, KOONTZ CL. The examination in the vascular laboratory. *Hand Clin.* 1993;9:5–13.

GELBERMAN RH, BLASINGAME JP. The timed Allen test. *J Trauma.* 1981;21:477–479.

Aids to Diagnosis

HOLDER LE, MERINE DS, YANG A. Nuclear medicine, contrast angiography, and magnetic resonance imaging for evaluation of vascular problems in the hand hand. *Hand Clin.* 1993;9:85–114.

HUTCHINSON DT. Color duplex imaging: applications to upper extremity and microvascular surgery. *Hand Clin.* 1993; 9:47–58.

KLEINERT JM, Gupta A. Pulse volume recording. *Hand Clin.* 1993;9:13–46.

KOMAN LA, SMITH BP, SMITH TL. Stress testing in the evaluation of upper extremity perfusion. *Hand Clin.* 1993;9:59–83.

Specific Conditions: Treatment and Outcome
Acute Injuries

Lacerations

FITRIDGE RA, RAPTIS S, MILLER JH, FARIS I. Upper extremity arterial injuries: experience at the Royal Adelaide Hospital, 1969–1991. *J Vasc Surg.* 1994;20:941–946.

GELBERMAN RH, BLASINGAME JP, FRONEK A, DIMICK MP. Forearm arterial injuries. *J Hand Surg.* 1979;4:401–408.

GELBERMAN RH, NUNLEY JA, KOMAN LA et al. The results of radial and ulnar arterial repair in the forearm: experience in three medical centers. *J Bone Jt Surg.* 1982;64A:383–387.

Amputations

SAIES AD, URBANIAK JR, NUNLEY JA, TARAS JS, GOLDNER RD, FITCH RD. Results after replantation and revascularization in the upper extremity in children. *J Bone Jt Surg.* 1994;76A: 1766–1776.

URBANIAK JR. To replant or not to replant? that is not the question. *J Hand Surg.* 1983;8:507–508.

URBANIAK JR, ROTH JH, NUNLEY JA, GOLDNER RD, KOMAN LA. The results of replantation after amputation of a single finger. *J Bone Jt Surg.* 1985;67A:611–619.

YAMARO Y. Repalntation of the amputated distal part of the fingers. *J Hand Surg.* 1985;10A:211–218.

Ring Avulsion Injuries

NISSENBAUM M. Class IIA ring avulsion injuries: an absolute indication for microvascular repair. *J Hand Surg.* 1989; 9A:810–815.

URBANIAK JR, EVANS JP, BRIGHT DS. Microvascular management of ring avulsion injuries. *J Hand Surg.* 1981;6:25–30.

Chronic Conditions

Ulnar Artery Thrombosis

KOMAN LA, URBANIAK JR. Ulnar artery insufficiency: a guide to treatment. *J Hand Surg.* 1981;6:16–24.

KOMAN LA, URBANIAK JR. Ulnar artery thrombosis. *Hand Clin.* 1985;1:311–325.

PERIS MD, TOMAINO MM. Ulnar artery thrombosis: evaluation and indications for operative treatment and surgical technique. *Am J Orthop.* 1996;26:685–689.

Vasospastic and Systemic Disorders

BUERGER L. Thromboangitis obliterans: a study of the vascular lesions leading to presenile spontaneous gangrene. *Am J Med Sci.* 1908;136:567–580.

JONES NF. Ischemia of the hand in ischemic disease: the potential role of microsurgical revasculariation and digital sympathectomy. *Clin Plast Surg.* 1989;16:547–556.

JONES NF. Acute and chronic ischemia of the hand: pathophysiology, treatment, and prognosis. *J Hand Surg.* 1991;16A:1074–1083.

MILLER LM, MORGAN RF. Vasospastic disorders: etiology, recognition, and treatment. *Hand Clin.* 1993;9:171–187.

SAMPLE QUESTIONS

1. The least appropriate amputation for attempted replantation is:
   (a) midpalmar
   (b) single digit through middle phalanx
   (c) trans-humeral
   (d) single digit through proximal phalanx
   (e) multiple digits through proximal phalanx

2. The most appropriate treatment for ulnar artery thrombosis with symptomatic cold intolerance is:
   (a) excision of the thrombosed artery and reverse interpositional vein grafting
   (b) intra-arterial thrombolytic therapy
   (c) calcium channel blockers
   (d) stellate ganglion block
   (e) microsurgical sympathectomy

3. When compared with normals, cold-stress testing in patients with Raynaud's phenomenon is characterized by:
   (a) lower resting temperature, less significant decrease in temperature with cooling, longer recovery to baseline
   (b) lower resting temperature, more significant decrease in temperature with cooling, longer recovery to baseline
   (c) higher resting temperature, more significant decrease in temperature with cooling, longer recovery to baseline
   (d) higher resting temperature, less significant decrease in temperature with cooling, longer recovery to baseline
   (e) similar resting temperature, similar decrease in temperature with cooling, longer recovery to baseline

4. The histological layer that plays the most significant role in the control of thrombogenesis is the:
   (a) intima
   (b) media
   (c) adventitia
   (d) internal elastic lamina
   (e) external elastic lamina

5. A ring avulsion injury with a severe, soft tissue degloving injury is best initially managed by:
   (a) irrigation, debridement, and delayed primary closure
   (b) microvascular reconstruction
   (c) neurovascular pedicled island flap
   (d) primary amputation and closure
   (e) tubed pedicle flap coverage

Chapter 31

Arthritis of the Wrist and Hand

Mark E. Baratz, MD and Adrienne J. Towsen, MD

Arthritis of the wrist and hand is a common problem that can cause significant disability. Advances in non-operative and surgical management can improve function and the quality of life for patients with arthritis. This review is designed to help the reader understand the pathological processes in arthritis of the wrist and hand, as well as the spectrum of options for treatment.

ETIOLOGY

Arthritis of the wrist and hand is usually the result of idiopathic osteoarthritis. Other less common causes include the inflammatory arthritides such as rheumatoid arthritis, gout and psoriatic arthritis. Fractures extending into the joint surface and complete ligament injuries can cause post-traumatic arthritis. Examples in the wrist include arthritis from an untreated scapholunate ligament tear (scapholunate advanced collapse [SLAC]) and arthritis from an ununited scaphoid fracture (scaphoid non-union advanced collapse [SNAC]).

BASIC SCIENCE

Pathomechanics of Scapholunate Instability

Disruption of the scapholunate ligament and surrounding ligamentous restraints leads to separation of the scaphoid and lunate. The scaphoid moves into a position of flexion causing the proximal pole to ride on the dorsal aspect of the scaphoid fossa. Arthritis will occur over the ensuing years, apparent in three stages on plain radiographs (Fig. 31–1). In stage I, there is wear between the proximal pole of the scaphoid and the radial styloid. In stage II, the arthritis extends to the entire scaphoid fossa. In stage III, the capitate migrates proximally, and wear occurs between the head of the capitate and the lunate. The lunate fossa is usually spared, even in cases of long-term scapholunate instability.

Pathomechanics of Rheumatoid Arthritis

Rheumatoid arthritis of the wrist involves proliferation of the synovium lining of the joint. Degradative enzymes and mediators of inflammation are released in and around the joint cavity. Enzymes such as collagenase degrade and create laxity of the extrinsic and intrinsic ligaments of the wrist. This leads to a variety of abnormal carpal positions. The carpus can shift into a more ulnar position on the radius. This shift is often accompanied by radial deviation of the carpus and metacarpals. Palmar subluxation and supination of the carpus may also occur. If there is attenuation of the scapholunate ligament, scapholunate dissociation will follow. Over time, the capitate migrates into the space between the scaphoid and lunate. This process is called carpal collapse and leads to arthritis throughout the wrist joint.

Orthopaedic Surgery: The Essentials. Edited by M.E. Baratz, A.D. Watson, and J.E. Imbriglia. Thieme Medical Publishers, Inc., New York © 1999

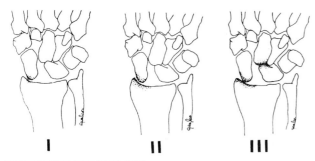

Figure 31–1 Schematic representation of the three stages of arthritis due to scapholunate instability. Reproduced with permission from Baratz ME, Towsen AJ. Midcarpal arthrodesis: four bone technique. In: *Techniques in Hand and Upper Extremity Surgery.* Vol 1, no 4. A: 1997;1:23.

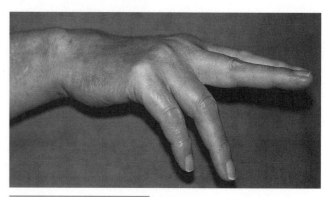

Figure 31–2 Loss of extension of the ring and small finger. This is due to attritional rupture from a dorsally subluxated ulnar head; the Vaughn-Jackson syndrome.

Synovitis in the distal radioulnar joint leads to dorsal subluxation of the ulnar head, referred to as caput ulnae. In this subluxed position, the extensor tendons of the fourth and fifth compartment can rub against the ulnar head. This leads to extensor tendon rupture of first the small, ring, and then the middle finger; a condition known as the Vaughn-Jackson syndrome (Fig. 31–2).

Synovitis of the metacarpophalangeal (MCP) joint can cause palmar subluxation and ulnar deviation of the proximal phalanx on the metacarpal head. Ulnar deviation of the fingers combined with radial deviation of the wrist and metacarpals is referred to as the Z-deformity (Fig. 31–3).

Inflammation of the proximal interphalangeal (PIP) joint can lead to the boutonniere deformity. Attenuation of the central slip of the extensor tendon will create flexion at the PIP joint combined with hyperextension of the distal interphalangeal (DIP) joint (Fig. 31–4). If the synovitis creates laxity of the palmar plate, a "swan-neck" deformity will occur with hyperextension at the PIP joint and flexion at the DIP joint (Fig. 31–5).

The boutonniere deformity of the thumb is the most common thumb deformity. The deformity consists of flexion at

the MCP joint and hyperextension of the interphalangeal (IP) joint. Subluxation of the metacarpal on the trapezium com-

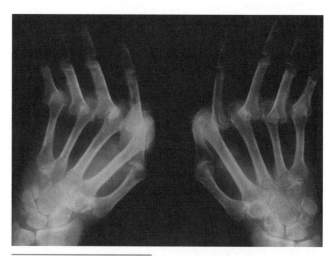

Figure 31–3 The Z-deformity. Ulnar deviation of the fingers with radial deviation of the wrist and metacarpals.

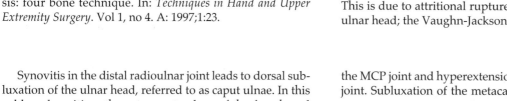

Attenuated
central slip

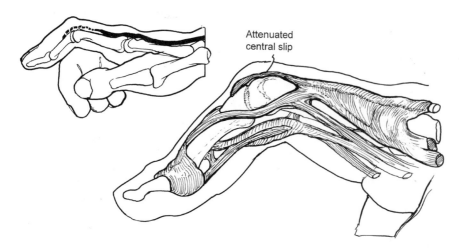

Figure 31–4 Boutonniere deformity. Reproduced with permission from Rizio L, Belsky MR. Finger deformities in rheumatoid arthritis. In: *Hand Clinics.*

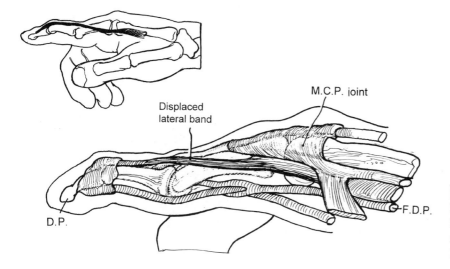

Figure 31–5 Swan-neck deformity. Reproduced with permission from Rizio L, Belsky MR. Finger deformities in rheumatoid arthritis. In: *Hand Clinics.* 1996;12:533.

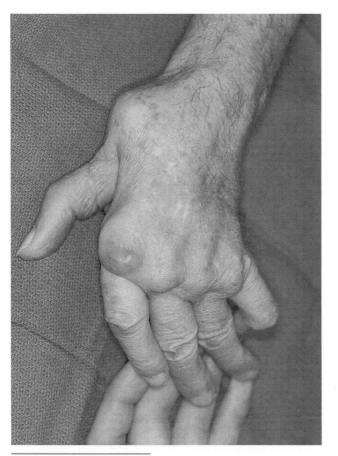

Figure 31–6 Swan-neck deformity of the thumb.

bined with hyperextension of the the MCP joint and flexion of the IP joint results in the swan-neck deformity (Fig. 31–6). This is the second most common thumb deformity in rheumatoid arthritis after the boutonniere deformity.

Silicone Synovitis

Silicone implants have been used to replace the scaphoid or lunate in scaphoid nonunion, SLAC wrist, and Kienbock's disease. In time, these carpal implants shed silicone particles into the joint. These particles incite an inflammatory response manifested by joint synovitis. This inflammatory response can cause extensive destruction of articular cartilage and resorption of bone. This process does not occur when silicone implants are used to replace MCP and IP joints. The loads across these joints are different than those which occur in the carpus. In addition, the joint has been resected so that there is no synovium to become inflammed and no articular cartilage to be destroyed.

Several studies have reported the incidence of silicone synovitis in patients with carpal implants. Late complications have been seen in patients since 1974. Symptoms of synovitis developed as early as 6 months and as late as 4 years after the implant surgery. Patients experienced pain, swelling, weakness, catching, and clicking. Radiographs demonstrated lytic lesions in the surrounding bones that progressed over time leading to increased bone destruction. Histologically, there is a multinuclear giant-cell reaction, associated with inflammation and fibrosis. The joint destruction may be eliminated by implant removal and synovectomy. It is recommended that patients who still have silicone implants be followed closely. The use of silicone implants remains controversial. The authors use them only for MCP and PIP joint arthroplasty.

Post-traumatic Arthritis

Degenerative arthritis can occur following a fracture that extends into the articular surface of the wrist joint. The factors thought to determine the onset of post-traumatic arthritis include the severity of the inital injury, the presence of residual incongruity in the joint surface, and associated ligament injuries affecting stability of the carpal bones.

ANATOMY
AND SURGICAL APPROACHES

Wrist Joint

Relevant Anatomy

Joint: The 8 bones of the wrist are bound together by interosseous ligaments and the joint capsule. The scapholunate interosseous ligament has 3 definable portions: palmar, dorsal and an intervening membranous portion. The dorsal and palmar portions confer the greatest stability to the scapholunate joint. The palmar capsule is more stout than the dorsal capsule. Its fibers are organized into bands that connect the carpal bones to each other and to the radius and ulna. The space of Poirer is a weak point in the center of the palmar capsule. It is through this weak point that the lunate extrudes following a lunate dislocation.

Nerves: The capsule of the wrist joint has extensive innervation by multiple nerve branches including the anterior and posterior interosseous nerves.

Tendons: Wrist extensors (extensor carpi radialis longus and brevis, extensor carpi ulnaris) and wrist flexors (flexor carpi radialis and ulnaris) cross the wrist joint. All insert into metacarpals except the flexor carpi ulnaris, which inserts into the pisiform.

Surgical Approach

The incision for a dorsal approach runs longitudinally along the dorsal aspect of the wrist to the mid-forearm. The subcutaneous tissues are elevated off the extensor retinaculum. The extensor retinaculum is divided between the tendons of the third and fourth extensor compartments. The extensor pollicis longus is released from its compartment and retracted toward the radial aspect of the wrist. The fourth extensor compartment can be elevated subperiosteally from the dorsal cortex (Fig. 31–7). Alternatively, the retinaculum over the fourth compartment can be opened with a Z-cut lengthening and the tendons retracted ulnarly.

Scaphotrapezialtrapezoid Joint

Relevant Anatomy

Joint: Strong intercarpal ligaments.

Nerves: Branches of radial sensory nerve pass directly over joint.

Tendons: Flexor carpi radialis longus passes directly beneath the joint en route to insertion at base of index metacarpal, middle finger metacarpal, and trapezial ridge.

Surgical Approach

An oblique or transverse incision is made over the scaphotrapezialtrapezoid (STT) joint. Identify, mobilize, and gently retract branches of the radial sensory nerve. Identify and cauterize the branch of radial artery crossing the STT joint (Fig. 31–8).

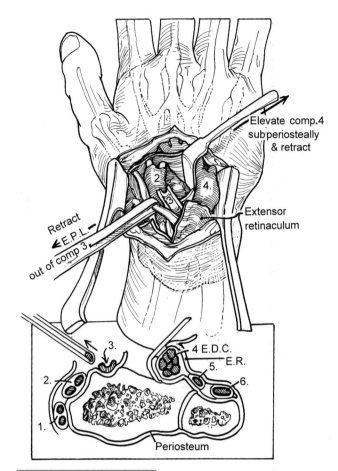

Figure 31–7   Dorsal approach to the wrist joint.

Thumb Carpometacarpal Joint

Relevant Anatomy

Joint: Saddle joint with 3 degrees of freedom. Primary static stabilizer is dorsal ligaments. The palmar "beak ligament" serves as a secondary stabilizer and pivot point during thumb rotation.

Nerves: Branches of the radial sensory and lateral antebrachial nerves course through the subcutaneous tissues at the base of the thumb. These branches innervate the dorsoradial aspect of the thumb and first web space.

Vessels: A dorsal branch of the radial artery passes over the capsule superficial to the scaphotrapezial joint. Three to four small branches supply the capsule. The artery then terminates in the deep arch of the hand (Fig. 31–9).

Tendons: The extensor pollicus brevis (EPB) and abductor pollicus longus (APL) pass through the first of six dorsal extensor compartments. The APL originates on the radius and interosseous membrane. Its multiple tendon slips insert on the thenar musculature and base of the thumb metacarpal. The EPB muscle orginates on the radius and interosseous membrane. Its tendon inserts on the base of the proximal phalanx. In approximately 50% of individuals, a septum will seperate the tendons of the EPB and APL in the first dorsal extensor compartment.

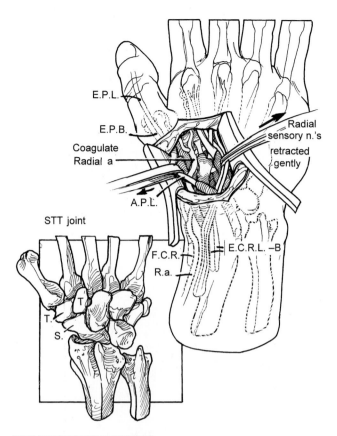

Figure 31–8 Dorsal radial approach to the STT joint. (Scaphotrapezialtrapezoid).

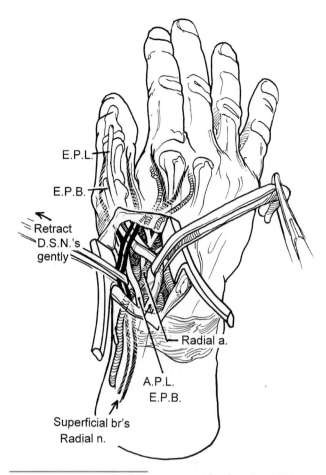

Figure 31–9 Dorsoradial exposure of the thumb CMC joint.

Surgical Approach

Dorsoradial approach (Fig. 31–10 A-D): Identify sensory branches. Release first dorsal extensor compartment. Approach joint capsule between EPB and multiple slips of APL. Identify and mobilize radial artery. Cauterize small branches to capsule. Reflect capsule to expose base of metacarpal, trapezium, and distal pole of scaphoid.

Metacarpophalangeal Joint
Relevant Anatomy

Joint: Metacarpal head is cam-shaped; as a result, collateral ligaments are lax with joint in extension, taut in flexion.

Nerves: The skin over the MCP joints is sparsely innervated. No major sensory nerves cross the MCP joint.

Vessels: Veins draining the fingers pass between the heads of the metacarpals.

Tendons: A single slip of the extensor digitorum communis (EDC) passes dorsal to the MCP joints of all four fingers, though anatomical variations occasionally occur (Fig. 31–11A). The index finger and small finger each have an additional tendon passing ulnar to the EDC tendon: the extensor indicis proprius (EIP) tendon to the index and the extensor digiti quinti (EDQ) to the small finger. Transverse fibers of the sagittal band pass from either side of the extensor tendon to the volar plate. These fibers help maintain the central position of the extensor tendon and are responsible for

extension of the proximal phalanx. Tendons of the lumbricals and interossei cross on either side of the MCP joint. The superficial head of the interossei insert on the base of the proximal phalanx. The deep head of the interossei and tendon of the lumbricals insert on the lateral bands of the extensor apparatus (see Fig. 31–11B).

Surgical Approach

Single joint: Use a dorsal longitudinal or transverse incision.

Multiple joints: Use a transverse incision. Divide the sagittal band on radial aspect of extensor tendon to expose capsule. Access to the MCP joint of the index and small fingers can be accomplished by dividing the extensor apparatus between the EDC and the EIP or EDQ tendons.

Proximal Interphalangeal and Distal Interphalangeal Joints
Relevant Anatomy

Nerves and vessels: Radial and ulnar digital nerves and arteries run along the palmar aspect of each finger, with the artery dorsal to the nerve. The nerve and artery divide into small terminal branches at the DIP joint.

Tendons: Three slips of the extensor apparatus pass dorsal to the PIP joint: the central slip and the radial and ulnar lateral bands. The central slip inserts on the base of the middle

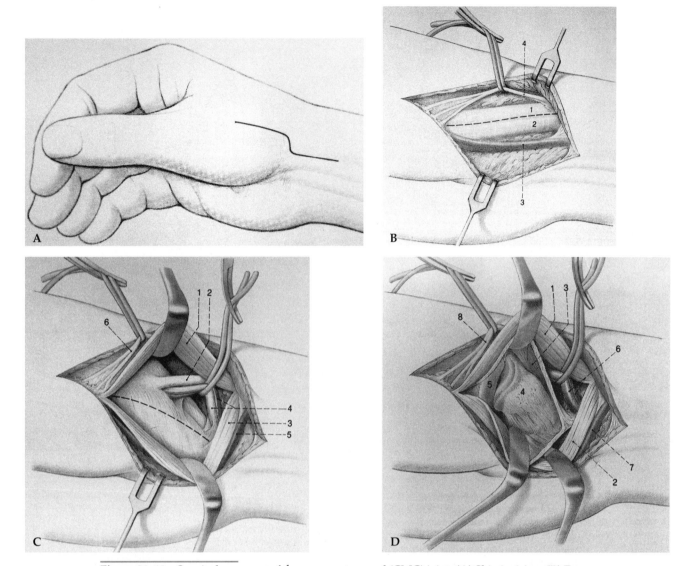

Figure 31–10   Surgical exposure of the carpometacarpal (CMC) joint. **(A)** Skin incision. **(B)** Exposure of superficial branch of radial nerve and splitting of tendon sheath. 1. Tendon of extensor pollicus brevis. 2. Tendon of abductor pollicus longus. 3. Cephalic vein of thumb. 4. Superficial branch of radial nerve. **(C)** The joint capsule is then opened over the CMC articulation of the thumb. 1. Extensor pollicus brevis. 2. Extensor carpi radialis longus. 3. Abductor pollicus longus. 4. Radial artery and vein. 5. Cephalic vein of thumb. 6. Superficial branch of radial nerve. **(D)** Open joint capsule. 1. Extensor pollicus brevis. 2. Abductor pollicus longus. 3. Capsule of CMC joint. 4. Trapezium. 5. Base of first metacarpal. 6. Radial artery and vein. 7. Cephalic vein of thumb. 8. Superficial branch of radial nerve. Reproduced with permission from Bauer R, Kerschbaumer F, Poisel S eds. *Operative Approaches in Orthopedic Surgery and Traumatology*. New York, NY: Thieme; 1987:305–306.

phalanx, allowing it to help maintain extension of the PIP joint. The lateral bands converge to form the terminal tendon just before it inserts on the distal phalanx. The terminal tendon works in conjuction with the spiral oblique retinacular ligament to extend the distal phalanx (Fig. 31–11A).

The finger has two tendons responsible for finger flexion, the flexor digitorum superficialis (FDS) and flexor digitorum profundus (FDP). The FDS tendon splits into two slips, each of which inserts on the base of the proximal phalanx. The FDP tendon inserts on the base of the distal phalanx. The flexor sheath condenses into a series of annular and cruciate

pulleys. Intact A2 and A4 pulleys are necessary to prevent bowstringing of the flexor tendons.

Surgical Approaches

Dorsal approach to the PIP joint: Adequate visualization can be achieved through a dorsal longitudinal incision combined with a longitudinal split in the extensor tendon over the PIP joint. During exposure for joint replacement, the insertion of the central slip on the base of the middle phalanx must be preserved.

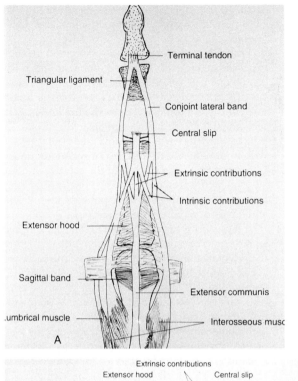

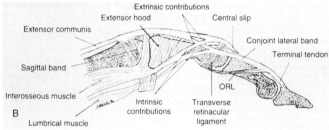

Figure 31–11 Dorsal view **(A)** and side view **(B)** of the extensor mechanism. Reproduced with permission from Rizio L, Belsky MR. Finger deformities in rheumatoid arthritis. In: *Hand Clinics.* 1996;12:532.

Palmar approach to the PIP joint: The skin is incised using a zigzag (Brunner) incision with the apex at the flexion crease of the PIP joint (Fig. 31–12). Both neurovascular bundles are identified and protected. The flexor sheath is opened between the A2 and A4 pulleys (Fig. 31–13). The FDS and FDP tendons are retracted to gain access to the palmar plate. The joint is opened by reflecting the proximal extension of the palmar plate.

Dorsal approach to the DIP joint: An H-shaped incision is made over the DIP joint. The distal extensions of this incision should stay a minimum of 5 mm from the nail fold. During exposure for DIP fusion, the transverse limb of the "H" can be carried through the terminal tendon to the joint. This avoids unnecessary undermining of the skin.

PEARL

Patients with STT arthritis often present with flexor carpi radialis tendonitis because the tendon passes directly palmar to joint.

EXAMINATION

While obtaining a history of wrist pain ask if it is related to remote or recent trauma. Wrist pain is usually worse with

use. Ask if the patient or his relatives have history of inflammatory arthritis. During the examination note deformity including malalignment at the wrist, metacarpophalangeal joints and fingers is essential to document joint motion particularly when considering joint replacement of the MCP or PIP joint.

PITFALL

The average MCP silicone arthroplasty results in 45 degrees of motion. The average PIP silicone arthroplasty results in 60 degrees of motion. Checking finger motion is an essential part of the initial examination for patients with inflammatory arthritis of the fingers.

Palpate for areas of tenderness and try to correlate this finding to the patient's complaints and radiographic findings. Provocative maneuvers can bring out areas of tenderness not apparent on the initial survey. For example the grind maneuver helps in the diagnosis of thumb CMC arthritis. This is performed by placing an axial load on thumb metacarpal while rotating the metacarpal or pushing the base dorsally and palmarly.

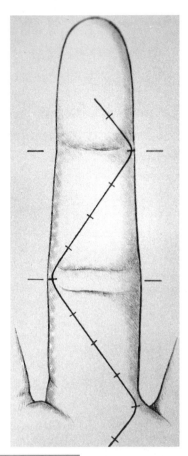

Figure 31–12 The Brunner zigzag incision. Reproduced with permission from Bauer R, Kerschbaumer F, Poisel S, eds. *Operative Approaches in Orthopedic Surgery and Traumatology.* New York, NY: Thieme; 1987:314.

AIDS TO DIAGNOSIS

Plain radiographs are the cornerstone of the evaluation for wrist and hand arthritis. Additional studies are rarely necessary. Tomograms may be helpful in determining extent of arthritis due to SLAC; information important to choosing the appropriate reconstructive procedure.

A bone scan is useful in a patient who has arthritic pain and normal radiographs. It is particularly helpful in identifying early thumb carpometacarpal (CMC) and STT joint arthritis. Relief of pain following a lidocaine injection into a joint suspected of being the source of painful arthritis can help confirm the diagnosis.

SPECIFIC CONDITIONS, TREATMENT, AND OUTCOME

Scapholunate Advanced Collapse

In the earliest stage of SLAC arthritis, wear occurs between the radial half of the scaphoid fossa and scaphoid. Radial styloidectomy may be considered in this situation. In a stage II SLAC wrist, the entire scaphoid fossa is degenerated, but there is no arthritis on the head of the capitate or lunate

fossa. At this stage, proximal row carpectomy or scaphoid excision with capitolunatetriquetral hamarte (CLTH) fusion are both viable options.

Proximal row carpectomy is performed through a dorsal exposure to the wrist. The head of the capitate is inspected to ensure that it is free of degenerative changes. The scaphoid is split in half and removed, followed by the lunate and triquetrum. The capitate rests on the lunate fossa. We do not recommended pinning the capitate to the radius. The capsule is closed, and the wrist is immobilized for 4 weeks. Pain relief with approximately 70 degrees of wrist motion is expected. Degenerative changes between the capitate and lunate fossa are evident in approximately 30% of patients at long-term followup, although most of these patients are not symptomatic and have not required further surgery.

If the arthritis has progressed to stage III with capitolunate joint degeneration, scaphoid exision with CLTH fusion is our treatment of choice. Through a dorsal approach, the articular surfaces are examined to confirm the extent of arthritis. The scaphoid is split, excised, and retained for use as bone graft. The articular cartilage and subchondral plate are removed from the articulating surfaces of the capitate, lunate, hamate, and triquetrum. At the lunotriquetral joint, only the distal half of the articulation is taken down to avoid damaging the remaining articulating surfaces of the radiocarpal joint. Prior to internal fixation, the capitate must be reduced on the lunate in two planes. In a stage III SLAC wrist, the capitate migrates proximally between the scaphoid and lunate. With the lunate in a dorsiflexed position, the capitate head is exposed when viewed from the dorsal surface; the "naked capitate" sign. Prior to fusion, the capitate must be moved directly over the lunate. The lunate can be reduced from its dorsiflexed position by pressing down on the neck of the capitate. Pins, screws, or staples can be used to provide internal fixation. Morselized scaphoid and distal radius bone graft, if necessary, are applied to the fusion site. The wrist is immobilized for 8 weeks. If plain radiographs are inconclusive to assess healing, tomograms are obtained. Average wrist motion after scaphoid excision and CLTH fusion is about 60 degrees. The nonunion rate should be less than 10%. Radiocarpal arthritis has been seen in less than 5% on long-term followup.

Total wrist fusion may be necessary for failed proximal row carpectomy or scaphoid excision with CLTH fusion, or in rare instances where the lunate fossa is degenerated. Rigid internal fixation combined with autogenous bone graft results in a high rate of union. The wrist should be positioned in approximately 10 degrees of dorsiflexion and 5 degrees of ulnar deviation.

Rheumatoid Arthritis (RA)

The initial evaluation of a person with rheumatoid arthritis should be used to characterize his disease, identify which structures will benefit from surgical care, and to determine the timing of surgery. The surgeon must document the onset and progression of the RA, as well as prior treatment. The surgeon should identify the most symptomatic joints. If possible, start with those operations with predictably good outcome such as tenosynovectomy and MP fusion.

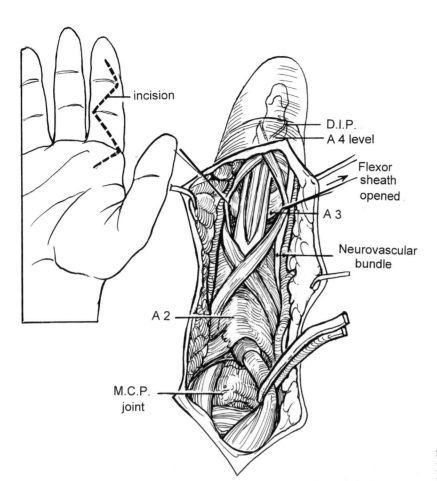

incision

D.I.P.
A 4 level

Flexor
sheath
opened

A 3

Neurovascular
bundle

A 2

M.C.P.
joint

Figure 31–1 Palmar approach to the PIP joint.

The Rheumatoid Wrist

Tenosynovitis

Synovectomy is recommended after 6 months of failed medical management. Extensor tendons are approached through a dorsal longitudinal incision. The dorsal retinaculum is Z-lengthened. Synovium is excised from around and within the tendons. Tendon edges are imbricated with a No. 4-0 nylon suture after exision of intratendinous synovitis. Prominent spicules are debrided from the dorsal aspect of the radius and the ulna. One limb of the retinaculum is repaired above and one below the EDC and extensor digiti minimi (EDM) tendons. The extensor pollicis longus (EPL) tendon is left free in the subcutaneous tissue.

Flexor tendons are approached through an extended, carpal tunnel incision including carpal tunnel release. Synovectomy is combined with debridement of spicules from the palmar aspect of wrist, for example, on scaphoid tubercle (Mannerfelt lesion).

Brown and Brown (1988) reported a 4% incidence of recurrent synovitis and a 2% incidence of rupture in previously intact tendons following synovectomy.

Tendon Rupture

Most tendon ruptures in rheumatoid arthritis are the result of chronic synovitis combined with abrasion against a prominent spicule of bone. As such, direct repair is impossible. Tendon grafting can be considered if the rupture was recent,

TABLE 31–1 Recommended tendons

Ruptured tendon	Tendon Transfer
Extensor pollicus longus	EIP
EDM and/or EDC	
One tendon	Side-to-side with EDC
Two tendons	Side-to-side with EDC for first, EIP for second
Three tendons	FDS or use wrist extensor (may need tendon graft)
Flexor pollicus longus	FDS transfer

leaving a functional motor. In chronic cases, tendon transfers are recommended using the tendons listed in Table 31–1.

Ertel et al (1988) reviewed the results of flexor tendon ruptures and observed the worst result with multiple ruptures in carpal canal, FDS and FDP ruptures in the same finger and in patients with advanced or aggressive rheumatoid arthritis.

Wrist Malalignment

Radial deviation of the carpus and metacarpal is a common deformity that must be corrected prior to addressing malalignment of the MCP joints. If the wrist is pain-free and has little or no arthritic changes, transfer of the extensor carpi radialis longus to the extensor carpi ulnaris can be used to reposition the wrist in slight ulnar deviation. Radiolunate fusion is second option, particularly when there is marked ulnar subluxation of the carpus.

Dorsal subluxation of the distal ulna (caput ulna syndrome) can result in pain, loss of forearm rotation, and attritional rupture of the overlying EDM and EDC tendons; the Vaughn-Jackson syndrome (Fig. 31–2). Two procedures have been commonly used to treat the dorsally subluxated ulnar head: resection of the distal ulna (Darrach procedure) or fusion of the ulna head to the radius with resection of a segment of ulnar diaphysis just proximal to the ulnar head (Sauve-Kapandji procedure). The Darrach procedure is simple to perform (Fig. 31–14). The Darrach procedure may be complicated by instability of the resected end of the distal ulna and ulnar subluxation of the carpus. The Sauve-Kapandji procedure carries the risk of nonunion, as well as instability of the resected end of the distal ulna. By preserving the ulnar head, the carpus should be supported and have less tendency toward ulnar subluxation.

Wrist Degeneration

Degeneration of the radiocarpal joint with a preserved midcarpal joint can be treated with a radioscapholunate fusion. Pancarpal arthritis is best treated in most instances with wrist arthrodesis. This can be accomplished with either pin or plate

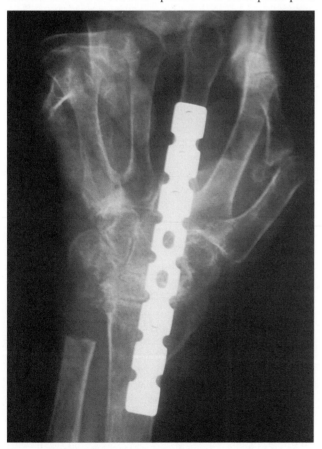

Figure 31–14 Fusion of the wrist combined with resection of the ulnar head; the Darrach resection.

fixation. We found equivalent fusion and complication rates using these two forms of fixation. With plates, it is easier to set and maintain wrist position. However, plates cannot be used in patients with very osteopenic bone or "tissue-paper skin," a situation often seen concurrently. Pins may migrate and cause local skin irritation or infections. However, they are easy to remove and can be used in patients with poor quality bone and skin.

Wrist arthroplasty may be considered in the low demand individual with a balanced wrist. It requires an intact extensor carpi radialis brevis tendon. The initial good results seen with wrist replacement seem to degenerate over time. Silicone implants may fracture and become symptomatic. Minimally constrained implants with metal stems have eroded through the metacarpal shaft. These same implants can loosen in a poorly balanced wrist.

Degeneration of the distal radioulnar joint is treated with either resection of the distal ulna or the Sauve-Kapandji procedure as described above.

Fingers: Metacarpophalangeal Joints

Synovitis

Synovitis of the MCP joints is managed initially with anti-inflammatory medications, splinting, and cortisone injections. When swelling persists after 6 months of medical treatment, synovectomy is recommended.

Malalignment

Joint malalignment consists of ulnar drift combined with palmar subluxation of the proximal phalanges on the metacarpal head. It may be associated with radial deviation of the carpus and metacarpal: the Z-deformity (Fig. 31–3). Failure to correct the radial deviation of the carpus can result in recurrent ulnar deviation of the phalanges. In MCP joints without advanced degeneration, it is possible to perform a soft-tissue realignment consisting of:

1. transverse incision across the metacarpal heads
2. synovectomy/joint debridement
3. release of palmar plate
4. centralization of tendon with reefing of radial extensor hood; release of junctura
5. intrinsic release with crossed intrinsic transfer

Metacarpophalangeal Joint Degeneration

If the joints are degenerated or impossible to reduce without shortening the metacarpal, then silicone arthroplasty is recommended (Fig. 31–15). Preoperative joint motion should be less than 45 degrees as this is the average motion after arthroplasty. The technique of silicone arthroplasty includes:

1. synovectomy and intrinsic release
2. release of collateral ligaments from metacarpal head
3. resection of metacarpal head at level of collateral ligament origin
4. clearing of metacarpal canal, placement of drill hole in radial aspect of metacarpal
5. release of palmar plate from proximal phalanx
6. creation of opening in base of proximal phalanx with burr

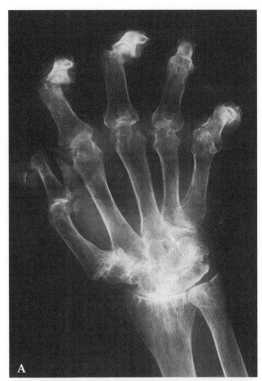

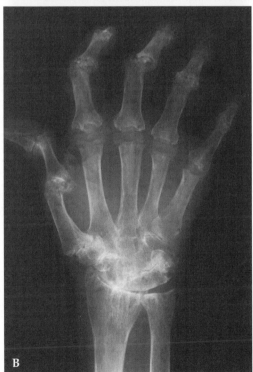

Figure 31–15 **(A)** Degenerated MCP joints due to rheumatoid arthritis. **(B)** The same hand after MCP joint arthroplasty.

7. trial implant. Must be able to fully extend without resistance. If can't, need to shorten metacarpal or use smaller implant.

8. irrigation and placement of implant

9. suturing of radial collateral ligament to radial aspect of metacarpal neck through small drill hole

10. centralization of tendon. May require release of radial half of extensor hood and junctura tendinae.

Postoperatively, a splint is applied in extension for 10 to 14 days. Use dynamic traction for 8 weeks, night splinting for 3 months. Kirschenbaum et al (1993) reported average motion of 45 to 55 degrees with a 15% rate of implant fracture at 8.5 years. Only 2% required revision. Pain relief, improved function, and improved appearance were consistently achieved. Loss of hand function over time was mostly related to deterioration of PIP joint motion.

The most challenging joints in our experience were those with marked palmar subluxation, especially with overriding of the proximal phalanx on the metacarpal head. In these individuals the surgeon may need to resect more of the metacarpal head and neck than usual. If resection is not adequate, the implant will fit tight and the proximal phalanx will palmarly subluxate. This will limit MCP joint extension and lead to premature implant failure.

Fingers: Interphalangeal Joints

Synovitis
Synovitis is managed the same as in the MCP joint.

Joint Malalignment and Degeneration
Two forms of joint malalignment are commonly seen in rheumatoid arthritis: boutonniere deformity and swan-neck deformity. The boutonniere deformity (see Fig. 31–4) includes the following:

1. attenuation of central slip

2. flexion of PIP joint

3. palmar subluxation of the lateral bands

4. hyperextension of the DIP joint

Nalebuff and Millender (1975) described three stages of boutonniere deformity:

Stage I: This is a mild deformity with an extension lag of < 15 degrees of the PIP joint. The deformity is passively correctable (the PIP joint can be passively extended) and there is no arthritis in the PIP joint. A stage I boutonniere can be treated with tenotomy of the extensor tendon just distal to the insertion of the central slip; the "Dolphin" or "Fowler" procedure.

Stage II: This is a moderate deformity with an extension lag < 40 degrees. The PIP joint is not passively correctable. Treatment consists of synovectomy with release of the transverse retinacular ligament to allow dorsal relocation of lateral bands. The lateral bands are sutured over the PIP joint. A Fowler tenotomy is used to improve DIP flexion.

Stage III: This is a severe deformity that is fixed with a degenerated PIP joint. The treatment is PIP joint fusion or arthroplasty. Arthroplasty is recommended in the ring and small finger. When done through a palmar approach the result seems to be more motion, sooner.

Kiefhaber and Strickland (1993) found that soft-tissue recontruction for severe boutonniere deformities was unpredictable and at best showed modest gains that deteriorated over time. Proximal interphalangeal fusion was recommended for joints with severe extensor lag or for any fixed deformity.

The swan-neck deformity can result from:

1. a chronic mallet deformity
2. an incompetent PIP joint palmar plate
3. intrinsic tendon tightness
4. metacarpophalangeal joint palmar subluxation + intrinsic tendon tightness

The deformity (see Fig. 31–5) consists of:

1. hyperextension at PIP joint
2. dorsal subluxation of lateral bands
3. loss of extensor tone at DIP joint; that is, extensor lag

Nalebuff and Millender (1975) described three types of swan-neck deformity:

Type I Swan-neck deformity: Supple. For the supple swan neck deformity there are 3 options depending on the location of the maximum deformity.

1. Distal interphalangeal fusion is performed if the deformity orginates at the DIP joint, and holding DIP joint in extension eliminates the swan-neck deformity.
2. Spiral oblique ligament reconstruction is used if the deformity began with loss of DIP extension and the DIP joint is not arthritic. A tendon graft is fixed to the extensor insertion on DIP joint. It is passed around the middle phalanx, dorsal to neurovascular bundle. The graft is then passed beneath the PIP joint palmar to the flexor sheath. The graft is then inserted into a bone tunnel in the midproximal phalanx. The graft is tensioned so that the DIP extends when the PIP joint is extended.
3. The "sublimis sling" can be used for swan neck deformity that begins with hyperextension at the PIP joint. One slip of the sublimis (flexor digitorum superficialis) is detached proximal to the A2 pulley. The tendon slip is passed through a slit in the A2 pulley and sutured to its insertion with PIP joint flexed about 30 degrees.

Type II Swan-neck deformity: Intrinsic tightness. This deformity is usually the result of MCP joint subluxation that causes secondary intrinsic tightness. Treatment begins with correction of the MCP joint deformity by either soft-tissue realignment or MCP arthroplasty. This is followed by an intrinsic release combined with DIP fusion or a sublimis sling procedure.

Type III Swan-neck deformity: Stiff without joint destruction. This deformity can be treated with joint manipulation or soft-tissue release combined with mobilization of the lateral bands. The PIP joint is pinned for 10 to 14 days.

Type IV Swan-neck deformity: Stiff with joint destruction. This deformity is treated with either PIP joint fusion or arthroplasty.

PEARL
Joint space narrowing without advanced joint destruction does not seem to preclude a successful soft-tissue procedure in treating swan-neck deformities.

Thumb

Synovitis
Synovitis is treated the same as in other joints.

Joint Malalignment and Degeneration
Nalebuff (1988) described five types of thumb deformity:

Type I Rheumatoid Thumb: Boutonniere deformity. This is the most common and has been divided into three stages:

Stage 1: This is a supple deformity that is passively correctable. It is treated with synovectomy of the MCP joint and repositioning of the extensor tendons dorsal to the MCP joint.

Stage 2: This boutonniere deformity has a fixed MCP joint and a supple interphalangeal (IP) joint. An MCP joint fusion can be performed if the carpometacarpal (CMC) and IP joints are not degenerated. If there is arthritis of the CMC and IP joints MCP arthroplasty can be performed.

Stage 3: In this deformity the MP and IP joints are fixed. The deformity can be corrected with an interphalangeal joint fusion and MCP arthroplasty.

Type II Rheumatoid thumb: Boutonniere deformity and CMC subluxation. This rare deformity consists of flexion at the MCP joint, extension at the IP joint and CMC joint subluxation. It is treated with CMC arthroplasty combined with boutonniere reconstruction as described above.

Type III Rheumatoid thumb: Swan-neck deformity (Fig. 31–6). This is the second most common deformity of thumbs affected by rheumatoid arthritis. The deformity consists of subluxation of the CMC joint, adduction of metacarpal, hyperextension of the MP joint, and flexion of the IP joint.

Nalebuff (1988) defined three stages of the swan-neck thumb deformity:

Stage 1. Carpometacarpal subluxation with no MCP hyperextension. This is treated with CMC arthroplasty.

Stage 2. Carpometacarpal subluxation with MCP hyperextension. A CMC arthroplasty is combined with advancement of the palmar plate of the MCP joint or MCP fusion if the joint is degenerated.

Stage 3. Swan deformity with web space contracture. Treatment is the same as in a stage 2 deformity with the addition of a web space release. The metacarpal bases may need to be resected to acheive adequate correction.

Type IV Rheumatoid Thumb: Gamekeeper's deformity. In this deformity the collateral ligament of the MCP joint is lax. The thumb proximal phalanx is radially deviated. In advanced cases there may be an associated adduction contracture of the metacarpal. It is treated with fusion of the MCP joint and, if necessary, a web space release.

Type V Rheumatoid Thumb: Metacarpophalangeal hyperextension with IP flexion. No CMC joint subluxation is present. This condition can be treated with MCP fusion and IP joint palmar plate advancement or MP arthroplasty with IP joint fusion.

SELECTED BIBLIOGRAPHY

Pathogenesis of Degenerative Arthritis of the Wrist

WATSON KH, RYU J. Evolution of arthritis of the wrist. *Clin Orthop.* 1986;202:57–67.

Pathogenesis of Post-traumatic Arthritis of the Wrist

BARATZ M, DES JARDINS J, ANDERSON D, IMBRIGLIA J. Displaced Intra-articular fractures of the distal radius: the effect of fracture displacement on contact stresses in a cadaver model. *J Hand Surg.* 1996;21A:183–188.

Silicone Synovitis

CARTER PR, BENTON LJ, DYSERT PA. A Study of the incidence of late osseous complications. *J Hand Surg.* 1986;11A:639–644.

PEIMER CA, MEDIGE J, ECKERT BS, WRIGHT JR, HOWARD CS. Reactive synovitis after silicone arthroplasty. *J Hand Surg.* 1986;11A:624–638.

SMITH RJ, ATKINSON RE, JUPITER JB. Silicone synovitis of the wrist. *J Hand Surg.* 1985;10A:47–60.

Proximal Row Carpectomy

CULP RW, McGUIGAN FX, TURNER MA, LICHTMAN DM, OSTERMAN AL, McCARROLL HR. Proximal row carpectomy: a multicenter study. *J Hand Surg.* 1993;18A:19–25.

IMBRIGLIA JE, BROUDY AS, HAGBERG WC, McKERNAN D. Proximal row carpectomy: clinical evaluation. *J Hand Surg.* 1990;15A:426–430.

WYRICK JD, STERN PJ, KIEFHABER TR. Motion-preserving procedures in the treatment of scapholunate advanced collapse wrist: proximal row carpectomy versus four-corner arthrodesis. *J Hand Surg.* 1995;20A:965–970.

Scaphoid Excision and Intercarpal Fusion

ASHMEAD D, WATSON K, DAMON C, HERBER S, PALY W. Scapholunate advanced collapse wrist salvage. *J Hand Surg.* 1994;19A:741–750.

KRAKAUER J, BISHOP AT, COONEY WP. Surgical treatment of scapholunate advanced collapse. *J Hand Surg.* 1994;19A:751–759.

Wrist Arthrodesis

BOLANO LE, GREEN DP. Wrist arthrodesis in post-traumatic arthritis: A comparison of two methods. *J Hand Surg.* 1993;18A:786–791.

Rheumatoid Tenosynovitis

BROWN FE, BROWN ML. Long-term results after tenosynovectomy to treat the rheumatoid hand. *J Hand Surg.* 1988;13A:704–798.

ERTEL AN, MILLENDER LH, NALEBUFF E, McKAY D, LESLIE B. Flexor tendon ruptures in patients with rheumatoid arthritis. *J Hand Surg.* 1988;13A:860–866.

Rheumatoid Wrist Malalignment and Degeneration

CLAYTON ML, FERLIC DC: Tendon transfer for radial rotation of the wrist in rheumatoid arthritis. *Clin Orthop.* 1974;100:176–185.

LINSCHEID RL, DOBYNS JH. Radiolunate arthrodesis. *J Hand Surg.* 1986;10A:821–829.

LOLLY SL, FERLIC DC, CLAYTON ML, DENNIS DA, STRINGER EA. Swanson silicone arthroplasty of the wrist in rheumatoid arthritis: a long-term followup. *J Hand Surg.* 1992;17A:142–149.

Rheumatoid Arthritis Involving the Distal Radioulnar Joint

DINGMAN PVC. Resection of the distal ulna (Darrach operation) an end-result study of 24 cases. *J Bone Jt Surg.* 1952;43A:893–900.

LESLIE BM, CARLSON G, RUBY LK. Results of extensor carpi ulnaris tenodesis in the rheumatoid wrist undergoing a distal ulnar excision. *J Hand Surg.* 1990;15A:547–551.

VINCENT KA, SZABO RM, AGEE JM. The Sauve-Kapandji procedure for reconstruction for the rheumatoid distal radioulnar joint. *J Hand Surg.* 1993;18A:978–983.

Rheumatoid Arthritis of the Metacarpophalangeal Joints

Ellison MR, Kelly KI, Flatt AE. The results of surgical synovectomy of the digital joints in rheumatoid disease. *J Bone Jt Surg.* 1971;53A:1041–1060.

Kirschenbaum D, Schneider LH, Adams DC, Cody RP. Arthroplasty of the metacarpophalangeal jointds with use of silicone-rubber implants in patients who have rheumatoid arthritis. Long-term results. *J Bone Jt Surg.* 1993;75A: 3–12.

Wood VE, Ichtertz DR, Yahiku H. Soft tissue metacarpophalangeal reconstruction for treatment of rheumatoid hand deformity. *J Hand Surg.* 1989;14A:163–174.

Rheumatoid Arthritis of the Interphalangeal Joints

Adamson GJ, Gellman H, Brumfield RH, Kuschner SH, Lawler JW. Flexible implant resection arthroplasty of the proximal interphalangeal joint in patients with systemic inflammatory arthritis. *J Hand Surg.* 1994;19A:378–384.

Keifhaber TR, Strickland JW. Soft tissue reconstruction for rheumatoid swan-neck and boutonniere deformities: long-term results. *J Hand Surg.* 1993;18A:984–989.

Nalebuff EA, Millender LH. Surgical treatment of the boutonniere deformity in rheumatoid arthritis. *Orthop Clin North Am.* 1975;6:753–763.

Nalebuff EA, Millender LH. Surgical treatment of the swan-neck deformity in rheumatoid arthritis. *Orthop Clin North Am.* 1975;6:733–752.

Rheumatoid Thumb

Nalebuff EA, Feldon PG, Millender LH. Rheumatoid arthritis in the hand and wrist. In: Green, ed. *Operative Hand Surgery.* New York, NY: Churchill Livingstone; 1988: 1744–1759.

SAMPLE QUESTIONS

1. Flexor carpi radialis tendonitis may be the presenting complaint of which form of wrist arthritis:
   - (a) thumb CMC
   - (b) stage II SLAC arthritis
   - (c) scaphotrapezialtrapezoid arthritis
   - (d) stage III SLAC arthritis
   - (e) stage IV Kienbock's disease

2. The swan-neck deformity of the thumb may consist of all of the following except:
   - (a) flexion of the IP joint
   - (b) subluxation of the metacarpal on the trapezium
   - (c) hyperextension of the MCP joint
   - (d) abduction of the thumb metacarpal
   - (e) thumb web space contracture

3. During resection of the trapezium during thumb CMC joint arthroplasty, the following structures should be identified:
   - (a) radial sensory nerve
   - (b) radial artery
   - (c) extensor pollicus longus tendon
   - (d) abductor pollicus longus tendon
   - (e) flexor carpi radialis longus tendon

4. A 57-year-old woman with rheumatoid arthritis has a fixed flexion deformity of her left ring finger PIP joint with hyperextension of her DIP joint. The treatment option with the most predictable outcome is:
   - (a) soft-tissue release with reconstruction of the extensor apparatus over the PIP joint
   - (b) proximal interphalangeal joint arthrodesis
   - (c) proximal interphalangeal joint arthroplasty
   - (d) extensor tendon tenotomy over the middle phalanx
   - (e) soft-tissue release with reconstruction of the extensor apparatus over the PIP joint with extensor tendon tenotomy over the middle phalanx

5. A 37-year-old accountant has arthritis of his right wrist due to SLAC arthritis. At the time of surgery, the degeneration is found to include the radioscaphoid and midcarpal joints. The procedure that will best eliminate the foci of his arthritis while preserving wrist motion is a:
   - (a) scaphotrapezialtrapezoid arthrodesis
   - (b) scaphotrapezialtrapezoid arthrodesis with radial styloidectomy
   - (c) proximal row carpectomy
   - (d) scaphoid excision with intercarpal fusion
   - (e) scaphoid replacement arthroplasty

Answers: 1) c; 2) d; 3) c; 4) b; 5) d

Pelvis, Hip, and Femur

Chapter 32

Pelvis, Acetabulum, and Hip Trauma

Matthew L. Jimenez, MD

Pelvis and acetabulum injuries often occur in the setting of high-energy trauma. These injuries are usually complex and require thorough evaluation for appropriate treatment planning in order to maximize functional outcome. Hip fractures are common in the ever-increasing elderly population. A thorough understanding of the patient's function and health and treatment that facilitates rapid mobilization optimizes the prognosis after hip fracture.

ETIOLOGY

Pelvic ring injury, acetabular fracture, hip dislocation, and femoral head fracture are typically due to high-energy trauma. Vital organ injury and blood loss are leading causes of morbidity and mortality.

Four different basic force patterns can cause pelvic injury. Anteroposterior (AP) force is commonly applied from anterior, externally rotates the hemipelvis, and opens the symphysis pubis. Greater force leads to progressive disruption including injury to the anterior and, ultimately, the posterior sacroiliac ligaments.

Lateral compression force is directed toward the lateral aspect of the pelvis or greater trochanter. Posteriorly directed lateral compression force causes cancellous impaction fracture of the sacrum. Anteriorly directed lateral compression force causes internal rotation of the hemipelvis. The typical result is pubic rami fracture or overlap and fracture of the anterior portion of the sacral ala.

External rotation force is usually applied to the pelvis through forced abduction of the lower extremity and is commonly associated with motorcycle accidents. It often results in complete disruption of the anterior pelvis, as well as the anterior and posterior ligaments of the posterior pelvis.

Shear forces are often due to vertical or oblique loading patterns. The force pattern is applied perpendicular to the bony trabeculae, and often leads to a fracture pattern that is both vertically and rotationally unstable.

Acetabulum fractures typically occur in motor vehicle accidents or in a fall from a height. The position of the leg, the direction of the force, and the associated pelvic injury determine the fracture pattern. Hip dislocation, femoral head fracture, or femoral neck fracture may accompany acetabular fracture.

Subtrochanteric and femoral shaft fractures are usually the result of high-energy trauma such as a motor vehicle accident or fall from a height. Acetabulum, pelvis, or femoral neck fractures may coexist.

Most femoral head fractures occur in motor vehicle accidents. Axial load of the femur applied at the foot or knee by the floorboard or dashboard, respectively, causes fractures of the femoral head from cleavage on the acetabular rim or avulsion from the ligamentum teres. Femoral head fractures are most commonly associated with hip dislocations.

Femoral neck and intertrochanteric hip fractures are low-energy injuries that occur in the elderly population and are the result of a fall. It is unclear whether the fracture occurs before, during, or upon impact. Femoral neck fractures in the young population are usually due to high-energy trauma. Axial loading of the femur by knee or foot impact with the dashboard or floorboard of a motor vehicle and axial loading of the femur from a fall from a height are common mechanisms.

BASIC SCIENCE

Evaluation and treatment of pelvis injuries are determined by pelvic stability; therefore, biomechanical considerations

467

Orthopaedic Surgery: The Essentials. Edited by M.E. Baratz, A.D. Watson, and J.E. Imbriglia. Thieme Medical Publishers, Inc., New York © 1999

define the injury and its treatment. Two analogies help illustrate pelvic stability. First, the pelvis can be considered a suspension bridge with the iliac wings as the bridge's pillars, and the interosseous and posterior sacroiliac ligaments as the suspension wires to prevent inferior sacral displacement. Second, the pelvis also behaves as an arch, with the sacrum as the keystone.

Biomechanical stability is defined as the ability of the pelvis to withstand normal physiologic loads without displacing. Vertical instability describes vertical displacement at the sacroiliac joint at physiologic loads. Rotational instability is present when the pelvis is free to open like a book or close so that the rami overlap.

ANATOMY AND SURGICAL APPROACHES

Anatomy

The pelvis is the bony link between the spine and the lower extremities. Significant forces are transmitted from the appendicular to the axial skeleton through the pelvis when ambulating and sitting.

The pelvic ring comprises the sacrum and two innominate bones. The two innominate bones are joined anteriorly at the pubic symphysis and posteriorly to the sacrum at the sacroiliac joints.

The pelvic brim is demarcated by the iliopectineal line, which divides the pelvis into the false pelvis above and the true pelvis below. The false pelvis consists of the sacral ala and iliac wings and contains the abdominal contents. The true pelvis comprises the ischiae and caudal sacrum and contains the major neurovascular structures and urogenital organs. The floor of the true pelvis consists of the coccyx and the coccygeal and levator ani muscles. The urethra, rectum, and vagina pass through the pelvic floor.

The anterior-inferior portion of the sacroiliac joint is predominantly cartilaginous. The posterior-superior portion is a strongly ligamentous syndesmotic joint between the sacrum and the posterior tuberosity of the ilium (Fig. 32–1). The symphysis pubis contains hyaline cartilage and fibrocartilage.

Anterior and posterior ligaments stabilize the sacroiliac joint. The posterior ligaments consist of short oblique and long longitudinal components. The posterior sacroiliac ligaments are stronger than the anterior sacroiliac ligaments and are the major stabilizers of the sacroiliac joint (Fig. 32–2). Transverse ligaments stabilize the symphysis pubis.

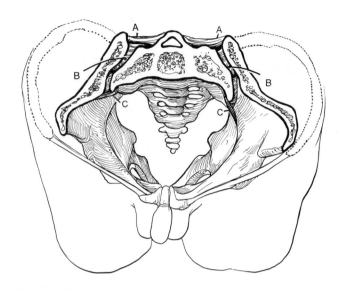

Figure 32–1 Cross section through the sacroiliac joints shows the direction of the interosseous sacroiliac ligaments. A = Iliolumbar ligament; B = Lateral lumbosacral ligament; C = Anterior sacroiliac ligament. Reproduced with permission from Tile M. Anatomy. In: Tile M, ed. *Fractures of the Pelvis and Acetabulum*. Baltimore, MD: Williams and Wilkins; 1995:15.

The sacrotuberous ligament connects the ischial tuberosity to the posterolateral aspect of the sacrum and the dorsal aspect of the posterior iliac spine. It maintains vertical stability of the pelvis. The sacrospinous ligament connects the ischial spine to the lateral margin of the sacrum and coccyx and lends fibers to the sacrotuberous ligament. It divides the greater and lesser sciatic notches and contributes to rotational stability of the posterior pelvis. The iliolumbar ligaments arise from the transverse processes of L-4 and L-5 and insert onto the posterior iliac crest and sacral ala. They help secure the spine to the pelvis (Fig. 32–2).

The acetabulum is formed by the confluence of the ilium, ischium, and pubis, joined at the triradiate cartilage. The triradiate cartilage fuses at skeletal maturity and the ilium, ischium, and pubis become one innominate bone. The acetabulum comprises the anterior and posterior columns that form an inverted "Y" (Fig. 32–3). The anterior column comprises the anterior border of the iliac wing, the pelvic brim, the anterior acetabular wall, and the superior pubic ramus. The posterior column comprises the ischial tuberosity, the lesser and greater sciatic notches, and the posterior acetabular wall.

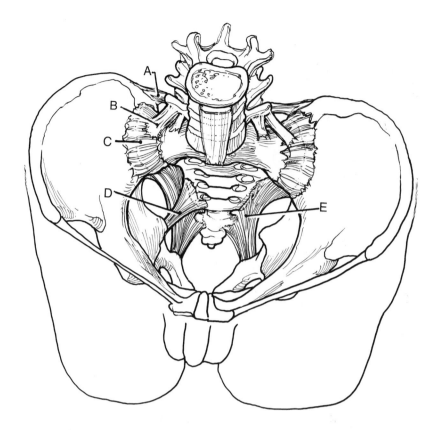

Figure 32–2 Anteroposterior (AP) view of the pelvis indicates that the sacrospinous ligament is a triangular strong ligament lying anterior to the sacrotuberous ligament, which is a strong, broad band extending from the lateral portion of the dorsum of the sacrum to the ischial tuberosity. Reproduced with permission from Tile M. Anatomy. A = Iliolumbar ligament; B = Lateral lumbosacral ligament; C = Anterior sacroiliac ligament; D = Sacrospinos ligament; E = Sacrotuberous ligament. In: Tile M, ed. *Fractures of the Pelvis and Acetabulum.* Baltimore, MD: Williams and Wilkins; 1995:16.

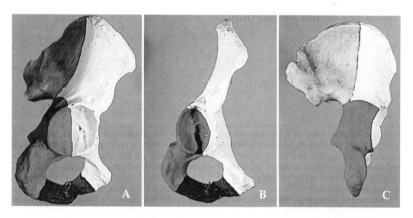

Figure 32–3 Columns of the acetabulum. **(A)** Lateral aspect. **(B)** Obturator-oblique view. **(C)** Iliac-oblique view. White: anterior column; dark grey: posterior column; black: the beam uniting inferior ends of the columns (ischio-pubic ramus). Reproduced with permission from Letournel E, Judet R. Anatomy of the acetabulum in Letournel E, ed. *Fractures of the Acetabulum.* NY: New York, Springer-Verlag; 1993:18.

Arterial supply of the femoral head comprises a branch of the medial femoral circumflex artery, the artery of the ligamentum teres, and a branch of the lateral femoral circumflex artery (Fig. 32–4). The most important contribution is the lateral epiphyseal artery, which arises from the medial femoral circumflex artery and is contained within the retinaculum of the femoral neck. The ascending branches of the medial and lateral femoral circumflex arteries can be injured by femoral head dislocation or fracture or femoral neck fracture. Femoral head dislocation also injures the artery of the ligamentum teres. Damage to the capsule and the blood supply is directly related to the degree of fracture displacement. Interruption

of the major blood supply to the femoral head increases the incidence of avascular necrosis (AVN), femoral head collapse, and post-traumatic hip arthrosis.

The average adult femoral neck-shaft angle is 130 to 135 degrees with 10 to 15 degrees of anteversion. Femoral head diameter varies between 40 and 60 mm. The calcar femorale is a vertically oriented condensation of bone radiating from the posteromedial aspect of the proximal femur toward the greater trochanter. It is continuous with the posterior femoral neck.

The intertrochanteric region of the hip comprises the region between the distal portion of the femoral neck to the

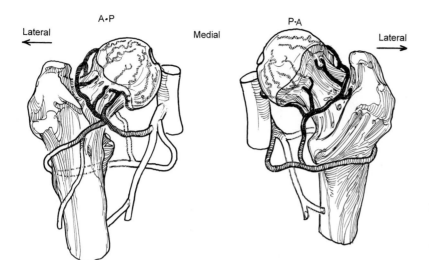

Lateral A-P Medial P-A Lateral

Figure 32–4 The lateral epiphyseal artery provides the predominant blood supply to the femoral head both anteriorly and posteriorly.

distal extent of the lesser trochanter. The intertrochanteric portion of the proximal femur is extracapsular and has a rich vascular network. Therefore, AVN of the femoral head and nonunion are rare after intertrochanteric hip fracture.

The femoral neck and intertrochanteric area comprise a dense network of cancellous bone organized along lines of tensile and compression stresses. Gradual loss of this network occurs with age because bone mass decreases. The Singh index (Levy at al., 1992) classifies osteopenia of the proximal femur (Fig. 32–5). Grade I represents severe osteopenia characterized by loss of all but a portion of the primary compression trabeculae. Grade VI represents normal bone density.

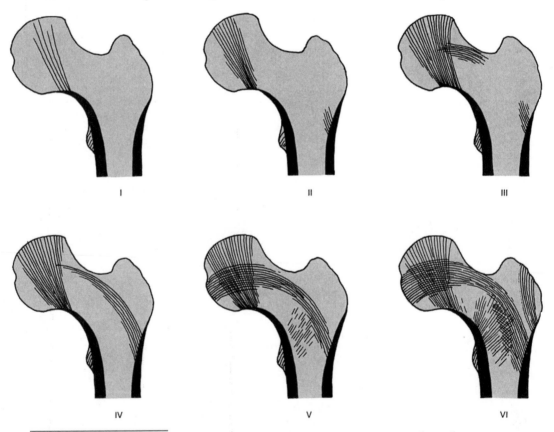

I II III

IV V VI

Figure 32–5 Singh classification of osteopenia of proximal femur. Grades I through III represent clinically significant osteopenia. Grade I: only primary compression trabeculae are present, and they are reduced in volume. Grade II: primary tension trabeculae are absent. Grade III: interruption of primary tension trabeculae in the greater trochanteric region. Grade IV: loss of secondary compression and tension trabeculae. Grade V: loss of trabecular bone in Ward's triangle. Grade VI: all primary and secondary trabecular groups are present including the region of Ward's triangle. Reproduced with permission from Levy RN, Capozzi JD, Mont MA. Intertrochanteric hip fractures. In: Browner BD, ed. *Skeletal Trauma*. Philadelphia, PA: WB Saunders; 1992;1445.

The intermediate grades represent varying degrees of loss of the primary and secondary compressive and tensile trabecular patterns. Fracture fixation stability correlates with proximal femoral bone density.

Kocher-Langenbeck Approach

The posterior approach to the hip is useful for posterior wall and posterior column acetabulum fractures, hip hemiarthroplasty, and some transverse and T-type acetabulum fractures. Either the prone or lateral position may be used with the hip extended and the knee flexed to reduce sciatic nerve tension during the procedure.

The incision begins at the posterior superior iliac spine (PSIS), extends over the greater trochanter, and continues distally parallel to the axis of the femur. The fascia lata and the gluteus maximus fascia is incised parallel to the incision, and the gluteus muscle is bluntly divided along its fibers. The sciatic nerve lies deep to the exposed pirifomis muscle and superficial to the more distal external rotators of the hip. The proximal portion of the gluteus maximus tendon insertion may be divided, if necessary, to improve exposure. The piriformis and obturator internus tendon insertions are divided, tagged with suture for later repair, and retracted posteriorly to protect the sciatic nerve and expose the greater and lesser sciatic notches (Fig. 32–6).

The common tendon of the superior and inferior gemelli and obturator internus may be divided, but dissection into the quadratus femoris should be avoided to minimize injury to the medial circumflex artery. The underlying gluteus medius and minimus muscles are retracted proximally to expose the joint capsule. Careful dissection between the gluteus minimus and joint capsule is essential to minimize vascular compromise of the joint. The origin of the hamstrings may be divided from the ischial tuberosity to expose the inferior portion of the posterior column. Capsular attachments to the fracture fragments should be preserved, but release of the capsule from the intact portion of the acetabulum may be necessary to improve exposure. A Schantz pin can be inserted into the femoral neck to apply lateral traction and distract the joint for exposure.

Subperiosteal dissection of the greater and lesser sciatic notches is necessary to expose the quadrilateral plate to facilitate reduction of posterior column, transverse, and T-type acetabulum fractures. Meticulous dissection, gentle retraction, and frequent release of retraction is necessary to protect the vulnerable sciatic nerve. A trochanteric osteotomy (Fig. 32–7) or partial release of the gluteus medius tendon may be necessary to improve visulatization.

Ilioinguinal Approach

Indications for this approach include all anterior wall and column fractures and some both-column, transverse, and T-type fractures with a large posterior column fragment. Anterior fractures with an associated posterior wall fracture are not amenable to an isolated ilioinguinal approach.

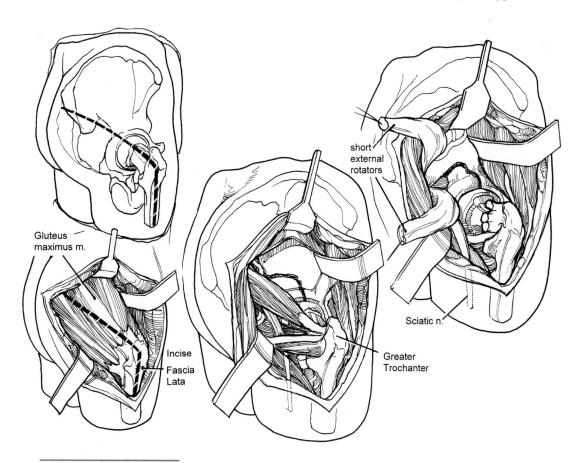

Figure 32–6 Posterior Kocher-Langenbeck approach.

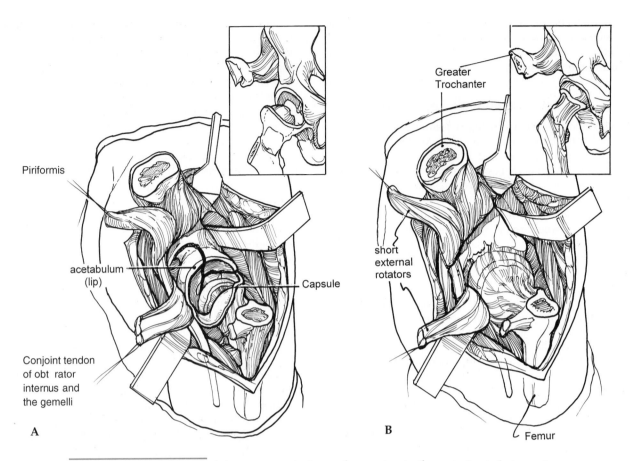

Figure 32–7 **(A)** Access of the greater sciatic notch anterior to the anterior inferior spine.
(B) Osteotomy of the greater trochanter allows for increased access to the superior portion of the
posterior column.

The patient is positioned supine unless a combined anterior and posterior approach is planned. The incision begins in the midline 2 cm superior to the symphysis pubis, extends to the anterior superior iliac spine (ASIS), and continues along the anterior and lateral iliac crest. It may be necessary to continue the lateral incision 5 cm cephalad to improve exposure of the iliac fossa and anterior sacroiliac joint.

The iliac crest periosteum is incised, and the iliopsoas muscle is elevated from the underlying iliac fossa with subperiosteal dissection. Posterior and inferior dissection exposes the anterior sacroiliac joint and pelvic brim.

The external ring of the inguinal canal is identified, and the spermatic cord or round ligament is isolated and retracted with a rubber drain. The external oblique aponeurosis is incised from the external inguinal ring laterally to 5 mm medial to the ASIS. The incision exposes the lateral femoral cutaneous nerve just medial to the ASIS.

The inguinal ligament is incised medial to lateral from its pubic attachment to the ASIS to release the transversalis fascia medially and the common origin of the internal oblique and the transversus abdominis laterally. This exposes the retropubic space medially, the iliac vessels and lymphatics centrally, and the psoas sheath laterally. The femoral nerve lies under the psoas fascia on the superior medial surface of the muscle.

The iliopectineal fascia is identified by sweeping medially with a finger placed on the medial surface of the iliopsoas muscle. It divides the lacuna muscularum, which contains the iliopsoas muscle and femoral nerve, from the lacuna vascularum, which contains the iliac artery and vein. The iliopectineal fascia also divides the true and false pelvis at its attachment on the pelvic brim. The femoral artery is adjacent to the medial surface of the iliopectineal fascia. Medial and lateral retraction with rubber drains of the contents of the lacuna vascularum and lacuna muscularum, respectively, exposes the iliopectineal fascia for safe division with blunt-tipped scissors to expose the quadrilateral plate.

Retraction of the iliac vessels exposes the obturator nerve and artery. An anomalous origin of the obturator artery (corona mortis), if present, requires ligation to prevent bleeding if it retracts into the pelvis during dissection. Subperiosteal dissection exposes the pelvic brim, superior pubic ramus, and quadrilateral plate. Division of the rectus abdominis sheath and muscle improve exposure of the symphysis pubis, retropubic space, and quadrilateral plate.

Medial retraction of the iliopsoas muscle defines the "lateral window" for access to the iliac fossa and the anterior sacroiliac joint. Knee flexion and external rotation and flexion of the hip decreases iliopsoas tension to improve exposure. The quadrilateral plate can be palpated but not visualized in the "lateral window".

Lateral retraction of the iliopsoas muscle and medial retraction of the vessels defines the "middle window" for access to the pelvic brim, superior pubic ramus, and quadrilateral plate. Lateral retraction of the vessels defines the "medial window" for access to the remainder of the superior pubic ramus, pubic symphysis, and quadrilateral plate (Fig. 32–8).

Combined Anterior and Posterior Approach

Complex acetabulum fractures often require more extensile exposures than either the anterior or the posterior approach can offer. Single extensile approaches are associated with heterotopic ossification and abductor weakness. Combining anterior and posterior approaches may provide adequate exposure with fewer complications.

The "floppy lateral" position is used. The patient is placed in the lateral decubitus position and maintained on the table so that he or she can be "rocked" forward or backward to facilitate posterior or anterior exposure, respectively.

Extended Iliofemoral Approach

This approach is essentially a lateral approach to the innominate bone that exposes the external surface of the iliac wing, posterior column, posterior wall of the acetabulum, and internal iliac fossa. It is useful for simultaneously exposing

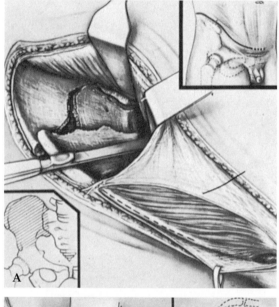

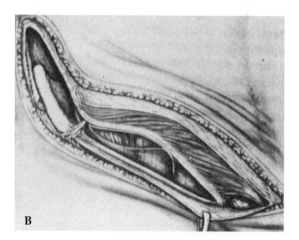

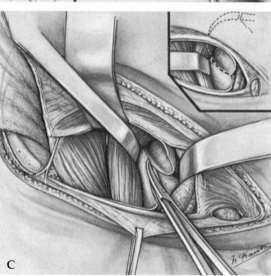

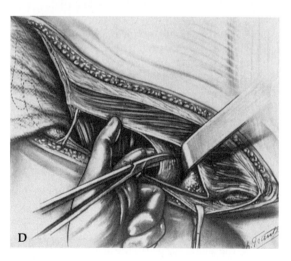

Figure 32–8   (A–H) The Ilio-inguinal approach. Reproduced with permission from Letournel E, Judet R. Surgical approaches to the acetabulum in Letournel E, ed. *Fractures of the Acetabulum.* New York, NY: Springer-Verlag; 1993;378–380.

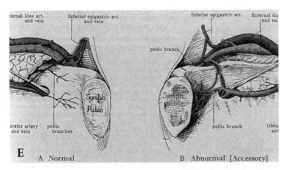

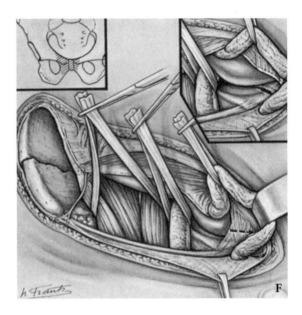

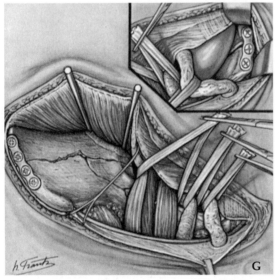

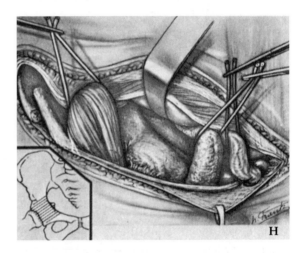

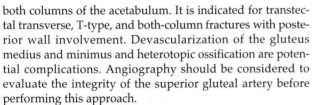

Figure 32–8   (continued)

both columns of the acetabulum. It is indicated for transtectal transverse, T-type, and both-column fractures with posterior wall involvement. Devascularization of the gluteus medius and minimus and heterotopic ossification are potential complications. Angiography should be considered to evaluate the integrity of the superior gluteal artery before performing this approach.

The lateral decubitis position is used. Hip extension and knee flexion is maintained throughout the procedure to protect the sciatic nerve. An inverted J-shaped incision begins along the posterior iliac crest, extends to the ASIS, and continues distally along the lateral thigh. The iliac crest periosteum is incised, the lateral surface of the iliac crest is exposed by subperiosteal elevation of the gluteus muscles. The fascia lata is incised along the length of the wound, and the tensor fascia lata muscle is retracted posteriorly to expose a fascia layer that separates it from the rectus femoris.

The rectus femoris is exposed, and the interval between it and the vastus lateralis is opened to expose the lateral femoral circumflex vessels, which are ligated. A fibrous layer that traverses the anterior aspect of the femur is divided to expose the greater trochanter. The gluteus minimus tendon insertion to the greater trochanter is divided, tagged with suture for later repair, and bluntly elevated from the underlying joint capsule. The gluteus medius tendon is divided and tagged with suture for later repair.

The underlying piriformis and conjoint short external rotator tendons are divided from their insertion and tagged with suture for later repair. Greater trochanter osteotomy can be performed instead to ensure appropriate reattachment of the gluteus and external rotator tendons. Posterior retraction of the piriformis and the conjoint short external rotator tendons protects the sciatic nerve and exposes the greater and lesser sciatic notches, ischial spine, and ischial tuberosity.

The reflected head of the rectus femoris is elevated to further expose the joint capsule. Incision and elevation of the capsule along the rim of the acetabulum exposes the interior of the hip joint. The origins of the sartorius and the rectus femoris can be divided from the ASIS and anterior inferior iliac spine (AIIS), respectively, to expose the anterior column and internal iliac fossa. Elevation of the iliopsoas muscle further exposes the internal iliac fossa. The superior portion of the anterior column is exposed, the portion medial to the pectineal eminence is not accessible (Fig. 32–9).

Triradiate Approach

The triradiate approach is an extensile approach to the lateral aspect of the ilium, posterior column, and posterior wall of the acetabulum. It is theoretically safer than the extended iliofemoral approach because collateral circulation to the gluteal muscles is preserved. It is useful for transtectal trasverse, T-type, and both-column fractures with posterior wall involvement. Heterotopic ossification is a potential complication.

The lateral position is used, and the hip is extended and the knee is flexed to decrease sciatic nerve tension. A Y-shaped incision that comprises a Kocher-Langenbeck incision with a second incision extending from the greater trochanter to the ASIS is performed. The Kocher-Langenbeck approach is performed with the exception that the fascia lata is reflected from the tensor fascia lata muscle. A greater trochanteric osteotomy is performed to permit proximal elevation and retraction of the gluteus medius and minimus and tensor fascia lata muscles (Fig. 32–10). The fascia lata may be release from the iliac crest to improve exposure of the iliac wing. The anterior arm of the Y-shaped incision can be extended medially across the lower abdomen and the iliopsoas muscle elevated to improve exposure of the inner wall of the innominate bone.

PITFALL

The extensile exposures (extended iliofemoral and triradiate) offer better visualization but have a higher complication rate.

EXAMINATION

The history for a patient who has sustained a high-energy injury should elucidate the mechanism, the patient's position at impact, and the direction of the force. These elements will help direct the physical exam and assist the examiner with determining specific injury patterns. Information from the emergency transport team is valuable, especially with obtunded patients.

The history and examination must consider life-threatening injuries that often accompany pelvis fractures and that can include head, chest, and abdominal injuries. Massive retroperitoneal bleeding is common with high-energy unstable pelvic fractures as well. Airway, breathing, and circulation must be assessed immediately and frequently.

In low-energy injuries, the history is important in determining the treatment and prognosis of femoral neck and intertrochanteric hip fractures. Antecedent cardiovascular, cerebrovascular, and pulmonary symptoms should be considered. Pre-injury function, activity, cognitive ability, and medical co-morbidities determine the short- and long-term prognoses. The presence of pre-injury groin pain that suggests degenerative arthritis should be determined.

Evaluation in the emergency department should begin with assessing airway, breathing, and circulation. A thorough physical examination should rule out associated head, neck, spine, and skeletal trauma. Neurologic and vascular examination should be performed, and the skin integrity should be assessed.

Hemodynamic instability and hypotension suggest massive intrapelvic bleeding. A rapid and logical search for the source of the hypotension must be initiated. The severity of the blood loss can be determined on the initial evaluation by assessing the pulse, blood pressure, and capillary refill. Polytraumatized patients may have multiple simultaneous causes of hypotension.

Physical examination, chest radiographs, and thoracic aspiration will detect the presence of intrathoracic blood loss. Supraumbilical peritoneal lavage and/or computed tomography (CT) can be used to assess the peritoneal cavity.

PEARL

If the peritoneal lavage is performed in a patient suspected of having a pelvic fracture, the entry point must be placed supraumbilical to avoid a false-positive lavage from inadvertent puncture of a large hematoma.

A complete examination of the perineal region must be performed. Open wounds must be palpated for communication with the underlying bony structures. Blood in the urethral meatus and a "high-riding" prostate on rectal exam suggest urethral trauma. A detailed neurologic examination is mandatory with particular attention to the motor and sensory distribution of the lumbosacral plexus. Table 32–1 provides a useful checklist for evaluating polytraumatized patients with a pelvis fracture.

The leg is often shortened and the thigh diameter increased when a subtrochantic crashaft femoral fracture is present. Significant blood loss into the thigh may occur. Compartment syndrome, though rare, is possible. Skin integrity must also be assessed

The affected leg is internally rotated with posterior hip dislocation and externally rotated with anterior dislocation. It is shortened and externally rotated with displaced femoral neck or intertrochanteric hip fracture. Hip motion is decreased and painful. Side-to-side "log-rolling" of the lower extremity or gentle tapping on the sole of the foot often causes pain when occult or undisplaced hip fractures are present.

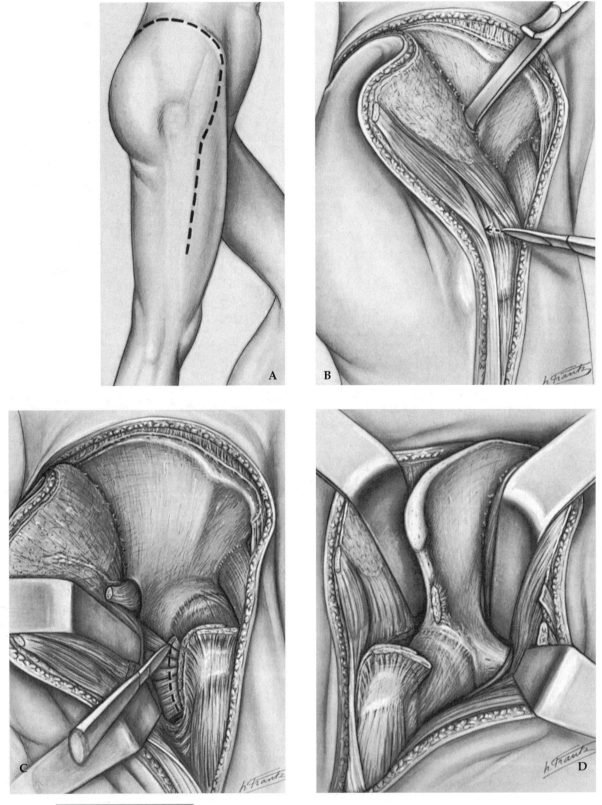

Figure 32–9   (A–D) Extended iliofemoral approach. Reproduced with permission from Letournel E, Judet R. Surgical approaches to the acetabulum in Letournel E, ed. *Fractures of the Acetabulum.* New York, Springer-Verlag, 1993;389–393.

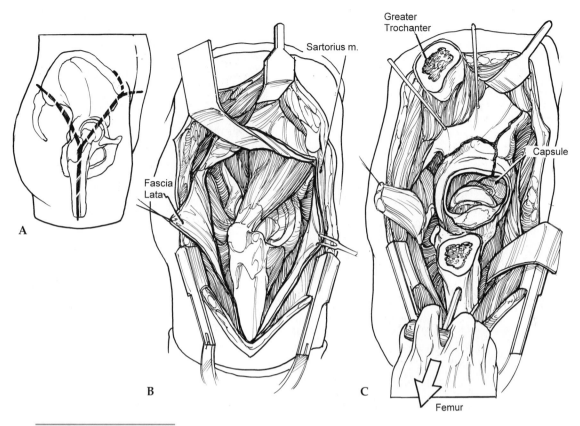

Figure 32–10   Triradiate transtrochanteric approach. **(A)** Incision. **(B)** Incision of the tensor fascia lata. **(C)** Trochenteric osteotomy and capsulorraphy of the hip joint.

TABLE 32–1   Pelvic Fracture Physical Exam

1. pain on palpation of injured region
2. unstable motion with AP or lateral compression
3. abnormal position of the lower extremity, rotational malalignment or leg-length discrepancy (significant pelvic displacement)
4. blood at the urethral meatus (possible urethral injury)
5. high-riding prostate on rectal exam (possible urethral injury)
6. scrotal or labial swelling and echymosis
7. massive flank or buttock swelling
8. neurologic exam (emphasis on lumbosacral plexus)

AIDS TO DIAGNOSIS

Initial radiographic evaluation of a polytraumatized patient includes chest, cervical spine, and AP pelvis films. Pelvic injury identified on the initial AP pelvis radiograph can be further radiographically evaluated with inlet and outlet radiographs of the pelvis. The inlet view images the sacral ala, AP displacement of the hemipelvis, and pubic ramus involvement. The outlet view images the sacrum, the sacral foramina, and vertical displacement of the hemipelvis (Fig. 32–11).

Radiographic signs of pelvic instability include displacement of the posterior sacroiliac complex more than 5 mm in any plane; posterior fracture diastasis, rather than impaction; and avulsion fracture of the transverse process of the fifth lumbar vertebra or the ischial spine attachment of the sacrospinous ligament. Computed tomography is useful for defining posterior injury.

An acetabular fracture identified on the AP pelvis radiograph requires obturator-oblique and iliac-oblique radiographs (Fig. 32–12). The obturator-oblique view evaluates the anterior column and posterior wall of the acetabulum. The beam is perpendicular to the obturator foramen and images the iliopectineal line, the anterior aspect of the obturator ring, and the posterior border of the acetabulum. The iliac-oblique view evaluates the posterior column and anterior wall. The beam is perpendicular to the plane of the iliac wing and images the iliac wing, the quadrilateral surface of the ischium, and the posterior border of the innominate bone.

Computed tomography helps define the fracture lines, intra-articular fragments, marginal impaction of the femoral head or acetabulum, posterior-wall fragment size, and concentricity of reduction. Newer three-dimensional CT scans can be helpful but are not necessary for routine evaluation of acetabular fractures. Signal averaging and step artifact can compromise the resolution and detail.

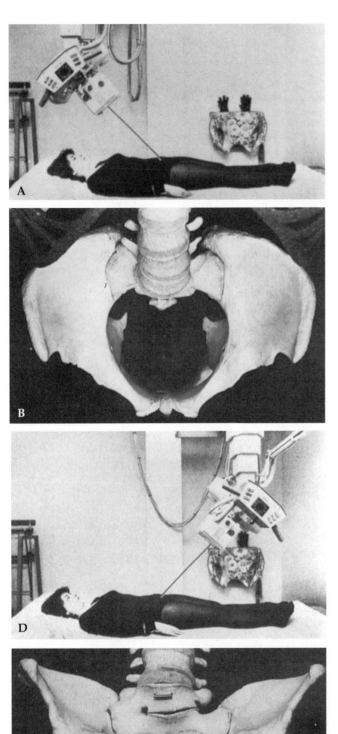

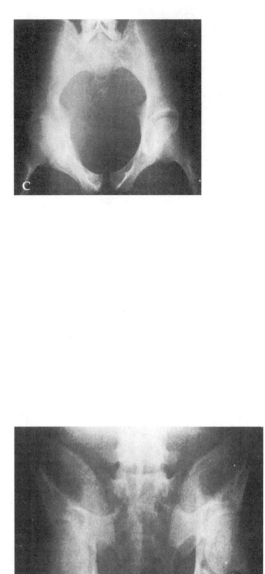

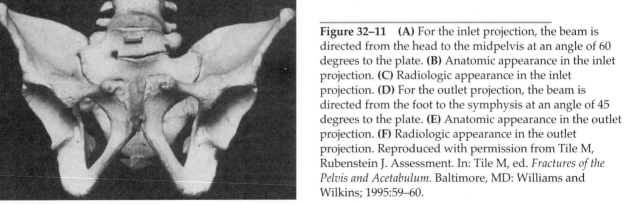

Figure 32–11 **(A)** For the inlet projection, the beam is directed from the head to the midpelvis at an angle of 60 degrees to the plate. **(B)** Anatomic appearance in the inlet projection. **(C)** Radiologic appearance in the inlet projection. **(D)** For the outlet projection, the beam is directed from the foot to the symphysis at an angle of 45 degrees to the plate. **(E)** Anatomic appearance in the outlet projection. **(F)** Radiologic appearance in the outlet projection. Reproduced with permission from Tile M, Rubenstein J. Assessment. In: Tile M, ed. *Fractures of the Pelvis and Acetabulum.* Baltimore, MD: Williams and Wilkins; 1995:59–60.

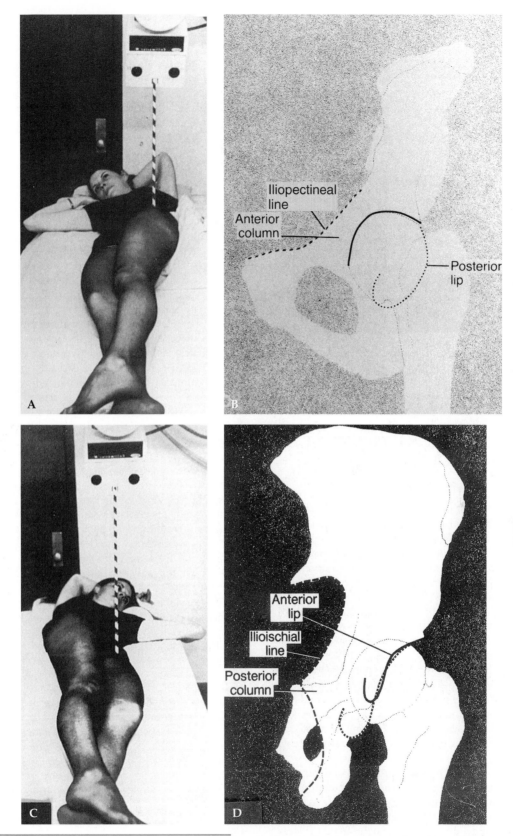

Figure 32–12 **(A)** The obturator-oblique view of the left hemipelvis is taken by elevating the affected hip 45 degrees from the horizontal by means of a wedge and directing the beam through the hip joint with 15 degrees upward tilt. **(B)** Various lines demonstrate important anatomic landmarks on the obturator-oblique view [including the anterior column, represented by the iliopectineal line; and the posterior lip of the acetabulum.] **(C)** The iliac-oblique view of the left hemipelvis is taken by rotating the patient into 45 degrees of external rotation by elevating the uninjured side on a wedge. **(D)** Anatomic landmarks of the left hemipelvis on the iliac-oblique view include the posterior column of the acetabulum, outlined by the ilioischial line, the iliac crest, and the anterior lip of the acetabulum. Reproduced with permission from Tile M, Rubenstein J. Assessment of acetabular fractures. In: Tile M, ed. *Fractures of the Pelvis and Acetabulum.* Baltimore, MD: Williams and Wilkins. 1995:307–308.

Femoral neck fracture is usually easily identified on AP pelvis and AP and lateral hip radiographs. Internal rotation AP radiograph of the hip may be necessary if routine radiographs appear normal but clinical suspicion suggests a femoral neck fracture. Internal rotation of the lower extremity brings the anteverted femoral neck into greatest profile. Computed tomography may be necessary to identify occult femoral neck fractures not visualized on routine or internal rotation radiographs when the history and physical findings suggest fracture.

Technetium 99m diphosphonate bone scanning is sensitive in detecting occult undisplaced fractures when plain radiographs are negative and femoral neck fracture is suspected. It is most sensitive 24 to 72 hours after injury. It is especially useful for identifying skeletal metastases if pathologic fracture is suspected. It may be prognostic for AVN of the femoral head and femoral neck nonunion.

The role of magnetic resonance imaging remains undefined, but it may be sensitive for diagnosis of femoral neck fracture during the first 24 hours after injury. Increased signal on T2 images consistent with marrow edema and a fracture line indicates occult femoral neck fracture. Magnetic resonance imaging also is a sensitive indicator of AVN of the femoral head.

SPECIFIC CONDITIONS, TREATMENT, AND OUTCOME

Pelvis Fractures

Pelvis injuries may result in significant long- and short-term disability. Stable fractures have a better prognosis than unstable fractures. Long-term pain and functional impairment occur more frequently in significantly displaced pelvic fractures.

Classification of the fracture pattern and the dominant injury force helps guide decision making and treatment. The Young-Burgess classification (1987) is based on the mechanism of injury. It proposes to help predict associated injuries and hemodynamic instability that may require resuscitation. The classification comprises *anteroposterior compression*, *lateral compression*, and *vertical shear* (Fig. 32–13).

Anteroposterior compression injuries are subdivided into three groups that reflect progressive anterior and posterior disruption. Lateral compression injuries are subclassified into three groups depending upon the point of application and direction of the force vector. Vertical shear injuries are due to a combination of forces that results in vertically unstable displacement.

The Tile classification (Tile 1988) proposes to determine prognosis and treatment options. It considers stability and mechanism of injury, and comprises three major groups. Type A injuries are stable without significant displacement. This group is further subdivided based on the anatomic location of the fracture. Type B injuries are rotationally unstable, but stable in the posterior and vertical directions. This injury pattern is further subdivided into external rotation instability, internal rotation instability, and bilateral rotationally unstable

injuries. Type C injuries are vertically, rotationally, and posteriorly unstable. This injury pattern is further subdivided into unilateral injury, bilateral injury with one side rotationally unstable and one side vertically unstable, and bilateral injury in which both sides of the pelvis are both vertically and rotationally unstable (Fig. 32–14).

Acute Management

Initial care of the polytraumatized patient with a pelvic fracture must address associated head, chest, abdominal and retroperitoneal injuries; hemodynamic instability; genitourinary injuries; life-threatening pelvic ring instability, and open fractures with gross contamination. Hemodynamic stability, prevention of septic sequelae, and stabilization of the fracture to allow early, safe patient mobilization are the immediate goals of pelvis fracture management.

Severe pelvic disruption can result in low-pressure bleeding from cancellous bone at the fracture sites or the retroperitoneal lumbar venous plexus, or it can result in high-pressure bleeding from pelvic arterial injury. Low-pressure bleeding is more common. Major arterial injury has been associated with only 20% of pelvic-hemorrhage-related deaths. The most frequent artery injured is the superior gluteal, followed by the internal pudendal, the obturator, and the lateral sacral artery, respectively. Figure 32–15 illustrates a useful algorithm for the initial management of pelvis fracture with and without hemodynamic instability.

Control of retroperitoneal hemorrhage consists of: (1) fracture stabilization to decrease blood loss from the fracture sites and lacerated soft tissue; (2) reduction and normalization of pelvic volume to tamponade retroperitoneal bleeding; and (3) therapeutic angiography or surgical exploration to identify and control arterial bleeding.

Definitive management of the pelvic injury is undertaken once the patient is hemodynamically stable and associated injuries are stabilized. Treatment is guided by pelvic stability, fracture location, and fracture pattern. Open wounds and neurovascular injury must also be considered when planning treatment.

External Fixation

Immediate external fixation of an unstable pelvis disruption provides immediate pelvic stability, reduces the pelvic volume, and creates retroperitoneal tamponade. Recently developed "resuscitation clamps" permit potentially rapid and effective pelvis stabilization in the emergency department. Continued, unexplained blood loss despite fracture stabilization and aggressive resuscitation mandates angiographic exploration.

Open Pelvic Fractures

Open fractues of the iliac wing and deep wound lacerations without significant contamination should be managed with early aggressive irrigation, debridement, and intravenous

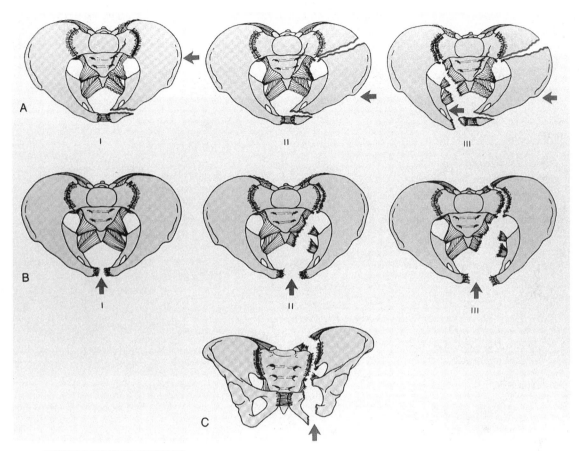

Figure 32–13 Young-Burgess classification. **(A)** Lateral compression fractures. Type I: The lateral force is applied posteriorly (arrow), causing a crush effect of the sacrum and fracture of the pubic rami. This is a stable injury because the ligaments remain intact. Type II: The lateral force is applied anteriorly (arrow), causing the typical anterior pubic rami fractures with an anterior sacral crush and either rupture of the posterior sacroiliac ligaments or fractures through the iliac wing. This is an ipsilateral injury. Type III: The force is directed anteriorly (arrow), causing internal rotation of the anterior hemipelvis and continuing through to the contralateral hemipelvis, which rotates externally. This results in a pattern of lateral compression on the ipsilateral side with apparent AP compression on the contralateral side, disruption of the posterior sacroiliac ligaments on the ipsilateral side and sacrospinous/sacrotuberous complex and anterior ligaments on the contralateral side. Alternatively, there may be an iliac wing fracture. **(B)** Anteroposterior compression fractures. Type I: The delivered force "opens" the pelvis, which remains stable due to intact posterior ligaments. Type II: The AP force causes further "opening" of the anterior pelvis with additional rupture of the anterior sacroiliac, sacrotuberous, and sacrospinous ligaments. This is rotationally unstable. Type III: Wide "opening" of the pelvis with complete disruption of all supporting ligament groups, including the posterior sacroiliac ligaments. **(C)** The injury force is vertically directed (arrow) to the supporting structures of the pelvis causing disruption along this line. Fractures of the pubic rami are usually seen anteriorly, whereas fractures of the sacrum or iliac wing are usually seen posteriorly. Fractures are vertical and are associated with vertical displacement of fragments. Injury to the posterior and anterior sacroiliac ligaments may be seen, as well as to sacrospinous/sacrotuberous, and possibly symphysis ligaments. Reproduced with permission from Young JWR. Burgess AR. *Radiologic Management of Pelvic Ring Fractures.* Baltimore, MD: Urban & Schwarzenberg; 1987:17, 22, 27, 42, 44, 48, 55.

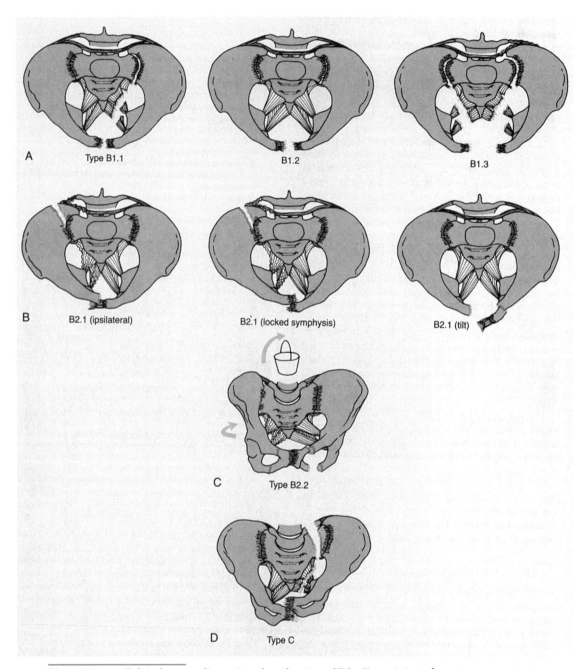

Figure 32–14   Pelvic fracture disruption classification of Tile. Type A (not shown) represents stable fractures of the pelvis not involving the ring or stable, minimally displaced fractures. **(A)** Type B represents rotationally unstable but vertically stable fractures. Type B1 injuries are external rotation or "open-book" injuries. **(B)** Type B2.1 represents internal rotation or lateral compression injuries on the ipsilateral side. **(C)** Type B2.2 represents lateral compression injuries with contralateral fracturing of the pubic rami and posterior structures. **(D)** Type C fractures are rotationally and vertically unstable and are represented here as a unilateral, unstable, vertically disrupted pelvis. Reproduced with permission from Tile, M. Pelvic Ring Fractures. Should they be fixed? *J Bone Jt Surg.* 1988:70B:1–12 and Kellam JF, Browner BD. Fractures of the pelvic ring. In: Browner BD, ed. *Skeletal Trauma.* Philadelphia, PA: WB Saunders; 1992:860.

antibiotics. Pelvic disruptions that communicate with the rectum, colon, vagina, or perineum are often grossly contaminated and require irrigation, debridement, and surgical repair. Early diverting colostomy is recommended for pelvic fractures that communicate with the colon, rectum, or perineum. Early detection by digital examination under general anesthesia and repair of vaginal laceration can minimize delayed formation of pelvic abscesses. Early and aggressive wound exploration and debridement, local packing to control hemorrhage, selected use of angiography, and immediate

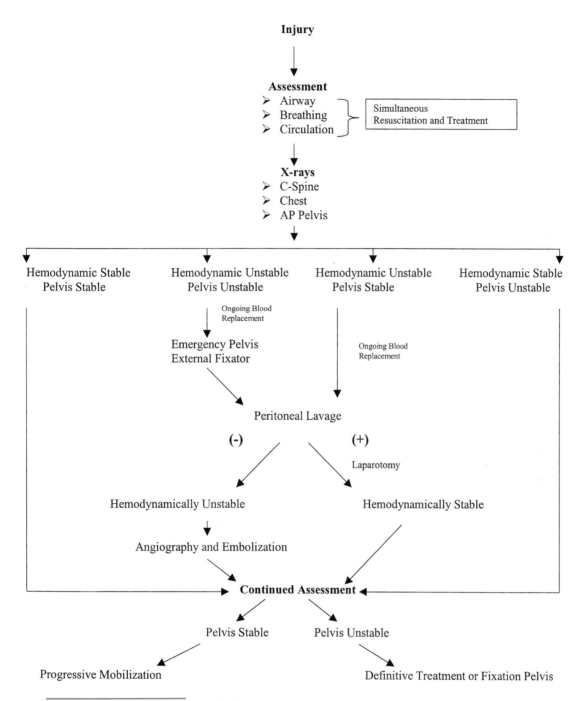

Figure 32–15   Initial treatment algorithm.

external fixation have significantly decreased the morbidity and mortality for open unstable pelvic disruptions.

Definitive Management

Low-energy pelvic fractures are typically stable and rarely require surgical intervention. Unstable pelvic disruptions require internal and/or external fixation. The injury pattern,

degree of displacement, and instability determine the fixation technique.

Symphysis Pubis Disruption

Pubic symphysis disruption can be due to anteroposterior compression, lateral compression, vertical shearing, and complex combined rotational forces. Closed management is recommended for isolated symphyseal diastasis less than 2.5 cm.

Internal or external fixation is necessary when diastasis exceeds 2.5 cm.

Pubic Ramus Fractures

Most pubic rami fractures are isolated injuries that may be treated nonoperatively. Anterior fixation may be necessary when unstable posterior pelvic ring injury accompanies pubic rami fractures. Internal fixation of superior pubic ramus fractures consists of plate and screw constructs or medullary screw techniques.

Iliac Wing Fractures

Iliac wing fractures are usually due to a direct blow to the iliac crest and rarely occur in isolation. Significantly displaced fractures, fractures associated with unstable pelvic disruptions, or displaced acetabular fractures require open reduction and internal fixation. An internal or external iliac exposure is used for open reduction of an iliac fracture. The internal iliac approach is the lateral portion of the ilioinguinal exposure (Fig. 32–8).

Sacroiliac Joint Dislocations

Open or closed anatomic reduction and internal fixation is recommended for unstable sacroiliac joint injuries. Surgical exposure, reduction technique, and fixation should be individualized to the injury pattern, patient body habitus, condition of the soft tissues, and experience of the surgeon.

Sacral Fractures

Isolated sacral fractures can typically be treated nonoperatively. Displaced fractures of the sacrum associated with instability or neurologic injury require reduction and fixation. Lumbosacral nerve root injuries fractures involve the sacral foramina. These nerve root lesions may be caused by stretch, compression from fracture comminution, or laceration. Commonly used fixation devices include posterior tension plates, sacral bars, and sacroiliac screw fixation.

Posterior Pelvic Fixation

Anterior fixation alone will not adequately stabilize the posterior pelvis in a vertically unstable injury because of the large forces that cross the sacroiliac joints. Anterior fixation alone is sufficient for rotational instability without vertical instability.

Acetabulum Fractures

Preoperative planning with thorough radiographic evaluation including AP and obturator and iliac oblique radiographs and CT is essential to determine the surgical approach, reduction techniques, and fixation constructs.

PEARL

Damage to the sciatic nerve may accompany posterior wall fractures or associated posterior hip dislocations. It can also be entrapped in the fracture site with posterior column and transverse fractures.

Reduction of associated hip dislocation should be attempted as soon as possible. Balanced skeletal traction is then applied. Open injuries and irreducible hip dislocations require emergent surgical treatment. The incidence of femoral head osteonecrosis increases significantly if reduction of fracture-dislocation is not accomplished within 6 to 12 hours after injury.

An alternative surgical approach should be considered when lacerations, abrasions, and degloving injuries exist because their presence increases the rate of infection. In the absence of other associated injuries and with minimal local soft-tissue injury, the incidence of infection is between 3 and 6%.

Acetabular fracture displacement results in joint incongruity, which leads to increased stress concentration in the articular cartilage of the femoral head and acetabulum. Increased peak stresses in articular cartilage increases the rate of post-traumatic arthrosis. The goal of surgical management for displaced acetabular fractures is restoration of articular congruence and anatomic reduction with stable internal fixation.

Letournel's modification of Judet's acetabular fracture classification (Matta, 1992) is useful for planning treatment. The classification defines the injury pattern based on pelvic anatomy and fracture biomechanics. The classification comprises five simple and five complex fracture patterns (Fig. 32–16).

The five simple fracture types include anterior wall, anterior column, posterior wall, posterior column, and transverse fractures of the acetabulum. The transverse fracture pattern can be further subdivided into transtectal, juxtatectal, and infratectal fractures based on the position of the fracture line relative to the dome (tectum) of the acetabulum (Fig. 32–17). Both-column fractures differ from the transverse fractures in that no portion of the superior weight-bearing dome remains attached to the iliac wing (Fig. 32–18).

The five complex fracture types combine at least two of the simple forms. These patterns include the T-type, posterior column and wall, transverse and posterior wall, anterior column with posterior hemitransverse, and associated both-column fractures. The five complex fracture types have a poorer prognosis because of the difficulty in independently restoring both columns.

Displaced acetabular fractures with more than 2 mm of articular surface displacement typically require open reduction and internal fixation. Nonoperative treatment is appropriate in the following situations:

- significant medical co-morbidity
- severe osteoporosis
- systemic or local infection
- undisplaced fractures
- some infratectal transverse and T-type fractures
- some both-column fractures with secondary congruence
- severe bony contamination of injury from bowel or genitourinary injury

Fracture configurations with congruency of most of the acetabular dome and femoral head may be treated nonoperatively. Congruency is determined by plain radiographs and CT.

Roof arc angles are measured on the plain radiographs to assess coverage of the femoral head by the dome of the acetabulum. (Fig. 32–19). Nonoperative management may be

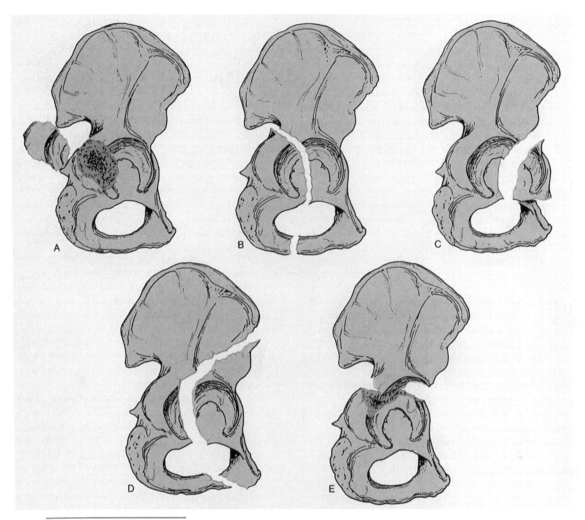

Figure 32–16 Classification of acetabulum fractures according to Letournel. **(A)** Posterior wall fracture, **(B)** posterior column fracture, **(C)** anterior wall fracture, **(D)** anterior column fracture, **(E)** transverse fracture.

appropriate when the medial, anterior, and posterior roof arc angles all are greater than 45 degrees. Balanced skeletal traction is applied for 8 weeks, at which point gradual mobilization and gait training is initiated.

Patients managed surgically are initially placed in balanced skeletal traction and undergo surgery 2 to 10 days after injury. Waiting at least 48 hours allows bleeding at the fracture surfaces to subside. Fracture mobilization becomes much more difficult after 2 to 3 weeks because of early, soft callus formation.

Posterior Wall Fractures

Posterior wall fractures can occur at any level of the posterior column, and constitute the most common acetabular fracture pattern. Associated difficulties include marginal impaction of the posterior wall, abrasions of the femoral head, and difficult timely closed reduction of the hip in acetabular fracture-dislocation. Computed tomography helps evaluate marginal impaction of the posterior wall fragments, joint congruency, and size of the posterior wall fragment.

The posterior Kocher-Langenbeck approach is best for posterior wall fracture. Marginal impaction of the acetabular articular cartilage must be recognized, elevated, and bone grafted. Large, posterior wall fragments should be stabilized with lag screw and buttress plates. Smaller fragments may be secured with spring plates.

Posterior Column Fracture

Posterior column fracture consists of complete detachment of the posterior column. Medial displacement of the femoral head, quadrilateral surface, and sciatic buttress into the true pelvis is apparent on the AP radiograph. Judet views demonstrate disruption of the ilioischial line and normal position of the roof of the acetabulum.

The Kocher-Langenbeck approach is best for isolated fractures of the posterior column. Reduction is facilitated by placing a 5-mm half-pin in the greater trochanter for joint distraction. A second half-pin is placed in the ischial tuberosity for rotational control of the posterior column. Fixation consists of 3.5-mm lag screws and reconstruction plates along the posterior column and sciatic buttress.

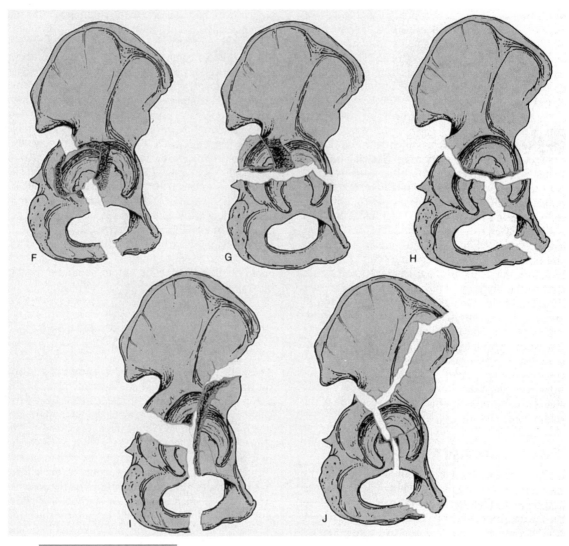

Figure 32–16 *(continued)* **(F)** associated posterior column and posterior wall fractures, **(G)** associated transverse and posterior wall fractures, **(H)** T-shaped fracture, **(I)** associated anterior column with posterior hemitransverse fractures and **(J)** fracture of both columns. Reproduced with permission from Matta J. Surgical treatment of acetabular fractures. In: Browner BD, ed. *Skeletal Trauma.* Philadelphia, PA: WB Saunders; 1992:902–903.

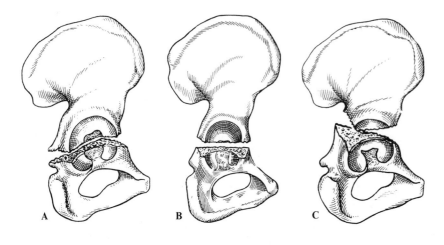

Figure 32–17   Schemes of transverse fractures. **(A)** Infra-tectal type, **(B)** juxta-tectal type, **(C)** trans-tectal type. Reproduced with permission from Letournel E, ed. *Fractures of the Acetabulum.* New York, NY: Springer-Verlag; 1993:142.

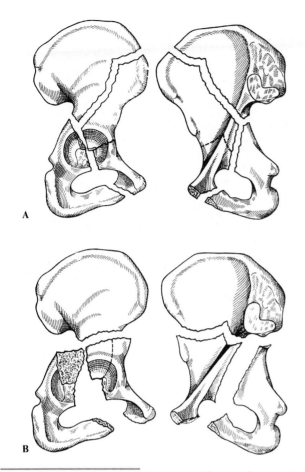

Figure 32–18 Both-column fractures. Schemes showing iliac component (**A**) extending to iliac crest (**B**) extending to the anterior border of the ilium. Reproduced with permission from Letournel E, Judet R, ed. *Fractures of the Acetabulum.* New York, NY: Springer-Verlag; 1993:253

Anterior Wall Fractures

The anterior wall fracture transects the acetabulum and detaches the anterior wall at the level of the AIIS. Obturator oblique radiographs demonstrate fracture through the iliopectineal line and the extent of superior weight-bearing dome involvement. The iliac-oblique view is often normal.

Either the anterior iliofemoral or ilioinguinal approach can be used. A half-pin in the greater trochanter is useful for joint distraction. Reconstruction plates along the pelvic brim provide stable fixation. Screw holes over the acetabular dome should not be used. External landmarks for screw "safe-zones" along the anterior column are the AIIS proximally and the iliopectineal eminence distally.

Anterior Column Fractures

The anterior column fracture is characterized by fracture that extends from distal to the iliopectineal eminence to any point along the anterior iliac wing proximal to the AIIS. The iliopectineal line is disrupted on the obturator oblique radiograph, and the ilioischial line is intact on the iliac oblique radiograph. The fracture is stabilized with lag screws and reconstruction plates through the ilioinguinal approach.

Transverse Fractures

Transverse fractures of the acetabulum occur in the sagittal plane and involve both columns of the acetabulum, but a portion of the weight-bearing dome remains attached to the ilium. Transtectal fractures pass through the weight-bearing dome. Juxtatectal fractures divide the anterior and posterior columns at the level of the cotyloid fossa, leaving a large portion of the roof segment intact. Infratectal fractures divide both columns well below the weight-bearing dome.

PEARL

A "floating acetabulum" occurs in both-column fractures and differentiates them from transverse fractures (Fig. 32–20).

The choice between ilioinguinal or Kocher-Langenbeck approach depends on the degree of displacement and location of the major fracture lines. Severe transtectal transverse fractures often require the extended iliofemoral approach or a combined ilioinguinal and Kocher-Langenbeck approach with the patient in the lateral decubitus position. The patient must be positioned "floppy lateral" so that he or she can be rocked back and forth when performing combined anterior and posterior approaches.

Complex Acetabular Fractures

Posterior Column with Posterior Wall and Transverse with Posterior Wall

These fracture patterns are combination injuries that are commonly associated with posterior hip dislocation or subluxation. Central hip dislocation may accompany the transverse with posterior wall pattern. Treatment for either pattern is similar to that for each pattern's components in isolation. Early recognition and reduction of posterior dislocations are important to minimize complications, such as osteonecrosis, nerve injury, and femoral head damage.

T-type fracture

This fracture type combines a transverse fracture with a vertical fracture best seen on the obturator oblique radiograph as obturator foramen interruption. Recognition of the vertical component of the fracture is critical for planning surgery. Unlike transverse fractures, the anterior and posterior columns are dissociated by the vertical fracture extending through the obturator foramen, and, therefore, often requires combined approaches or an extended iliofemoral approach.

Anterior Column with Posterior Hemitransverse

An anterior wall or column fracture is accompanied by a transverse fracture of the posterior column. An anterior approach is adequate when there is little or no displacement of the hemitransverse component. Significant displacement of the hemitransverse component requires a posterior approach.

Associated Both-column

A "floating acetabulum" wherein no portion of the acetabular articular surface is in continuity with the ilium accompanies a fracture through the anterior and posterior columns. The

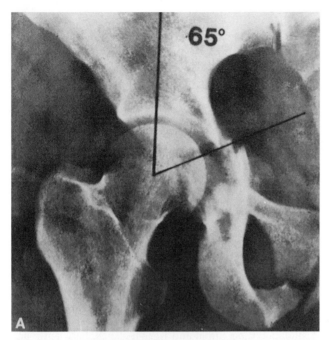

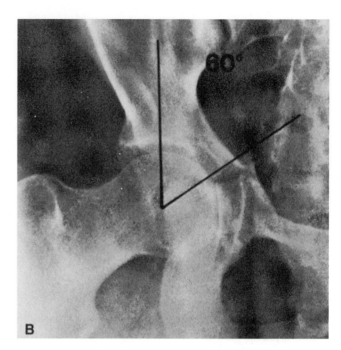

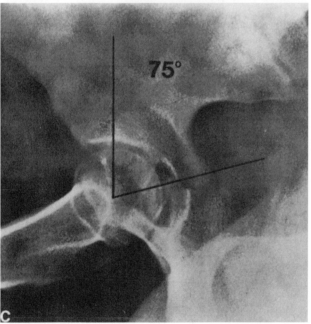

Figure 32–19 **(A)** The AP view, **(B)** the obturator-oblique view, and **(C)** the iliac-oblique view of a T-shaped fracture showing congruence of the femoral head out of traction and adequate roof arc measurements. Closed treatment is indicated. Reproduced with permission from Matta J. Operative indication and choice of surgical approach for fractures of the acetabulum. *Tech. Orthop.* 1996;1:18.

"spur sign" on the obturator oblique radiograph is pathognomonic for a both-column fracture, and represents the intact ilium protruding beyond the medially displaced acetabulum (see Fig. 32–20).

The ilioinguinal approach is appropriate for both-column fractures, especially within the first 3 to 5 days after injury when the fragments are mobile. Significant dome comminution, posterior wall involvement, or fractures managed late often require combined or extensile approaches.

Femoral Head Fractures

The Pipkin classification (Fig. 32–21) (Pipkin, 1957) is useful for treatment planning and differentiates femoral head fractures by anatomic location as follows:

I.   hip dislocation with a fracture of the femoral head caudad to the fovea

II.   hip dislocation with a fracture of the femoral head cephalad to the fovea

III. type I or type II fracture associated with a fracture of the femoral neck

IV. type I or type II fracture associated with a fracture of the acetabulum

Urgent closed reduction of the femoral head should be attempted in the emergency department after resuscitation and thorough radiographic evaluation. Closed reduction in the operating room under general anesthesia should be attempted if the attempt in the emergency department is unsuccessful. Failed closed reduction in the operating room mandates open reduction. Plain radiographs of the pelvis and CT of the hip with 2- to 3-mm cuts through the acetabulum and femoral head are repeated after successful reduction to ensure concentric reduction and to rule out intra-articular fragments and associated fractures.

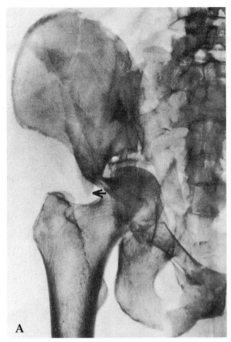

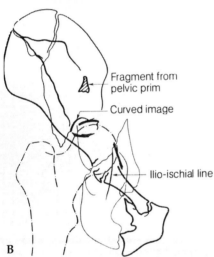

Figure 32–20 Both-column fracture. **(A)** Anteroposterior radiograph; Black arrow showing the "spur sign" **(B)** diagram. Reproduced with permission from Letournel E, ed. *Fractures of the Acetabulum.* New York, NY: Springer-Verlag; 1993:271.

Isolated Pipkin type I and II femoral head fractures with less than 1 to 2 mm of displacement can be managed with 4 weeks of non–weight-bearing, followed by 4 weeks of touch-down weight bearing, and progression to full weight bearing by the end of 10 weeks. Fracture displacement greater than 1 to 2 mm requires surgery. Fragments large enough to acco-modate internal fixation should be anatomically reduced and internally fixed. Smaller fragments should be excised.

Pipkin type III fractures require surgery. Anatomic reduction and internal fixation should be attempted in younger patients. Older patients should undergo hemiarthroplasty because of an increased risk of AVN of the femoral head, subsequent collapse, and degenerative arthritis. The risk of AVN increases with prolonged time from hip dislocation to reduction and with the degree of femoral head and neck fragmen-

tation and displacement. Pipkin type IV femoral head fractures require anatomic reduction and stable fixation of the femoral head fracture at the same time as operative treatment of the acetabular fracture.

Femoral Neck Fractures

The Garden classification (Garden, 1961) is an anatomic classification that groups femoral neck fractures by fracture pattern and displacement to predict prognosis and guide treatment because the risk of AVN increases with increasing displacement (Fig. 32–22). Type I fractures comprise an incomplete valgus impacted fracture of the femoral neck. Type II fractures are nondisplaced, complete femoral neck fractures. Partially and completely displaced complete femoral neck fractures define types III and IV, respectively.

The Garden type I fracture pattern is usually stable due to impacted cancellous bone and the mechanically favorable valgus alignment. The Garden Type II fracture pattern is rare and usually unstable. Garden types III and IV fracture patterns are often difficult to distinguish radiographically. The lateral radiograph is most useful and demonstrates colinearity of the femoral head trabeculae and acetabular trabeculae in Garden type IV.

The long-term outcome of Garden types I and II fractures are similar, as are the results of Garden III and IV fracture patterns. Therefore, it is probably more useful to classify femoral neck fractures as displaced or nondisplaced.

Initial hospital management of femoral neck fracture is Buck's traction for comfort. Alternatively, the lower extremity may be elevated on a pillow and allowed to rest in a comfortable position. The heel must be protected to prevent skin breakdown. Frequent side-to-side repositioning is essential to prevent sacral and gluteal skin pressure necrosis.

Surgical management and early mobilization is indicated for all patients able to tolerate surgery. Early mobilization decreases the risk of deep venous thrombosis, decubitus ulcers, atelectasis, and pneumonia. There is a 10 to 30% incidence of fracture displacement when nondisplaced femoral neck fractures are treated nonoperatively.

Nondisplaced Femoral Neck Fractures

The lateral epiphyseal vessels are seldom injured in nondisplaced femoral neck fractures. Thus, femoral neck nonunion and AVN are rare. Internal fixation with three parallel partially threaded cannulated cancellous screws placed parallel to the femoral neck is indicated to restore and maintain stability while healing and permit early mobilization.

Displaced Femoral Neck Fractures

Injury to the lateral epiphyseal vessels is more likely with displaced femoral neck fracture. Thus, femoral neck nonunion and AVN of the femoral head are likely. Young patients should undergo reduction and fixation as in undisplaced fractures with full disclosure of the prognosis. Reduction and fixation can be attempted in elderly individuals; however, poorly tolerated protected weight-bearing is often necessary postoperatively. Hemiarthroplasty is usually a better option. Indications for hemiarthroplasty for displaced femoral neck fractures in the elderly include medical co-morbidities that affect bone such as chronic renal failure, rheumatoid arthritis, and long-term corticosteroid use, significant osteoporosis, and fracture comminution.

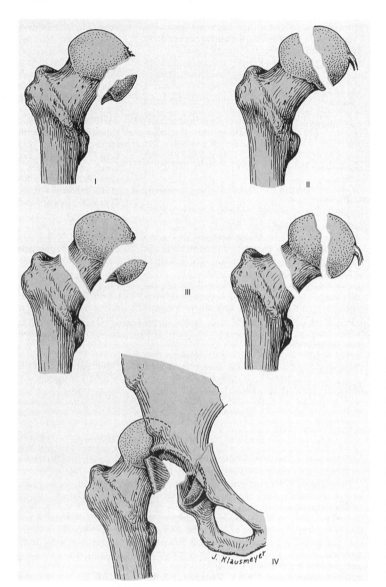

Figure 32–21 Pipkin's classification of femoral head fractures. Pipkin's type I is a fracture fragment below the ligamentum teres; type II is a fracture fragment above the ligamentum. Type III is either of these with an associated femoral neck fracture—a combination with a significantly poorer patient prognosis. Type IV is either of these with an associated acetabular fracture. Reproduced with permission from Swiontkowski MF. Intracapsular hip fractures. In: Browner BD, ed. *Skeletal Trauma.* Philadelphia, PA: WB Saunders; 1992:1373.

Fatigue Fractures of the Femoral Neck

Fatigue fractures of the femoral neck are due to cyclical loading. Normal cyclical loading of mechanically compromised bone as in osteoporosis can cause fatigue fracture. Fatigue fractures may also occur in patients with normal bone who increase the stress on the femoral neck by acutely increasing activity. Prognosis depends on whether the fatigue fracture is a tension or compression type, which can be determined by the anatomic location of the fracture.

Tension fatigue femoral neck fractures are best demonstrated on an internal rotation AP radiograph of the hip; which images the femoral neck in full profile. The fracture line begins at the superior aspect of the femoral neck. Tension fractures are at risk for further displacement, nonunion, and AVN.

Compression fatigue fractures of the femoral neck are best demonstrated as increased bone density at the inferior aspect of the femoral neck on an internal rotation AP radiograph of the hip. There is little risk of fracture displacement.

Intertrochanteric Fractures

The Evans classification (Guans, 1949) is useful for guiding prognosis and treatment. It is based on the number, orienta-

tion, and displacement of the fracture (Fig. 32–23). The primary fracture line extends from proximal-lateral to distal-medial between the greater and lesser trochanters. Undisplaced and displaced two-part fractures define types I and II, respectively. Types III and IV are displaced three-part fractures. There is greater trochanter comminution in type III and lesser trochanter and posteromedial femur comminution in type IV. Type V is a displaced four-part fracture with comminution of both the greater and lesser trochanters.

The *reverse oblique intertrochanteric fracture* is a separate type defined by a primary fracture line that extends from proximal-medial to distal-lateral originating at or above the lesser trochanter. Lateral cortex comminution is common (Fig. 32–24).

Type I and type II fractures can usually be anatomically reduced and fixed in a stable configuration. Types III, IV, and V are more difficult to reduce anatomically and are less stable after reduction. Fracture instability increases with comminution, fracture displacement, and osteopenia. Displacement during the postoperative period is more likely with unstable patterns.

The goal of treatment for intertrochanteric hip fracture is early mobilization and restoration of pre-injury functional capacity. Early reduction and surgical stabilization with a

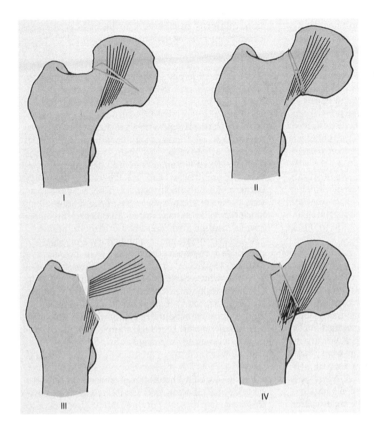

Figure 32–22 The Garden classification for femoral neck fractures. Grade I is an incomplete, impacted fracture in valgus malalignment (generally stable); grade II is a nondisplaced fracture; grade III is an incompletely displaced fracture in varus malignment; grade IV is a completely displaced fracture with no engagement of the two fragments. The compression trabeculae in the femoral head line up with the trabeculae in the acetabular side. Displacement is generally more evident on the lateral view in grade IV. For prognostic purposes, these groupings can be lumped into nondisplaced/impacted (grades I and II) and displaced (grades III and IV), as the risks of nonunion and aseptic necrosis are similar within these grouped stages. Reproduced with permission from Swiontkowski MF. Intracapsular hip fractures. In: Browner BD, ed. *Skeletal Trauma*. Philadelphia, PA: WB Saunders 1992;1390.

sliding screw-plate or screw-rod device permits more rapid mobilization than does bedrest and traction and, thus, minimizes the risk of thromboembolism, pneumonia, skin breakdown, urinary tract infections, and prolonged hospital stay.

Indications for nonoperative management include significant medical co-morbidities or cognitive disabilities that preclude surgery and rehabilitation and pre-injury nonambulatory function.

The sliding hip screw device is the most common implant used for surgical stabilization of Evans types I to V intertrochanteric hip fractures. The fracture fragments settle into a stable configuration as the screw slides within the barrel of the plate. Screw cut-out is less likely with sliding devices than with older fixed-angle one-piece designs. Most fracture patterns can be stabilized with a 130- to 150-degree four-hole plate and screw construct. Sliding of the screw within the plate barrel and fracture impaction is easier with higher angle devices, but the proximal femoral anatomy may require a lesser angle.

The screw should enter the lateral cortex at or slightly inferior to the level of the lesser trochanter and should be placed centrally in the femoral neck and head. Central placement of the screw minimizes the risk of screw cut-out, especially in unstable fracture patterns.

The direction and angle of the reverse oblique fracture pattern precludes the use of the standard plate-screw construct. Fracture distraction and displacement occur as the screw slides within the barrel of the plate. A 95-degree condylar compression plate-screw construct or a 95-degree fixed-angle blade plate is preferable. The length of the side plate is determined by the distal most extent of the fracture.

Postoperative weight bearing remains undefined. Patients with stable fracture patterns, restoration of the posteromedial buttress, and adequate bone stock can begin weight bearing as tolerated with an assistive device. Highly unstable fracture patterns in patients with severe osteoporosis should be protected from full weight bearing until radiographic evidence of union is apparent. Early mobilization should be instituted regardless of the weight-bearing status.

The ultimate outcome and eventual ambulatory status after intertrochanteric hip fracture are influenced by the patient's nutritional status, cognitive status, emotional health, chronologic and physiologic age, social network, and pre-injury functional capacity.

SUBTROCHANTERIC FRACTURES

Fractures of the femoral diaphysis that occur between the lesser trochanter and 8 cm distal to the lesser trochanter are subtrochanteric femur fractures. The high bending stresses and predominance of cortical bone in this region, the frequent comminution, and the frequent presence of associated femoral neck, intertrochanteric, and/or diaphyseal fractures combine to make subtrochanteric fractures difficult to treat.

Many classification systems have been proposed. It is most useful to describe the fracture in terms of its relationship to the lesser trochanter, associated fractures, comminution, and involvement of the posteromedial cortex, greater trochanter, and piriformis fossa.

The goal of treatment is rapid mobilization to minimize the complications of prolonged bedrest. Balanced skeletal traction may be necessary for a multiply injured patient to maintain length and alignment until the patient can tolerate surgery.

The choice of fixation device depends on the fracture pattern. Low subtrochanteric fractures (2 cm or more distal to

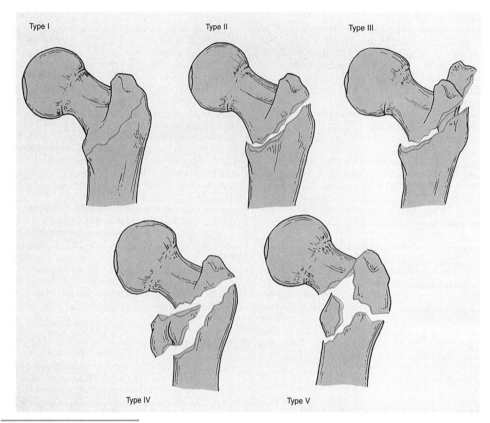

Type I

Type II

Type III

Type IV

Type V

Figure 32–23 Evans classification of intertrochanteric fractures. The primary fracture line runs between the lesser and greater trochanters. Increasing comminution, involving the greater and/or lesser trochanteric region, increases instability and thus the fracture grade. A small lesser trochanteric fragment is conventionally ignored. Type I: undisplaced two-part fracture. Type II: displaced two-part fracture. Type III: displaced three-part fracture with posterolateral comminution. Type IV: displaced three-part fracture with large posteromedial comminuted fragment. Type V: displaced four-part fracture with comminution involving both trochanters. Reproduced with permission from Levy RN, Capozzi JD, Mont MA. Intertrochanteric hip fractures. In: Browner BD, ed. *Skeletal Trauma*. Philadelphia, PA: WB Saunders; 1992:1448.

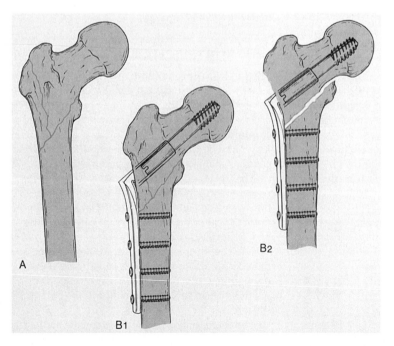

A

B1

B2

Figure 32–24 **(A)** Reverse oblique intertrochanteric fracture. Lateral comminution is common. **(B)** Telescoping of the sliding hip screw does not promote interfragmentary compression because of the orientation of the fracture plane. Stability requires secure impaction of the fracture with either osteotomy of the distal piece to provide mechanical engagement or an implant that resists progressive medial displacement of the shaft. Reproduced with permission from Levy RN, Capozzi JD, Mont MA. Intertrochanteric hip fractures. In: Browner BD, ed. *Skeletal Trauma*. Philadelphia, PA: WB Saunders; 1992:1449.

the lesser trochanter) without intertrochanteric, piriformis fossa, or femoral neck fracture are amenable to statically locked intramedullary nailing. A second generation intramedullary nail or supplemental screw fixation may be necessary when intertrochanteric or femoral neck fracture is present. Intramedullary nailing is contraindicated when the fracture involves the piriformis fossa.

High subtrochanteric fractures (within 2 cm of the lesser trochanter) can be treated with a sliding hip screw and side plate construct like that used for intertrochanteric hip fractures. A long side plate is necessary if the fracture extends into the diaphysis. Bone grafting is necessary when posteromedial cortex comminution is present. A high subtrochanteric fracture with diaphyseal extension but no fracture of the piriformis fossa can be treated with second generation intramedullary nailing.

Subtrochanteric femur fractures are typically unstable and often take longer to unite than intertrochanteric hip fractures. Therefore, protected weight-bearing is necessary until callus formation becomes radiographically apparent. Range of motion and strengthening exercises can often begin in the early postoperative period.

FEMORAL SHAFT FRACTURES

Femoral shaft fractures typically occur in high-energy trauma, therefore, initial evaluation and treatment of the patient is directed at life-threatening injuries to the head, thorax, abdomen, and pelvis. The leg should be realigned by closed reduction, and longitudinal traction or a plaster splint should be applied. Open wounds should be identified and a sterile dressing applied.

Definitive treatment of the fracture should be undertaken as soon as possible to minimize the risk of respiratory distress syndrome. The goal of treatment is to allow mobilization of the patient as soon as is safely possible. Treatment options include balanced skeletal traction, external fixation, intramedullary nailing, and plate and screw fixation.

Complications of balanced skeletal traction include complications of prolonged bedrest, malunion, nonunion, and knee stiffness. It may be useful in patients who cannot undergo surgery soon after injury, in patients who cannot tolerate surgery, or when appropriate fixation devices are not available.

External fixation may be necessary when severe soft tissue injuries are present or rapid stabilization is needed such as for repair of a vascular injury. The sizable soft tissue envelope makes it difficult to achieve stable fixation, and pin tract infections may occur. Nevertheless, external fixation may provide temporary stabilization until internal fixation can be performed.

PEARL

External fixation should be converted to intramedullary nailing as soon as possible, preferably within three weeks of external fixation, to minimize the risk an infected intramedullary nail.

Plate and screw fixation requires direct exposure of the femoral shaft and fracture site. This allows anatomic reduction but entails significant soft tissue stripping. Complications include nonunion, plate failure, and deep infection.

Intramedullary nailing results in a very high union rate with an extremely low complication rate. Closed reduction without exposure of the femoral shaft and fracture site minimizes the risks of nonunion and infection. The nail provides stable, though not rigid, fixation to maximize the union rate and permit early mobilization.

The Winquist classification (Winquist, 1980) describes the extent of comminution. Rotational malunion and shortening are associated with greater degrees of comminution. Type O femoral shaft fractures have no comminution. Type I fractures include a single butterfly fragment that comprises less than 50% of the femoral shaft diameter. A single butterfly fragment comprises between 50 and 100% of the femoral shaft diameter in Type II fractures. The butterfly fragment in Type III fractures is itself comminuted and comprises 50 to 100% of the femoral shaft diameter. Segmental comminution is present in Type IV fractures.

The patient can be positioned supine or lateral decubitus on a flouroscopic operating table or on a fracture table. A femoral distracter may be necessary to help achieve reduction if the fracture table is not used. The nail can be placed antegrade through an entry point at the piriformis fossa or retrograde through the intercondylar notch of the knee.

PITFALL

Excessive traction on the fracture table can result in pudendal nerve palsy.

Reaming of the intramedullary canal permits placement of a larger diameter nail; however, reaming compromises the endosteal blood supply and increases embolization of intramedullary fat and marrow elements. Pulmonary injury is a relative contraindication of reamed intramedullary nailing of the femur.

PEARL

The bending stiffness of an intramedullary nail increases by the fourth power of the radius of the nail.

The proximal femur must be carefully evaluated before proceeding with fixation of femoral shaft fractures. A coexisting femoral neck fracture requires closed or open reduction and fixation with parallel screws prior to treatment of the femoral shaft fracture. Fixation options include parallel screws for the femoral neck followed by antegrade or retrograde nailing, second generation nailing, which is technically difficult and risks displacing the femoral neck fracture, or parallel screws for the femoral neck and plate fixation of the femur.

SELECTED BIBLIOGRAPHY

Evans EM, The treatment of trochanteric fractures of the femur. *J Bone Jt Surg.* 1949;31B:190–203.

Ganden RS, Low-angle fixation in fractures of the femoral neck. *J Bone Jt Surg.* 1961;43B:647–663.

Jimenez ML, Vrahas MS. Surgical approaches to the acetabulum. *Orthop Clin North Am.* 1997;28:419–434.

Judet R, Judet J, Letournel E. Fractures of the acetabulum: classification and surgical approaches for open reduction. *J Bone Jt Surg.* 1964;46A:1615–1638.

Kellam JF, Browner BD. Fractures of the pelvic ring. In: Browner BD, ed. *Skeletal Trauma.* Philadelphia, PA: WB Saunders; 1992:860.

Kellam JF. The role of external fixation in pelvic disruptions. *Clin Orthop.* 1989;241:66–82.

Kellam JF, McMurtry RY, Tile M. The unstable pelvic fracture. *Orthop Clin North Am.* 1987;18:25–41.

Letournel E, Judet R, ed. *Fractures of the Acetabulum.* 2nd ed. New York, NY: Springer-Verlag; 1993.

Levy RN, Capozzi JD, Mont MA. Intertrochanteric hip fractures. In: Browner BD, ed. *Skeletal Trauma.* Philadelphia, PA: WB Saunders; 1992:1445.

Matta J. Operative indications and choice of surgical approach for fractures of the acetabulum. *Tech Orthop.* 1986;1:13–22.

Matta J. Surgical treatment of acetabular fractures. In Browner BD, ed. *Skeletal trauma.* Philadelphia, PA: WB Saunders; 1992:902–903.

Matta J, Anderson L, Epstein H, Hendrick P. Fractures of the acetabulum: a retrospective analysis. *Clin Orthop.* 1986;205:220–240.

Matta J, Letournel E, Browner B. Surgical management of acetabular fractures. *Instruct Course Lect.* 1986;35:382–397.

Mears DC, Rubash H. *Pelvic and acetabular fractures.* Thorofare, New Jersey: Slack; 1986.

Pennal GF, Tile M, Waddell JP, Garside H. Pelvic disruption: assessment and classification. *Clin Orthop.* 1980; 151:12–21.

Pipkin G. Treatment of grade IV fracture dislocation of the hip. A review. *J Bone Jt Surg.* 1957;39A:1027–1042.

Swiontkowski MF. Intracapsular Hip Fractures. In: Browner BD, ed. *Skeletal Trauma.* Philadelphia, PA: WB Saunders; 1992:1370.

Tile M. Pelvic ring fractures: should they be fixed? *J Bone Jt Surg.* 1988;70B:1–12.

Tile M, ed. *Fractures of the Pelvis and Acetabulum.* 2nd ed. Baltimore; MD: Williams and Wilkins; 1995.

Tile M, Rubenstein J. Assessment of acetabular fractures. In: Tile M, ed. *Fractures of the Pelvis and Acetabulum.* Baltimore, MD; Williams and Wilkins. 1995:307–308.

Winquist RA, Hensen ST Jr. Comminuted fractures of the femoral shaft treated by intramedullary, nailing. *Orthop Clin North Am.* 1980;11:633–648.

Young JWR, Burgess AR. *Radiological Management of Pelvic Ring Fractures.* Baltimore; MD: Urban & Schwarzenberg; 1987.

SAMPLE QUESTIONS

1. The principle blood supply to the adult femoral head is the:
   (a) lateral femoral circumflex artery
   (b) lateral epiphyseal artery
   (c) medial epiphyseal artery
   (d) artery of the ligamentum teres
   (e) obturator artery

2. Treatment of a Pipkin type III femoral head fracture in a 32-year-old male consists of:
   (a) closed reduction, balanced skeletal traction for 7 to 10 days, then open reduction and internal fixation
   (b) hip hemiarthroplasty
   (c) total hip arthroplasty
   (d) immediate, single attempt at closed reduction, followed by emergent anatomic reduction and internal fixation

3. The iliac-oblique radiograph images the:
   (a) sacrum, sacroiliac joints, and symphysis pubis
   (b) iliopectineal line, anterior obturator ring, and posterior border of acetabulum
   (c) anterior column and posterior wall
   (d) iliac wing, quadrilateral surface of the ischium, and posterior border of the innominate bone
   (e) pelvic inlet

4. The pelvis fracture injury pattern most likely to be unstable is characterized by:
   (a) symphysis pubis disruption less than 2.5 cm
   (b) bilateral superior and inferior pubic ramus fractures with overlap, and unilateral posterior sacral ala fracture
   (c) bilateral sacroiliac joint dislocation with superior migration of left hemipelvis, symphysis pubic disruption, and left superior and inferior pubic ramus fractures
   (d) left iliac wing fracture, anterior column fracture, and left sacral ala fracture

5. The hip radiographs of a 63-year-old female with a 3-week history of left groin pain are normal. An internal rotation AP hip radiograph demonstrates increased bone density at the inferior femoral neck. Treatment should be:
   (a) hip pinning with three parallel partially threaded cancellous screws
   (b) hip pinning with compression screw and side plate
   (c) core decompression
   (d) observation
   (e) protected weight-bearing with a cane in the right hand

Chapter 33

Pelvis, Hip, and Femur Reconstruction

Ray C. Wasielewski, MD

Outline

Total hip arthroplasty (THA) will be detailed in this chapter. The pitfalls and special considerations will be emphasized. The technical aspects of hip replacement surgery remain the same regardless of the etiology of the arthropathy. However, special considerations are needed in conditions that affect the size and shape of the acetabulum or femur. For example, developmental dysplasia of the hip, SCFE, and the metabolic bone diseases such as scurvy and acromegaly will influence the surgical procedure. Additionally, the treatment of AVN will be discussed as the outcome of this disease process has been favorably affected by recent surgical innovations.

ETIOLOGY

Reconstruction of the adult hip is frequently required to treat a variety of arthropathies.

osteoarthritis
avascular necrosis (AUN)
ankylosing spondylitis
Reiter's arthropathy
psoriatic arthropathy
rheumatoid arthritis
gout
pseudogout
hemophilia
post-traumatic arthritis
Paget's arthropathy
developmental dysplasia of the hip (DDH)
Perthes' arthropathy
slipped capital femoral epiphysis (SCFE)
synovial proliferative disorders

BASIC SCIENCE

Characteristics of Materials Used in Total Hip Arthroplasty

Stainless steel, cobalt-chrome-molybdenum and titanium-vanadium-aluminum stems have performed well as arthroplasty materials. Because of fatigue-related failures of stainless steel stems, cobalt- and titanium-based stems are the preferred materials for cementless THA. Both show an ability to accommodate bone ingrowth. Titanium stems have a decreased modulus of elasticity compared with cobalt chrome, and they have desirable bone ingrowth characteristics. The lower modulus may provide for better loading of the femur and decreased stress shielding. This may result in less thigh pain. One disadvantage of titanium is that it is

Orthopaedic Surgery: The Essentials. Edited by M.E. Baratz, A.D. Watson, and J.E. Imbriglia. Thieme Medical Publishers, Inc., New York © 1999

more notch sensitive than cobalt chrome. This limits its use in small sizes, particularly when porous coated. Titanium is less favorable for cemented use because it strains much more than the cement mantle with loading. Cement does not tolerate these strains, resulting in debonding at the cement implant interface. Few cemented stems are now made of titanium, most are cobalt-based alloys. Cobalt-chrome stems can tolerate more extensive porous coating, even in small sizes. However, in larger sizes cobalt stems may cause excessive stress shielding and thigh pain. Because stress shielding is due to the rigidity of the implant (not just modulus), one of the best ways to decrease structural rigidity is to slot the stem or have a cut-out area. These modifications allow the implant to have a flexibility and stiffness closer to that of bone.

EXAMINATION

History

The most frequent chief complaint of the patient with hip arthritis is groin pain. A small number of patients will complain of knee pain. If the patient has radiographic evidence of knee as well as hip pathology, then a lidocaine injection of the knee may be required to isolate the component of pain originating from the hip.

PEARL

If pain is acute in onset but not related to trauma, consider avascular necrosis (AVN) in the differential diagnosis.

If the patient makes a sweeping motion through the groin, suspect radicular pain from the upper lumbar spine. If the patient has pain on pressing on the groin, suspect an inguinal adenopathy or hernia or an occult superior rami fracture. Lateral thigh pain is often called hip pain by patients and referring doctors; however, it frequently represents only hip bursitis or iliotibial band irritation. Although buttock pain can represent pain of acetabular origin, it is most commonly sciatic pain or radicular pain.

PEARL

Pain at rest and pain relief only with narcotics are strong indicators for operative intervention.

Review of Systems

Ongoing infections should be sought out. Patients with poor dentition should get a panorex view before surgery to rule out occult abscesses. Urinary tract infections require 7 to 10 days of antibiotic treatment prior to surgery for patients with white blood cells and leukoesterase present on urinalysis. A culture with sensitivity should be sent for in all patients with a positive urinalysis before the start of empiric antibiotics. Cultures should be re-evaluated prior to surgery to identify cases of resistant or fastidious organisms. Areas of skin breakdown or ulcerations need to be completely healed prior to surgery. Diverticular disease or diverticulitis should be evaluated and treated prior to surgery.

Physical Examination

The exam begins with observation. Watch patients walk into the examining room. Ask them to move from the chair to the examining table to evaluate the difficulty they have getting up out of a chair. Assess for an antalgic or Trendelenburg gait. Neurologic gait abnormalities causing foot drop or recurvatum deformity secondary to quadriceps weakness can be suspected after watching gait. An unstable gait may indicate a balance disorder or spinal stenosis.

Palpate for areas of tenderness. The groin should not be tender. If there is groin tenderness, one should suspect an occult fracture of the superior pubic ramus, arterio-venous malformation after an invasive procedure, or inguinal adenopathy. Often there is tenderness over the greater trochanter from irritation of the iliotibial band due to abnormal gait or joint mechanics.

Range of motion (ROM) including flexion, extension, adduction, and abduction should be measured. Pain at the extreme of internal rotation will occur in most patients needing THA. Joint contractures need to be quantitated. An adductor tenotomy may be required at the beginning of hip replacement surgery if adduction contractures are present. If flexion contractures are diagnosed with the Thomas test, then an anterior lateral approach may be needed. External rotation contractures rarely require correction.

When a preoperative leg length discrepancy (LLD) is present, its etiology must be identified. Only discrepancies due to the hip joint pathology can be corrected by hip joint surgery. Failure to make the appropriate determination may result in technical problems during surgery and a poor outcome.

The *actual* leg length discrepancy is measured from the anterior superior iliac spine (ASIS) to the medial malleolus of the ankle. A short limb is most commonly due to loss of hip joint cartilage and acetabular bone or femoral head collapse. However, knee osteoarthritis, ankle pathology, old fractures or congenital limb length discrepancies can also be present. A long cassette film of the entire extremity should be ordered whenever the leg length discrepancy is greater than that expected from joint pathology.

The *apparent* leg length discrepancy is measured from the umbilicus to the medial malleolus of ankle. Apparent LLD can be due to multiple causes. Consider adduction contractures or spinal deformity as the cause of a difference between apparent and actual leg. Discuss this with the patient prior to surgery as hip surgery will often not correct these discrepancies.

A careful neurovascular exam should be performed. Ankle-brachial indicies (ABIs) are indicated if no palpable dorsalis pedis or posterior tibialis pulses can be felt. A baseline examination of sciatic nerve, tibial, and peroneal divisions should be recorded. If the history suggests that the patient has spinal stenosis or spinal claudication, then this should be evaluated by magnetic resonance imaging (MRI), computed tomography (CT), or CT-myelogram.

AIDS TO DIAGNOSIS

Radiographs

Radiographs should be done with marker balls so that the magnification is known. Knowledge of the exact magnification of the x-rays relative to the templates allows the femur and acetabulum to be correctly sized for implantation. The anteroposterior (AP) pelvis film is valuable to measure leg length discrepancies and to compare the uninvolved hip for templating. The AP hip film is taken with the extremity in slight internal rotation to accurately determine the diameter, shape, and proximal metaphyseal configuration. The lateral view of the hip and femur demonstrates the diameter of the femoral canal and the AP bow of the femur.

Several features of the standard hip radiographs need to be evaluated. The degree of radiographic osteopenia should be noted as it may indicate osteoporosis. Joint space and bony architecture should also be noted. Template the radiograph

and select a prosthesis to maximize stability while minimizing leg length increase.

PEARL
To maximize stability and minimize leg length increase, a slightly more offset prosthesis than the templates would indicate may be best suited for the patient with mild joint space narrowing.

With moderate (5–10 mm) joint space narrowing, a prosthesis that matches the offset of the patient works best. If the normal opposite hip is available, match the proximal femoral configuration as closely as possible.

If there is severe (> 10 mm) joint space narrowing, make at least two determinations of leg length discrepancy prior to surgery (i.e., clinical and radiographic). Compare templated measurements with the normal hip. Consider maneuvers to protect or monitor the sciatic nerve as leg length discrepancy and the anticipated lengthening approaches 3 cm.

The direction of joint space narrowing is also noted. Superior joint space narrowing usually indicates osteoarthritis and occasionally represents AVN. Patients with medial joint space narrowing may have a tendency towards protrusio; therefore, consider under-reaming the acetabulum 3 mm (for normal bone quality) or 4 mm (for osteoporotic bone) less than the

TABLE 33–1 Differential diagnosis (severe "hip" pain)

Diagnosis	Groin Pain	Lateral Pain	Buttock Pain
Spinal stenosis	✓	✓	
Hip bursitis		✓	
Synovitis	✓		
AVN	✓		
Radicular pain		✓	✓
Meralgia paresthetica		✓	
Gout ➢ Hip aspiration and serography	✓		
Pseudogout ➢ Hip aspiration	✓		
Occult fracture hip or rami ➢ Pathologic ➢ Metabolic	✓		
Tumor	✓		✓
Inguinal adenopathy	✓		
Vascular claudication	✓		
External iliac or femoral AV Malformation	✓		

TABLE 33–2   Preoperative assessments/outcome measurement

1. Harris hip score (100 points)
   A. Pain: 44 points
   B. Function: 47 points
   C. Absence of Deformity: 4 points
   E. Range of Motion: 5

2. Short form 36 (SF 36): This instrument is accepted by the medical community as a proven measure of outcome. It can be broken down into physical and mental components.

3. Classifying patients A, B, or C*
   A. Class A patients:
      1. Unilateral arthropathy
      2. No significant medical comorbidity
   B. Class B patients:
      1. Other joint in need of THA
      2. Other unsuccessful or failing THA
   C. Class C patients:
      1. Advanced inflammatory arthropathy
      2. Multiple joints in need of total joint arthroplasty
      3. Multiple unsuccessful or failing THA
      4. Significant medical comorbidity
      5. Significant psychological impairment

4. Anesthesia severity assessment patient anesthesia classification: Patients with a rating of 3 or greater are at significant increased risk of perioperative morbidity. These patients often have longer lengths of hospital stays with higher hospital charges.

5. AAHKS (American Association of Hip and Knee Surgeons) evaluation forms.

* In Bibliography

planned acetabular component size. Concentric joint space narrowing is usually a sign of inflammatory arthropathy.

The acetabulum may demonstrate cyst formation, sclerosis, or osteophytes. Cysts may need to be grafted with either acetabular reamings or bone substitutes. Sclerosis may cause reamers to be pushed inferiorly resulting in inferior acetabular component placement. Consider saving the transverse acetabular ligament to give some resistance to this tendency during reaming. Osteophytes must be removed to prevent impingement and subsequent hip instability. If hypertrophic osteophytes are present, then consider prophylactic treatment for heterotopic bone formation.

Lumbosacral spine films are indicated in patients with low back pain, suspected spinal stenosis, or in patients with a pelvic obliquity due to scoliosis.

Cervical spine films must be obtained in all rheumatoid patients. After initial AP and lateral views, some patients require flexion-extension C-spine radiographs. Evidence of C1-2 subluxation may necessitate fiber optic intubation. When there is severe subluxation at this level or at a subaxial level, spine surgery consultation prior to hip surgery is indicated.

Magnetic Resonance Imaging

Magnetic resonance imaging is seldom indicated. In a patient with severe hip pain and normal radiographs, an MRI may be helpful. Magnetic resonance imaging is the best imaging modality for evaluating AVN in the early stages.

Bone Scan

A three-phase bone scan may be useful to evaluate for the presence of infection or AVN. A bone scan is also indicated in cases in which x-rays are normal and there is some concern about the possible origin of the pain being from the sacroiliac joint, lumbusacral region at a ligament or tendon enthesis.

Computed Tomography Scan

Computed tomography may be useful to evaluate the bone dimension and configuration prior to joint arthroplasty. Sagittal and coronal sections through the canal may assist in selecting prosthesis type and geometry. A CT scan is indicated to assess anteversion in congenital dysplasia of the hip or retroversion in slipped capital femoral epiphysis anomalies so that the appropriate femoral component can be selected. Anteversion is determined by making distal cuts through the femoral condyles at the knee and proximal cuts through the neck. The cuts are then compared to quantitate the angulation of the proximal femur relative to the posterior aspect of the distal condyles.

For patients with suspected loosening of their femoral implants, a CT rotation study is helpful in definitively demonstrating that a component is loose. This study is similar to the aforementioned anteversion study, but done with the leg first in maximal external rotation followed by maximal internal rotation. Proximal and distal cuts are made in each extreme. A loose stem will change its proximal angulation relative to the posterior condyles

Injections

Provocative injections are utilized to make determinations of the origin of "hip pain." Lidocaine alone should be utilized as adding steroids may have an undesired effect on contiguous sources of pain.

Technique: Intra-articular Hip Joint Injection

The intra-articular hip joint injection is best done under fluoroscopic guidance. The starting point can be grossly located as being 3 finger breaths caudal to the ASIS and 2 finger breaths medial. Examine the hip prior to injection for pain inducing maneuvers or positions. Repeat the exam after the injection to check for alleviation of symptoms. The injection should not start too far medial so as to avoid injection of the femoral nerve. A knee immobilizer can be temporarily used in all cases where this complication occurs.

Technique: Hip Bursal Injection

The hip bursal injection is performed in the lateral decubitus position. The midportion of the trochanter and the vastus tubercle are palpated and marked at the locations of greatest pain. Two separate injection sites are preferable as they optimize the likelihood of success. One should utilize a 22-gauge 3 inch needle, as the most common reason for failure is not having adequate needle length to get completely down to the trochanter; in rare circumstances a 5-inch needle should be used if the patient is obese. The spinal needle should be advanced to the fascia lata, where pain is usually felt by the patient. You should be easily able to feel as the needle is advanced through the fascia (particularly if it is inflamed and thickened). When doing two injections, the sites are most commonly located at the midportion of the trochanter and just over the vastus tubercle. The injection should be deposited just after penetration through the fascia is felt. Almost immediately after injection, the patient should feel pain relief. (Lidocaine portion of injection).

Technique: Saocioiliac Joint Injection

The technique for SI injection is best demonstrated by looking at a skeleton immediately prior to the injection so that you can see the angle necessary to enter this oblique joint. Palpate along the iliac crest medially to the start of the sacrum. Proceed caudal about 2.5 cm to the starting point. This is generally 2 cm lateral to where the sacrum can be palpated at the medial most aspect of the ilium. The needle (22 gauge × 3 inches = 8.89 cm) is directed from lateral to medial at about a 45-degrees angle until a pop is felt as the needle passes through the superficial posterior ligaments. Two to four cc of solution are injected into the joint.

GENERAL PREOPERATIVE PLANNING

Autologous Blood Donation

Donation of two units of packed red cells will almost eliminate the need for postoperative banked blood transfusions. Cell-saver use during revision surgery is recommended in patients with a decreased preoperative hemoglobin or in a large anticipated operative blood loss. Erythopoetin should be considered in patients with anemia, particularly those with renal abnormalities. Additionally, this is of great value in Jehovah's Witness patients, who do not accept perioperative blood products.

Somatosensory Evoked Potentials

Somatosensory evoked potentials (SSEPs) should be available to monitor all patients at risk for sciatic nerve injury. Specific indications include patients with leg length discrepancies greater than 5 cm or occasionally patients with abnormal spinal conditions on electromyographic (EMG) or nerve conduction study testing.

Templating

Accurate templating helps ensure success. Radiographs with marker ball magnification are essential. The standard AP and lateral hip radiographs are minimum requirements. The AP radiograph of the pelvis should be obtained to evaluate the opposite normal hip and provide important insight into reconstructing the involved side to approximate the uninvolved hip.

Acetabular Templating

When placing the acetabular templates over the AP radiography, first, measure the distance between the marker balls and compare this with the known distance between these radiopaque balls (usually 10 cm). The actual magnification of the x-rays is determined and compared with the magnification of the templates. Typically, manufacturers use the same magnification on all their hip templates (15 to 20% magnification depending on manufacturer). Sizing the acetabulum on an orthogonal lateral view of the acetabulum will provide additional insight on sizing, particularly in the nonhemispheric acetabulae.

The acetabular template should be medialized almost to the base of the fovea. Fully hemispheric implants (180 degrees) obtain optimal coverage in patients with a deep acetabulum and 170-degree implants are best in patients with a shallow acetabulum. When utilizing 170-degree implants, one may not want to medialize to the base of the fovea, as this may result in bone overhang and impingement. Other reasons to avoid overmedialization include patients with osteoporosis or RA (protrusio diathesis) or in very young patients in which bone conservation is mandatory to preserve bone stock for future revision surgery.

In general, when templating for acetabular implant abduction/adduction, the cup should be angled so as to intersect the midpoint of the obturator foramen. This inclination will often cause a small overhang superiorly beyond the lateral edge of the acetabulum. A more horizontal cup position is desired because it improves hip stability, improves femoral head coverage, and may decrease linear polyethylene wear.

Templating for Femoral Arthroplasty

The varus/valgus angulation of the femoral stem template should be matched as closely as possible to the proximal femoral canal. The neck angulation should be as similar as possible to achieve anatomic reproduction of the patients offset and length. When available, the template should be overlaid on the uninvolved hip to compare it with the normal femoral geometry. These measurements on the normal hip are often the most accurate because the affected side has geometric changes due to the pathology that can adversely influence templating. The most common problem is excessive hip external rotation on x-rays (evident by a prominent lesser trochanter) that gives the appearance of more valgus than is actually present. Slightly internally rotating the leg when taking x-rays in patients with external rotation contractures will rectify this problem. Adduction contractures also greatly distort the geometry, making it difficult to template the affected hip. A CAT scan may be indicated when distortion is severe.

Indications for Cemented Femoral Arthroplasty

The hybrid THA utilizing a cemented femoral stem and cementless acetabular component represents the "gold standard" and National Institutes of Health consensus. Remember, any shape femur can be cemented whereas there are many configurations that preclude cementless femoral arthroplasty

Shape of femoral canal

Trumpet-shaped femora do not template well for cementless femoral arthroplasty because it is difficult to obtain contact between the subchondral bone and the ingrowth surface of proximally porous coated femoral stems.

Age

All patients older than 60 years of age should be considered for cemented arthroplasty.

Bone quality

Patients with poor bone quality should be considered for cemented femoral arthroplasty.

Anteversion/retroversion

Excessive anteversion or retroversion makes it difficult to accommodate cementless prosthesis.

Varus/valgus

Patients with excessive varus or valgus are the best candidates for cemented arthroplasy unless special cementless stems are available.

Size: small/large

Patients with very small or very large femoral canals are best suited for cemented femoral arthroplasty.

Techniques for Templating

Whether templating the femur for cemented or cementless arthroplasty, it is critical that a good AP film be obtained (14×17 inch cassette) in slight internal rotation. Most patients have external rotation contractures that tend to make the femur appear more anteverted than is actually the case.

The femur should be reconstructed with a femoral component of similar offset and neck/shaft angulation. Templating off of the normal side provides verification of the stem geometry needed.

After matching the template to the geometry and configuration of the femur, select the actual size that will most likely be required. In cementless implants, this will be the size that causes a tight fit within the intrameoullary canal distal to the lesser trochanter. After this "diaphyseal" sizing, see how the proximal configuration matches. If the prosthesis does not approximate against the subchondral bone of the proximal metaphysis, select a more extensively coated prosthesis whose ingrowth surface reaches the subchondral bone. Fully coated prostheses may be required in cases in which adequate contact does not occur until the metaphyseal/diaphyseal junction. A cemented prosthesis may be a better option in these cases, particularly in primary THA.

In sizing for a cemented femoral stem, err on the side of undersizing. Leave a 1- to 1.5-mm space between prosthesis

and subchondral bone of the diaphysis and metaphysis. Most templates for cemented femoral components have this built-in (usually depicted by a dotted border).

The depth that the implant assumes within the femur is determined by several factors. Foremost is the position that most closely reconstructs the patients original offset and leg length. A critical objective of THA is to reconstruct offset to maximize the abductor moment arm and stability.

Remember the real value of templating is in its predictive value. When you template, you can see the type of implants that are necessary to accommodate bone deformities, curvatures of the femur, and abnormal bone configuration and shape.

Selection of Femoral Stems

One of the major factors affecting implant selection is bone quality. As bone quality decreases, the indications for cemented THA increases unless a special cementless prosthesis is utilized. A stem that is porous coated only on the proximal third can be used in a patient with normal anatomy and good bone quality. A more fully porous coated ($\frac{5}{8}$) can be used in patients who have osteopenia or other metabolic conditions that diminish bone quality (post-transplant or a seronegative or seropositive arthropathy). More extensively coated femoral stems are used in young patients with "champagne-fluted" femoral canals. These patients may require stems with more porous surface to adequately contact the endosteal femoral surface (usually at the level of the lesser trochanter). Only rarely are fully coated stems indicated in primary THA cases. These stems may be indicated if osteotomies are necessary to correct proximal metaphyseal deformities. Young patients with CDH and small canal geometries may require fully coated cementless stems to maximize area contact of the porous surface with subchondral bone to optimize the chances of bone ingrowth. Cemented stems are used in patients with significant medical problems, inflammatory arthropathies, in transplant patients, or in patients on chronic steroids.

Stem Selection in Abnormal Proximal Canal Geometry

1. Significant varus (coxa varus):

    Cemented stem: Iowa (1320),(Zimmer, Warsaw, Indiana) High Offset Endurance (DePuy, Warsaw, Indiana)

    Cementless stem: anatomic medullary locking (standard), DePuy, Warsaw, Indiana) Replica (large: 1250) (DePuy, Warsaw, Indiana)

2. Significant valgus (CDH, etc.):

    Cemented stem: Precoat (Zimmer, Warsaw, Indiana), Valgus Iowa (1400)

    Cementless stem: [should be used with extreme caution in patients with valgus necks as varus prostheses may act like a wedge causing fracture] anatomic medullary locking (modified medial aspect)-DePuy

ANATOMY AND SURGICAL APPROACHES

Anterior Lateral Approach (Modified Hardinge)—Total Hip Arthroplasty
Indications

Recent investigations suggest that both the anterolateral and posterior approach yield similar hip stability and acceptably low rates of hip dislocation. The anterior lateral approach is advantageous for cases in which a flexion contracture exists because contracted tissues are released as part of the dissection. It is the approach of choice when doing the case without assistance. You do not need a leg holder during femoral preparation, as the leg is simply externally rotated and placed in a hip pocket across the field.

Technique (Anterolateral Approach)

Caveats:

1. When dividing the gluteus medius in the proximal deep dissection, do not cheat too far anteriorly in an attempt to preserve the abductor muscle insertion, as the opposite may result.

2. In cases in which flexion contractures exist, an extensive capsular release down the anterior femur beyond the intertrochanteric line is often required. The dissection may need to be carried medially and posterior to the lesser trochanter and then distally to address adduction contractures.

3. The femur is retracted posteriorly in the anterolateral approach for acetabular preparation. Dividing the inferior capsule down to the transverse acetabular ligament enhances this exposure by allowing the femur to be more easily retracted posterior.

4. Anterior acetabular exposure is optimized by placing a blunt AuFranc Cobra retractor over the anterior column. Preparing the site for retractor insertion is accomplished by utilizing the electrocautery to make a 2-cm incision through the capsule just anterior to the labrum. The Cobra retractor is easily inserted over the anterior column directly against bone and is pulled medially to retract the anterior tissues. In a similar fashion a retractor can also be placed inferiorly through a slit made over the transverse acetabular ligament. This inferior retractor also provides sufficient retraction of the femur posteriorly. When needed, a posterior retractor can be placed against the posterior column between the labrum and capsule. Avoid using posterior retractors whenever possible to minimize the likelihood of injury to the sciatic nerve.

Contemporary technique suggests that the acetabulum should be reamed 1 to 4 mm less than the acetabular component size to afford maximum rim interference fit. The correct amount of underreaming should just allow contact of the dome of the component with the medial acetabular bone plate.

When using an anterolateral approach, the cup anteversion is only 15–20 degrees. This position will often leave some bone overhang posteriorly. If the cup is overanteverted (most often caused by trying to match the bony borders of the acetabulum), an elevated lip liner placed anteriorly will help improve hip stability (by improving anterior coverage). How-ever, it is always better to change the position of the cup into less anteversion.

The femoral stem should not be over anteverted as this may also result in a dislocation. When using an anterolateral approach, use stems without anteversion to increase anterior stability. Most of the time when an anterior dislocation occurs after an anterior lateral approach, it is due to impingement on the posterior capsular tissues or bone. Complete posterior capsular resections and removal of any posterior bony prominence may improve hip stability.

Posterior Approach—Total Hip Arthroplasty
Indications

Certain preoperative variables make this approach more desirable for primary hip replacement. These include: CDH (excessive femoral anteversion), slipped capital femoral epiphysis (femoral head is located posteriorly), cases in which trochanteric osteotomy may be indicated, and when posterior column defects are present. The posterior approach may be preferable in cases of severe acetabular perimeter osteophytes (particularly if protrusio is present). Exposure of the sciatic nerve is easier to accomplish through the posterior approach for cases in which leg lengthening will be substantial and release of the piriformis and gluteal sling is needed to decrease the tension on the sciatic nerve.

Technique

Position the patient in the lateral decubitus position using either a beanbag or pelvic positioner. Do not allow the patient to be flexed at the hip as this will make alignment of the acetabular component difficult. Make sure to have the ASIS easily palpable for use as a landmark during the placement of transacetabular screws. Make sure that the hip is easily flexed to 90 degrees without impingement on the pelvic positioner, as this will affect the ability to determine hip stability during component trialing.

The skin incision is centered over the greater trochanter with equal extension distally in line with the femur and proximally, curved posteriorly in line with the gluteus maximus fibers. Divide the fascia lata in line with the skin incision. Locate the posterior border of the gluteus medius tendon. Locate the superior aspect of the deep interval by identifying the piriformis tendon directly beneath the tendon of the gluteus medius. To improve exposure, in muscular or obese patients, it is often helpful to make a cut above the piriformis tendon through the minimus. Place an AuFranc Cobra retractor up over the piriformis between the minimus and the capsule and retract anteriorly. This exposes the superior aspect of the hip area. Divide and tag (No. 5 Ticron suture) the posterior structures: the piriformis, obturator internus and gemelli, obturator externus, and capsule. Continue down the femur elevating the quadratus and dividing the gluteal sling when needed to improve exposure. The tagged capsule and external rotators can be reflected posteriorly to protect the sciatic nerve.

Acetabular bone preparation is done as previously described in the section on anterolateral approach. Acetabular implant alignment and position are slightly different because the acetabular anteversion should be increased about

10 to 15 degrees more than is built into most acetabular alignment jigs. This extra anteversion will usually result in about 20 to 35 degrees of acetabular version. Most of the time this alignment will be very similar to that of the contour of the acetabular rim. Most commonly, there will be slight overhang of the implant superiorly and posteriorly. Under no circumstances should the acetabular implant be visible above the anterior column bone as this indicates inadequate anteversion of the acetabular implant.

When placing transacetabular screws to augment acetabular shell fixation, the tendency is to place these screws in the more anterior quadrants when exposure is through a posterior approach. However, the safe zone for screw placement are in the posterior regions (quadrants) of the acetabulum. Access to the posterior bone is improved by adequately retracting the femur anteriorly with an aufranc retractor placed over the anterior column. During screw placement, remove the inferior Aufranc Cobra retractor to help get the drill properly aligned to drill posterior-superior and posterior-inferior screw holes.

For femoral preparation through the posterior approach, make sure to adequately antevert the femoral implant. Because the hip is internally rotated, it is easy to get confused with the orientation. As the lesser trochanter is a posterior structure, angulation away from this bony prominence is anteversion. The exact amount of version should be at least the amount in the femoral canal (usually 20 to 25 degrees). Select a cementless femoral stem that has anteversion built into it when using the posterior approach. This will augment posterior stability.

When closing the posterior soft tissue dissection, reapproximate the external rotators, and capsule and to the trochanter through drill holes in the bone with no. 5 Ticron sutures. Tie these sutures under tension with the hip in external rotation to decrease the ability of the hip to internally rotate, further augmenting posterior stability. If the hip cannot be externally rotated at least 15 degrees, do a release of the gluteus minimus along its undersurface (see internal rotation contractures below). Check to see that the knee can be extended with the hip in full extension. If this is not possible, release the flexion contracture (see below).

Special Surgical Exposures and Releases
Flexion Contractures

Hip flexion contractures are frequently due to contracture of the anterior capsular tissues and rectus musculature. The anterolateral approach is the best approach to address flexion contractures because the anterior capsular structures (iliofemoral ligament) are released as part of the approach. Also the reflected head of the rectus can be released through this approach. Occasionally, if significant hip lengthening is done the psoas muscle becomes excessively taut resulting in a flexion (and external rotation) contracture. The tendinous portion of the piriformis can be tenotomized just distal to the point it crosses over the pelvic brim, leaving the muscular portion intact to maintain muscular continuity. After adequate release of a hip flexion contracture, the knee should bend to 90 degrees with the hip in the fully extended position.

Adduction Contractures

Adequate hip abduction is important for adequate THA function and stability. Excessive hip adduction is a position of hip instability regardless of the surgical approach. Adduction contractures are corrected by making a separate medial groin incision to subcutaneously release the contracted adductor tendons. This should be done before starting the THA. After tenotomy, make sure that the hip can be adducted to at least neutral. Through an anteriolateral approach, the adductor release is continued by releasing anteriorly and medially across the intertrochanteric line. The inferior and anterior capsular regions should also be released.

Internal Rotation Contractures

Internal rotation contractures are common after total hip arthroplasty when the gluteus minimus muscle become tight when the hip is lengthened. It is important to correct internal rotation contractures if a posterior approach to the hip is done, otherwise a tendency toward hip internal rotation and posterior hip dislocation will result. It may be necessary to release the undersurface of the gluteus minimus from caudad to cephalad. A complete anterior and medial capsulectomy should also be performed. Occasionally the gluteus medius will need to be released along its superior attachment at the outer iliac crest. This is most commonly needed when leg lengthening greater than 3 cm is required, such as with congenitally dysplastic hips.

Cementless Acetabular Preparation—Special Considerations: Posterior Approach

The exposure for acetabular arthroplasty is optimized by placing retractors anteriorly (between the labrum and capsule over the anterior column), inferiorly (over the transverse acetabulum) and only occasionally posteriorly. If the posterior capsular tissues are blocking exposure, a cerebellar self-retaining retractor can be placed between the trochanter and the posterior tissues. This should provide adequate exposure while decreasing the likelihood of causing damage to the sciatic nerve. If the femur still does not adequately retract anteriorly, the inferior capsule and then the gluteal sling should be released. In very rare cases in which this exposure needs to be increased—possibly because of a severe acetabular defect or posterior superior defect that needs bulk allograft (bringing a CDH down to the normal anatomic location)—a trochanteric osteotomy may be necessary. The posterior approach does allow for this option.

The only way to be assured that the acetabular component is properly seated against good host bone is to remove all of the periacetabular soft tissues. The labrum needs to be removed as well as the tissues from the fovea. Leave the transverse acetabular ligament intact. It should be kept in place to prevent the reamer from being forced inferiorly when the bone is sclerotic superiorly. The opposite is true if there is osteopenic bone superiorly. In these cases, the transverse acetabular ligament can have a detrimental affect by tending to force the acetabular reamer superiorly.

Start acetabular reaming by selecting a reamer size 1 cm smaller than templated. Begin by reaming medially to the base of the fovea (slightly less if a 170° cup is used). Any ossification should be removed by this small reamer during medialization, exposing the true base of the fovea. When the acetabulum is sufficiently reamed medially, antevert and adduct the reamer into the final position the acetabular implant will assume. Periodically remove the reamer to assess the anterior and posterior columns to ensure that equal amounts of bone are being reamed. Concentrically expand the acetabulum to a size 1 to 4 mm less than the acetabular component size. The correct amount of underreaming is that which provides maximum rim interference fit while just allowing contact of the dome of the component with the medial acetabular bone plate.

Adequate reaming of the anterior and posterior columns has been obtained when there is good bleeding bone around the entire circumference. The author recommends 1 mm of underreaming in patients who have sclerotic bone, 2 mm in the normal patient, and 3 mm in the osteopenic patient. Consider underreaming 3–4 mm in patients for which it is essential that the cup not be medialized (protrusio). Only 1 mm of underreaming is necessary in patients for whom additional fixation is utilized (such as screw fixation, fins, or peg fixation). Cups with holes in the superior dome optimize the ability to ascertain that the cup is well seated. This is particularly important when you are impacting the cup into an undersized reamed acetabulum. Utilize 170° cups for shallow acetabulums and 180° cups for deep acetabulums.

Screws should be used where suboptimal acetabular fit occurs. The theoretical disadvantages to using screws, such as increased wear debris formation, should not overshadow potential early failures that would occur if screws are not used. When placing transacetabular fixation screws to augment cup fixation use the acetabular quadrant system. Screws should be placed in the posterior superior quadrants where bone depth and safety are optimized. Posterior inferior quadrant screws can be used with palpation of the posterior column (Figs. 33–1 and 33–2).

SURGICAL TECHNIQUE
Cemented Femoral Arthroplasty

Preparation of the femoral canal for cemented arthroplasty involves adequate exposure of the proximal femur. Position the opening in the proximal femoral canal in the middle of the incision. The femoral shaft should also line up with the incision. This allows for use of intramedullary instruments while avoiding their impingement on the walls of the incision. Pack a lap sponge in the acetabulum under the proximal femur to move the proximal femur up out of the wound. Apply a downward pressure on the knee to raise the proximal femur further out of the incision. Finally, place a two-pronged wooden handled retractor under the femur at the level of the lesser trochanter. Remove the remnants of the

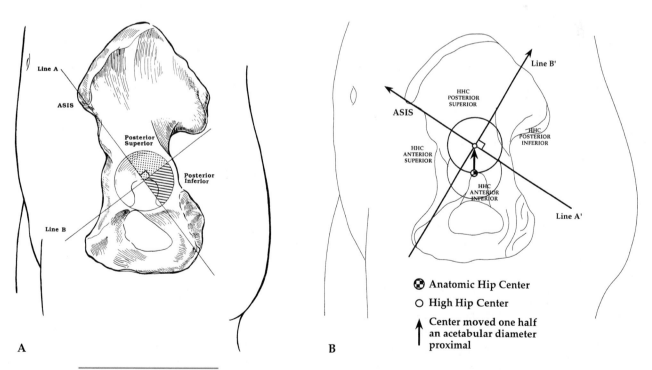

Figure 33–1 **(A)** The quadrant system at the normal (anatomic) hip center. The posterior inferior and posterior superior quadrants are recommended for transacetabular fixation screws in total hip arthroplasty. **(B)** Schematic diagram illustrating the high hip center (HHC) quadrant system superimposed one half of an acetabular diameter proximal to the original anatomic acetabular quadrant system.

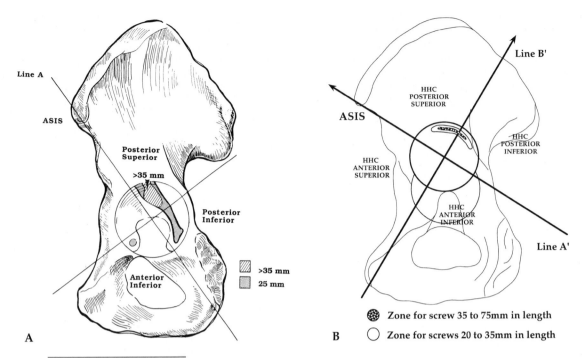

Figure 33–2 **(A)** Bone depth within the quadrants. The central region of the posterior inferior and posterior superior quadrants provide the best bone stock for screw purchase. **(B)** Topographic map of the acetabular bone depth showing a zone in the peripheral HHC posterior quadrants where screws 25 mm, to greater than 35 mm, can be placed up into the ilium.

obturator externus and internus, gemelli, and piriformis from the trochanteric region to improve visualization of the intramedullary canal.

Enter the canal with a T-awl. Often, this awl will only go partially down the canal. This occurs because of impingement against the lateral subchondral bone because the awl is in varus. If this is not recognized, the implant will also be placed in varus. To fully insert the awl down into the intramedullary canal of the femur requires adequate lateralization. Use a conical reamer to lateralize into this typically sclerotic bone. Do not proceed with reaming or broaching of the femoral canal until the awl freely goes down the canal.

Excessive reaming of the femoral canal results in premature failure of cemented implants. This is because reaming removes the interstices from the subchondral bone that allow for cement intercalation. To varify adequate lateralization it is appropriate to ream once down the intramedullary canal with a small reamer (8 or 9 mm). Broaching should always begin with the smallest broach. If the broach easily advances to the level of the neck cut, countersink the broach before going up to the next size. If the broach cannot be countersunk, consider the possibility that the prosthesis is in varus or you have templated wrong. An intra-operative radiograph with the broach in the femoral canal should be obtained whenever there is any doubt. Do not oversize the femoral stem as a good cement mantle is important for a successful long-term result.

The last two broaches must be inserted in the correct varus/valgus alignment and anteversion. Calcar ream once the final broach is in place to obtain a good, flush calcar fit. If the calcar has not been cut appropriately, it can affect implant version. For instance, if the posterior aspect of the calcar is prominent relative to anterior, a collared stem will tend to move into retroversion during insertion.

Stability testing can be difficult because the cemented femoral trial frequently fits loosely in the canal. Wrap a sponge around the prosthesis to stabilize it during trial reduction. Trial reduction should be done with the patient paralyzed to relax the soft tissue and provide a conservative measure of hip stability. Accept no more than 5mm of hip pistoning on passive pull. Also check this with retraction removed from the fascial edges. The hip should be difficult to dislocate when reproducing the motion needed for activities of daily living.

Once the implant size and alignment have been determined, prepare the femoral canal for cementing. Remove cancellous bone from the medial, anterior, and posterior aspect of the proximal femur down to the lesser trochanter. Do not remove lateral trochanteric cancellous bone. This may lead to excessive cement intercalation into the trochanter, weakening the bone and increasing the chance of postoperative fracture. Plug the canal distally. Dry the canal with lap sponges that do not leave lint in the canal.

Inject cement in a retrograde fashion from distal to proximal. Pressurize the cement using a proximal pressurizer or by using your thumb. Cement should extrude through the blood vessel canals of the proximal femoral metaphysis. This is best accomplished by having cement of sufficiently low viscosity.

Initially insert the prosthesis in slight varus to preserve the lateral cement mantle. Approximately half way down into the canal, bring the prosthesis into the appropriate valgus. Use a centralizer for the stem. Utilize preoperative templating and intra-operative findings to optimize the position of the prosthesis collar to the calcar. If the collar overlapped the calcar, try to reproduce this overlap intraoperatively. Stabilize the prosthesis while allowing the cement to polymerize, firmly fixing the implant to bone. Remove excess cement prior to polymerization.

Cementless Femoral Arthroplasty

It is important that the preliminary neck cut is as close as possible to the pre-templated level (usually 1–2 cm proximal to the lesser trochanter). A long neck cut will make it difficult to get an appropriate fit of the implant. A short neck cut will require the prosthesis be left proud or that an extended neck length will be needed. Additionally, a long neck cut will decrease offset and a short neck cut will increase offset.

Enter the femoral canal with a T-awl. If the T-awl does not go easily down the intramedullary canal of the femur, it is usually due to the awl impinging on the lateral subchondral bone (too much varus). In the cementless case, do not lateralize with a conical reamer because this reamer has a diameter that is often greater than the lateral dimension of the cementless prosthesis. Taking too much lateral bone will prevent the porous surface of the implant from being apposed to host bone, making bone ingrowth less likely. Instead, use a small straight reamer. Lateralize with an 8- or 9-mm reamer until it easily goes down the canal (12–16 cm). Ream the intramedullary canal by half millimeter sizes until there is chattering from contact with the subchondral bone. If this occurs at a smaller size than templated, get a radiograph to assess if the reamer is in varus or if the femoral bow is affecting size.

Broach the femoral canal starting with the smallest size. When the broach advances easily to the level of the calcar, attempt to countersink the broach. Make sure that the broach advances with each stroke of the hammer. When the strokes achieve a high-pitched sound, stop. An inability to countersink the broach indicates the correct size. If smaller than the anticipated size, get an intra-operative radiograph. Usually this occurs when the broach is in too much varus or if the broach has a greater metaphyseal flare than the femoral canal. If the metaphyseal flare has been misjudged, the broach may actually be in valgus. This is a dangerous situation that will result in fracture if not quickly identified and rectified. Consider using an implant design with a narrow flare and more valgus Medial Modified Anatomic (DePuy Orthopaedics, Warsaw, IN) in cases of a valgus proximal canal. If a crack does develop during broaching, remove the broach and utilize a cable grip system to anatomically reduce the fracture before the split has extended down the canal. Place one wire above and below the lesser trochanter. Consider going to a 5/8 coated stem to increase the likelihood of getting proximal apposition of the ingrowth surface to the subchondral metaphyseal bone. Often the crack will open slightly on impacting of the prosthesis down to the calcar. If the crack widens before the implant hits the calcar, consider a cemented implant rather than downsizing to a smaller size

cementless implant. Cracks that develop during placement of the final implant are either missed fractures that occur during broaching or fractures that result from the femoral component being advanced beyond the depth broached.

> ### PEARL
> A good rule is to never advance the implant beyond the point broached to avoid intra-operative fracture of the femur.

SPECIAL CASES

Developmental Dysplasia of the Hip
Preoperative Evaluation

The physical examination is the key in identifying several important features of DDH that will need to be addressed at arthroplasty. Excessive internal hip rotation suggests excessive femoral anteversion. Patients with DDH are often unable to abduct the involved extremity past neutral, suggesting the need for an adductor release at arthroplasty. It is important that the *actual* LLD be determined and correlated with the *apparent* leg length. If the actual LLD is greater than 3 cm and there is a desire to increase the length of the leg at least 3 cm, SSEP monitoring is indicated. Patients with DDH who have severe adduction contractures will frequently have an apparent LLD as this is compensated for by pelvic obliquity to allow for ambulation.

It is important that marker balls be used on all radiographs to determine the exact magnification for templating. The canal diameter needs to be measured to assure that small enough stem sizes can be ordered for surgery. Whenever a question remains about canal size, a CT scan should be done to determine the exact dimensions. A CT scan provides important information in cases in which there is significant metaphyseal dysplasia, such as excessive femoral anteversion. Femoral anteversion can be determined by comparing sagittal cuts at the level of the posterior condyles (knee) with sections at the level of the femoral neck. If anteversion is greater than 30 degrees, cemented stem backups should be made available. Other important radiographic findings include whether or not a tear drop is present. If present, this suggests that at some time the femoral head was within the acetabulum. It will be possible to ream at the anatomic hip center to reconstruct the hip at the original acetabular location. If the tear drop is absent leaving only a shallow false acetabulum, place the hip at the high hip center (HHC) or use a structural allograft to reconstruct the acetabulum. The patient's own femoral head and neck can be used. It may be necessary to have special acetabular cages that can be screwed in place, into which all-polyethylene acetabular components can be cemented.

Special Equipment

Somatosensory evoked potentials monitoring is critical if the leg is to be lengthened more than 3 cm. Templating will demonstrate the need for size 22 femoral heads, particularly if the acetabulum is going to be smaller than 44 to 46 mm. Cemented acetabular implants work well smaller sized if there is a large acetabular defect that will require a bulk allograft precluding the use of a cementless cup.

Surgery

The technical requirement of THA in the DDH patient varies depending on the extent of contractures, bony deformity, and surgical objectives. A posterior approach is recommended in patients with DDH. The excessive femoral anteversion makes the anterolateral approach less stable unless one retroverts a cemented stem within the canal. The posterior approach also preserves the gluteus minimus and medius, whose fascia must frequently be released during lengthening. The Hardinge approach and subsequent lengthening may compromise the musculature. The posterior approach allows the posterior column to be well visualized, particularly if structural allograft and plating are needed for acetabular arthroplasty. When doing the posterior approach, release the gluteal sling. This makes anterior retraction of the femur and wide acetabular exposure possible. This will also protect the sciatic nerve during leg lengthening by releasing one of the possible points where the nerve can become taut. Release of the piriformis may have the same effect, particularly if it is bifurcate, with the nerve passing between the two heads.

There are many contractures about the congenitally dysplastic hip. Some of these do not become apparent until the leg has been lengthened. Severe adduction contractures should be addressed at the start of the THA through subcutaneous release and during arthroplasty by capsular and periarticular tissue release. Complete capsular removal may be necessary to bring the leg out to length. It is often necessary to release the piriformis at its musculotendinous junction to address flexion and adduction contractures. This is done by removing the entire inferior capsule. The musculotendinous junction is found at the point where the piriformis tendon passes into the pelvis over the brim of the acetabulum and anterior column. It may also be necessary to do an extensive release of the tensor fascia lata and gluteus medius origin along the lateral wing of the ilium if abduction contractures occur with lengthening.

Acetabular Arthroplasty Highlights

Acetabular reaming should be done with caution as maximum bone preservation is critical. Because it is common to be left with a shallow acetabulum after reaming, 170-degree acetabular components are recommended. If cementless acetabular implants are to be successful, adequate stability and apposition against host bone are required for ingrowth. Usually there will be adequate bone apposition provided by the anterior and posterior columns with a defect superiorly. If the superior defect is large, it should be addressed by bulk autograft or by placing the cup at the HHC. The final cup size is usually small (size 42 or less), necessitating that size 22 heads be available. Supplemental screw fixation is frequently required to optimize cementless cup stability. Be careful during screw placement because bone depth is diminished, particularly in the HHC. Screw placement in the HHC is much more dangerous as the size of the safe zone narrows (Figs. 33–1 and 33–2). Consider cementing the acetabular implants

if inadequate apposition of porous coating against the host bone of the acetabulum is present. Have cages available for all cases with significant preoperative acetabular dysplasia

Femoral Arthroplasty Highlights

If greater than 3 cm of lengthening is anticipated, a femoral shortening should be done to protect the sciatic nerve and bring the leg out to length. Some femoral deformity can also be corrected at the same time. It is critical to recognize and address the excessive valgus and anteversion in the femur of the DDH patient. Trying to place a stem with too large a metaphysis into the small DDH canal will result in femoral fracture that is difficult to reconstruct. If fracture occurs, first the fracture fragments need to be anatomically reduced with wires or cables. The fracture line inside the canal needs to be closed by a thin layer of applied polymethylmethacrylate so cement will not extrude during cementing, and a small cemented stem is inserted. The proximal femoral configuration usually precludes the use of cementless femoral devices except those that are specially designed for DDH femora.

PEARL

Small cemented stems are the mainstay for femoral arthroplasty for developmental dysplasia of the hip (DDH). High energy rate forged CoCrMo stems are preferred because maximum material strength is needed in these typically small implants.

Perthes' Arthroplasty

The preoperative workup should include a physical examination measuring the magnitude of any external rotation contracture or LLD. Both the actual and apparent LLD should be determined. Radiographs will often demonstrate an "AVN-like" appearance with secondary osteoarthritis. Coxa magna (enlarged femoral head) may also be present. The hip is shortened with a LLD of usually more than 1cm. An AP pelvis view is usually adequate to determine the amount of shortening that has occurred with this disease process. Femoral neck dysplasia (retroversion) can be demonstrated on a true lateral radiograph or CT scan. Comparing sagittal sections at the level of the posterior condyles of the knee with cuts through the neck will quantitate the magnitude of the retroversion.

Special Equipment

These patients are usually young, so a cementless femoral arthroplasty is desired. However, cemented stems should be available in cases in which cementless arthroplasty is precluded by the abnormal architecture of the proximal femur.

Surgical Approach

The hip with Perthes' arthropathy is best addressed through the posterior approach. The external rotation contracture is partially released as the rotators are removed. Reattach these structures with the hip in neutral rotation to allow the patient to freely internally rotate after surgery. If lengthening of greater than about 1.5 cm is required, release the gluteal sling and perform a complete capsulectomy to optimize exposure.

Acetabular Preparation

There may be a large acetabular defect in Perthes' patients with coxa magna. An oversized acetabular component is usually sufficient to address these defects. Morselized graft from the femoral head may be needed to fill acetabular defects. The resected femoral head should be saved until its use for bone graft is assessed. Larger defects may require bulk autograft reconstruction with a portion of the femoral head.

Femoral Preparation

The canal version should be assessed at the time of femoral arthroplasty. Determine the orientation after the neck resection cut because this will affect the amount of anteversion placed in the acetabular component.

If the proximal metaphysis is in mild retroversion, consider a cementless prosthesis with anteversion built in. If significant retroversion is present, consider doing a derotational osteotomy if the patient is in his or her 40s and compliant. The patient will need prolonged protected weight bearing. These stems should be fully porous-coated and 8 inches long to bypass the osteotomy and enhance stability and bone ingrowth. It is preferable to use a cemented stem whenever there is significant malformation of the femur. Consider a slightly undersized stem (forged CoCrMo) that can be rotated into appropriate anteversion despite the proximal metaphyseal retroversion deformity. If sufficient anteversion is not possible, place the acetabular implant in slightly more anteversion to compensate for this and improve stability against posterior dislocation. An elevated lip liner, placing the elevation directly posterior may be sufficient in some cases.

Paget's Arthropathy

Paget's disease can cause several problems at arthroplasty due to large femoral canal diameter and excessive bleeding. Control of Paget's should be optimized prior to surgery. Monitoring of serum alkaline phosphatase and urinary hydroxyproline will help. Nonsteroidal anti-inflammatory drugs should be stopped 2 weeks prior to surgery. Autologous blood donation is recommended. Patients should be warned that they will probably need perioperative banked blood and should be typed and crossed for 4 units of blood. A cell-saver should be used intra-operatively.

Cemented implants should be used. This will decrease the postoperative bleeding. Peroxide or epinephrine helps control hemostasis when drying the bone surfaces for cementing. The cement should be slightly more viscous to aid cement intercalation. Use of drains with sterile collecting systems to reinfuse postoperative bleeding may minimize the need for transfusions.

Seropositive Arthropathy

Patients with seropositive arthropathy should be in remission prior to surgery. When both hips have severe arthropathy, consider doing bilateral total hip replacements.

Most patients with seropositive arthropathies have osteopenia with proximal metaphyseal flaring (trumpet-shaped femurs). These features may preclude the use of cementless femoral implants, except in patients less than 40 years old. Acetabular arthroplasty is complicated by soft tissue and bone deformities: patients have synovitis that needs to be excised for adequate acetabular visualization. The labrum is redundant requiring complete circumferential excision. If there is no tissue within the fovea, beware of protrusio; the hip has eroded medially, removing these tissues. If protrusio is present, do not medialize the acetabulum, particularly in osteopenic bone. Start with a reamer almost as large as templated. Ream the peripheral rim only. Clean the base of acetabulum with a Cobb elevator until the bone begins to bleed. The medial defect should be grafted with the acetabular reamings or autograft from the femoral head. After placing the graft, reverse ream with the last reamer to contour the grafted acetabulum. Impact an oversized cup into place (2–4 mm greater than reamed). In cases of severe osteopenia or protrusio, underream the acetabulum up to 4 mm to get adequate rim fit and prevent recurrent protrusio. Supplemental screw fixation is recommended if there is any question about stability. Select a nonhemispheric acetabular component, as most patients will have a shallow acetabulum. Use cemented acetabular implants in patients over the age of 70.

Reconstruction after Hip Fracture

Patients with femoral neck fractures requiring hip replacement surgery should have their surgery done within 24 to 48 hours of injury.

Edema in the periarticular tissues about the fracture can make exposure difficult and can also make it difficult to get the leg out to length. Determine the relationship of the center of the head to the tip of the trochanter to give an estimate of how much lengthening is needed: From the opposite hip or an old pelvic film. Technical aspects of removing the femoral head include: "T-ing" the capsule posteriorly, making a preliminary femoral neck cut before removing the femoral head, and placing an AuFranc Cobra retractor over the anterior column between the labrum and the capsule. The head is easily removed with a corkscrew or Cobb elevator to cut the ligamentum teres.

A cemented bipolar arthroplasty is recommended in patients with femoral neck fractures. Often these patients are osteopenic and the wedge effect of cementless implants can cause late femoral fracture. This was common after placement of implants such as the Austin-Moore. Cemented stems allow immediate weight bearing.

Bipolar hip reconstruction should be a treatment alternative for severe intertrochanteric fractures in osteopenic patients. Bipolar arthroplasty provides a stable construct for early weight bearing and rehabilitation. Calcar replacement prostheses are excellent for these cases because there is frequently bone loss down to the lesser trochanter. These stems tend to be longer than normal cemented stems.

PEARL
When cementing into the fractured femur seal the anatomically reduced edges on the inside with cement to prevert cement from entering the fracture during pressurization.

Anatomically reduce the trochanter to the femur with a cable grips system. Seal the inside fracture line with a fine layer of cement before cementing the stem. This prevents cement from extruding between the fracture fragments. Bipolar constructs may be preferable to hip pinning because patients can ambulate the day after surgery without the risk of construct failure and reoperation.

Ankylosing Spondylitis

Patients with ankylosing spondylitis (AS) can have severe hip contractures and spinal deformities that make ambulation almost impossible. The examination should quantitate hip motion and contracture. Most patients with AS need pulmonary function tests prior to surgery due to restrictive lung disease from thoracic spine ankylosis.

Patients with AS often have adduction contractures that should be treated with subcutaneous tenotomies before beginning THA. When both hips are affected, bilateral replacements are recommended. Contracted hips are best addressed through an anterior lateral approach to release the anterior (flexion) contracture. The reflected head of the rectus should be released as well. The iliopsoas needs to be tenotomized at the musculotendinous junction as the tendon crosses over the anterior acetabular lip. Release down the anterior and medial femur if needed to address adduction contractures. Avoid overlengthening as this may worsen contractures.

Cementless stems do extremely well in patients with AS. The stem should not have built in anteversion if the anterolateral approach is utilized. Postoperative irradiation is highly recommended to decrease heterotopic ossification. Valium may be used to help patients with spasm and maintain hip motion. Patients should lie flat on their stomachs for about a half hour—5 minutes at a time—at least twice a day, to help decrease the amount of residual hip flexion contracture. With the addition of aggressive physical therapy, patients usually end up with 10 to 20 degrees of contracture.

REVISION TOTAL HIP ARTHROPLASTY

Evaluation

The following radiographs should be obtained:

1. Anteroposterior pelvis, AP and lateral of the hip on a 14 × 17-cassette
2. Judet radiographs (obturator oblique, iliac oblique) in all patients requiring acetabular revision
3. bone scan; evaluate for loosening or infection
4. computed tomography scan (three dimensional reconstructions): severe defects
5. contrast enhanced CT: screws or cement contiguous to vessels

The hip in need of revision usually has one of the following pain types or locations:

1. types: constant (infection), start-up (femur)
2. locations: groin (femoral), buttock (cup), thigh (femoral), knee (referred from femur)

Try to eliminate the back as a possible etiology by history and examination. The arterial system can be eliminated by documenting good peripheral pulses. Hip bursitis is frequently at the top of the differential, particularly with a radiographically normal THA. Lateral thigh pain is the hallmark of hip bursitis. If the patient has significant lateral trochanteric pain on palpation and this pain reproduces the patients "hip pain," inject this site with bupivacaine hydrochloride (Marcaine) to see if the patient's pain subsides. Many patients with a failing THA will have hip bursitis, as this can be due to a secondary change in hip biomechanics. The injection will demonstrate to the patient the portion of the pain coming from the bursa versus the failing hip. Intra-articular injections are seldom indicated except in patients with back pathology.

Lucent zones around cemented prostheses are highly suggestive of loosening. Another common finding of loosened femoral stems is that they are retroverted on the lateral radiograph. Because the stem was not likely implanted in that position, this often signifies that it has subsided into retroversion. This subsidence may not be evident on the AP radiographs because it has a greater rotational component as compared to subsidence caudally down into the femoral canal. In cases in which it is not clear if the stem is loose, a CT rotation study can also be performed (see Selected Bibliography). A bone scan may also help in determining whether there is femoral or acetabular loosening.

Evaluating the stability of the cementless femoral stem can be difficult. Look for calcar resorption that is typical of a well-fixed cementless prosthesis. Refractory thigh pain may require a thigh corset for 3–12 months as the bone remodels. Look for radiographic evidence of stem loosening such as caudal or rotational subsidence of the cementless stem. Lucencies around the distal prosthesis (zones 3, 4, 5) do not necessarily indicate that the stem is loose. Some cementless prostheses will have slightly increased uptake at the tip of the stem despite being well fixed. This is particularly true in some slotted prostheses, which have less structural rigidity and tend to bend more with loading. Rule out infection prior to hip revision. Radiographs may demonstrate periosteal reaction and bone destruction. Bone scans help but are not specific for infection. The infected hip acutely is constantly painful with no time free of pain. Most infected hips are painful even at rest. Aspirate any failed THA in a patient with an elevated sedimentation rate (ESR). This includes patients with seronegative and seropositive spondylarthropathies because the ESR cannot differentiate infection from the underlying medical condition. Any patient with fever of unknown origin or any patient who has recurrent hip dislocations should have a hip aspiration.

Revision Acetabular Arthroplasty

Radiographic assessment of acetabular deficiency

1) Protrusio of acetabular implant (beyond iliopectineal line)—indicates medial wall deficiency.
2) Iliac oblique—shows posterior column discontinuities and deficiencies
3) Obturator oblique—shows anterior column discontinuities and deficiencies—pelvic discontinuity

Patients who have cemented acetabular implants may have exceptionally large defects that are not apparent on radiographs. When revising any acetabular implant, be prepared to cement an all-polyethylene cup; use acetabular containment rings and large cementless implants with screws. Expanding the acetabulum greater than one third the acetabular diameter (i.e., reaming a size 54 acetabulum beyond a size 72) will risk creating a pelvic discontinuity. Excessive reaming of the columns will also decrease the available bone for screw purchase. Reaming one quarter of the acetabular diameter is safe (i.e., reaming a size 56 acetabulum to a size 70), preserving 50% of the cross-sectional area of the anterior and posterior columns.

Surgical Technique

1. Press-fit Acetabular Ingrowth Implant
   A. 75% cup coverage with host bone
   B. Consider using screw fixation to supplement stability
2. Press-fit Acetabular Ingrowth Implant with Morselized Autograft
   A. 50–75% coverage with host bone
   B. Graft with acetabular reamings (supplement with coral or allograft);
   C. Reverse ream to contour acetabulum
   D. Use screw fixation to supplement stability
3. Press-fit Acetabular Ingrowth Implant with Bulk Autograft
   A. If >50% coverage with host bone cup can be cementless
   B. Graft fixation with countersunk screws and plating
   C. Always augment fixation with transacetabular screws
4. Cemented Acetabular Implant with bulk autograft
   A. If <50% coverage with host bone, cup must be cemented
   B. Graft fixation with countersunk screws and plating
   C. Seal host-graft junction prior to cementing cup with thin layer of cement.

5. Cemented Acetabular Implant with Morselized Autograft
   A. Morselized allograft reversed ream with small reamer
   B. Impaction graft morselized allograft with larger circular impactor
   C. Cement cup into morselized graft bed
   D. Prolonged immobilization
6. Antiprotrusio Cage (APC)
   A. Morselized allograft or coral graft
   B. Screw fixation of APC to host bone
   C. Cement cup in place

Revision Femoral Arthroplasty

Femoral revision arthroplasty can be a complex operation requiring extensive exposure. Choose the posterior approach because it offers the greatest versatility. Remove long-stem femoral implants (cemented and cementless) by doing long Wagner osteotomies rotating the lateral femur up on a vascularized pedicle of the vastus lateralis to preserve its blood supply. A longitudinal osteotomy of the femoral shaft can be added down to the knee to remove long bowed stems. When the canal is pried open, even the longest implants can be removed from the canal.

In most revision surgeries, the bone in the proximal third of the femur has been damaged by the prior arthroplasty. Long, extensively coated implants are optimal because they ensure bone ingrowth into the undisturbed diaphyseal bone. These implants work well when revising cemented stems, because patients undergoing revision surgery have smooth canals that are difficult to intercalate with cement. These canals also have extensive membranes that must be removed. Lights placed down into the canal will verify that adequate removal has occurred. The Ultra-drive (Biomet, Warsaw, Indiana) can be used to remove distal cement and the plug. This device will minimize bone loss and the likelihood of bone perforations. Other helpful instruments for cement

TABLE 33–3   Femoral defect classification and treatment options

Defect	Characteristics	Treatment
Type I	Similar to femur in primary THA Metaphysis intact Partial loss of calcar Minor anterior/posterior bone loss Diaphysis intact	Older patient: cemented stem Younger patient: proximally to fully coated stem
Type II	More extensive metaphyseal bone loss Metaphysis not intact Complete absence of calcar Major anterior/posterior bone loss Diaphysis intact	Older patient: long cemented stems down into diaphysis (200 mm+) Younger patient: fully coated stem; impaction grafting
Type III	Extensive metaphyseal and some diaphyseal bone loss Structurally incompetent metaphysis Complete absence of calcar Diaphysis not fully intact	Older patient: Very long cemented stems down through diaphysis (250 mm+) Younger patient: fully coated stem (curved); allograft prosthetic composite (APC)

removal include the Moreland cement removing instruments. Revising large diameter femoral stems can be challenging. In younger patients, impaction grafting to replace bone loss should be considered. In older patients with limited life expectancy, use long-stem cemented devices that reach into the undisturbed diaphyseal bone. Adequately lavage and dry the entire femoral canal to prevent catastrophic hypotension that occurs during insertion of the femoral stems. This occurs secondary to embolization of the intramedullary elements that are not adequately removed prior to cementing.

PITFALL

When a stem loosens, it tends to move into retroversion causing remodeling of the proximal femur. When trying to place a cementless femoral revision prosthesis into this irregular proximal geometry, there is a large defect posteriorly. This is managed by wedging a bone graft into the defect to augment rotational stability.

Sciatic Nerve Neurolysis

Sciatic nerve neurolyses are frequently necessary for complex THA revision procedures, particularly when multiple posterior approaches have previously been performed. When these cases also involve lengthening the leg, the nerve is at risk even when an anterolateral approach is done. When posterior column defects need to be repaired and extensive exposure of this region is necessary, locating the sciatic nerve is important. Expose the nerve by following the tendon of the piriformis to the sciatic notch. This nerve is beneath the piriformis. Follow the nerve distally and expose it through the gluteal sling. While in most cases the nerve is accessible proximally, after previous proximal dissections the nerve may be more safely located at the gluteal sling. The nerve runs under the sling about 2 cm from the femur. After dividing the gluteal sling, the nerve can be found 1 cm under its proximal edge.

Dividing the gluteal sling helps decompress the sciatic nerve, as does dividing the piriformis. If leg lengthening is anticipated, dissect out the nerve. During trial reductions assess nerve tension. If excessive tension is present, decrease the neck length. If this results in instability, consider using a constrained acetabular component. It is essential to have constrained acetabular components available in all cases in which the sciatic nerve is at risk.

Somatosensory evoked potentials monitoring of the sciatic nerve should be considered in congenital dislocation of the hip, revision surgery with expected limb lengthening <3 cm, and in patients with spinal stenosis or spinal dysplasias who may have sensitized peripheral nerves. Spontaneous EMG is an alternative to SSEP that has been evaluated for its efficacy in avoiding nerve injury during revision and complex total hip arthroplasty. This technique detects sustained EMG activity during retractor placement and extremity positioning that might threaten the sciatic nerve.

Acetabular Quadrants

The anatomic (Fig. 33–1a) and HHC (Fig. 33–1b) quadrants can be used to locate the safe zones for the transacetabular placement of screws. The quadrants can be used as a guide for retractor placement, for drilling acetabular screw holes for graft fixation, or to estimate bone depth in a specific acetabular zone.

The external iliac vessels lie opposite the anterior superior quadrant, and the obturator neural and vascular structures lie opposite the anterior inferior quadrant. The medial acetabular zone is opposite the external iliac vein and obturator nerve, artery, and vein that course along the superior quadrilateral surface. The sciatic nerve and the superior gluteal nerve and vessels course opposite the posterior superior quadrant, and the inferior gluteal and internal pudendal structures are opposite the posterior inferior quadrant. Screws and anchoring holes can be placed safely in these posterior zones. The sciatic notch is easily palpable and the superior gluteal nerve and vessels can be protected. The central region of the posterior superior and posterior inferior quadrants have the greatest bone depth for transacetabular screw placement (Fig. 33–2a).

The quadrants for a HHC acetabulum are different than those formed at the normal anatomic acetabulum. The peripheral one half of the posterior superior and posterior inferior HHC quadrants contain the best available bone stock (Fig. 33–2b) and are relatively safe for transacetabular screw placement. The entire anterior superior and anterior inferior HHC quadrants, as well as the central half of the posterior superior and posterior inferior quadrants, should be avoided due to the close proximity of intrapelvic structures and the paucity of protective musculature on the inner wall of the pelvis opposite these zones.

POSTOPERATIVE CARE AND EXPECTED OUTCOME

Infection Control

Administer intravenous (IV) antibiotics (cefazolin sodium [Ancef] every 8 hours) for 24-36 hours after a routine primary arthroplasty. After a revision arthroplasty, IV antibiotics are given for 7 days or until the final intra-operative culture results. Intravenous antibiotics are not discontinued in any patient who has continued wound (incisional) drainage or an indwelling Foley catheter.

Deep Venous Thrombosis Prophylaxis

Patients are given 2.5 to 5 mg of warfarin sodium (coumadin) the evening of surgery. Patients with a deep venous thrombosis (DVT) diathesis get Coumadin the night before surgery. Patients get daily prothrombin time, partial thromboplastin time, and international normalized ratio labs. Hemoglobin (Hgb) measurements can be discontinued on postoperative day 3 if the Hgb is greater than 10. Stools guaiac determinations should be done at least once during the hospitalization. The INR should be maintained between 1.5 and 2.5. If the INR is greater than 3.0, physical therapy is held and the patient is placed at bed rest. Autologous fresh frozen plasma is given. If the drain is still in place, it should not be discontinued until the INR is less than 2.0. If the drain was already discontinued, the wound is watched for signs of hematoma. Occasionally, a hip spica ace wrap is used as a compressive dressing. The most effective DVT prophylaxis is early post-op patient mobilization

Hemovac Drains

Drains are frequently discontinued on postoperative day 2. The drain is not discontinued until 2 consecutive 8 hour nursing shifts with outputs less than 50cc. Continue antibiotic prophylactic coverage until the drains are discontinued. If drainage is heavy, increase the frequency of dressing changes to every 2 to 4 hours.

Foley Catheter

Foley catheters are frequently discontinued on postoperative day 1. The Foley is left in place while an epidural catheter is being utilized and then discontinued 6 hours after the epidural has been discontinued. A straight catheterization order must be written to prevent urinary retention from causing excessive bladder distension. Antibiotic prophylactic coverage is continued until the Foley is discontinued.

Activity Protocols

Total hip arthroplasty patients should attempt to get out of bed the day of surgery. A gentle motion and active assistive strengthening program should be started on postoperative day 1. Patients should not be given a rigorous strengthening program until 6 weeks postoperatively. The main focus initially is safe ambulation with a walker or crutches. Patients are discharged when they can state their hip precautions, their wound has minimal drainage, and they are safe with ambulation and stair-climbing.

Weight-bearing status is generally based on the type of femoral component. Because the forces incurred getting on and off of a bed pan are far greater than those of touch down weight bearing (TDWB), all compliant patients are permitted at least TDWB. Patients with an uncomplicated hybrid hip replacements (a cemented femoral stem and a cementless cup) weight bear as tolerated. Protected weight-bearing should be considered when a significant amount of medial bone graft has been placed in cases of protrusio or in cases in which a large acetabular defect has been reconstructed with cancellous bone or a bulk allograft. A cemented acetabular construct can tolerate greater stresses than a similar construct that utilizes a cementless component.

Patients with cementless femoral stems can be TDWB for 3 weeks followed by partial weight bearing of 10 to 50 pounds for the next 3 weeks. At 6 weeks, release the patient to full weight-bearing, but have the therapist advance this slowly under observation. Start aggressive abduction and major strengthening exercises at 6 weeks.

Followup should occur at 3 weeks, 6 weeks, 3 months, 6 months, 1 year, and each year thereafter. At yearly checkups, give the patient an assessment of the predicted implant longevity. There is a 97% chance of having a cemented femoral stem in place 10 years after surgery. The data on cementless femoral stems range from 80–95% success rates at 10 years. Obese patients, young patients, and active patients should all be told to expect diminished implant longevity.

TREATMENT OF AVASCULAR NECROSIS OF THE HIP

Etiology

Most cases of AVN have a clear etiology. Avascular necrosis can be due to prolonged use of steroids (RA), high-dose steroids, or to only a short course of low-dose steroids (medrol dose pack). Alcohol is a common cause of bilateral AVN. In patients with unilateral disease, trauma is a likely cause.

Core Decompression

Core decompression can be an effective modality in delaying the need for THA. Although most patients gradually progress radiographically, their pain is often mitigated. Important variables in predicting success are the extent of femoral head involvement and head sphericity. Less head involvement and better sphericity increase success. A young patient with femoral head collapse or a patient with a significant subchondral fracture are also candidates for core decompression. These patients often progress radiographically even when their symptoms are mitigated, suggesting that core decompression delays but does not prevent the need for eventual THA. In patients with bilateral hip AVN, perform a core decompression on the most involved side, reserving a newer procedure, free fibula transplantation, for the less involved femoral head.

Free Fibula Transfer

Free fibular transfers revascularize the avascular segment of the femoral head. Free fibula transplantation works best in patients who have a spherical head at the time of transplantation. Once collapse has occurred, the hip will deteriorate even if revascularization is successful.

Technique for Free Fibula Transfer

The patient is placed in the lateral decubitus position on a beanbag. A skin incision is made over the trochanter similar to the anterolateral approach to the hip. Two thirds of the incision is carried distally from the trochanter in line with the femur, and one third of the incision is carried proximally curving slightly posterior. The fascia is divided in line with the skin incision, and the edges are retracted with a Charnley retractor. The vastus tubercle is identified and the vastus lateralis is split 5 cm distal in line with the fiber direction. The incision is "T'd" at the vastus tubercle to create an anterior trough for the vessel anastomoses. The vastus lateralis is spread to expose the lateral femur just distal to the trochanter for reaming. Under fluoroscopic guidance, a Steinmann pin is placed into the femoral head within the avascular lesion and is overreamed in half-millimeter increments to a dimension of 1 to 2 mm greater than the anticipated diameter of the harvested fibula. An AP of the leg with marker balls will help determine the diameter of the fibula graft. The first part of the reamings from the normal femoral neck are saved for use as autogenous bone graft. The femoral head is reamed within 6 to 10 mm of the subchondral bone. If a subchondral fracture is present, err on the side of being slightly further away from the subchondral bone to mitigate the likelihood of later collapse. The portion of the lesion not removed with the reaming is removed with a Hall bur under fluoroscopy. This leaves a cauliflower-shaped defect within the femoral head to be filled with the free fibula and bone graft.

A 10-cm segment of the fibula is harvested with one artery and both veins (Fig. 33–3). The fibula should be harvested simultaneously with preparation of the proximal femur and while the proximally vessels are being exposed. These proximal vessels are found by following the interval between the

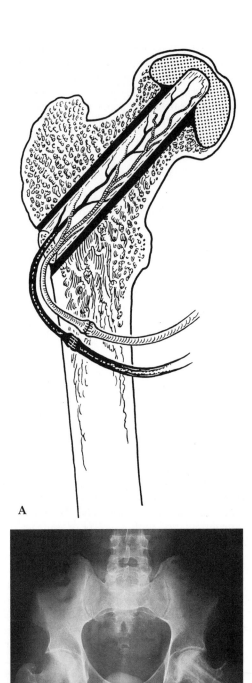

A

B

Figure 33–4 **(A)** Schematic showing free fibula placed within the femoral neck and avascular portion of the femoral head. **(B)** Radiograph illustrating placement of a free vascularized fibula within the femoral head.

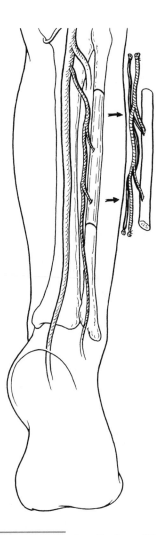

Figure 33–3 Schematic of a free fibula graft being harvested from the midportion of the fibula.

vastus medialis and the gluteus medius medial to the fascia under the rectus. The ascending branch of the profundus femoris artery and the accompanying vein can be easily identified. The bone graft and free fibula are placed into the prepared femoral neck up into the head (Fig. 33–4). The fibula is secured with a 2.5-mm screw or Steinmann pin. The vessels are anastomosed using No. 9 nylon suture under the microscope. The wound is closed in layers. The split in the vastus is closed as well as the posterior T, and the anterior T is left open to accommodate the anastomosed vessels. The fascia lata is closed over a drain. The subcutaneous tissues and skin are closed. The patient is placed on dextran for 72 hours and chlorpromazin (Thorazine) to decrease vessel spasm. Bone scans are done at 6 weeks to assess the graft viability.

Keep patients non–weight-bearing (TDWB 10 lbs. if compliant) for 6 weeks followed by an additional 6 weeks of grad-

ual progression to weight bearing as tolerated (WBAT). The patients with a larger femoral head defect must be protected for 3 additional months to avoid fracture. Patients with a free fibula on one side and a core decompression on the other should use a wheelchair for 6 weeks, followed by an additional 6 weeks of protected weight bearing. Encourage all patients to begin a water exercise program at 12 weeks and to continue this for 6 months postoperatively. Encourage swimming beginning at 12 weeks to optimize rehabilitation.

SELECTED BIBLIOGRAPHY

BERGER R, FLETCHER F, DONALDSON T, WASIELEWSKI R, PETERSON M, RUBASH H. Dynamic test to diagnose loose uncemented femoral total hip components. *Clin Orthop.* 1996;330:115–123.

BROWER AC. Appendicular arthropathy. *Orthop Clin North Am.* 1990;21:405–422

D'ANTONIO JA. Preoperative templating and choosing the implant for primary THA in the young patient. Instruct course lect *Instructional Course Lectures.* 1994;43:339–346.

HARRIS WH. Traumatic arthritis of the hip after dislocation and acetabular fractures; treatment by mold arthroplasty: an end-result study using a new method of result evaluation. *J Bone Jt Surg.* 1969;51A:737–755.

HOPPENFIELD, S, DE BOER P. *Surgical Exposures in Orthopaedics.* Philadelphia, PA: Lippincott; 1984.

INSALL JN, DORR LD, SCOTT RD, SCOTT WN. Rationale of the Knee Society clinical rating system. *Clin Orthop Rel Res.* 1989;248:13–14.

MALLORY TH. *The Anterolateral Approach in Primary and Revision Total Hip Arthroplasty.* [video Classic #27102] American Academy of Orthopaedic Surgeons, Rosemont, IL.

PAPROSKY WG, BRADFORD MS, JABLONSKY WS. Acetabular reconstruction with massive acetabular allografts. *Instruct Course Lect.* 1996;45:149–159.

WASIELEWSKI RC. Limitations in expanding the acetabulum during acetabular arthroplasty. (unpublished data, Ohio State University, 1996.)

WASIELEWSKI RC, COOPERSTEIN LA, KRUGER MP, RUBASH HE. Acetabular anatomy and the transacetabular fixation of screws in total hip arthroplasty. *J Bone Jt Surg.* 1990;72A:501–508.

WASIELEWSKI RC, COOPERSTEIN LA, RUBASH HE. Radiographic analysis of intrapelvic transacetabular screws after acetabular arthroplasty. AAOS 58th Annual Meeting Poster Exhibit #E44. Anaheim, CA. March 11, 1991.

SAMPLE QUESTIONS

1. A 25 year old male patient with systemic lupus is seen in your office having been referred by his rheumatologist with the diagnosis of bilateral hip AVN. He has been on steroids for the past 10 years. His SLE is relatively well controlled with occasional flare-ups once to twice every year. He walks with a cane with an antalgic gait. He has mild right hip pain and moderate left hip pain. He is a security guard and has difficulty when he is up on his feet for more than one hour. MRI films demonstrate 50% head involvement on the right and 75% head involvement on the left. X-rays demonstrate Stage IV AVN on the left and Stage I AVN on the right. The most appropriate treatment for this patient would be:

(a) Core decompression, bilaterally.
(b) Free fibula replacement on the right and core decompression on the left.
(c) Free fibula replacement on the right and total hip replacement on the left.
(d) Core decompression on the right and total hip replacement on the left.

2. A 32 year old patient with ankylosing spondylosis walks into your office in a crouched over position with bent

knees (30 degrees) and his hips flexed 60 degrees. Physical examination demonstrates that he has 60 degree of hip flexion contractures bilaterally. He has hip adduction contractures bilaterally measuring 15 degrees that prevent him from abducting his hips. He has severe hip arthropathy with significant peri-articular osteophyte formation. He has moderate protrusio in both hips. The most appropriate surgical management is:

(a) Total hip replacement on the right side followed in six months by a total hip replacement on the left side.
(b) Bilateral total hip replacements, bilateral adductor tenotomies followed by post-operative irradiation of both hips to prevent heterotopic ossification through anterio-lateral approaches.
(c) Bilateral total hip replacements through posterior approaches with post-operative irradiation.
(d) Total hip replacements separated by 3 months through anterior lateral approach and post-operative irradiation with abductor tenotomies.

3. A colleague of yours calls you to refer a patient with total hip replacement done 10 weeks prior. This primary arthroplasty was complicated by peri-operative drainage and

now the patient has a grossly infected hip replacement with gram positive cocci present on an aspirate done the previous day. You admit the patient to your service for operative intervention the following day. The patient's ASA level is 4. Physical exam demonstrates the patient has exquisite pain on any range of motion. X-rays demonstrate a cemented femoral stem. The cement is well intercalated into the femur and extends about 3 cm. past the tip of the stem. A cementless acetabular implant has complete surrounding radiolucencies in zones 1 through 3. The anticipated operative procedure would include the following:

(a) Irrigation, debridement and complete synovectomy.

(b) Removal of the prosthesis by interrupting the cement implant interface with osteotomies, removing the stem and then removing the cement in a proximal to distal fashion, piece by piece.

(c) Wagner osteotomy for stem and cement removal and circulage wire fixation of the femur.

(d) Irrigation and debridement of the hip with prosthetic retention.

4. Pelvic disassociations encountered at revision acetabular arthroplasty are best addressed by:

(a) Posterior pelvic plating across the disassociation followed by rigid cup fixation with cement or ingrowth fixation with multiple screws.

(b) Allograft placement with cementing of the cup into place.

(c) Large cementless cup fixation placing transacetabular screws on both sides of the disassociation.

(d) Cemented acetabular arthroplasty.

5. A 65 year old patient with osteoporosis and coxa varus is best treated by:

(a) Use of a high offset varus stem, such as Iowa, (Zimmer) cemented in place.

(b) CDH type stem.

(c) Cementless stem with a varus option (AML).

(d) Osteotomy to correct the varus position of the hip.

Answers 1) b; 2) b; 3) c; 4) c; 5) a.

Knee and Leg

Knee and Leg Trauma

Barry Riemer, MD

Outline

Fractures of the tibia can be associated with substantial morbidity. Articular fractures can lead to joint stiffness and posttraumatic arthritis. Proximal metaphyseal fractures can create compartment syndrome. Tibial shaft fractures are at risk of non-union. This chapter is designed to offer the reader a system for evaluating and treating this difficult class of fractures.

ETIOLOGY

Tibial Plateau Fractures

Most unicondylar tibial plateau fractures occur from varus/valgus stressing, with lateral plateau fractures predominating. The classic "bumper" fracture occurs from a direct blow to the lateral knee in a pedestrian-motor vehicle accident, crushing the lateral articular surface and fracturing the lateral metaphyseal cortex. Similar injuries can occur in falls and sports. Eccentric loading from high-energy mechanisms such as motorcycle and motor vehicle accidents are also common. Medial fractures from varus forces occur infrequently.

Bicondylar Fractures

Bicondylar fractures occur from axial loading. Forces can be dissipated by comminuting the joint or proximal tibial metaphysis. Proximal tibia metaphyseal fractures with minimal joint extension are usually from a high-energy direct blow to the upper tibia.

Tibial Shaft Fractures

Most low-energy fractures from sports are rotational and tend to be spiral in geometry. High-energy fractures, generally from motor vehicle accidents, motorcycle accidents, or falls from a significant height fragment the tibia by a direct blow or high-energy varus/valgus stressing. Fracture lines tend to be transverse (often with a "butterfly" fragment), segmental, or highly comminuted. Transverse fractures from either a direct blow or varus/valgus forces tend to break the fibula at the same level of the tibia, further destabilizing the construct.

Pilon Fractures

Pilon fractures can occur from rotational forces or axial load. Rotational fractures occur from low-energy falls and sports injuries, skiing in particular. The talus rotates within the mortise, fragmenting the tibial plafond. The ankle is broken into a few large fragments. Crush is minimal. High-energy fractures from axial load are most frequently seen following motor vehicle or motorcycle accidents and significant falls

Orthopaedic Surgery: The Essentials. Edited by M.E. Baratz, A.D. Watson, and J.E. Imbriglia. Thieme Medical Publishers, Inc., New York © 1999

where the patient lands on the feet. The tibial plafond is broken by the talus being driven vertically. The metaphysis is crushed, and severe comminution is common. Articular segments are broken into multiple small pieces.

SELECTED BASIC SCIENCE

Tibial Plateau Fractures

Tibial plateau fractures occur as combinations of depression of the articular surface with a metaphyseal crush and shearing of one or both condyles (Figs. 34–1 through 34–3). Tibial condyles are much wider than the shaft, creating a cantilevered effect. When condyles are broken, they can displace in two directions, outward and longitudinally. Outward (lateral or medial) displacement of a condyle occurs from the impact of the blow. Vertical displacement is possible because there is no shaft below the fragment. This allows a shear vector. Stabilization of the lateral or medial displacement is simply understood; lag screws are inserted. To stabilize the shear or longitudinal forces, the buttress principle must be utilized. This involves a screw or, more generally, a plate that controls the apex of the fracture (Figs. 34–1 and 34–2).

> ## PEARL
> When applying a plate to stabilize a unicondylar plateau fracture, the plate must be molded so that it contacts the apex of the fracture. In a simple shear fracture with no depression, horizontal lag screws close to the knee are usually adequate.

Bicondylar tibial plateau or proximal tibia fractures are mechanically difficult to stabilize. The problem is stabilization of a wide, soft (metaphyseal) bone. Unilateral fixation, such as a single plate, dissipates its hold before reaching the contralateral side. If the contralateral cortex cannot be perfectly reduced, the fracture will remain unstable and tend to collapse into an angular deformity (Fig. 34–4). Fixation that has both medial and lateral support is often necessary.

> ## PEARL
> Biomechanical considerations are secondary to biology. The soft tissues often cannot tolerate a second incision, so a supplemental cast can be utilized.

Stabilization of these fractures can be in the form of bilateral plates or hybrid external fixation. Bilateral plates consist of one large plate on the side of greatest instability and the best soft tissue covering, with a small contralateral plate applied through a limited incision. Hybrid external fixation can be in the form of a circular wire fixator or a unilateral plate with a unilateral external fixator below the joint (Fig. 34–5). Circular wire fixators gain support by divergent small wires near the subchondral bone. This creates a broad stable "mesh" below the joint, allowing control of both medial and lateral cortices. An upper ring can be attached to either a lower tibial ring or, more generally, unilateral half-pin external fixation.

Tibial Shaft Fractures

Union of tibial shaft fractures is highly influenced by biomechanical stresses. The forces that are most likely to produce union are controlled, limited, axial vectors. Immobilization or fixation that allows angular or rotational movement without axial loading tends to produce nonunion. Weight bearing is often used as an adjunct to allow axial loading of the fracture.

Tibial cortical blood flow is primitive, with few venous valves. Blood flow is centrifugal and is influenced by hydraulic pressures generated by muscle action. This is potentiated by total contact casting or braces that concentrate the pumping action of muscles, improving tibial cortical vascularity while bearing weight. "PTB" (patellar tendon bone) casting delivers its effect not by unloading the tibia, as originally thought, but by creating an hydraulic cylinder that improves cortical blood flow with weight bearing.

Grading of Soft Tissue Injuries: Closed and Open

Several soft tissue grading systems have been reported. Systems that grade closed fractures have not been sufficiently reliable for clinical relevance. Gustilo graded open fractures by increasing severity. Grade I are open 1 cm or less, with grades II and IIIA fractures having progressively greater soft tissue injuries. Any fracture that is associated with a high-energy mechanism or severe comminution automatically is classified as IIIA without regard to wound. Interobserver reliability has been fair. In reality, very little difference exists between the infection rates for these categories of open fractures, provided initial wound care is appropriate. Grades IIIB and IIIC open fractures have a much worse prognosis. Significant soft tissue stripping has occurred, and the fracture requires flap coverage to reconstruct avulsed skin and muscle. Grade IIIC fractures have a sufficient arterial injury such that vascular reconstruction is mandated for limb preservation. Interobserver reliability differentiating grades IIIB and IIIC from the rest of open fractures has been good.

Pilon Fractures

Pilon fractures from rotational forces create large metaphyseal joint fragments with very little crush. Lag screws and the buttress principal are applied, utilizing lag screws to compress fragments together with ancillary fixation at the apex of a fragment with either a plate or screws (Fig. 34–6). Most fractures, however, occur from axial loading with crush of the distal tibial metaphysis. The biomechanical problem is restoring stability to a wide, soft, crushed bone. This can be accomplished with bilateral plates, usually with one on the fibula and another on the tibia. Hybrid external fixation can be applied with circular wire fixators, creating a small wire mesh just above the ankle joint. Another alternative is unilateral external fixation. First the fibula is fixed, and this is augmented by a medial unilateral fixator gaining purchase in the tibia, talus, and calcaneus. This creates a ligamentotaxis effect across the medial joint, opening metaphyseal defects and helping to align articular fragments (Fig. 34–7). The metaphyseal defect can be bone grafted. The plafond can be approached through limited incisions for screw fixation.

ANATOMY AND SURGICAL APPROACHES

Tibial Plateau Fractures

Most fractures occur as combinations of shear and depression of the lateral plateau. The lateral cortical rim is usually broken as one large piece. The weight bearing portion of the lateral plateau is depressed. The depressed segment is elevated by exposing the distal portion of the condyle, making a drill hole, and tapping the fragment upwards (Fig. 34–1). The lateral condylar fracture is stabilized by lag screws and either a plate or an ancillary screw at the apex of a fracture (Figs. 34–1 and 34–2). To stabilize the lateral plateau, a longitudinal incision 1 cm lateral to the crest of the tibia is made. The fascia is incised, and the anterior compartment is reflected from Gerdy's tubercle. At least 5 mm of the iliotibial band is maintained in continuity with the anterior compartment fascia for repair over the implant.

The dissection over Gerdy's tubercle is carried sufficiently posterior towards the fibular head to accommodate an appropriate plate. The lateral meniscus is large, so an arthrotomy will not allow visualization of the joint. The joint can be seen by elevation of the capsule off the proximal tibia, allowing visualization beneath the meniscus. Meniscal tears are rare, but avulsions are common and easily repaired. A hole can

then be placed under the cantilevered lateral plateau for elevation of the depressed segment and for bone grafting. Autogenous graft can be harvested from the lateral femoral condyle through the same longitudinal incision (Fig. 34–8).

Medial Plateau Fractures

Most medial fixation is performed as an adjunct to lateral plating. Very little exposure is needed. A posteromedial incision is made, the pes anserinus tendons are elevated, and the plate is slid underneath. In cases of a major medial plateau fracture, a longitudinal incision 1 cm off the tibial crest is utilized. Because the medial meniscus is small, an arthrotomy can be utilized to view the joint. The pes anserinus tendons are reflected, and the plate is applied underneath (Fig. 34–9).

Shaft Fractures

The tibia is a two-bone weight bearing system. In low-energy injuries, the interosseus membrane is minimally stripped from the bone. This is a dense, leatherlike structure that can bear weight. When a rotational deformity is reduced, the interosseus membrane is tightened. An oblique fracture that, radiographically, would seem unstable becomes quite stable because the interosseus membrane, not the bone, can bear weight. Fractures tend not to shorten significantly after reduction, even if early weight bearing is utilized.

Most tibial diaphyseal fixation is performed by intramedullary nailing. Access to the shaft is through an incision around the knee. The author prefers incising the patellar tendon in line with the crest of the tibia, allowing linear access to the medullary canal. Alternatives are either medial or lateral incisions, retracting the tendon. Locking screws are inserted from medial to lateral to avoid penetration of the anterior compartment muscles (Fig. 34–10).

When external fixation is utilized, stab wounds are made just medial to the tibial crest. Pins are inserted in an approximately 30-degree orientation to the shaft (Fig. 34–13) Circular, wire fixator pins are placed close to the knee joint through minimal incisions (Fig. 34–5). The capsular reflection over the upper tibia ranges between 10 and 14 mm. When possible, pins should be at least 14 mm below the knee. The tibiofibular joint communicates with the knee in some patients. Pins crossing this joint can lead to knee infections.

The crest and medial surface of the tibia are subcutaneous. Incisions in these areas should be avoided due to poor healing. Approaches to the shaft for plate fixation elevate some of

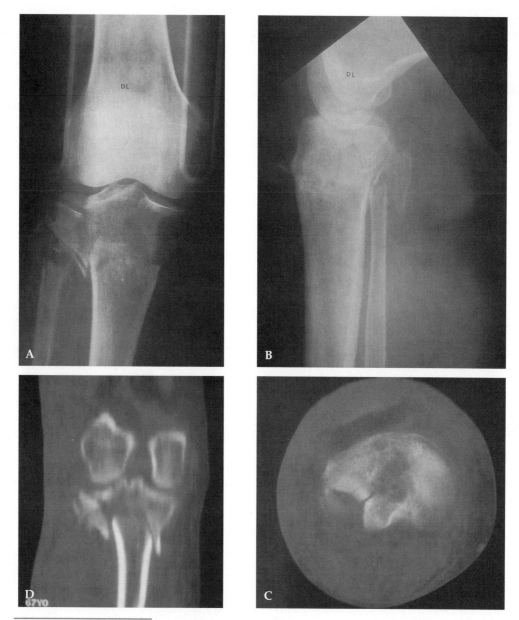

Figure 34–1 A highly comminuted bicondylar tibial plateau fracture. The lateral plateau is comminuted with elements of shear and depression. **(A,B)** Anteroposterior (AP) and lateral radiographs showing a severely comminuted lateral tibial plateau fracture with a mildly comminuted transverse metaphyseal extension. The lateral plateau is both split and depressed. The location and degree of depression cannot be accurately determined from these radiographs. **(C)** Computed tomography (CT) scan demonstrates that the fracture involves two thirds of the lateral plateau and that the depressed segment is posterolateral. **(D)** Tomographic reconstruction of the CT scan shows the fracture well. Computer "averaging" and the small size of the image can obliterate some of the fine fracture lines.

the remaining precarious periosteal blood supply to the diaphysis, either lateral or posterior. An alternative to "open plating" is indirect reduction technique (Fig. 34–6). An incision is made above the fracture, generally medially. A plate is slid subcutaneously, across from the fracture site. A second incision is made distal to the fracture; the proximal and distal screws are inserted, avoiding exposure of the fracture site.

Each distal tibial surface is not axially aligned with the shaft. The lateral distal tibia, in particular, rotates 30 degrees relative to the shaft, and the medial side rotates approximately 15 degrees. Plates must be accurately contoured or iatrogenic deformity can develop.

Pilon Fractures

Because fixation of pilon fractures is highly determined by fracture geometry and soft tissue injury, no specific

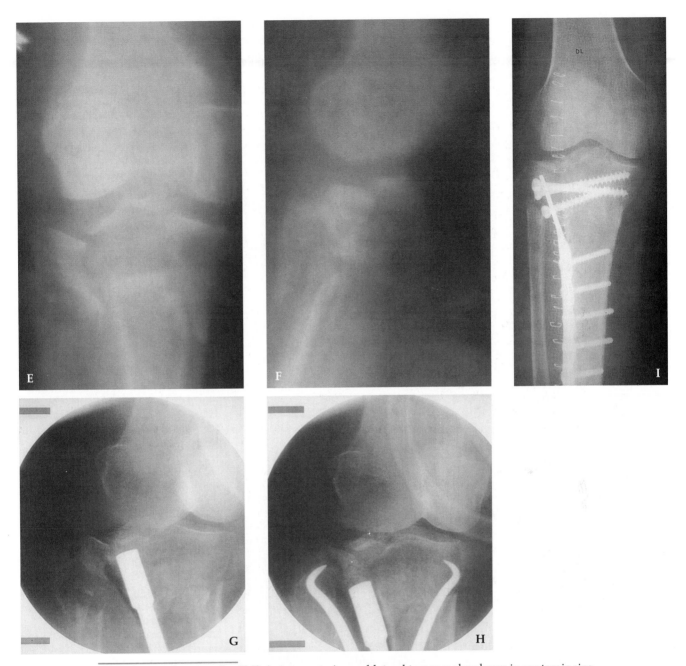

Figure 34–1 *(continued)* **(E,F)** Anteroposterior and lateral tomography shows in anatomic size the degree of depression and comminution of the fracture. **(G)** To repair this fracture, the posterolateral depressed segment must be elevated and the lateral cortex buttressed. Soft tissue swelling precluded the application of a ancillary medial plate. Under fluoroscopic control, the bone impacter has been inserted through a window under the lateral plateau. The depressed segments are identified and elevated. **(H)** Clamps are applied across the fracture to stabilized the elevated fragment. **(I)** The fracture is stabilized with plates and screws. Bone graph has been harvested from the lateral femoral condyle to replace crushed metaphyseal bone under the segment that was surgically elevated. The plate is contoured to the apex of the lateral cortical fragment, the buttress principle.

approaches exist for fixation of all fractures. When fibula fixation is needed, a lateral approach is utilized, and a plate can be applied.

Tibial internal fixation can be either limited or open. Limited fixation often involves an additional incision for bone grafting. This is centered over the metaphyseal crush. Percutaneous screws are inserted through stab wounds that allow fixation across the midportion of a fragment. One to two centimeters of incision is sometimes needed to "tease" a fragment back into place with a small hook or instrument (Fig. 34–7).

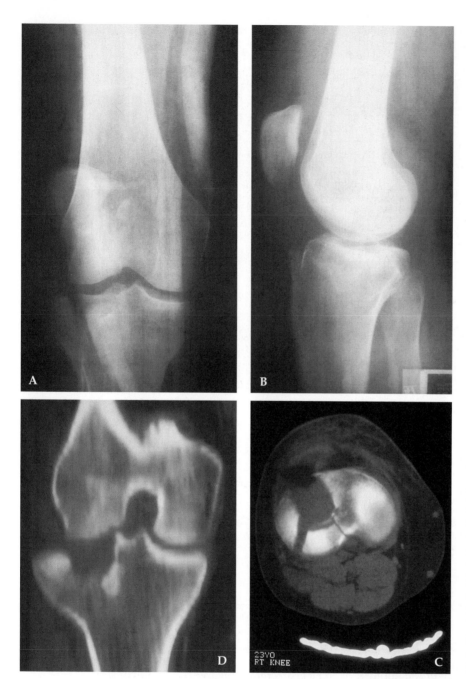

Figure 34–2 A split depression fracture of the lateral tibial plateau. **(A,B)** Anteroposterior and lateral radiographs of the knee showing a split depression fracture of the lateral plateau. The degree of depression and displacement cannot be determined from these radiographs. **(C)** Computed tomography scans shows a large defect; the location of depression and the size of the split piece can be identified, but the degree of depression cannot. This does not help for preoperative planning. **(D)** Tomographic reconstruction of a CT scan, in this case, shows the degree of depression. The orientation of joint fragments cannot be well identified.

When open reduction internal fixation (ORIF) with plates is indicated, generally with rotational injuries, most fractures can be reduced through an incision 1 cm lateral to the tibial crest, curving gently towards the medial malleolus. This allows visualization of the entire anterior ankle joint. Antero-medial or lateral plates can be applied (Fig. 34–14). Medial plates cannot be safely applied through this approach. Wound complications are common, and this approach mini-mizes the potential for exposed bone (Fig. 34–6).

PEARL

The distal tibia is obviously metaphyseal. When purchase is precarious, screws or external fixator pins can be inserted into the distal fibula, which is more diaphyseal bone. Violation of this syn-desmosis can lead to a synostosis, which is of little consequence compared to the magnitude of pilon fractures.

EXAMINATION

Tibial Plateau Fractures

Pedestrian-motor vehicle accidents should make a physician suspect a tibial plateau fracture.

Once diagnosed, the knee must be examined for a liga-mentous injury. Differentiating a medial collateral ligament

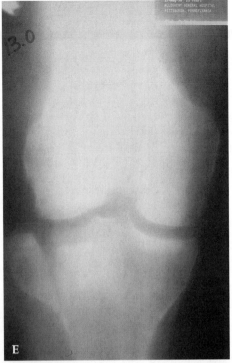

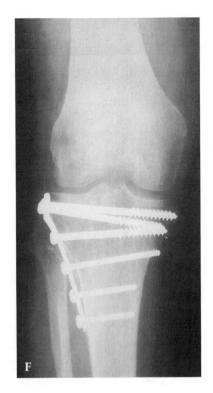

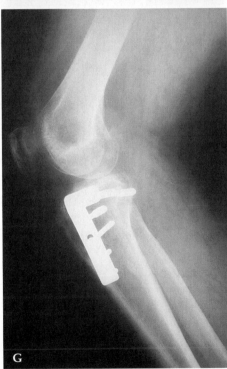

Figure 34–2 *(continued)* **(E)** Tomography shows the orientation and size of the depressed fragments and bones and split fragment. **(F,G)** The fracture has been repaired and is united. The capsule was elevated from the lateral plateau and an avulsed meniscus was repaired. Bone graft was harvested from the lateral femoral condyle through the same logintudinal incision.

PEARL

Nothing in one leg stops a car, and attention is often drawn to the most dramatic injuries. Contralateral knee dislocations and tibial plateau fractures can be overlooked in the presence of dramatic distracting injuries.

injury from a depressed plateau fracture with valgus stressing can be difficult. If a plateau is not depressed, apparent instability is due to ligamentous injury and must be documented. Integrity of the cruciate ligaments must also be documented.

Neurovascular compromise is infrequent. Fractures that involve the fibular neck are associated with peroneal nerve palsies. Unicondylar fractures infrequently are associated with vascular injuries. Bicondylar fractures or fractures that dissociate the knee from the shaft, however, often injure the

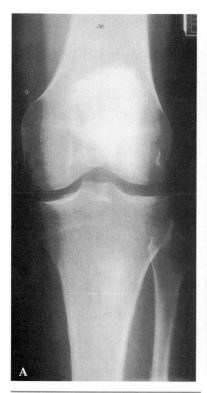

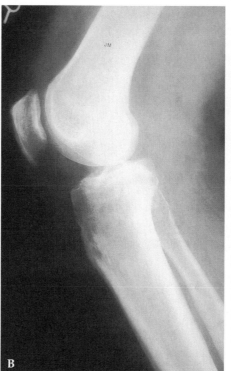

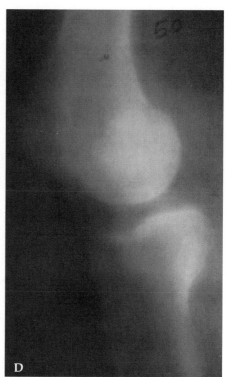

Figure 34–3   A mildly displaced lateral tibial plateau fracture diagnosed by magnetic resonance imaging (MRI) scanning, but with surgical planning by tomography. **(A,B)** Anteroposterior and lateral radiographs of a 54-year-old male struck at his lateral knee by a car. A tense effusion is present. Radiographs are negative. **(C)** An MRI scan was obtained. The only abnormality was an apparent fracture of the lateral plateau. Note the extent of the fracture and cortical margins cannot be identified. Bone ends cannot adequately be differentiated from subchondral injury. **(D)** Tomography showed a localized area of depression in the anterior half of the lateral plateau. Sufficient depression was not present for internal fixation. Magnetic resonance imaging scanning diagnosed the fracture but did not provide sufficient definition for operative planning. Although on MRI scanning a large zone of injury was visible, tomography showed the bony depression to be minimal.

trifurcation of the popliteal artery (Fig. 34–5). Either angiography or serial examinations are needed. It is rare to have an arterial injury in the presence of intact pulses. Pulses, however, can be lost; therefore, serial examinations are needed.

Shaft Fractures

The soft tissue envelope of the tibia must be assessed. Both the degree and nature of swelling are critical. Tense compartment swelling must be differentiated from soft tissue swelling. The ends of the bones must be examined. If injury is suspected, radiographs centered on the knee and ankle must be obtained (Fig. 34–12).

Open fracture grading according to the system of Gustilo should ideally be performed following debridement and initial stabilization. Location and size of wounds, obviously, are documented. It is also critical to clinically assess the degree of soft tissue stripping. This is done by direct examination of the wound, but it also can be inferred by the intrinsic stability of the fracture. A tibia that bends 90 degrees when elevated has sustained a major soft tissue injury, irrespective of the degree of open wound. Wounds that have occurred with potential for extreme contamination must be identified. In particular,

farm or immersion injuries are at risk for serious contamination without regard to the size of open wounds.

Pilon Fractures

Pilon fractures frequently occur from falls. Suicide attempts are a common etiology. A psychiatric evaluation can assist in patient management and selecting realistic treatment alternatives.

The rapid deceleration of a fall can cause associated injuries. The thoracolumbar junction is particularly vulnerable. Standard radiographs center on the midthoracic and lumbar spines leaving the thoracolumbar junction as a "watershed" area that can be overlooked. Radiographs centered at T12 are critical.

Deformity of the distal tibia can make radiographs of the foot (the talus and calcaneus in particular) difficult to obtain. Following initial reduction, repeat radiographs or ancillary studies must be performed.

The nature and degree of soft tissue injury must be assessed. Blistering is frequent. Closed fractures can become secondarily opened by skin breakdown. Initial management of the soft tissue injury of even closed fractures, therefore, is

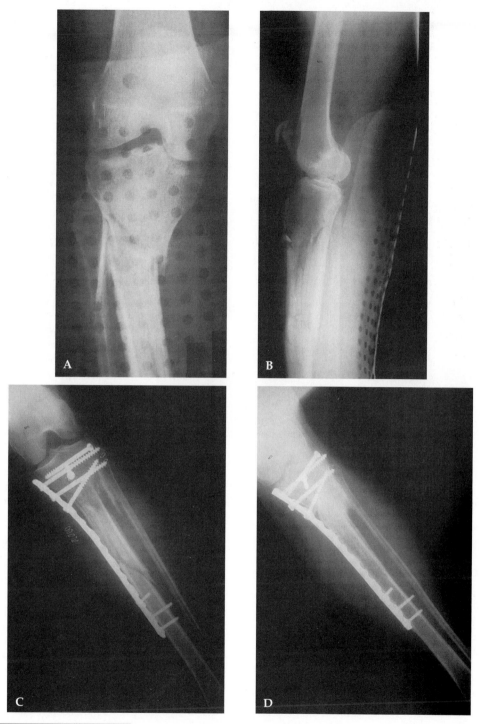

Figure 34–4 Comminuted proximal tibial metaphyseal fracture with a minor joint extension treated with indirect reduction technique with a medial subcutaneous plate. **(A,B)** Anteroposterior and lateral radiographs of a highly comminuted closed proximal tibial metaphyseal fracture with joint extension. **(C)** Immediate postoperative radiograph showing indirect reduction technique fixation. Note the proximal medial staple line. A tunnel was created along the subcutaneous border of the tibia. A plate was slid under the skin. Stab wounds were used for distal screw purchase. The joint was repaired with ancillary percutaneous screws. **(D)** The fracture is united. Because of the lateral cortical defect, a long, leg cast was applied for the first several weeks. The intact fibula also acted as an ancillary strut to the medial plate.

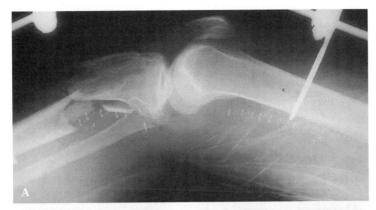

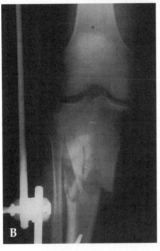

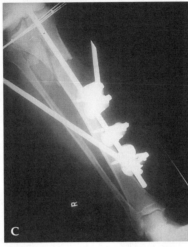

Figure 34–5 Proximal tibial metaphyseal fracture with joint extension associated with an arterial injury. Application of an emergency femoro-tibial frame, replaced by circular, wire fixator. **(A,B)** A direct blow caused a severely comminuted proximal tibia metaphyseal fracture with a longitudinal split into the knee joint. An arterial injury was present. A femoral tibial fixator was applied as an "emergency frame." The ability of such a frame to control the proximal tibial fragments is inconsistent. In this case, the fracture repeatedly displaced into an apex anterior deformity. **(C)** Because the articular fragments were large and comminution in the peri-articular area was not great, a circular, wire fixator was applied. Note the olive wires to compress the fragments. This is attached to a frame of half pins in the distal tibia. This construct allows circumferential support, protecting against varus/valgus as well as AP deformation. The crossing wires in the upper tibia allow axial motion, which promotes healing.

critical. Because of the axial load applied to the limb to create a pilon fracture, compartment syndromes are relatively frequent. Vascular injuries are rare.

AIDS TO DIAGNOSIS

Tibial Plateau Fractures

Both Schatzker and AO classify tibial plateau fractures (Muller et al., 1990). For treatment considerations, unicondylar fractures can be divided into components of depression of an articular segment and splitting of a condyle. In bicondylar fractures, both condyles are dissociated from the tibial shaft. Diagnosing a fracture is simple on plain radiographs. Determining operative indications involves CT scanning, tomography (plain or CT reconstruction), magnetic resonance imaging (MRI) scanning, and arthroscopy (Figs. 34–1 and 34–3).

Computed Tomography Scanning

Computed tomography scanning shows the cross-sectional anatomy of the fracture. If percutaneous techniques are to be utilized, the orientation and size of fragments can be seen. The location of a depressed segment can also be identified, occasionally of clinical significance (Fig. 34–1).

Tomography

Tomography is useful to show both the degree of depression and articular step-offs. Localization of depressed fragments

for elevation can also be identified. Tomographic reconstruction of CT scans are also helpful. Computer "averaging" can sometimes obliterate fracture lines or radiographically coalesce small displaced fragments (Fig. 34–1).

Magnetic Resonance Imaging

Magnetic resonance imaging scanning has been infrequently reported with tibial plateau fractures. The scans present an excellent view of ligamentous structures. Some meniscal injuries can be identified, though fracture displacement can mask a meniscal injury. A plateau fracture can be easily diagnosed on MRI scanning by edema in the subchondral bone. Fracture geometry, determining the exact degree of displacement or step-off, however, may not be accurately determined (Fig. 34–3).

Arthroscopy

Arthroscopy can be helpful in questionable cases. The menisci can be elevated, and the plateau underneath can be examined. It is also an accurate way of determining the integrity of the cruciate ligaments. An articular segment can be traumatically evenly depressed without a step-off or split, and arthroscopy can underestimate the degree of depression. Operative fluoroscopy can assist.

Shaft Fractures

Diagnosing diaphyseal fractures is simple by plain radiographs. Care must be taken to evaluate the ends of the bone.

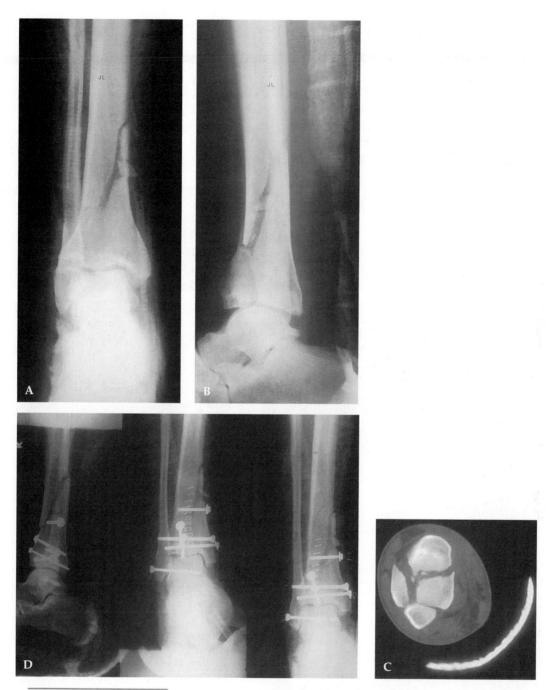

Figure 34–6   A rotational pilon fracture caused by rotation of the talus within the mortise. The plafond is fragmented into large pieces. Classified as type C, with the joint dissociated from the shaft. **(A,B)** Anteroposterior and lateral radiographs of the ankle showing a rotational pilon fracture. The number and orientation of fragments cannot be identified. **(C)** A CT scan shows that the distal tibia is fragmented, broken into three main pieces. The orientation and size of the fragments can be identified. **(D)** An anterior incision exposed the fracture. A screw was placed from the tibia into the talus to maintain the length and orientation of the talus relative to the fibula. This was removed prior to allowing the patient to ambulate. Percutaneous lag screws repaired the articular fragments. Note the intact bone of the fibula was used to anchor screws for better purchase. Note the most proximal screw helps to prevent shear of the large, medial malleolar fragment.

This is particularly important with fractures in the proximal or distal thirds. Undisplaced articular fragments can displace with surgical manipulation. In particular, closed nailing technique can displace tibial plateau or plafond fragments. Computed tomography scanning might be indicated to determine the plane of large fragments for prophylactic percutaneous lag screw fixation to prevent displacement during surgical manipulation (Figs. 34–12 and 34–13).

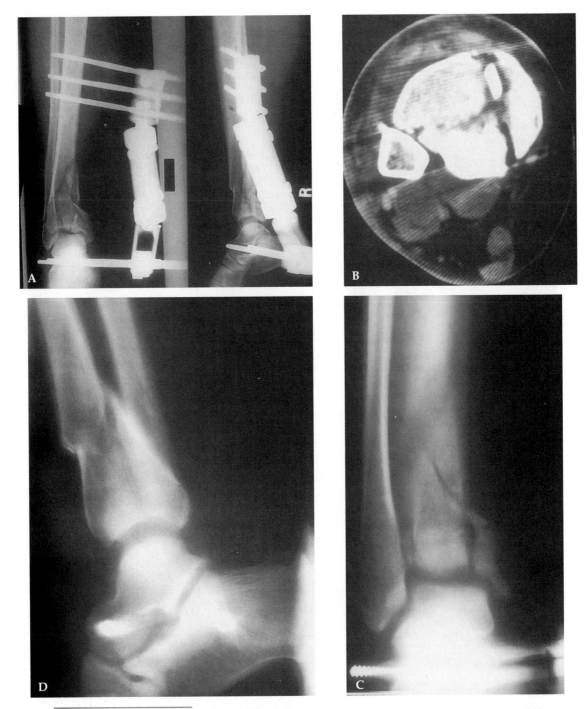

Figure 34–7   A comminuted closed-type C pilon fracture with severe soft tissue injury. **(A)** To control the soft tissues, an external fixator was applied to a displaced type C pilon fracture. Ligomentotaxis has partially reduced the fracture. **(B)** Computed tomography scan through the distal articular surface shows multiple fragments. The size and orientation of fragments is identified. **(C,D)** Tomography demonstrates the degree of epiphyseal comminution and helps orient fragments.

Pilon Fractures

AO has described three classes of pilon fractures, A, B, and C. Type A fractures are extra-articular. Type B fractures have a segment or articular cartilage that is attached to an intact strut of the tibial shaft. Type C fractures have completely dissociated the joint from the shaft.

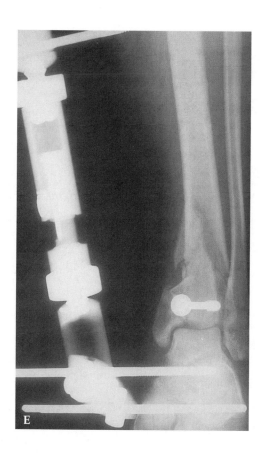

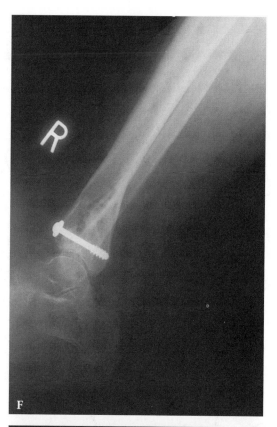

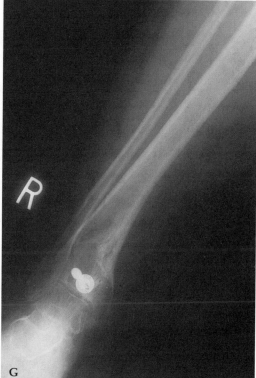

Figure 34–7 *(continued)* **(E)** With a combination of limited internal fixation and ligomentotaxis, the fracture is reduced. The metaphyseal defect is bone grafted. **(F,G)** The fracture has united in an anatomic reduction with good maintenance of the joint space.

Type A Extra-articular Fractures

Type A extra-articular fractures are easily diagnosed, once a joint injury has been excluded. Computed tomography scan-ning or tomography is helpful in confirming that there is no intra-articular extension. The metaphysis is commonly crushed. Appreciation of the magnitude of the defect is often seen following reduction.

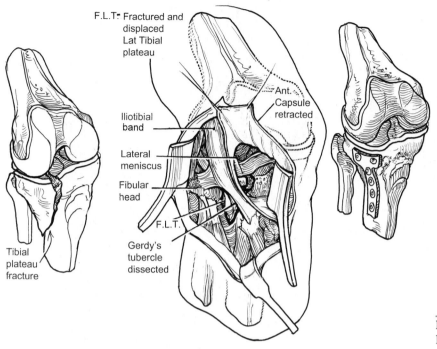

F.L.T: Fractured and displaced Lat Tibial plateau

Ant. Capsule retracted

Iliotibial band

Lateral meniscus

Fibular head

F.L.T.

Gerdy's tubercle dissected

Tibial plateau fracture

Figure 34–8   Schematic illustrating a lateral buttress plate.

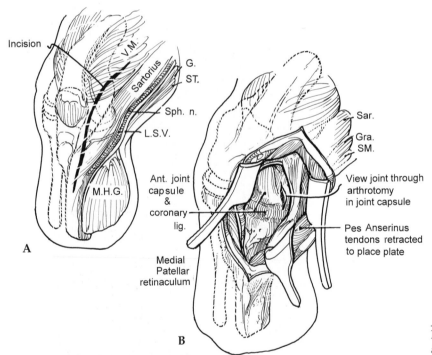

Incision

V.M.

Sartorius

G.
ST.

Sph. n.

L.S.V.

M.H.G.

Ant. joint capsule & coronary lig.

Medial Patellar retinaculum

A

Sar.

Gra.
SM.

View joint through arthrotomy in joint capsule

Pes Anserinus tendons retracted to place plate

B

Figure 34–9   (A,B) Anteromedial approach to a medial tibial plateau.

Type B Fractures

Type B fractures with a piece of articular cartilage remaining in continuity with an intact strut of bone must be differentiated from type C fractures (Fig. 34–7). On initial radiographs, the talus is usually subluxed anteriorly. The talus must be perfectly reduced to the intact strut of articular cartilage. Computed tomography scanning is helpful in identifying the location and orientation of the intact strut of bone. Tomography or tomographic reconstructions of CT scanning can help identify the degree of articular comminution.

Type C Fractures

Type C fractures, where the joint is dissociated from the shaft, have problems with both joint incongruity and metaphyseal crush. In rotational injuries, where the joint is fragmented into large pieces, a large fragment of plafond is usually attached to the tibiofibular synostosis. Identification of the location and size of this fragment is critical for open reduction and internal fixation. This is well seen on CT scanning. Occasionally, tomography or tomographic CT reconstruction is helpful (Fig. 34–6).

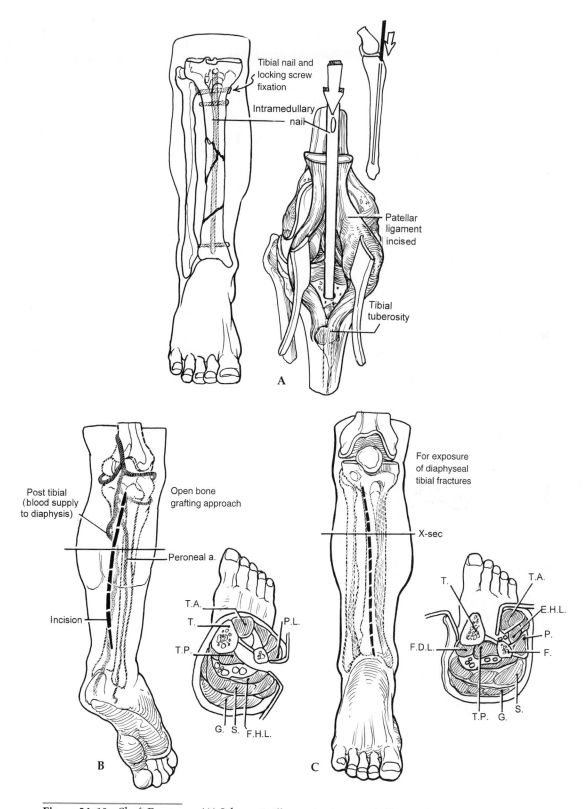

Figure 34–10 Shaft Fractures. **(A)** Schematic illustrating intramedullary nailing. **(B)** Posterolateral approach. **(C)** Anterior approach.

In type C crush injuries, the metaphysis is usually severely crushed, and the plafond has been displaced vertically. As in rotational injuries, a portion of the tibial plafond is frequently attached to the tibiofibular synostosis, but the fragment is often small (Fig. 34–7). This fragment still should be identified with CT scanning. Tomography or tomographic

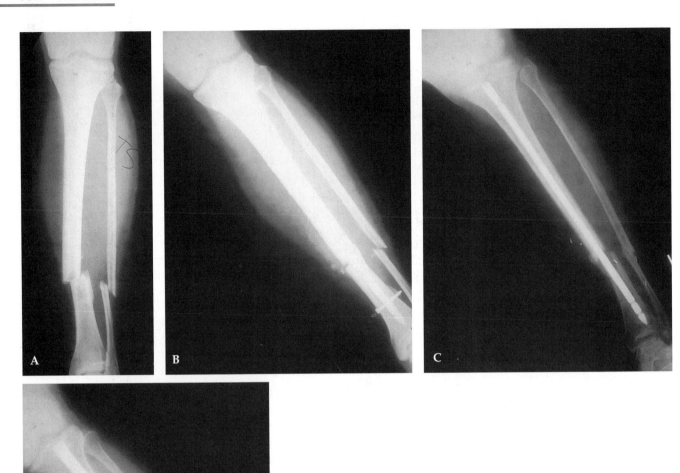

Figure 34–11   An open tibia fracture treated by immediate debridement and nonreamed nailing. An inappropriate dynamization led to deformity that was reconstructed by a reamed nail. **(A)** Grade III open distal third tibia fracture. **(B)** Immediate debridement and stabilization with a nonreamed, static, locked tibial nail. Note the extra length of cross-locking screws to facilitate extraction if the screws break. **(C)** A nonunion was treated by distal dynamization, allowing the fracture to deform into varus. The proximal locking screw should have been removed to allow union but prevent deformity. **(D)** A reamed nail has been used to achieve union and correct the deformity.

CT reconstructions are very helpful to identify the degree of articular impaction, as well as the degree of the metaphyseal defect.

SPECIFIC CONDITIONS, TREATMENT, AND OUTCOME

Indications: Unicondylar Fractures

Specific indications for fixation do not exist. All authors agree that 1 cm of depression is an absolute indication for ORIF.

Most authors believe that a 4 mm depression is an indication for surgery. A split fracture that causes a step-off as opposed to a smooth depression may indicate internal fixation at 2 mm.

Treatment: Unicondylar Fractures
Plate and Screw Fixation

Split depression unicondylar plateau fractures are managed by plate and screw ORIF (Fig. 34–2). This involves elevation of the depressed segment, bone grafting the metaphyseal defect from the lateral femoral condyle or iliac crest, and the

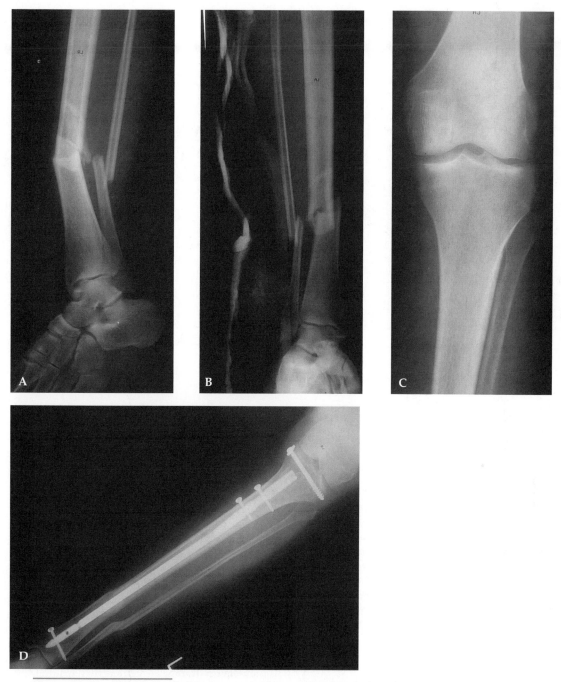

Figure 34–12   Closed distal tibia fracture with an undisplaced plateau fracture. Treatment with percutaneous fixation of a plateau and closed nonreamed nailing of the tibial shaft. **(A,B)** Radiographs of a closed distal third tibial fracture in a blunt polytrauma patient. Associated injuries included a contralateral closed tibia fracture and severe chest injury. Associated injuries mandated internal fixation. **(C)** A tense knee fusion is present. Radiographs showed a questionable longitudinal split through the tibial plateau. Because of clinical suspicion, the leg was rotated under fluoroscopic control, and an undisplaced fracture line was identified. **(D)** To prevent splitting of the tibial plateau, a percutaneous screw was prophylactically placed across the subchondral bone of the knee to hold the upper tibia in place. The locked nail was inserted into the tibia and the fracture united. Note the locking screws are slightly too long. If the screws fatigue, removal will be simplified.

application of a lateral plate. The depressed articular segment is not stabilized by the bone graft but by subchondral screws. This provides sufficient stability for early motion. Internal fixation of tibial plateau fractures usually requires image inten-

sification. This prevents intra-articular screw penetration and ensures adequate restoration of the joint. If a meniscus is avulsed, it should be repaired. Outcome is determined by articular damage that occurs at the time of the injury, associ-

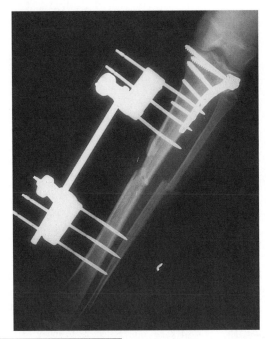

Figure 34–13 A unilateral anteromedial fixator has been applied to a grade IIIB open tibia fracture with an associated ipsilateral tibial plateau fracture.

ated major ligamentous injury, and the adequacy of restoration of the joint.

Percutaneous Screws

If a condyle is broken as one large piece (shear fracture), percutaneous lag screws can restore the joint. Computed tomography scanning will show the orientation of the fragment. Alternatively, under fluoroscopy, the leg can be rotated so the fracture line is perfectly visible with no overlap. Screws can then be placed perpendicular to the fracture line lagging the fragments together. Ideally, two screws near the joint and the third screw at the apex of the fracture (buttress principle) are optimal. Dissecting the anterior compartment to insert an apical screw is frequently not needed.

Arthroscopy

Reports of arthroscopic-assisted tibial plateau fixation are preliminary and selective. Arthroscopy is most useful when a large condylar segment is present, and the fracture is amenable to percutaneous fixation. Arthroscopy can be a valuable tool in diagnosing cruciate and meniscal injuries. Shear fractures can be easily visualized and reduced arthroscopically and then repaired with percutaneous screws. Depressed segments, in contrast, can be more difficult to visualize. Step-offs are easily seen arthroscopically, but depressed plateau fractures frequently displace as a gently sloped concavity, making determinations of the degree of depression or elevation difficult. Fluoroscopy is, therefore, often needed. A small incision under the plateau can be used to elevate a depressed segment and, again, percutaneous screws can be used. If open surgery is needed for fixation, arthroscopy is of very little benefit.

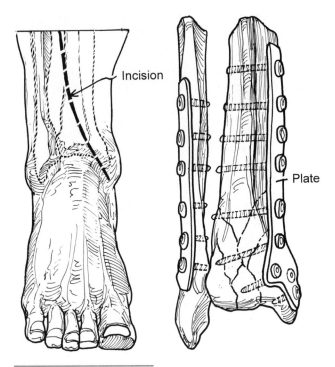

Figure 34–14 Pilon Fractures: open reduction internal fixation with plates.

Indications: Bicondylar Tibial Plateau Fractures

Indications for fixation include those for unicondylar fractures but also include metaphyseal diaphyseal instability.

Treatment Bicondylar: Tibial Plateau Fractures

Associated soft tissue injuries and degree and location of comminution determine treatment options. If large fragments are present, options include plate and screw fixation or circular, wire fixators with hybrid frames. If the medial or lateral cortices can be opposed, a unilateral plate is sufficient (Figs. 34–1 and 34–4). If significant metaphyseal comminution exists, either bilateral plates, cast supplementation, or circular, wire fixators are indicated. Serious open wounds, vascular injuries and compartment syndromes, are common in high-energy trauma. An emergency femoral tibial fixator is often needed (Fig. 34–5). This often does not control the proximal fragment, allowing displacement. Delayed reconstruction is often necessary. The timing and technique are indicated by the status of the soft tissues and bony defects.

Treatment: Closed, Low-energy Tibial Shaft Fractures

Most low-energy fractures can be well managed by functional bracing. Bracing is indicated for fractures that have shortened less than 1 cm and are not associated with massive swelling or major wounds. Fifty percent of the cortices must be in contact.

Contraindications to the use of functional bracing include polytrauma patients, associated orthopaedic injuries, (ipsilateral lower extremity, in particular), obesity, and significant soft tissue injuries, open or closed. The fracture is initially splinted and elevated to reduce swelling. Within the first 4 weeks, a prefabricated molded brace is applied, and the patient is encouraged to bear weight on the limb. The ankle is left free or hinged with a shoe insert for additional support. Fractures generally heal within 3 months. Patients can be functional while fractures are uniting. Though excellent results have been reported, the attrition rate in many studies has been as high as 20%, and studies have selected for only the lowest energy fractures.

Treatment: High-energy Closed, Grade I, II, and IIIA Open Fractures

Treatment for all of these injuries are similar with the exception of wound management. Open wounds are taken to surgery and debrided. Fixation is generally applied on admission. High-energy closed fractures can be treated more electively.

External fixation is most often reserved for open fractures but can also be applied to high-energy closed injuries. Unilateral frames are applied with three pins above and three below the fracture along the medial surface of the tibia out of the crest (Fig. 34–13). Pins in the tibial crest are associated with high rates of pin-tract infection and stress fractures after removal. Weight bearing is encouraged. This increases the risk of pin-tract infection but significantly improves rates of union. Frames are maintained until fractures have united and are followed by either full weight bearing or functional bracing for a short interval. Union rates of 90% can be anticipated. The problem with external fixation is reconstruction. Malunions and nonunions following external fixation, especially when a pin-tract infection has been present, have a high incidence of sepsis postreconstruction.

Reamed, locked nailing will reliably heal tibial fractures provided adequate purchase in the proximal and distal metaphyses can be obtained. Union in 20 weeks can be anticipated. Because the nails are strong, early weight bearing can be allowed in most cases. Malunions are infrequent. Delayed unions have been reported in some studies and can be treated by dynamization following fibular union or exchange nailing. A significant concern is iatrogenic compartment syndromes. Fracture tables must be avoided as longitudinal traction has been shown to significantly increase compartment pressures. The force of reaming and the bulk of a wide nail might provoke a compartment syndrome. Reamed nailing should not be performed until traumatic swelling has begun to subside.

Nonreamed nailing is a rapid and effective way of acutely stabilizing tibia fractures (Figs. 34–11 and 34–12). The chances of precipitating a compartment syndrome are low. Because the nails are small, weight bearing must be restricted to avoid implant fatigue. Malunions have been rare, but delayed and nonunions have been commonplace, especially with static nailing. Reconstructive procedures, either dynamizations or

exchanged nailings, are frequently indicated (Fig. 34–11). Some authors have recommended routine dynamization following fibular union to increase the rate of union and decrease the interval to union. Union in 20 to 30 weeks can be anticipated.

Treatment: Grade IIIB and IIIC Open Fractures

Grade IIIB open fractures by definition have a major wound that requires flap coverage. Soft tissues are therefore missing. Virtually all grade IIIC open fractures have a similar wound but are complicated by an arterial injury that requires reconstruction. Patients are taken immediately to surgery for thorough wound debridement. The bone edges are delivered into the wound for debridement of fracture surfaces. Early fracture stability helps soft tissue healing by reducing movement, which causes fluid build up. "Second look" operations are often needed. This is especially important when a dependent pocket of tissue can collect fluid that is not amenable to dressing changes. Many studies have shown that early coverage reduces the rate of late sepsis. In the author's institution, however, no such correlation has been seen.

Nonreamed nailing is the current treatment of choice in most trauma centers, though indications and results are still evolving. Static locking is necessary to stabilize soft tissues. Because the nails are thin, weight bearing must be restricted. Following fibular union, dynamization can be performed if union is not proceeding adequately. Another salvage would be exchange nailing. An alternative to late reconstruction is routine early posterolateral bone grafting (Fig. 34–11).

External fixation is an established technique. As among lesser open fractures, a unilateral frame is applied, early weight bearing is encouraged, and the frame is maintained until union. An alternative is to remove the frame following soft tissue healing. This shortens the interval of fixation, and obviously reduces the risk of pin-tract infection. The rates of malunion, however, increase. The problem of external fixation is late reconstruction. Early removal is probably associated with an increased rate of reconstructions with their attendant risk of infectious complications.

Tibial reconstructions after external fixation should not be performed with reamed, intramedullary nailing. Closed nonreamed nailing and open plating with bone grafting have recently been reported with at least preliminary good successes. Posterolateral bone grafting is rarely an option after a grade IIIB open tibia because soft tissue planes have been obliterated. Neurovascular structures cannot be identified or protected adequately. Fibulectomies are indicated only as an adjunct to other forms of fixation. Fibulectomy alone allows tibias to deform.

Plating grade IIIB open tibia fractures should be avoided. It is only indicated when a fracture is so severe that it extends to a joint, or when no other forms of fixation are possible due to rare fracture patterns or associated injuries.

Circular, wire fixators are, likewise, rarely indicated acutely for tibial diaphyseal fractures.

Fractures that extend from the diaphysis through the metaphysis might be indications for hybrid frames or circular, wire fixators. Soft tissue reconstructions around large bulky fixators can be difficult unless plastic surgeons are highly experienced in working around these frames.

Amputation Versus Salvage:
(Severe IIIB and IIIC Open Fractures).

PEARL

If amputation is a serious possibility, fixation that does not jeopardize a below-knee prosthesis should be utilized. Intramedullary nails can cause a painful scar over the patellar tendon. External fixators and unilateral or circular, wire fixators can cause painful scars around the upper tibia. The choice of fixation must be individualized.

No absolute indications for amputation exists. In general, fractures that lacerate the posterior tibial nerve or destroy all vessels to the foot should be considered for amputation. The issue is not only whether the neurovascular structures can be acutely reconstructed but extent of the the soft tissue injury to the rest of the leg. It is rare that a IIIC fracture or one associated with a laceration to the posterior tibial nerve occurs without extraordinary damage to the rest of the limb. A dysvascular foot or a stiff foot and ankle with incomplete sensation on the sole leads to chronic pain and poor function.

The author has successfully salvaged rare fractures with these neurovascular injuries but only when a spike of bone happened to selectively cut these structures without extraordinary, associated, soft tissue injury.

Treatment: Pilon Fractures

Pilon fractures are rare and severe injuries. Multiple techniques have been described for treatment, all with advantages and drawbacks. Soft tissue injury often dictates treatment option. Because pilon fractures are so rare, it is difficult to gain experience with every technique. It is more important to utilize the technique with which the surgeon is familiar.

Type A Pilon Fractures

Type A fractures are extra-articular pilon fractures. The problem is metaphyseal crush, not articular extension. These fractures are too distal for a nail. If the fibula is broken, restoration of the fibula with plates or intramedullary nailing can restore axis and length. Ancillary support either as a cast or, more generally, a plate or medial external fixation will help maintain alignment. Circular, wire fixators are an excellent alternative, allowing both medial and lateral stability in a

wide, soft bone. Bone grafting the metaphyseal defect is often necessary if medial soft tissues will tolerate an incision.

Type B Pilon Fractures

Type B fractures have a portion of the articular surface attached to an intact strut of tibial bone (Fig. 34–15). Almost always, the anterior tibial lip is fractured, and the tibia has subluxed anterior. Reconstruction must begin by reducing the talus perfectly to the remaining intact strut of tibial bone and molding the balance of the anterior tibial lip to the dome of the talus. This often requires at least provisional K-wire fixation of the tibia to the talus. Depending on the size of the fragments and the soft tissue injury, either internal or external fixation can be utilized. When the talus has subluxed anteriorly, often the capsule and the ligamentous structures about the ankle have been seriously disrupted. Even after anatomic reduction and fixation, the talus still has the ability to sometimes sublux anteriorly.

External fixators have not been adequate to hold the talus perfectly in place. In these cases, even after anatomic fixation, K-wire fixation of the tibiotalor joint may be necessary.

Type C Pilon Fractures

Type C have the joint completely dissociated from the tibial shaft. Fracture geometry as well as the soft tissue envelope determine treatment. In rotational fractures, the tibial plafond is broken into large fragments (Fig. 34–6). The soft tissue envelope is generally fairly well restored. When the soft tissues accommodate an incision, ORIF is the preferred method of treatment. An alternative is circular, wire fixation as a hybrid frame to tibial half pins above. Medial external fixation with minimal internal fixation can also be employed (see Fig. 34–6).

More commonly in American trauma centers are axial load or crush-type fractures. The tibial plafond is severely fractured so that plate and screw purchase is precarious, and the soft tissue envelope is severely disrupted. Unilateral external fixation with limited internal fixation following fibular fixation is a commonly used technique. The fibula is fixed with either an intramedullary nail or with plates and screws. This restores length and rotation. A medial external fixator is applied, creating a medial buttress and ligamentotaxis of the articular segment. Under fluoroscopic control and using preoperative CT scanning for orientation, the articular segments are lagged together with cannulated screws (Fig. 34–7). Occasionally, ORIF can be utilized, as well as circular, wire fixators with hybrid frames.

Outcome of Pilon Fractures

All pilon fractures have potential for permanent ankle and subtalar joint stiffness. All intra-articular pilon fractures can be associated with significant degenerative changes. Treatment should be geared toward optimal results. Extra-articular fractures should not be associated with degenerative changes but still have potential for subtalar and ankle joint stiffness due to soft tissue injury. In addition to hind foot stiffness, intra-articular fractures, types B and C, are frequently associated with degenerative arthritis. This can develop even

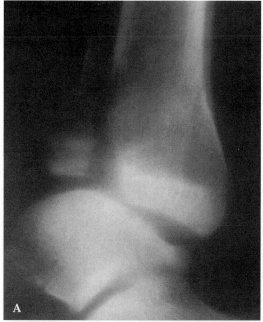

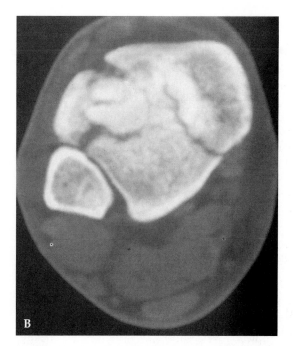

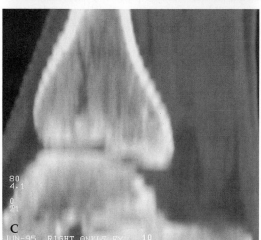

Figure 34–15   Type B pilon fracture. Closed with a moderate soft tissue injury. Treated with limited internal fixation and a transfibular pin. **(A)** Lateral radiograph showing a type B pilon fracture. Note the posterior articular surface is attached to a strut of intact tibial and the talus has subluxed anterior. **(B)** A CT scan shows the size and orientation of fragments. **(C)** Computed tomography reconstruction "averaging" has obliterated some of the fracture geometry.

in the face of anatomic reduction. The degree of radiographic change and functional impairment are extremely variable.

Infection, either as a wound or pin-tract complication, is a serious problem. Hybrid unilateral frames can lead to calcaneal or talar osteomyelitis. Infections of circular, wire-fixator pins can leak bacteria into the ankle joint. Open reduction and internal fixation incisions through thin, damaged skin can lead to exposed plates requiring extensive, soft tissue reconstructions. All techniques have the potential for complications so severe that amputation can ensue. It is imperative to select treatments that address maintenance of bone stock and the soft tissue envelope. If the soft tissue injury is severe, articular reconstruction may be secondary.

SELECTED BIBLIOGRAPHY

BONAR SK, MARSH JL. Unilateral external fixation for severe pilon fractures. *Foot Ankle.* 1993;14:57–64.

BREHRENS F, SEARLS K. External fixation of the tibia: basic concepts and prospective evaluation. *J Bone Jt Surg.* 1986; 68B:246–254.

GUSTILO RB, MEDOZA RM, WILLIAMS DN. Problems in the management of type III open (severe) fractures: a new classification of type III open fractures. *J Trauma.* 1984;24:742–746.

KOVAL KJ, SANDERS R, BORRELLI J, et al. Indirect reduction and

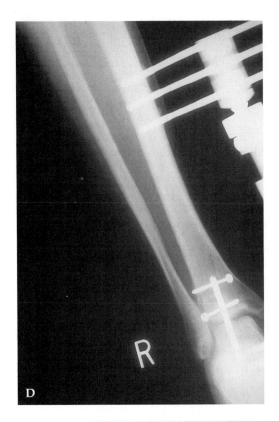

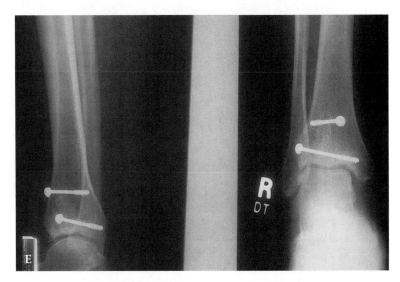

Figure 34–15 *(continued)* **(D)** An open reduction internal fixation has been performed; the fracture is anatomically reduced. A combination of limited internal fixation and ligamentotaxis has held the fracture. Note the K-wire through the calcaneus fixing the talus to the posterior strut of the tibia. Following reduction and stabilization, even with the external fixator in place, the tibia subluxed forward on the weight of the calcaneus resting on a mattress. Even though an anatomic reduction had been performed, and an external fixator applied, the fracture remained unstable. **(E)** Final reduction, the joint space has been preserved. The soft tissue injury, however, mandated residual stiffness of the ankle.

percutaneous screw fixation of displaced tibial plateau fracture. *J Orthop Trauma.* 1992;6:340–346.

MARSH JL, NEPOLA JV, WUEST TK, et al. Unilateral external fixation until healing with the dynamic axial fixator for severe open tibial fractures. *J Orthop Trauma.* 1991;5:341–348.

MULLER ME, NAZARIAN S, KOCH P, SCHATZKER J. The comprehensive classification of fractures of long bones. Berkin. Springer. Verlay, 1990:148–191.

NICOLL EA. Fractures of the tibial shaft: a survey of 705 cases. *J Bone Jt Surg.* 1964;46B:373–387.

RIEMER B, BUTTERFIELD SL. A comparison of reamed and nonreamed solid core nailing of the tibial diaphysis after external fixation. *J Orthop Trauma.* 1993;7:279–285.

RIEMER B, DICHRISTINA D, COOPER A, SHAUL S, et al. Nonreamed nailing of tibial diaphyseal fractures in blunt polytrauma patients. *J Orthop Trauma.* 1995;9:66–75.

RIEMER B, MIRANDA M, BUTTERFIELD S, BURKE C. Nonreamed nailing of closed and minor open tibial fractures in patients with blunt polytrauma. *Clin Orthop Rel Res.* 1995;320:119–124.

RUEDI TP, ALLGOWER M. The operative treatment of intraarticular fractures of the lower end of the tibia. *Clin Orthop.* 1979;138:105–110.

SARMIENTO A, GERSTEN LM, SOBOL PA, SHANKWILER JA, VANGSNESS LT. Tibial shaft fractures treated with functional braces: Experience with 780 fractures. *J Bone Jt Surg.* 1989;71B:602–609.

SCHATZKER J, MCBROOM R, BRUCE D. Tibial plateau fractures: the Toronto experience 1968–1975. *Clin Orthop.* 1979;138:94–104.

WEINER LS, KELLEY M, YANG E, et al. The use of combination internal fixation and hybrid external fixation in severe proximal tibial fractures. *J Orthop Trauma.* 1955;9:244–250.

SAMPLE QUESTIONS

1. A low-energy spiral geometry tibial fracture is:
   (a) likely to shorten considerably with weight-bearing
   (b) associated with a higher incidence of compartment syndromes then open fractures of the tibia
   (c) best treated by an intramedullary nail
   (d) best treated by functional bracing and early weight-bearing

2. Alternatives for treatment for grade III open tibia fractures include all but:
   (a) unilateral external fixation, early weight-bearing, with the fixator maintained to union
   (b) immediate nonreamed nailing with restricted weight-bearing, accepting a high rate of nonunions
   (c) immediate plate fixation
   (d) external fixation maintained until soft tissues have healed, followed by casting and weight-bearing

3. Rotational pilon fractures:
   (a) are associated with a high degree of metaphyseal crush
   (b) are commonly seen following high-energy motor vehicle or motor cycle accidents
   (c) are the pilon fractures most commonly treated by ORIF
   (d) have an excellent prognosis for normal function

4. Unicondylar, split-depression-type tibial plateau fractures:
   (a) are rarely associated with ligamentous injuries
   (b) are frequently associated with tears of the meniscus
   (c) a 4-mm articular step-off associated with an 8-mm depressed segment is a clear indication for internal fixation
   (d) is best treated by hybrid external fixation

5. All of the following statements are true concerning a bicondylar tibial plateau fracture with severe metaphyseal comminution and large articular fragments except:
   (a) Unilateral plate fixation and early range of motion is an acceptable treatment.
   (b) Unilateral femoral tibial fixation will reliably stabilize the fracture.
   (c) Hybrid external fixation is an excellent alternative for treatment.
   (d) A decision to apply bilateral plates is based more on the soft tissue injury than biomechanical considerations.

Answers: 1) d; 2) c; 3) c; 4) c; 5) a

Chapter 35

Soft Tissue Problems of the Knee

Brian J. Cole, MD, Lucio S. Ernlund, MD and Freddie H. Fu, MD

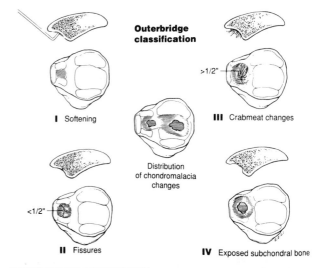

Figure 35–1 Outerbridge classification of chondromalacia. Grade I: softening and swelling. Grade II: fragmentation and fissuring in an area less than 1/2 inch. Grade III: the area is greater than 1/2 inch. Grade IV: cartilage erosion to bone. Reproduced with permission from Tria AJ, Klein KS. *An Illustrated Guide to the Knee.* New York, NY: Churchill Livingstone; 1992: 142.

35–1). It should not be used as a synonym for anterior knee pain or PF symptoms.

ANTERIOR KNEE PAIN AND PATELLOFEMORAL DISORDERS

Patellofemoral (PF) disorders encompass a large differential diagnosis including but not limited to nonarthritic (non-PF) causes of anterior knee pain, PF malalignment, and PF arthritis. Diagnosis and treatment of non-PF causes of anterior knee pain is challenging. Patellofemoral malalignment and arthritis require accurate diagnosis to formulate a treatment plan. Rehabilitation focusing on the extensor mechanism, when unsuccessful, may lead to one of several realignment-type procedures. The term chondromalacia patella as described by Outerbridge (1961) describes the pathologic changes often occurring concomitantly with PF pain (Fig.

> **PITFALL**
>
> **Chondromalacia is often used as a synonym for anterior knee pain and should only be used when describing the gross pathology of the articular cartilage.**

Basic Science
Biomechanics

Normal function of the PF joint depends on the balance between lower extremity alignment as well as static (retinaculum, bony anatomy, Q [quadriceps] angle) and dynamic

541

---

vastus medialis obliquus (VMO) stabilizers. The patella increases the moment arm (the distance between the extensor mechanism to the center of the knee) and thereby increases quadriceps strength by one third to one half. Large forces are generated across the PF joint:

walking: $0.5 \times$ body weight

stair climbing: $3.3 \times$ body weight

deep squats: $7 \times$ body weight

The lateral and inferior articular surfaces normally contact the trochlea at 10 to 20 degrees of flexion. As flexion increases, the contact site moves medial (45 degrees) and proximal (90 degrees) with the odd facet coming into contact last (135 degrees). With patella alta, sites of contact occur at higher degrees of flexion.

Coronal (lateral) plane contact forces are greatest at low flexion angles ($<$ 30 degrees). In general, sagittal (posterior) plane PF contact forces increase with knee flexion between 0 degrees and 90 degrees. These increases are partly mitigated by increasing PF contact area at higher flexion angles (pressure = force/area). Normally, after 90 degrees, the quadriceps tendon contacts the trochlea, resisting increases in PF contact pressure. Patellofemoral contact pressures vary with testing conditions. During open-chain (nonweight-bearing) extension exercises, the flexion moment arm increases and PF contact pressure peaks at terminal extension. During closed-chain exercises (weight-bearing), PF contact pressure peaks as the flexion angle increases.

PEARL

From 0 to 45 degrees, closed-chain exercises are recommended, and from 45 to 90 degrees, open-chain exercises are recommended to minimize PF reaction forces during PF rehabilitation.

The Q angle is defined in extension as the angle between the line of pull of the quadriceps (anterior superior iliac spine to center of patella) and patellar tendon (center of patella to center of tibial tubercle) (Fig. 35–2). Angles greater than 20 degrees are considered abnormal, reflecting a net lateral moment during quadriceps contraction. The lateral moment is normally counteracted by the VMO and static restraints. Measuring the tubercle-sulcus Q angle (the relative position of the tibial tubercle to the inferior pole of the patella at 90 degrees) is preferred by many, as it accounts for the effects of malalignment. Angles greater than 8 to 10 degrees are consistent with a lateralized distal patella vector primarily due to malalignment.

PITFALL

By itself, the Q angle is insufficient to determine the source or treatment of PF pain.

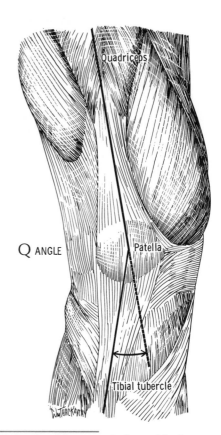

Figure 35–2   Quadriceps angle formed by intersection of the quadriceps tendon vector and the patellar tendon vector. More than 20 degrees is considered abnormal. Reprinted with permission from Insall JN. *Surgery of the Knee.* New York, NY: Churchill Livingstone, 1984: 195.

Anatomy
Embryology

The patella is the largest of the sesamoid bones and forms within the quadriceps muscle as early as 7.5 weeks gestation. The trochlear groove forms before fetal knee motion and is thought to be primarily genetically determined.

Articular surface

The patella has the thickest articular surface in the body. It is divided into medial and lateral facets by a central ridge or crest. The medial facet has a separate, odd (vertically oriented) facet with limited trochlear contact during flexion. The larger, lateral facet is concave in both the longitudinal and transverse planes.

Synovium

The plica synovialis mediopatellaris is an embryologic remnant of the medial-based synovial fold extending from the suprapatellar pouch around the patella to the fat pad distally.

Soft tissue stabilizers

These circumferentially converge on the patella, including:

1. cephalad: quadriceps tendon

2. distal: patellar tendon
3. medial: VMO, retinaculum and PF ligament
4. lateral: vastus lateralis tendon, retinaculum, and iliotibial band (ITB)

The medial PF ligament is the major restraint to lateral displacement (53%). Capsular thickenings, called patellomeniscal ligaments (Kaplan's ligaments), are thought to be the cause of referred joint line pain in PF disorders.

Vascular and Arterial Supply

Circumferential anastomoses of the four genicular, the supreme genicular, and the medial and anterior tibial recurrent arteries comprise the majority of the arterial supply. Venous drainage is by the popliteal and internal saphenous veins.

Innervation

Nocioceptive pain fibers within the lateral retinaculum are believed to be a cause of anterior and PF knee pain.

Examination
History

Mechanism
Ask the patient about specific patellar trauma, subluxation, or dislocation.

Pain
Patients with PF disorders often have poorly localized dull ache exacerbated by prolonged sitting ("movie sign") or stair climbing. This is often bilateral and of insidious onset. Locations most commonly include anteromedial, retropatellar, and posterior. Pain in long-standing PF disease may be from soft tissue contractures, lateral retinacular pain fibers, and arthrosis.

Giving Way
Patellofemoral "giving way" may represent patellar instability or occur secondary to painful quadriceps inhibition unlike that which occurs secondary to ligamentous instability where the knee "comes apart."

Crepitus
Crepitus is often bothersome to the patient, not commonly associated with pain, and not to be overtreated. Sources include malalignment, synovial impingement, quadriceps tendon, and chondrosis.

Locking
A patient may have a catching sensation that occurs during extension under load (stair-climbing or chair-rising), unlike meniscal pathology where the knee "locks up."

Swelling
Swelling is less common in PF disorders. It suggests intra-articular pathology. Peripatellar soft tissue swelling can also occur.

PEARL
Bilateral complaints of pain of insidious onset exacerbated by prolonged sitting with the knee in a flexed position or while negotiating stairs is relatively common in PF disease.

Physical Examination

In addition to tests specific for PF disorders (below), the exam should include tests necessary to establish other pathologic conditions that may exist.

Observation
Evaluate for foot pronation, external tibial torsion, genu valgum, femoral anteversion (hip internal rotation) and valgus, gynecoid pelvis, flexion contractures, patellar subluxation and Q angle measured in extension and flexion.

Palpation
Effusion
Use distally directed pressure on the suprapatellar area with the palm of one hand while balloting the patella medially with the other hand.

Tenderness
Palpate for tenderness in all anterior knee structures including entire extensor mechanism, medial/lateral patellar facets, retinaculum, epicondyles, ITB, pes anserinus, joint line, and fat pad.

Flexibility and Strength
Evaluate quadriceps (prone knee flexion), hamstrings (supine popliteal angles), and ITB for abnormal flexibility and strength.

Crepitus
Apply posteriorly directed patellar pressure during active and passive range of motion (ROM). Note the presence of pain and where in the flexion arc it occurs.

Percussion
Evaluate for neuromas at prior surgical sites.

Special Tests
Lateral Pull Sign
Test for VMO insufficiency leading to disproportionate superolateral pull of the patella with quadriceps contraction with the knee in extension.

J Sign
Persistent lateral patellar movement with flexion (J sign) rather than inferomedial may occur with PF malalignment.

Extensor Lag
Passive range of motion (PROM) greater than active range of motion (AROM) is consistent with quadriceps insufficiency.

Patellofemoral crepitus

This is often indicative of chondromalacia. It is graded: none (0^+), mild (1^+), moderate (2^+), and severe (3^+). Patellofemoral joint compression with the palm of the hand may recreate symptoms. Crepitus alone does not confirm PF dysfunction.

Passive Patellar Tilt

This test is performed with the knee in full extension to assess side-to-side differences in the ability to elevate the lateral edge of the patella (Fig. 35–3). Zero degrees = normal (parallel), < 0 degrees = tight lateral retinaculum (negative tilt).

Patellar Glide

Perform this test with the knee in 30-degree flexion to engage patella into trochlear groove (Fig. 35–3b). Normal: 2-quadrant displacement medial or lateral without pain or apprehension (subjective feeling that the patella will dislocate). Abnormal: apprehension with > 2-quadrant lateral displacement with the ability to nearly or completely dislocate the patella (> 4 quadrants); reduced medial displacement with excessive lateral compression syndrome (ELCS) or a tight lateral retinaculum.

Aids to Diagnosis

Radiographic Evaluation

Standard Anteroposterior View

Use this extension weight-bearing radiograph to evaluate for soft tissue abnormalities, fractures, joint space narrowing, osteochondritis dissecans (OCD), loose bodies (from medial facet/lateral femoral condyle), and overall alignment.

Posteroanterior View (45 degrees) (Rosenberg, 1988)

A 45-degree posteroanterior (PA) flexion weight-bearing radiograph (x-ray parallel to tibial plateau, centered at joint line) is sensitive for early joint space narrowing, OCD, and evaluation of notch.

Lateral View

Use a lateral decubitus radiograph with knee flexed 30 to 45 degrees, placing the patellar tendon under tension. Evaluate subchondral sclerosis and patellar alta/baja (limitations) based on the Blumensaat line (knee must be flexed 30 degrees), the Insall-Salvati index, and the Blackburne and Peel index often associated with PF dysfunction (Fig. 35–4). Look for fragmentation of the inferior pole of the patella (Sinding-Larssen-Johanssen) or tibial tubercle (Osgood-Schlatter).

Patellar Views (Axial Views)

Wiberg (1941) described different facet configurations according to the ratio of the size of the medial and lateral facets (I: 24%, II: 57%, III: 19%) (Fig. 35–5). Type III is associated with a wide, lateral PF ligament, a predominant lateral facet (3:1), and lateral instability. Lateral displacement of the patella may be normal from 0 to 20 degrees of flexion. Excessive patellar

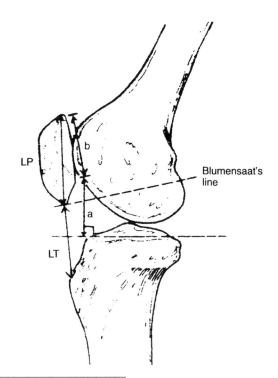

Figure 35–4   Composite illustration of three popular methods of evaluating patellar alta/baja. 1. Blumensaat's Line: With the knee flexed 30 degrees, the lower pole of the patella should lie on a line extended from the intercondylar notch. 2. Insall-Salvati index: Patella tendon length (LT) to patella length (LP) should be 1.0 cm. An index greater than 1.2 is patella alta, an index less than 0.8 is patella baja. 3. Blackburne and Peel index: The ratio of the distance from the tibial plateau to the inferior articular surface of the patella (a) to the length of the patella articular surface (b) should be 0.8. An index greater than 1.0 is considered patella alta. Reproduced with permission from Harner CD, Miller MD, Irrgang JJ. Management of the stiff knee after trauma and ligament reconstruction. In: Siliski JM, ed. *Traumatic Disorders of the Knee*. New York, NY: Springer-Verlag; 1994:364.

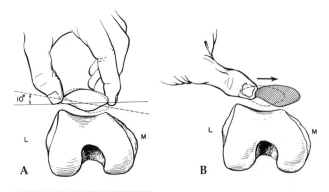

Figure 35–3   Special tests for patellar mobility. **(A)** Patellar tilt is based on a neutral position parallel to the horizontal plane (solid line). A negative tilt is associated with tight lateral restraints. **(B)** Patellar glide is measured based on the number of quadrants the patella can be passively translated medially (M) or laterally (L). Reproduced with permission from Fu FH, Maday MG. Arthroscopic lateral release and the lateral patellar compression syndrome. *Orthop Clin North Am.* 1992, 23:603.

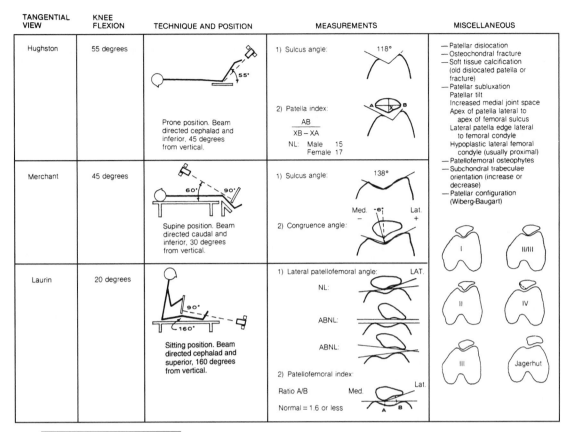

TANGENTIAL VIEW	KNEE FLEXION	TECHNIQUE AND POSITION	MEASUREMENTS	MISCELLANEOUS
Hughston	55 degrees	Prone position. Beam directed cephalad and inferior, 45 degrees from vertical.	1) Sulcus angle: 118° 2) Patella index: $\dfrac{AB}{XB-XA}$ NL: Male 15 Female 17	— Patellar dislocation — Osteochondral fracture — Soft tissue calcification (old dislocated patella or fracture) — Patellar subluxation Patellar tilt Increased medial joint space Apex of patella lateral to apex of femoral sulcus Lateral patella edge lateral to femoral condyle Hypoplastic lateral femoral condyle (usually proximal) — Patellofemoral osteophytes — Subchondral trabeculae orientation (increase or decrease) — Patellar configuration (Wiberg-Baugart)
Merchant	45 degrees	Supine position. Beam directed caudal and inferior, 30 degrees from vertical.	1) Sulcus angle: 138° 2) Congruence angle: Med. −6 Lat.	
Laurin	20 degrees	Sitting position. Beam directed cephalad and superior, 160 degrees from vertical.	1) Lateral patellofemoral angle: LAT. NL: ABNL: ABNL: 2) Patellofemoral index: Ratio A/B Med. Lat. Normal = 1.6 or less	

Figure 35–5 Patellofemoral (PF) measurements on plain tangential radiographs. Reproduced with permission from Carson WG et al. Patellofemoral disorders; physical and radiographic evaluation. Part I: physical examination. *Clin Orthop*. 1984;185:126.

tilt is best demonstrated at 20 to 30 degrees using Laurin's view. Subluxation decreases from 0 to 30 degrees of flexion and is best measured using the Mercer-Merchant view at 45 degrees flexion. Lateral facet arthrosis is seen as subchondral sclerosis, cyst formation, perpendicular trabeculae, facet collapse, lateral margin patellar osteophytes, or fractures and calcification within the lateral retinaculum. Medial facet osteoporosis may be present from relative unloading.

Sunrise View

In this view, the knee is flexed 60 to 90 degrees and the beam is tangential to the PF joint. One can see more of the femoral condyles than on other to views described below. The sunrise view is good for patellar fractures, dislocations, loose bodies and articular irregularities but not for malalignment measures.

Mercer-Merchant View

The knee is flexed 45 degrees, and the X-ray is angled caudad 30 degrees in this view (Fig. 35–6). The sulcus angle (Normal: 140 degrees ± 5 degrees) and the congruence angle (Normal: −6 degrees ± 11 degrees) are formed between lines bisecting the sulcus and median crest, reflecting patellar centralization and/or subluxation. Normally, the median crest bisector (solid line) is medial to the sulcus bisector (broken line) and is considered negative by convention. A congruence angle greater than 16 degrees is diagnostic of lateral subluxation.

Laurin View

This is a 20-degree tangential view. The lateral PF tilt angle is the intersection of the line connecting the peaks of the femoral

Figure 35–6 A typical Merchant's view suggesting lateral patellar subluxation. Only the anterior one-third of the condyles are imaged compared to a sunrise view demonstrating most of the femur. Note lateral subluxation and tilt of the left patella.

condyles with a line along the lateral facet reflecting patellar tilt. The medial opening reflects tilt.

PEARL

Subluxation is best measured using Mercer-Merchant view (congruence angle), whereas tilt is better evaluated using Laurin's view (PF tilt angle).

PITFALL

A tight, lateral retinaculum causing medial rotation of the central ridge may suggest medial subluxation, which is actually only tilt without subluxation. Medial subluxation without previous surgery is extremely rare.

Computed Tomographic Scan

Detection of PF malalignment is more sensitive earlier in flexion before it engages in the trochlea. Midpatellar transverse computed tomography (CT) scans performed in 15, 30, and 45 degrees of flexion prevent image overlap or distortion seen in plain radiographs. Subluxation (congruence angle with central ridge of patella well medial to bisected trochlea) and tilt (lateral PF tilt angle > 12 degrees) is more accurately referenced from the posterior condyles of the femur.

Magnetic Resonance Imaging

Kinematic axial magnetic resonance imaging (MRI) is investigational. Articular or osseous lesions may be identified as well as other intra-articular pathology.

Bone Scan (Technetium Scintigraphy)

A bone scan differentiates articular from soft tissue sources of pain. In reflex sympathetic dystrophy (RSD), typically uptake is diffuse. In PF disorders, the patella is "hotter" than the distal femoral diaphysis.

PITFALL

Imaging studies alone cannot be used definitively to make diagnosis of painful dysfunction of the PF joint.

Specific Conditions, Treatment, and Outcome

Nonpatellofemoral Causes of Anterior Knee Pain

Common to the many etiologies of anterior and PF pain are quadriceps atrophy, weakness, and chronic effusions. Radiographic evaluation is used to rule out malalignment and unsuspected bony pathology. Evaluation and treatment is problem specific as described in this section.

Plica

A diagnosis of exclusion, especially in the presence of notching ("kissing lesion") of the medial femoral condyle related to contact with the plica at 30 to 40 degrees of flexion. Patients present with a history of overuse, trauma, or prior surgery. Palpation reveals a tender band along the medial peripatellar retinaculum. Injection or arthroscopic resection is usually curative.

Tendonitis

Patellar tendonitis ("jumper's knee") presents with distinct tenderness at the origin of the patellar tendon. Relaxation and extension facilitates deep palpation. Treatment includes correction of training errors, rest, progressive strengthening and stretching, multimodality physical therapy, injection and patellar tendon strapping. Surgical exploration and excision is rarely required. Quadriceps tendonitis is less common and similarly treated.

Bursitis

Prepatellar bursitis ("housemaid's knee") presents as a spectrum ranging from acute, swollen, boggy, and tender inflammation to chronic, thickened skin anterior to the patella. Acutely, infection must be ruled out. Surgical excision is rarely required. Inflamation of the pes anserinus is diagnosed by palpation of the sartorius, gracilis, and semitendinosus common tendon insertion along the proximal anteromedial tibial metaphysis. Treatment is similar to tendonitis.

Fat Pad Syndrome

A direct blow or hyperextension injury may traumatize the anterior or infrapatellar fat pad. Symptoms resolve with symptomatic treatment. Hoffa's disease, chronic infrapatellar fat pad fibrosis and calcification, may result from recurrent trauma. Surgical excision or release is often necessary.

Chronic Effusion

Generalized synovitis secondary to intra-articular pathology or inflammatory disease may cause quadriceps inhibition resulting in increased PF joint stress. Treatment is directed toward the specific condition.

Iliotibial Band Friction Syndrome

Overuse may lead to painful inflammation in the region of the lateral femoral epicondyle as the ITB flexes and extends the knee. Risk factors include genu varum, internal tibial torsion, and excessive pronation. Treatment is similar to tendonitis, emphasizes stretching, and occasionally requires partial ITB excision.

Tumorous Conditions

Quadriceps hemangiomas, synovial chondromatosis, osteoid osteoma, and osteochondroma are some of the tumorous conditions that may cause effusion and anterior knee pain. Appropriate suspicion, radiographic evaluation, and lesion-directed excision is required.

Referred Pain

Examination of the back, hips and ankle for age-specific pathology may reveal a remote source of anterior knee pain.

Patellar Osteochondritis Dissecans

This condition rarely may occur along the lateral facet. It is diagnosed best by lateral and axial radiographs. Treatment is determined by the stage of the lesion, including immobilization or drilling (stage I), drilling and fixation (stages II and III), and abrasion chondroplasty with excision (stage IV).

Saphenous Neuralgia and Varices

The inferomedial arthroscopic portal or trauma may damage the infrapatellar branch of the saphenous nerve or peripatellar tissues. Patients complain of numbness or burning along the anterior knee that remains symptomatic at rest. Discrete tenderness is relieved by injection of 1% lidocaine (Xylocaine). Neuroma excision is usually curative. Anterior saphenous varices present with activity-related swelling about the medial side of the knee that decreases with elevation. Vascular consultation and ligation may be curative.

Cruciate Ligament Insufficiency

Cruciate insufficiency, treated conservatively or with reconstruction, may present with anterior knee pain. Some reports on the use of hamstring rather than patellar tendons for anterior cruciate ligament (ACL) reconstruction have demonstrated decreased rates of PF pain.

Adolescent Anterior Knee Pain

This is a broad category and includes PF malalignment, excessive lateral compression syndrome, patella alta/baja, muscle imbalance, Sinding-Larssen-Johanssen disease, Osgood-Schlatter's disease, and hypermobility of the patella secondary to excessive ligamentous laxity. Most of these conditions are treated with conservative modalities (i.e., physical therapy and relative rest) and rarely require surgery.

Reflex sympathetic dystrophy

Patients with reflex sympathetic dystrophy have histories of trauma leading to severe anterior knee pain even at rest, atrophy, skin changes (shiny, red, warm, alopecia) and symptoms out of proportion to the inciting event. Radiographs may show diffuse osteopenia. Bone scans show a "hot" PF joint. Treatment includes desensitization, physical therapy, and sympathetic blockade.

Patellofemoral Disorders

The term patellar instability is specific to patients with a history of lateral subluxation or dislocation, but it may also include patients with ELCS. Articular damage is a common sequelae of long-standing tilt and recurrent instability. A history of trauma, effusion, and crepitus with reproduction of symptoms with PF compression is common.

Operative treatment assumes that at least 3 months of nonoperative treatment have failed. Treatment of PF instability includes lateral release (LR), proximal realignment, and medial tubercle transfer. Treatment of articular degeneration includes chondroplasty, tubercle elevation, patellectomy, and arthroplasty. In general, tubercle elevation reduces sagittal plane forces; and LR, proximal realignment, and medialization of the tubercle reduces coronally directed forces. Combinations of the above procedures should be utilized when appropriate.

Excessive Lateral Compression Syndrome (isolated patellar tilt)

Definition

The definition of ELCS is chronic lateral tilt and compression of the patella from lateral retinacular tightness without instability, hypermobility, or abnormal Q angle.

History

The patient will have a history of activity-related bilateral anterior knee pain with stairs or sitting.

Physical Findings

On examination one finds negative patellar tilt, decreased medial patellar glide, loss of flexibility, facet and retinacular tenderness, positive lateral pull and J signs.

Radiologic Findings

Radiologic workup shows abnormal lateral PF tilt angle, normal or nearly normal congruence angle, and patellar arthrosis.

Treatment

Treatment comprises arthroscopy, chondral debridement, and LR. High-grade arthrosis may require additional anteromedialization of the tubercle.

Patellar Instability

Definition

Patellar instability is a spectrum ranging from patellar subluxation to frank dislocation.

History

There will be a history of patellar slipping with cutting maneuvers and a possible history of trauma.

Physical Findings

Apprehension, increased lateral patellar glide, and negative patellar tilt with lateral retinacular tightness are often present.

Radiologic Findings

Abnormal congruence angle and abnormal lateral PF angle with tilt are found.

Treatment

Treatment comprises LR only with normal alignment; medial tubercle transfer with evidence of malalignment and low-grade arthrosis. High-grade arthrosis requires anteromedialization of the tubercle.

Patellar Arthrosis

Definition

Varying degrees of arthritis due to trauma and/or malalignment define patellar arthrosis.

History

There will be a history of pain primarily with stairs and extension and, possibly, a remote history of trauma.

Physical Findings

There is no significant malalignment and retropatellar crepitus exacerbated by palmer pressure, or facet tenderness and effusion are typically present.

Radiologic Findings

Findings include patellar arthrosis and positive bone scan.

Treatment

Treatment comprises arthroscopic debridement, anteromedialization of the tibial tubercle, patellectomy, or arthroplasty.

Nonoperative Treatment

Most patients with PF malalignment can be treated with nonoperative means. Individualized and pain-free rehabilitation should be attempted for at least 3 months before surgical intervention is considered. Variations of this protocol are used for postoperative rehabilitation with relative protection of surgical reconstructions.

Phase I

Reduce inflammation and effusion, improve VMO control of patellar tracking, improve flexibility, and institute soft tissue stretching and McConnell taping techniques to correct soft tissue imbalances. Patellar sleeves or dynamic braces are controversial, but sometimes helpful.

Phase II

Isotonic eccentric and concentric strengthening with emphasis on muscle endurance and adduction facilitating VMO contraction is introduced. Institute closed-chain exercises in extension and open-chain exercises in flexion. Avoid isokinetics.

Phase III

Introduce proprioceptive and sport-specific functional training. Use plyometrics, aquatics, running, and agility drills.

Operative Treatment

Fig. 35–7 represents a three-arm algorithm (adapted from Post, 1994) for surgical decision making should conservative measures fail to resolve the patient's symptoms. Procedures are chosen based upon the degree of articular arthrosis and the presence of PF malalignment.

Diagnostic Arthroscopy

Goals

Define the specific pathology to facilitate treatment.

Indications

Adjunct to additional procedures.

Techniques

View surgical site superolaterally or superomedially with a 30-degree scope. The patella should articulate laterally at 10 to 20 degrees, centralize and articulate medially at 30 to 40 degrees.

Results and Complications

These are dependent on the specific pathology.

Arthroscopic Chondral Debridement

Goals

The goal of this procedure is the removal of unstable chondral flaps; abrasion chondroplasty to stimulate fibrocartilage formation is of questionable benefit.

Indications

Use arthroscopic chondral debridement with traumatic chondral flaps or as an adjunct to a realignment procedure.

Techniques

Basket forceps and a rotary shaver are used to excise fronds and fibrillations. Beveling of normal cartilage should be avoided.

Results

This procedure does not prevent progression of underlying disease. Results are best with isolated patellar chondromalacia or traumatic lesions.

Complications

Damage to normal cartilage may occur.

Lateral Release

Goals

Relieving posterolateral tether and tilt, decreasing lateral facet stress, improving congruence in combination with other realignment procedures, and improving dynamic VMO function are the goals of LR. By itself, LR will not affect subluxation.

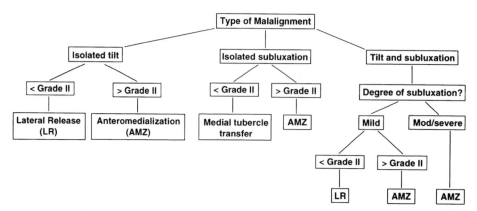

Figure 35–7 Algorithm for surgical treatment of PF malalignment. Reproduced with permission from Post WR. Surgical decision making in patellofemoral pain and instability. *Oper Tech Sports Med*. 1994;2:280.

Indications

Indications comprise pain greater than instability, ELCS, minimal subluxation, low-grade arthrosis (grade I or II), minimal hypermobility, and nearly normal Q angle.

Techniques

Arthroscopic, subcutaneous, and mini-open techniques are employed. Use a retinacular release 1 to 2 cm lateral to the patella from the joint line to the distal most portion of the vastus lateralis (Fig. 35–8). After LR, the patella should be able to be passively tilted 80 degrees.

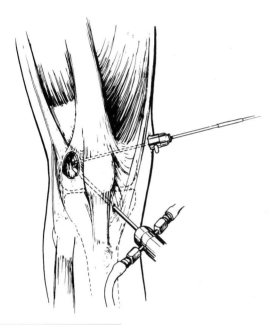

Figure 35–8 Arthroscopic technique for the lateral release (LR). Inferomedial portal for viewing and inflow and superomedial portal 3 to 6 cm proximal to superior pole of patella for intra-articular release using electrocautery. Reproduced with permission from Fu FH, Maday MG. Arthroscopic lateral release and the lateral patellar compression syndrome. *Orthop Clin North Am.* 1992;23:608.

Results

Success rates of 85 to 90% can be achieved in properly chosen patients. Long-term results deteriorate with higher grades of chondrosis (stage III or IV), patellar instability, and hypermobility.

Complications

Complications can include hemarthrosis, infection, RSD, arthrofibrosis, neuroma, medial subluxation of the patella, and worsened pain without evidence of tilt. Greater contact on the distal medial facet in the presence of articular lesions may cause crepitus after LR.

PEARL

After a lateral release (LR), obtain hemostasis at the level of the superior pole (lateral superior geniculate artery) and lateral joint line (lateral inferior geniculate artery) to prevent postoperative hemarthrosis.

Proximal Realignment

Goals

Increased static posteromedial restraint to limit subluxation. The Q angle is not altered, but patellofemoral incongruence is corrected.

Indications

A need for greater static restraint in the presence of lateral tilt when LR alone is felt to be insufficient.

Techniques

A proximal medial VMO imbrication with lateral release is used (Fig. 35–9).

Results

Combined with lateral release, proximal realignment offers no clear benefit to LR alone.

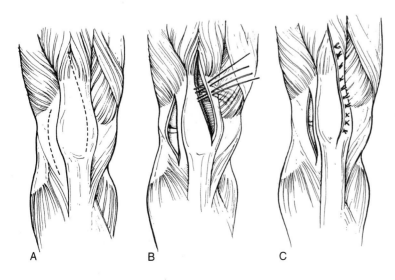

Figure 35–9 Proximal realignment. **(A)** After exposure of the quadriceps, two incisions are made. The first enters the knee joint through a medial parapatellar arthrotomy at the margin of the vastus medialis and the second is a LR. **(B)** Realignment is accomplished by advancing the medial flap laterally and distally in line with the fibers of the vastus medialis obliquus. **(C)** After suturing, the incision lies in a straight line across the front of the patella, and the ER should open widely. Reproduced with permission from Miller MD, Cooper DE, and Warner JP. *Review of Sports Medicine and Arthroscopy.* Philadelphia, PA: WB Saunders; 1995:58.

A   B   C

Complications

Possible complications include quadriceps dysfunction, phlebitis, hematoma, arthrofibrosis, recurrent instability, and potentially increased medial PF contact stress, if performed alone.

Distal Realignment Procedures

Medial tibial tubercle transfer

Goals:

Decreasing the lateral quadriceps vector and the tendency to subluxate.

Indications:

Recurrent instability with minimal pain, low grade arthrosis and increased Q angle.

Techniques:

Roux-Elmslie-Trillat procedure: LR, proximal realignment, and straight medial displacement of the tibial tubercle.

Results:

In properly indicated patients, 80% good to excellent results can be expected.

Tibial tubercle anteromedialization

Goals:

Decreasing sagittal and coronal plane PF contact forces. Moving the tubercle anteriorly unloads, distal and lateral facets; moving the tubercle medially improves Q angle and instability.

Indications:

Recurrent instability, patellar tilt with moderate to severe pain, and high-grade arthrosis (> II), especially with distal medial or central lateral facet arthrosis.

Techniques:

Oblique anteromedial to posterolateral osteotomy resulting in anterior (> 10 mm) and medial translation (> 8 mm) (Fig. 35–10). Combine osteotomy with LR.

Results:

Even with high grade (III or IV) arthrosis, results are 70 to 90% excellent or good.

Tibial tubercle elevation

Goals:

Decreasing the distal sagittal plane PF contact force with load shifting away from distal articular lesions to proximal articular surface is the goal of tibial tubercle elevation.

Indications:

Pain with high-grade arthrosis without malalignment or instability in patients who are not candidates for athroplasty or patellectomy.

Techniques:

The tibial tubercle is elevated 2 cm on the distal-based shingle and a tricortical, iliac crest bone graft is used. Alternatively, an oblique osteotomy will reduce the required size of the iliac crest bone graft.

Results:

PF joint reaction force is reduced 50%. Results are best in post-traumatic arthrosis (> 90% satisfactory).

Distal realignment complications:

Inadvertent posterior displacement increasing PF contact force and arthrosis may occur following a Hauser procedure. Anteromedialization may cause proximal medial patellar pain, if lesions exist there. Inadequate correction, nonunion, infection, arthrofibrosis, recurrent instability, skin necrosis (if elevated > 2 cm) and growth arrest in skeletally immature patients may occur.

Patellectomy

Goals:

Relief of pain with relative improvement in overall function.

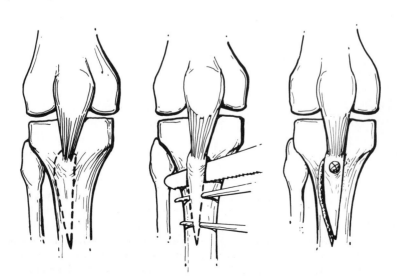

Figure 35–10 Anteromedial transfer as described by Fulkerson. Reproduced with permission from Walsh WM. Patellofemoral joint. In: DeLee JC, Drez D Jr, eds. *Orthopaedic Sports Medicine: Principles and Practice.* Philadelphia, PA: WB Saunders; 1994;1233.

Indications:

Severe pain from extensive articular lesions limiting quadriceps function that are not amenable to realignment or anteriorization.

Techniques:

Longitudinal side-to-side repair, "purse-string" imbrication, and transverse proximal-to-distal repair are techniques employed. They can be combined with LR and proximal realignment.

Results:

At follow up of more than 5 years, results are 33 to 60% excellent.

Complications:

A strength deficit of 30 to 50% with symptoms of giving way may occur.

Patellofemoral Arthroplasty

Goals:

Relief of pain with relative improvement in overall function.

Indications:

Isolated PF arthritis in elderly or low-demand individuals.

Techniques:

Patellar resurfacing or total PF replacement is employed.

Results:

The best results are achieved when malalignment is addressed: up to 85% good or excellent at 2 to 12-year followup.

Complications:

Loosening, wear, and infection can occur.

Summary

Anterior knee pain may have a variety of causes, only some of which are due to PF disorders. Diagnosis and treatment is difficult and is predicated on a systematic history and physical examination. Radiographic evaluation may offer additional information to diagnose and treat PF disorders. Chondromalacia should not be used as a substitute term to describe anterior knee or PF pain. Performing a LR as a panacea to treating all conditions presenting with anterior knee pain is to be condemned. Rigorous attempts at rehabilitation are usually successful. In the event that surgical intervention is required, malalignment (i.e., tilt, instability) and arthrosis must be completely evaluated and addressed by the chosen procedure.

ANTERIOR CRUCIATE LIGAMENT INJURIES

Ligamentous injuries to the knee account for 25 to 40% of all knee injuries. The incidence of ACL tears varies widely depending on the population studied. While sprains of the medial collateral ligament (MCL) are more common, the ACL is the most frequently disrupted ligament of the knee and is injured 9 times more frequently than the posterior cruciate ligament (PCL). In more than 70% of patients who present with an acute traumatic hemarthrosis of the knee, the ACL is at least partially torn. Annually in the United States, more than 250,000 patients are diagnosed as having torn their ACLs. The highest rate of injury appears to be in those age 10 to 19 years old who engage in high risk sports such as football, baseball, soccer, skiing and basketball. It is estimated that more than 25% to 30% of all ski-related knee injuries involve the ACL. In college football, 42 per 1000 players are at risk per year. There is a 16% chance of injuring the ACL over a typical 4-year college career, which is 100 times the risk of the general population. Associated injuries are common, with the classic triad described by O'Donoghue (1955, ACL-MCL-medial meniscus) being less common than a ACL-MCL-lateral meniscus triad.

Basic Science

Biomechanics

Kinematics

The ACL is the primary restraint (86%) to anteroposterior (AP) translation. It also provides restraint to internal rotation (IR), external rotation (ER), and hyperextension. Secondary stabilizers to AP translation include the MCL and medial meniscus. The ACL and PCL regulate the "screw-home" mechanism of the knee during the final 20 degrees of extension, with the tibia externally rotating on the femur 15 degrees at terminal extension. The ACL and PCL cross at the instant center of rotation, which moves posteriorly during flexion. A combination of rolling and gliding occurs at the articular surface during knee flexion. Ligament stress is greatest at 0 to 45 degrees, and translation is greatest at 20 to 30 degrees.

Strength and Load

The ACL normally encounters 400 to 500 N of force during walking. Cutting and changes in acceleration can increase this to 1700 N. The ultimate tensile strength (maximum stress before failure) ranges between 1730 N (Noyes, 1984) and 2500 N (Woo, 1990). The ACL is about half as stiff and strong as the MCL.

Anatomy

Embryology

The cruciate ligaments are first recognized at 7 to 8 weeks gestation as a condensation of vascular synovial mesenchyme.

Histology

The ACL is an intracapsular but extrasynovial structure. The ACL is primarily composed of type I (90%) and III (10%) collagen with variable amounts of elastin and reticulin. As in all ligaments, the ultrastructure is composed of fibrils which form fibers, which form subfascicular units, which are arranged into fascicles, and, finally, the ligament.

Functional anatomy

Fascicles of the ACL are divided into three functional groups:

1. anteromedial band (AMB): tight in flexion
2. posterolateral band (PLB): tight in extension
3. central band: functional over entire range of motion. In reality, tension develops along a continuum of fibers during ROM.

Surgical Anatomy

Origin

The ACL originates at the posteromedial lateral femoral condyle as a crescent averaging 23 mm in length (Fig. 35–11).

Insertion

The ACL inserts anterior to the medial tibial eminence 15 mm posterior to the anterior horn of medial meniscus as an oval

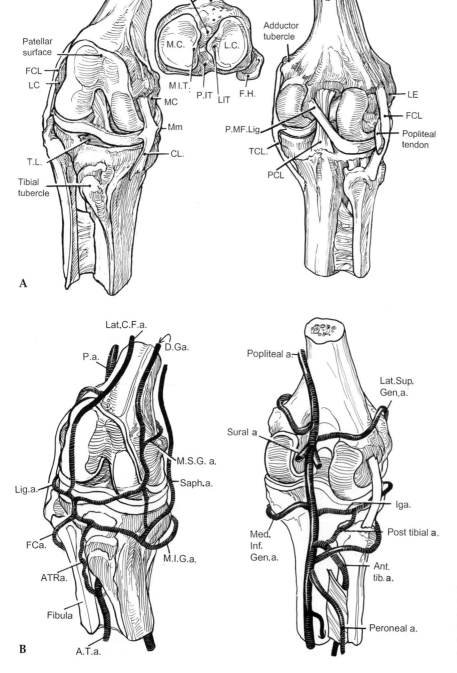

Figure 35–11 **(A)** Anterior view in flexion and posterior view in extension of the bones, ligaments, and menisci of the knee. **(B)** Vascular anatomy about the knee.

averaging 38 mm in length. The average ACL flexion length is 31 ± 3 mm, and average width is 11 mm.

Vascular supply

The ACL vascular supply is primarily from the middle geniculate via the periligamentous synovial sheath, and the medial and lateral inferior geniculate arteries via the fat pad.

Innervation

Primarily innervation is from the tibial nerve via the periligamentous vessels. Mechanoreceptors (proprioceptive) include the Ruffini end-organs, Pacinian corpuscles and free nerve endings. Reflex hamstring (HS) contraction pulling the tibia posteriorly may occur to protect the ACL during excessive load during anterior tibial translation.

Examination
History

Mechanism

This is most commonly a combination of forces at low velocity without contact during deceleration. Mechanisms include:

1. valgus/ER
2. hyperextension $\pm$ IR
3. direct valgus load
4. hyperflexion (rare)

A pure valgus stress may only cause an isolated MCL tear. Combined ACL-MCL injuries are commonly produced by valgus/ER tearing the posterior oblique ligament (POL), ACL, and MCL, in that order.

Symptoms

Acutely, 30 to 90% of patients experience a "pop" or "snap." Other symptoms include hemarthrosis (up to 75%), inability to bear weight or return to play, instability as if the knee "comes apart," and locking due to the ACL stump or a torn meniscus (35–75% in acute and 75–98% in chronic). Not all meniscal tears, however, require treatment. Chronically, patients may complain of instability ("two fist sign"), giving way with cutting or pivoting, and intermittent swelling or pain due to meniscal pathology and/or arthrosis.

PITFALL

Buckling or giving way is not pathognomonic for anterior cruciate ligament (ACL) deficiency. It occurs with patellofemoral (PF) instability, meniscal pathology, or painful inhibition of the quadriceps.

Physical Examination

The examination is optimally performed after the original injury, before pain and swelling develop. This is less important in the chronically ACL-deficient knee. Evaluation of the meniscus, collateral ligaments, cartilage surface, and posterolateral corner should also be undertaken, as these areas are commonly involved at the time of injury.

Inspection

Observe for effusion (may be delayed 12–24 hours), ecchymoses, antalgic gait, atrophy, and limited ROM. Combined ACL-MCL injuries may demonstrate a medial-based soft tissue swelling. Patients often demonstrate a "quadriceps avoidance" gait to reduce the risk of anterior tibial translation.

Palpation

Tenderness may exist with associated injuries (i.e., collaterals, meniscus, osteochondral injury).

Motion

Motion may be decreased due to HS spasm, meniscal pathology, effusion, ACL stump impingement, and pain.

Special Tests
Lachman Test

Acutely, this is the most sensitive test for ACL deficiency (Fig. 35–12). It is performed in 20 to 30 degrees of flexion with an anterior force applied to the proximal tibia. Assess the endpoint (i.e., soft or firm) and the amount of displacement with

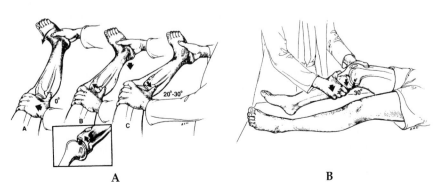

A   **B**

Figure 35–12   Common tests used for the diagnosis of an anterior cruciate ligament (ACL) tear. **(A)** The pivot shift test. Begin with the knee in full extension and internal tibial rotation with a valgus stress applied at the knee. The anteriorly subluxated tibia will reduce as the knee is flexed 20 to 30 degrees and the iliotibial band drops behind the knee's center of rotation. **(B)** The Lachman test. An anterior force is applied to the proximal tibia with the knee in 30 degrees of flexion. Reproduced with permission from Tria AJ, Klein KS. *An Illustrated Guide to the Knee.* New York, NY: Churchill Livingstone; 1992:50, 52.

side-to-side comparison (i.e., > 3 mm is considered patho-logic). The test is graded: grade I (1–4 mm), grade II (5–10 mm), and grade III (> 10 mm). Letters further define the grade: A = solid endpoint, B = soft endpoint.

Anterior Drawer Test

A less reliable test compared to the Lachman test due to the effects of hamstring spasm, meniscal buttressing, effusion, and kinematic condylar restriction. The test is performed and graded as the Lachman test, with knee in 90 degrees of flexion.

Pivot Shift Test

This test is pathognomonic of ACL deficiency, especially when performed under anesthesia. It represents subluxation-reduction of the anterior tibia when the knee is brought from 0 to 20 to 30 degrees of flexion with the foot in slight IR, with slight valgus and axial load placed upon the knee. The posterior pull of the ITB is thought to assist in the reduction of the anteriorly subluxated tibia as it passes behind the knee's center of rotation with flexion. The test is graded: 0 (absent), 1+ (glide), 2+ (jump), and 3+ (transient locking). Sensitivity is improved with hip abduction and ER of the tibia. False negatives occur with displaced menisci or MCL deficiency.

Collateral Ligament Evaluation

Medial collateral ligament/lateral collateral ligament inser-tional tenderness may exist, accurately pointing to the site of injury. During collateral ligament evaluation (Fig. 35–13) the lateral collateral ligament (LCL) can be felt as a distinct band with the leg in a figure-four position. Additionally, stress test-ing can be performed and graded as in the Lachman test.

Abduction Stress Test

The abduction stress test is performed at full extension and 30 degrees of flexion. A gradual abduction stress is applied to the leg of the supine patient while the lateral knee is sup-ported with one of the examiner's hands. The ankle is grasped with the other hand while applying a gentle valgus

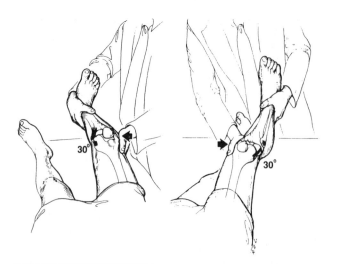

Figure 35–13   Valgus (**B**) and varus (**B**) stress testing in 30 degrees of flexion to test the medial collateral ligament and lateral collateral ligament, respectively. Reproduced with per-mission from Tria AJ, Klein KS. *An Illustrated Guide to the Knee.* New York, NY: Churchill Livingstone; 1992: 49, 50.

stress. The thigh can simply rest on the table surface, or the examiner can support the thigh to better palpate the joint line.

Adduction Stress Test

This test is similar to the abduction stress test, except the examiner places the hand on the medial knee to resist a varus stress applied at the ankle.

Interpretation

Isolated tears of the MCL or LCL are associated with valgus or varus laxity at 30 degrees. An opening at both 30 degrees and 0 degrees implies additional injury. Significant valgus laxity at 0 degrees implies injury to the posteromedial cap-sule (including the POL) and possibly injury to the PCL and or ACL. Mild (< 5 degrees) varus laxity at 0 degrees and 30 degrees can represent isolated LCL injury; but with grade 2+ to 3+ opening, posterolateral capsule and/or concomitant PCL injury may exist.

External Rotation Test

The anterior drawer test can be performed with the foot in 30 degrees IR to tighten lateral structures and 15 degrees ER to tighten medial structures. Anterior subluxation of the medial tibia in the ER position may indicate MCL and possi-bly ACL injury.

Instrumented Laxity Testing

Various devices such as the KT-1000/2000 (MED-metric; San Diego, CA) objectively measure pre- and postoperative side-to-side differences in knee laxity while simulating a Lachman test. Maximal manual translation greater than 10 mm, maxi-mal manual side-to-side difference greater than 3 mm, or a compliance index greater than 2 mm is highly suggestive of ACL deficiency.

Aids to Diagnosis
Radiographic Evaluation

Complete radiographic evaluation is discussed above in Anterior Knee Pain and Patellofemoral Disorders. Specific findings related to the ACL are emphasized in this section. In general, an AP, lateral, axial and 45 degree PA flexion weight-bearing radiograph should be obtained.

Standard Anteroposterior View

Use an extension weight-bearing view. Evaluate for soft tis-sue abnormalities, joint space narrowing, and overall align-ment. Segond fracture (lateral tibial capsular avulsion in up to 7% of ACL injuries) may occur secondary to IR with AP translation (Fig. 35–14). Exclude tibial eminence fractures in adolescents. Chronic ACL deficient knees may demonstrate peaked tibial eminences, degenerative joint disease (DJD), narrowing of the intercondylar notch with osteophytes, and Fairbank's changes due to meniscal deficiency (squaring of the condyle, ridging, and joint space narrowing with DJD). Chronic MCL injury may appear as a calcification near the femoral origin of the MCL (Pellegrini-Stieda lesion). Lateral collateral ligament avulsion fractures may also be seen off of the fibula.

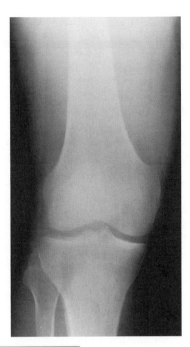

Figure 35–14 Anteroposterior radiograph demonstrating a Segond fracture or lateral tibial capsular avulsion.

Valgus and Varus Stress Anteroposterior View
Suspicion of concomitant collateral ligament injury will demonstrate widening of the respective joint space on these views performed with the knee in 15 to 20 degrees flexion.

Lateral View
Deepening of the sulcus terminalis of the lateral femoral condyle may be seen.

Magnetic Resonance Imaging
Excellent accuracy (78–97%), sensitivity, and specificity (90–95%) can be obtained with MRI. Bone bruises seen on MRI of acute ACL injuries due to bony impaction occur most commonly in the posterolateral tibial plateau and anterior lateral femoral condyle. An MRI is useful to assess for associated pathology (e.g., collaterals, menisci, cartilage) (Figs. 35–15 and 35–16).

Bone Scan (Technetium Scintigraphy)

Bone scans are not routinely used in the acute setting. Chronically, increased osseous metabolic activity in the medial, lateral, and PF compartments (in that order) that may decrease after ACL reconstruction can be seen.

Specific Conditions, Treatment, and Outcome

The decision regarding treatment depends on a thorough understanding of the clinical and functional attributes of a torn ACL. Several studies report unacceptable functional performance in sports and activities that require deceleration and directional change on an ACL deficient knee. The absolute indications for ACL reconstruction are not clearly determined based on the literature. There is abundant evidence suggesting that ACL deficiency places the knee at high

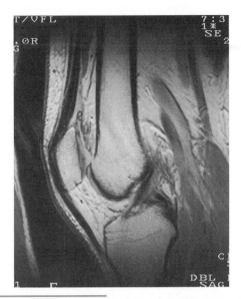

Figure 35–15 Magnetic resonance imaging scan demonstrating a normal ACL.

risk of damaging otherwise normal structures, such as the meniscus and articular cartilage, with recurrent episodes of instability over time. Ultimately, chronic ACL deficiency may lead to a higher incidence of irreparable meniscal tears and late degenerative changes in the knee. The patient's age, activity level, degree of instability, associated injuries, and ability to comply with a therapeutic program are important components of any algorithm predicating a treatment plan for the ACL deficient knee (Fig. 35–17).

Nonoperative Treatment

Reports on the true natural history of nonoperatively treated ACL injuries are flawed by several factors including, but not limited to, undocumented or missed ACL injuries, biased patient selection for nonsurgical treatment, mixing of acute

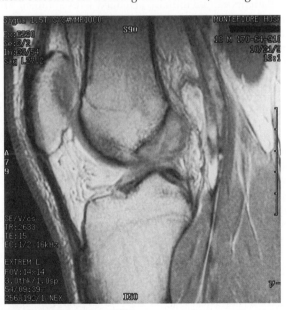

Figure 35–16 Magnetic resonance imaging scan demonstrating a complete tear of the ACL.

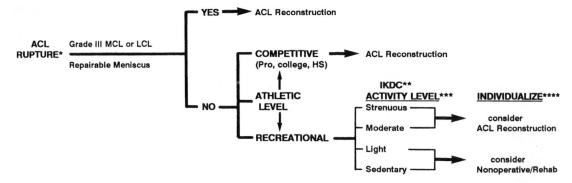

Figure 35–17 Algorithm for patient selection for ACL reconstruction based on associated collateral ligament and meniscal injury and anticipated future physical demands on the knee. *Midsubstance. **IKDC, International Knee Documentation Committee. ***Activity levels: strenuous (jumping or pivoting as in football and basketball), moderate (heavy manual work as in skiing), light (light manual work as in running), sedentary (activities of daily living). ****Individualize: Consider age, arthritis, occupation, activity modification and co-existing medial conditions. Reproduced with permission from Fu FH, Harner CD, Vince KG. *Knee Surgery*. Philadelphia, PA: Williams and Wilkins; 1994:652.

and chronic injuries, patients who are lost to followup, associated injuries, not accounting for age and activity level, and the variability in nonsurgical treatment and reporting of results. "Noyes' Rule of 3s" commonly quoted as "one third of the patients will compensate, one third will compensate with symptoms, and one third will do poorly" is often an inaccurate estimation of the results of nonoperative treatment (Noyes et al 1983). The majority of patients report worsening of their symptoms as subsequent giving-way episodes ensue. As indicated by the algorithm in Fig. 35–17, consideration of associated injury and activity level are perhaps the most important treatment determinants. In the presence of a pivot shift, despite only partial tearing of the ACL, the knee should be considered functionally as ACL deficient.

Acutely, emphasis on control of edema, analgesia, motion, quad control, and early weight-bearing as tolerated are critical. Patients can be initially managed with a hinged knee brace, crutches, cryotherapy, compression, elevation, and progressive ROM and isometric strengthening. Aseptic aspiration of a hemarthrosis may be diagnostic (e.g., blood and fat may indicate osteochondral injury) and therapeutic, allowing a more accurate physical examination.

Initially, nonoperative treatment is recommended for all patients including operative candidates prior to surgical reconstruction to reduce the incidence of knee stiffness. Nonoperative treatment only is indicated in those patients with an isolated injury and a willingness to modify their lifestyle. This should include a multimodality approach emphasizing resolution of inflammation, ROM, endurance, strengthening (especially HS and gastrocnemius), functional training, bracing, and patient education towards lifestyle modification. The goal is to obtain full ROM and return the muscle function to within 90% as compared with the normal side. Open-chain exercises provide isolated exercise for the HS and quadriceps. Closed-chain strengthening, isometrics, and cycling are frequently employed to minimize patellofemoral stresses. Dynamic stability is enhanced by gaining neuromuscular control through enhanced proprioception. Brace efficacy is controversial and is most useful in enhancing proprioception and in controlling anterior translation at low loads and rates of load application.

Operative Treatment

As previously indicated, several considerations are germane to the decision to surgically intervene.

Indications

Patient Age

No upper age limit for ACL reconstruction has been defined. Older patients may have equally as high or greater activity level expectations as their younger counterparts. Adolescents with open growth plates may be better candidates for HS reconstruction than bone-patellar tendon-bone (BPTB) reconstruction, although the latter is preferred by several authors and does not necessarily cause growth disturbances.

Partial Anterior Cruciate Ligament Tears

Operative treatment is recommended in high-demand patients with a partial ACL tear greater than 50% and the presence of a pivot shift.

Meniscal Tears

Combined ACL tears and "bucket-handle" meniscal tears causing a mechanical block must be addressed acutely. Simultaneous meniscal repair and ACL reconstruction have meniscal healing rates between 80 and 94% as opposed to meniscal repair in the ACL deficient knee where healing rates vary between 50 and 87%.

Anterior Cruciate–Medial Collateral Ligament Injuries

Combined ACL-MCL repair is commonly associated with postoperative loss of motion. The general consensus is that combined ACL-MCL injuries are managed by first nonoperatively treating the MCL injury with a hinged knee brace and early ACL reconstruction after ROM and muscular control are achieved. It is not unusual to wait an additional 2 to 3 weeks to attain normal ROM compared with an isolated ACL tear. Combined chronic ACL-MCL insufficiency may require an advancement procedure if laxity persists after ACL reconstruction

Surgical Considerations

Timing

It is largely believed that allowing the edema to resolve and initiating preoperative rehabilitation to regain ROM are important factors in reducing the incidence of postoperative arthrofibrosis. Thus, the commonly quoted window of waiting 3 weeks before reconstruction is not a rigid criteria.

Primary Repair

Unlike the MCL, the ACL does not heal well. Most surgeons agree that there is no longer a place for primary repair. Repair of a bony avulsion, especially in adolescents with tibial eminence fractures, may be an exception to this rule if the ligament is viable without significant intrasubstance failure.

Extra-articular Reconstruction

Several procedures (i.e, Ellison, Losee) developed to tenodese the ITB may reduce the pivot shift, but do not reliably limit anterior translation. These procedures do not have significant benefits over intra-articular reconstruction alone.

Intra-articular Reconstruction

This procedure is now considered the "gold standard" for active patients with ACL deficiency. After the decision to preceed with operative treatment has been discussed with the patient, the type of graft must be selected. Factors to be considered include availability, morbidity, structural properties, fixation, risk of disease transmission, surgeon familiarity, and cost.

Graft Selection

Possible grafts include autograft (BPTB, HS, ITB, quadriceps tendon), allograft (BPTB, Achilles tendon), synthetics (e.g., GoreTex, Dacron), and combined (biological with ligament augmentation device).

Bone-patellar tendon-bone grafts are typically used in the acute or chronic ACL-deficient knee in a high-level competitive or recreational athlete without PF problems. Hamstring grafts are typically used in cases with a significant history of PF problems, adolescents, and, possibly, lower-demand patients. Results comparing BPTB to HS grafts in the general population appear to be similar. Allografts, although preferred by some in the acute setting, are most commonly used in revisions, older patients, combined ligament reconstruction, or where no other graft source is available. Freshfrozen allografts exposed to less than 2.5 Mrads of radiation (minimizing decline in strength) are commonly used. Of note, the risk of acquired immunodeficiency syndrome (AIDS) transmission using radiated fresh-frozen allografts has been reported to be 1:1,667,700. Iliotibial band, quadriceps tendon, and synthetic grafts are infrequently used. Advantages and disadvantages are listed in Table 35–1.

Structural Properties of Anterior Cruciate Ligament Graft

The ultimate tensile strength (UTS) of ACL grafts are: Normal ACL, 2160 N; 14 mm BPTB autograft, 164%; 10 mm BPTB, 107%; single semitendinosus (ST), 70%; single gracilis (G), 49%; and doubled ST-G, estimated as 250% of normal ACL UTS.

Stiffness: Stiffer grafts may be more vulnerable to early failure as they assume load before secondary restraints engage. The BPTB autograft is 3 times, and the ST-G autograft is approximately equal to, the normal ACL stiffness.

Graft Healing

Originally, the transplanted graft functions as a nonvascularized, free graft. Grafts undergo avascular necrosis, cellular repopulation, and revascularization during a process of "ligamentization" that is initiated between 1 and 3 months after surgery. Remodeling occurs in response to stress over the next 3 to 12 months. Graft tensile strength is weakest during the initial phase of avascular necrosis, retaining about 50% of its original tensile strength at 3 to 6 months and about 80% at 9 to 12 months. At 12 months, the graft may be only about 50% as strong as the native ACL. Complete maturation may take between 1 to 3 years and somewhat longer with BPTB allografts. Bone healing within tibial and femoral tunnels takes at least 6 to 8 weeks in normal bone, but may take up to 6 months. Stable ingrowth of ligament into bone in animal studies takes about 8 to 12 weeks after implantation.

TABLE 35–1   Graft Advantages and Disadvantages

		Advantages	Disadvantages
Autografts	BPTB	High UTS, early bone-to-bone healing, strong and flexible fixation, availability, accessible, technically forgiving	High stiffness, extensor morbidity, more anterior knee pain, difficult placement, patellar fracture, PT rupture
	HS	Less stiffness, less extensor morbidity, less anterior knee pain, high UTS with multiple strands, comparable results with BPTB	Lower UTS, less effective fixation, soft-tissue-to-bone healing, technically difficult, HS muscle weakness up to 1 year
Allografts		No donor site morbidity, technically forgiving, availability	Cost, sterility considerations, recipient biological response, bony tunnel reabsorption, disease transmission, delayed incorporation

Graft Fixation

Initially, the points of fixation are the weakest portion of the repair and must tolerate between 50 and 250 N during controlled rehabilitation. Numerous devices are available for fixation including metal and biodegradable interference screws, Endobutton (Acuflex Microsurgical; Mansfield, MA) with polyester tape, sutures around a post, screw/washer over a tendon, staple over a bone block, or tendon and sutures through a button. The most common construct, an interference screw against a bone block within a tunnel, has the following biomechanical characteristics: minimal contact length of 12.5 mm, minimal divergence of 15 degrees, 7×20-mm screw with a gap of 1 to 2 mm or 9×20-mm screw with a gap of 3 to 4 mm, and an insertion torque of 8 to 12 pounds. Other fixation devices with their respective estimated failure loads are listed in Table 35–2.

Graft Placement

Isometry is a condition in which there exists little to no change in the distance between the ligament graft-attachment sites through ROM. Graft diameter and attachment site size preclude "ideal isometry" as do changes in loads and flexion angles. The best one can achieve is anatomic placement of the graft to minimize graft length change during ROM ($\leqq 2$ mm or $\leqq 10\%$ change over 30 mm)(Table 35–3).

TABLE 35–2   Fixation device and estimated failure loads

Fixation Device	Estimated Failure Load
9-mm interference screw	400–500 N
No. 2 suture/No. 5 suture	64 N/150–450 N
Endobutton (Acuflex Microsurgical; Mansfield, MA)	250–500 N
Screw/washer on HS	160–200 N
Double-loop HS around screw/washer	821 N
Staples	100–240 N

TABLE 35–3   Errors in graft placement with resulting graft tension

		Too Posterior	Too Anterior
Femur Position	Extension	Tight	Loose
	Flexion	Loose	Tight
Tibial Position	Extension	Tight	Loose
	Flexion	Loose	Tight with impingement

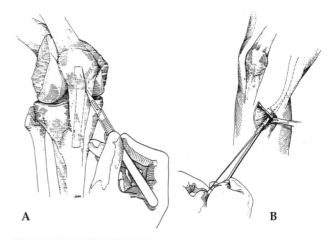

Figure 35–18   Graft harvesting. **(A)** Bone-patellar tendon-bone harvesting with the knee at 90 degrees of flexion. **(B)** Hamstring harvesting. The tendon stripper is advanced parallel to the semitendinosus using a back and forth or rotary type motion. Reproduced with permission from Fu FH, Harner CD, Vince KG. *Knee Surgery.* Philadelphia, PA: Williams and Wilkins; 1994:670, 671.

Surgical Technique
Graft Harvesting

Central third BPTB: A tourniquet may be used, but infiltration with 1:300,000 epinephrine solution may be satisfactory and limits ischemic morbidity including subclinical neuropraxia and muscle contractile dysfunction (Fig. 35–18). A 7 to 9-cm longitudinal skin incision is made 1 cm medial to the midline of the patellar tendon (PT). Alternatively, single or mini-double transverse incisions are preferred by some because of improved cosmesis. Subcutaneous flaps are developed, and the paratenon is reflected to expose the medial and lateral borders of the PT. Proximal extension is achieved with knee extended. While the knee is flexed, mark the distal pole of the patella and the center of the PT insertion onto the tibial tubercle with a sterile marking pen. A central 9 to 11-mm section of the PT is incised using a sawing-type motion with a No. 10 blade. Care is taken to stay parallel to the fibers of the PT as they deviate laterally toward the tibial tubercle.

The tibial tubercle and the patellar bone blocks are also outlined using a No. 10 blade. Although techniques may vary, a 5 to 6-mm in depth and 20 to 25-mm in length trapezoidal, bone plug (avoiding the joint surface) is harvested from the patella using an oscillating saw and 1/4 inch osteotome. Similarly, a bone plug in the shape of an equilateral triangle (maximizing bone beneath the remaining PT) is harvested from the tibial tubercle. Carefully dissect the fat pad from the patellar tendon with Metzenbaum scissors from distal to proximal. Contour the bone blocks into a cylinder and place 1 to 3 No. 5 nonresorbable sutures through each block after predrilling with a .062-inch K-wire. Oblique or parallel passage of the sutures minimizes the likelihood of suture laceration with an interference screw. Alternatively, an Endobutton may be used for fixation over the anterolateral femur.

Hamstrings: A figure-of-four position may be helpful to initially identify and harvest the HS tendons from the pes anserinus (Fig. 35–18b). Through a 5-cm longitudinal incision located 4 cm medial and 3 cm distal to the tibial tubercle, layer 1 (the sartorius fascia) is identified. The G (more proximal) and ST tendons are palpated as two small bumps beneath layer 1, which is then incised parallel to these tendons. Care is taken not to violate layer 2, the superficial MCL. The G and ST tendons are found and retrieved from the undersurface of layer 1 using a right-angle clamp and Penrose drain. The infrapatellar branches of the saphenous nerve crossing the gracilis must be protected.

A tendon stripper can be used with tendon insertions left intact (slotted tendon stripper) or detached (closed tendon stripper). Mobilization requires release of fascial bands between the G and ST tendons. Connections between the ST and medial head of the gastrocnemius must be released 7 cm proximal to the insertion of the ST tendon. Additionally, a sling of tissue from the semimembranosus to the ST tendon may need to be released. At the time of distal release of the tendons, a running, baseball whip stitch with No. 2 or No. 5 nonabsorbable suture is placed in the free end of each tendon. The tendon stripper is advanced parallel to the tendon using a slow and steady, back and forth motion up into the thigh until the tendon is freed from its muscle-tendon junction. Each tendon is prepared by first stripping residual muscle from the tendon substance and doubling them to create a quadruple stand graft of 26 to 32 cm in length and 8 to 9 cm in diameter. The free ends are prepared as before using nonabsorbable suture. Depending on the femoral fixation system used a large polyester tape or No. 3 to No. 5 nonabsorbable sutures are used within the looped ends of the G and ST tendons.

Graft Placement

Anterior cruciate ligament reconstruction can be performed with a one-incision (endoscopic) or two-incision (arthroscopically assisted or mini-arthrotomy) technique. The femoral tunnel is prepared either inside-out (one-incision) or outside-in (two-incision). Examination under anesthesia with side-to-side comparison and diagnostic arthroscopy through anteromedial and anterolateral portals is performed in either technique to address associated pathology.

One-incision endoscopic technique: The contralateral limb is placed in a well-leg holder and the operative limb in a leg holder placed over a thigh-high tourniquet. The foot of the bed is lowered for circumferential access to the operative leg. After the graft is harvested, the intercondylar notch and ACL stump are debrided using a full-radius resector and basket rongeur. The goal is to expose the intercondylar wall of the lateral femoral condyle and the insertion site on the tibial eminence. Care must be taken not to injure the PCL or the intermeniscal ligament. A notchplasty (widening of the intercondylar notch) is performed from anterior to posterior. Only enough bone to aid in visualization and protect the graft from abrasion is removed. The "over-the-top" position must be identified and not confused with "resident's ridge," a prominence along the medial wall of the lateral femoral condyle located only two thirds of the way back posteriorly often mistaken as the most posterior aspect of the lateral femoral condyle.

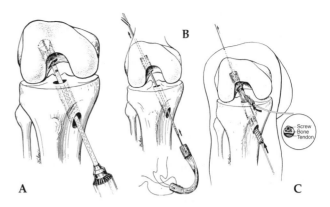

Figure 35–19 **(A)** Femoral tunnel preparation through the tibial tunnel. **(B)** Graft passage. **(C)** Graft fixation with interference screw. Reproduced with permission from Miller MD, Fu FH. Arthroscopic allograft anterior cruciate ligament reconstruction. *Op Tech Sports Med.* 1995;1:116.

With the arthroscope in the inferolateral portal, the tibial tunnel is started at a point midway between the tibial tubercle and the posteromedial edge of the tibia (Fig. 35–19). An ACL drill guide is set at 50 to 55 degrees for the BPTB graft and 45 to 50 degrees for the HS graft. The guide is placed through the inferomedial portal to place a guide pin into the center of the ACL tibial attachment site, erring slightly posteriorly (staying just anterior to Humphry's ligament). An appropriately sized cannulated reamer is used to overdrill the guide pin.

The femoral tunnel site is chosen such that the center of the hole will be located approximately at the 11-o'clock position in a right knee and at the 1-o'clock position in a left knee. Using a guide pin and appropriately sized cannulated reamer, the femoral tunnel is drilled through the tibial tunnel with the knee flexed 90 degrees, leaving a 1- to 2-mm posterior cortical rim. The intra-articular edges of both tunnels are debrided of remaining soft tissue and bone to minimize the potential to develop a soft tissue "cyclops" lesion and to prevent graft abrasion. Using the sutures attached to the graft end, the graft is passed retrograde through the tibial tunnel into the femoral tunnel and fixed within the femoral tunnel. The knee is flexed and extended several times while placing tension on the graft before the graft is fixed to the tibia with the knee in nearly full extension.

Two-incision arthroscopically assisted technique: The tibia tunnel is prepared as in the one-incision technique. The femoral tunnel is prepared using a 4-cm incision made in the midline of the lateral supracondylar area of the femur at the level of the proximal pole of the patella. The ITSB is split in line with its fibers, and the vastus lateralis elevated and retracted anteriorly. The lateral superior geniculate vessels are identified and electrocauterized. The femoral tunnel is prepared from outside-in using a drill guide placed intraarticularly and through the incision at the supracondylar region, meeting a point at a similar notch location as in the one-incision technique. The BPTB graft is passed and fixed in the lateral cortex from outside-in using an interference screw. The HS is fixed with a staple or screw and washer technique. The graft is fixed at the tibia as in the one-incision technique.

PEARL

In the event that the graft is too short to secure to the tibia, the sutures can be transfixed around a screw and washer. If a bone-patellar tendon-bone (BPTB) graft is too long, a bone staple can be used, impacting the graft into a trough prepared to seat the bone plug.

Rehabilitation

Following ACL reconstruction, rehabilitation must respect initial graft strength, fixation, and biological healing. Postoperative rehabilitation emphasizes control of inflammation, progressive weight-bearing, restoration of motion including full extension, quadriceps exercises, and restoration of normal gait. Cold and compression are used in the first week to control inflammation and pain. Full weight-bearing is achieved as tolerated and assistive devices are eliminated when the patient demonstrates a normal gait. Full extension symmetric to the noninvolved side is achieved within 2 to 3 weeks, and full flexion within 8 weeks after surgery. Bracing in extension for the first week, unlocking it only for exercises, is preferred by some to minimize notch scarring. Patellar mobilization is gently performed.

Some surgeons advocate avoiding quadriceps loading from 45 degree flexion to full extension for 2 to 3 months because of concerns of placing excessive stress on the graft. Closed-chain minisquats (muscle co-contraction) exercises are utilized to minimize anterior tibial translation in this functional range. Open-chain quad sets can be performed in full extension minimizing ACL stress.

Proprioceptive activities are initiated to regain neuromuscular control. Accelerated rehabilitation can return an athlete to full sports participation in 4 to 6 months, in some instances. More commonly, it takes 6 to 9 months to return to sports. A functional brace may be recommended for the first 1 to 2 years after surgery.

Results

The goals of surgical reconstruction of the ACL-deficient knee are to first restore ligamentous stability and delay or prevent articular and meniscal damage. Ideally, a painless knee with full motion and normal strength and coordination is desirable. The lack of a uniform grading system for reporting the results of ACL reconstruction makes comparisons between studies difficult.

Reports of BPTB and HS autografts or allografts show good and excellent results in greater than 90% of patients at intermediate-term followup. Synthetic ligaments have had unacceptable rates of failure in most medium or long-term reports. Prospective, randomized long-term followup is still lacking, and controversy remains regarding the effects of ACL reconstruction on the future degeneration of articular surfaces.

Complications

The most common complication following ACL reconstruction is loss of motion, especially extension, due to quadriceps weakness and PF problems. A flexion contracture greater than 10 degrees or flexion less than 130 degrees may lead to a functional deficit. Stiffness may occur as a result of operating while the patient is still recovering from the inflammation of the initial injury. Patients with loss of motion should be evaluated for notch scarring or capsulitis. Treatment may include arthroscopic debridement and prolonged rehabilitation. Other causes of poor motion include prolonged immobilization, a "cyclops" lesion (residual tissue anterior to an ACL graft) blocking full extension, aberrant tunnel placement, inadequate notchplasty, improper graft tensioning, infrapatellar contracture syndrome, and generalized arthrofibrosis.

Anterior knee pain, often attributed to harvesting of the BPBT autograft, is not necessarily less frequent following HS reconstruction, especially when accelerated rehabilitation programs are used. The reported incidence ranges from 5 to 50%. Preoperative PF crepitus may be a risk factor for postoperative anterior knee pain.

Other less common complications include patella fracture, patellar tendonitis, graft rupture from impingement, failure of fixation, accelerated degenerative arthritis, ankylosis, fat pad fibrosis, recurrent effusion, deep vein thrombosis, heterotopic ossification, septic knee, and skin problems.

Future Directions

In the near future, improvements in current techniques, including graft fixation, the development of a three-dimensional arthroscopic visualization system, and robotic surgical procedures may enhance the outcome of ACL reconstruction. In the distant future, resorbable stents and growth factors may induce ACL healing. Full restoration of an ACL-deficient knee may be achieved through genetic manipulation, including tissue regeneration.

POSTERIOR CRUCIATE LIGAMENT INJURIES

Although more common than once believed, injuries to the PCL account for between 3 and 20% of all knee ligament injuries. It is estimated that 40% of all PCL injuries are isolated tears. The true incidence is probably much greater than this because many isolated tears remain undetected. Most injuries occur in young males involved in motor vehicle-related accidents ("dashboard injury") and contact sports.

Basic Science
Biomechanics

Kinematics

The PCL is the primary restraint (95%) to posterior tibial translation at 90 degrees of flexion. The PCL and ACL regulate the screw-home mechanism of external tibial rotation in terminal extension. The PCL also acts as a secondary restraint to ER of the tibia in combined posterolateral complex (PLC) injuries and to varus/valgus stability. The meniscofemoral ligaments provide a secondary restraint to posterior tibial translation by tightening with IR and flexion of the tibia. Other secondary restraints to posterior translation include the posterior medial and lateral capsules, the PLC, the MCL and LCL, and central portion of the medial capsule. A significant increase in medial compartment and PF contact pressures occurs after sectioning of the PCL. This has important implications for the development of arthritis in chronic PCL deficiency as well as for rehabilitation of the PCL-injured knee.

Strength and Load

The PCL is not twice as strong as the ACL, as commonly quoted. The anterolateral band (ALB) is about as strong as the entire ACL. The ALB is about twice as strong (about 1200 N versus 450 N) and stiff as the posteomedial band (PMB) and meniscofemoral ligaments.

PEARL

Restoration of the anterolateral band (ALB) and accurate placement of the femoral origin are anatomically and biomechanically the most important consideration in reestablishing normal kinematics in the PCL-deficient knee.

Anatomy
Embryology

The cruciate ligaments are first recognized at 7 to 8 weeks gestation as a condensation of vascular synovial mesenchyme. At about 22 weeks gestation, the PCL resembles an adult ligament.

Histology

Like the ACL, the PCL is considered an intracapsular but extrasynovial structure. The histology is as described in Anterior Cruciate Ligament Injuries.

Functional Anatomy

Fascicles of the PCL are divided into two functional (not microscopic) groups

1. anterolateral band: larger, tightens in flexion
1. posteromedial band: smaller, tightens in extension

Additionally, there are two variably present (70 to 100%) meniscofemoral ligaments: the anterior (ligament of Humphrey) and posterior (ligament of Wrisberg) (Fig. 35–11).

Surgical Anatomy

The PCL is located near the central axis of the knee, being more vertical in extension and horizontal in flexion. The cross-sectional area of the PCL decreases from proximal to distal, averaging 11 mm in width at its midsection.

Origin

The origin of the PCL is in an anteromedial direction off of the anterolateral medial femoral condyle as a semicircle averaging 32 mm in width.

Insertion

The PCL inserts in a lateromedial direction onto the intra-articular upper surface at the tibial fovea (approximately 1 cm below the tibial surface) as a rectangle averaging 13 mm in width (Fig. 35–11).

The meniscofemoral ligaments take origin from the posterior horn of the lateral meniscus and "sandwich" the PCL as they insert onto the anterior and posterior aspects of the posterior PCL near its femoral insertion.

Vascular supply

As in the ACL, the vascular supply of the PCL is primarily from the middle geniculate artery.

Innervation

Innervation is primarily from the posterior articular branches of the tibial nerve. Similar mechanoreceptors as in the ACL have been identified, concentrated at the femoral origin for proprioceptive function.

Examination

The diagnosis is often missed at initial examination unless gross instability is present. Attention to the history and physical examination is paramount to determine the nature and extent of the often complex injury patterns associated with PCL tears.

History

Mechanism
Isolated PCL tears are most commonly caused by:

1. direct trauma to the proximal tibia with the foot plantar flexed ("dashboard injury")
2. downward-directed force to the thigh with the knee in hyperflexion (landing from a jump)

Severe hyperextension injuries are often associated with PCL and posterior capsule injury after the ACL is torn. Posterior cruciate-PLC injuries occur with ER, and a posteromedial varus-directed force causing varus and ER knee instability. Isolated varus or valgus stress can injure the PCL after the respective collateral ligament tears.

Symptoms
Acutely, patients with an isolated sport-related PCL tear may consider it as a minor event and return to play. A mild to moderate effusion or hemarthrosis may develop, but this is less common and severe as after ACL tears. Complaints of instability occur during rapid directional change, as well as with less demanding activities in patients with combined injuries. Pain tends to worsen over time, commonly localizing to the PF area or medial compartment. In chronic PCL-deficiency, up to 70% of patients complain of pain associated with ambulation and 50% with descending stairs.

Physical Examination

Inspection

Observe for mild effusion, anterior tibial contusion, or popliteal ecchymoses. The presence of a varus-thrust gait with or without hyperextension should call attention to the PLC.

Palpation

Tenderness may exist in areas of direct trauma.

Motion

Forceful passive ROM beyond 90 degrees may produce pain.

Special Tests (Figure 3–1)

Posterior Drawer Test

The most sensitive test for PCL insufficiency (Fig. 35–20). The test should be performed with the hip and knee flexed to 45 and 90 degrees, respectively, and the foot in neutral or ER to reduce the secondary restraining effects of the menisco-femoral ligaments and PLC. Grading is identical to the Lachman test described above in Anterior Cruciate Ligament Injuries. Grade II (+ 5 to 10 mm) instability exists when the tibial condyle is flush with the femoral condyle, and it often represents an isolated injury amenable to nonoperative treatment. Grade III instability exists when the tibia is displaced more than 10 mm posteriorly and often represents a combined injury requiring operative treatment. The endpoint (i.e., A = solid and B = soft) may return to normal in the chronically PCL-deficient knee.

PEARL

The medial tibial plateau should be at least 10 mm anterior to the medial femoral condyle when the knee is flexed to 90 degrees in a normal knee. The injured knee should always be compared with the normal knee.

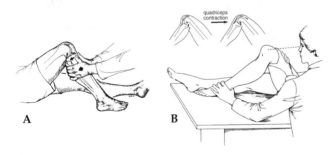

Figure 35–20 Special tests for posterior cruciate ligament (PCL) tears. **(A)** The posterior drawer test is the most sensitive test used to diagnose a PCL tear. Reproduced with permission from Tria AJ, Klein KS. *An Illustrated Guide to the Knee.* New York, NY: Churchill Livingstone; 1992: **(B)** The quadriceps active test. As viewed from the side, as the quadriceps contracts, the posterior sag is reduced. Reproduced with permission from Andrews JR, Edwards JC, Satterwhite YE. Isolated posterior cruciate ligament injuries. *Clin Sports Med.* 1994; 13:525, 53.

Posterior Sag Sign

The hips and knees are flexed to 90 degrees while the examiner grasps and lifts the heels of the supine patient. The position of the tibia is compared as viewed from the side. Gravity causes the PCL-deficient knee to rest in the posteriorly subluxated position. This test is more sensitive in chronic injuries.

Quadriceps Active Test

The affected hip and knee are flexed to 90 degrees, and the foot is stabilized in neutral on the table (Fig. 35–20b). Voluntary quadriceps contraction reduces the posteriorly subluxated tibia anteriorly. An active posterior drawer test is performed with voluntary HS contraction from this position.

Lachman Test

A Lachman test will show anterior translation to the level of the normal side with a firm endpoint, and examiners often confuse this finding with ACL-deficiency.

Reverse Pivot Shift Test

Beginning at 90 degrees, the knee is held in ER and passively extended, whereby a shift occurs at 20 to 30 degrees of flexion as the posteriorly subluxated lateral tibial plateau reduces anteriorly. This test has low specificity and can be falsely positive in the normal knee under anesthesia or with generalized ligament laxity. False negatives can occur with biceps femoris spasm.

Collateral Evaluation

Varus laxity at 30 degrees of flexion indicates LCL and possibly PLC injury. Slight opening at 0 degrees may indicate this combined injury, whereas severe opening may indicate additional PCL and, possibly, ACL injury. Increased valgus opening at 30 degrees flexion indicates MCL injury.

Posterolateral Complex Evaluation

Subtle changes in rotation during examination may be found by performing the following maneuvers:

Increased posterior translation, ER, and varus angulation at 30 degrees of knee flexion that decreases at 90 degrees indicates isolated PLC injury. Should these findings increase at 90 degrees, then a combined PCL-PLC injury should be suspected.

Prone passive ER test: Forceful increases in ER beyond 10 degrees (compared with the noninjured knee) of the medial border of the foot in the prone patient at 30 and 90 degrees of knee flexion is interpreted as above.

Posterolateral drawer test: Increased ER of the lateral tibial plateau when performing the posterolateral drawer test in 15 degrees of ER is a less specific test for combined PCL-PLC injury.

ER recurvatum test: This is performed by grasping the great toes of the supine patient with the knee in extension. If the knee falls into varus, hyperextension, and ER, it may indicate isolated PLC injury. Excessive varus and hyperextension may indicate ACL and, possibly, PCL injury.

Instrumented laxity testing: The KT-1000/2000 (Med-metric; San Diego, CA) is not accurate (70% confidence) for the

PCL and has less than 33% sensitivity for a grade I PCL tear and 86% sensitivity for grades II to III tears.

PITFALL

Missing a combined PCL-PLC injury will have a deleterious effect on the outcome of the PCL reconstructed knee.

Aids to Diagnosis

Radiographic Evaluation

Complete radiographic evaluation is discussed in Anterior Knee Pain and Patellofemoral Disorders. Specific findings associated with PCL tears are emphasized in this section. An AP, lateral, axial, and 45 degree PA flexion weight-bearing radiograph should be obtained.

Standard Anteroposterior View

Obtain this study for evidence of avulsion fractures of the PCL, as these should be fixed acutely even if minimally displaced. Check for avulsion fractures of the fibular head (LCL, biceps femoris) and of Gerdy's tubercle (ITB). Chronic injuries need to be evaluated for arthrosis, especially in the PF and medial compartments.

Forty-five Degree Posterolateral View

This view is helpful in identifying subtle joint space narrowing.

Patellar Views (Axial Views)

A Merchant's view is helpful to identify PF arthrosis.

Long Cassette Lower-extremity View

Rule out varus alignment requiring valgus high-tibial osteotomy (HTO) prior to considering PCL reconstruction.

Magnetic Resonance Imaging

Magnetic resonance scanning is both sensitive and specific (100%) in the diagnosis of acute complete tears and somewhat less reliable in identifying partial PCL tears (Figs. 35–21 and 35–22). Meniscal tears (less common than with ACL tears), chondral injury, and PLC injuries are evaluated. Operative treatment of associated pathology (i.e., meniscus, cartilage) can be planned despite nonoperative PCL treatment.

Bone Scan (Technetium Scintigraphy)

Bone scans will show increased activity due to early arthritis, especially in medial and PF compartments in the chronically PCL-deficient knee.

Specific Conditions, Treatment, and Outcome

The goal of treatment in PCL injuries is to relieve symptoms and prevent the development of degenerative arthritis. Treatment options depend on the findings at physical examination, the site of the tear, the presence of associated ligamentous injuries, and the patient's activity level. Most surgeons

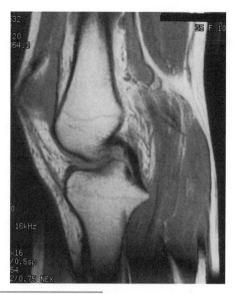

Figure 35–21 Magnetic resonance imaging scan demonstrating a normal PCL.

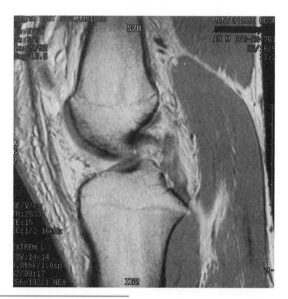

Figure 35–22 Magnetic resonance imaging scan demonstrating a complete tear of the PCL.

agree that nonoperative treatment is appropriate for acute, isolated PCL injuries. Typically, these are patients who present with less than grade III laxity without associated injuries. An algorithm for the treatment of acute PCL injuries other than those associated with avulsion fractures is presented in Fig. 35–23.

Nonoperative Treatment

The natural history of acute and chronic PCL injuries is still a matter of debate. Additionally, the long-term results of PCL reconstruction have not been adequately studied. It is generally accepted that isolated PCL injuries will do relatively well and combined injuries will do poorly when treated nonoperatively. Injuries occurring during athletics tend to do

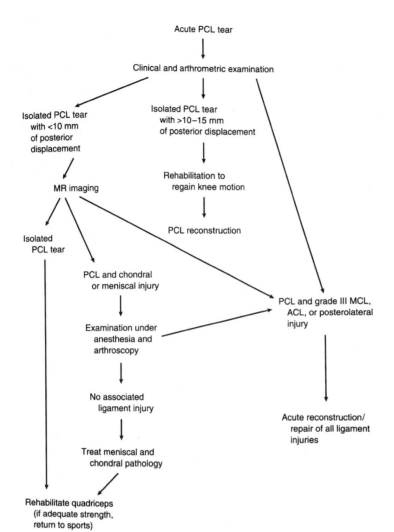

Acute PCL tear

Clinical and arthrometric examination

Isolated PCL tear
with <10 mm
of posterior
displacement

Isolated PCL tear
with >10–15 mm
of posterior displacement

Rehabilitation to
regain knee motion

MR imaging

PCL reconstruction

Isolated
PCL tear

PCL and chondral
or meniscal injury

PCL and grade III MCL,
ACL, or posterolateral
injury

Examination under
anesthesia and
arthroscopy

No associated
ligament injury

Acute reconstruction/
repair of all ligament
injuries

Treat meniscal and
chondral pathology

Rehabilitate quadriceps
(if adequate strength,
return to sports)

Figure 35–23 Treatment algorithm for suggested management of acute PCL tears. Copyright © 1993 American Academy of Orthopaedic Surgeons. Reproduced with permission from the *Journal of the American Acadamy of Orthopaedic Surgeons: A Comprehensive Review* 1993;1:72.

much better than those resulting from motor vehicle accidents or falls. Compensatory quadriceps contraction may help patients adapt to PCL-deficiency. It appears that less than 10% of patients with isolated PCL tears will progress to post-traumatic arthritis. The development of pain and degenerative arthritis is more common in patients with combined PCL injuries.

A few long-term studies suggest that the natural history of isolated PCL tears includes three phases:

1. functional adaptation (3 to 18 months)
2. functional tolerance (15 to 20 years)
3. progressive disabling arthritis after 25 years

The rate or extent of this progression depends on several factors including degree of instability, rotatory laxity, menisectomy, quadriceps muscle weakness, and PF problems.

Nonoperative treatment for isolated PCL tears with less than 10 mm of posterior displacement is not the same as nontreatment. Acutely, isolated PCL injuries should be managed with splinting in extension until motion is tolerated, progressive weight-bearing, and cold therapy with compression. Rehabilitation emphasizes closed-chain strengthening (minisquats, leg presses) until 90% of the quadriceps and HS strength on the normal side is achieved. The patient can

return to athletic activity usually within 3 to 4 weeks. Yearly followup for the development of pain or disability from instability or arthritis should be performed.

Operative Treatment

Surgical reconstruction is generally reserved for:

1. acute bony avulsions
2. symptomatic, chronic PCL-deficiency
3. acute or chronic combined ligament injuries and
4. isolated PCL tears in active young patients with less than 10 mm laxity on posterior displacement testing who complain of instability or pain

Reconstruction in patients with moderate to severe osteoarthritis is not recommended. In the chronic, PCL-deficient patient, evaluation for a varus thrust and chronic PLC deficiency must be undertaken. If the patient does not have a varus thrust, then PCL-PLC reconstruction can be performed (see below). If a patient has a varus thrust, a valgus HTO is indicated with PCL-PLC reconstruction after a 3 to 6 month recovery period. Acute combined PCL-MCL-ACL or PCL-MCL injures may need all components reconstructed in contrast to ACL-MCL injuries where usually only the ACL is reconstructed. Combined chronic PCL-MCL insufficiency may require an advancement procedure if laxity persists after PCL reconstruction.

Bony Avulsions

Radiographs document the presence and size of the avulsion fracture. Approached posteriorly, large fragments are secured with screws. Some recommend nonoperative treatment for small avulsions when the posterolateral drawer test is less than 10 mm. If operative treatment is necessary, small fragments are repaired using sutures through drill holes. Primary repair of interstitial PCL tears has been unsuccessful.

Intra-articular Reconstruction of Isolated PCL Injuries

After the decision to reconstruct the PCL has been made, graft selection must be determined. Autograft BPTB or HS and allograft BPTB or Achilles tendon are currently used in PCL reconstruction. The advantages and disadvantages are similar to those listed for ACL reconstruction (see Table 35–1). It is the authors' preference to use fresh-frozen Achilles' tendon allograft because it is technically easier to pass through bone tunnels, affix to the tibia, and has no donor site morbidity. Compared with the HS, it provides higher ultimate tensile strength and better initial fixation. The theoretical risk of human immunodeficiency virus transmission is estimated at 1:1,667,700.

If a grade III MCL, ACL, or PLC injury occurs in association with a PCL injury, reconstruction of all ligaments should be performed. When a knee dislocation has been suspected, appropriate neurovascular evaluation must be performed. Although delaying PCL reconstruction with an associated ACL tear may be appropriate to prevent postoperative arthrofibrosis, it is not recommended for associated PLC injuries as delayed repair is associated with relatively poor results (see below).

Our current arthroscopic technique recreates the ALB of the PCL using a fresh-frozen 11-mm Achilles' tendon allograft (Fig. 35–24). As in ACL reconstruction, examination under anesthesia with side-to-side comparison followed by diagnostic arthroscopy is performed to address associated pathology. The PLC should be evaluated by performing the tests described above. Arthroscopic PCL reconstruction follows six steps as outlined below.

Step 1. Preparation of the notch and ligament insertion sites: A 30 and 70 degree arthroscope through the anterolateral portal is helpful to visualize and prepare the tibial PCL insertion site. A posteromedial portal is made 1 cm above the joint line at the posteromedial edge of the medial femoral condyle. This portal is established by transilluminating the area with the arthroscope placed through the notch along the lateral portion of the medial femoral condyle. It may be helpful to elevate the posterior capsule at the PCL attachment site.

Step 2. Tibial tunnel preparation: A PCL arthroscopic drill guide is inserted through the anteromedial portal and directed through the intercondylar notch over the tibial "footprint," erring slightly lateral to the center of this site. The entrance site along the anteromedial tibia is located about 1 cm below and 2 to 3 cm medial to the tibial tubercle with the guide set at

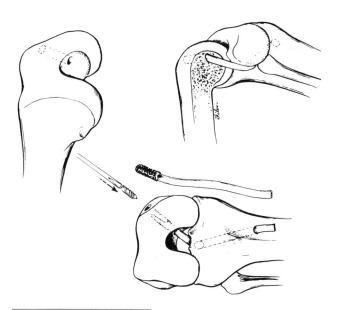

Figure 35–24 Schematic of PCL reconstruction using the Achilles tendon allograft. Reproduced with permission from Harner CD, Miller MD. Graft tensioning and fixation in posterior cruciate ligament surgery. *Op Tech Sports Med.* 1993; 1:116.

45 to 55 degrees. The appropriate-sized cannulated reamer is used over a Kirschner wire under direct visualization.

Step 3. Femoral tunnel placement: A 3-cm longitudinal, medial parapatellar incision is made midway between the medial femoral condyle and the medial patellar edge. The arthroscopic drill guide is set at 30 degrees and inserted through the anteromedial portal with the knee flexed at 90 degrees. The guide is positioned over the anterior portion of the PCL located 8 to 10 mm behind the articular cartilage edge of the medial femoral condyle.

Step 4. Preparation of Achilles tendon graft: An 11-mm wide × 25- to 30-mm long, bone plug is fashioned at the calcaneal insertion. The soft tissue end is trimmed and tubularized with No. 2 nonabsorbable sutures. Two retention sutures (No. 5 nonabsorbable) are placed through the bone plug.

Step 5. Graft passage: A looped 18-gauge wire is passed through the tibial tunnel and retrieved outside the knee through the femoral tunnel. The graft is drawn into the knee (tendon portion first) by passing the free ends of the No. 2 sutures through the looped end of the wire and drawing it back through the tibial tunnel below.

Step 6. Graft fixation: Femoral fixation is from outside-in with an interference screw (7- 9-mm × 20 mm). Tension is placed on the tibial end of the graft and the knee is cycled (flexed and extended). Tibial fixation is performed with the knee flexed 70 to 80 degrees and an anteriorly directed force placed upon the back of the tibia; fixation is performed at the anteromedial tibia using a screw and spikewasher.

Reconstruction of Combined Ligament Injuries

Posterior Cruciate Ligament and Posterolateral Complex

The PLC has been variably defined to include the following structures: LCL and the PLC (arcuate ligament, popliteal tendon, popliteofibular ligament, fabellofibular ligament and posterolateral capsule) Compared with PCL or ACL tears, isolated injuries to the PLC are uncommon and more frequently seen with combined ligament injuries (ACL or PCL). As already indicated, the disability (pain, instability) of these injuries is far greater than isolated PCL or ACL deficiency. If the PLC is not addressed at the time of PCL (or ACL) reconstruction, it may contribute to early PCL (or ACL) failure and persistent instability. Additionally, the results of late PLC reconstruction are comparatively poor.

If it is determined that there is an associated injury to the PLC, then it should be reconstructed as described above. Some recommend delaying the tibial fixation until after the PLC is reconstructed. Using a curvilinear lateral incision, the PLC is exposed and evaluated. The surgical options include primary repair, advancement or recession, and augmentation or reconstruction. In the chronic setting, it is critical to evaluate limb alignment and to assess for varus thrust during the stance phase of gait. If necessary, a valgus HTO may be performed before or in combination with reconstruction.

Posterior Cruciate Ligament and Anterior Cruciate Ligament

The combination of PCL-ACL injuries should raise the possibility of an acute knee dislocation with spontaneous reduction. Evaluation for neurovascular injury is performed, which can include side-to-side differences in pulses, arteriogram, Doppler ultrasound, or MRI vascular study. Treatment of acute, combined PCL-ACL injuries are delayed for 1 to 3 weeks to watch for vascular injuries and to regain knee motion. As in acute ACL reconstruction, there is a risk for postoperative arthrofibrosis if surgery is performed before motion is regained and significant inflammation has not resolved. We recommend PCL reconstruction first (Achilles tendon allograft or BPTB autograft) followed by ACL reconstruction (BPTB or HS autograft).

PEARL

The normal step-off of the medial tibial plateau (> 10 mm) must be recreated before the posterior cruciate ligament (PCL) graft is secured at the tibia.

Posterior Cruciate Ligament and Medial Collateral Ligament

This is the least common PCL combined injury. In the presence of grades I and II MCL injury, isolated PCL reconstruction should follow the usual protocol (Fig. 35–23). A grade III MCL tear should be addressed by primary repair, advancement, reinforcement, or reconstruction if medial instability remains after PCL reconstruction.

Rehabilitation

The goal of postoperative rehabilitation is to protect the graft from excessive forces until bone-to-bone or tendon-to-bone healing has occurred. This is more easily accomplished by performing exercises in the prone position to pull the tibia anteriorly, maintaining extension in the brace during the early phase of rehabilitation and avoiding open-chain HS exercise.

The following may be used as a rehabilitation guide:

1. Weight bearing: Partial weight-bearing with crutches for 6 weeks for isolated PCL reconstruction and up to 3 months for combined injury reconstruction.

2. Hinged brace: Locked in extension for 1 week, unlocked for ROM excercises for 6 weeks, and then unlocked continuously until normal gait is established.

3. ROM excercises: Passive knee-flexion exercises are advanced slowly over the first 6 weeks. About two thirds of patients will regain full flexion within 3 to 6 months, and one third will take 9 to 1 2 months to regain full flexion.

4. Gait: After 6 weeks, the brace is unlocked and emphasis is placed on establishing normal gait. Closed-chain exercises (biking, leg-press, pool) are begun.

Ultimately, muscle strength should be at least 90% of that on the noninjured side. Emphasis is then placed on sport-specific agility and proprioceptive skills by a trained therapist. It is usually 8 to 12 weeks before patients are walking without assistive devices and 8 to 12 months before patients are allowed to return to normal activities.

Results

Most studies reporting the results of PCL reconstruction suffer from the same limitations as those reporting the results of ACL reconstruction, namely, heterogeneous patient-population, varied injury patterns, diverse timing (acute vs. chronic), and varied techniques. Our results show that about 50% of patients can be converted from grade III to II laxity, 35% can achieve a laxity pattern similar to the uninvolved knee, and laxity is not improved at all in 15%. Subjectively, 70% to 80% of the patients noted improvement. In summary, the results of PCL surgery lag behind those of ACL surgery. Adherence to the treatment algorithm and addressing associated pathology at the time of reconstruction is likely to yield the best results.

Complications

Immediate complications are similar to ACL surgery, but specifically include neurovascular injury (pins and drilling) and neuropraxia (prolonged tourniquet use). Vascular injury must be addressed immediately by a vascular surgeon, and most neuropraxias will resolve by 18 months. Late complications include postoperative increases in laxity (usually from technical error or failure to treat associated ligament injury), loss of motion due to excessive graft tensioning or inadequate rehabilitation, and rarely, avascular necrosis of the medial femoral condyle due to femoral tunnel preparation.

Future Directions

A better understanding of the natural history of PCL injuries is needed. Research in the areas of anatomy, biomechanics, and kinematics will help to more accurately reconstruct the PCL. Advancements in graft materials and fixation techniques continue to evolve as research yields new technologies.

MENISCAL INJURIES

The meniscus is an important structure maintaining homeostasis within the knee joint by assisting in load transmission, stabilization, lubrication, nutrition, and proprioception. Meniscal tears represent about 50% of all knee injuries that ultimately require surgery. The male to female ratio is 2.5:17 with the peak incidence in males occurring between age 31 and 40 and the peak incidence in females occurring between age 11 and 20. The incidence is 61 per 100,000 people. In general isolated medial meniscus tears are more frequent than lateral meniscus tears. Degenerative tears are found in 60% of cadaver knees more than 65 years old.

Two patterns of meniscal injury are seen: traumatic and degenerative. Degenerative tears are typically complex and not amenable to repair Traumatic tears are often associated with ACL injuries are usually amenable to repair. The incidence of meniscal tears rises significantly with the chronicity of the ACL tear, ranging from 65% in acute injuries to 90% in chronic injuries. The lateral meniscus is more frequently torn in the acute ACL injury due to rotary forces. The medial meniscus is more frequently torn in chronic ACL-deficiency (3:1) due to repeated episodes of instability and its relative lack of mobility.

Basic Science
Biomechanics

Meniscal motion
Using three-dimensional MRI, meniscal motion has been shown as the knee is moved from 0 to 120 degrees (Fig. 35–25). The medial mensicus has an overall excursion of 5.1 mm compared with 11.2 mm for the lateral mensicus. Both posterior horns are less mobile relative to their respective anterior horns, and the medial mensicus is less mobile than the lateral meniscus due to its greater soft tissue and bony constraints.

Load transmission
The development of "hoop stress" within the meniscus depends on intact anterior and posterior attachments. Hoop stress also relies on the conversion of axial load into tensile strain through intact longitudinally oriented collagen fibers. Loads normally transmitted to articular cartilage are partially borne by the menisci transmitting 50% of the knee load in extension and 85% with flexion during weight-bearing. The posterior horns carry more load than the anterior horns. About 50% of this load is borne by the medial mensicus, and 70% is borne by the lateral mensicus.

The paucity of radial fibers make menisci susceptible to splits in the longitudinal and horizontal direction. As the size of the meniscus decreases, the contact stress borne by the articular cartilage increases. Total meniscectomy decreases tibia-femoral contact area by 50% and increases peak loads nearly fourfold. One study showed that total meniscectomy decreased contact area by 75% and increased peak contact stress by 235%. Others have shown that a partial meniscectomy of 15 to 34% increases peak loads by more than 350%. Results after partial excision of the lateral mensicus are less favorable than partial excision of the medial mensicus.

Joint stability and congruity
The concave menisci increase the congruity and conformity of the tibio-femoral joint. The medial meniscus is a secondary AP stabilizer only in the ACL-deficient knee. Their viscoelasticity provides a shock-absorbing capacity in intact knees that is about 20% greater than knees that have undergone complete meniscectomy.

Joint lubrication and nutrition
Microcanals within the meniscus transport fluid for joint nutrition and lubrication. Following meniscectomy, there is a 20% increase in the coefficient of friction.

Joint proprioception
Mechanoreceptors provide a feedback mechanism for sensing joint position.

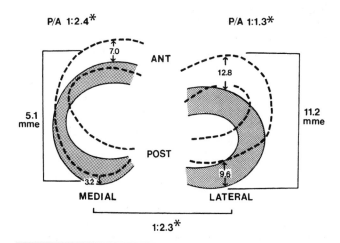

Figure 35–25   Diagram of mean meniscal excursion (in millimeters) along the tibial plateau, ANT, anterior; POST, posterior; mme, mean meniscal excursion; P/A, ratio of posterior to anterior meniscal translation during flexion; *, $p < 0.05$ by Student *t*-test analysis. Reproduced with permission from Thompson WO, Thaete FL, Fu FH, Dye SF. Tibial meniscal dynamics using three-dimensional reconstruction of magnetic resonance images. *Am J Sports Med*. 1991; 19:214.

PEARL

Because the posterior horn of the medial meniscus is the least mobile, it is more susceptible to shear stress in the anterior cruciate ligament (ACL)-deficient knee leading to a high incidence of tears with repeated episodes of instability.

Meniscal Healing

Injuries that extend into the peripheral vasculature (red-red tear) heal similar to other vascularized connective tissue. Tears in the border zone (red-white) have good potential for healing. Tears in the avascular zone (white-white) have poor healing potential without supplemental techniques. The perimeniscal capillary plexus provides substrate (fibrin clot), vessels, and cells for this healing response. A synovial pannus forms from the synovial fringe over the area of injury, providing vessel ansastamoses with the perimeniscal capillary plexus. By 10 weeks, fibrovascular scar has formed that is modulated to normal appearing fibrocartilage of indeterminate strength over the next several months. Red-white and possibly some white-white tears can have their healing enhanced by techniques that extend vascularity such as vascular access channels, synovial abrasion, and fibrin clot.

Vascular access channels

Creating access of peripheral vessels to avascular regions by a channel (i.e., trephination) allows the avascular portion of the menisci to heal through proliferation of fibrous scar. Some authors are wary of this technique; it requires disruption of some of the circumferential fibers.

Synovial abrasion

Parameniscal abrasion with a meniscal rasp of tibial and femoral surface synovial fringe encourages vascular extension to avascular regions via formation of vascular synovial pannus.

Exogenous fibrin clot

A clot precipitated on a sterile glass surface and placed within the defect within the vascular zone can promote healing. It provides a scaffold of adhesive, chemotactic (i.e., platelet derived growth factor), and mitogenic factors for cellular migration, proliferation, and matrix production that eventually (6 months) modulates into fibrocartilage.

Anatomy
Embryology

The menisci appear as distinct structures between the 8th and 10th week of gestation. They arise as a condensation of the intermediate mensenchyme and form attachments to the surrounding joint capsule and cruciates.

Histology

The meniscus is composed of fibrocartilage and extracellular matrix (ECM). Chondrocytes and fibroblasts are responsible for synthesis and maintenance of the ECM. The ECM is primarily composed of an interlacing network of type I collagen (55–65% of dry weight) and minor amounts of types II, III, V, and VI collagen. The collagen is arranged in a circumferential orientation with an intermingling of radially oriented fibers acting as ties. The radial fibers help convert compressive forces into tensile forces ("hoop stress"). Within this network of collagen are small amounts of elastin, proteoglycans, and glycoproteins helping to resist compressive forces.

Functional anatomy

The menisci are semilunar cartilages that act as anatomical extensions of the tibial plateau, effectively increasing the congruity with the femoral condyles (Fig. 35–26). They are triangular in cross section, being thicker peripherally where they

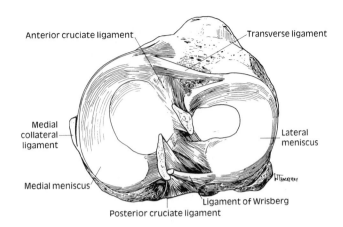

Figure 35–26 Drawing of tibial plateau showing the shape and attachments of the lateral and medial menisci in relationship to the cruciate ligaments. Reproduced with permission from Nicholas JA, Hershman EB. *The Lower Extremity and Spine in Sports Medicine.* St. Louis, MO: CU Mosby; 1995: 687.

attach to the joint capsule and tibia through the coronary ligaments. Anteriorly, they are interconnected by the transverse intermeniscal ligament. They are firmly attached at their horns anteriorly and posteriorly.

Medial Meniscus

The medial mensicus is semicircular covering about 64% of the area of the medial tibial plateau. It is broader posteriorly than anteriorly. The anterior and posterior horns attach anterior to the ACL and PCL tibial insertion sites within the intercondylar fossa, respectively. Peripherally, the medial mensicus is firmly attached to the joint capsule and to the deep MCL.

Lateral Meniscus

The lateral meniscus is circular, covering approximately 84% of the area of the lateral tibial plateau. It has a uniform width throughout. The horns attach in close proximity to one another. The anterior horn inserts adjacent to the anterior half of the ACL. The posterior horn inserts slightly more medial at the posterior border of the ACL, in front of the posterior horn of the medial mensicus. Peripherally, it is loosely attached to the capsule, except at the popliteal hiatus. At the hiatus, it is only attached to an aponeurotic extension from the popliteus and portions of the arcuate and meniscofemoral ligaments.

Vascular Supply

During the transition from prenatal to postnatal development, the vascular supply recedes to the outer region of the meniscus. Peripherally, it is supplied by branches of the lateral, medial, and middle geniculate arteries, forming a perimeniscal capillary plexus. The peripheral 10 to 30% of the mensicus in the adult is vascular. The remaining portions receives nutrition via diffusion enhanced by joint loading. Energy production is principally through anaerobic glycolysis. Three zones exist based on decreasing vascular supply from the periphery to the center: red-red, red-white, and white-white, with decreasing capacity to heal after injury.

Innervation

The peripheral two thirds of the meniscus is innervated by myelinated and unmyelinated nerve fibers supplied by the posterior tibial, obturator, femoral, and peroneal nerves. Primarily concentrated in the anterior and posterior horns, mechanoreceptors (Ruffini, Golgi, and Pacini) and free nerve endings have proprioceptive and nociceptive functions.

Examination

History

Commonly associated with a twisting injury to the knee. Patients often complain of pain localized to the joint line. Typically, the location is posterior to the collateral ligaments. Older patients may present with an insidious onset of pain. Hyperflexion (e.g., squatting) may exacerbate the pain. Swelling may be present. Peripheral acute tears may present with an insidious onset of a hemarthrosis. Chronic tears that become dislodged or that are associated with arthritis may cause effusions. Mechanical locking, catching or giving way from a displaced fragment may also occur.

Physical Examination

Observation

Observe for antalgic gait, effusion, decreased active or passive ROM, and thigh atrophy from feedback inhibition to the quadriceps due to pain.

Palpation

Palpate for effusion (50% of patients), joint line tenderness (77–86% of patients), extensor mechanism pathology, and for associated ligament insufficiency. Collateral ligament tenderness is commonly present at the joint line, but will extend proximal or distal over the course of the ligament.

Range of motion

Mechanical blocking may cause a decrease in active or passive motion.

Special Tests

McMurray's Test

This test is performed on the supine patient beginning with the knee flexed to 90 degrees, axially loaded and slowly extended with IR and ER forces applied to the tibia. The addition of a varus or valgus stress can help delineate medial meniscus or lateral meniscus tears, respectively. A positive test is a palpable click along the joint line often associated with pain.

Apley's Test

Perform this test on the prone patient with the knees flexed to 90 degrees and axially loaded through the heels with IR and ER. A positive test is pain relieved with distraction. Pain not occurring during compression but occurring with distraction may indicate collateral ligament injury.

Steinmann Test

Performing a brisk tibial rotation of the flexed knee elicits pain.

Squat Test

In this test, asking the patient to squat repetitively or to "duck walk" elicits symptoms or inability to perform in the presence of meniscal tears.

PEARL

Clinical examination accuracy is about 82% for medial meniscus tears and 76% accurate for lateral meniscus tears.

Aids to Diagnosis

Radiographs

Complete radiographic evaluation is discussed in Anterior Knee Pain and Patellofemoral disorders. In general, an AP, lateral, axial and 45 degree PA flexion weight-bearing radiograph should be obtained. Specifically, a history of prior meniscectomy may lead to early degenerative changes including those described by Fairbank (1948, squaring of the femoral condyles, marginal ridging, and joint space narrowing) and peaked eminences and notch osteophytes thought to be related to chronic ACL-deficiency with repeated episodes of instability.

Magnetic Resonance Imaging

Accuracy in MRI has improved significantly over the last few years and is slightly greater for medial meniscus (93–98%) than lateral meniscus tears (90–96%). Signal grading comprises: grade I; intrameniscal ovoid or globular signal; grade II; linear signal not reaching the articular surface and, grade III; intrameniscal signal communicating with the articular surface. Only a grade III signal coincides with tears with an accuracy of up to 90%. Grades I and II probably represent mucinous degeneration and are present in asymptomatic patients past age 30 who do not have evidence of meniscal tears. Following meniscal repair, an abnormal signal may persist for as long as 3 to 6 years postoperatively.

Sagittal images offer the most information concerning the meniscus. Normally, the meniscus has a uniform, low signal on T1- and T2-weighted images. A torn meniscus imbibes fluid and is seen well on T2-weighted images. Common pitfalls exist when reading the MRI. The transverse intermeniscal ligament can mimic a tear of the anterior horn of the lateral meniscus. The superior recess above the posterior horn of the medial meniscus can mimic a partial-thickness tear of the medial meniscus. The popliteal tendon sheath and meniscofemoral ligament can be misinterpreted as a tear of the posterior horn of the lateral meniscus.

Arthrography

Double contrast arthrography has an accuracy of at least 83 to 93%. This invasive test is used mostly in areas where the MRI is not available and to evaluate the results of meniscal repair.

Classification

Location

Based on vascularity, tears are located in the peripheral vascular zone (red-red), middle zone (red-white), and central avascular zone (white-white). Other geographic classifications exist to describe the radial and circumferential extent of the tear. One method divides the medial meniscus into three radial zones (A, B, and C) from the posterior third to the anterior third, and the lateral meniscus into three radial zones (D, E, and F) from the anterior third to the posterior third. These are subclassified into four circumferential zones (0, 1, 2, and 3) from the meniscal synovial junction (0), outer third (1), central third (2), and inner third (3). Zones 0 to 1 correspond to the red-red zone, zones 1 to 2 correspond to the red-white zone, and zones 2 to 3 correspond to the white-white zone.

Orientation and Appearance

Figure 35–27 describes various tears. In general, it is best to document the length, location, and tear pattern. Tears can be vertical, longitudinal oblique or flap, degenerative or complex, radial, and horizontal cleavage. They can be acute or chronic. The ability to displace the tear by greater than 3 mm with an arthroscopic probe is used to determine stability.

Specific Conditions, Treatment, and Outcome

Total meniscectomy, once the standard of care, leads to the development of arthritis. Attempts to preserve the meniscus are now the rule rather than the exception. When a meniscus

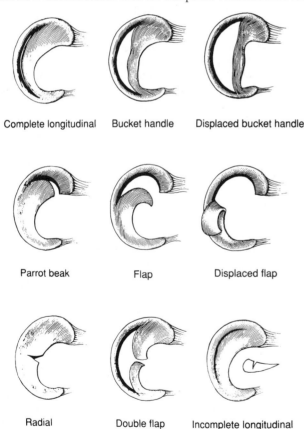

Complete longitudinal   Bucket handle   Displaced bucket handle

Parrot beak   Flap   Displaced flap

Radial   Double flap   Incomplete longitudinal

Figure 35–27   Gross anatomy of the most common meniscus tears. Reproduced with permission from Tria AJ, Klein KS. *An illustrated Guide to the Knee.* New York, NY: Churchill Livingstone; 1992: 100.

tear is not amenable to repair, partial meniscectomy is the preferred treatment.

Nonoperative Treatment

Nonsurgical treatment for meniscal tears may be suitable for asymptomatic tears, older patients who are willing to change their lifestyle, and those at high risk for surgery. All patients should be initially managed with rest, ice compression, elevation, and NSAIDs. Rehabilitation emphasizing painless, full ROM and strengthening is performed.

Meniscal tears found at the time of arthroscopy that do not require repair may be stimulated to heal faster by performing parameniscal abrasion. This includes:

1. partial-thickness splits
2. full-thickness vertical or oblique tears less than 5 mm in length, if stable
3. short radial or minor inner-rim tears
4. degenerative tears in osteoarthritics without mechanical symptoms
5. stable tears with inability to displace the central portion by greater than 3 mm.

It has recently been suggested that tears of the lateral meniscus posterior to the popliteal hiatus need only parameniscal abrasion and do not require excision or repair. Additionally, some authors report longitudinal tears of less than 1.5 cm can also be left alone, if deemed stable at arthroscopy.

Operative Treatment

Surgical intervention is recommended for those patients with a history of persistent pain, catching or locking, and a physical examination consistent with a meniscal tear. More than 90% of athletes with symptomatic meniscal tears are unable to return to sports at the same level unless treated. Operative treatment includes (1) total meniscectomy, (2) partial meniscectomy, (3) meniscal repair, and (4) meniscal transplantation.

Total Meniscectomy

Early literature on the short-term followup following total meniscectomy showed a high incidence of good results. Long-term followup, however, at intervals of 10 to 22 years, demonstrated significant increases in the incidence and severity of degenerative arthritis following total meniscectomy. In 1948, Fairbank was the first to suggest that degenerative changes after meniscectomy resulted from increased joint reactive forces. Given our present understanding of the biomechanical importance of the meniscus, procedures that preserve the meniscus have significant long-term advantages.

Partial Meniscectomy

Partial meniscectomy will significantly increase forces across the articular cartilage, and maximizing meniscal preservation should minimize the incidence and severity of degenerative change over time. Removal of only the torn or unstable portion (flaps, complex tears, degenerative and central/radial tears) with subsequent contouring of the remaining meniscus is recommended. Use of an arthroscopic basket forceps and motorized shaver are helpful to accomplish these goals.

PEARL

Irreparable bucket-handle tears should be reduced, detached posteriorly, partially detached anteriorly, and avulsed from the residual attachment.

Meniscal Repair

Our present understanding of meniscal vasculature and healing potential has resulted in an increased popularity of meniscal repair. It is important to evaluate the meniscus for the location, extent, and stability of the tear. Using the modified Gillquist approach, one can view the posterior horn of the medial meniscus by passing the 30- and 70-degree arthroscope between the medial femor condyle and PCL. The site is prepared using a meniscal rasp or motorized shaver. At present, the most common criteria for meniscal repair include the following.

Criteria for repair

Location

This is possibly the most important factor. Peripheral tears (10–30%) with good vascular access (red-red and red-white) are optimal. If bleeding is not evident, it has been suggested that tears within 3 mm of the periphery are presumed vascular, and tears greater than 5 mm from the periphery are presumed avascular. Tears 3 to 5 mm from the periphery have variable vascularity and results may be improved by the use of vascular extension techniques.

Stability

Stable tears include partial-thickness (< 50% of height of meniscus) and full-thickness oblique or vertical tears less than 10 mm in length with inability to displace the central portion with a probe greater than 3 mm. Unstable tears should be resected or repaired.

Length

Stable tears less than 10 to 15 mm in length can be left alone or treated with parameniscal abrasion. Radial tears less than 5 mm in length can also be left alone. Longer tears (> 4 cm) may have lower healing rates, especially when isolated repair is performed

---

PEARL

Combining length and stability factors yields the recommendation that stable tears greater than 10 to 15 mm in length *or* tears that are any length and unstable (displaced by > 3 mm) to probing are amenable to partial meniscectomy or repair.

Tear pattern

Peripheral, vertical, longitudinal tears represent the ideal situation for repair. Chronic bucket-handle tears often have radial components, making them less amenable to repair. Complex bucket-handle tears, flap tears, degenerative, complex, and radial tears often perform poorly with repair and are more often amenable to excision. Horizontal cleavage tears are not repairable, and the unstable leaf should be excised, leaving up to 3 mm of the leaf.

Patient age

Age by itself does not affect the ability of the meniscus to heal. Although some recommend that a patient under the age of 50 should be considered a candidate for repair if the tear is repairable, probably any tear amenable to repair should be considered for repair.

Chronicity

Both acute and chronic tears can be repaired, but acute tears less than 8 weeks old have better healing potential, probably because they are less likely to be complex or degenerative.

Ligament stability

Anterior cruciate ligament deficiency must also be corrected simultaneously to prevent instability and retearing. Because of relatively poor results following removal of the lateral meniscus versus the medial meniscus, some authors maintain that aggressive salvage of the lateral meniscus regardless of the status of the ACL is warranted. Repairable meniscus tears in ACL-stable knees are less common and often associated with complex or degenerative tears. On the other hand, repairable tears are usually part of a complex that includes a torn ACL. Compared with the ACL-deficient knee, the PCL-deficient knee has a lower incidence of associated meniscal pathology.

PEARL

The ideal candidate for repair is the young patient with an acute longitudinal tear in the periphery of the meniscus that is 1 to 2 cm in length that is repaired in conjunction with an ACL reconstruction.

Technical aspects of meniscus repair

Suture placement

Anatomic coaptation of the edges is the desired result. Most authors recommend a separate suture every 3 to 5 mm of tear and that the entrance site be 2 to 3 mm from the tear margin to prevent cutting out. Only polydioxanone sutures (PDS) (Ethicon, Inc.; Somerville, NJ) and nonabsorbable sutures retain significant strength beyond 6 weeks. The choice of suture material is technique dependent. If support is desired beyond 6 weeks of healing, then nonabsorbable sutures should be used. Arthroscopically, one can use either the ipsilateral or contralateral portal for suture placement, as long as the neurovascular structures are protected. Ideally, sutures should be placed perpendicular to the tear surface. Vertical, matress sutures have the highest tearing stress, as such a suture catches more circumferential fibers within the loop. It is best to have the two suture ends near one another and then diverge for optimal strength and coaptation. If it is not possible to place a vertical matress, a horizontal matress is considered second best. With a horizontal matress, sutures may need to be placed on the tibial and femoral surface for maximal coaptation. Horizontal sutures require a minimum meniscal bridge between the two suture arms of 2 to 4 mm.

On the lateral side, sutures are passed with the knee in the figure-four position with 70 to 90 degrees of knee flexion. On the medial side, the knee is placed in 10 to 30 degrees of flexion for optimal visualization and to avoid capturing the posteromedial capsular recess.

Incisions

Depending on the technique utilized, a longitudinal incision centered at the joint line may be required to facilitate repair or to tie sutures against the capsule. Repairs performed arthroscopically will not require a capsulotomy, and only subcutaneous dissection is required. For the medial meniscus, a posteromedial incision is utilized. The pes tendons, saphenous nerve and its intrapatellar branch are retracted posteriorly. An oblique capsular incision is made as needed, just posterior to the trailing edge at the MCL.

For the lateral meniscus, a posterolateral incision is used in line with the posterior border of the fibular head with the knee flexed to 90 degrees. The posterior border of the ITB is incised and retracted posteriorly with the biceps femoris to protect the peroneal nerve. At times, the lateral head of the gastrocnemius must also be retracted posteriorly. An oblique capsular incision is made as needed parallel to the posterior border of the popliteus tendon.

Open meniscal repair

This technique provides limited access to the meniscus and is most indicated for peripheral posterior third tears. It is performed through lateral- or medial-based longitudinal incisions as described above, often using a double-armed suture and vertical matress for anatomic repair.

Inside-out arthroscopic repair

Long, flexible Keith needles are passed through a curved, single- or double-barrel cannula placed through the arthroscopic portal (Fig. 35–28, left). A single-barrel cannula allows vertically oriented suture placement, but a double barrel cannula may be quicker. Nonabsorbable No. 2-0 or absorbable No. 2-0 PDS sutures are used and placed from posterior to anterior as a vertical or horizontal mattress. Outer mini-incisions are made (as described above) to prevent entrapment of subcutaneous nerve branches as the sutures are tied over the capsule.

Outside-in arthroscopic repair

An 18-gauge spinal needle is placed as a cannula to pass a No. 0 PDS suture through the tear from the outside-in (Fig.35–28). The sutures are retrieved from within the knee through the arthroscopic portal and a large "mulberry" knot is tied outside of the knee and subsequently drawn back into the knee. Separate 1- to 2-cm incisions or a single, long incision can be made to tie adjacent sutures to one another against the capsule without capturing subcutaneous nerves.

All-inside arthroscopic repair

A special cannulated suture hook is used to perforate both sides of the tear. Sutures are passed through the lumen of the hook, and a knot pusher is used to secure them into place. No additional incisions are required.

Enhancement of meniscal healing

As described above, promotion of neovascularization can be accomplished by perimeniscal abrasion, placement of exogenous fibrin clot, and creating vascular access channels. Most commonly, perimeniscal abrasion is used. Although fibrin clot is believed to occur spontaneously during ACL reconstruction or with peripheral tears, it is especially useful during the repair of isolated tears extending into the white-red zones. Fibrin clot is prepared by stirring 50 to 75 ml of the patient's venous blood with a glass rod, rinsing the clot through a sponge, and arthroscopically suturing it into the defect. Vascular access channels can be prepared with an 18-gauge spinal needle.

Allograft meniscal transplantation

The rationale of meniscal transplantation is to prevent degenerative changes in the postmeniscectomy patient. Young patients who have undergone even partial meniscectomy, especially of the lateral meniscus, are undoubtedly at significant risk for developing arthritis. At present, the most

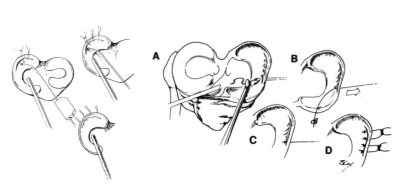

Figure 35–28 Two of the most common meniscal repair techniques. Left: the inside-out technique. Reproduced with permission from Fu FH, Harner CD, Vince KG. *Knee Surgery*. Philadelphia, PA: Williams and Wilkins; 1994: 623. Right: the outside-in technique. **(A)** Sutures are placed from outside-in through a spinal needle. **(B)** Knot is tied. **(C)** Suture is pulled back. **(D)** Sutures are tied together outside the capsule. Reproduced with permission from Hanks GA, Kalenak A. Alternative arthroscopy techniques for meniscal repair: a review. *Orthop Rev.* 1990; 19:29.

accepted indications for meniscal transplantation are patients less than age 45 with pain and discomfort associated with early osteoarthritis (less than grade IV) of the involved compartment without ACL-deficiency or significant malalignment. Contraindications include age greater than 60 or patients with bony architectural changes, prior infection, significant malalignment, or instability. Meniscal allografts are considered "immunologically privileged," and clinical rejection has not been a problem. Several graft preservation techniques are available including fresh, fresh freezing, cryopreservation, and freeze drying. Secondary sterilization with radiation of less than 2.5 MRad minimizes mechanical degradation while sterilizing all but the most virulent bacterial and viral pathogens. Techniques include arthrotomy, arthroscopy, or combined approaches and are beyond the scope of this discussion. Long-term followup is limited with success rates ranging between 60 and 100% at 8 to 48 months.

Meniscal Cyst

Meniscal cysts more commonly involve the lateral meniscus than the medial meniscus (3 to 10:1). They have an incidence of less than 1 to 22% and are associated with meniscal tears in 18 to 100% of cases. They usually involve a horizontal cleavage tear of the peripheral, middle third of the lateral meniscus. The peak incidence is in males in the second or third decade. Patients complain of a dull ache along the joint line and have a tender, rubbery mass that may change size with flexion. Magnetic resonance imaging is helpful to confirm the diagnosis. Meniscal cysts usually contain a gelatinous fluid. Treatment of symptomatic cysts with a meniscal tear includes partial meniscectomy with arthroscopic cyst decompression. When no tear is identified, en bloc resection may be required.

Discoid Meniscus

The incidence of discoid meniscus involving the lateral meniscus is about 0.4 to 7% and 0 to 0.3% for the medial meniscus. Less than 10% are bilateral. These lesions have been classified by Watanabe as (1) complete, (2) incomplete, and (3) Wrisberg-ligament type (absent posterior coronary ligament) with normal shape and excessive hypermobility. Only the first two types have been found in the medial meniscus. Radiographically, the first two types may demonstrate a widened joint space, squaring of the condyle, cupping of the tibial plateau, and a hypoplastic tibial spine that are all found on the lateral side. Magnetic resonance imaging is helpful to confirm the diagnosis. Complete and incomplete types are disc-shaped, and if found incidentally are left alone. When torn and symptomatic, saucerization (central partial meniscectomy) is performed to trim the meniscus back to a stable 6 to 8-mm rim.

The Wrisberg-ligament type commonly presents as the "snapping knee syndrome" in children or adolescents who complain of lateral joint line pain. An audible clunk with terminal extension may occur because the posterior horn is tethered by only the ligament of Wrisberg (not the tibial plateau), and thus, is excessively mobile. No radiographic changes occur. A symptomatic Wrisberg-ligament type should be treated by repair of its hypermobile posterior horn.

Rehabilitation

Rehabilitation protocols following meniscal repair have evolved as our understanding of meniscal biomechanics and healing has improved. During the first 8 weeks, weight bearing as tolerated in a hinged knee brace locked in extension and unlocked only for therapeutic exercise is performed. Motion begins in the initial phase, but flexion beyond 90 degrees is avoided for 6 months. After 8 weeks, patients are weaned from crutch and brace use, and greater emphasis is placed on strengthening and proprioception. Terminal, knee extension exercises and open-chain, kinetic exercises are avoided for the first 3 months. Sport-specific training or work hardening begins at about 6 months, taking an average of about 9 months to return to full activities. Variations of this protocol are in use with greater acceptance of accelerated rehabilitation protocols. Meniscal repair in conjunction with ACL reconstruction follows a protocol similar to the ACL rehabilitation guidelines.

Results

Results of partial meniscectomy are better than total meniscectomy in the short-term. In the degenerative, ACL-deficient knee, results of partial meniscectomy are satisfactory if mechanical meniscal symptoms are the presenting complaint.

Overall healing rates range from 78 to 95%. Isolated meniscal repair in the ACL-deficient knee has a failure rate of 40 to 50%. More recent reports show even higher healing rates, and this is believed to be related to more appropriate patient selection and improved techniques. Meniscal repair in conjunction with ACL reconstruction has a healing rate in excess of 90 to 95%. This has been related to the postoperative hemarthrosis and to the knee stability conferred by the reconstruction.

Complications

The overall complication rate is around 2.5%. The most common complication following meniscal repair is a failure to heal or a retear occurring in as many as 50% of those with unstable knees and as little as 0 to 5% in stable knees. Not all failures, however, are symptomatic. Repeat surgery rates for partial meniscectomy and repair are each about 25%. Neurovascular injury most commonly involving the infrapatellar branch and the saphenous nerve ranges from 2 to 28%, most of which resolve before 4 months. Stiffness occurs in 6 to 12%, with loss of extension being more common than loss of flexion, especially with medial meniscus repair or concomitant ACL reconstruction. Other complications include arthrofibrosis, infection, thrombophlebitis, and RSD.

Future Directions

Future trends include improved repair techniques and the use of synthetic meniscus implants. New meniscal repair techniques include the use of a bioresorbable implant for easier all-inside meniscal repair, but long-term results are lacking. Recently, the use of a bovine collagen meniscus implant fabricated as a meniscus replacement has been reported in animal models. The template is slowly resorbed as it induces and supports the ingrowth of host cells and matrix. Clinical studies are in preliminary stages.

SELECTED BIBLIOGRAPHY

General References

FU FH, HARNER CD, VINCE KG. *Knee Surgery*. Baltimore, MD: Williams and Wilkins; 1994.

MERCHANT AC, MERCER RL, JACOBSEN RJ, COOL CR. Roentgenographic analysis of patellofemoral congruence. *J Bone Jt Surg*. 1974;56A:1391–1396.

MILLER MD, COOPER DE, WARNER JP. *Review of Sports Medicine and Arthroscopy*. New York, NY: WB Saunders; 1995.

OUTERBRIDGE RE. The etiology of chondromalacia patellae. *J Bone Jt Surg*. 1961;43B:752–757.

ROSENBERG TD, PAULOS LE, PARKER RD, COWARD DB, SCOTT SM. The forty-five degree posteroanterior flexion weight-bearing radiograph of the knee. *J Bone Jt Surg*. 1988;70A:1479–1983.

WIBERG G. Roentgenographic and anatomic studies on the femorapatellar joint. *Acta Orthop Scand*. 1941;12:319–410.

Anterior Knee Pain and Patellofemoral Disorders

DREZ D, DELEE JC. Patellofemoral joint surgery. *Op Tech Sports Med*. 1994;2:238–334.

FU FH, MADAY MG. Arthroscopic lateral release and the lateral patellar compression syndrome. *Orthop Clin North Am*. 1992;23:601–612.

FULKERSON JP. Patellofemoral pain disorders: evaluation and management. *J Am Acad Orthop Surg*. 1994;2:124–132.

FULKERSON JP, HUNGERFORD DS. *Disorders of the Patellofemoral Joint*, 2nd ed. Baltimore, MD: Williams and Wilkins; 1990.

POST WR. Surgical decision making in patellofemoral pain and instability. *Oper Tech Sports Med*. 1994;4:273–284.

Anterior Cruciate Ligament Injuries

BALDERSTON RA. Surgery of the anterior cruciate ligament. *Op Tech Orthop*. 1996;6:125–180.

DREZ D, DELEE JC. Anterior cruciate ligament injuries. *Op Tech Sports Med*. 1993;1:1–83.

FU FH. The anterior cruciate ligament. *Clin Sports Med*. 1993;12:625–852.

HARNER CD. Failed anterior cruciate ligament surgery. *Clin Orthop Rel Res*. 1996;325:1–139.

LARSON RL, TAILLON M. Anterior cruciate ligament insufficiency: principles of treatment. *J Am Acad Orthop Surg*. 1994;2:26–35.

NOYES FR, BUTLER DL, GROOD ES et al. Biomechanical analysis of human ligament grafts used in knee-ligament repairs and reconstruction. *J Bone Jt Surg*. 1984;66A:344–352.

NOYES FR, MATTHEWS DS, MOOAR LA, GROOD ES. The symptomatic ACL deficient knee. II. The results of rehabilitation, activity modification and counseling on functional disability. *J Bone Jt Surg*. 1983;65A:163–174.

O'DONOGHUE DH. An analysis of end results of surgical treatment of major injuries to the ligaments of the knee. *J Bone Jt Surg*. 1955;37A:1–12.

WOJTYS EM. *The ACL Deficient Knee*. Am Acad Orthop Surg Monograph Series. Rosemont, IL; 1994.

WOO SLY, ADAMS DJ. The tensile properties of human ACL and ACL graft tissues. In: Dale D et al, eds. *Knee Ligaments. Structure, Function, Injury and Repair*. New York: Raven Press; 1990.

Posterior Cruciate Ligament Injuries

COVEY DC, SAPEGA AA. Injuries of the posterior cruciate ligament. *J Bone Jt Surg*. 1993;75A:1376–1386.

SEEBACHER J. INGLIS A, MARSHALL J, WARREN RF. The structure of the posterolateral aspect of the knee. *J Bone Jt Surg*. 1982;64A:536–541.

VELTRI DM, WARREN RF. Isolated and combined posterior cruciate ligament injuries. *J Am Acad Orthop Surg*. 1993;1:67–75.

Meniscus

BELZER JP, CANNON WD. Meniscus tears: treatment in the stable and unstable knee. *J Am Acad Orthop Surg*. 1993;1:41–47.

CANNON WD, DEHAVEN KE. Meniscus repair. *Sports Med Arthroscop Rev*. 1993;1:103–176.

DEHAVEN KE. Decision-making factors in the treatment of meniscus lesions. *Clin Orthop Rel Res*. 1990;252:49–54.

DREZ D, DELEE JC. Meniscal surgery. *Op Tech Sports Med*. 1994;2:152–235.

FAIRBANK TJ. Knee joint changes after meniscectomy. *J Bone Jt Surg*. 1948;30B:664–670.

SHERMAN OH. Meniscal repair. *Clin in Sports Med*. 1996;15:445–630.

SAMPLE QUESTIONS

1. Patellar tilt is best evaluated radiographically using the:
   (a) Merchant's view
   (b) Laurin's view
   (c) sunrise view
   (d) 45-degree PA view
   (e) lateral view

2. A 25-year-old female presents with a history of anterior bilateral knee pain made worse during negotiation of steps. Upon evaluation, it is determined that she has lateral retinacular tightness and a normal Q angle. The best initial management of this problem is:
   (a) physical therapy with quadriceps strengthening using open-chain exercises from 0 to 45 degrees

(b) physical therapy with quadriceps strengthening using closed-chain exercises from 45 to 90 degrees

(c) physical therapy with quadriceps strengthening using closed-chain exercises from 0 to 45 degrees

(d) arthroscopic lateral release

(e) distal realignment

3. During ACL reconstruction, placing the femoral tunnel too far anterior will result in:

(a) excessive graft tension in flexion and looseness in extension

(b) excessive graft impingement in flexion

(c) excessive graft tension in extension and looseness in flexion

(d) excessive graft tension in flexion and extension

(e) excessive graft looseness in flexion and extension

4. During the physical examination for a PCL injury, it was noted that there was an increase in external tibial rotation at 30 degrees that increased even further at 90 degrees compared with the contralateral side. This is most consistent with:

(a) isolated PCL injury

(b) combined PCL and LCL injury

(c) combined PCL and posterolateral corner injury

(d) combined PCL, ACL and posterolateral corner injury

(e) isolated LCL injury

5. Which of the following meniscal tears is most optimal to repair?

(a) a vertical peripheral lateral meniscus tear 10 mm in length posterior to the popliteal hiatus in combination with ACL reconstruction

(b) a vertical peripheral lateral meniscus tear 8 mm in length that is displaced 3 mm into the joint with probing in combination with ACL reconstruction

(c) a complex bucket-handle tear involving the entire medial meniscus in an ACL-deficient knee without ACL reconstruction

(d) a horizontal lateral meniscus tear 12 mm in length extending to the periphery

(e) a radial tear 5 mm in length of the medial meniscus in combination with ACL reconstruction

Answers: 1) b; 2) c; 3) a; 4) c; 5) b

Chapter 36

Knee Reconstruction

Robert Hube, MD, Nicholas G. Sotereanos, MD, David Hungerford, MD,
and Hugh P. Chandler, MD

Outline

Knee arthritis results in more than 250,000 operative procedures per year in the United States, of which 100,0000 are total knee arthroplasties (TKAs). This chapter reviews the spectrum of non-operative and surgical management for arthritis of the knee.

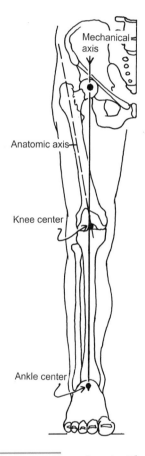

Figure 36–1 Knee axes. Reproduced with permission from Rohr WL: *Primary total knee arthroplasty.* In: Chapman's, Operative Orthopaedics. Philadelphia: Lippincott-Raven, 1988:718.

BASIC SCIENCE

Knee Biomechanics

The mechanical axis of the tibiofemoral joint is defined by a line passing from the center of the femoral head to the center of the ankle's tibial plafond (Fig. 36–1). This axis is measured using plain radiographs with a long cassette while the patient is standing. The femoral shaft axis averages 5 degrees valgus for men and 7 degrees valgus for women. With a normal mechanical axis, 60% of the load is transmitted through the medial compartment of the knee and 40% through the lateral compartment. The magnitude of the load through the joint varies with activity, but ranges from two to four times body weight. In single leg stance, the patella-femoral forces can exceed four times body weight. A change in the mechanical axis through trauma or joint degeneration will alter the load distribution.

Osteoarthritis is frequently associated with medial compartment degeneration and a varus knee. Patients with rheumatoid arthritis may often develop a valgus deformity producing joint laxity and degeneration in the lateral compartment. Wedge osteotomies of the tibia or femur may be used to restore the mechanical axis and unload a compartment of the knee with unilateral osteoarthritis. In patients undergoing knee replacement, the mechanical axis must be

Orthopaedic Surgery: The Essentials. Edited by M.E. Baratz, A.D. Watson, and J.E. Imbriglia. Thieme Medical Publishers, Inc., New York © 1999

restored through bone cuts, soft tissue balancing and choice of implant.

Knee Kinematics

An important concept in TKA is the difference between posterior translation and roll back. Roll back is a normal phenomenon in which the femoral condyle rotates or rolls posteriorly on the tibial plateau during knee flexion. This motion is controlled by the posterior cruciate ligament (PCL). The loss of normal kinematics, that is roll back, can result in loss of knee motion. It may also weaken the knee by compromising the mechanical advantage of the quadriceps. Posterior translation has the further adverse effect of increased shear forces at the tibiofemoral articulation. Posterior translation can be prevented in TKA by the use of an implant that permits preservation of the PCL. Posterior translation can also be controlled by using an implant with posterior support, such as the "roller in trough" design or a posterior stabilized knee. Fluoroscopic cineography studies show that even with retention of the PCL, the tibia often subluxes anteriorly. This is opposite to normal motion, in which the tibia should move posteriorly.

AIDS TO DIAGNOSIS

Plain Radiographs

Plain radiographs are the most important diagnostic study in the evaluation of knee arthritis. An anteroposterior (AP) view on a long cassette while the patient is standing provides information on mechanical axis and degree to which the medial and lateral compartments have degenerated (Fig. 36–2A). The flexion weight-bearing view is taken with the knee flexed 45 degrees. This view may show medial or lateral compartment wear not visible on an AP view taken with the knee extended. The lateral view shows the position and degree of wear on the patella (Fig. 37–2B). A skyline view shows the condition of the medial and lateral facets of the patella, as well as patellar subluxation. This view is taken with patient prone, knee flexed back at an angle 35-40 degrees caudad. The central ray is directed at the patella.

Bone scans, computed tomography, and magnetic resonance imaging are rarely necessary in the evaluation of the arthritic knee.

ANATOMY AND SURGICAL APPROACHES

Anatomy

In the knee joint, the femur articulates with the tibia through the cartilage-covered surfaces of the femoral condyles. The fibula lies on the lateral side of the tibia and connects to it via the interosseous membrane. The patella is a sesamoid bone contained within the quadriceps tendon. The patella has two facets that articulate with the two femoral condyles. The quadriceps and patella attach to the tibia via the patellar tendon.

Ligaments of the knee joint can be distinguished as external and internal (Fig. 36–3). The external ligaments include

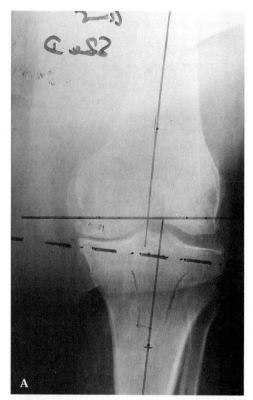

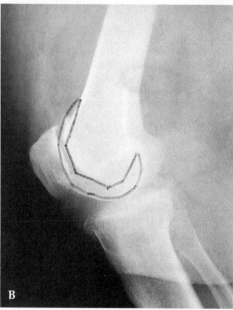

Figure 36–2 **(A)** Anteroposterior (AP) and **(B)** lateral radiograph of a 65-year-old man with osteoarthritis secondary to varus deformity in the left knee (templated for a total knee arthroplasty [TKA]).

the ligamentum patellae, the patellar retinacula, and the collateral ligaments. The broad medial patellar retinaculum runs medial to the patella and attaches to the tibial tubercle. Fibers of the iliotibial tract, fibers from the rectus femoris muscle, and the vastus lateralis form the lateral patellar retinaculum prior to its insertion on the lateral aspect of the tibial tuberosity. The round fibular collateral ligament connects the head of

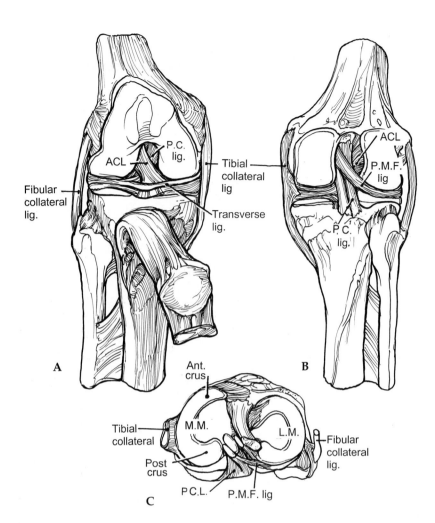

Figure 36–3 **(A)** Right knee joint, anterior view of cruciate ligaments. **(B)** Right knee joint posterior view of cruciate ligaments. **(C)** View of upper surfaces of the menisci.

the fibula to the lateral epicondyle of the femur. The medial collateral ligament is firmly attached to the joint capsule and to the medial meniscus.

The intracapsular ligaments consist of the cruciate ligaments, which are separated from the joint cavity by a synovial membrane. The anterior cruciate ligament (ACL) descends from the medial surface of the lateral condyle of the femur to the anterior intercondylar area of the tibia. It prevents the tibia from sliding anteriorly in relation to the femur. The stronger PCL prevents the tibia from translating posteriorly in relation to the femur. The PCL passes from the lateral surface of the medial femoral condyle to the posterior intercondylar area of the tibia.

The menisci are C-shaped wedges of fibrocartilage. The lateral meniscus is more circular and uniform in width. The medial meniscus is semicircular in shape and unlike the lateral meniscus, attaches to the medial collateral ligament. The two menisci are connected anteriorly by the transverse ligament (ligament of Humphrey). The posterior meniscofemoral ligament passes behind the PCL (ligament of Weisberg), from the lateral meniscus to the inner surface of the medial femoral condyle. The anterior meniscofemoral ligament occasionally forms a connection between the posterior end of the lateral meniscus with the medial condyle of the femur in front of the PCL.

The quadriceps femoris is composed of four parts. The straight head of the rectus femoris arises from the anterior

inferior iliac spine and the upper margin of the acetabulum to insert at the tibial tuberosity. The vastus lateralis arises from the greater trochanter and lateral lip of linea aspera. The vastus intermedius arises from the anterior surface of the femoral shaft and radiates into the capsule of the knee joint. The vastus medialis arises from the medial lip of linea aspera and the distal portion of the intertrochanteric line. The four muscles join to form a common tendon that inserts into the patella (Fig. 36–4). The semimembranosus muscle is the strongest flexor of the knee joint and the most effective internal rotator. It arises from the ischial tuberosity and continues to the medial tibial condyle and oblique popliteal ligament. The long head of the biceps femoris originates at the ischial tuberosity, the short head originates at the posterior surface of the femur, and both unite to insert into the head of the fibula. The biceps femoris functions as an external rotator of the leg when the knee joint is flexed. The semitendinosus muscle arises from the ischial tuberosity and runs medially toward the tibial tuberosity to join the pes anserinus. The medial and lateral gastrocnemius originate just proximal to their respective femoral condyles. Some of the fibers from both heads also arise from the knee joint capsule. They join the tendon of the soleus to form the Achilles' tendon, which inserts on the calcaneal tuberosity. The popliteal muscle arises from the lateral femoral condyle and inserts on the posterior surface of the tibia to flex the knee joint and medially rotate the leg.

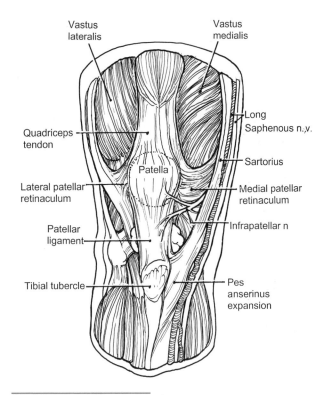

Figure 36–4 Outer layer of the knee joint.

The knee joint is vascularized by branches of the femoral, popliteal, anterior tibial, and posterior tibial arteries. The femoral artery runs through the adductor canal and passes through the adductor hiatus to the popliteal fossa. It becomes the popliteal artery on the dorsal side of the thigh. The popliteal artery lies immediately behind the posterior joint capsule in the midline and is adjacent to the medial head of the gastrocnemius. It gives off branches to flexors near the knee joint and supplies the knee joint with five genicular arteries. It is accompanied by the paired popliteal veins.

Nerve branches to the knee joint arise from the fibular nerve, which supplies the short head of the biceps femoris and the tibial nerve, which supplies the long head of the biceps femoris, the semitendinosus, semimembranosus, both heads of the gastrocnemius, the popliteus; the saphenous nerve; and the common peroneal nerve. The common peroneal nerve descends superficially anterior to the biceps femoris tendon. It crosses over the lateral head of the gastrocnemius distally and winds around the neck of the fibula.

Surgical Approaches
Medial Parapatellar

A midline longitudinal incision is used starting several inches proximal to superior the pole of the patella and extending 2-3 inches distal to the knee joint. A medial parapatellar incision is then made. The rectus tendon is divided longitudinally and the capsule is incised medial to the patella and patellar tendon. Access to the knee joint is possible through

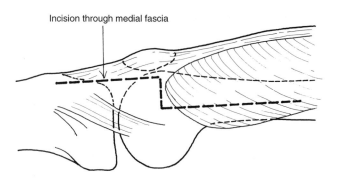

Figure 36–5 Medial parapatellar incision used for subvastus approach.

eversion of the patella. Eversion can be facilitated by a proximal release of the lateral quadriceps. Eversion should be done carefully to avoid avulsion of the patellar tendon, a devastating complication of TKA.

Midvastus

The midvastus approach is an alteration of the standard midline approach leaving the quadriceps tendon intact and splits the vastus medialis muscle. It also has the advantage of stability of the patellofemoral joint.

Subvastus

Several advantages of the subvastus approach are that there is less pain and quadriceps inhibition and the patella tracking is improved. An anterior longitudinal skin incision is used.

A medial parapatellar incision is made from the tibial tubercle to 1 cm distal to the insertion of the vastus medialis. The dissection is extended posteriorly, through the retinaculam over to the vastus medialis insertion (Fig. 36–5). The vastus is elevated from the intermuscular septum and anterior surface of the femur. With lateral retraction the anterior surface of the knee is exposed (Fig. 36–6).

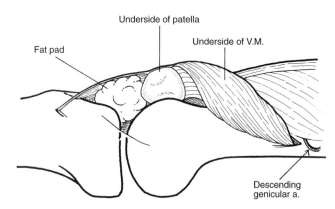

Figure 36–6 Elevation of vastus off the anterior surface of the femur exposing the knee joint.

Tibial Tubercle Osteotomy

Osteotomy of the tibial tubercle may be helpful when extensive exposure is necessary. It is also useful when realignment of the quadriceps mechanism is necessary for patellar tracking problems. Osteotomy should be considered any time that the patellar tendon is at risk of avulsion from the tibial tubercle during eversion of the patella.

The periosteum is elevated off of the medial aspect of the tibial tubercle. Using a small, straight osteotome, a transverse cut is made in the anterior cortex of the tibia just proximal to the insertion of the patellar tendon (Fig. 36–7). This cut provides a buttress to prevent proximal migration of the osteotomized tibial tubercle. An oscillating saw is used to create an osteotomy fragment approximately 2 cm wide, 1 cm thick, and at least 7 cm long (Fig. 36–7b). The osteotomy is completed distally with a curved osteotome. Care is taken to leave the periosteum attached to the distal aspect of the fragment and the muscles of the anterior compartment are left

attached to the lateral margin of the fragment (Figs. 36–7c and 36–7d). At the completion of the arthroplasty, the tubercle fragment is positioned for optimal tracking of the patella and temporarily fixed with an obliquely placed K-wire. Permanent fixation is accomplished with two 6.5-mm titanium cancellous screws engaging the posterior cortex (Fig. 36–7e). Alternatively, a cerclage wire or cable can be passed around the proximal portion of the osteotomized fragment (Fig. 36–7f).

SPECIFIC CONDITIONS, TREATMENT, AND OUTCOME

Osteoarthritis

The management of the osteoarthritic knee begins with activity modification including low-impact exercise, weight loss, and use of a cane on the contralateral side. Oral nonsteroidal

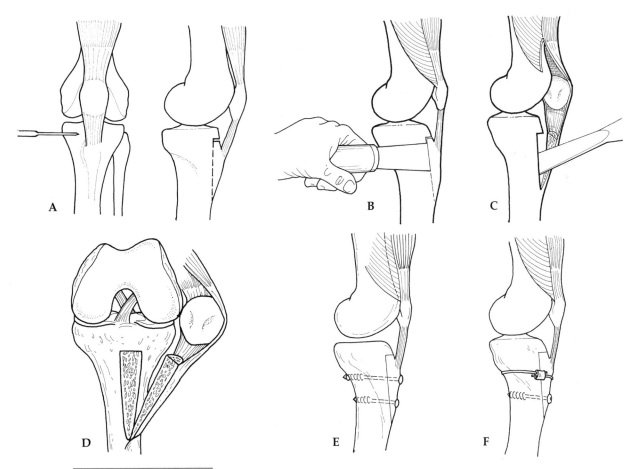

Figure 36–7 Technique for osteotomy of tibial tubercle. **(A)** Transverse cut in anterior cortex of tibia. **(B)** Oscillating saw creates longitudinal component of osteotomy. **(C)** Osteotome used to elevate tibial tubercle. **(D)** Patella everted leaving periosteum and muscle attached laterally and distally. **(E)** Fixation of tibial tubercle with two 6.5-mm cancellous screws. **(F)** Fixation of tibial tubercle with cable and cancellous screw.

anti-inflammatory agents or intra-articular injections of steroids may provide substantial pain relief. Physical therapy may help maintain a functional range of motion and adequate muscle tone. Full arc extension exercises should be avoided. Terminal arc exercises (20 degrees flexion to full extension), straight leg raising, and isometric quadriceps exercises can strengthen the quadriceps without exacerbating patello-femoral symptoms.

Injection of hyaluronic acid is a relatively new form of treatment for osteoarthritis at an early stage (Adams et al, 1995). These supplements address the pathophysiology affecting the joint, thus relieving pain. They may restore elasticity and improve viscosity by mimicking the physical properties of normal synovial fluid. The patient who fails nonoperative management may be offered one of the forms of treatment listed below.

Arthroscopic Debridement

In cases of moderate degenerative diseases, athroscopic debridement may provide pain relief. A simple arthroscopic debridement includes joint lavage, removal of meniscal fragments, and loose debris. Extensive procedures, such as drilling of subchondral bone and abrasion arthroplasty are unpredictable. The clinical outcome in patients with severe arthritis is poor.

Osteotomy

The aim of an osteotomy of the femur or tibia is to transfer weight-bearing loads to an uninvolved tibiofemoral joint surface and to realign the anatomical axis of the limb. Osteotomy is indicated in young, active patients with selected mild to moderate unicompartmental degenerative arthritis and with good motion of the knee.

Medial Compartment Disease

Valgus osteotomy of the proximal tibia is indicated for medial compartment osteoarthritis with less than 15 degrees of a fixed varus deformity and an intact lateral compartment. Contraindications include flexion contracture of > 15 degrees, flexion less than 90 degrees, and lateral subluxation of the tibia on the femur greater than 1 cm. A relative contraindication is the patient who is physiologically older than 60 years. Different techniques of osteotomy fixation have been reported. The standard method is the lateral closing wedge osteotomy with staple fixation but cast immobilization without staples or internal fixation with plates are also acceptable options. External fixators have recently been reported. Opening wedge osteotomy from the medial side is helpful if the extremity is short or the collateral ligament is lax (Fig. 36–8). The goal is an overcorrection of the tibiofemoral axis to 7 to 10 degrees.

Complications include over or undercorrection, penetration of the articular tibia surface, nonunion, compartment syndrome, patella infera, and peroneal nerve palsy. TKA may be more difficult following osteotomy because of patella baja.

Despite the success of total knee replacement, the high tibia osteotomy maintains an important role in the management of osteoarthritis of the knee in the active young adult. Good results are maintained in about 60% of patients with an average 10-year followup.

Lateral Compartment Disease

A closing wedge osteotomy of the distal femur is usually performed for unicompartmental osteoarthritis involving the lateral compartment. Indications for femoral varus osteotomy include a tibiofemoral axis greater than 12 degrees and 10 degrees deviation of the knee joint from the horizontal. Contraindications are a poor range of motion, geriatric patients, and morbid obesity.

Unicompartmental Arthroplasty

Unicompartmental arthroplasty can be performed in cases with single compartment arthritis, when high tibial osteotomy is not indicated. Superior results of this procedure depend on the right patient selection (Fig. 36–9).

Compared with total knee replacement, the advantages of the "uni" are the preservation of bone stock and cruciate ligaments, leaving the knee with nearly normal kinematics. A decreased recovery time and a full range of motion is another advantage. Contraindications to the procedure are younger patients, obesity, extreme deformities of the tibiofemoral axis, ACL sufficiency, a severely decreased range of motion, and inflammatory arthritis. Technically, the tibial implant should be placed at right angles to the tibia axis. The mechanical axis should fall over the implant. Complications include polyethelene wear debris and loosening.

Total Knee Arthroplasty

Total knee arthroplasty is indicated in cases of symptomatic arthritis that involves at least two compartments. Contraindications include a failed extensor mechanism, active sepsis, prior surgical fusion, and a neuropathic knee. The goals of a TKA are the restoration of the anatomic and mechanical axis, a horizontal joint in stance phase of gait, an

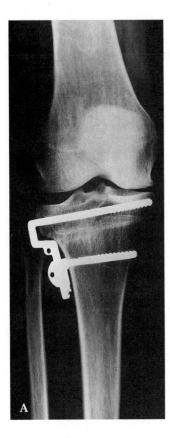
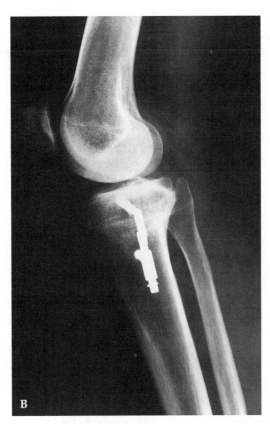

Figure 36–8 **(A)** An AP and **(B)** lateral radiograph of the right knee following high tibia osteotomy of a 47-year-old man.

equal flexion and extension gap, ligament balance, and a proper patellar tracking.

To achieve these goals, certain implant designs have been developed. The most common are the unconstrained "resurfacing" implants that either allow preservation or substitution ("posterior stabilized") of the PCL. Retaining the PCL has potential advantages and disadvantages. The PCL maintains the normal kinematics of the knee and its proprioception function. However, if the PCL has been preserved and is tight in flexion it can cause polyethylene wear. Soft tissue balancing is technically easier in PCL-substituting implants because of exposure and goal of balanced flexion and extension gaps. Constrained implants are used in unstable knees especially after failed TKAs. Constrained implants are associated with an increased rate of tibial or femoral loosening (because of increased stress at the bone-cement interface), polyethylene wear, and higher infection rates.

Preoperative planning of TKA must include an exact templating using a full-length radiograph of the lower extremity. To achieve anatomic alignment, the tibia may be cut at 0 degrees with a slight slope and the femur at 5 to 7 degrees of valgus. A notch of the anterior femoral cortex should be avoided. Maximal coverage of the tibial plateau is essential to get cortical support. If the patella is resurfaced, the original thickness should be restored. Patellar alignment is enhanced by placing the femoral component in slight external rotation, and the tibial tray in external rotation (thus internally rotating the tibial tubercle). After the surfaces have been cut, trial components should be inserted to check the alignment, the flexion and extension gap, soft tissue balancing, patellar tracking, and the range of motion. An increased flexion gap (tight in

extension and loose in flexion) can be corrected by re-cutting the distal femur and using a thicker tibial component. If the knee is stable in full extension, but is tight in flexion, the tibia may be cut with more posterior slope, the posterior cruciate recessed more, and use of a smaller femoral component. It may be necessary to excise the posterior cruciate and substitute a PCL substituting knee. In cases in which the joint is tight in both positions, an additional cut of the proximal tibia should be made. If the patella tracks laterally, a lateral release has to be done. To prevent avascular necrosis of the patella with the risk of patella fractures, the superolateral geniculate artery should ideally be preserved. In cases of deficient bone stock or excessive defects, bone grafting is indicated. Complications of TKA include polyethylene wear (insert should be thicker than 8 mm), component loosening, abnormal patellofemoral tracking, decreased range of motion, supracondylar fracture, peroneal nerve palsy, and skin necroses.

Revision Arthroplasty

Pain following TKA has many causes. Identifying the source of pain is essential before considering revision surgery. Table 36–1 lists reasons for failure of TKA. Malalignment of knee replacement components may lead to failed arthroplasty by placing excessive loads on the components and the surrounding tissues (Table 36–2). Malalignment of the prosthesis warrants special consideration as it is a preventable and potentially correctable cause of failed TKA. Each component has the potential of 6 degrees of malposition; therefore, many combinations of malalignment are possible. Malrotated or translated components are the frequent offenders (see Table 36–3).

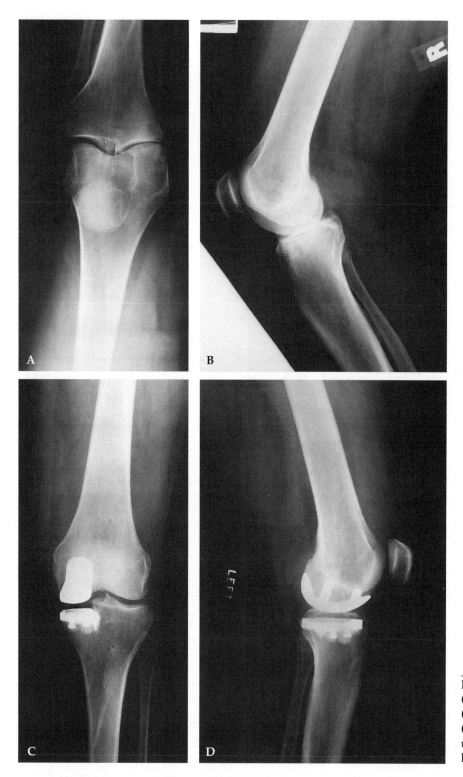

Figure 36–9   (A) Preoperative AP, **(B)** Preoperative lateral, **(C)** postoperative AP, and **(D)** postoperative lateral of a unicompartmental arthroplasty on the left knee of a 63-year-old woman.

It is essential to evaluate bone stock and the soft tissues such as the status of the extensor mechanism and ligaments. The original joint line should be restored if possible. Small bone defects can be filled with component spacer blocks and wedges. Large defects require bone grafts (Fig. 36–10). If the collateral ligaments are intact, a nonconstrained prosthesis can be used. Constrained implants are associated with higher failure rates secondary to implant loosening. In planning the surgical approach, parallel skin incisions should be avoided. A standard midline incision may not provide an appropriate approach to the joint. Alternative approaches may be necessary.

Arthrodesis

Indication for arthrodesis includes failed TKA joint destruction with severe damage of ligaments and extensor mechanism, uncontrollable septic arthritis, and neuropathic joint disease. The fusion should be performed in 10 to 15 degrees

TABLE 36–1   Potential causes of failed total knee arthroplasty

Infection (0.5–1%)
Aseptic loosening (1–10%)
Malalignment
Knee instability (0–5%)
Polyethylene Wear (0.5%/year)
Painful neuroma
Stiffness

TABLE 36–2   Deleterious effects of a malaligned total knee prosthesis.

Bone overload
Ligament overload
Polyethylene overload
Knee instability

TABLE 36–3   Common types of malaligned knee replacement components.

Femoral component in flexion
Femoral component internally rotated
Tibial component in varus
Tibial component anteriorly sloped
Tibial component internally rotated
Tibial component medially displaced
Patella laterally displaced

of flexion and 0 to 7 degrees of valgus. Techniques for fixation include intramedullary fixation or an external fixator. Fusion rates are higher after a failed constrained implant than after a hinged implant. Complications include malunion and nonunion.

Synovectomy

Synovectomy is most commonly used in knees with rheumatoid arthritis. Indications are chronic synovial proliferation with swelling and pain without arthritic changes. The results are superior when the procedure is performed at an early stage without severe joint deconstruction. Good results have been achieved with both open and arthroscopic techniques. Advantage of the arthroscopic approach is the decreased recovery time.

PEARL

The most common cause of malaligned components is poor exposure, varus orientation and internal rotation of the tibial component.

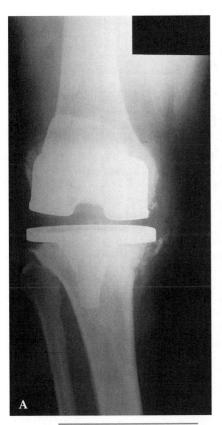
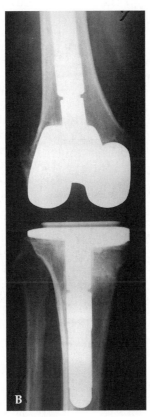
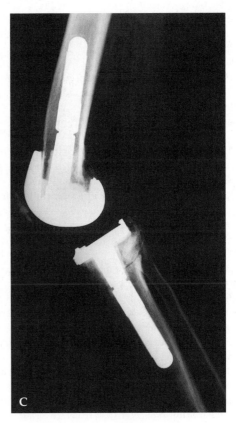

Figure 36–10 **(A)** AP radiograph of a right knee with a loosened TKA of a 71-year-old woman. **(B)** An AP and **(C)** lateral radiograph of the TKA revision with bone grafting of tibia defect using a femoral head.

SELECTED BIBLIOGRAPHY

ADAMS ME, ATKINSON MH, LUSSIER AJ, SCHULZ JI, SIMINOVITCH KA, WADE JP, ZUMMER M. The role of viscosupplementation with hylan G-F 20 (Synvisc) in the treatment of osteoarthritis of the knee: a Canadian multicenter trial comparing hylan G-F 20 alone, hylan G-F 20 with nonsteroidal anti-inflammatory drugs (NSAIDs) and NSAIDs alone. *Osteoarthritis Cartilage.* 1995;3:213–225.

ASP JP, RAND JA. Peroneal nerve palsy after total knee arthroplasty. *Clin Orthop.* 1990;261:233–237.

BAUMGAERTNER MR, CANNON WD Jr, VITTORI JM, SCHMIDT ES, MAURER RC. Arthroscopic debridement of the arthritic knee. *Clin Orthop.* 1990;253:197–202.

BAYLEY JC, SCOTT RD, EWALD FC, HOLMES GB Jr. Failure of the metal-backed patellar component after total knee replacement. *J Bone Jt Surg.* 1988;70A:668–674.

BERMAN AT, BOSACCO SJ, KIRSHNER S, AVOLIO A Jr. Factors influencing long-term results in high tibial osteotomy. *Clin Orthop.* 1991;272:192–198.

BOOTH RE Jr, LOTKE PA. The results of Spacer Block Technique in revision of infected total knee arthroplasty. *Clin Orthop.* 1989;248:57–60.

BURGER RR, BASCH T, HOPSON CN. Implant salvage in infected total knee arthroplasty. *Clin Orthop.* 1991;273:105–112.

COLLIER JP, McNAMARA JL, SURPRENANT VA, JENSEN RE, SURPRENANT HP. All polyethylene patellar components are not the answer. *Clin Orthop.* 1991;273:198–203.

COLLIER JP, MAYOR MB, McNAMARA JL, SURPRENANT VA, JENSEN RE. Analysis of the failure of 122 polyethylene inserts from uncemented tibial knee components. *Clin Orthop.* 1991;273:232–242.

COLLINS DN, HEIM SA, NELSON CL, SMITH P III. Porous-coated anatomic total knee arthroplasty: a prospective analysis comparing cemented and cementless fixation. *Clin Orthop.* 1991;267:128–136.

COVENTRY MB. Upper tibial osteotomy for osteoarthritis. *J Bone Jt Surg.* 1985;67A:1136–1140.

DiGIOIA AM III, RUBASH HE. Periprosthetic fractures of the femur after total knee arthroplasty: a literature review and treatment algorithm. *Clin Orthop.* 1991;271:135–142.

DORR LD, BOIARDO RA. Technical considerations in total knee arthroplasty. *Clin Orthop.* 1986;205:5–11.

ELIA EA, LOTKE PA. Results of revision total knee arthroplasty associated with significant bone loss. *Clin Orthop.* 1991;271:114–121.

ENGLAND SP, STERN SH, INSALL JN, WINDSOR RE. Total knee arthroplasty in diabetes mellitus. *Clin Orthop.* 1990;260:130–134.

ENIS JE, GARDNER R, ROBLEDO MA, LATTA L, SMITH R. Comparison of patellar resurfacing versus nonresurfacing in bilateral total knee arthroplasty. *Clin Orthop.* 1990;260:38–42.

FIGGIE HE III, GOLDBERG VM, FIGGIE MP, INGLIS AE, KELLY M, SOBEL M. The effect of alignment of the implant on fractures of the patella after condylar total knee arthroplasty. *J Bone Jt Surg.* 1989;71A:1031–1039.

FIGGIE MP, GOLDBERG VM, FIGGIE HE III, HEIPLE KG, SOBEL M. Total knee arthroplasty for the treatment of chronic hemophilic arthropathy. *Clin Orthop.* 1989;248:98–107.

FRIEDMAN RJ, HIRST P, POSS R, KELLEY K, SLEDGE CB. Results of revision total knee arthroplasty performed for aseptic loosening. *Clin Orthop.* 1990;255:235–241.

FRIEDMAN RJ, FRIEDRICH LV, WHITE RL, KAYS MB, BRUNDAGE DM, GRAHAM J. Antibiotic prophylaxis and tourniquet inflation in total knee arthroplasty. *Clin Orthop.* 1990;260:17–23.

GOLDBERG VM, FIGGIE MP, FIGGIE HE III, HEIPLE KG, SOBEL M. Use of a total condylar knee prosthesis for treatment of osteoarthritis and rheumatoid arthritis: long-term results. *J Bone Jt Surg.* 1988;70A:802–811.

GOLDBERG VM, FIGGIE MP, FIGGIE HE III, SOBEL M. The results of revision total knee arthroplasty. *Clin Orthop.* 1988;226:86–92.

HOLDEN DL, JAMES SL, LARSON RL, and SLOCUM DB. Proximal tibial osteotomy in patients who are 50 years old or less: A long-term follow-up study. *J Bone Jt Surg.* 1988;70A:977–982.

INSALL JN and KELLY M. The total condylar prosthesis. *Clin Orthop.* 1986;205:43–48.

LANDY MM and WALKER PS. Wear of ultra-high molecular weight polyethylene components of 90 retrieved knee prosthesis. *J Arthroplasty.* 3(suppl):1988;573–585.

LOTKE PA, FARALLI VJ, ORENSTEIN EM, ECKER ML. Blood loss after total knee replacement: effects of tourniquet release and continuous passive motion. *J Bone Jt Surg.* 1991;73A:1037–1040.

LUSSIER A, CIVIDINO AA, McFARLANE CA, OLSZYNSKI WP, POTASHNER WJ, DE MEDICIS R. Visculosupplementation with hylan for the treatment of osteoarthritis: findings from clinical practice in Canada. *J Rheum.* 1996;23:1579–1585.

LYNCH AF, BOURNE RB, RORABECK CH, RANKIN RN, DONALD A. Deep-vein thrombosis and continuous passive motion after total knee arthroplasty. *J Bone Jt Surg.* 1988;70A:11–14.

MARQUEST P. Mechanics and osteoarthritis of the patellofemoral joint. *Clin Orthop.* 1979;144:70–73.

McDERMOTT AG, FINKLESTEIN JA, FARINE I, BOYNTON EL, MACINTOSH DL, GROSS A. Distal femoral varus osteotomy for valgus deformity of the knee. *J Bone Jt Surg.* 1988;70A:110–116.

OGILVIE-HARRIS DJ, BASINSKI A. Arthroscopic synovectomy of the knee for rheumatoid arthritis. *Arthroscopy* 1991;7:91–97.

PADGETT DE, STERN SH, INSALL JN. Revision total knee arthroplasty for failed unicompartmental replacement. *J Bone Jt Surg.* 1991;73A:186–190.

PICETTI GD III, McGANN WA WELCH RB. The patellofemoral joint after total knee arthroplasty without patellar resurfacing. *J Bone Jt Surg.* 1990;72A:1379–1382.

PRODROMOS CC, ANDRIACCHI TP, GALANTE JO. A relationship between gait and clinical changes following high tibial osteotomy. *J Bone Jt Surg.* 1985;67A:1188–1194.

RANAWAT CS, PADGETT DE, OHASHI Y. Total knee arthroplasty for patients younger than 55 years. *Clin Orthop.* 1989;248:27–33.

RAND JA, ILSTRUP DM. Survivorship analysis of total knee

arthroplasty: cumulative rates of survival of 9200 total knee arthroplasties. *J Bone Jt Surg.* 1991;73A:391–409.

RAND JA. Alternatives to re-implantation for salvage of the total knee arthroplasty complicated by infection. *Instruct Course Lect.* 1993;42:341–347.

RITTER MA, FECHTMAN RA. Proximal tibial osteotomy: a survivorship analysis. *Arthroplasty.* 1988;3:309–311.

ROSENBERG TD, PAULOS LE, PARKER RD, COWARD DB, SCOTT SM. The 45-degree posteroanterior flexion weight-bearing radiograph of the knee. *J Bone Jt Surg.* 1988;70A: 1479–1483.

RUDAN JF, SIMURDA MA. High tibial osteotomy: a prospective clinical and roentgenographic review. *Clin Orthop.* 1990; 255:251–256.

SCHNEIDER R, ABENAVOLI AM, SOUNDRY M, INSTALL J. Failure of total condylar knee replacements: correlation of radiographic, clinical, and surgical findings. *Radiology.* 1984; 152:309–315.

SCHOIFET SD, MORREY BF. Treatment of infection after total knee arthroplasty by debridement with retention of the components. *J Bone Jt Surg.* 1990;72A: 1383–1390.

SCOTT RD, SANTORE RF. Unicondylar unicompartmental replacement for osteoarthritis of the knee. *J Bone Jt Surg.* 1990;63A:536–544.

SCOTT RD, COBB AG, McQUEARY FG, THORNHILL TS. Unicompartmental knee arthroplasty; eight- to twelve-year follow-up evaluation with survivorship analysis. *Clin Orthop.* 1991;271:96–100.

SCUDERI GR, INSALL JN, WINDSOR RE, MORAN MC. Survivorship of cemented knee replacements. *J Bone Jt Surg.* 1989; 71B:798–803.

SHOJI H, YOSHINO S, KAJINO A. Patellar replacement in bilat-

eral total knee arthroplasty: a study of patients who had rheumatoid arthritis and no gross deformity of the patella. *J Bone Jt Surg.* 1989;71A:853–856.

SMITH BE, ASKEW MJ, GRADISAR IA Jr, GRADISAR JS, LEW MM. The effect of patient weight on the functional outcome of total knee arthroplasty. *Clin Orthop.* 1992;276:237–244.

STAEHELI JW, CASS JR, MORREY BF. Condylar total knee arthroplasty after failed proximal tibial osteotomy. *J Bone Jt Surg.* 1987;69A:28–31.

STERN SH, INSALL JN. Total knee arthroplasty in obese patients. *J Bone Jt Surg.* 1990;72A:1400–1404.

VINCE KG, INSALL JN, KELLY MA. The total condylar prosthesis: ten- to twelve-year results of a cemented knee replacement. *J Bone Jt Surg Br.* 1989;71B:793–797.

WANG J, KUO KN, ADRIACCHI TP, GALANTE JO. The influence of walking mechanics and time on the results of proximal tibial osteotomy. *J Bone Jt Surg.* 1990;72A:905–909.

WILSON MG, KELLEY K, THORNHILL TS. Infection as a complication of total knee replacement arthroplasty: risk factors and treatment in 67 cases. *J Bone Jt Surg.* 1990;72A: 878–883.

WINDSOR RE, INSALL JN, VINCE KE. Technical consideration of total knee arthroplasty after proximal tibial osteotomy. *J Bone Jt Surg.* 1988;70A:547–555.

WINDSOR RE, INSALL JN, URS WK. Two-stage reimplantation for the salvage of total knee arthroplasty complicated by infection: further follow-up and refinement of indications. *J Bone Jt Surg.* 1990;72A:272–278.

WRIGHT J, EWALD FC, WALKER PS. Total knee arthroplasty with the kinematic prosthesis: results after 5 to 9 years: a follow-up note. *J Bone Jt Surg.* 1990;72A:1003–1009.

SAMPLE QUESTIONS

1. After high tibial osteotomy, complications when performing subsequent total knee arthroplasty commonly include:
   (a) elevation of joint line
   (b) medial collateral ligamentous instability
   (c) patella baja
   (d) patella alta
   (e) a, b, and c

2. To facilitate tracking of the patella during total knee arthroplasty, components should be positioned as follows:
   (a) centering of femoral component
   (b) medialization of patellar component
   (c) external rotation of tibial tray
   (d) medialization of patella
   (e) a and d

3. When performing a high tibial osteotomy correction, the anatomic axis should near:
   (a) 6 degrees valgus

   (b) 9 degrees valgus
   (c) 10 to 13 degrees valgus
   (d) 7 degrees of varus from the mechanical axis

4. When performing a cruciate retaining TKA with a tight flexion gap and loose extension gap, the surgeon should:
   (a) insert smaller polyethelene tray
   (b) release posterior cruciate ligament
   (c) insert smaller femoral component
   (d) resect posterior condyles of the tibia
   (e) resect more distal femur

5. Contraindications to high tibial osteotomy include:
   (a) patellar femoral arthrosis
   (b) 5 degrees flexion contracture
   (c) anterior cruciate disruption
   (d) age greater than 50
   (e) lateral meniscal tear

Answers: 1) c; 2) c; 3) b; 4) b; 5) c

Foot and Ankle

Section

XI

Chapter 37

Foot and Ankle Trauma

John T. Campbell, MD and Lew C. Schon, MD

Foot and ankle trauma is common in nearly any orthopaedic surgeon's practice. These injuries may be due to motor vehicle crashes, industrial accidents, sporting activities, penetrating trauma, and even low-energy twisting injuries. Historically, such injuries have been managed nonoperatively. In addition, attention to cranial, thoracic, abdominal, and long-bone fractures in the multiply injured patient may result in delayed or "missed" diagnosis. Foot and ankle trauma can result in substantial long-term morbidity with impairment of work, daily living, and recreational activities. Thus, recent trends in foot and ankle trauma include heightened diagnostic awareness and more aggressive, operative care to minimize such morbidity.

This chapter intends to provide practical information about selected topics to assist the orthopaedic surgeon in managing foot and ankle injuries. Evolving attitudes in treatment modalities will be emphasized.

FOREFOOT

Fractures of the metatarsals and phalanges are common entities due to the exposed position of these structures and the low amount of energy required to cause their injury. Both metatarsal and phalangeal fractures can occur by indirect mechanism, such as twisting injuries, but most result from direct trauma such as dropping a heavy object onto the foot. High-energy injuries, as those from motor vehicle accidents or close-range gunshots, occur less often. High-energy and crush injuries may cause substantial superficial and deep soft-tissue injury.

Treatment of metatarsal fractures depends on the degree of fracture displacement. Displacement must be assessed both clinically and radiographically. Nondisplaced or minimally displaced fractures can be treated with a short-leg cast or a hard-sole shoe with progressive weight-bearing over several weeks. Substantial displacement (> 2 mm) or angulation (> 10 degrees) may require reduction to minimize complications such as malunion, clawtoes, or stress-transfer metatarsalgia due to redistribution of weight-bearing on the metatarsal heads. Displacement or angulation may be less well tolerated in the first and fifth metatarsal and may pose shoe-wearing problems. Closed reduction can be performed using finger traps to realign the fractured metatarsal. If the reduction remains stable, immobilization will complete the treatment; however, an unstable reduction requires percutaneous pinning. If closed reduction is unsuccessful or if multiple metatarsals are fractured, overall alignment of the foot can be restored through open reduction and internal fixation (ORIF) with Kirschner wires (K-wires) or screws and plates (Fig. 37–1). For severe crush injuries or open fractures, percutaneous pinning or small external fixation frames can maintain the bony architecture and allow soft-tissue healing.

Fractures of the base of the fifth metatarsal constitute a unique subset of metatarsal fractures and typically result

Orthopaedic Surgery: The Essentials. Edited by M.E. Baratz, A.D. Watson, and J.E. Imbriglia. Thieme Medical Publishers, Inc., New York © 1999

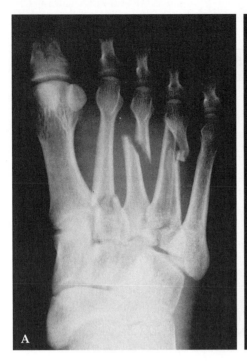
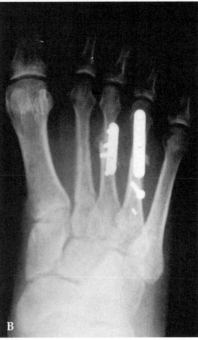

Figure 37–1 Preoperative **(A)** and postoperative **(B)** anteroposterior (AP) views of multiple displaced metatarsal fractures stabilized with mini AO plates and screws. [Reproduced with permission from Schon LC, Marks RM: The management of neuroarthropathic fracture-dislocations in the diabetic patient. *Orthop Clin North Am* 1995;26:375–392.]

from a twisting injury. Avulsion fractures of the fifth metatarsal tuberosity can be managed with immobilization in a short-leg walking cast or a hard-sole shoe. Nonunions are rare, and typically asymptomatic. Surgical management of these injuries should be considered in the high-performance athlete with a severely displaced fracture or a symptomatic nonunion. Simple excision of the fragment is sufficient.

Fracture of the metadiaphyseal region of the fifth metatarsal, with extension into the metatarsocuboid or intermetatarsal joint, is notoriously prone to delayed union or nonunion and can result in prolonged morbidity. Nondisplaced fractures in this region can be successfully treated by strict non–weight-bearing in a short-leg cast. Displaced fractures or delayed union may require intramedullary screw fixation or open bone grafting.

Distal phalanx fractures are usually treated nonoperatively with the use of a hard-sole shoe. These fractures may present with nail bed laceration and subungual hematoma. Treatment involves a digital block with local anesthetic, removal of the nail plate, debridement, reduction of the fracture site, closure of the nail-bed laceration, and placement of the nail plate or nonadherent dressing as a stent into the nail fold. Nondisplaced middle and proximal phalanx fractures can be treated by immobilization with "buddy-taping" to an adjacent digit. Displaced fractures are managed with closed reduction and buddy-taping. Intra-articular fractures or the rare displaced middle or proximal phalanx fracture that remains unstable after reduction may require K-wire pinning to maintain reduction.

TARSOMETATARSAL JOINTS

Etiology

Injuries of the tarsometatarsal joints can occur by both high- or low-energy indirect or direct mechanisms. Examples of indirect, low-energy injuries include:

1. twisting of the forefoot, such as in a simple mis-step, with supination/pronation or abduction/adduction forces applied to the forefoot;
2. an axial load applied to the posterior hindfoot while the forefoot is held in extreme plantarflexion. This disrupts the dorsal soft tissues and permits dorsal dislocation of the joints (common, for example, among athletes such as a football lineman, when another player lands on the posterior heel while the ball of the foot is held by the turf).

An indirect, high-energy injury can be produced in a motor vehicle accident when the foot is held plantarflexed against the floorboard at the moment of impact, and an additional axial load is applied. Direct injuries are usually low-energy injuries such as those that occur when a heavy object is dropped on the dorsum of the foot. Industrial accidents, high-velocity gunshot injuries, and lawn-mower injuries are examples of high-energy direct injuries.

Anatomy, Surgical Approaches, and Selected Basic Science

The three-dimensional osseous anatomy of the tarsometatarsal joints is complex (Fig. 37–2). The bases of the metatarsals and their corresponding tarsal bones form a transverse arch with a dorsal apex centrally. The bones that make up this transverse arch are wider dorsally than plantarly to confer stability. The second tarsometatarsal joint is more proximal than the neighboring first and third joints. This "keystone" formation of the second metatarsal base makes the joint more rigid than the other tarsometatarsal joints.

The plantar tarsometatarsal, intertarsal, and intermetatarsal ligaments and joint capsules are stronger than their dorsal counterparts. Noteworthy among these is Lisfranc's ligament, which attaches to the medial cuneiform and the base of the second metatarsal. This structure stabilizes the base of the second metatarsal in its mortise and to the first

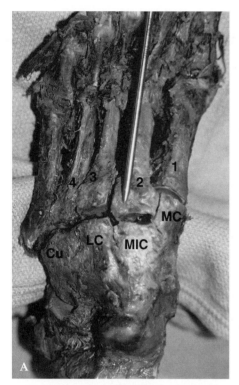

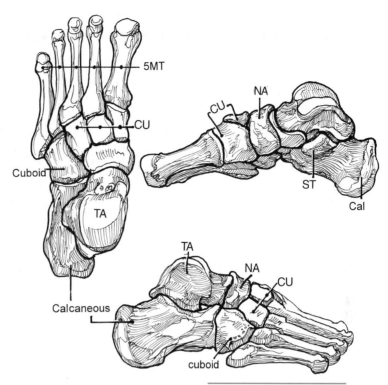

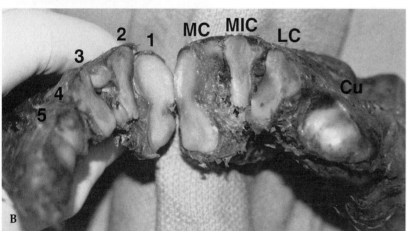

Figure 37–2 Dissected Lisfranc (tarsometatarsal) joint complex. 1, first metatarsal; 2, second metatarsal; 3, third metatarsal; 4, fourth metatarsal; 5, fifth metatarsal; MC, medial cuneiform; MIC, middle cuneiform; LC, lateral cuneiform; Cu, cuboid. **(A)** Left: Dorsal perspective with metal probe demonstrating the keystone configuration of the second metatarsal base. Right: Osseous anatomy of tarsometatarsal meant joints; MT, metatarsal; CU, cuneiform; TA, talus; NA, navicular; ST, sustentaculum tali; Cal, calcaneus. **(B)** Lateral view demonstrating the tarsometatarsal articulations.

ray. There is no direct ligamentous stabilization of the first and second metatarsal bases to each other. The plantar fascia and the intrinsic flexor musculature are secondary stabilizers. The clinical consequence of the tarsometatarsal bony and ligamentous anatomy is that tarsometatarsal disruption typically includes dorsal subluxation of the metatarsals and diastasis between the first ray and the complex of lesser rays.

PEARL

Lisfranc's ligament is a strong plantar ligament that connects the base of the second metatarsal to the medial cuneiform.

Several local structures can be jeopardized by tarsometatarsal injuries. The deep peroneal artery, a continuation of the anterior tibial artery from the leg, crosses the ankle and midfoot to plunge between the bases of the first and second metatarsals. In this location it may be injured during tarsometataursal dislocation. Severe dislocation can produce traction or compression injuries to the deep peroneal, sural, saphenous, and superficial peroneal nerves. Finally, the anterior tibialis tendon can become entrapped in the first metatarsal-cuneiform joint, preventing closed reduction attempts.

Surgical approaches are centered over the tarsometatarsal joint level. A midline medial incision can provide excellent exposure of the first metatarsal-cuneiform joint. Sharp dissection through the skin and subcutaneous tissues is carried out, protecting crossing branches of the saphenous nerve. The superficial fascia of the abductor hallucis muscle is incised, and the muscle fibers are bluntly reflected plantarward, revealing the underlying deep muscle fascia and the periosteal-capsular sleeve. Dissection should follow the path of the hematoma down to the bones and joint for reduction and fixation. Dorsal incisions can be made between the first and second metatarsals and between the third and fourth metatarsals. Full-thickness flaps are raised carefully to avoid undermining, which may result in skin necrosis. The extensor retinaculum is incised, and the tendons are carefully retracted. The neurovascular bundle is identified coursing from deep to the extensor hallucis brevis tendon toward the interval between the first and second metatarsals. It is protected during the remainder of the exposure. The joint capsules are incised, and subperiosteal dissection is performed to reveal the fracture-dislocation. These incisions can be combined as dictated by the particular fracture pattern.

Examination

A patient with a midfoot fracture-dislocation typically presents with a grossly deformed foot and marked swelling (Fig. 37–3). A minimally displaced sprain can present with more subtle symptoms and little malalignment or instability. The clinician should check for open wounds, evaluate the neurovascular status of the foot, and assess sensation in each of the peripheral nerves of the foot. Tendons should be palpated and evaluated for function.

It is imperative to examine for the presence of compartment syndrome, which may be manifested by tense swelling of the foot, pain out of proportion to the injury pattern, and severe pain with passive motion of the involved muscle compartments. Vascular or neurological impairment occurs late in compartment syndrome. Measurement of intracompartmental pressures may serve as a useful adjunct, particularly for the unconscious, intoxicated, or multiply injured patient. Compartment syndrome requires emergent fasciotomy to minimize complications due to ischemia.

PEARL
Compartment syndrome of the foot presents as swelling and severe pain that is exacerbated with passive stretch of the muscle compartment involved.

More subtle tarsometatarsal sprains should be suspected in a patient with midfoot pain or swelling, a history that

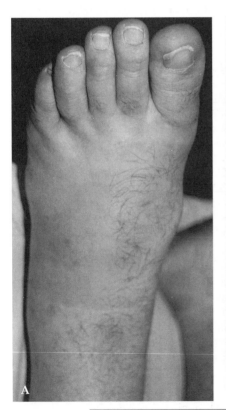 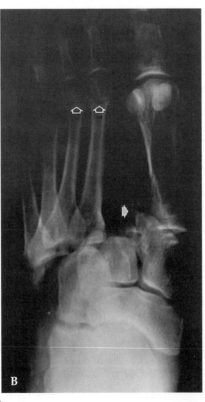 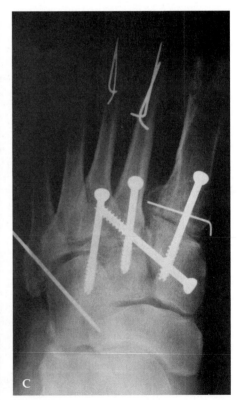

Figure 37–3 This 38-year-old male presented with a swollen left foot secondary to fracture-dislocations of the tarsometatarsal joints. **(A)** Clinical photograph. **(B)** AP radiograph. The solid arrow indicates the "fleck sign" of fracture fragment off the base of the second metatarsal. The open arrows indicate displaced second and third metatarsal neck fractures. **(C)** AP radiograph demonstrating 4.5-mm cannulated screw fixation of the first, second, and third metatarsal cuneiform joints; pinning of the fifth metatarsocuboid joint; and cross-pin fixation of the second and third metatarsal neck fractures.

describes one of the common mechanisms of injury, and tender tarsometatarsal joints. The pronation-abduction test, wherein the examiner pronates and abducts the forefoot relative to the midfoot, will reproduce pain when an acute ligamentous injury is present.

While the patient is waiting for radiographic evaluation and definitive treatment, the injured extremity should be immobilized in a splint and elevated with ice applied. Any gross deformity should be reduced to preserve the circulation to the foot, even if radiographs have not yet been obtained.

Aids to Diagnosis

Radiographs are essential in the diagnosis and treatment of injuries to the tarsometatarsal joints. A standard radiographic series includes anteroposterior (AP), oblique, and lateral views. Gross displacement is usually evident. If not, the films should be carefully examined to ensure that the cortical surfaces of the metatarsal bases are collinear with the cortical surfaces of their respective tarsal bones.

The AP view is the best view to show the bases of the first and second metatarsals, the medial and middle cuneiforms, the intermetatarsal joint, and the intertarsal joint. A "fleck" sign may be present, representing a small fragment of bone avulsed from the base of the second metatarsal by the strong, Lisfranc's ligament (see Fig. 37–3B). Even if the second metatarsal base is aligned within its bony mortise, the presence of a fleck sign implies a spontaneously reduced second tarsometatarsal dislocation. There may be a fracture of the second metatarsal base that occurred as it remained locked securely in its mortise while the remainder of the forefoot was abducted or adducted. Isolated injury to the first metatarsal-cuneiform joint with otherwise intact tarsometatarsal joints may also be present.

The oblique view allows visualization of the lateral tarsometatarsal joints. The medial cortex of the base of the fourth metatarsal should align exactly with the medial cortex of the cuboid. The oblique view may demonstrate a crush-type fracture of the cuboid ("nutcracker" injury) that results from compression of this primarily cancellous bone by an abducted forefoot. The lateral view is used to evaluate the degree of dorsal subluxation or dislocation of the metatarsal bases and to check for malalignment of the metatarsal heads in the sagittal plane.

Tarsometatarsal joint injuries can be very subtle, without dramatic deformity or radiographically obvious fractures. Weight-bearing x-rays may demonstrate subluxation or diastasis in subtle injuries, but stress radiography may be necessary to document instability. Local or general anesthesia improves the examiner's ability to apply stress.

Computed tomography (CT) scanning is rarely necessary but may be useful in diagnosing subtle fracture-dislocations of the tarsometatarsal joints. It may also identify small intra-articular fracture fragments that are not evident on plain radiographs. Persistent joint incongruence or degenerative changes indicate past trauma in patients with chronic midfoot pain.

Bone scans and magnetic resonance imaging (MRI) may be helpful in diagnosing an occult injury or in evaluating chronic symptoms after a traumatic episode, but is not routinely used. Magnetic resonance imaging may have a role in research but is rarely useful in evaluating tarsometatarsal injuries.

Specific Conditions, Treatment, and Outcome

Several classification systems of tarsometatarsal injuries have been used. Hardcastle et al (1982) described three categories: total incongruity, partial (either medial or lateral) incongruity, and divergent injuries. Myerson and colleagues (1986) refined this system to encompass additional fracture-dislocation patterns. These classifications attempt to correlate the mechanism of injury with the radiographic pattern. The classifications were also devised to facilitate treatment planning. It is not yet known if they provide any prognostic information.

The most reliable predictor of outcome is the adequacy of reduction of the tarsometatarsal joints. Although chronic disability and post-traumatic arthritis can occur after an anatomic reduction, poor results are far more common after inadequate initial reduction or loss of reduction. The treatment goal is congruent, anatomic reduction of the tarsometatarsal joints with restoration of the bony architecture.

Nondisplaced, unstable injuries of the tarsometatarsal joints are uncommon, but may present as "ankle sprains." Many represent soft-tissue sprain injuries, especially in athletes. Stress radiography frequently demonstrates instability. Recently, treatment of nondisplaced tarsometatarsal injuries has evolved from non–weight-bearing immobilization to operative treatment to accelerate the rehabilitation course and decrease the risk of chronic symptoms. Operative treatment consists of closed manipulation and compression screw fixation of the unstable joints. Postoperative treatment includes non–weight-bearing for 3 to 4 weeks followed by progressive weight-bearing in a walker boot. The boot can be removed for daily range-of-motion exercises. Approximately 12 to 16 weeks after the initial surgery, the screw can be removed.

Nondisplaced or minimally displaced fracture-dislocations can be treated with immobilization in a short-leg cast, particularly in the debilitated patient who is not a surgical candidate. Close clinical followup, including frequent radiographs, is necessary to ensure that displacement and loss of position do not occur in the cast. Casting must be carefully monitored in such patients, as it can cause skin ulcerations. Cast immobilization and non–weight-bearing are continued for 6 to 8 weeks, followed by removable, walker boot brace. Progression to full weight-bearing takes place over another 6 weeks.

Displaced fracture-dislocations of the tarsometatarsal joints require anatomic reduction to optimize long-term results. Closed reduction can be attempted and, in some cases, will be adequate. Often, however, small fracture or chondral fragments or soft tissues can become entrapped in the joint space and block anatomic reduction. Open reduction is frequently necessary to remove interposed tissues, to ensure anatomic reduction, and to examine the articular surfaces for chondral damage.

Open reduction is performed through dorsal incisions or a medial incision as dictated by the fracture pattern. Full-thickness flaps minimize the risk of skin slough and wound complications. Following the planes created by the injury, the fracture-dislocation is exposed. The second metatarsal is usually the key to reduction of the entire forefoot. It is approached through an incision between the first and second metatarsals. Small, bony fragments and interposed soft tissues are removed. The second metatarsal base is reduced into the mortise of the middle cuneiform. Provisional fixation is provided via a bone-holding clamp, a K-wire, or a guide pin from a cannulated screw set. Next, the first tarsometatarsal joint is approached and reduced either through the same incision or a medial incision. The first tarsometatarsal joint is usually reduced easily after the second tarsometatarsal joint has been reduced; otherwise, it can be manipulated under direct vision and provisionally fixed. The remaining lesser metatarsals, if involved, can then be addressed.

Maintenance of the reduction is paramount. Open reduction followed by casting was a common approach in the past, but it resulted in an unacceptably high rate of redisplacement, often 1 to 2 weeks after reduction as edema subsided. Current recommendations are to use internal fixation such as K-wires or compression screws. Percutaneous K-wires are more user-friendly but have several disadvantages such as skin problems and infections, necessitating early removal and late displacement.

We join many others in preferring screw fixation. Screws are placed longitudinally across the involved tarsometatarsal joints, as well as between disrupted first and second metatarsal bases and divergent medial and middle cuneiforms. The medial rays are the key to midfoot stability, and the lateral rays are more mobile; therefore, the fourth and fifth tarsometatarsal joints are usually fixed with K-wires (see Fig. 37–3C), which are removed at 6 to 8 weeks.

Postoperatively, the patient is non–weight-bearing in a bulky dressing with plaster posterior and coaptation splints. The sutures are removed after 10 to 14 days, and a cast or walker boot is applied. Partial weight-bearing in a removable walker boot begins 6 weeks after surgery. The patient advances to full weight-bearing 12 weeks after surgery. As foot edema decreases, the screws may become prominent and can be removed if they cause symptoms. Removal should be delayed at least 12 to 16 weeks after surgery, as late redisplacement has been reported with premature screw removal. Some authors believe the screws may remain in place indefinitely because it may not be possible to restore tarsometatarsal motion after screw removal.

Open fracture-dislocations require emergent irrigation and debridement. Open injuries without substantial contamination are managed with immediate ORIF. Severely contaminated wounds are managed with external fixation or percutaneous pins. Serial debridements are performed every 48 hours. Delayed wound closure, skin grafting, local flaps, or free-tissue transfer is performed once the wounds are stable, usually within 7 days. Compartment syndrome requires immediate fasciotomy to prevent the sequelae of muscle ischemia, nerve injury, contractures, and clawtoes. Fasciotomies can be performed through the same incisions used for ORIF. The wounds are initially left open, followed by delayed closure or skin grafting at 5 to 7 days.

The best predictor of successful outcome is the adequacy of reduction. Other factors, such as injury pattern, age, and type of fixation, do not have as clear an impact on the result. A stable, plantigrade foot that fits in a shoe can be expected in most patients when an anatomic reduction is achieved. Persistent pain and edema are not uncommon in the first 6 to 12 months after such an injury. This can limit a patient's return to strenuous activities and manual labor. In most cases, these symptoms subside and the patient can then resume regular activities.

Early complications associated with these injuries include wound-healing problems and infections. Careful technique and vigilance minimize these risks. The major late complication encountered is post-traumatic arthritis. Although it does not correlate with injury type or fixation technique, it may be related to overall severity of the injury. It is more difficult to obtain an acceptable reduction in more severe injuries, and articular damage worsens with increasing severity of injury. Long-term radiographic studies of patients with tarsometatarsal injuries often demonstrate degenerative changes, but they do not necessarily correlate with outcome. The development of symptomatic, post-traumatic arthritis can be treated effectively with nonoperative measures, such as an orthotic, or with tarsometatarsal arthrodesis and resection arthroplasty of the fourth and fifth tarsometatarsal joints, if involved. Transfer metatarsalgia can occur due to malunion or malalignment and is treated by orthotics. Recalcitrant cases may require metatarsal osteotomy.

OS CALCIS

Etiology

Os calcis fractures can be intra-articular, where the fracture line extends into the subtalar joint, or extra-articular. Extra-articular fractures are generally low-energy injuries produced by twisting or muscular contraction that results in avulsion of a bony fragment (Fig. 37–4). An inversion injury of the foot

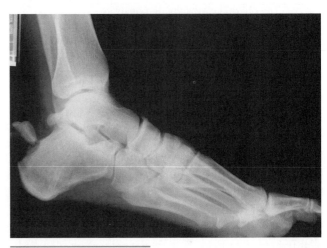

Figure 37–4 Extra-articular calcaneal fracture involving the dorsal aspect of the posterior tuberosity of the calcaneus. Fragment displacement is due to the pull of the Achilles tendon.

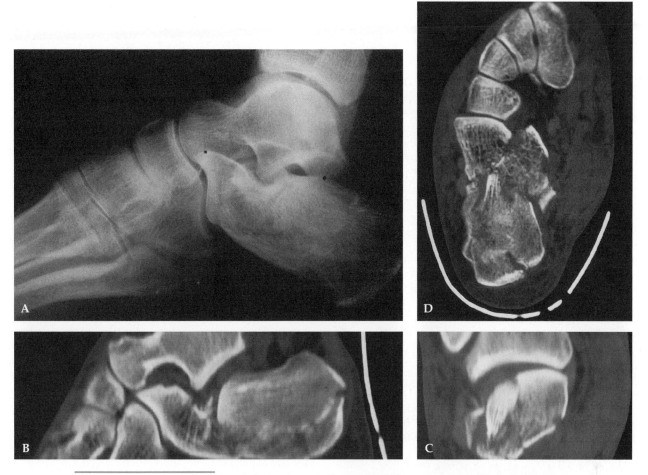

Figure 37–5 Preoperative views of an intra-articular calcaneal fracture. **(A)** Radiograph. **(B)** Sagittal CT image. **(C)** Coronal CT image of the posterior subtalar facet. **(D)** Axial CT image.

can cause the strong, bifurcate ligament to avulse the anterior process of the os calcis. Similarly, a strong contraction of the triceps surae can result in an avulsion of the posterior aspect of the tuberosity.

Intra-articular fractures of the calcaneus typically involve higher energy (Fig. 37–5). An axial load during a fall from a height or a motor vehicle accident forces the talar body into the weaker cancellous bone of the os calcis. The fracture may split the os calcis into anteromedial and posterolateral fragments. This fracture may also involve the articular surface of the calcaneocuboid joint. A secondary fracture may occur based on the direction of the force. A purely axial force will produce a secondary fracture exiting the tuberosity posteriorly. This creates the classic Essex-Lopresti "tongue-type" fracture. A more horizontally directed force causes a secondary fracture that exits the superior surface of the os calcis just posterior to the joint surface: the classic Essex-Lopresti "joint-depression" fracture. With greater energy, a lateral fracture fragment displaces laterally, or "blows out," and the subtalar fragment rotates into the body of the os calcis. The fracture comminution increases as the energy imparted to the

foot rises. High-energy os calcis fractures result in significant soft-tissue injury and swelling. On rare occasions, intra-articular fractures may occur from low-energy injuries, particularly in patients with severe osteopenia.

Anatomy, Surgical Approaches, and Selected Basic Science

The os calcis is an irregularly shaped, roughly rectangular bone (Fig. 37–6). It is composed of cancellous bone with a thin cortical shell. The rounded tuberosity sits posteriorly and provides the attachment site for the Achilles' tendon as well as the origin of the thick plantar fascia. The sustentaculum tali is a dense bony prominence that protrudes medially and supports the talar body (Fig. 37–7). The three facets of the subtalar joint lie superiorly, with the anterior and middle facets separated from the posterior facet by the sulcus calcaneus and the obliquely oriented sinus tarsi. The anterior process articulates with the cuboid and is the attachment site for the calcaneocuboid dorsal ligament, joint capsule, and bifurcate ligament that attaches to both the cuboid and navicular.

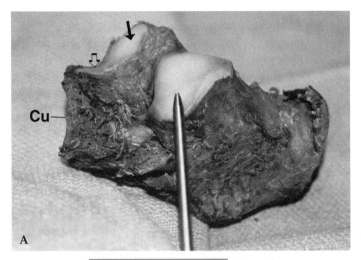

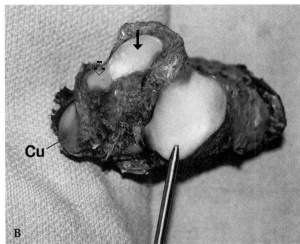

Figure 37–6   Lateral **(A)** and dorsal **(B)** views of the dissected calcaneus demonstrating posterior (probe), middle (solid arrow), and anterior (open arrow) facets and the facet for the cuboid (Cu). Notice the typical confluence of the middle and anterior facets.

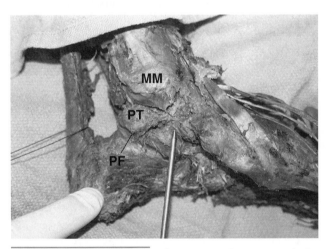

Figure 37–7   Medial view of the dissected hindfoot with the medial tendons and neurovascular bundle removed. The metal probe indicates the middle facet and the supporting sustentaculum tali. The suture encircles the insertion of the Achilles tendon. PF-posterior facet; MM-medial malleolus; PT-posterior talus.

Laterally, the angle of Gissane is formed by the anterior portion of the posterior facet and the superior border of the anterior process.

The peroneal tendons course along the lateral wall of the calcaneus and continue distally toward the midfoot. The calcaneofibular ligament (CFL) is closely apposed to the deep aspect of the peroneal tendon sheath and provides lateral stability to the subtalar joint. The sural nerve and lesser saphenous vein are usually posterior to the peroneal tendons. Medially, the posterior tibialis and flexor digitorum longus tendons course medial to the sustentaculum tali. The flexor hallucis longus passes inferior to this bony process. The posterior tibial artery and vein and the tibial nerve course through the tarsal tunnel along the medial side of the os calcis in the interval between the flexor digitorum longus and flexor hallucis

longus. The branching pattern of the tibial nerve, which gives rise to the medial plantar nerve, the lateral plantar nerve, and the medial calcaneal branch, is highly variable. Posteriorly, the Achilles tendon attaches to the tuberosity of the os calcis by way of a fibroperiosteal sheet that continues plantarly as a continuous layer to give origin to the plantar fascia.

A recent study (Manoli and Weber, 1990) on the osseofascial compartments of the foot described a deep calcaneal compartment, which consists of the quadratus plantae muscle, the lateral plantar nerve, and, occasionally, the medial plantar nerve. The deep calcaneal compartment is tightly apposed to the anterior aspect of the os calcis. Os calcis fractures can result in substantial bleeding and hematoma formation in this limited osseofascial space. It has been postulated that a deep calcaneal compartment syndrome can occur that may cause severe pain acutely and long-term morbidity.

The heel pad is located plantar to the calcaneal tuberosity. It is composed of fibrofatty tissue that absorbs the impact of heel strike. The heel pad consists of vertically oriented fibrous septa that attach to the periosteal layer of the tuberosity and the thick skin of the heel. Fat globules reside within each of these fibrous cells to provide a honeycomblike structure of cushioning material. The remainder of the os calcis is covered with a thin sleeve of neurovascular and musculotendinous structures, subcutaneous tissue, and skin. This limited soft-tissue envelope must be considered when planning treatment of an os calcis fracture.

Normal walking requires normal hindfoot mechanics, which are a function of subtalar and transverse tarsal joint (talonavicular and calcaneocuboid joints) anatomy. The larger posterior facet of the subtalar joint occupies a different plane than the anterior and middle facets, resulting in a complex three-dimensional relationship. The subtalar joint is intricately coupled with the transverse tarsal joints. Because the function of these three joints is so clearly interdependent, many authors speak of them as the subtalar complex.

The subtalar complex has a critical role during gait. The subtalar joint and heel are everted at heel-strike and during early stance. Hindfoot eversion renders the axes of the talon-avicular and calcaneocuboid joints parallel, making the transverse tarsal joints mobile. The result is a supple foot that can absorb the heel-strike impact and accommodate to the terrain. As stance phase progresses to heel off, the subtalar joint and heel invert. The talonavicular and calcaneocuboid joint axes become nonparallel, and the transverse tarsal joints become locked or rigid. The result is a rigid foot that provides a rigid lever arm to increase ankle plantarflexion torque for propulsion. Injury or deformity of any of the subtalar complex can destabilize the elegant biomechanics and cause limitation of motion and gait.

PEARL

When the talonavicular joint and calcaneocuboid joint are parallel, the foot is supple and can accommodate to travel on uneven ground. In a normal foot, this occurs during hindfoot eversion. A calcaneous fracture that heals in varus will lock the subtalar joint in inversion, creating a rigid transverse tarsal joint.

Biomechanical study (Sangeorzan et al, 1995) of the subtalar joint in models of os calcis fractures supports recent trends in the management of these injuries. Specimens with articular surface displacement of more than 2 mm demonstrated significantly decreased contact areas compared with control specimens or those with nondisplaced fracture lines. Specimens with residual displacement greater than 5 mm showed significant increases in subtalar contact pressures. These results support anatomic reduction of intra-articular calcaneal fractures with 2 mm of incongruity.

Historically, open surgical procedures for os calcis fractures were associated with major complications and wound-healing problems. Recently, acceptable results have been consistently obtained with open approaches. Lateral and medial approaches have been described; the extensile lateral approach is more commonly applicable.

The patient with a unilateral fracture is positioned in lateral decubitus and supported by a deflatable beanbag. Bilateral fractures can be approached in one operation by laying the patient in a prone position. A lateral L-shaped incision (Fig. 37–8) is made with the posterior limb 1 cm anterior to the border of the Achilles' tendon. The incision extends distally to the lateral heel and gently curves toward the base of the fourth metatarsal, allowing access to the calcaneocuboid joint. The apex of the incision is located at the junction of the thin lateral skin and the thickened plantar skin of the heel. Blunt dissection of the subcutaneous tissue is performed in the proximal and distal ends of the incision to protect the sural nerve and peroneal tendons. Sharp dissection is used to elevate a full-thickness flap from the lateral aspect of the os calcis, taking care to handle the skin and soft tissues gently (Fig. 37–9). The CFL, the peroneal tendons and sheath, and the sural nerve are reflected anteriorly within the flap to reveal the subtalar joint and sinus tarsi. The flap can be gently retracted anteriorly by inserting multiple K-wires into the lateral malleolus and talar neck and bending them proximally. This "no-touch" technique is thought to minimize wound complications. The peroneal tendons and sural nerve can be mobilized either superiorly or inferiorly to provide adequate access to the anterior process of the calcaneus and the calcaneocuboid joint.

PITFALL

Skin edges that are undermined during dissection or vigorously retracted are at risk of necrosis with skin slough.

A medial approach to the os calcis may be necessary to supplement the lateral approach. A gently curving vertical incision is made midway between the medial malleolus and

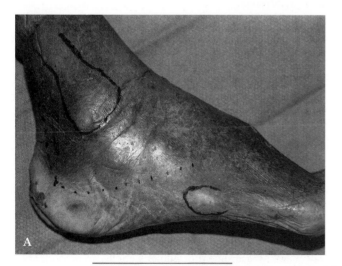

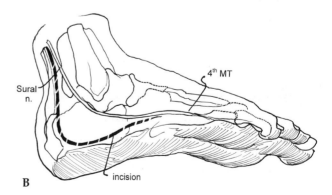

Figure 37–8 **(A)** Lateral incision for calcaneal fracture reduction and stabilization. The fibula and the base of the fifth metatarsal are outlined. **(B)** Lateral L-shaped incision. MT, metatarsal.

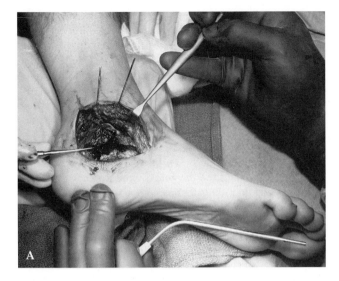

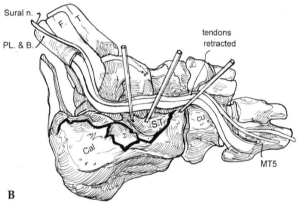

Figure 37–9 **(A)** Intra-operative photograph of the lateral approach with exposed lateral calcaneal wall. **(B)** No-touch technique.

the anterior border of the Achilles' tendon. The incision parallels the flexor tendons and the neurovascular structures (Fig. 37–10A). Cautious dissection is essential, as displacement of the fracture can elevate the neurovascular structures toward the skin. It is imperative to be wary of the highly variable branching pattern of the tibial nerve. After anterior mobilization of these structures, deeper dissection to the medial wall of the calcaneus is performed, revealing the sustentaculum tali and the medial cortical exit of the fracture line (Fig. 37–10B). Reduction and fixation can be performed based on exposure of this fracture line.

PITFALL

A displaced fracture of the calcaneus can displace the tibial nerve toward the skin, placing it at risk during a medial approach.

Examination

The typical deformity of the os calcis fracture includes longitudinal and axial shortening, as well as heel widening with varus. The foot with an intra-articular fracture of the os calcis is typically ecchymotic and swollen. Tenderness and crepita-

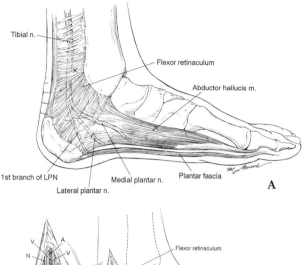

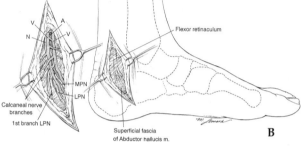

Figure 37–10 **(A)** Skin incision for medial approach to the oscalcis. **(B)** Deep dissection medial approach to the os calcis.

tion may be noted over the tuberosity, lateral wall, and calcaneocuboid joints. The remainder of the foot is palpated to exclude other injuries. Careful neurovascular evaluation includes palpation or Doppler examination of the dorsalis pedis and posterior tibial pulses and a sensory examination of the deep and superficial peroneal, sural, and tibial nerves. Pain out of proportion to the injury, pain with passive motion of the small muscles of the foot, and a tensely swollen foot suggest compartment syndrome. Intracompartmental pressure testing is a useful adjunct for evaluating foot compartment syndrome.

Axial load injuries that cause os calcis fractures can also produce lumbosacral, hip, pelvis, and/or proximal tibial fractures. Patients with os calcis fractures should be examined for pain and tenderness in the lower back, pelvis, and extremities.

Aids to Diagnosis

Radiographs confirm the os calcis fracture and provide some indication of the fracture type and severity. Standard radiographs include AP, external oblique, and lateral views of the foot. The AP and external oblique views can demonstrate involvement of the calcaneocuboid joint and anterior process of the os calcis and can identify other injuries in the foot.

The lateral view shows the posterior facet and tuberosity. It is difficult to reliably image the posterior facet of the subtalar joint because it occupies a plane that is oblique to the x-ray beam. Measurement of Bohler's angle can help identify depression of the subtalar joint, though, when compared with the contralateral foot. This angle is created by drawing a line from the superior corner of the posterior tuberosity to the highest point of the posterior facet and a line from the anterior process to the highest point of the posterior facet. This angle normally ranges from 20 to 40 degrees, and will be decreased with posterior facet depression. The crucial angle of Gissane, the angle formed by the projection of dense subchondral bone under the posterior facet and the upward slope of the anterior process, usually ranges from 125 to 140 degrees. It will increase with posterior facet depression.

Although standard radiographs are helpful in recognizing fractures of the os calcis, they do not provide adequate information about the subtalar joint. An axial heel view can demonstrate posterior facet involvement, heel widening, and hindfoot varus. Multiple Broden oblique views—taken with the foot internally rotated 15 to 20 degrees and the x-ray tube at angles of 10, 20, 30, and 40 degrees cephalad—can also image various portions of the posterior facet.

Computed tomography scanning has dramatically improved imaging of the complex anatomy of the subtalar joint and its deformation in fractures of the os calcis. A semicoronal CT image is obtained with the foot plantigrade on the gurney and the gantry angled perpendicular to the posterior facet on the scout film. This view will show fracture extension into the joint, comminution, lateral wall extrusion, and varus malalignment of the tuberosity fragment. It may also show impingement of the peroneal tendons. An axial CT scan, along the plane of the plantar aspect of the foot, shows the calcaneocuboid joint. Fracture classifications based on CT scanning appear to provide a useful analysis of this complicated fracture and prognostic information for nonoperative and operative treatment.

Specific Conditions, Treatment, and Outcome

Extra-articular os calcis fractures typically result from low-energy mechanisms. Bony avulsions are common. The goals of treatment for such fractures include reduction of deformity, bony healing, restoration of motion, and resumption of functional activities. Closed treatment is usually sufficient to achieve such goals; surgical intervention is only rarely necessary.

Anterior process fractures, caused by avulsion from tension on the bifurcate ligament, are often mistaken for simple inversion sprains of the ankle. Precise palpation and careful x-ray evaluation identify the true site of injury. Closed reduction and immobilization of the foot in slight eversion is sufficient in most cases. A short-leg walking cast is applied for 4 to 6 weeks, at which point weight bearing is advanced as tolerated. Nonunions are rare and usually asymptomatic. If a symptomatic nonunion does occur, a small fragment can be excised; larger fragments may be reduced and stabilized.

Open reduction and internal fixation may be necessary in open fractures, in high-performance athletes, or when there is substantial calcaneocuboid joint displacement. A longitudinal incision is centered over the calcaneocuboid joint and careful subcutaneous dissection is performed to avoid injury to branches of the sural nerve and peroneal tendons. The extensor digitorum brevis muscle is reflected to reveal the anterior process and calcaneocuboid joint. The fracture is reduced and stabilized with a standard or cannulated cancellous screw. Postoperatively, a short-leg non–weight-bearing cast is used for 4 to 6 weeks, followed by progressive, weight bearing out of the cast.

In general, fractures of the anterior process have a good outcome if treated in a timely manner. Pain relief and return of motion are usually good, and most patients can return to their pre-injury activity level, including athletics. Complications include sural neuritis, peroneal tendonitis, and hardware prominence.

Extra-articular fracture of the tuberosity is caused by avulsion of the Achilles' tendon. It can consist of a small piece with little displacement or a large fragment resulting in proximal retraction of the tendon. If the fragment is small, closed reduction and immobilization in plantarflexion for 4 to 6 weeks followed by immobilization in decreasing degrees of equinus for another 4 to 6 weeks is effective. Closed reduction and percutaneous fixation or even ORIF with a cancellous screw may be necessary for a larger fragment with Achilles tendon retraction. A posterior oblique incision is made either medially or laterally, depending on displacement and fragment size. Care is taken to protect the posterior tibial neurovascular bundle or the sural nerve. One advantage of internal fixation compared with percutaneous K-wire fixation is fewer skin problems and superficial infections that may require percutaneous pin removal before bony union. In addition, secure internal fixation permits early rehabilitation after immobilization in slight equinus for approximately 4 weeks.

The clinician should be aware that, although unusual, tenting of the posterior skin of the heel can be caused by retraction of the tuberosity fragment by the Achilles tendon. Such pressure can rapidly result in full-thickness skin compromise and slough, converting a major injury into a disastrous one. This circumstance is a surgical emergency that requires immediate ORIF to relieve the pressure on the soft tissues and restore their viability.

Intra-articular fractures of the calcaneus are substantially more challenging. Historically, they have been devastating injuries, often relegating a young laborer to a sedentary life of severe pain, disability, and deformity. In this century, great advances have been made in understanding the pathomechanics and pathoanatomy of these fractures, which has led to improved diagnostic techniques and treatment alternatives. Treatment goals include restoration of a congruent articular surface and reduction of deformities, which typically include varus tilt, lateral impingement, and longitudinal and axial shortening (Fig. 37–11). Achieving these goals produces a stable, plantigrade foot, and allows early range of motion, facilitating the return to daily activities.

Various classification schemes have been described to guide treatment and determine prognosis. Essex-Lopresti (1952) described a radiographic classification system of intra-articular fractures. The first category is a "joint depression" fracture where the primary fracture exits just posterior to the posterior facet. The articular fragment typically rotates plantarly and posteriorly into the cancellous body of the calcaneus; the calcaneocuboid joint may be involved. The second category is a "tongue-type" fracture wherein the primary fracture exits the tuberosity posteriorly. The articular fragment may rotate plantarly into the body; the calcaneocuboid joint may be involved. The third category comprises comminuted fractures with no distinguishable pattern.

Crosby and Fitzgibbons (1990), as well as Sanders et al (1993) have developed more detailed classification systems based on CT scanning of the posterior facet. Both base their fracture classifications on the number of fragments and

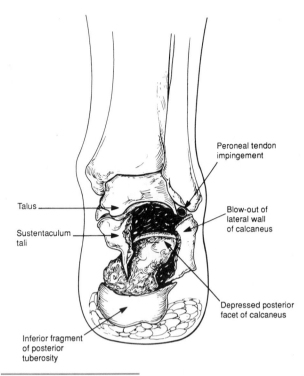

Talus

Sustentaculum tali

Inferior fragment of posterior tuberosity

Peroneal tendon impingement

Blow-out of lateral wall of calcaneus

Depressed posterior facet of calcaneus

Figure 37–11 Drawing illustrating calcaneus fracture with varus, shortening, widening, and peroneal impingement.

degree of displacement of the posterior facet. Both have also been shown to provide prognostic information, with more severe fractures demonstrating worse long-term outcomes for both nonoperative (Crosby and Fitzgibbons) and operative treatment (Sanders et al).

Intra-articular os calcis fractures are considered nondisplaced if articular displacement is less than 2 mm. Historically, cast immobilization was recommended for such injuries. Recent evidence suggests that early range-of-motion and rehabilitation exercises may allow a faster return to function and better ultimate results than rigid immobilization for 2 to 3 months. Initial treatment is with a well-padded posterior and coaptation short-leg splint until the initial swelling and pain have improved, usually 2 weeks. An ankle-foot orthosis at 90 degrees or a walker boot brace is then used for immobilization and strict non–weight-bearing for 6 to 8 weeks. The patient is encouraged to remove the brace for daily sessions of ankle and hindfoot active range-of-motion exercises. Depending on patient compliance and bone quality, gradual weight-bearing is begun 8 weeks after injury. At 12 weeks, most patients have resumed full weight-bearing in the walker boot brace. The patient is weaned from the brace to a standard shoe, and may require a slightly larger shoe than the pre-injury size due to persistent edema and residual deformity. Some patients will also require an orthotic insert and an extra-depth shoe for residual deformity.

Most patients with nondisplaced intra-articular fractures treated in this manner will have an acceptable outcome, with 80% or more of their pre-injury subtalar motion. There may be residual pain, swelling, and difficulty with shoe-wearing, but most patients will have satisfactory results with return to most activities. Post-traumatic arthritis can still occur, even if articular displacement remains less than 2 mm. This may be due to

altered joint stresses due to residual deformity of the heel or chondral damage suffered at the time of injury. Post-traumatic arthritis can be treated with subtalar arthrodesis or triple arthrodesis if the transverse tarsal joints are also symptomatic.

Treatment of displaced intra-articular os calcis fractures is controversial. These fractures can be either the tongue-type or joint depression variants. Proposed treatments include closed manipulation and immobilization, closed manipulation and percutaneous pin fixation, open reduction and pinning, ORIF, and primary arthrodesis. Numerous studies have reported success with each method. However, it is difficult to compare these series because of differences in injury severity, length of followup, and patient populations. In addition, series reported before the 1980s did not include CT-scan evaluation of the subtalar joint.

Most displaced intra-articular fractures are treated with ORIF (Fig. 37–12). Exceptions include patients with substantial comorbidity such as diabetes or severe peripheral vascular disease. Elderly patients are also generally treated less aggressively; however, this patient population is poorly represented in most reported studies of os calcis fractures. The multiply injured patient who is unable to undergo operative treatment may be managed with closed measures, although it is possible to perform surgery for these fractures up to 3 weeks after injury. Displaced intra-articular os calcis fractures that cannot undergo ORIF can be managed with closed manipulation and immobilization. Patients must be informed that the fracture may redisplace and result in a malunion. Closed reduction and percutaneous K-wire or Steinmann pin fixation may be a better alternative because it provides at least a few weeks of temporary fixation before pin removal. Tongue-type fractures are more amenable to this method than joint depression fractures. Open reduction is favored for healthy, active patients. Surgery is preferably performed within 12 hours of injury, before the onset of severe swelling. Early surgery should not preclude appropriate trauma care and diagnostic imaging of the injured os calcis. If ORIF cannot be performed within 12 hours, the patient is admitted and the foot is elevated. A pneumatic foot pump may help reduce edema and allow earlier surgery. Once dorsiflexion of the ankle produces dorsal skin wrinkles (the "wrinkle test"), the edema is sufficiently resolved to allow surgery.

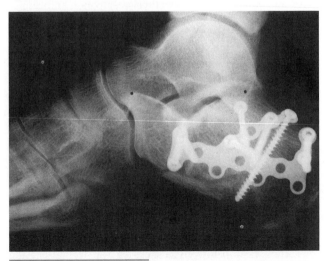

Figure 37–12 Postoperative radiograph of patient in Figure 37–5.

The extensile lateral approach is used. After exposure, the lateral wall fragments are reflected to reveal the depressed articular fragment. A Schanz screw can be placed into the tuberosity fragment to assist reduction. The articular surface fragments are reduced to the medial sustentaculum fragment and provisionally fixed with K-wires. Standard or cannulated screws replace the provisional K-wires to fix the lateral articular fragments to the sustentaculum piece and support the overlying joint surface. The tuberosity is manipulated and provisional K-wires are inserted to maintain the reduction. The anterior process and calcaneocuboid joint are reduced and provisionally fixed with K-wires. A medial exposure may be added if reduction is not possible laterally, or if there is compromise of the neurovascular bundle.

Various plates have been developed for os calcis fixation. Each type should be available in the operating room to select the one that best fits the anatomy of the patient. The plate is fixed with a combination of cortical and cancellous screws along the lateral wall of the calcaneus. The provisional K-wires and Schanz screw are removed after the plate is applied. A drain is placed and the lateral incision is closed in layers. A well-padded plaster posterior and coaptation short-leg splint is applied. The stitches are removed at 2 to 3 weeks. The patient is placed in a walker boot brace, which is removed 3 to 4 times a day for active range-of-motion exercises. The patient remains non–weight-bearing for 6 to 8 weeks postoperatively and is advanced to achieve full weight-bearing at 12 to 16 weeks. The patient is then weaned from the boot to a standard shoe.

Displaced intra-articular fractures with severe comminution have a substantially worse prognosis regardless of treatment method. ORIF with immediate subtalar arthrodesis has become popular in healthy, active patients. In theory, patients with severe intra-articular comminution develop disabling subtalar degenerative joint disease regardless of their treatment. Combined ORIF and immediate subtalar arthrodesis reduces deformity, minimizes lateral impingement, and eliminates the theoretically inevitable degenerative joint disease. Elderly patients or those with diabetes, peripheral vascular disease, or sedentary lifestyles are managed with closed methods. Articular comminution is now routinely studied on preoperative CT scanning. If bony comminution or severe chondral damage is appreciated at the time of ORIF, immediate subtalar arthrodesis should be considered.

The extensile lateral exposure is used. After reduction maneuvers and provisional fixation, the subtalar joint surface is denuded of its cartilage with hand or power instruments. The heel is positioned in 5 to 7 degrees of valgus, and a large cannulated cancellous screw is inserted from the posterior non–weight-bearing point of the heel across the subtalar joint into the talar neck. ORIF is performed as described above. The foot is immobilized in a non–weight-bearing short-leg cast or walker boot brace for 12 weeks until clinical and radiographic fusion are evident. Weight-bearing is progressed to full weight-bearing over another 3 to 4 weeks.

This treatment algorithm for displaced intra-articular fractures has yielded satisfactory results in 70 to 80% of patients. Most undergoing ORIF regain between 25 and 75% of their subtalar motion and have little pain. Many studies report that most patients return to work and daily activities, although the results in workers' compensation or liability cases generally are less satisfactory.

Complications of these fractures include lateral wall impingement, post-traumatic subtalar arthritis, and malunion. Nonunion is relatively rare, perhaps because of the large cancellous component of the calcaneus. Treatment options for symptomatic nonunion include open bone grafting and subtalar arthrodesis. Malunion may result in either a varus heel or lateral wall impingement. Varus malunion alters weight-bearing mechanics. Lateral wall impingement comprises a spectrum of syndromes, including peroneal tendon or sural nerve compression and painful abutment against the medial aspect of the lateral malleolus. Lateral wall decompression may relieve these symptoms but has produced relatively disappointing results unless combined with subtalar arthrodesis.

Subtalar post-traumatic arthritis can be treated with anti-inflammatory medications, shoe modifications or accommodative inserts, and corticosteroid injections. Subtalar arthrodesis produces the most reliable, long-term solution with excellent pain relief and function. It is common for radiographically evident transverse tarsal joint degenerative arthritis to be asymptomatic. Only when it is symptomatic should triple arthrodesis be considered.

TALUS

Etiology

Talus fractures typically occur in motor vehicle accidents or falls from a height. Ankle dorsiflexion with impingement of the talar neck on the anterior tibia leads to a talar neck fracture. The displacement increases with the force of injury. Ankle, subtalar, or talonavicular dislocation may also occur.

Talar body fractures occur with axial load and may accompany distal tibia or ankle fractures. Talar head fractures likewise occur in high-energy injuries to the midfoot and result from bending or torsional injury.

Posterior process of the talus fracture typically involves the lateral tubercle and is referred to as a Shepherd's fracture. Proposed mechanisms include avulsion by the posterior talofibular ligament and posterior impingement on the tibia in extreme plantarflexion.

A fracture of the lateral process of the talus is often misdiagnosed as an ankle sprain. The mechanism is believed to be dorsiflexion and inversion. Recent reports document an increased incidence of this fracture in snowboarders.

Anatomy, Surgical Approaches, and Selected Basic Science

The talus is a complex bone with no muscle attachments. The talar body consists of the tibiotalar articular surface superiorly (talar dome) and the subtalar articular surface inferiorly. The talar dome is wider anteriorly and has a longitudinal sulcus that corresponds to a longitudinal ridge on the tibial articular surface. This sulcus is thought to increase mediolateral stability. The lateral process is a pyramidal projection of the lateral talar body, with the apex lateral and inferior, that articulates with the angle of Gissane of the calcaneus. The superolateral surface of the lateral process of the talus articulates with the fibula. The posterior process of the talus comprises the medial and lateral tubercles that protrude posteriorly from the talus in an interval between the tibiotalar and subtalar articular surfaces. The flexor hallucis longus tendon occupies the groove between the medial and lateral tubercles of the posterior process of the talus. An accessory ossicle, the os trigonum, may be present posterior to the lateral tubercle in 3 to 8% of patients. The talar neck extends distally from the body to the talar head, which articulates with the navicular. The talar neck angulates medially 24 degrees and inferiorly 24 degrees, on average.

The talus has multiple ligament attachments that influence its movement because there are no direct muscle attachments to the talus. The anterior talofibular ligament (ATFL) arises from the anterior margin of the distal fibula and inserts onto the lateral surface of the talar neck. The posterior talofibular ligament (PTFL) arises from the posterior aspect of the distal fibula and inserts onto the lateral tubercle of the posterior process of the talus. There is a variable origin of the deep deltoid ligament from the distal medial malleolus and a variable insertion onto the medial wall of the talus. There are lateral, posterior, and medial talocalcaneal ligaments that span the subtalar joint. The lateral talocalcaneal ligament parallels the overlying CFL. The posterior and medial talocalcaneal ligaments arise from the lateral and medial tubercles of the posterior process, respectively, and course inferolaterally and inferomedially to insert on the lateral calcaneus and sustentaculum tali, respectively. The cervical ligament arises from the inferior surface of the talar neck to insert in the interval between the posterior and middle facets of the calcaneus. The talonavicular ligament is a dorsal thickening of the talonavicular joint capsule. The calcaneonavicular, or "spring" ligament does not attach to the talus, but forms part of the talonavicular articulation.

The blood supply of the talus has important implications in talar neck fractures. The artery of the tarsal canal is a branch of the posterior tibial artery. It courses inferior to the talar neck from medial and supplies the central portion of the talar body. The artery of the sinus tarsi can be a branch of the peroneal or anterior tibial artery. It courses inferior to the talar neck from the sinus tarsi laterally to anastomose with the artery of the tarsal canal. It supplies the lateral portion of the talar body and the inferior portion of the talar neck. Deltoid branches of the posterior tibial artery supply the medial portion of the talar body. Superior neck vessels that branch from the anterior tibial artery supply the talar head and superior talar neck. Intraosseous anastomoses are variable and may not be sufficient if extraosseous vascular injury occurs.

Medial or lateral longitudinal incisions are useful to expose talar neck fractures. Medial incisions permit direct visualization of the medial cortex to minimize varus deformity, but they can jeopardize the deltoid branches of the posterior tibial artery, which may be the only remaining vascular supply to the talus. Lateral incisions preserve the deltoid branches and improve visualization of the subtalar joint.

Anterolateral, anteromedial, or medial ankle arthrotomy is necessary for ORIF of talar body fractures. The anterolateral approach begins with a longitudinal skin incision lateral to the peroneus tertius. Blunt dissection through the subcutaneous tissue is necessary to protect the superficial peroneal nerve, which branches at the syndesmosis. The extensor tendons are retracted medially, and a longitudinal capsulotomy is performed.

The skin incision is made medial to the tibialis anterior tendon for an anteromedial approach. The saphenous nerve is protected with blunt subcutaneous dissection. The tibialis anterior tendon is retracted laterally to enable a longitudinal capsulotomy.

A direct medial approach with a medial malleolus osteotomy may improve medial exposure. The osteotomy is fixed with a compression screw. It is helpful to drill for the screw before making the osteotomy. A chevron osteotomy improves the fixation stability and increases the surface area for healing.

A sinus tarsi approach with a bell-shaped incision over the sinus tarsi that extends posteriorly to the tip of the fibula is used to expose the lateral process of the talus. The sural nerve, branches of the superficial peroneal nerve, and peroneal tendons must be protected. The sinus tarsi, lateral process, and lateral wall of the calcaneus are exposed by subperiosteal dissection after elevation of the extensor digitorum brevis from its bed.

The posterolateral approach is used for compression screw fixation of the lateral tubercle of the posterior process fractures or talar neck fractures or for excision of posterior process nonunion. A skin incision is made in the interval between the Achilles' tendon and posterior border of the fibula. Blunt dissection through the subcutaneous tissue is necessary to protect the sural nerve. Blunt dissection is continued in the interval between the peroneal tendons and the Achilles' tendon until the posterior process of the talus is identified. Frequently, the flexor hallucis longus tendon is an easier landmark to identify. It can be followed to its groove between the lateral and medial tubercles of the posterior process of the talus.

A three-dimensional analysis (Daniels et al, 1996) of displaced talar neck fractures demonstrated a significant decrease in the subtalar arc of motion in cadaveric specimens with varus malalignment of the talar neck. There was also increased hindfoot varus, forefoot varus, and forefoot adductus when varus malalignment of the talar neck was created.

A biomechanical study (Swanson et al, 1992) of talar neck fracture fixation demonstrated that screws provided more rigid fixation than K-wires. Screws placed from posterior to anterior provided more rigid fixation than screws placed from anterior to posterior. A recent anatomic study (Ebraheim et al, 1996) demonstrated that a 4.5-mm screw could be easily placed from the lateral tubercle, but a second screw placed lateral to the first may injure the PTFL.

Examination

The history should determine the mechanism of injury, location of pain, presence of neurovascular deficit, and symptoms of compartment syndrome. The mechanism will suggest the extent of bony and soft-tissue injury. The location of pain may help determine the fracture site when x-rays are equivocal.

Physical examination requires evaluation of deformity. Gross deformity should be reduced before x-rays are obtained. Inspection of the skin is necessary because talar neck fractures with subluxation or dislocation can compromise the skin by stretch or pressure. Palpation or Doppler examination of the posterior tibial and dorsalis pedis pulses is essential. Compartment syndrome must be suspected when pain with passive motion accompany a tensely swollen foot.

Aids to Diagnosis

Radiographic evaluation includes AP, lateral, and medial and lateral oblique views of the foot and AP, lateral, and mortise views of the ankle. The AP and medial views show the talar neck and talar head. The lateral oblique view shows the talar neck and head as well as the lateral process. The lateral view should be examined for subtalar or tibiotalar subluxation. The lateral process and posterior process are also imaged on the lateral view. The talar body and dome are imaged on the ankle views. The ankle views are examined for tibiotalar subluxation or dislocation. Medial malleolus fractures often accompany talus fractures.

Hawkins (1970) described a classification of talar neck fractures that helps guide treatment and prognosis. Type I talar neck fractures are nondisplaced. Type II fractures are displaced with subtalar subluxation or dislocation. Type III fractures are displaced with subtalar and tibiotalar subluxation or dislocation. Type IV fractures were not originally described by Hawkins but are displaced fractures with subtalar, tibiotalar, and talonavicular subluxation or dislocation. Hawkins proposed that the risk of avascular necrosis after talar neck fracture increases with each type. Hawkins also described the radiographic finding of a linear subchondral lucency that appears 6 to 8 weeks after a talar neck fracture and signifies a positive prognosis that avascular necrosis will not occur. Absence of the "Hawkins' sign" does not imply avascular necrosis will occur.

PEARL

The "Hawkins' sign" is a linear subchondral lucency beneath the dome of the talus. It is thought to result from bone resorption during a hyperemic state during healing of a talar neck fracture. The presence of the Hawkins' sign suggests a low risk of avascular necrosis.

Canale and Kelly (1978) described a special radiograph to more clearly image the talar neck. The x-ray is taken with the foot maximally plantarflexed and pronated 15 degrees. The beam is aimed 75 degrees cephalad. This view is useful to ensure that a nondisplaced talar neck fracture is indeed nondisplaced. It is also useful intra-operatively to confirm anatomic reduction. Another view useful to image this fragment is an AP of the foot with the leg internally rotated 15 degrees and the foot plantarflexed 30 degrees.

Computed tomography scanning is useful to evaluate intra-articular involvement or comminution. It may also be useful in equivocal lateral process or posterior process frac-

tures. A CT scan will also provide better detail of an equivocally nondisplaced talar neck or talar body fracture.

Magnetic resonance imaging and bone scans are rarely used except to confirm avascular necrosis. Technetium bone scans may be useful to rule out a nonunion when a patient has chronic posterior or lateral ankle pain after posterior or lateral process fracture. Relief after an injection of lidocaine about the nonunion confirms that the nonunion is the source of discomfort.

Specific Conditions, Treatment, and Outcome

Hawkins type I nondisplaced talar neck fractures can be treated with a non–weight-bearing cast with the foot in slight equinus for 4 to 6 weeks. This is followed by weight bearing in a short-leg walking cast for 4 to 6 weeks. Range-of-motion exercises and activity progression begin after 8 to 12 weeks of immobilization. Nondisplaced talar neck fractures are rare; therefore, thorough radiographic evaluation is essential before treating the fracture as nondisplaced. Percutaneous screw fixation can be considered to begin range-of-motion exercises sooner; however, operative treatment risks fracture displacement and avascular necrosis.

Displaced talar neck fractures require urgent treatment to restore articular congruity and minimize the risk of avascular necrosis. A lateral or medial exposure may be used, but medial exposures should be avoided when there is significant displacement and subluxation because the medial deltoid branches of the posterior tibial artery may be the only remaining vascular supply to the talus. The subluxed or dislocated joint(s) should be reduced, and then the talar neck can be reduced. Careful intra-operative radiographs as described by Canale and Kelley (1978) are essential to avoid varus malunion of the talar neck. Cancellous screws or K-wires can be used for fixation. Posteriorly placed screws provide more rigid fixation, but they require a separate exposure and are more difficult to place accurately. The screw heads may also cause posterior ankle impingement.

Nondisplaced talar body fractures are treated with cast immobilization and non–weight-bearing that is advanced 4 to 6 weeks after the fracture. Talar body fractures with 2 or more mm of articular displacement require ORIF to restore tibiotalar and subtalar congruity. Thorough preoperative planning is essential to select the most appropriate approach for fracture reduction and fixation. Surgical access to these fractures may be challenging, often requiring osteotomy of the medial malleolus.

Fractures of the posterior process of the talus are treated with a non–weight-bearing cast for 1 week followed by a walker boot for 2 to 6 weeks. The walker boot is removed periodically for range-of-motion exercises. Ambulatory walker boots may need to be continued for an additional 4 to 6 weeks as symptoms warrant. Chronic, posterior ankle pain 6 or more months after injury should be evaluated with a bone scan. A positive scan indicates nonunion, which is amenable to excision via a posterolateral approach.

Nondisplaced fractures of the lateral process are treated with non–weight-bearing casts with the foot and ankle in eversion for 4 weeks. This is followed by weight bearing as tolerated in a walker boot for 2 to 4 weeks. Displaced fractures require ORIF or excision depending on fragment size and comminution. After ORIF, a non–weight-bearing walker boot is used for 4 to 6 weeks. Range-of-motion exercises are begun 2 to 4 weeks postoperatively and weight bearing is advanced when the fracture is clinically united. Range-of-motion and exercises weight bearing can begin 2 to 3 weeks postoperatively if excision is performed. Early recognition and treatment of lateral process of the talus fractures is essential for a good outcome.

A complication of talar body, talar neck, or lateral process fractures is post-traumatic arthritis. Inadequate reduction, malunion, and chondral damage at the time of injury can result in post-traumatic arthritis. Avascular necrosis may complicate a talar neck fracture and progress to collapse, articular incongruity, and post-traumatic arthritis. The incidence of avascular necrosis after talar neck fracture is less than 5% in Hawkins type I, 0 to 13% in type II, 20 to 50% in type III, and 80 to 100% in type IV. To prevent collapse and subsequent post-traumatic arthritis, patients with avascular necrosis should be non–weight-bearing until radiographic healing is evident. Symptomatic post-traumatic arthritis may require ankle or subtalar arthrodesis. Pseudoarthrosis of an attempted ankle arthrodesis is more likely when avascular necrosis is present.

Talar neck and talar body nonunion are rare and may require revision ORIF with bone grafting. Talar neck malunion is more common than nonunion and typically is a varus and dorsiflexion deformity. Opening wedge osteotomy with corticocancellous bone graft has been described to correct talar neck malunion. Symptomatic nonunion of the lateral talar process or posterior talar process may require excision. Both can be prevented by early recognition and treatment.

ANKLE TRAUMA

Etiology

Ankle sprains are commonly caused by an inversion injury. The anterior talofibular ligament (ATFL) is injured when the foot is plantarflexed. The CFL is injured when the foot is in neutral or dorsiflexion. Internal rotation of the foot and ankle often accompanies the inversion stress and may injure either the ATFL or CFL regardless of foot position. External rotation of the ankle can cause syndesmotic sprain with injury to the anterior inferior tibiofibular ligament (AITFL). Additional injuries occur in approximately 40% of ankle sprains and may include osteochondral lesions or peroneal tendon tears.

Low-energy ankle fractures typically occur from a twisting injury, such as a misstep off a curb. The most common mechanisms were described by Lauge-Hansen (1950), who categorized them by the position of the foot at the time of injury and the direction of the deforming force. The classification includes supination-adduction, supination-external rotation, pronation-abduction, and pronation-external-rotation. High-energy ankle injuries cause more substantial fracture displacement, may be open and can occur from motor-vehicle and industrial accidents. High-energy pilon fractures are often the result of an axial load such as a fall from a height or a motor-vehicle accident.

Anatomy, Surgical Approaches, and Basic Science

The ankle joint comprises the articulation of the tibia, fibula, and talus. The distal tibial articular surface, or plafond, is trapezoidal in shape and is buttressed by the medial malleolus, which projects more distally than the plafond. The distal tibia articulates posterolaterally with the fibula via the incisura fibulare. The distal extent of the fibula is composed of the lateral malleolus, a wide, bulbous segment of bone. The dome of the talus is covered by articular cartilage and is wider anteriorly than posteriorly, with a shallow groove in the center. This sulcus conforms to the articular surface of the tibial plafond and confers stability to the articulation. Even minimal subluxation of the talus causes substantial articular incongruence, resulting in dramatically decreased contact area and increased articular contact pressure.

The ankle ligaments confer additional static stability. The lateral ligament complex includes the ATFL, the CFL, and the PTFL (Fig. 37–13). The ATFL resists anterolateral rotatory subluxation of the talus, and its strain is highest in plantarflexion. The CFL resists subtalar and tibiotalar inversion, and its strain is highest in dorsiflexion. The PTFL resists posterior subluxation. The ATFL and CFL work in concert to resist inversion of the ankle.

The deltoid ligament complex restrains the talus medially to prevent lateral subluxation and rotation. The superficial deltoid arises from the anterior colliculus of the medial malleolus and inserts on the medial navicular and calcaneus. The deep deltoid ligament originates from the posterior colliculus and intercollicular groove and inserts onto the medial talus.

The syndesmotic ligaments, including the ATFL, the PTFL, and the interosseous membrane, stabilize the tibiofibular articulation. These ligaments influence the complex rotatory and longitudinal motion of the fibula that occurs with ankle motion and weight-bearing. The ankle joint capsule is a secondary soft-tissue restraint.

The peroneus longus and brevis pass posterior to the lateral malleolus and dorsiflex and evert the foot. The also provide dynamic lateral ankle stability. The tibialis anterior, extensor hallucis longus, extensor digitorum longus, and peroneus tertius tendons course over the dorsum of the ankle. All can dorsiflex the ankle. The tibialis posterior, flexor digitorum longus, and flexor hallucis longus pass posteromedially and can plantarflex and invert the foot and ankle. The Achilles' tendon is directly posterior and plantarflexes and inverts the foot and ankle.

The sural nerve and the lesser saphenous vein course along the superficial posterolateral ankle. The sural nerve has multiple small branches to the lateral side of the heel and hindfoot. The peroneal artery branches in the deep soft tissues of the posterolateral ankle but is only at risk with procedures that involve the syndesmosis. The superficial peroneal nerve pierces the deep fascia in the leg and crosses the anterolateral ankle near the syndesmosis. The deep peroneal nerve and dorsalis pedis artery cross the ankle between the extensor hallucis longus and extensor digitorum longus tendons at the level of the joint. The saphenous nerve and vein are located on the anteromedial aspect of the ankle. The posterior tibial artery and vein travel with the tibial nerve in the interval between the tendons of the flexor digitorum longus and

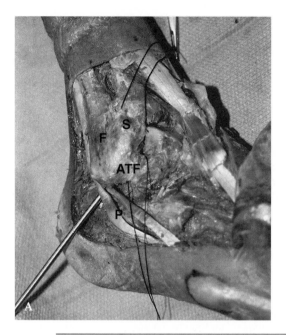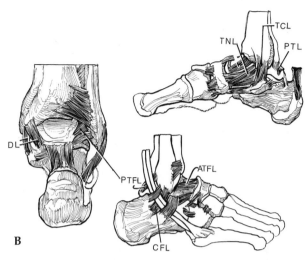

Figure 37–13 **(A)** Dissected exposure of the lateral aspect of the ankle. F, fibula; S, syndesmotic ligaments (encircled by suture); ATF, anterior talofibular ligament (encircled by suture); P, peroneal tendons. The probe tip demonstrates the course of the calcaneofibular ligament. **(B)** Schematic illustrating ligaments of the ankle.

flexor hallucis longus. The nerve can have variable branching patterns.

Surgical approaches to the fibula are relatively uncomplicated. A straight lateral approach is centered over the lateral malleolus, in a plane between the sural and superficial peroneal nerves. This incision can be positioned more posteriorly on the fibula to allow access to the posterior portion of the tibia or more anteriorly near the syndesmotic ligaments. After incision through the skin and subcutaneous tissue, subperiosteal elevation is performed over the fracture site. The exposure can be extended proximally, taking care to protect the superficial peroneal nerve as it exits through the deep fascia of the lateral compartment. A recent cadaveric study (Huene and Bunnell, 1995) has demonstrated that the superficial peroneal nerve branches cross a distal fibula incision in 22% of specimens.

A longitudinal medial incision can expose the distal extent of the medial malleolus to allow reduction and fixation of fractures. Curvilinear incisions located more anteromedial allow access to the malleolus and the anteromedial corner of the tibiotalar joint. This approach facilitates reduction of the medial malleolus, allows inspection of the joint, and permits removal of loose bony fragments or chondral pieces. The saphenous nerve and vein must be protected from injury during subcutaneous dissection. Subperiosteal dissection exposes the malleolus fracture site.

Examination

The history should detail the mechanism of injury, previous foot and ankle injuries, other musculoskeletal complaints, and medical history. The precise location of pain helps differentiate sprains from subtle fractures when radiographs are equivocal.

Precise palpation of each of the lateral and medial ligaments and the bony prominences helps differentiate an ankle sprain from a subtle fracture. If an ankle sprain is suspected, the ATFL is examined with an anterolateral drawer maneuver where the examiner stabilizes the leg in one hand and places the other hand on the heel. The plantarflexed foot is pulled anteriorly with internal rotation and translation. The test is positive when the anterolateral talar dome becomes apparent subcutaneously. There may also be an anterolateral skin dimple. The CFL is evaluated by inverting the dorsiflexed foot. Both maneuvers should be performed on the contralateral ankle for comparison. Both may be difficult to perform acutely because of patient discomfort.

Gross deformity should be reduced immediately even if radiographs are not yet obtained. The skin and soft tissues must be examined for open wounds, ischemia, and fracture blisters. Neurovascular evaluation includes palpation or Doppler examination of the posterior tibial and dorsalis pedis pulses. The sensory distribution of each peripheral nerve must be evaluated. Tendons should be palpated and actively tested. Compartment syndrome of the foot or leg should be suspected when severe pain with a tensely swollen foot or leg is present.

Aids to Diagnosis

Radiographic assessment of the ankle begins with AP, mortise, and lateral views. The AP and mortise views are useful for identifying lateral and medial malleolus fractures and for diagnosing diastasis or disruption of the syndesmosis ligament complex. On both AP and mortise views, the clear space between the lateral edge of the posterior tibia and the medial border of the fibula measured 1 cm above the joint level should be less than 6 mm. In addition, the amount of overlap between the anterior tibial tubercle and the fibula should be more than 6 mm on the AP view and more than 1 mm on the mortise view. Asymmetry of the joint space or widening of the medial clear space between the medial malleolus and talar dome of more than 4 mm usually signifies disruption of the restraints to talar subluxation. The lateral view can demonstrate subluxation of the talus and fractures of the posterior malleolus and fibula. Full-length AP and lateral views of the tibia and fibula are necessary to rule out a more proximal fracture of the fibula (Maissoneuve fracture) in patients with a medial ankle sprain or an abnormal mortise view but no obvious lateral malleolus fracture.

Two classification schemes have been described for ankle fractures. The Danis-Weber (Mueller et al, 1979) classification categorizes these injuries by the level of the fibula fracture. Type A fractures are distal to the tibiotalar joint and the syndesmotic ligaments, type B fractures (Fig. 37–14) start at the level of the ankle joint and may involve the syndesmotic ligaments, and type C fractures are located proximal to the syndesmosis and imply disruption of the ligaments. This system is easy to apply. It does not describe injuries to the medial malleolus or deltoid ligament and may, therefore, be limited in describing the pathoanatomy of many injuries. The Lauge-Hansen (1950) classification describes the mechanism of fracture and may assist in determining appropriate reduction methods. It is not always useful for determining whether ORIF is necessary. Each fracture pattern is named for the position of the foot at the time of injury and the force applied. Each pattern is numerically staged according to the degree of injury.

Axial CT scanning of the ankle with sagittal and coronal reconstructions may be useful in complex injuries with intraarticular injury or associated fractures. It may also be useful in the patient with a previous sprain with chronic pain who may have osteochondritis dissecans.

Stress radiographs may be useful to document an ankle sprain. Local or general anesthesia improves the examiner's ability to apply stress. Stress radiographs should include a lateral view with anterior drawer to test the ATFL, a mortise view with inversion to test the CFL, and another mortise view with external rotation to test the syndesmotic ligaments. Stress views may also be useful in chronic lateral ligamentous instability (Fig. 37–15).

Technetium bone scans are used only rarely for acute injuries but may be of use for stress fractures or late presentation of occult injuries. Magnetic resonance imaging is used primarily for evaluation of chronic pain after ankle injuries.

Specific Conditions, Treatment, and Outcome

Ankle sprains are treated nonoperatively with functional bracing. Casts are occasionally used for more severe sprains. Sprains are classified as grade I, II, or III. Grade I sprains are partial tears without instability. Grade II sprains are believed to comprise complete tears of the ATFL and partial tear of the CFL. There may be mild to moderate anterolateral rotatory instability but no inversion instability. Grade III sprains manifest complete tears of both the ATFL and CFL with anterolateral rotatory and inversion instability.

Grade I and II sprains are treated with 1 to 2 weeks of rest, ice compression, and elevation. A functional brace that permits dorsiflexion and plantarflexion but limits inversion and eversion is used for 4 to 6 weeks from the time of injury. Weight-bearing is advanced as tolerated. Active range-of-motion exercises are essential during the bracing period.

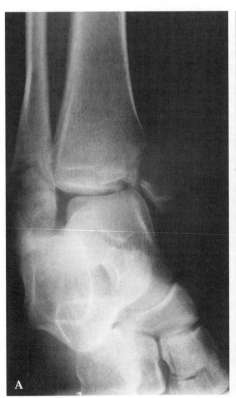
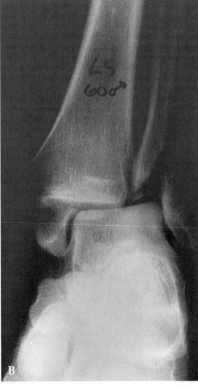

Figure 37–14 AP radiographs of **(A)** a displaced Danis-Weber type A supination/adduction ankle fracture pattern and **(B)** a displaced Danis-Weber type B ankle fracture pattern with medial malleolar fracture.

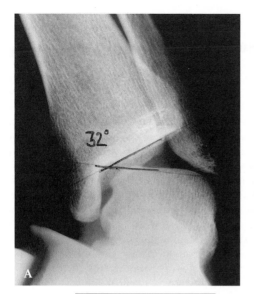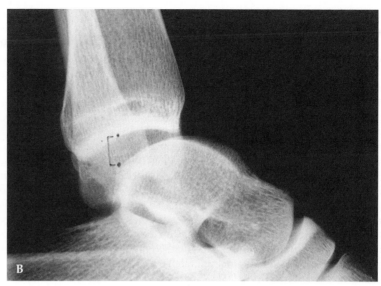

Figure 37–15 Ankle instability demonstrated by AP **(A)** and lateral **(B)** stress radiographs.

Once the brace is discontinued, physical therapy for proprioceptive retraining and strengthening is initiated with an emphasis on the peroneal muscles. Straight-line running on a level surface may begin when the patient is comfortable, but unlevel ground and turns should be avoided until physical therapy is complete.

Grade III sprains may be managed with a short-leg walking cast for 4 to 6 weeks or functional bracing as for Grade I and II injuries. Better range-of-motion and strength are reported benefits of functional bracing, but patients with these severe injuries may be more comfortable in a cast. Physical therapy, weight-bearing, and activity are prescribed in the same manner as for Grade I and II sprains.

The goal of treatment for ankle fractures includes reduction of the tibiotalar joint to restore congruency, restoration of bony and ligamentous stability, and early range-of-motion and weight-bearing. Operative treatment is indicated only when these goals cannot be achieved nonoperatively.

Ankle fractures should be treated as early as possible. When severe swelling and fracture blisters are present, the limb must be elevated for 10 to 14 days to minimize skin problems before cast immobilization or surgical intervention. Gross deformity should be reduced immediately, even if radiographic studies are not yet available, to alleviate pressure or stretch injury to the skin and neurovascular structures.

Fractures can often be reduced and stabilized as late as 3 weeks after injury. Ankle fractures that present after 3 weeks may be better managed with continued nonoperative methods because open or closed reduction becomes exceedingly more difficult. Late symptomatic malunion can be managed with osteotomy or arthrodesis.

Open ankle fractures require immediate irrigation and debridement. ORIF can be performed at the same sitting in grade I, II, and possibly IIIA open fractures. Regardless of the grade of the soft-tissue injury, ORIF should be delayed if there is gross contamination. A repeat irrigation and debridement may be necessary in 48 hours.

Nonoperative treatment is appropriate for stable injuries or when stability can be obtained with closed methods. Isolated fractures of either the lateral or medial malleolus do not destabilize the tibiotalar joint unless ligamentous injury has occurred on the opposite part of the ankle. An isolated fracture of the lateral malleolus without injury to the medial malleolus or deltoid ligament is a stable injury. This is because the intact medial malleolar-deltoid ligament complex restrains the talus from displacing. The patient will have lateral ankle pain and tenderness but no medial ankle pain or tenderness. There may be displacement of the fibula fracture, but there is no asymmetry of the mortise or talar subluxation on plain radiographs. This injury would be classified as either a Danis-Weber type A or B (depending on the level of the fracture) or an early-stage Lauge-Hansen supination-adduction or supination-external rotation injury.

Closed reduction and a short-leg cast with non–weight-bearing for 4 weeks is necessary if the lateral malleolus fracture is displaced. Weight-bearing and progression to a walker boot and shoe are guided by clinical and radiographic evidence of healing. Weight-bearing in a walker boot is appropriate if there is no displacement. The walker boot is removed during the day for range-of-motion exercises. Physical therapy may be necessary for proprioceptive retraining, range of motion, and strengthening.

Frequent radiographs should be compared with the original postreduction films to ensure that displacement has not occurred, especially in weight-bearing patients. Redisplacement or lateral talar subluxation implies an occult injury to the deltoid ligament with loss of stability. In this instance, operative treatment becomes necessary.

An isolated fracture of the medial malleolus is far less common and may represent an early-stage Lauge-Hansen pronation-abduction or pronation-external rotation mechanism. Closed reduction and immobilization as described above is appropriate for nondisplaced or minimally displaced transverse medial malleolar fractures.

ORIF of isolated medial malleolus fractures is necessary whenever closed reduction is not possible. An injury that will likely require ORIF is the vertically oriented shear fracture of the medial malleolus. This fracture is prone to displacement due to the orientation of the fracture plane. Other indications for surgery include interposed bone or soft tissue such as the posterior tibialis tendon and free osteochondral fragments from intra-articular comminution.

Open reduction is performed through an anteromedial incision as described previously. The medial malleolus is reduced and fixed with two partially threaded cancellous or cannulated cancellous screws. Alternative fixation methods such as K-wire fixation and tension-band wiring can be utilized in osteopenic bone. Non–weight-bearing in a short-leg cast or walker boot is used for 2 to 6 weeks, with gradual return to full weight-bearing initiated 6 to 12 weeks after surgery.

A bimalleolar fracture involving both the lateral and medial malleoli is inherently unstable because there are no restraints to talar displacement. These injuries correspond to Danis-Weber type B or C and to Lauge-Hansen higher stage supination-external rotation, pronation-abduction, or pronation-external rotation injuries. Unless there are medical contraindications, these injuries undergo ORIF of both sides of the ankle. The fibula is exposed as described previously. Soft tissue and hematoma that might block reduction are debrided. The fibula fracture is reduced and held with a bone clamp. Spiral or oblique fractures without comminution can be stabilized with one or two interfragmentary screws. Lag screws can rarely be used in transverse or short oblique fractures. A one-third tubular plate is contoured to the lateral surface of the fibula. The plate is fixed with bicortical screws proximal to the level of the tibiotalar joint and with unicortical, cancellous screws distal to the level of the tibiotalar joint to avoid intra-articular penetration (Fig. 37–16). Rigid screw

and plate fixation may be difficult to achieve when severe comminution is present. Supplemental fixation with small K-wires may be necessary. Intramedullary fixation with a Rush rod has been described (Pritchett, 1993) for comminuted fractures of the lateral malleolus in osteopenic bone. After reduction and fixation of the lateral malleolus, the medial malleolus undergoes ORIF as described above. Postoperative management includes a non–weight-bearing short-leg cast for 4 to 6 weeks followed by a walker boot, range-of-motion exercises, and advancement of weight-bearing as clinical and radiographic healing progresses.

A "bimalleolar equivalent" fracture pattern, with fracture of the lateral malleolus and disruption of the deltoid ligament, is also an unstable injury pattern because of the loss of medial ligamentous restraint. Diagnostic evidence of this injury includes medial ankle joint widening an asymmetric mortise or talar subluxation. A thorough physical examination and review of the x-rays are imperative because ORIF will be necessary to restore tibiotalar stability.

Operative management of the bimalleolar equivalent ankle fracture consists of ORIF of the lateral malleolus as described. Intra-operative radiographs are then obtained. If the reduction is congruent, the deltoid ligament does not need to be repaired. If the reduction is not congruent, exploration of the medial ankle is necessary to remove the block to reduction. Deltoid repair is then performed. The postoperative regimen is the same as that for bimalleolar fractures.

Trimalleolar or "trimalleolar-equivalent" fractures are bimalleolar or bimalleolar-equivalent fractures accompanied by fracture of the posterior malleolus of the distal tibia. The principles of treatment are the same as those for bimalleolar

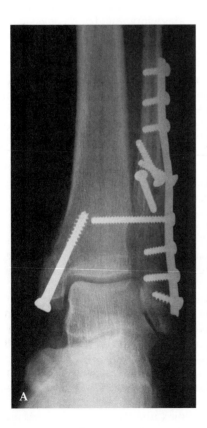 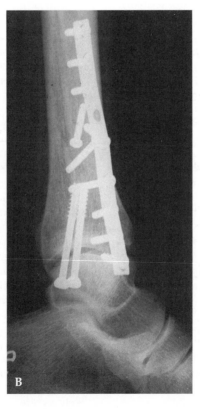

Figure 37–16 Fixation of a bimalleolar comminuted Danis-Weber type C ankle fracture. **(A)** Anteroposterior radiograph demonstrating medial and lateral fixation, including interfragmentary and syndesmotic screws. **(B)** Lateral radiograph.

fractures. Open reduction and internal fixation of the posterior malleolus is recommended when the fragment constitutes at least 25% of the articular surface as seen on the lateral radiograph. One study (Harper and Hardin, 1988) suggests that fixation is not necessary in fragments comprising more than 25% of the joint surface as long as less than 2 mm of posterior articular displacement remains after fixation of the lateral and medial malleoli. Any evidence of tibiotalar instability due to a displaced posterior malleolus fracture is an indication for internal fixation.

Open reduction and internal fixation of posterior malleolus fractures requires that the lateral incision be placed more posteriorly to improve exposure of both the lateral malleolus and posterior tibia. The posterior malleolus is exposed and reduced, and a cancellous screw is inserted either through the fragment to engage the anterior tibia or from anterior to engage the posterior malleolus fragment. Cannulated screws may be useful to ensure appropriate internal fixation position. Extreme care is essential to avoid injury to the peroneal tendons, sural nerve, and anterior neurovascular bundle.

Syndesmotic ligament and interosseous membrane injury may accompany an ankle fracture as in a Danis-Weber type C or Lauge-Hansen pronation-external rotation injury. They can also occur in isolation as in a "high" ankle sprain. (Fig. 37–17). In either case, syndesmotic ligament injury can result in instability between the tibia and fibula, leading to chronic pain and possibly talar subluxation. The Danis-Weber classification helps predict syndesmotic injury. No syndesmotic injury occurs in type A fractures. Type B ankle fractures may or may not have syndesmotic involvement. Syndesmotic injury is presumed if tibiotalar instability is evident in type B

ankle fractures. Unstable type B ankle fractures require ORIF because of medial and lateral injury and syndesmotic stability can be assessed intra-operatively. Type C fractures have injury of the syndesmotic ligaments (AITFL and PITFL) and interosseous membrane to the level of the fracture and thus require ORIF including syndesmotic fixation.

Syndesmotic stability is assessed intra-operatively after fixation of the lateral and medial malleoli restores stability to the joint. The fibula is grasped with a bone reduction clamp and pulled laterally. Another method uses "live" flouroscopic imaging of the ankle while applying an external rotation force to the foot and ankle. Mortise asymmetry or widening of the tibiofibular overlap suggests syndesmotic instability. There are no guidelines as to how much translation, asymmetry, or widening is acceptable and how much represents instability. It is likely better to "overtreat" syndesmotic injuries than to "undertreat" them.

Syndesmotic fixation consists of a 3.5 or 4.5-mm cortical screw transfixing both cortices of the fibula and the lateral cortex of the tibia 1 to 2 cm proximal to the tibiotalar joint line. It may be necessary to engage the medial cortex of the tibia if purchase is poor. More proximal fibula fractures suggest more extensive syndesmotic injury and may require two screws. The fibula is fixed to the tibia at the level of the syndesmosis (approximately 1 to 2 cm above the tibiotalar joint line) with one or two screws. The screw(s) enter the posterolateral fibula and are directed anteromedially into the tibia, parallel to the joint line. The screw(s) can be inserted through a lateral neutralization plate or around it. Lag technique is not used because it could result in compression of the syndesmosis and narrowing of the ankle mortise. This will block

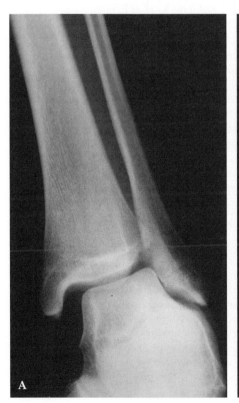
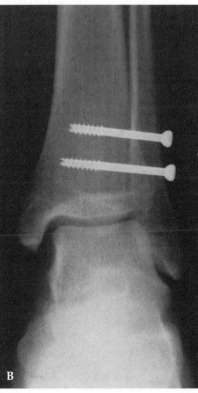

Figure 37–17 This 18-year-old man was run over by a bus, sustaining a syndesmotic injury. **(A)** Preoperative AP radiograph. **(B)** Postoperative radiograph demonstrating insertion of two 4.5-mm cannulated screws after reduction of syndesmosis.

full dorsiflexion of the ankle because the talar dome is wider anteriorly. Similarly, it is important to maximally dorsiflex the ankle during syndesmotic screw insertion to avoid narrowing of the ankle mortise. Direct repair of the ligaments is rarely necessary.

Postoperative care after syndesmotic fixation is undefined. Historically, the patient was non–weight-bearing until the syndesmotic screw was removed after 6 to 8 weeks. Reports of syndesmotic displacement after early screw removal prompted some to recommend waiting 12 to 16 weeks. Reports indicate there has been no increase in the incidence of screw breakage. We recommend leaving syndesmotic screws in place with the understanding that they will eventually break. We remove the screws 8 to 12 weeks postoperatively in athletes or in individuals who do not regain full dorsiflexion.

Of patients with ankle fractures, 80 to 90% will achieve pain-free function with restoration of alignment, stability, and range of motion. Factors that worsen the prognosis include severe comminution, medical comorbidity, and failure to obtain an anatomic reduction. Potential complications include infection, nonunion of the fibula or medial malleolus, malunion, sural or superficial peroneal nerve injury, and post-traumatic arthritis. The estimated incidence of post-traumatic arthritis is unknown because there are few natural history studies. Post-traumatic arthritis may correlate with failure to obtain anatomic reduction and may necessitate ankle arthrodesis for relief of symptoms.

CONCLUSIONS

Then have been major advances in understanding, recognizing, and treating foot and ankle trauma in the last two decades. Early diagnosis based on detailed clinical and radiographic examinations, occasionally supplemented by special radiographic views, CT scans, and/or MRI, facilitates care and optimizes long-term outcome. The goal of any treatment for foot and ankle trauma is early range of motion, weight bearing, and muscle strengthening. This allows early return to work and minimizes the harmful sequelae of immobilization. The treating physician must be able to recognize, understand, and distinguish injuries that require operative care from those that can be treated nonoperatively.

SELECTED BIBLIOGRAPHY

AITKEN AP, POULSON D. Dislocations of the tarsometatarsal joint. *J Bone Jt Surg.* 1963;45A:246–260.

ARNTZ CT, VEITH RG, HANSEN ST, Jr. Fractures and fracture-dislocations of the tarsometatarsal joint. *J Bone Jt Surg.* 1988;70A:173–181.

CANALE ST, KELLY FB Jr. Fractures of the neck of the talus: long-term evaluation of 71 cases. *J Bone Jt Surg.* 1978; 60A:143–156.

CROSBY LA, FITZGIBBONS T. Computerized tomography scanning of acute intra-articular fractures of the calcaneus: a new classification system. *J Bone Jt Surg.* 1990;72A:852–859.

DANIELS TR, SMITH JW, ROSS TI. Varus malalignment of the talar neck: its effects on the position of the foot and on subtalar motion. *J Bone Jt Surg.* 1996;78A:1559–1567.

DELEE JC. Fractures and dislocations of the foot. In: Mann RA, Coughlin MJ, eds. *Surgery of the Foot and Ankle.* 6th ed. St. Louis, MO: Mosby Year Book; 1993;1465–1703.

EBRAHEIM NA, MEKHAIL AO, SALPIETRO BJ, MERMER MJ, JACKSON WT. Talar neck fractures: anatomic considerations for posterior screw application. *Foot Ankle Int.* 1996;17: 541–547.

ESSEX-LOPRESTI P. The mechanism, reduction technique, and results in fractures of the os calcis. *Br J Surg.* 1952;39: 395–419.

FRANKLIN JL, JOHNSON KD, HANSEN ST Jr. Immediate internal fixation of open ankle fractures: report of 38 cases treated with a standard protocol. *J Bone Jt Surg.* 1984;66A: 1349–1356.

HARDCASTLE PH, RESCHAUER R, KUTSCHA-LISSBERG E, SCHOFFMANN W. Injuries to the tarsometatarsal joint: incidence, classification and treatment. *J Bone Jt Surg.* 1982;64B: 349–356.

HARPER MC, HARDIN G. Posterior malleolar fractures of the ankle associated with external rotation–abduction injuries. *J Bone Jt Surg.* 1988;70A:1348–1356.

HAWKINS LG. Fractures of the neck of the talus. *J Bone Jt Surg.* 1970;52A:991–1002.

HUENE DB, BUNNELL WP. Operative anatomy of nerves encountered in the lateral approach to the distal part of the fibula. *J Bone Jt Surg.* 1995;77A:1021–1024.

LAUGE-HANSEN N. Fractures of the ankle; II: combined experimental-surgical and experimental-roentgenologic investigation. *Arch Surg.* 1950;60:957–985.

MANOLI A, WEBER TG. Fasciotomy of the foot: an anatomical study with special reference to release of the calcaneal compartment. *Foot Ankle.* 1990;10:267–275.

MUELLER ME, ALLGOWER M, SCHNEIDER R, WILLENEGGER H. *Manual of Internal Fixation. Techniques Recommended by the AO Group.* 2nd ed. New York, NY: Springer-Verlag; 1979.

MYERSON MS, FISHER RT, BURGESS AR, KENZORA JE. Fracture dislocations of the tarsometatarsal joints: end results correlated with pathology and treatment. *Foot Ankle.* 1986;6:225–242.

PEREIRA DS, KOVAL KJ, RESNICK RB, SHESKIER SC, KUMMER F, ZUCKERMAN JD. Tibiotalar contact area and pressure distribution: the effect of mortise widening and syndesmosis fixation. *Foot Ankle Int.* 1996;17:269–274.

PRITCHETT JW. Rush rods versus plate osteosystheses for unstable ankle fractures in the elderly. *Orthop Rev.* 1993;22:691–696.

RAMSEY PL, HAMILTON W. Changes in tibiotalar area of contact caused by lateral talar shift. *J Bone Jt Surg.* 1976; 58A:356–357.

SANDERS R. Intra-articular fractures of the calcaneus: present state of the art. *J Orthop Trauma.* 1992;6:252–265.

SANDERS R, FORTIN P, DIPASQUALE T, WALLING A. Operative treatment in 120 displaced intra-articular calcaneal fractures: results using a prognostic computed tomography scan classification. *Clin Orthop.* 1993;290:87–95.

SANGEORZAN BJ, ANANTHAKRISHNAN D, TENCER AF. Contact characteristics of the subtalar joint after a simulated calcaneus fracture. *J Orthop Trauma.* 1995;9:251–258.

SWANSON TV, BRAY TJ, HOLMES GB Jr. Fractures of the talar neck: a mechanical study of fixation. *J Bone Jt Surg.* 1992;74A:544–551.

SAMPLE QUESTIONS

1. Lisfranc's ligament:
   - (a) is a dorsally located ligament stabilizing the first to the second metatarsal
   - (b) is a dorsally located ligament stabilizing the medial cuneiform to the second metatarsal
   - (c) is a dorsally located ligament stabilizing the middle cuneiform to the first metatarsal
   - (d) is a plantarly located ligament stabilizing the medial cuneiform to the second metatarsal
   - (e) is a plantarly located ligament stabilizing the middle cuneiform to the first metatarsal

2. The middle facet of the subtalar joint:
   - (a) is located laterally and is supported by the posterior tuberosity
   - (b) is located laterally and is confluent with the posterior facet
   - (c) is located medially and is supported by the posterior tuberosity
   - (d) is located medially and is supported by the sustentaculum tali
   - (e) is located medially and is confluent with the posterior facet

3. The typical deformity that results after a calcaneal fracture consists of all the following except:
   - (a) varus alignment
   - (b) posterior tibial tendon impingement
   - (c) shortening of calcaneal height
   - (d) peroneal tendon impingement
   - (e) calcaneal widening

4. Severe talar neck fractures may result in all of the following except:
   - (a) 50% ankle arthritis, 33% subtalar arthritis
   - (b) 33% ankle arthritis, 50% subtalar arthritis
   - (c) 20 to 50% avascular necrosis for type II fractures
   - (d) 80 to 100% avascular necrosis for type III fractures
   - (e) 10% delayed union, 5% nonunion

5. Ankle injuries that are likely to be accompanied by syndesmotic injury include:
   - (a) tip of the fibula avulsion
   - (b) vertical medial malleolus fracture
   - (c) bimalleolar ankle fracture with talar subluxation
   - (d) Maissoneuve fracture
   - (e) c and d

Chapter 38

Foot and Ankle Reconstruction

Anthony D. Watson, MD and Keith L. Wapner, MD

Outline

Foot and ankle disorders comprise a wide spectrum of pathology including overuse tendon injury, arthritis, compression neuropathy, forefoot deformity, and diabetic complications. Thorough history and physical examination are often sufficient for diagnosis. Nonoperative treatment is often successful. Operative treatment is indicated when nonoperative treatment fails, and it requires a thorough understanding of the pathophysiology and relevant anatomy.

ETIOLOGY

Tendon Injuries

All of the tendons that cross the ankle are subject to injury, but the most commonly injured are the Achilles, posterior tibial, and peroneal tendons. Most tendon injuries are traumatic, but degenerative tears are not unusual. Posterior tibial tendon (PTT) injuries in particular are typically attritional tears without a history of injury.

Posterior tibial tendon insufficiency due to attritional, degenerative tears is associated with Painful Adult Acquired Flatfoot Deformity. It typically occurs in the middle-aged patient. It is unclear whether attritional rupture leads to synovitis or primary synovitis weakens the tendon and predisposes it to attritional tears and eventual rupture.

Achilles' tendon ruptures are the third most frequent major tendon disruption behind rotator cuff and extensor mechanism ruptures. Acute rupture occurs most commonly 2 to 3 cm proximal to the calcaneal insertion in physically active men with sedentary jobs between the ages of 30 and 50. Diagnosis is missed in as many as 25% of cases.

Direct injuries are less common than indirect and can be either closed or open injuries. Closed injuries are the result of a direct blow to the tensioned tendon. Open ruptures are the result of sharp lacerations or severe crush injuries.

Indirect rupture of the Achilles' tendon occurs when tendon tension exceeds the ultimate strain of 7 to 15% and ultimate strength, which may be as high as 400 kiloPascals. Three indirect loading mechanisms have been described and include pushing off with the weight-bearing forefoot while simultaneously extending the knee, sudden unexpected dorsiflexion of the ankle accompanied by strong contraction of the Achilles as may occur in falling forward, and violent dorsiflexion of the plantarflexed foot. Although most mechanisms require rapid loading of a taut tendon, ruptures may also occur with normal walking or running.

615

Chronic tears of the Achilles' tendon may be the result of inadequately diagnosed or treated acute ruptures. A large tendon gap results from rapid tendinous degeneration and retraction of the proximal tendon stump. Secondary contraction and fibrosis of the Achilles tendon complex may occur. Chronic ruptures may also be due to an overuse syndrome or degenerative tendinosis. Microtears from cumulative trauma from overuse cause cyclic partial rupture and scarring. Degenerative tendinosis can result in lengthening and fusiform swelling of the tendon and insufficiency of the Achilles tendon complex.

Isolated peroneal tendon injury is rare, but peroneal tendon injury may accompany as many as 20% of all lateral ankle injuries. Isolated tendon injuries include tendon dislocation and attritional tears due to repetitive overuse. The incidence of peroneal tendon dislocation decreased markedly when more rigid ski boots that fit above the ankle were introduced. Forced eversion, dorsiflexion, and external rotation can dislocate the peroneal tendons. Peroneal tendinitis and attritional tears are likely due to overuse and have been found in 11% of ankles examined at autopsy.

Chronic recurrent peroneal tendon subluxation can complicate both acute peroneal tendon dislocation and lateral ankle sprains. The superior peroneal retinaculum (SPR) may become attenuated after either peroneal tendon dislocation or lateral ankle sprain. The posterolateral ridge of the fibula may also avulse. Either can predispose to peroneal tendon instability.

Peroneal tendon injury that accompanies an acute lateral ankle sprain is often underappreciated because of the more easily recognizable ankle sprain. Inversion, plantarflexion, and external rotation can stretch the peroneal tendons. Healing of the resulting microtears induces inflammation. Rehabilitation of lateral ankle sprains includes peroneal tendon strengthening, which can aggravate the inflammation and cause tendinitis and attritional tears. The peroneus brevis tendon may impinge against the posterior edge of the fibula and develop longitudinal attritional tears that cause "splaying" and thickening of the tendon.

Arthritis

Degenerative arthritis of the ankle, subtalar, and transverse tarsal joints are most commonly post-traumatic. Articular incongruity after intra-articular injury causes uneven pressure distribution and pathologic joint mechanics. Chondral injury at the time of injury may initiate a degenerative process that will occur regardless of perfect articular congruity. Extra-articular malunions may alter joint reaction forces and pressure distribution. Chronic ankle and/or hindfoot instability due to recurrent ankle sprains or chronic midfoot instability due to Lisfranc sprain can lead to degenerative arthritis because of abnormal joint kinematics.

Idiopathic degenerative arthritis may occur without antecedent trauma or instability but is very rare. Inflammatory arthritis is not unusual in the ankle and hindfoot and is most commonly rheumatoid arthritis. Rheumatoid arthritis most commonly affects the forefoot, the talonavicular joint, the subtalar joint, and the ankle, in that order. Seronegative inflammatory arthropathies more commonly affect the forefoot but can involve the subtalar joint.

Nerve Disorders

Tarsal tunnel syndrome is caused by compression of the posterior tibial nerve or one of its branches. The etiology can be identified in approximately half of the cases. Described etiologies include ganglion cyst, lipoma, exostosis due to fracture, tarsal coalition, enlarged venous plexus, hemangioma, anomalous or accessory muscle, and severe hindfoot pronation.

Interdigital neuroma, traditionally known as Morton's neuroma, also appears to be an entrapment neuropathy with secondary intraneural deposition of amorphous eosinophillic material. The most common etiology is narrow shoewear. Acute trauma, a space-occupying mass, or compression by the transverse metatarsal ligament may also cause interdigital neuroma. Interdigital neuromas most commonly occur in the third web space at the level of the transverse metatarsal ligament (Fig. 38–1). Rarely, interdigital neuromas are found in the second web space. The preponderance of third web space interdigital neuroma suggests a predisposing anatomic factor.

Forefoot Deformities

Deformities of the hallux and lesser toes are most commonly due to ill-fitting shoewear. Hallux valgus, mallet toes, and hammertoes are rare in cultures that do not wear shoes. Narrow toe-box shoes crowd the toes and force them into deformed postures (Fig. 38–2). High heels exacerbate the problem as the foot "slides down the ramp into a funnel."

Hallux valgus deformity is caused by a deforming force that causes lateral subluxation of the first metatarsophalangeal joint with valgus angulation of the great toe and varus angulation of the first metatarsal. The great toe pronates and the first metatarsal head subluxes medially relative to the sesamoids. The flexor hallucis longus (FHL) and extensor hallucis longus (EHL) tendons bowstring laterally and further deform the great toe at the metatarsophalangeal joint (Fig. 38–2a). Postulated deforming forces include pes planus deformity, Achilles' tendon contracture, cystic degeneration of the medial capsule of the first metatarsophalangeal joint due to inflammatory disease, obliquity of the first metatarsocuneiform joint that results in metatarsal primus varus, and first metatarsocuneiform joint instability and hypermobility. The increased pronation of the foot with pes planus or Achilles' tendon contracture increases valgus force on the great toe and eventually leads to deterioration of the medial capsule of the first metatarsophalangeal joint.

Other postulated etiologies include congenital predisposition to deformity, which often causes juvenile hallux valgus deformity, amputation of the second toe, and generalized joint hyperelasticity. Rheumatoid arthritis typically causes hallux valgus and lesser toe hammertoe deformities with metatarsophalangeal dislocation.

Mallet toe and hammertoe deformities are typically a consequence of ill-fitting shoewear. Clawtoe deformity may also be due to ill-fitting shoewear, but neurologic causes such as Charcot-Marie-Tooth disease, diabetic neuropathy, and Volkmann's ischemia after compartment syndrome must all be considered, especially when all toes are involved.

Hammertoe deformity may be due to metatarsophalangeal synovitis and instability. Metatarsophalangeal synovitis and instability are most common in the second toe,

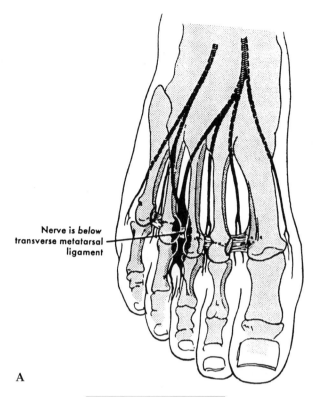

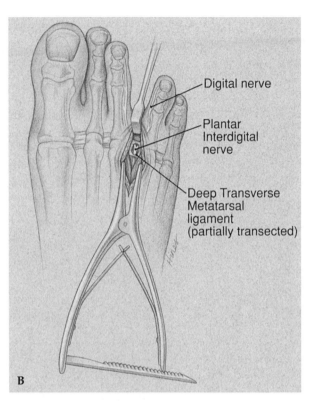

Figure 38–1 **(A)** Interdigital neuroma demonstrated in the third web space plantar to the transverse metatarsal ligament. Reproduced with permission from Mann RA, Baxter DE. Diseases of the nerves. In: Mann RA, Coughlin MJ, eds. *Surgery of the Foot and Ankle.* 6th ed. St. Louis, MO: Mosby Year Book, 1993:546. **(B)** Resection of an interdigital neuroma via dorsal approach. Reproduced with permission from Reynolds JC. Surgical treatment of interdigital neuroma. *Op Tech Orthop.* 1992;2:200.

especially when the second metatarsal is longer than the first metatarsal. Typically, activity leads to synovitis, which causes preferential attenuation of the lateral collateral ligament and plantar plate of the metatasophalangeal joint. The toe angulates into varus and eventually subluxes or dislocates at the metatarsophalangeal joint. This causes intrinsic-extrinsic imbalance and a hammertoe deformity (Fig. 38–3).

Diabetic Foot Disorders

Peripheral vascular disease, neuropathy, or both underlay all diabetic foot disorders. Sensory, motor, and autonomic nerves are all affected by neuropathy. The cause of vascular disease is unknown; however, it is typically more severe in diabetics than in nondiabetics. Proposed causes of neuropathy include ischemia due to vasonervorum disease caused by either sorbitol accumulation or intraneural accretion of glycosylation products.

Peripheral vascular disease compromises perfusion of the foot. Wound healing may be delayed or may not occur at all. Severely compromised perfusion may lead to gangrene. The metabolic demand of a diabetic foot infection can lead to gangrene when the compromised vascular supply cannot be increased.

Autonomic neuropathy causes dry skin, which can callus and crack easily allowing skin flora to gain entry into the deeper tissues. Unrecognized skin wounds and bony injuries can occur in sensory neuropathy. Motor neuropathy weakens the intrinsic muscles of the foot.

Intrinsic-extrinsic motor imbalance leads to clawtoe deformities and bony prominences that may develop ulcers because of unrecognized pressure due to sensory neuropathy.

Charcot neuroarthropathy develops when neuropathy is present and adequate perfusion of the foot remains. Multiple, unrecognized microfractures of the bones of the foot develop and induce the hyperemic response necessary for bony healing. The hyperemia causes bone resorption, which weakens the bones. However, the patient feels no pain because of sensory neuropathy, and continues standing and walking on the mechanically compromised foot, which causes progressive fracture and eventually deformity.

PEARL

Charcot neuroarthropathy occurs only in the setting of poor sensation and good circulation.

ANATOMY, SURGICAL APPROACHES, AND BASIC SCIENCE

Tarsal Tunnel

The tarsal tunnel is defined by the medial malleolus, sustentaculum tali, medial wall of the calcaneus, deltoid ligament, and flexor retinaculum. The contents from anteromedial to

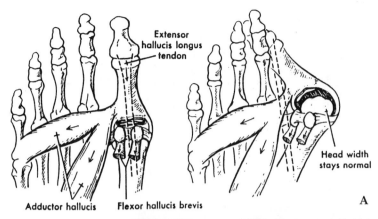

Extensor
hallucis longus
tendon

Head width
stays normal

Adductor hallucis   Flexor hallucis brevis

A

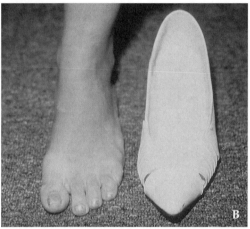

B

Figure 38–2 (A) Pathomechanics of
hallux valgus deformity. Valgus
angulation and lateral translation of the
proximal phalanx forces the metatarsal
head medially to cause varus angulation
of the metatarsal. The medial joint
capsule attenuates and contracture of the
lateral soft tissues develops. Reproduced
with permission from Mann RA,
Coughlin MJ. Adult Hallux Valgus. In:
Mann RA, Coughlin MJ, eds. *Surgery of
the Foot and Ankle.* 6th ed. St. Louis, MO:
Mosby Year Book, 1993:184.
(B) Difference in shape and size of a
typical foot and woman's dress shoe.

posterolateral include the PTT, flexor digitorum longus (FDL)
tendon, posterior tibial artery, tibial nerve, and FHL tendon.
The medial malleolus functions as a pulley for the PTT and
FDL tendon and the sustentaculum tali functions as a pulley
for the FHL tendon. The FHL tendon is immediately posterior to the ankle and posteromedial to the subtalar joint.

Posterior Tibial Tendon

The posterior tibial muscle is in the posterior compartment
of the leg. The myotendinous junction is proximal to the
tarsal tunnel. The PTT proceeds through the tarsal tunnel
posterior to the medial malleolus. The tendon passes through
a sheath, which begins at the medial malleolus and extends to
the insertion of the navicular (Fig. 38–4). Its major insertion is
into the proximal pole of the navicular. There are additional
insertions onto the plantar aspect of the cuneiforms and first
metatarsal.

Achilles' Tendon

The Achilles' tendon is the common tendon of the gastrocnemius and soleus muscles. The gastrocnemius muscle comprises a lateral head and larger medial head, which arise just
proximal to their respective femoral condyles. The soleus
originates from the oblique line of the tibia, the middle third
of the lateral tibial surface, and the back of the proximal third
of the posterior fibula. The aponeuroses of both muscles combine to form the Achilles' tendon, which is 10 to 15 cm in
length and inserts onto the middle third of the posterior surface of the calcaneus. The Achilles' tendon is surrounded by

a paratenon, which provides blood supply. The orientation
of the tendon fibers rotates 90 degrees internally as it courses
toward its insertion so that the proximal lateral fibers are
directly posterior and superficial distally.

Peroneal Tendon

The peroneal muscles originate along the proximal fibula.
The musculotendinous junction of both is proximal to the
ankle, but the peroneus brevis musculotendinous junction is
typically distal to that of the peroneus longus. The tendons
course posterior to the lateral malleolus, deep to the SPR and
superficial to the calcaneofibular ligament within the common tendon sheath, where the peroneus brevis lies deep to
the peroneus longus (Fig. 38–5). The peroneus brevis proceeds distally to the base of the fifth metatarsal. The peroneus
longus courses along the lateral calcaneus posterior and inferior to the peroneus brevis, passes medially plantar to the
cuboid, and continues medially to insert on the base of the
first metatarsal and the medial cuneiform.

Topographic Nerve Anatomy

Sensory nerves are easily jeopardized during foot and ankle
surgery. The superficial peroneal nerve pierces the deep fascia of the lateral compartment 10 to 15 cm proximal to the
ankle. It courses distally along the anterolateral leg and
crosses the ankle joint in the area of the syndesmosis. It typically branches proximal to the ankle joint. The intermediate
dorsal cutaneous branch passes lateral to the syndesmosis
and branches over the dorsal forefoot. The medial cutaneous

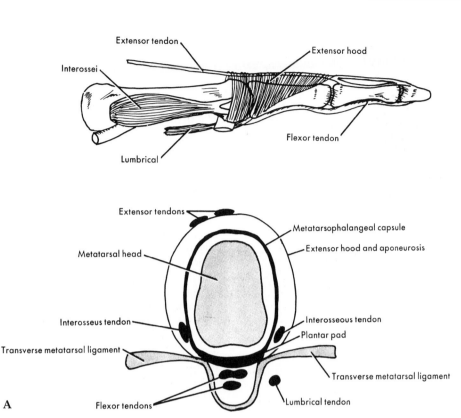

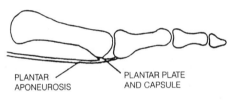

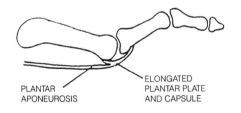

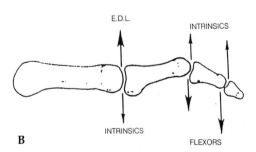

Figure 38–3 **(A)** Lateral and cross-section views of a lesser toe metatarsal head. **(B)** Attenuated plantar plate allows dorsiflexion of metatarsophalangeal joint when extrinsic motors overpower intrinsic motors. Reproduced with permission from Coughlin MJ, Mann RA. Lesser toe deformities. In: Mann RA, Coughlin MJ, eds. *Surgery of the Foot and Ankle.* 6th ed. St. Louis, MO: Mosby Year Book, 1993:347–348.

branch passes medial to the syndesmosis and branches over the dorsal forefoot. Its most medial branch is the dorsal medial hallucal nerve, which can be jeopardized by first metatarsophalangeal joint surgery.

The sural nerve courses posterolaterally along the posterior leg and is lateral to the Achilles' tendon. It continues distally along the course of the peroneal tendons and is distributed along the lateral forefoot. A lateral calcaneal sensory

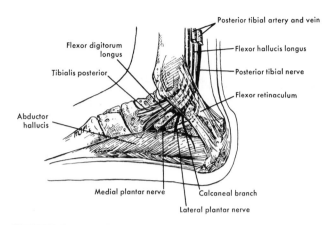

Figure 38–4 Anatomy of the tarsal tunnel. Reproduced with permission from Mann RA, Baxter DE. Diseases of the nerves. In: Mann RA, Coughlin MJ, eds. *Surgery of the Foot and Ankle.* 6th ed. St. Louis, MO: Mosby Year Book, 1993:554.

branch arises proximal to the ankle. The sural nerve and the lateral calcaneal sensory branch can be jeopardized by Achilles' tendon, peroneal tendon, and sinus tarsi approaches.

There are three major branches of the tibial nerve. The medial calcaneal sensory branch arises proximal to the tarsal tunnel. The medial and lateral plantar branches arise in the tarsal tunnel. Both branch in the plantar forefoot to provide digital branches. An anastomosis between the medial and lateral plantar branches in the third web space has been hypothesized as an etiology for Morton's neuroma.

The saphenous nerve and deep peroneal nerve are rarely clinically significant. The saphenous nerve crosses the medial ankle joint and provides limited dorsal sensation. The deep peroneal nerve accompanies the anterior tibial and dorsalis pedis artery and continues into the forefoot, where it becomes superficial in the dorsal first web space where it provides sensation.

First Metatarsophalangeal Joint

The first metatarsophalangeal joint is stabilized by medial and lateral collateral and sesamoid ligaments. A thick fibrocartilaginous plantar plate is formed by confluence of the two flexor hallucis brevis tendons and incorporates the sesamoid bones. The abductor hallucis muscle inserts onto the medial sesamoid and the base of the proximal phalanx. The two heads of the adductor hallucis insert onto the lateral sesamoid and the base of the proximal phalanx. The plantar aponeurosis also inserts onto the joint capsule. The cristae of the metatarsal head divides the plantar aspect into two facets, which articulate with the sesamoid bones.

The extensor hallucis longus and extensor hallucis brevis tendons balance the FHL and flexor hallucis brevis tendons in the sagittal plane. The abductor hallucis balances the adductor hallucis in the transverse plane.

The main blood supply to the first metatarsal is a nutrient artery that enters the mid-diaphysis and extends distally and proximally. The proximal metatarsal receives additional blood supply from the epiphyseal artery. Additional blood supply to the metatarsal head arises from the metatarsophalangeal joint capsule.

PITFALL

Compromise of the dual blood supply of the metatarsal head by distal osteotomy and soft tissue release can lead to avascular necrosis of the metatarsal head.

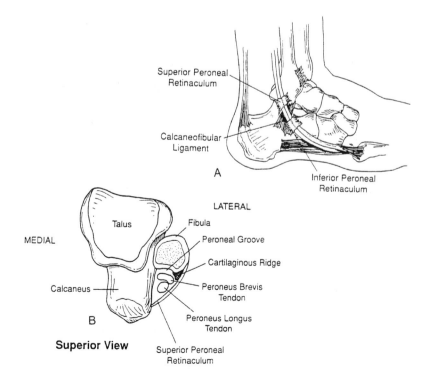

Superior View

Figure 38–5 Lateral **(A)** and transverse **(B)** views of peroneal tendon anatomy. The calcaneofibular ligament is deep to the peroneal tendons, which are contained within a fibro-osseous tunnel defined by the superior and inferior peroneal retinacula and the fibula and its osseo-cartilaginous posterolateral ridge. Reproduced with permission from Clanton TO, Schon LS. Athletic Injuries to the soft tissues of the foot and ankle. In: Mann RA, Coughlin MJ, eds. *Surgery of the Foot and Ankle.* 6th ed., St. Louis, MO: Mosby Year Book; 1993:1169.

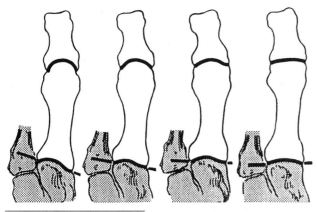

Figure 38–6 Variations in the shape of the first metatarsal head and the orientation of first metatarso-cuneiform joint can contribute to development of hallux valgus deformity. An oblique first metatarso-cuneiform joint predisposes to metatarsus primus varus, and a rounded metatarsal head predisposes to hallux valgus. Reproduced with permission from Mann RA, Coughlin MJ. Adult hallux valgus. In: Mann RA, Coughlin MJ, eds. *Surgery of the Foot and Ankle.* 6th ed. St. Louis,MO: Mosby Year Book; 1993:178.

The shape of the first metatarsal head and metatarso-cuneiform joint is quite variable (Fig. 38–6). Patients with a rounded first metatarsal head have a less stable joint and are more susceptible to progressive deformity. Patients with a flattened metatarsal head have a higher incidence of hallux rigidus.

Lesser Toe Flexor-Extensor Mechanism

The flexor-extensor mechanism of the lesser toes resembles that of the fingers. Appreciation of this mechanism clarifies lesser toe deformities (Fig. 38–3). The extrinsic extensors are the extensor digitorum longus and extensor digitorum brevis (EDB). Together they form the extensor expansion over the proximal phalanx and extend the metatarsophalangeal joint. The extensor digitorum longus continues distally and trifurcates to form the central slip, which inserts onto the middle phalanx, and the lateral bands, which insert onto the base of the distal phalanx. These extensions of the extensor digitorum longus extend the interphalangeal joints when the metatarsophalangeal joint is neutral or plantarflexed.

The extrinsic flexors of the toe are the FDL and the flexor digitorum brevis. The former flexes the distal interphalangeal joint, whereas the latter flexes the proximal interphalangeal joint (PIP).

The interossei muscles and lumbricals constitute the intrinsic motors of the toes. These structures lie plantar to the metatarsophalangeal joint, and their tendons course dorsally as they continue past the metatarsophalangeal joint. The intrinsic tendons coalesce with the lateral bands of the extensor digitorum longus, and, thus, flex the metatarsophalangeal joint and extend the interphalangeal joints.

Surgical Approaches

Most operations for the foot and ankle use direct approaches to the anatomic structure(s) of interest. Each approach will be discussed with its corresponding procedure. The sinus tarsi approach to the subtalar joint will be described here.

The sinus tarsi approach can be extended to include the calcaneocuboid, ankle, and even the talonavicular joints. A bell-shaped curvilinear incision extends from the tip of the fibula to the base of the fourth metatarsal. It curves in its midportion dorsally towards the toe extensor tendons. Blunt subcutaneous dissection is used to approach the fascia of the EDB muscle so as to protect branches of the sural and superficial peroneal nerves. A distally-based U-shaped EDB muscle flap is elevated from the underlying sinus tarsi and anterior process of the calcaneus. A soft tissue cuff should be left for later repair during wound closure. Continued distal elevation of the flap will expose the calcaneocuboid joint. The fatty tissue in the sinus tarsi can be removed to expose the anterior portion of the posterior facet of the subtalar joint. Subperiosteal dissection can be started on the lateral talar neck and continued dorsally, medially, and distally to expose the talonavicular joint.

EXAMINATION

Posterior Tibial Tendon

The patient most often does not remember a history of an acute trauma but rather an insidious onset of pain and swelling of the posterior medial aspect of the ankle. With time, the patient will note loss of the medial longitudinal arch and progressive difficulty in activities involving push-off.

Tenderness along the course of the PTT from the medial malleolus to the insertion of the navicular is present when there is tenosynovitis. The sheath will often be boggy. Plantarflexion and inversion may be weak and painful in tenosynovitis and may be absent with complete rupture. Standing examination will reveal a "collapsed" arch and forefoot abduction manifested by the "too many toes sign" when viewing the feet from behind the patient (Fig. 38–7). The patient will be unable to perform a single heel rise, and

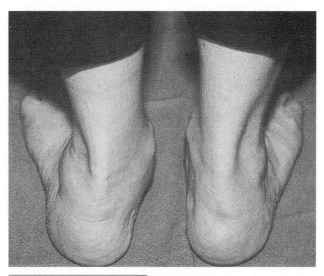

Figure 38–7 Talonavicular sag and "too many toes" sign in a patient with pes planovalgus deformity of the left foot due to posterior tibial tendon rupture and insufficiency.

the heel will remain in a valgus posture. Sinus tarsi and sub-fibular pain and tenderness may develop with progressive deformity.

Achilles' Tendon

Achilles' tendon rupture typically occurs in male patients between the ages of 30 and 50 while participating in an athletic activity. Patients usually recall hearing a "pop" after jumping, pushing off, or landing after a jump. There is sudden pain in the calf posterior to the ankle. Walking and ascending or descending stairs is difficult. The intensity of the pain may vary and patients who experience little or no pain may delay seeking medical attention.

Gait is abnormal and may include foot paradoxical drop. Swelling and ecchymosis may be present. A defect in the tendon, or "hatchet strike defect," is usually palpable. Active plantarflexion may be weak; however, the presence of active plantarflexion does not rule out an Achilles' tendon rupture because the tibialis posterior and FDL can plantarflex the ankle.

A more sensitive sign of Achilles' tendon rupture is the Thompson's test (Fig. 38–8). The patient lies in the prone position on the exam table with the feet hanging over the edge of the table. The calf is squeezed just distal to its maximum circumference. The absence of passive plantarflexion is a positive Thompson's test and indicates a complete Achilles' tendon rupture.

Persistent pain in the Achilles' tendon and/or weakness are present in chronic Achilles' tendon rupture resulting from

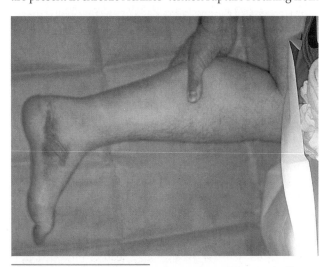

Figure 38–8 The Thompson's test is positive, or indicates Achilles tendon rupture, when squeezing the calf fails to passively plantarflex the ankle.

missed or untreated acute Achilles' tendon rupture. A careful history will usually document an acute injury after which the symptoms began. Gradual onset of Achilles' tendon pain and weakness suggest chronic Achilles' tendon rupture due to overuse or degenerative tendinosis. A history of transient or repeated episodes of pain in a runner's Achilles' tendon may indicate chronic, partial rupture. A limp and/or plantarflexion weakness may be present. A tender nodule, fusiform swelling within the tendon, or a defect in the tendon may be palpable. Thompson's test is often negative due to partial healing and scarring.

Peroneal Tendon

The patient's history may or may not include a significant acute event, but peroneal tendon injury should be suspected in any lateral ankle injury. A history of multiple ankle sprains is not uncommon and is especially suggestive. It is imperative that the patient precisely define the location of pain.

Warmth and swelling may be present along the tendon and in the fibular groove. Peroneal tendon tenderness approximately 1 to 2 cm proximal to the distal tip of the fibula may be present. Pain with active eversion of the ankle implicates peroneal tendon injury. Subluxation of the peroneal tendons can be palpated with one or two fingers resting on the posterior ridge of the fibula while the patient actively everts the ankle. Ankle stability should be assessed with anterolateral rotatory drawer and inversion.

Arthritis

Patients with degenerative arthritis typically complain of insidious onset of progressive stiffness and pain that diffusely involves a joint and is worse with activity. Ankle arthritis is typically painful anteriorly. Subtalar arthritis causes sinus tarsi pain, which is aggravated when walking on gravel or unlevel ground. The talonavicular and calcaneocuboid joints are painful at the location of the involved joint. Multiple joint involvement with morning stiffness suggests inflammatory arthritis.

Findings on physical examination include painful and decreased range of motion, crepitus, and palpable osteophytes. Deformity may be present. Precise palpation is necessary to accurately determine the involved joint. Observation of gait is useful to help determine functional disability.

Nerve Disorders

Patients with compressive neuropathy complain of burning and tingling pain in the distribution of the affected nerve. Night pain and rest pain are common. Pain may radiate proximally. Pain proximal to the calf suggests a higher lesion such as a lumbar radiculopathy.

Pain occurs over the course of the tibial nerve and into the sole of the foot and toes in tarsal tunnel syndrome and between the third and fourth toes in interdigital neuroma. Interdigital neuroma pain is relieved by removing shoes and is worsened by narrow, high heel shoes. Patients with interdigital neuroma often describe a sensation of their socks being "balled up" under their toes even when they are not wearing socks.

The tibial nerve is frequently tender in tarsal tunnel syndrome. There may also be tenderness at the origin of the abductor hallucis where the medial and lateral plantar nerves pass deep to enter the midfoot. Tinel's sign may be positive over the tarsal tunnel. Decreased 2-point discrimination has been described in tarsal tunnel, but the resolution of 2-point discrimination is not as great in the foot as it is in the hand.

The web space between the metatarsal heads is tender and often reproduces the symptoms of interdigital neuroma. It is essential to differentiate web space tenderness from plantar or articular metatarsal head tenderness. Squeezing the forefoot from medial and lateral may reproduce pain and may also produce a Moulder's click, which occurs when the neuroma is squeezed from between two metatarsal heads. Thorough neurologic evaluation is essential in nerve disorders of the foot to rule out peripheral neuropathy, more proximal neurologic lesions, instability and synovitis of the metatarsophalangeal joint, and metatarsalgia.

Forefoot Deformities

Patients with forefoot deformities often complain of pain due to pressure on the deformity from the shoe. Hard corns will indicate areas of increased extrinsic pressure. Plantar calluses suggest increased pressure on the metatarsal head of a dislocated metatarsophalangeal joint due to hammer toe or claw toe.

Mallet toe deformity is flexion of the distal interphalangeal joint. Hammer toe deformity comprises flexion of the PIP and extension of the metatarsophalangeal joint. Claw toe deformity consists of flexion of the proximal and distal interphalangeal joints and hyperextension of the metatarsophalangeal joint. Lateral or medial deviation at the metatarsolphalangeal joint may accompany hammer toe or claw toe (Fig. 38–9).

The flexibility of the deformity must be assessed to plan treatment. Flexible lesser toe deformities may be amenable to tendon transfer and/or capsular release, but rigid deformities require bony procedures. Adductor tightness in hallux valgus may limit the amount of correction that can be achieved with soft tissue or distal osteotomy procedures.

Range of motion, pain with motion, and sesamoid tenderness should be assessed in the first metatarsophalangeal joint. Degenerative joint disease or sesamoid tenderness may require arthrodesis for adequate symptom relief. First metatarsocuneiform joint mobility must be assessed because it may require arthrodesis to correct hallux valgus.

Diabetic Foot Disorders

Pulses should be palpated and sensation tested with Semmes-Weinstein monofilament. A foot that is insensate to the 5.07 monofilament has lost protective sensation. Calluses must always be pared because underlying ulcers are often present. The ulcer must be probed to accurately determine its depth. The foot should be carefully inspected for wounds. An isolated gangrenous toe suggests a web space abscess.

Acute Charcot neuroarthropathy presents with warmth, redness, and swelling. It is commonly misdiagnosed as infection. Diabetic foot infections are rare when perfusion is adequate and there is no portal of entry for skin flora. The typical deformity in chronic Charcot neuroarthropathy is pes planovalgus with prominence of the talar head medially or even a rocker-bottom foot deformity.

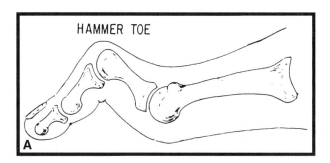

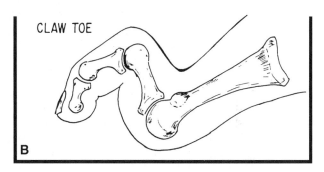

Figure 38–9 **(A)** Hammer toe. **(B)** Claw toe. Reproduced with permission from Brahms MA. Deformities of the Toes. In: Jahss MH, ed. *Disorders of the Foot and Ankle.* Philadelphia, PA: WB Saunders, 1991:1189.

PITFALL

The red, warm, swollen foot with sensory neuropathy, palpable pulses, and no wounds or ulcers should be suspected of having acute Charcot neuroarthropathy. Treatment of Charcot neuroarthropathy is often delayed because infection is suspected and Charcot neuroarthropathy is not considered.

AIDS TO DIAGNOSIS

Tendon Injuries

Plain radiographs are useful to rule out degenerative joint disease and to document talonavicular subluxation in PTT insufficiency. They may be necessary to rule out associated fractures, bony avulsion, or intratendinous calcification suggesting chronic degenerative tendinosis. A small avulsion fracture of the fibula by the SPR may accompany peroneal tendon dislocation or subluxation.

Various radiographic angles to evaluate PTT insufficiency have been described including the talocalcaneal, lateral talar-first metatarsal, and talar head coverage angles. None have been prognostically significant, but they are useful for determining the adequacy of radiographic correction of the deformity.

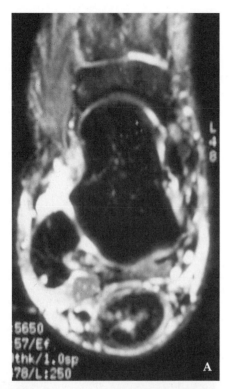

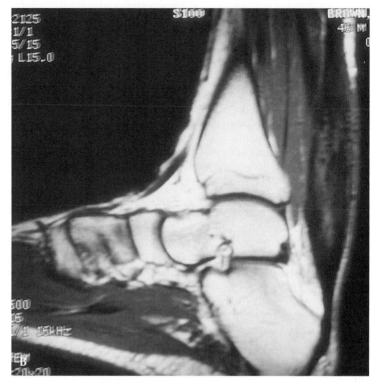

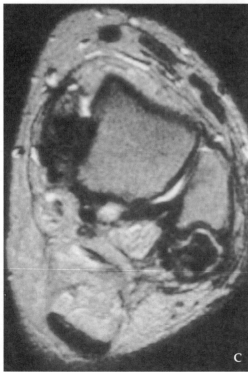

Figure 38–10   (A,B) Magnetic resonance imaging of chronic Achilles' tendinosis demonstrating thickening of the tendon and increased intra-tendinous signal intensity. **(C)** Similar findings in the peroneal tendons.

Ultrasound and magnetic resonance imaging (MRI) may be useful in equivocal cases of tendon injury. An MRI staging classification of PTT insufficiency has been proposed but has little prognostic or therapeutic value. Magnetic resonance imaging is useful in the diagnosis of chronic ruptures because it can demonstrate the extent of damage to the tendon, differentiate between complete and partial tears, and identify areas of intrasubstance degeneration not palpable on examination (Fig. 38–10).

Arthritis

Standing radiographs are essential to evaluate alignment. Decreased joint space, osteophyte formation, articular incongruity, and subchondral sclerosis are consistent with degenerative change (Fig. 38–11). Findings are similar in inflammatory arthritis except that articular erosions may be present and osteophyte formation is unusual.

Laboratory studies including rheumatoid factor, antinuclear antibody, and erythrocyte sedimentation rate are useful to rule out inflammatory arthritis. Joint aspiration can be analyzed for cell count and differential, crystals, protein, and glucose. Injections of local anesthetic and steroid may be useful to differentiate involved joints from uninvolved joints.

Nerve Disorders

Well-performed and interpreted electromyographic studies can be useful to diagnose tarsal tunnel syndrome. Terminal latency of the medial plantar nerve should be less than 6.2 milliseconds and terminal latency of the lateral plantar nerve should be less than 7.0 milliseconds. Magnetic resonance

imaging may also be useful to rule out a space-occupying mass such as a ganglion, lipoma, or anomalous muscle.

Forefoot Deformities

Weight-bearing anteroposterior (AP) and lateral radiographs of the feet are essential to accurately evaluate deformity. The hallux valgus angle is described by the angle between the longitudinal axes of the proximal phalanx and first metatarsal. The intermetatarsal angle is subtended by the longitudinal axes of the first and second metatarsals. The distal metatarsal articular angle is formed by the line connecting the lateral and medial extents of the metatarsal head articular surface and the longitudinal axis of the metatarsal. The position of the sesamoids and congruency of the metatarsophalangeal joint should be determined to facilitate preoperative planning.

Degenerative joint disease should be evaluated because arthrodesis is likely to be the only satisfactory procedure to control symptoms. Dorsal osteophytes are apparent at the first metatarsophalangeal joint in hallux rigidus. An oblique radiograph demonstrates the plantar two thirds of the metatarsophalangeal joint. Cheilectomy is sufficient when the plantar two thirds of the metatarsophalangeal joint is normal in spite of dorsal degenerative changes. Joint space narrowing or overlapping of the proximal phalanx on the metatarsal head in the lesser toes on the AP view suggests subluxation or dislocation at the metatarsophalangeal joint.

Diabetic Foot Disorders

Radiographs are necessary to diagnose Charcot neuroarthropathy (Fig. 38–12) and to rule out osteomyelitis. Osteomyelitis is rarely radiographically apparent until 3 to 4

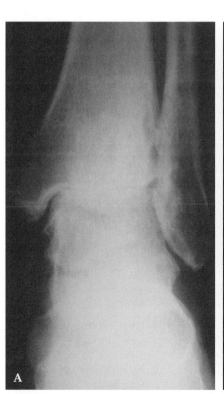
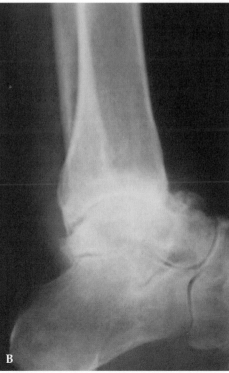

Figure 38–11 Radiographic degenerative joint disease of the ankle (**A**) and subtalar joint (**B**).

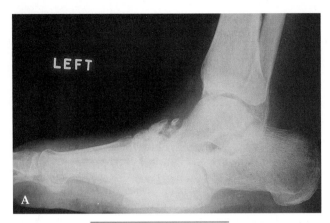 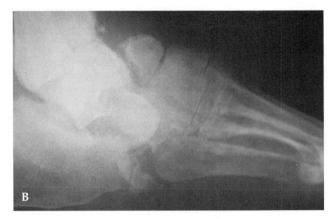

Figure 38–12 Radiographs of Charcot neuroarthropathy of the midfoot (**A**) and hindfoot (**B**).

weeks after the onset. Simultaneous technetium bone scan and white blood cell tagged indium scan can be useful for diagnosing osteomyelitis when radiographs are negative. Increased uptake in the same area of a bone on both scans suggests osteomyelitis. Marrow edema on MRI also suggests osteomyelitis.

Venous Doppler scanning and transcutaneous oxygen measurements are useful for determining adequacy of perfusion. The ankle-brachial index (ABI) is the ratio of the pressure in the foot to that in the arm. It must be greater than 0.45 for a diabetic to heal a foot wound. An ABI greater than 1 is not uncommon in diabetics with incompressible, calcified vessels. When the ABI is greater than 1, a triphasic waveform or a transcutaneous oxygen measurement greater than 30 demonstrates adequate perfusion. Total lymphocyte count greater than 1500 and serum albumin greater than 3.0 indicate adequate nutritional status to combat infection and heal wounds.

SPECIFIC CONDITIONS, TREATMENT, AND OUTCOME

Posterior Tibial Tendon

The Johnson classification has been proposed to guide treatment. Tenosynovitis without deformity describes stage I insufficiency. Stage II disease comprises planovalgus deformity with weakness or rupture of the PTT. Fixed pes planovalgus deformity occurs in stage III.

Nonoperative treatment options for stage I PTT insufficiency include cast immobilization, anti-inflammatory medication, or a longitudinal arch support with a medial heel wedge orthotic. Operative debridement of the tendon may be indicated if symptoms do not improve in 2 to 3 months. The entire tendon must be inspected for longitudinal tears, which should be debrided and repaired. A FDL tendon transfer may be necessary to restore function if a degenerative rupture is impending or present.

Nonoperative treatment of stage II deformity consists of a UCBL orthosis or a hinged or fixed AFO that stabilizes the foot and ankle. The patient must understand that nonoperative

treatment is palliative and will not correct the deformity. The deformity may progress and become fixed in spite of bracing.

Surgical treatment of stage II insufficiency remains undefined. Excellent results have been reported with FDL transfer in patients without forefoot deformity (Fig. 38–13). However, the results of isolated tendon transfers in stage II deformities have been less satisfactory. Various bony procedures in isolation or combination have been proposed to supplement FDL tendon transfer and include medial displacement calcaneal osteotomy, lateral column lengthening with interposition iliac crest bone graft either in the anterior calcaneus or in the calcaneocuboid joint (Fig. 38–13), or subtalar arthrodesis.

Patients with fixed deformity (stage III) or degenerative arthritis require accomodative shoewear and bracing. If nonoperative measures fail, double or triple arthrodesis to realign and stabilize the hindfoot may be necessary.

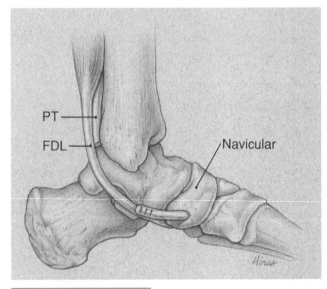

Figure 38–13 Flexor digitorum longus tendon transfer for posterior tibial tendon rupture. Reproduced with permission from Deland JT. Posterior tibial tendon insufficiency: soft-tissue reconstruction, *Op Tech Orthop.* 1992;2:159.

Achilles' Tendon

The goal of treatment is restoration of normal Achilles' tendon complex length and tension. Treatment can be either operative or nonoperative. Chronic Achilles tendon ruptures are more complex.

Nonoperative treatment of acute Achilles' tendon ruptures typically consists of either a short leg or long leg cast with the foot in gravity equinus, which is the relaxed position the foot assumes when the patient is sitting on a table with the knees flexed over the edge. No plantar flexion force is applied to the foot. Immobilization is maintained for 8 to 12 weeks. The patient is non–weight-bearing for the first 4 weeks. A 2.5-cm heel lift is used for 4 weeks after the cast is removed. It is not clear whether a short leg or long leg cast is better. The most common complications of nonoperative treatment is rerupture and tendon lengthening.

Operative repair can be performed open and percutaneously. Numerous open techniques have been described and include simple end-to-end suture, plantaris weave reinforcement, peroneus brevis reinforcement, fascial augmentation, and pullout wire techniques.

Surgical repair is traditionally performed with the patient in the prone position. A medial approach avoids the sural nerve. The incision should be made through skin and subcutaneous tissue onto the paratenon to create full-thickness skin flaps and minimize wound-healing complications (Fig. 38–14). The paratenon is incised parallel to the incision. The rupture is identified. Midsubstance ruptures are most common, but proximal and distal ruptures can occur. The paratenon is elevated off of the Achilles' tendon, and the rupture and tendon ends are inspected. The tendon ends typically resemble a mop. All frayed ends of the tendon must be debrided (Fig. 38–15). Heavy, nonabsorbable suture is used to perform an end-to-end repair. A Bunnell or Kessler tendon-grasping suture technique is essential to avoid suture pullout.

A tear at the myotendinous junction is often difficult to repair because of inadequate purchase of suture material in the proximal tissues. Tendon strips may be raised from the long distal portion of the tendon and inverted proximally to

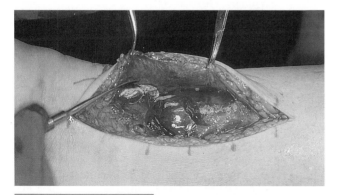

Figure 38–14 Repair of ruptured Achilles' tendon. Dissection is performed deep to the paratenon, which is held by hemostats to avoid injury to the vascular supply to the overlying skin.

PEARL

It is useful to prep and drape both legs. The position of the ankles should be approximately symmetric after repair to ensure that the length-tension relationship of the injured Achilles' tendon has been restored.

reinforce the repair (Fig. 38–15). Weaving these strips into the proximal tissues effects a continuous repair.

Repair of tendon avulsion from its calcaneal insertion requires placing drill holes transversely through the calcaneus. The ends of Bunnel or Kessler grasping sutures placed in the tendon can be brought through these drill holes and tied over the bony bridge to secure fixation of the tendon to the underlying bone (Fig. 38–15).

When the plantaris tendon is present, it is often useful to weave this tendon through the repair to augment the repair strength. The paratenon must be carefully closed to help prevent scarring of the tendon to the overlying soft tissues and skin.

A short-leg cast with the foot in gravity equinus is applied for four weeks of non–weight-bearing. A removable, walker boot with a dorsflexion block at 10 degrees of plantarflexion may be applied 4 weeks postoperatively in reliable patients. Otherwise, a second short-leg cast with the ankle in less plantarflexion is applied for 2 weeks and changed to a third cast with less plantarflexion for 2 more weeks. In either case, weight bearing is advanced as tolerated. After casting is completed, a walker boot is used.

Strengthening begins 8 weeks postoperatively, and the walker boot is discontinued when the patient can initiate active heel rise and has pain-free dorsiflexion of 10 degrees. A small heel lift may be used for 3 to 4 weeks after completion of ambulatory immobilization. Complications of surgical treatment include infection, skin slough, rerupture, and sural nerve injury. The incidence of rerupture after surgical repair is approximately half that after nonoperative treatment.

Nonoperative treatment of chronic Achilles' tendon ruptures typically does not improve function because the tendon has healed lengthened or with a large fixed gap. Patients who do not want surgery generally obtain adequate pain relief with an AFO.

Surgical treatment requires excision of the fibrotic scar between the tendon ends. End-to-end repair of the tendon is often impossible because of the resulting gap. Transfer of the FHL or FDL tendon is a useful technique to bridge the gap (Fig. 38–16). Postoperative treatment after surgical reconstruction for chronic Achilles' tendon rupture is similar to that for acute rupture, although prolonged immobilization may be necessary to protect a tenuous reconstruction.

Peroneal Tendon

Nonsurgical treatment includes immobilization in a short-leg walking cast to allow the inflammatory process to become quiescent. Immobilization is unlikely to be effective

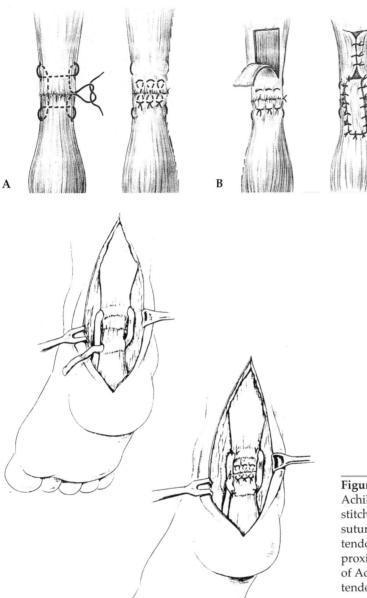

A

B

C

Figure 38–15 **(A)** Direct repair of Achilles' tendon rupture with Kessler stitch reinforced with figure-of-eight sutures. **(B)** Reinforcement of Achilles' tendon repair with turn-down flap of the proximal aponeurosis. **(C)** Reinforcement of Achilles' tendon repair with plantaris tendon weave. Reproduced with permission from Shereff MJ. *Atlas of Foot and Ankle Surgery.* Philadelphia, PA: WB Saunders, 1993:309–311.

if tears are present. A brace that limits inversion and eversion of the hindfoot may control peroneal tendon subluxation. Physical therapy may be useful to restore normal strength and proprioception if the tendons are intact and after cast immobilization.

Surgical repair is indicated when nonoperative measures fail. An incision is made along the course of the peroneal tendons (Fig. 38–17). Blunt dissection of the subcutaneous tissue is necessary to protect the sural nerve. The SPR is exposed and examined for tears or laxity. It is then released a few millimeters off the posterior fibula so as to leave a soft tissue cuff

for later repair. The peroneal sheath is then incised longitudinally and the peroneal tendons are exposed.

Both tendons should be examined on all surfaces because tears are often encountered on the deep surface of the peroneus brevis tendon. A low-lying peroneus brevis muscle belly, a peroneus quartus tendon, and proliferative inflammatory tissue must be excised to decompress the fibular groove.

The frayed tissue alongside full- and partial-thickness longitudinal tears of the peroneus brevis tendon should be excised, and the tear should be repaired with a running No. 6-0 nylon suture. The tendon should also be tubularized

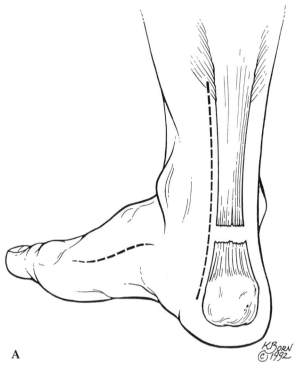

A

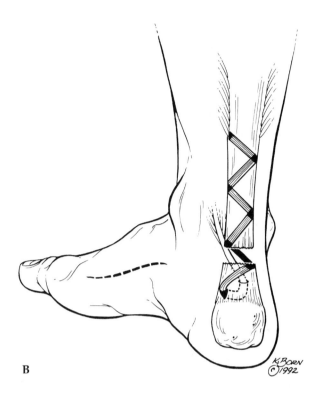

B

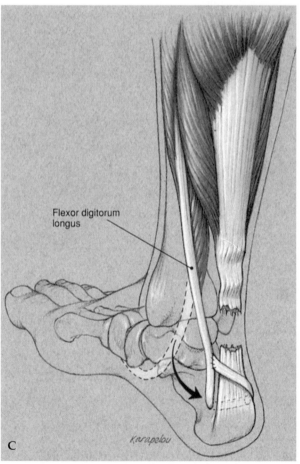

Flexor digitorum longus

C

Figure 38–16 **(A)** Flexor hallucis longus (FHL) tendon is harvested via incisions. **(B)** Then the FHL is placed from lateral to medial through a transverse drill hole in the posterosuperior calcaneus and weaved through the Achilles' tendon stumps. Reproduced with permission from Wapner, KL, Pavlock, GS et al. Repair of chronic Achilles' tendon rupture with flexor hallucis longus tendon transfer. *Foot Ankle.* 1993;14:445–447. **(C)** The same incisions are used to harvest the FDL tendon for reconstructing a chronic Achilles' tendon rupture. Reproduced from Mann RA. Achilles' tendon reconstruction using the flexor digitorum longus. *Op Tech Orthop.* 1994;4:139.

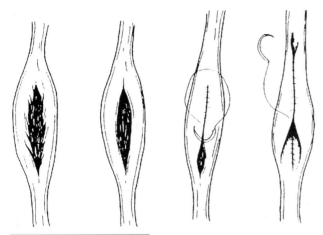

Figure 38–17 Debridement, tubularization, and repair of peroneal tendon tear. Reproduced with permission from Yodlowski M, Mizel MS. Reconstruction of peroneus brevis pathology. *Op Tech Orthop.* 1994;4:150.

using a running No. 6-0 nylon suture (Fig. 38–14). The frayed tissue alongside a peripheral tear can be excised and the remaining edge contoured smooth. Multiple frayed tears or severe degeneration beyond repair require excision of the pathologic section and tenodesis of the proximal and distal ends of the peroneus brevis to the peroneus longus tendon.

A sharp posterior ridge of the fibula should be smoothed with a rongeur and rasp. The tendons are reduced and the SPR repaired. Subluxing peroneal tendons often require deepening of the posterior fibular groove with a gouge. The SPR must be repaired with sufficient tension to prevent tendon subluxation or dislocation but must be lax enough to allow free motion of the tendons. Tendon stability should be assessed through a full range of ankle motion with two fingers along the posterior ridge of the fibula and over the tendons.

A short-leg cast is applied and the patient is non–weight-bearing for 2 weeks. A short-leg walking cast is then applied for 4 weeks. An ankle brace that limits hindfoot inversion and eversion is then used for 4 weeks after which gentle strengthening and range-of-motion exercises are commenced.

Staged reconstruction with the FHL tendon may be necessary if both peroneal tendons must be sacrificed because of tumor, trauma, or degeneration. The tendons are excised and a Hunter tendon rod is inserted in the first stage. A pseudosynovial sheath forms around the Hunter tendon rod, which is removed approximately 3 months later. The FHL tendon is then transferred through the pseudosynovial sheath to insert onto the base of the fifth metatarsal. Postoperative care is similar to that for a tendon repair.

Arthritis

Nonoperative treatment for ankle arthritis consists of AFO brace immobilization and a SACH heel and/or rocker-bottom shoe modification. Symptomatic subtalar and transverse tarsal joint arthritis may be relieved with a UCBL orthosis. Cortisone injections may provide temporary relief. Arthrodesis is indicated when nonoperative treatment fails to relieve disabling pain.

Ankle arthrodesis is performed through a transfibular approach. A lateral incision is made over the distal fibula and extending toward the base of the fourth metatarsal. The distal fibula is exposed subperiosteally. An oblique osteotomy of the distal fibula is begun at the lateral cortex proximal to the tibial plafond and is directed distally and medially to exit at the level of the tibial plafond. The distal fibula is removed and split longitudinally, and the cancellous bone is harvested for bone graft. A laminar spreader can be placed within the joint to assist in visualization. The tibial and talar subchondral bone is removed with either curettes or a sagittal saw. The exposed cancellous bone is "feathered" with a small osteotome to increase the surface area for fusion.

The optimum position for arthrodesis is neutral dorsiflexion, slight external rotation, and 5 degrees of valgus. A variety of fixation techniques have been described, but we recommend two parallel screws directed either antegrade or retrograde from the lateral inferior talus to the medial tibia (Fig. 38–18). A third screw placed from the lateral tibia just anterior to the fibula into the medial talus may occasionally be necessary. A short-leg cast is applied postoperatively and is changed periodically until fusion is radiographically evident. The patient is non–weight-bearing for 4 to 6 weeks at which time weight-bearing is advanced as tolerated. Shoe modification with a SACH heel and/or rocker-bottom sole facilitates essentially normal gait.

The sinus tarsi approach is used for subtalar arthrodesis. Visualization is improved by releasing the interosseous ligaments and placing a laminar spreader between the talar neck and dorsal calcaneus near the middle facet portion of the subtalar joint. An osteotome is used to remove the remaining cartilage and subchondral bone. Care must be taken to avoid

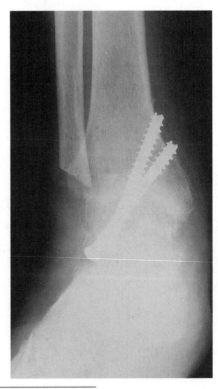

Figure 38–18 Postoperative radiograph of ankle arthrodesis.

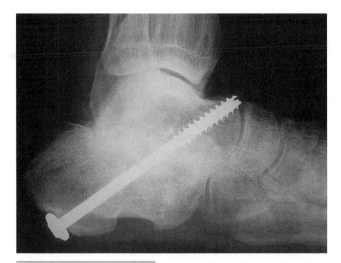

Figure 38–19 Postoperative radiograph of subtalar arthrodesis.

injury to the FHL tendon medially. The exposed cancellous bone should be feathered with a small osteotome. One or two compression screws are placed from the inferior posterior aspect of the calcaneus, across the arthrodesis site, and into the anterior body of the talus or talar neck (Fig. 38–19). A short-leg cast is applied and the patient is non–weight-bearing for 4 weeks. Weight bearing is advanced as tolerated in a short-leg walking cast for 4 weeks, and the patient is advanced as tolerated into regular shoewear.

The sinus tarsi approach is also used for triple arthrodesis by extending the incision distally to include the calcaneocuboid joint. The talonavicular joint can be approached by continuing subperiosteal dissection medially and dorsally; however, it is usually easier to make a medial longitudinal incision directly over the joint. The subchondral bone of all three joints should be removed with osteotomes and the exposed cancellous bone "feathered" with a small osteotome. Compression screw or staple fixation can be used for the calcaneocuboid joint, and compression screw fixation can be used for the talonavicular and subtalar joints (Fig. 38–20). A short-leg cast is applied in which the patient is non–weight-

bearing for 6 weeks. Weight-bearing is advanced as tolerated in a short-leg walking cast, which is discontinued when arthrodesis is radiographically evident.

Tarsal Tunnel Syndrome

Nonoperative treatment includes nonsteroidal anti-inflammatory medication, ambulatory immobilization, and orthotic devices to decrease pronation. Low-dose neurotropic medication such as amitryptaline may be useful.

Surgical decompression of the tarsal tunnel is indicated for disabling symptoms that fail to improve with nonoperative treatment. A skin incision is made along the course of the tibial nerve beginning proximal to the medial malleolus and extending distally to the origin of the abductor hallucis. The entire flexor retinaculum is incised, and the superficial and deep fascia of the origin of the abductor hallucis are both released to decompress the terminal branches (Fig. 38–21). Meticulous hemostasis is essential to minimize postoperative bleeding, scar formation, and symptomatic recurrence. The patient is non–weight-bearing for 4 weeks, then is progressively mobilized. The prognosis for surgery is better if a space-occupying mass is identified; otherwise, symptom resolution occurs in only 60 to 75% of patients.

Interdigital Neuroma

Nonoperative treatment includes a wide toe-box, flat shoe with a soft, metatarsal support orthotic that ends just proximal to the metatarsal heads (Fig. 38–1). The orthotic transfers pressure from the location of the neuroma and elevates and spreads the metatarsal heads to decrease the compression of the interdigital neuroma. Nonsteroidal anti-inflammatory medications may be useful. A single steroid injection into the web space is successful in 60% of patients but should be avoided in patients who have a thin, plantar fat pad. Multiple injections are unlikely to be successful if the first injection was not successful. Furthermore, multiple injections should be avoided to prevent plantar fat pad atrophy.

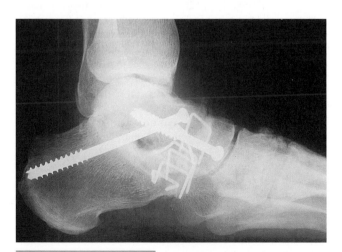

Figure 38–20 Postoperative radiograph of triple arthrodesis.

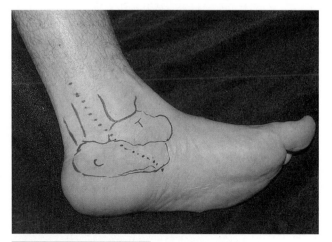

Figure 38–21 Incision for tarsal tunnel release.

Surgical excision of the neuroma is indicated when nonoperative treatment options have been exhausted. A dorsal skin incision is centered in the web space, and blunt dissection of the subcutaneous tissue is used to approach the transverse metatarsal ligament (Fig. 38–1). The transverse metatarsal ligament is incised and a self-retaining retractor is placed between the metatarsal heads to spread the metatarsals and improve visualization of the neuroma. The neuroma and the nerve branches are identified and divided distally. The nerve can then be grasped and pulled distally to facilitate dissection of the nerve well proximal to the weight-bearing surface of the forefoot. The nerve is transected well proximal to the weight-bearing surface of the forefoot, and the foot is forcibly dorsiflexed to allow the remaining nerve to retract. Heel-touch weight-bearing is permitted for 2 weeks postoperatively, and then weight-bearing is advanced as tolerated. Satisfactory symptom relief occurs in approximately 80% of patients.

PITFALL

The nerve must be transected as far proximal as possible to minimize the risk of recurrence. It is imperative to thoroughly dissect and identify the nerve and any branches in the web space to minimize the risk of recurrence.

Recurrent interdigital neuromas are symptomatically similar to primary interdigital neuromas. Nonoperative treatment is similar, and if unsuccessful, revision surgery with either a dorsal incision or a plantar longitudinal incision in the web space that extends proximally to the proximal plantar fascia is indicated. With either incision, it is imperative to dissect and transect the nerve well proximal to the recurrent neuroma and to bury the stump in the interossei muscle. Symptomatic relief will occur in approximately 80% of patients.

Hallux Valgus

Nonoperative treatment consists of education about proper shoewear. Shoes with a straight last and a rounded toe-box will often relieve discomfort. Pointed, narrow toe-box shoes will be painful and cause progression of the deformity. A simple, transferable, longitudinal arch support may also be helpful, especially when metatarsalgia or ball-of-foot pain, is present.

Surgical treatment may be indicated for disabling pain unrelieved by nonoperative treatment. Patients must understand that hallux valgus surgery is for pain relief and not for cosmesis. Narrow, pointed toe-box shoes are not permitted after surgical correction of hallux valgus because recurrent deformity will occur.

The first metatarsophalangeal joint may be congruent or incongruent. When a hallux valgus deformity is present, and a distal metatarsal articular angle demonstrates that the cartilage cap of the first metatarsal head is oblique, the joint may be congruent. This must be recognized preoperatively so that surgical correction does not lead to incongruency of the joint.

The presence of a lateral facet at the base of the first metatarsal may require an osteotomy for adequate reduction.

More than a hundred surgical procedures have been described for hallux valgus correction. Selection of the appropriate procedure requires consideration of the magnitude of hallux valgus and metatarsus primus varus deformity, great toe pronation, sesamoid position, adductor tightness, condition and congruency of the metatarsophalangeal joint, and functional demands of the patient. A radiographic classification of hallux valgus has been proposed to guide preoperative planning; however, it fails to fully consider clinical parameters.

Mild bunion deformities are amenable to the modified McBride procedure or the distal Chevron osteotomy. The modified McBride procedure is indicated for mild hallux valgus deformity (hallux valgus angle < 30 degrees) with metatarsophalangeal incongruency and without metatarsus primus varus, tibial sesamoid subluxation lateral to the crista, great toe pronation, and degenerative joint disease in active adults. It includes medial eminence resection and medial capsular plication via a medial incision, and release of the adductor tendon, transverse metatarsal ligament, and fibular sesamoidal ligament via a dorsal first web space incision (Fig. 38–22).

A midline medial skin incision is made, and blunt dissection of the subcutaneous tissue is performed to raise dorsal and plantar flaps and to identify and protect the sensory nerves. Capsulotomy is performed by excising redundant medial capsule defined by two parallel incisions perpendicular to the longitudinal axis of the metatarsal. The incisions should converge dorsally at the superior surface of the medial eminence and plantarly at the tibial sesamoid. A second incision is then made along the dorsomedial capsule over the medial eminence and elevated subperiosteally from the underlying medial eminence and metatarsal head. Another option is a V-Y capsulotomy with the base of the Y over the medial metatarsal diaphysis and the intersection of the limbs at the proximal margin of the medial eminence. The medial eminence is resected at the level of the sagittal sulcus on a plane parallel with the medial border of the foot.

A longitudinal skin incision is then made in the dorsal first web space and blunt dissection through subcutaneous is performed to identify the adductor hallucis tendon. It is isolated and transected. The underlying fibular sesamoidal ligament, which connects the fibular sesamoid and metatarsal head, is then divided. Finally, the transverse metatarsal ligament is divided. Lateral metatarsophalangeal joint capsule contracture should be released by manually pulling the toe into varus and not by complete transection of the lateral capsule. The adductor tendon may be reattached to the lateral metatarsophalangeal joint capsule. Redundant medial capsule tissue is excised to allow repair of the hallux in neutral position.

The indications for distal chevron osteotomy are similar to those for the modified McBride procedure except that more lateral subluxation of the tibial sesamoid can be corrected, but adductor tightness must not be present (Figs. 38–22d through 38–22f). Distal chevron osteotomy compromises intramedullary vascular supply of the metatarsal head. Therefore, distal osteotomy with lateral soft tissue release may completely compromise the metatarsal head vascular supply and cause avascular necrosis.

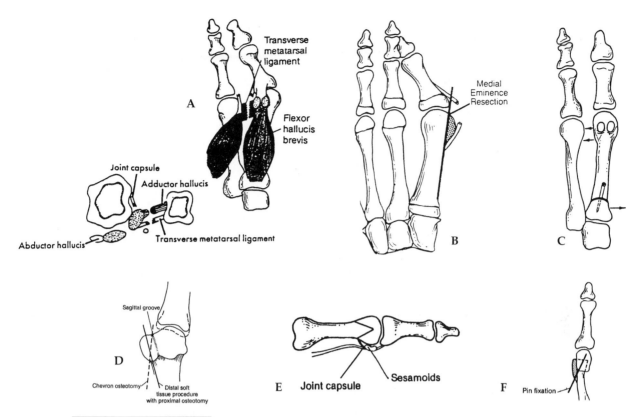

Figure 38–22 **(A,B)** Distal soft tissue release. **(C)** Proximal first metatarsal crescentic osteotomy. **(D)** The plane of medial eminence resection is along the solid line for the modified McBride procedure and along the dashed line for distal chevron osteotomy. **(E)** The configuration of the chevron osteotomy. **(F)** Lateral translation of the metatarsal head and pin fixation. Reproduced with permission from Mann RA, Coughlin MJ. Adult hallux valgus. In: Mann RA, Coughlin MJ, eds. *Surgery of the Foot and Ankle.* 6th ed. St. Louis, MO: Mosby Year Book; 1993:207, 222, 230, 322.

The medial midline approach is used. Capsular elevation from the metatarsal head should be minimized to protect the capsular vascular supply. The medial eminence is resected at or just medial to the sulcus along a plane parallel with the medial border of the foot. A chevron osteotomy is performed with a thin sagittal saw with the apex distal and located in the center of the head. The head fragment is translated laterally 4 to 5 mm. A smooth 0.045-inch Kirschner wire (K-wire) transfixes the osteotomy and is removed 4 to 6 weeks postoperatively. A bunion dressing that maintains the corrected position of the hallux is applied, and heel-touch weight bearing is permitted in a wooden-soled shoe until the osteotomy is healed. Normal shoe wear is permitted when swelling has decreased.

More severe hallux valgus with great toe pronation, metatarsus primus varus, and/or adductor tightness requires proximal osteotomy (Fig. 38–22c). Medial eminence resection, medial capsular plication, and lateral soft tissue release are performed as in the modified McBride procedure. Crescentic osteotomy of the proximal first metatarsal is then performed with a special curved saw after subperiosteal exposure of the base of the first metatarsal via a dorsal longitudinal incision. The crescentic osteotomy should be made concave proximally. The osteotomy must be perpendicular to the plantigrade plane to avoid plantar-flexion or dorsiflexion of the first metatarsal. Proximal chevron osteotomy has been proposed

to facilitate fixation and minimize the risk of inadvertent plantar-flexion or dorsiflexion of the first metatarsal. It is performed via extension of the medial incision proximally over the base of the first metatarsal.

Keller resection arthroplasty of the base of the proximal phalanx may be adequate in an older, sedentary patient with degenerative arthritis (Fig. 38–23). A medial or dorsal exposure is used. The medial eminence of the first metatarsal head is removed at the sulcus on a plane parallel to the medial border of the foot. Subperiosteal dissection is performed to expose the base of the proximal phalanx and the proximal 1 cm is removed with a sagittal saw. This procedure must not be used in young or active patients because transfer metatarsalgia, cock-up deformity, and recurrent hallux valgus will occur with time.

First metatarsophalangeal joint arthrodesis is more appropriate in young or active patients with degenerative arthritis. The joint is exposed with either a dorsal or medial approach. The cartilage and subchondral bone are removed. The metatarsal head and base of the proximal phalanx are fashioned into a ball and socket, respectively, either by hand or with powered reamers. The underlying cancellous bone is feathered to maximize surface area. The metatarsophalangeal arthrodesis is positioned in 15 degrees of valgus and 15 degrees of dorsiflexion relative to the plantar surface of the foot (Fig. 38–23d). Screws, pins, or a plate and screws can be

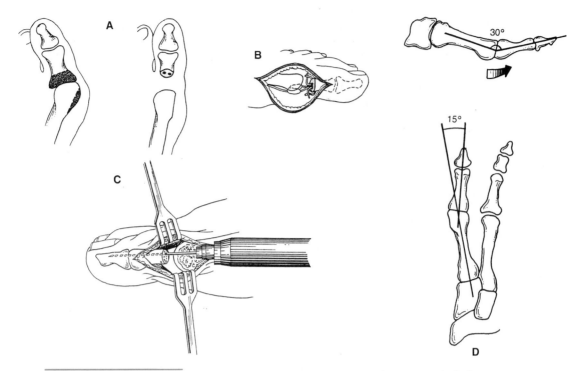

Figure 38–23 **(A)** The plane of medial eminence resection in Keller proximal phalanx resection arthroplasty is parallel to the medial metatarsal cortex and the proximal third of the proximal phalanx is excised. **(B)** The plantar plate and MTP joint capsule are repaired to the residual proximal phalanx. **(C)** A 5/64-inch smooth Kirschner wire (K-wire) placed longitudinally for fixation while soft tissue scarring occurs in the joint space. **(D)** The optimum hallux position for first metatarsophalangeal joint arthrodesis. Reproduced with permission from Mann RA, Coughlin MJ. Adult hallux valgus. In: Mann RA, Coughlin MJ, eds. *Surgery of the Foot and Ankle.* 6th ed. St. Louis, MO: Mosby Year Book. 1993:245–251.

used for fixation. Accurate positioning of the arthrodesis is important to maintain an adequate lever arm, minimize vaulting gait, and permit most shoewear. Patients will not be able to wear heels higher than one inch. Reported union rates are greater than 90%, and patient satisfaction is greater than 85%. Half of pseudoarthroses are actually symptomatic.

Hallux Rigidus

Hallux rigidus should be distinguished from degenerative arthritis of the first metatarsophalangeal joint (Fig. 38–24a). Hallux rigidus comprises degenerative arthritis limited to the dorsal one-third of the metatarsophalangeal joint. Pain is due to dorsal impingement with dorsiflexion and pressure from

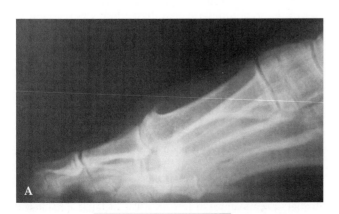

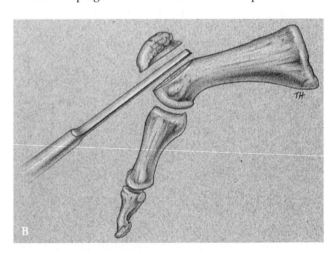

Figure 38–24 **(A)** Hallux rigidus with metatarsal head dorsal osteophyte. **(B)** Cheilectomy with removal of the osteophyte and dorsal one third of the metatarsal head. Reproduced with permission from Clanton TO, Durham-Smith G. *Op Tech Orthop.* 1992;2:186.

shoes on the dorsal osteophyte. Nonoperative treatment for either hallux rigidus or degenerative arthritis includes shoes with a toe-box of adequate depth, injections, and limiting first metatarsophalangeal joint motion with either a full-length, rigid orthotic or by stiffening of the sole of the shoe.

Cheilectomy is effective when nonoperative treatment fails (Fig. 38–24b). A dorsal or medial exposure is performed and the dorsal one-third of the metatarsal head and any accompanying osteophytes of the first metatarsal head and/or proximal phalanx are removed. The dorsal approach facilitates excision of lateral osteophytes, but the medial approach minimizes extensor hallucis longus contracture. Immobilization should be discontinued 1 week postoperatively, and the patient should begin aggressive active and passive range of motion of the toe 5 to 6 times a day.

Patients with degenerative arthritis who fail nonoperative treatment should consider first metatarsophalangeal arthrodesis. The technique and positioning are the same as when the procedure is performed for hallux valgus deformity with degenerative arthritis.

Lesser Toe Deformities

Nonoperative treatment of lesser toe deformities is palliative and often successful. A wide toe-box shoe of adequate depth relieves pressure on bony prominences. Selective stretching of the shoe over a painful bony prominence can effectively relieve discomfort. A sling of tape can be placed over the proximal phalanx of a hammertoe or clawtoe and then taped to the plantar surface of the foot to reduce flexible deformities. Corn pads and sleeves with a silicone pad are also useful.

Surgical treatment is necessary when nonoperative methods fail. The choice of procedure depends on the type of deformity, the flexibility of the deformity, and the stability of the metatarsophalangeal joint.

Flexible mallet toe deformity is often amenable to percutaneous release of the FDL insertion onto the base of the distal phalanx. Internal fixation is usually unnecessary.

Distal interphalangeal joint resection arthroplasty corrects rigid mallet toe deformity. An elliptical incision is made over the distal interphalangeal joint through skin, tendon, and joint capsule directly to bone. It is imperative to avoid injury to the germinal matrix of the nail. The head of the middle phalanx is exposed by circumferentially releasing the joint capsule, collateral ligaments, and plantar plate. A sagittal saw or bone biter is used to resect the head of the middle phalanx at the phalangeal neck. Sharp bony edges are contoured with a rongeur. A smooth 0.045- or 0.062-inch K-wire is placed longitudinally into all three phalanges with the interphalangeal joints in neutral extension. The patient is allowed to bear weight as tolerated in a wooden-soled shoe until the pin is removed 4 to 6 weeks postoperatively.

Flexible hammertoe or clawtoe deformity can be corrected with Girdlestone-Taylor flexor-to-extensor tendon transfer (Fig. 38–25). The FDL is percutaneously released from the distal phalanx, retrieved from a second plantar incision at the base of the toe, and split along its raphe. A dorsal longitudinal incision is made over the proximal phalanx. The medial and lateral halves of the FDL are passed along the medial and lateral cortices of the proximal phalanx and delivered into the dorsal wound. A 0.045- or 0.062-inch smooth K-wire longitu-

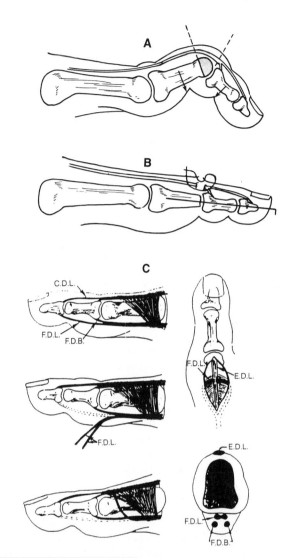

Figure 38–25 **(A)** Proximal interphalangeal joint resection arthroplasty. **(B)** Smooth K-wire fixation placed longitudinally. **(C)** Girdlestone-Taylor flexor-to-extensor tendon transfer. Reproduced with permission from Coughlin MJ, Mann RA. Lesser toe deformities. In: Mann RA, Coughlin MJ, eds. *Surgery of the Foot and Ankle.* 6th ed. St. Louis, MO: Mosby Year Book; 1993:355,359–360.

dinally transfixes the phalanges with the interphalangeal joints in neutral extension and is passed into the metatarsal with the metatarsophalangeal joint in plantarflexion and the ankle in neutral dorsiflexion. The transferred tendon halves are repaired to the extensor hood. An unsplit FDL can also be routed plantar to dorsal through a drill hole in the proximal phalanx. Flexible claw toe deformity may also require percutaneous or open release of the metatarsophalangeal joint. Heel-touch weight bearing in a wooden-sole shoe is permitted until the pin is removed 4 to 6 weeks postoperatively.

Rigid hammertoe or clawtoe deformity requires PIP joint resection arthroplasty (see Figs. 38–25a and 38–25b). An elliptical or longitudinal incision is made over the PIP joint. The head of the proximal phalanx is exposed by circumferential release of the joint capsule, collateral ligaments, and plantar plate. A sagittal saw is used to resect the head of the proximal phalanx at the phalangeal neck, and sharp edges are contoured with a rongeur. A smooth 0.062-inch K-wire transfixes the phalanges with the interphalangeal joints in neutral extension. The patient is permitted to bear weight as tolerated in a wooden-sole shoe. The pin is removed in 4 to 6 weeks.

Extensor tenotomy, dorsal capsulotomy, or metatarsophalangeal joint arthroplasty may need to be added to PIP resection arthroplasty in rigid clawtoe to correct metatarsophalangeal hyperextension. A dorsal longitudinal incision over the metatarsophalangeal joint is made. The metatarsal head is exposed by release of the joint capsule. A 2-mm thick sliver of cartilage and subchondral bone is removed along a plane perpendicular to the longitudinal axis of the metatarsal. Some authors have suggested that plantar condylectomy should also be performed to induce plantar plate contracture and prevent recurrence. A longitudinal, smooth 0.045- or 0.062-inch K-wire that transfixes the phalanges with the interphalangeal joints in neutral extension is used for fixation, but it is advanced into the metatarsal. Heel-touch weight-bearing in a wooden-soled shoe is permitted until the pin is removed 6 weeks postoperatively.

Rheumatoid arthritis of the forefoot characteristically causes hallux valgus and hammertoe deformities with dorsal dislocation of the lesser metatarsophalangeal joints (Fig. 38–26). Dislocation of the lesser metatarsophalangeal joints causes the plantar fat pad to migrate distally off the weight-bearing surface of the forefoot.

Extra-depth accommodative shoes with soft leather uppers and molded plastizote inlays that support the metatarsals and relieve the metatarsal heads are effective. First metatarsophalangeal arthrodesis and resection of the lesser metatarsal heads at the metatarsal necks via longitudinal dorsal web space incisions provides reliable pain relief when nonoperative management fails (Fig. 38–26). The procedure restores weight-bearing to the first ray, improves great toe push-off during gait, and reduces the distal migration of the plantar fat pad.

Diabetic Foot Disorders
Ulcers

A classification of diabetic foot ulcers has been proposed to guide treatment. Skin compromise without ulceration defines grade 0. Grade I ulcers are through the epidermis but not through the subcutaneous tissue (Fig. 38–27). Tendons and deep soft tissues are exposed in Grade II ulcers. Bone is exposed in grade III ulcers. Grade IV and V ulcers are associated with local and entire foot gangrene, respectively (Table 38–1).

Accommodative shoewear and total contact plastazote inserts with relief over the ulcer are adequate treatment for grade 0 ulcers. Grade I ulcers are treated with a total contact cast. Normal saline wet-to-dry dressing changes, office debridement, and total contact casting once the wound is clean are used to convert grade II ulcers to grade I ulcers. Surgical debridement and bony resection are often necessary to convert grade III ulcers to grade II ulcers. Amputation is necessary in grade IV and V ulcers. Forefoot ulcers have a better prognosis for healing and limb salvage than hindfoot ulcers.

Total contact casts permit ambulatory weight-bearing while healing a grade I or clean grade II ulcer. The effectiveness of total contact casting is attributed to edema control,

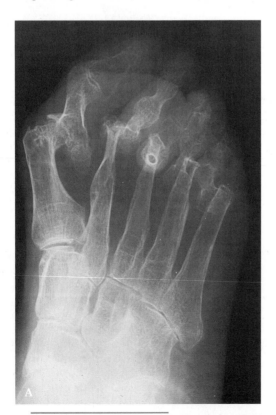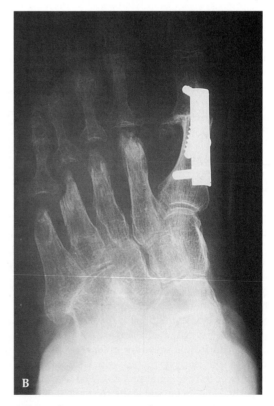

Figure 38–26 **(A)** Rheumatoid arthritis. **(B)** First metatarsophalangeal joint arthrodesis and lesser metatarsal head resection arthroplasty.

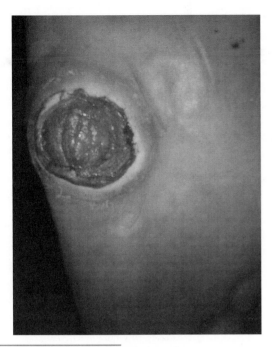

Figure 38–27 Grade I diabetic foot ulcer.

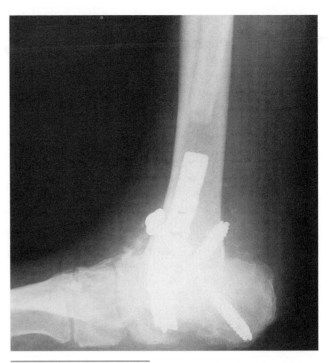

Figure 38–28 Hindfoot realignment arthrodesis for Charcot neuroarthropathy deformity.

redistribution of weight bearing, and minimization of shear stresses on the plantar skin. Very little cast padding is used except over bony prominences, which are padded with felt or foam. Some authors limit toe motion by enclosing the toes in the cast. The first layer of cast material is an elastic gauze plaster (Orthoflex)™, and the remaining layers can be fiberglass. The cast should be changed every 1 or 2 weeks to control edema and monitor the skin.

Charcot Neuroarthropathy

Acute Charcot neuroarthropathy requires immediate management. Total contact casting is used to prevent progressive deformity. The cast is changed every 2 weeks until redness, warmth, and swelling have resolved. Swelling can be quantified by having the patient place his or her foot into a container of water and measuring the amount displaced. Swelling has resolved when the measured volume of water displaced plateaus.

After total contact casting is completed, the patient wears an accomodative shoe with a total contact plastizote insert and double-upright locked ankle brace with a calf lacer or a plastizote-lined molded AFO. Bracing can occasionally be discontinued after the bones have radiographically consolidated, typically after 6 to 9 months, but most patients require lifelong bracing to prevent recurrent collapse and progressive deformity. The shoe and insert are worn for the rest of the patient's life.

Exostectomies and realignment osteotomies and arthrodeses may be necessary to heal refractory ulcers or to facilitate shoe and brace wearing (Fig. 38–28). Surgery should not be performed in Charcot neuroarthropathy until consolidation has occurred. Surgery should never be attempted in acute Charcot neuroarthropathy even if there is progressive deformity. Internal fixation will fail in the actively resorbing bone, and deformity progression will be accelerated.

TABLE 38–1   Diabetic Foot Ulcer Classification

Grade	Description
0	Skin compromise without ulcer, previous ulcer, at-risk deformity and neuropathy
I	Superficial ulcer extending to or into subcutaneous tissue without infection
II	Deep ulcer through subcutaneous tissue exposing tendon or other deep soft tissue other than bone
III	Deep ulcer with exposed or infected bone and/or abscess
IV	Any ulcer with ischemia and/or local gangrene
V	Any ulcer with ischemia and diffuse foot gangrene

SELECTED BIBLIOGRAPHY

ARNER O, LINDHOLM A. Subcutaneous rupture of the Achilles tendon. *Acta Chir Scand.* 1959;239(Suppl.):1–51.

COUGHLIN MJ, MANN RA. Deformities of the lesser toes. In: Mann, RA, Coughlin, MJ, eds. *Surgery of the Foot and Ankle.* 6th ed. St Louis, MO: Mosby Year Book, 1993;341–412.

DALTON GP. Chronic achilles tendon rupture. *Foot Ankle Clin.* 1996;1:225–237.

GRAVES SC, MANN RA, GRAVES KO. Triple arthrodesis in older adults: results after long term followup. *J Bone Jt Surg.* 1993;75A:355–362.

JONES DC. Tendon disorders of the foot and ankle. *J Am Acad Orthop Surg.* 1993;1:87–94.

MANN RA, COUGHLIN MJ. Adult hallux valgus. In: Mann RA, Coughlin MJ, eds. *Surgery of the Foot and Ankle.* 6th ed. St. Louis, MO: Mosby Year Book; 1993:167–296.

MANN RA, REYNOLDS JC. Interdigital neuromas: a critical analysis. *Foot Ankle.* 1983;3:238–243.

MANN RA, THOMPSON FM. Rupture of the posterior tibial tendon causing flat foot: surgical treatment. *J Bone Jt Surg.* 1985;67A:556–561.

MANN RA, VAN MANEN WJ, WAPNER KL, MARTIN J. Ankle arthrodesis. *Clin Orthop.* 1991;268:49–55.

MIZEL MS, MICHELSON JD, WAPNER KL. Diagnosis and treatment of peroneus brevis injury, *Foot Ankle Clin.* 1996;1: 343–354.

THOMPSON FM, MANN RA. Arthritides. In: Mann RA, Coughlin MJ, eds. *Surgery of the Foot and Ankle.* 6th ed. St Louis, MO: Mosby Year Book; 1993:615–672.

WAPNER KL. Acute repair of achilles tendon. In: Johnson KA, ed. *Master Techniques in Orthopaedic Surgery, the Foot and Ankle.* New York, NY: Raven Press; 1994:299–309.

WAPNER KL, PAVLOCK GS, HECHT PJ et al. Repair of chronic achilles tendon rupture with flexor hallucis longus tendon transfer. *Foot Ankle Clin.* 1993;14:445–447.

YODLOWSKI M, MIZEL MS. Reconstruction of peroneus brevis pathology. *Op Tech Orthop.* 1994;4:146–151.

SAMPLE QUESTIONS

1. A 62-year-old female complains of medial ankle pain. She is unable to perform a single-limb toe raise. She has a pes planovalgus deformity that is passively correctable. Which of the following is the best initial treatment:
   (a) operative exploration and debridement
   (b) flexor digitorum longus tendon transfer
   (c) short articulated AFO
   (d) cortisone injection
   (e) lateral column lengthening and FDL tendon transfer

2. Hammertoe deformity is due to:
   (a) neurologic deficit
   (b) intrinsic-extrinsic imbalance
   (c) narrow shoes
   (d) a and b
   (e) b and c

3. The most reliable operation to correct hallux valgus in a 35-year-old female with minimal metatarsus primus varus, no degenerative joint disease, an incongruent metatarsophalangeal joint, and no adductor tightness is:
   (a) modified McBride procedure (lateral soft tissue release, medial eminence resection, and medial capsular plication)
   (b) distal chevron osteotomy
   (c) proximal crescentic osteotomy
   (d) keller resection arthroplasty
   (e) first metatarsophalangeal joint arthrodesis

4. A 57-year-old male with non–insulin-dependent diabetes mellitus and sensory neuropathy has a 4-week history of midfoot warmth, redness, and swelling that has not responded to treatment with first-generation cephalosporin antibiotics. Pulses are palpable. Appropriate management at this time includes:
   (a) broad spectrum antibiotics
   (b) magnetic resonance imaging of the foot
   (c) bone biopsy for cultures
   (d) total contact cast
   (e) low-dose amitryptaline

5. A 28-year-old female flight attendant complains of burning forefoot pain that is worse in high heel shoes and relieved when she takes off her shoes midflight. She is tender in the third web space. There are no plantar calluses. Appropriate initial management includes:
   (a) electromyogram/nerve conduction velocity
   (b) wider shoes
   (c) corticosteroid injection
   (d) third and fourth metatarsal dorsiflexion osteotomy
   (e) third and fourth metatarsal head plantar condylectomy

Answers: 1) c; 2) e; 3) b; 4) d; 5) b

Pediatrics

Pediatric Fractures

B. David Horn, MD

Outline

Fractures are common in the pediatric age group and fortunately, most heal without difficulty or complication. Complications however, do occur, and children do not "grow out of" all malunions. A thorough understanding of the unique qualities of the child's musculoskeletal system is an essential prerequisite to successful management of pediatric fractures. In addition, children often sustain fractures not seen in adults, and treatment for pediatric fractures must be undertaken with respect for the future development of the child.

ETIOLOGY

A variety of mechanisms may account for pediatric fractures. Accidental injury accounts for most fractures, but there are some types of fractures that are commonly seen and have an etiology unique to children and adolescents. These include birth injuries, child abuse, and pathological fractures. The treating physician needs to be aware of these conditions to provide optimal treatment for the patient.

Birth injuries should be suspected in the neonate with fractures. Risk factors for birth injuries include obstetrical maneuvers during delivery, breech delivery, prolonged labor, and a large birth weight. Even though birth injuries are predominantly associated with vaginal deliveries, they also may occur during cesarean section. The clavicle, humerus, and femur are most commonly fractured. Epiphyseal injury may occur at birth and most commonly involve the proximal humerus, distal femur, distal humerus, and proximal femur. Infants with birth fractures commonly present with pseudoparalysis of the extremity, edema, crepitus, and pain with motion of the limb. Diagnosis of these injuries may be difficult and is made on the basis of physical examination and imaging studies. While radiographs will document metaphyseal and diaphyseal fractures, they may appear normal in infants with physeal injuries. Where there is a clinical suspicion of a birth fracture and plain radiographs are negative, ultrasound, magnetic resonance imaging, and bone scintigraphy may be of value in detecting these injuries. Concomitant injuries including plexopathy, spinal cord injury, and muscle injury should be suspected in infants with birth fractures.

Child abuse should be suspected when a long bone fracture is present in a child less than 1 year of age. Other signs suggestive of child abuse include a described mechanism of injury that does not fit the physical findings, an unreasonable delay in treatment following injury, a history of similar injuries, and the presence of fractures or soft tissue injuries at different stages of healing. Certain fracture patterns may also lead one to suspect child abuse, although no single fracture pattern is absolutely diagnostic for intentional injury. Posterior rib fractures; symmetrical physeal separations; and spiral, long bone fractures, particularly of the femur and humerus, are highly suggestive of child abuse. State laws mandate that suspected child abuse be reported to social wel-

Orthopaedic Surgery: The Essentials. Edited by M.E. Baratz, A.D. Watson, and J.E. Imbriglia. Thieme Medical Publishers, Inc., New York © 1999

fare agencies. Many hospitals have multidisciplinary teams to evaluate and treat the complex medical and social needs of these patients and their families.

Pathological fractures occur in abnormal bone and are usually low-energy injuries. Metabolic bone diseases, skeletal dysplasias, defects in collagen synthesis, and a variety of benign or malignant neoplasms can weaken bone. Treatment includes diagnosis of the underlying problem and care of the fracture.

BASIC SCIENCE

Children's Bones

There are significant anatomic, biomechanical, and physiological differences between immature and mature bones. These differences account for many of the unique fractures seen in children.

Immature bone is a composite of cartilage and bone. In comparison with mature bone, immature bone is more porous, less dense, has a lower modulus of elasticity, and is surrounded by a thick periosteum. These factors have several clinical implications. Children's fractures are often associated with less swelling, are more stable, and are often less comminuted than similar fractures in adults. The decreased modulus of elasticity results in an increased incidence of plastic deformation and a lower energy to failure in children's bone than in adult bones. The periosteum found in immature bone is loosely applied to the diaphysis but is adherent at the metalphyseal-epiphyseal region, where it helps stabilize the growth plate. The thick periosteum supports the bone in tension and serves as an aid to reduction of fractures. Periosteal new bone formation may develop as early as 2 days after fracture and contributes to rapid healing.

The biomechanical characteristics of immature bone result in several fractures that are unique to children. The first is the torus or buckle fracture, which represents compression failure of the cortex and is seen at the metaphyseal-diaphyseal junction (Fig. 39–1). This junction represents a region of differential cortical strength where the more rigid diaphyseal cortex is compressed into the weaker trabecular metaphysis.

A second injury unique to immature bone is plastic deformation, in which a series of microfractures occurs along the compression side of a bone resulting in permanent deformation of the bone. No visible fracture develops and because subperiosteal hematoma formation is minimal, little, if any, periosteal reaction is noted on radiographs. If significant, plastic deformation of bones needs to be corrected.

A third injury unique to children is the greenstick fracture, which represents a failure of the tension side of bone with plastic deformation of the compression side. Due to the tendency of the intact cortex to increase the deformity of the fracture, effective management of the greenstick fracture may require completion of the fracture.

Growth Plate

The growth plate, or physis, is a highly specialized cartilaginous structure at the end of long bones that is responsible for longitudinal growth of the bones. Some circumferential growth of the bones is also accomplished by the peripheral portion of the physis. Histologically, the physis consists of

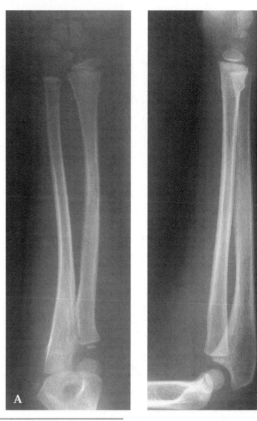

Figure 39–1 Anteroposterior **(A)** and lateral **(B)** radiographs of a 6-year-old boy with a buckle fracture of his distal radial metaphysis.

three zones (Fig. 39–2). The first is the reserve zone, which is located adjacent to the secondary center of ossification. The reserve zone is characterized by a sparse distribution of chondrocytes surrounded by abundant matrix. The cells of the reserve zone are thought to be active in matrix production, although their exact function is unknown. The proliferative zone is represented by longitudinal columns of flattened cells that are involved in matrix production, cellular proliferation, and longitudinal growth. The hypertrophic zone consists of columns of hypertrophied chondrocytes that prepare the matrix for calcification. The last region of the hypertrophic zone is the zone of provisional calcification, where the cartilage matrix becomes calcified. Adjacent to the zone of provisional calcification is the primary spongiosa, where bone is formed on the calcified cartilage. At the secondary spongiosa, the primary spongiosa is remodeled with removal of cartilage bars and replacement of the woven bone with lamellar bone. Although physeal fractures are thought to occur through the hypertrophic zone of the growth plate, they have been histologically identified throughout the various zones of the growth plate.

Physeal Fractures

Physeal fractures account for 20 to 30% of pediatric fractures. The diagnosis of these injuries is often made difficult by the fact that the physis is radiolucent. Radiographs may only reveal soft tissue swelling. Physeal fractures have a bimodal distribution with peak incidences in infancy and adolescence.

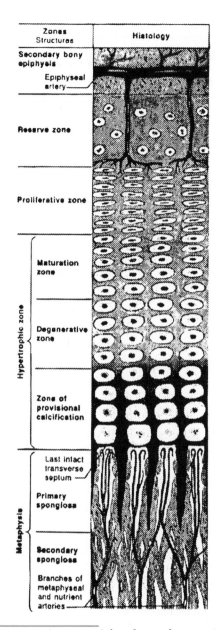

Figure 39–2 A diagram of the physis showing the reserve zone, proliferative zone, and hypertrophic zone.

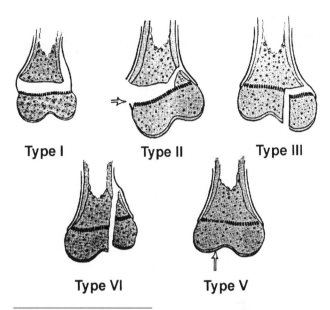

Figure 39–3 Salter-Harris classification of fractures.

The classification system popularized by Salter and Harris (1963) is used widely and relies upon the radiographic appearance of the fracture (Fig. 39–3).

Salter-Harris type I injuries are transverse fractures through the physis with no involvement of the metaphysis or epiphysis. These fractures are produced by shear or tensile forces and occur most commonly in early childhood when the physis is thick. The fracture line is principally through the lower hypertrophic zone. The reserve and proliferative zone remain attached to the epiphysis. The prognosis for continued growth is generally excellent, although early closure may occur. Salter-Harris type II fractures are characterized by a fracture through the physis with involvement of a metaphyseal bone fragment. This injury is also the result of shear or tensile forces. The metaphyseal fragment, known as the Thurston-Holland fragment, is located on the compres-

sion side of the fracture and indicates where there is intact periosteum. Salter-Harris type II fractures represent 75% of physeal fractures, and like the type I fractures, the reserve and proliferative zones usually remain vascularized with the epiphysis. The prognosis for continued growth is good, but early closure of the physis is not possible. Salter-Harris type III fractures consist of a fracture through the physis that extends through the epiphysis into the joint. If the alignment of the articular surface and the physis are anatomically restored, the prognosis is good. The initial forces may destroy a portion of the physis resulting in progressive deformity. Salter-Harris type IV fractures traverse the epiphysis, physis, and continue across the metaphysis. Salter-Harris type V fractures result from a crushing injury to the growth plate.

Anatomic reduction of the fracture is required to minimize growth arrest. The force of the initial injury may be severe enough to destroy a portion of the physis. This may result in a growth arrest despite surgical restoration of anatomic alignment.

ANATOMY AND SURGICAL APPROACHES

The skeletally immature elbow and knee pose special problems regarding the anatomy and radiographic appearance. Much of the developing skeleton is cartilaginous and radiolucent, so a knowledge of normal pediatric radiographic anatomy is needed to make an accurate diagnosis in children. In addition, many pediatric fractures are treated by percutaneous techniques with radiographic guidance, so an appreciation of the unique characteristics of the growing skeleton is needed to optimize treatment.

The elbow consists of the humeroulnar joint, which has a single axis of rotation; a proximal radiocapitellar joint, which provides for pronation and supination; and a proximal radial ulnar articulation. As the distal humeral diaphysis broadens into the metaphysis, it forms a medial and lateral column of bone separated by the coronoid fossa on the anterior aspect and the olecranon fossa posteriorly. The medial and lateral columns support of the distal humerus and provide for regions of secure fixation.

PEARL

Ossification of the distal humerus: *c*apitellum, *r*adial head, *m*edial epicondyle, *t*rochlea, *o*lecranon, and *l*ateral epicondyle (CRMTOL) occurs at ages 2, 4, 6, 8, and 10, respectively.

There are five ossification centers to the elbow. Except for the medial and lateral epicondyles, these are all intra-articular. They tend to appear at characteristics ages, and knowledge of their appearance is important to avoid confusing them with fractures. The ossification center of the capitellum usually appears at 2 years of age, the radial head at 4 years of age, the medial epicondyle at 6 years of age, the trochlea at 8 years of age, the olecranon at 10 years of age, and the lateral epicondyle at 10 years of age. By about 12 years of age, the lateral epicondyle, trochlea, and capitellum join to form a single epiphysis. The angle formed between the arm and the forearm is known as the carrying angle. This varies from individual to individual, but tends to average about 7 to 10 degrees and is symmetric. One goal of treatment of pediatric elbow fractures is the maintenance of equal carrying angles. Comparison radiographs of the uninjured side may be useful to interpret elbow radiographs.

The brachial artery and median nerve are anterior to the elbow joint, whereas the ulna nerve is positioned behind the medial epicondyle and the radial nerve courses anterior-laterally, over the elbow. These structures are vulnerable to injury secondary to fractures.

Irregular ossification centers occur in the young knee and make radiographic evaluation difficult. Knee ossification irregularities are typically located posterior to a line along the posterior shaft of the femur, whereas ossification defects anterior to this line may represent fracture.

The examiner must also be aware of patterns of referred pain from the hip. Hip pathology in children and adolescents frequently radiates to the thigh or knee, so any patient with a complaint of thigh or knee pain must have a hip examination. Any asymmetry in hip motion should be further investigated with appropriate imaging studies.

EXAMINATION

The diagnosis of fractures in the pediatric age group is not always straightforward. Certainly the majority of fractures are preceded by trauma, but even trivial trauma may result in significant injury. Children may be unable to give an accurate history, so the physical examination is important. Physical findings suggestive of a fracture include tenderness, swelling, deformity, pain, and loss of function. Due to the mechanical characteristics of immature bone and its thick, adherent periosteum, fractures may not always present with swelling or deformity. Palpation of the extremity is essential to discover areas of point tenderness, which are most consistent with the presence of a fracture. Many Salter-Harris type I physeal fractures are nondisplaced and are diagnosed solely on the physical finding of point tenderness at the physis.

Certain fractures in children (particularly supracondylar fractures of the humerus and proximal fractures of the tibial physis) are associated with neurovascular injury or compartment syndrome. A thorough neurovascular examination should be performed and recorded for all patients. The earliest sign of compartment syndrome is pain with passive stretch of the affected muscle followed by pallor, pulselessness, and paralysis. Each child with a fracture must be examined for signs of compartment syndrome. If there is a clinical evidence of compartment syndrome, fasciotomy of the compartment is indicated. If the patient is unable to cooperate with the physical examination, or if there is uncertainty in diagnosis, compartment pressures may be obtained. Caution should be observed when fractures are accompanied by a concomitant nerve palsy, which may mask the pain associated with a compartment syndrome. For example, median nerve palsy in association with supracondylar fracture of the humerus may mask compartment syndrome of the forearm until the process becomes irreversible.

AIDS TO DIAGNOSIS

Radiographs of the injured extremity must include the joint above and below the injured bone. This is particularly important in the forearm, where radial head dislocations or fractures may occur along with ulna fractures (The Monteggia fracture). Irregular ossification may be mistaken for a fracture. Comparison views are helpful in differentiating a fracture from a normal variation in ossification. Soft tissue signs, such as the anterior and posterior fat pad signs around the elbow, are useful when seen on plain radiographs to raise the suspicion of a fracture.

In infants, ultrasound is helpful in imaging cartilage and can detect physeal fractures. Magnetic resonance imaging is useful in imaging nonosseous tissues and may be the most accurate way to demonstrate the extent of a fracture through the physis and cartilaginous anlage. Computed tomography is useful in assessing intra-articular fractures and assessing the extent of a bony injury. Bone scintigraphy can be used to detect concurrent fractures in patients with multiple trauma or child abuse.

SPECIFIC CONDITIONS, TREATMENT, AND OUTCOME

Fractures of the Proximal Humerus

Fractures of the proximal humerus may be physeal or metaphyseal in nature. Salter-Harris type I fractures occur most commonly in patients up to 5 years of age, whereas, Salter-Harris type II occur in patients older than 11 years of age. Metaphyseal fractures of the proximal humerus occur most frequently between 5 and 11 years of age. Neonates and young children may demonstrate "pseudoparalysis," which is an inability to move the fractured arm. Most of these fractures can be treated nonoperatively. Some angulation may be accepted in the injuries as there is a large amount of growth and remodeling present at the proximal humeral physis. With large amounts of fracture angulation, the greater tuberosity or distal fragment may impinge upon the acromion with abduction of the shoulder. This is a situation where a reduction needs to be performed.

Surgical Technique

Closed reduction and percutaneous pinning of these injuries is rarely required. When indicated, the reduction is obtained by flexing the distal fragment 90 degrees, abducting the arm 70 degrees, and providing slight external rotation. The reduction is checked with the fluoroscope. If it is acceptable, two slightly divergent smooth Kirschner wires (K-wires) are used to fix the fracture. They should enter the proximal humeral shaft in its anterior lateral margin and be advanced so they engage the proximal fragment. Care must be taken to avoid damaging the axillary nerve with this technique. The pins are left outside the skin and may be removed after 3 weeks.

Postoperative Care

Postoperatively, the patient should be placed in a shoulder immobilizer or a Velpeau's bandage. After the pins are removed, mobilization of the shoulder may begin.

Expected Outcome

Most fractures of proximal humerus heal uneventfully. Any shortening that may occur is rarely of functional significance. Residual disability from these injuries is unusual.

Fractures of the Humeral Shaft

Humeral shaft fractures commonly occur as a result of birth trauma and may also be injured as result of child abuse in infants. In older children, direct trauma is usually the cause of humeral shaft fractures. Most of these fractures can be treated closed. Indications for open reduction and internal fixation include inability to obtain a satisfactory reduction, an open fracture, the multiply injured patient, and fractures associated with vascular injury.

Children up to 3 years of age may be treated with a sling and swathe or Velpeau's splint. Older children can usually be treated with coaptation splints along with a Velpeau's bandage. Younger children generally heal in about 3 to 4 weeks, whereas adolescents may take as long as 8 weeks to heal.

Most patients do well with this injury. There may be some resultant shortening or overgrowth of the humerus, but this is usually well tolerated. Nonunion of the humeral shaft is unusual in children and adolescents. Angulation and rotational malalignment are also well tolerated because of the large range of motion available through the shoulder joint. Nerve injuries in children are less common than in adults. The radial nerve is the most commonly injured nerve with humeral shaft fractures. This is usually a neuropraxia that recovers within 8 to 12 weeks after injury.

Transepiphyseal Fractures of the Distal Humerus

Transepiphyseal fractures of the distal humerus are typically Salter-Harris type I or II fractures that occur through the distal humeral physis. These injuries usually occur in children less than 2 years of age and may occur as a result of birth trauma. Typically, the child will present with a swollen and painful elbow with deformity suggesting an elbow dislocation. Plain radiographs of a transepiphyseal distal humerus fracture will show a normal relationship between the proximal radius and the capitellum and between the distal humerus and olecranon, with an apparent shifting of the entire elbow joint. A flake of metaphyseal bone may be also be seen on plain radiographs with Salter-Harris type II injuries. If radiographs are nondiagnostic, ultrasound of the elbow may be useful to confirm the diagnosis. Stable fractures may be treated with closed reduction and casting with the elbow in flexion and the forearm in pronation. Unstable fractures may require percutaneous pin fixation.

Surgical Technique

The fracture is reduced with a reduction maneuver similar to that used for supracondylar humerus fractures (see below). Unstable injuries should undergo percutaneous pinning. Care must be taken in inserting the medial pin to avoid impaling the ulnar nerve. Fractures more than 5 days old should not be reduced, and their position should be accepted. Postoperatively, the patient is placed in a long arm splint, and the pins are left in for 3 weeks. Range-of-motion exercises can be instituted after pin removal.

Remodeling with this injury can be expected, although significant varus and valgus angulation may not remodel and should be avoided if possible. Restoration of a normal range of motion should be obtained after treatment.

Supracondylar Humerus Fractures

Supracondylar humerus fractures represent about 60% of elbow fractures in children and most commonly occur between ages 3 and 10. Supracondylar fractures are classified as to the position of the elbow at the time of injury. Flexion-type supracondylar fractures result from a fall onto a flexed elbow and account for about 3% of these injuries. The majority of supracondylar fractures are extension type and result from a fall onto an extended elbow. Extension-type injuries account for about 97% of supracondylar fractures and are further classified according to the Gartland classification system (1959). Gartland type I fractures are nondisplaced. Type II injuries are angulated posteriorly with an intact posterior cortex. Type III fractures have no cortical contact between fragments and are completely displaced (Fig. 39–4).

Type I injuries and stable type II injuries may be treated by closed means. This usually consists of splinting or casting in about 110 to 120 degrees of elbow flexion with the forearm pronated. Three weeks of immobilization is usually sufficient for fracture healing. Some type I injuries, particularly in children between 2 and 4 years of age, may have a component of varus deformity secondary to impaction and buckling of the medial column of the distal humerus. These injuries may

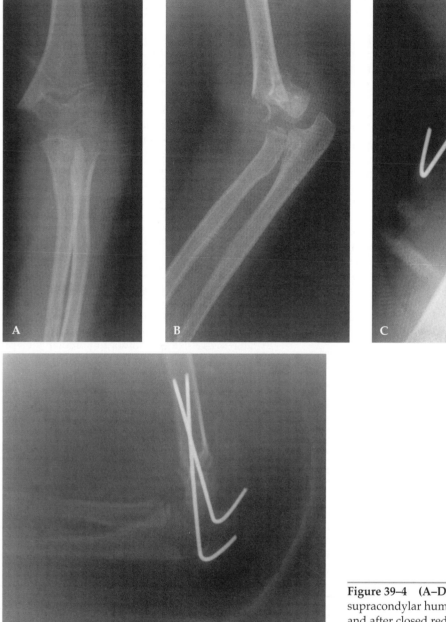

Figure 39–4 (A–D) Type III
supracondylar humerus fracture, before
and after closed reduction and internal
fixation.

require a closed reduction and percutaneous pinning to prevent varus deformity of the elbow. Unstable type II fractures and most type III supracondylar fractures should be treated with closed reduction and percutaneous pinning. This is accomplished under general anesthesia.

Surgical Technique

Longitudinal traction is applied to the extremity with the elbow extended and the forearm supinated. An assistant provides counter-traction to the upper arm. The elbow is hyperextended to disengage the fracture fragments. Next, any medial or lateral translation should be corrected and checked with a fluoroscope. The elbow is then flexed with the thumb placed over the olecranon to provide an anteriorly directed

force. Once full flexion is achieved, the forearm is pronated. The reduction is again checked with a fluoroscope in both the anteroposterior (AP) and lateral planes. If a satisfactory reduction is achieved, the elbow should be pinned. Smooth pins are used and should be inserted with a power drill. Either crossed medial-lateral pins or two lateral pins may be used. Children age 5 and under usually require 0.062 inches pins. Older children may require larger, smooth Steinmann pins. On the lateral side, the insertion site is lateral to the ossific nucleus of the capitellum with the pin directed proximally, medially, and posteriorly angulated about 10 degrees. The pin should engage the medial cortex of the proximal fragment at least 2 cm from the fracture site. If two lateral pins are to be used, they should not cross at the fracture site, as this will allow the fracture to rotate. Care must be taken in inserting the first pin to allow sufficient room for the second. When placing a medial pin, the surgeon should exercise caution to avoid damage to the ulnar nerve, which lies behind the medial epicondyle. Swelling may obscure the medial epicondyle, making accurate pin placement difficult. The edema can be displaced by gentle massage of the tissues overlying the medial epicondyle so that the bony prominence can be palpated. It may be necessary to make a small incision over the medial epicondyle to permit direct palpation. The medial pin should be directed laterally, proximally, and 5 to 10 degrees anteriorly to engage the lateral cortex of the proximal fragment at least 2 cm from the fracture site. Following pin insertion, the elbow should be extended and the carrying angle of the elbow examined and compared. Varus deformity of the elbow should not be accepted. The reduction should be checked in the AP and lateral planes. The pins are then bent, cut short, and left outside of the skin. The elbow is then flexed until the pulse is obliterated. At this point, the elbow should be extended 10 degrees and a posterior splint applied. Patients are observed overnight with neurovascular checks.

Patients with vascular injury, open fractures, or with fractures that can not be reduced closed may require open reduction. Flexion type supracondylar fractures also commonly require open reduction.

Postoperative Care

Postoperative care consists of splinting or casting for about 3 weeks, after which the pins may be removed and motion begun. Expected outcome includes almost full range of motion of the elbow, near symmetric elbow carrying angles, and full return of function.

> ### PEARL
> Neuropraxia of the anterior interosseous branch of the median nerve is a relatively common complication of supracondylar humerus fractures.

Complications

Supracondylar humerus fractures are notorious for their high complication rate. Nerve injury occurs in about 7% of fractures. The anterior interosseous branch of the median nerve AIN is the most commonly injured nerve. The function of this nerve is checked by asking the patient to flex the interphalangeal joint of the thumb and the distal interphalangeal joint of the index finger. Most nerve injuries are neuropraxias and spontaneous recovery can be expected in 12 to 16 weeks. Further diagnostic studies may be needed if the nerve does not recover in that time span.

Vascular injuries may occur with supracondylar humerus fractures. Controversy exists as to the proper way to treat supracondylar fractures with associated vascular injuries. If the patient does not have a radial pulse and the hand is ischemic, initial treatment in the emergency department should consist of splinting the elbow in extension. Immediate reduction and fixation of the fracture should be performed in the operating room and the elbow extended. If the pulse is detectable either on exam or with a Doppler probe and the

hand is vascularized, the patient should be closely observed. If the pulse is absent but the hand is viable, the patient may be observed for signs of ischemia. Often, the brachial artery may be in spasm, and a pulse may not be detectable for 20 to 30 minutes after a closed reduction and pinning of the fracture. If the hand is ischemic, immediate exploration of the brachial artery at the fracture site should be performed. If surgical treatment of a vascular injury is needed, a surgeon trained in small vessel repair should be available to perform the surgery. Intra-operative angiography may be of value in the treatment of these injuries, but treatment of an ischemic injury after a supracondylar fracture should not be delayed for an angiogram in the angiography suite.

Compartment syndrome is a feared complication of supracondylar humerus fractures. Signs of an impending compartment syndrome include severe pain, pain with passive stretch, pallor, pulselessness, and parasthesias. The most important early findings are deep forearm pain, pain with passive stretch, and pain requiring large amounts of narcotics. A normal pulse or a normal level of oxygen blood saturation detected by pulse oximetry does not exclude a compartment syndrome, as these may be normal in a patient with a compartment syndrome. If the physical exam is in question, compartment pressures should be measured. Special care needs to be taken in patients with nerve injuries. These patients may not have normal pain sensation, and, therefore, may be at risk for an undiagnosed compartment syndrome.

Lateral Condyle Fractures

Lateral condyle fractures constitute about 20% of elbow fractures in children. These commonly occur after a fall on an outstretched arm with resultant forearm varus resulting in an avulsion of the lateral condyle. These injuries are Salter-Harris type IV fractures and involve the metaphysis, the capitellum, and the trochlea, which in children is primarily cartilage. Historically, these injuries have been difficult to heal, and, particularly in displaced fractures, nonunion of the lateral condyle has been a problem. These injuries have been classified according to the degree of displacement and fracture instability. Stage I injuries are nondisplaced, the fracture line does not extend entirely through the cartilaginous portion of the trochlea, and the articular surface is intact. Stage II injuries have a complete fracture through the articular surface but are nondisplaced or minimally displaced. Stage III injuries are displaced and rotated. Nondisplaced fractures may be treated with casting with the elbow flexed at least 90 degrees and the forearm supinated. These injuries require frequent radiographs to check for displacement. Nondisplaced fractures generally take longer to heal than supracondylar fractures and usually require between 4 and 6 weeks of immobilization.

Any fracture that displaces requires fixation. Fractures that are minimally displaced may be percutaneously pinned following a closed reduction. If there is rotation or displacement of more than 4 mm, the fracture should undergo an open reduction followed by pinning (Fig. 39–5).

Surgical Technique

The open reduction is performed through a direct lateral incision. A Kocher approach is used with the plane of dissection

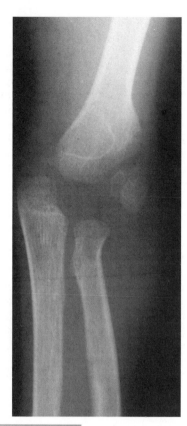

Figure 39–5 Displaced and rotated lateral condyle fracture requiring an open reduction and internal fixation as treatment.

between the triceps posteriorly and the brachialis muscle anteriorly. The fracture usually causes a large amount of soft tissue stripping, and the fracture hematoma will serve as a guide to the fracture site. Care should be taken to not dissect posteriorly on the lateral condyle as the blood supply to the fragment is derived from the posterior soft tissues. After the approach is made, the anterior aspect of the elbow joint can be visualized and palpated. Following a satisfactory reduction of the fracture, two smooth K-wires can be used to fix the fragment. After 4 weeks of immobilization, the patient may be placed in a splint and motion begun. When healing is evident on radiographs, the pins may be removed.

The goals of the surgery are to obtain union of the fracture and to restore full motion of the elbow. This is usually accomplished. There may be a residual prominence over the lateral condyle because of overgrowth of the condyle. The other significant complication is nonunion leading to cubitus valgus and tardy ulnar nerve palsy. This complication is best treated by avoidance: Nondisplaced fractures need frequent follow-up to ensure that no displacement occurs. Any fracture that displaces should undergo fixation.

Fractures of the Medial Epicondyle

Fractures of the medial epicondyle account for 5 to 10% of elbow fractures in children. These are extra-articular fractures frequently seen in association with elbow dislocations. The majority of medial epicondyle fractures can be treated with casting. Indications for fixation include fracture displacement

more than 2 cm, medial elbow instability, and an associated elbow dislocation.

Surgical Technique

Fixation is performed by making a small incision over the medial epicondyle and using blunt dissection to reach the bony prominence of the medial epicondyle. This is done to avoid injury to the ulnar nerve. In younger patients, pin fixation may be used. Older patients may benefit from the improved stability and the ability for early motion provided by screw fixation. The pin or guide wire for a cannulated screw is inserted under x-ray guidance after reduction of the medial epicondyle. The fracture position and fixation can be checked with the fluoroscope. If satisfactory, a screw is inserted over the wire.

Postoperative Care

Postoperative care consists of immobilization with either a splint or cast. Patients with an associated elbow dislocation should begin motion 7 to 10 days after injury to help avoid elbow stiffness. Healing of these fractures usually occurs in 3 weeks. Loss of extension is common, and patients with concomitant elbow dislocations lose more motion than patients with isolated epicondyle fractures. Early, active, elbow motion exercises should be instituted to help prevent stiffness.

Radial Neck Fractures

Radial neck fractures are typically Salter-Harris type I or type II injuries resulting from a fall onto an outstretched arm. Fractures with more than 45 degrees of angulation and more than 50% displacement require reduction. This may be attempted by rotating the forearm with pressure directed laterally over the radial head. Alternately, a smooth K-wire may be used percutaneously as a "joystick" to reduce the fracture. An open reduction through a Kocher approach may be required for treatment of these injuries when the fracture is completely displaced or when a closed reduction cannot be obtained. When performing an open reduction and internal fixation, a pin transfixing the radiocapitellar joint should not be used because of the risk of pin breakage and subsequent difficulty in pin removal.

Postoperative Care

These injuries require immobilization for 3 weeks, after which there is usually sufficient healing to begin motion.

Forearm Fractures

Forearm fractures are the most commonly seen fractures in children. Midshaft forearm fractures may be unstable and require fixation. Indications for operative stabilization include open fractures, fractures with associated neurovascular injury, fractures in which a closed reduction can not be satisfactorily maintained, and fractures with associated upper extremity injuries such as elbow dislocations, where early motion is desirable.

Surgical Technique

A reduction is obtained by closed or open techniques utilizing standard orthopaedic approaches. In many cases, intramedullary pin fixation is a satisfactory method of fracture fixation. The bone that is most easily aligned should be stabilized first. For the ulna, a stab wound is made over the tip of the olecranon. A drill hole is made into the tip of the olecranon, and a small, smooth wire is introduced under C-arm guidance down the shaft of the ulna. The radial pin is inserted 2 cm proximal to the distal radial physis. A small incision is made over the insertion site, with care taken to avoid injury to the sensory branch of the radial nerve. The cortex is opened with a small hand drill and a small, smooth wire is inserted under C-arm guidance. The proximal tip of the wire should be distal to the proximal radial physis. The pins may be bent and left out of the skin or buried. These intermedullary wires act as splints rather than rigid fixation and must be supplemented by cast immobilization (Fig. 39–6).

Distal radial metaphyseal fractures, particularly when there is not a corresponding ulna fracture, may be difficult to reduce and once reduced, may be unstable. A general anesthetic may be required to reduce these fractures, and, if unstable, percutaneous pinning may be required to maintain the reduction. A single pin across the fracture is usually satisfactory for these injuries. Distal radial physeal fractures are also commonly seen. Often these can be reduced in an outpatient setting but again, redisplacement, is a problem. If displacement occurs within 1 week after injury, a second closed reduction may be performed. If reduction is lost more than 1 week after injury, the fracture is best left alone because of the risk of further injury to the growth plate. Management of this injury may also be aided by a percutaneous wire fixation.

Postoperative Care

The pins should be maintained until the fracture heals, usually within 6 weeks. Once the fracture is stabilized, early motion can begin. Frequent postoperative radiographs are needed to ensure maintenance of reduction.

Complications

Complications include loss of reduction and loss of motion.

Hip Fractures

Pediatric hip fractures are unusual, representing less than 1% of all pediatric femur fractures. Most of these are high-energy injuries, although child abuse may be a cause, particularly in children less than 3 years of age.

The most widely used classification is Canale's modification of Delbet's classification (Canale, 1977). Type I fractures are transphyseal, type II fractures are transcervical, type III fractures occur through the base of the femoral neck (cervicotrochanteric), and type IV fractures are intertrochanteric.

Infants with nondisplaced type I fractures may be treated in a spica cast. If the fracture is displaced, the child may be placed into skin traction for reduction followed by casting. Frequent followup is necessary to ensure that loss of reduction does not occur. If the fracture displaces, the fracture should be reduced and fixed with smooth pins. In children more than 4 years of age, nondisplaced fractures should be pinned with smooth pins. If the fracture occurs with a dislocation of the femoral head, a single attempt at a closed reduction may be performed. If this is not successful, open reduction and internal fixation should be performed. If the head is dislocated posteriorly, a posterior approach should be used.

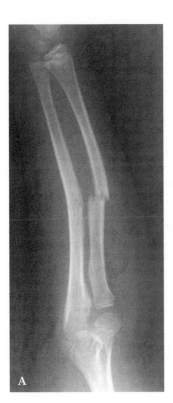
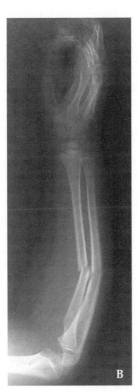
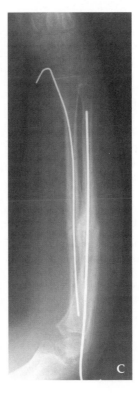

Figure 39–6 **(A)** Preoperative x-ray depicting fracture of radius and ulna. These fractures required open reduction and internal fixation for definitive treatment. Preoperative **(B)** and postoperative **(C)** radiographs of a radius and ulna fracture that underwent open reduction and internal fixation.

If the dislocation is anterior, an anterior approach should be used. After reduction, the hip should be pinned with smooth pins and a spica cast applied. Pins may be removed after the fracture heals.

Type II fractures account for about half of all pediatric proximal femur fractures. Children with these fractures should have the fracture reduced and pinned. If a satisfactory closed reduction can not be obtained, an open reduction should be performed.

Type III fractures that are nondisplaced may be treated with an abduction spica cast. Displaced cervicotrochanteric fractures should undergo a closed or open reduction followed by pin fixation.

Type IV fractures are intertrochanteric fractures of the proximal femur. Nondisplaced fractures may be treated with a spica cast. If the fracture is displaced, it should be reduced and a spica cast applied. If a satisfactory reduction cannot be maintained, closed reduction followed by internal fixation should be performed. Primary internal fixation of type IV fractures should be performed in older patients because of the difficulties in maintaining these fractures in a spica cast.

PITFALL

Fractures of the proximal femur are associated with a high incidence of complications including avascular necrosis, varus malunion, and nonunion.

Expected Outcomes

Treatment of proximal femur fractures in children is rife with complications. Avascular necrosis of the femoral head occurs about 40% of the time, with the incidence decreasing as the fracture line becomes more distal. Fracture displacement also increases the incidence of avascular necrosis. If it occurs, avascular necrosis may involve the entire femoral head, a portion of the femoral head, or the proximal femoral metaphysis.

Premature closure of the upper femoral physis may also occur following these injuries and may be related to internal fixation and avascular necrosis. Varus malunion, resulting in a coxa vara, occurs between 10 to 40% of the time following femoral neck fractures in children. Accurate reduction and the use of internal fixation may reduce the incidence of this complication. Nonunion following femur neck fractures may also occur. This is usually related to varus malalignment of the fracture and is best avoided by an accurate reduction of the fracture and the use of internal fixation.

Femoral Shaft Fractures

Femoral shaft fractures can be one of the most challenging fractures to treat in the pediatric age group. They represent about 1.6% of pediatric fractures, with peak incidences occurring at 2 to 3 years of age and in late adolescence. In infants and toddlers, child abuse should be suspected. Certain principles need to be understood to successfully treat femoral shaft fractures in children. First, children between the ages of 2 and 10 generally will experience 1 to 2 cm overgrowth of the fractured femur. Second, the femur in children has some capacity to remodel. The amount of remodeling that can be expected is dependent on the age of the child and the location and direction of the angulation. In general, younger children have a better capacity for remodeling than older children, and AP deformity will remodel better than varus or valgus angulation. Deformity close to the distal femoral physis will remodel better than deformity located away from the growth plate. Minor amounts of rotational malalignment (up to 10 degrees) may also slowly remodel. Third, children possess a thick, biologically active periosteum about their femurs.

Children up to 5 years of age with less than 2 cm of fracture shortening and less than 20 degrees of angulation can be treated with immediate spica casting. Frequent followup radiographs are required. Fractures with a greater amount of initial displacement should be placed in skin or skeletal traction for 10 to 14 days followed by a spica cast. Children older than age 6 with fracture displacement less than 2 cm and angulation less than 20 degrees may also be treated by immediate spica casting. Fractures with greater amounts of displacement should be treated by initial traction followed by spica casting. Children older than age 6 may also be treated by operative means (Fig. 39–7). The advantages of operative treatment include more rapid mobilization of the child and more reliable maintenance of fracture alignment.

Surgical Technique

External fixation may be performed according to standard techniques. Overgrowth does not seem to occur as readily with external fixation as it does with cast treatment, so the fracture should be anatomically reduced, if possible. Flexible, retrograde, intramedullary nailing of femoral shaft fractures is another excellent option for patients older than age 6. The fracture is reduced with the patient on a fracture table and the position checked with fluoroscopy. The rod length is then determined by holding up the flexible nail against the femur and checking the length with fluoroscopy. Medially, the nail should extend to the greater trochanter and laterally to the middle of the femoral neck. The insertion site both medially and laterally for the nails is 3 cm proximal to the distal femoral physis. Laterally, the approach is made by splitting the iliotibial band longitudinally and elevating the vastus lateralis to expose the distal femur. Medially, the vastus medialis is exposed and retracted anteriorly, exposing the medial distal flare of the femur. The periosteum is incised, and a drill is used to make an entry point for the nails. The nails are then inserted and driven across the fracture site while monitoring the fracture and nail position in AP and lateral planes with the fluoroscope. The tips of both nails should be bent at about a 30 degree angle to facilitate insertion and passage across the fracture site. The first nail should be bent in a "C" configuration and the second nail should be bent in a "S" shape to obtain three points of fixation with each nail. After surgery, the patient is placed in a single spica cast for 3 weeks. Toe-touch weight bearing is allowed when the spica is removed. At 6 weeks, full weight bearing may be begun. The rods are typically removed 3 to 6 months after insertion.

Adolescents with femur fractures who are skeletally mature may be treated as adults with antegrade reamed femoral nailing. This technique should be used cautiously in individuals with open growth plates because of the risk of avascular necrosis of the femoral head.

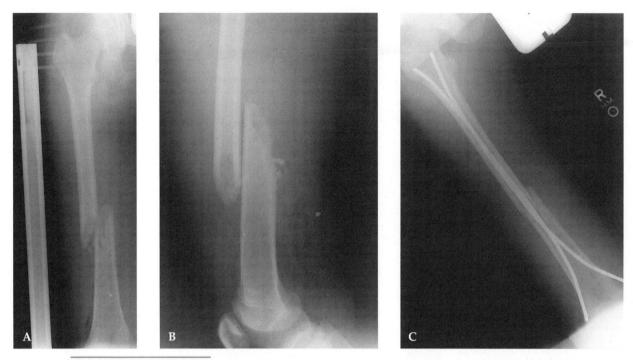

Figure 39–7   (**A,B**) Radiographs of the femur of a twelve year old girl who sustained a gunshot wound to her femur. (**C**) The fracture after closed reduction and retrograde intermedullary fixation.

Expected Outcome

Diaphyseal femoral fractures in children heal readily and generally have a satisfactory result. Limping may persist for up to 1 year after injury. The most significant complications revolve around residual angulation and limb length discrepancy. Care must be taken in the treatment of these injuries to avoid unacceptable femoral shortening or angulation.

Distal Femoral Physeal Fractures

These injuries represent about 15% of lower-extremity physeal injuries. The distal femoral physis is the largest and fastest growing physis in the body, contributing 70% of the length of the femur and 38% of the length of the entire limb. Although the physis is extra-articular, Salter-Harris type III and IV injuries involving the distal femoral physis also involve the knee joint. In addition, the popliteal artery runs posterior to the physis and may be damaged when there is posterior displacement of the distal femoral metaphysis. Nondisplaced fractures may be casted until healing with either a long-leg cast or hip spica cast. Displaced Salter-Harris type I and II injuries should be reduced and pinned. Salter-Harris type I fractures should have cross-pinning with smooth wires. These wires should be removed in 3 weeks to help minimize the risk of physeal damage. Salter-Harris type II fractures with a large metaphyseal fragment should be stabilized with a pin or screw through the metaphyseal fragment, and the fixation should be augmented by casting.

Displaced Salter-Harris type III and IV fractures require either a closed or open reduction to accurately realign the physis and knee joint, followed by internal fixation of the fracture (Fig. 39–8A,B).

These injuries usually heal in 3 weeks, at which point percutaneous fixation can be removed and knee motion begun.

> ## PITFALL
>
> **Growth arrest occurs in as high as 70% of pediatric patients following distal femoral physeal fractures.**

Expected Outcome

These fractures heal readily, but complications are common. Vascular injuries may occur after displaced femoral physeal fractures. These occur when the physis is displaced anteriorly, and the distal femoral metaphysis is posteriorly displaced against the popliteal artery. For this reason, these injuries require emergency reduction. Growth arrest also frequently occurs following distal femoral physeal fractures, with an incidence of up to 70%.

Keys to minimizing growth arrest are accurate reduction of the physis and avoidance of the growth plate with fixation, if possible. If this is not feasible, smooth pins only should be used to cross the physis, and these should be removed after 3 weeks. The family should be informed of the possibility of growth disturbance of the distal femur at the time of injury. Patients with these injuries require long-term followup to evaluate the status of the growth plate.

Proximal Tibial Physis Injury

Proximal tibial physis fractures represent about 1% of all physeal injuries. Most are Salter-Harris types I and II fractures. The popliteal neurovascular bundle is tightly bound to the proximal tibial epiphysis, so it is vulnerable to injury with

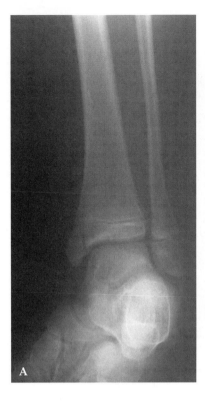

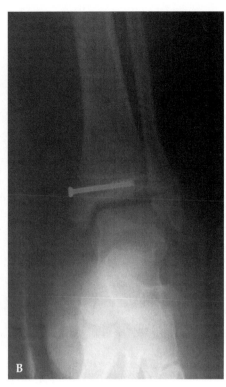

Figure 39–8 Preoperative **(A)** and postoperative **(B)** radiographs after closed reduction and screw fixation of a Salter-Harris type III fracture of the medial malleolus. Note how the screw does not cross the physis.

these fractures. Patients with proximal tibial physeal fractures require careful assessment for neurovascular injury such as ischemia, nerve damage, or compartment syndrome.

PITFALL

Fractures of the proximal tibial physis may be accompanied by injury to the popliteal artery.

Treatment

Treatment for these injuries consist of either a closed or open reduction followed by casting. Pin fixation may be required for unstable injuries, avoiding the physis, if possible. After the fracture is reduced, the patient may require hospital admission for frequent neurovascular examinations.

The most serious complications from this injury are neurovascular. Growth arrest may also occur following these fractures. Patients with these injuries need to be followed with serial radiographs.

Tibial Spine Fractures

Fractures of the tibial spine usually occur secondary to a fall, usually off of a bicycle or during sports. The most common

mechanism injury is valgus and external rotation of the tibia on the femur. The epiphyseal bone of the tibial eminence is biomechanically weaker than the tendinous substance of the anterior cruciate ligament, so a fracture of the tibial eminence results from the injury rather than an anterior cruciate ligament, rupture. The ligament may stretch and undergo plastic deformation prior to fracture of the tibial spine, but complete disruption of the ligament does not occur. The residual laxity from the plastic deformation of the ligament is rarely clinically significant. Meyers and McKeever (1959) have classified these fractures into three types. Type I fractures are nondisplaced, type II fractures are elevated anteriorly with an intact posterior hinge, and type III injuries are complete separations of the tibial spine from the tibial epiphysis.

Treatment

Type I fractures are treated with a long-leg cast for 6 weeks. The knee should be fully extended. Type II injuries can be reduced by extension of the knee. With knee extension, the femoral condyles reduce the elevated tibial spine and serve to maintain fracture reduction. Conscious sedation or general anesthesia is frequently needed to perform the reduction, and knee aspiration may facilitate reduction. The knee is casted for 6 weeks in full extension. Type III injuries may be treated by an attempt at closed reduction. If unsuccessful, type III fractures require either an arthoscopic or an open reduction with internal fixation. Following reduction, the fracture should be stabilized with internal fixation. Sutures, smooth pins, or screws are commonly used to provide fixation for these fractures.

Postoperative Care

Patients generally require immobilization for 6 weeks, followed by rehabilitation to recover motion and strength. The functional outcome from these injuries is usually good despite residual laxity of the anterior cruciate ligament.

Tibial Tuberosity Fractures

Tibial tuberosity fractures occur in patients close to skeletal maturity. Three types of fractures have been described. Type I injuries are small fractures through the distal portion of the tibial tuberosity. Type II fractures involve the epiphyseal fragment of the tibial tubicle and do not extend into the knee joint. Type III fractures extend from the tibial tuberosity through the primary ossification center of the proximal tibia and into the knee joint.

Treatment

Patients with this injury should be carefully examined for signs and symptoms of compartment syndrome. Nondisplaced fractures can be treated in a long-leg cast with the knee extended. Displaced Type II and III injuries need an accurate anatomic reduction followed by internal fixation for optimal results. Type II injuries can be treated by closed reduction and internal fixation, whereas type III injuries require visualization of the knee joint to ensure accurate reduction of the fracture. A medial parapetellar incision can be used for exposure. The menisci are elevated by transecting the anterior portion of the meniscotibial ligament. The fracture is reduced and fixed with screws or wires. If the fracture fixation is stable, patients are immobilized for 7 to 10 days, after which progressive motion is begun.

Expected Outcome

The expected outcome after tibial tubercle fractures is full knee motion. In children less than 11 years of age who sustain this injury, growth arrest of the anterior portion of the proximal tibial physis may occur leading to a progressive genu recurvatum. This complication is unusual because this injury tends to occur in older individuals as the tibial tubercle growth plate is beginning to close. Compartment syndromes have also been reported after these injuries, particularly after type III fractures.

Tibial Shaft Fractures

Most tibial shaft fractures in children occur from low-energy injuries such as sports or falls. Tibia fractures in children less than 1 year of age may indicate child abuse. In addition,

patients with tibial fractures should be examined for signs of compartment syndrome. Patients may require admission to the hospital for close observation. Most tibia fractures can be treated with a long-leg cast as long as an acceptable reduction is maintained. In children 8 years or less, up to 10 degrees of recurvatum and 5 degrees of coronal plane angulation may be accepted. In addition, 1 cm of shortening may be acceptable in children 5 years old and younger. Children more than 5 years of age should have no more than 5 mm of shortening. Rotation of the two tibias should be within 5 degrees of each other. For patients in whom an acceptable reduction can not be maintained by closed reduction and casting, supplemental percutaneous pin fixation or external fixation may used.

Complications

Most closed tibia fractures heal within 8 to 12 weeks. Proximal tibial metaphyseal fractures may develop a post-traumatic tibia valga. This deformity results from overgrowth of the medial aspect of the tibia and may be distressing for both the physician and parents. Parents should be warned of the possibility of valgus overgrowth at the time of initial treatment. To help prevent this complication, valgus reduction of proximal tibial metaphyseal fractures should be avoided. If post-traumatic tibia valga occurs, the extremity should be observed. The peak amount of valgus usually occurs 12 to 18 months after injury, after which resolution of the deformity may occur. Residual deformity may be corrected by osteotomy when the patient is more than 10 years of age.

Distal Tibial Physeal Fractures

Three types of distal tibial physeal fractures will be discussed. First are the Salter-Harris type III and IV injuries involving the medial malleolus. These involve both the growth plate and the joint surface and require an accurate reduction to help minimize the chance of a secondary growth disturbance and articular incongruity. Fractures that are nondisplaced may be treated by a long-leg cast with frequent radiographs to check for displacement. Displaced fractures should be treated by open reduction followed by internal fixation. If the physis is crossed by the fixation device, smooth pins should be used to minimize damage to the growth plate.

Surgical Technique

An anteromedial ankle arthrotomy is performed, and the anterior portion of the ankle joint is visualized. The fracture is reduced and fixed. If possible, the physis should not be violated by the fixation. In larger children, a cannulated screw or pin can be placed across the epiphysis, parallel to the physis (Fig. 39–8). If fixation can not be obtained without crossing the growth plate, smooth pins should be used, and they should be removed as soon as union has occurred.

Postoperative Care

After fixation, the leg should be immobilized in a long-leg cast. These fractures usually heal within 6 weeks. Physical therapy is usually helpful after healing.

Even with accurate alignment of the fracture, post-traumatic growth problems may occur. This should be discussed with the family at the initiation of treatment. It should be emphasized that accurate reduction of the fracture helps minimize but does not eliminate the chance of growth disturbance. Long-term followup is needed after these injuries to assess the growth of the distal tibia.

Juvenile Fracture of Tillaux

This fracture occurs in adolescents who are approaching skeletal maturity. The juvenile Tillaux fracture represents an avulsion of the anterolateral distal tibial epiphysis caused by an external rotation of the foot in the ankle. The anterolateral aspect of the distal tibial epiphysis is avulsed by the pull of the anterior tibiofibular ligaments, resulting in a Salter-Harris type III fracture of the distal tibia.

The distal tibial physis first closes its central portion, then its medial. The lateral portion of the distal tibial physis is the last portion of the distal tibial physis to close. Because of this unique pattern of closure, the lateral distal tibial epiphysis remains vulnerable to fracture until complete closure of the distal tibial physis has occurred. Because injury occurs close to skeletal maturity, growth deformity is infrequent. The main concern with this fracture is that it is intra-articular. Fractures with more than 2 mm of displacement require reduction. Following reduction, a cast or internal fixation is used to maintain the reduction.

Closed reduction is performed by inverting and internally rotating the foot. If this does not result in a satisfactory reduc-

tion, an open reduction can be performed through a small anterolateral arthrotomy. After the fragment is reduced, fixation is performed with either pins or cannulated screws.

Postoperative Care

A long-leg cast is applied for 6 weeks when fracture healing occurs. After cast removal, physical therapy is often useful for obtaining complete rehabilitation. Significant complications from these injuries are rare.

Triplane Fracture

Like the juvenile Tillaux fracture, this fracture occurs in adolescents nearing the end of their growth. The triplane fracture is a complex fracture that has the appearance of a Salter-Harris type III fracture on an AP radiograph (similar to a juvenile Tillaux fracture) and the appearance of a Salter-Harris type II fracture of the distal tibia on the lateral radiograph. Because this fracture is intra-articular, accurate alignment of the joint is required. If this can be obtained by closed means, the patient can be treated in a long-leg cast for 6 weeks. If an accurate reduction cannot be obtained closed, then open reduction and internal fixation should be performed. The reduction of the intra-articular fragment is performed in a similar manner to that for a juvenile Tillaux fracture. If the tibial metaphyseal component needs to be reduced, this can be performed with percutaneous fixation from a posterolateral approach.

Patients with this injury should be held in a long-leg cast for 6 weeks. Rehabilitation can be begun after fracture healing has occurred. This fracture occurs in people who are close to skeletal maturity, so significant growth problems are unusual after this injury.

SELECTED BIBLIOGRAPHY

CANALE ST, BOURLAND WL. Fracture of the femoral neck and intertrochanteric region of the femur in children. *J Bone Jt Surg.* 1977;59A:431–443.

GARTLAND J. Management of supracondylar fractures in children. *Surg Gyn Obst.* 1959;109–145.

JAKOB R, FOWLES JV, RANG M, KASSAB, MT. Observations concerning fractures of the lateral humeral condyle in children. *J Bone Jt Surg.* 1975;57B:430–436.

KING J, DIEFENDORF D, APTHORP J, NEGRETE VF, CARLSON M. Analysis of 429 fractures in 189 battered children. *J Pediatr Orthop.* 1988;8:585–589.

KLING TF Jr, BRIGHT RW, HENSINGER RN. Distal tibial physeal fractures in children that may require open reduction. *J Bone Jt Surg.* 1984;66A:647–657.

MEYERS MH, MCKEEVER FM. Fracture of the intercondylar eminence of the tibia. *J Bone Jt Surg.* 1975;52A:1677–1684.

OGDEN JA, TROSS RB, MURPHY MJ. Fractures of the tibial tuberosity in adolescents. *J Bone Jt Surg.* 1980;62A:205–215.

PIRONE AM, GRAHAM HK, KRAJBICH JI. Management of displaced extension-type supracondylar fractures of the humerus in children. *J Bone Jt Surg.* 1988;70A:641–650.

RISEBOROUGH EJ, BARRETT IR, SHAPIRO F. Growth disturbances following distal femoral physeal fracture-separations. *J Bone Jt Surg.* 1983;65A:885–893.

SALTER RB, HARRIS WR. Injuries involving the epiphyseal plate. *J Bone Jt Surg.* 1963;45A:587–622.

SHELTON WR, CANALE ST. Fractures of the tibia through the proximal tibial epiphyseal cartilage. *J Bone Jt Surg.* 1979;61A:167–173.

SPIEGEL PG, MAST JW, COOPERMAN DR, LAROS GS. Triplane fractures of the distal tibial epiphysis. *Clin Orthop.* 1984;188:74–89.

SAMPLE QUESTIONS

1. Compared with adult bone, the bone in children is:
   (a) denser than adult bone
   (b) has an increased modulus elasticity
   (c) is surrounded by a thicker periosteum
   (d) is less likely to undergo plastic deformation than adult bone
   (e) has a higher energy to failure than adult bone

2. A 9-month-old child presented to the emergency department with a nondisplaced spiral fracture of the right femur. Treatment should consist of:
   (a) Bryant's traction for 2 weeks followed by spica casting
   (b) immediate spica casting, skeletal survey, and social work consultation
   (c) skeletal traction for 5 days followed by spica casting
   (d) long-leg cast
   (e) skin traction for 4 weeks

3. A 5-year-old girl sustained a type III extension supracondylar humerus fracture of her nondominant left arm. Upon examination, she is unable to flex the interphalangeal joint of her thumb and the distal interphalangeal joint of her index finger. She has intact sensation over her left upper extremity. The nerve most likely injured is the:
   (a) radial nerve
   (b) posterior interosseous nerve
   (c) ulnar nerve
   (d) anterior interosseous nerve
   (e) musculocutaneous nerve

4. A 10-year-old boy fell off his bicycle and presents with a swollen knee. Radiographs show type II tibial spine fracture. Initial treatment should consist of:
   (a) open reduction internal fixation through median parapatella approach
   (b) arthroscopic examination and screw fixation of the fragment
   (c) aspiration of the knee followed by reduction of the fracture by extension of the knee
   (d) casting in 30 degrees of knee flexion for 6 weeks
   (e) application of a hinged knee brace blocking the terminal 30 degrees of flexion for 6 weeks

5. The sequence of closure of the distal tibial physis is as follows:
   (a) central portion, medial portion, lateral portion
   (b) posterior portion, lateral portion, medial portion
   (c) lateral portion, central portion, medial portion
   (d) anterior medial portion, central portion, posterior medial portion, lateral portion
   (e) anterior lateral portion, posterior lateral portion, medial portion, central portion

Answers: 1) c; 2) b; 3) d; 4) c; 5) a

Chapter 40

Congenital Anomalies of the Upper Extremity

Scott H. Kozin, MD and Joseph J. Thoder, MD

Outline

Congenital anomalies of the upper extremity are usually sporadic in occurrence and shocking to the parents. The family needs to be counseled with reference to the cause, treatment, and prognosis. The treating physician must have a knowledge of basic embryogenesis, normal developmental milestones, and the classification of congenital malformations to understand this complex array of deformities. In addition, an awareness of associated syndromes is mandatory as they often impact treatment and outcome. Upper extremity anomalies vary greatly with regards to incidence. The most common congenital anomalies are syndactyly and polydactyly. These entities are well understood and appear to be caused by abnormalities of the apical ectodermal ridge. They are succinctly classified and have specific treatment algorithms. Less common malformations, such as macrodactyly, are poorly understood and have more general treatment recommendations.

The beginning section of this chapter will discuss the embryology of the upper limb, describe the development of hand function, and present the classification of congenital limb anomalies. The remainder of the text will concentrate on the individual anomalies as defined by the classification schema. Pertinent points that are fundamental to the diagnosis and treatment will be highlighted.

BASIC SCIENCE

Embryology

Embryogenesis of the upper extremity begins with formation of the upper limb bud on the lateral wall of the embryo at 4 weeks after fertilization. Most congenital deformities occur during embryogenesis, when the limb is rapidly forming. The limb bud is formed by the migration and multiplication of the dorsal somatopleure (ectoderm and underlying undifferentiated somatic mesoderm) from the eighth to tenth somites to the lateral wall. A thickened layer of ectoderm condenses over the limb bud and is known as the apical ectodermal ridge (AER). This specialized ectoderm guides the underlying mesoderm to differentiate into appropriate structures. Without the AER, the mesoderm fails to differentiate into the proper limb components.

> **PEARL**
>
> The apical ectodermal ridge (AER) is a thick layer of ectoderm lying on the limb bud. The AER has been implicated in coordinating limb development. Defects in the AER may lead to a cleft hand, syndactyly, or polydactyly.

The limb develops in a proximal to distal direction, with the arm and forearm appearing before the hand plate. Condensation of the mesoderm forms the skeletal anlagen, which will eventually undergo chondrification and then ossification. By 5 weeks gestation, the hand segment has appeared in the form of a paddle covered by the AER. Cell death and interdigital necrotic zones are crucial to finger separation. This web space formation is a combined effort of cells destined to die (programmed cell death) and cells induced to undergo necrosis. The AER fragments around the hand paddle. Interspace formation occurs in areas not covered by the AER. The AER appears critical to limb development and potential malformations may be explained by alterations in the AER. For example, failure of the ridge to separate may lead to syndactyly. Localized hypoplasia of the AER may cause an underlying cleft hand. Hyperplasia of the AER may lead to polydactyly.

The ingrowth of vessels and nerves into the developing extremity occurs during the fifth to eighth week. Joint formation occurs with condensation of the precursors to chondrocytes to form dense plates between future bones. Subsequent joint cavitation further defines the articulation. However, proper joint development requires motion for final modeling of the joint surface. By the eighth week, embryogenesis is

Orthopaedic Surgery: The Essentials. Edited by M.E. Baratz, A.D. Watson, and J.E. Imbriglia. Thieme Medical Publishers, Inc., New York © 1999

complete and all limb structures are present with mobile joint cavities and periosteal bone formation. Subsequently, the fetal period commences with differential growth of the existing structures and continues until birth.

PEARL

Embryogenesis of the upper extremity commences at 4 weeks and is complete 8 weeks after fertilization, at which time all limb structures are present.

Growth and Development

At the time of birth, all major systems in the hand are fully developed except the nervous system. Myelination of peripheral nerves is not complete until approximately 2 years of age. Skeletal maturation shows great variability between sexes and races in normal development. Secondary ossification centers tend to occur earlier in girls than in boys and earlier in black children than in white children. Children with congenitally abnormal hands will show delayed ossification centers compared with their normal hands or those of their peers. From the time of birth to skeletal maturity, a child's head will double in size, the trunk triple, the arms quadruple in length, and the legs increase by a factor of 5. Hand size increases rapidly over the first 4 years of life.

Function of the hand is divided into two categories. The first is the unspecialized, passive, force transmitter for the mobile limb. The second is the skilled mobile object manipulator. This second category progresses through unique stages of development to achieve the level of the functioning human hand. The most primitive form of grasp is referred to as hook grip. It is employed when demand calls for prolonged power without the need for precision. The fingers are flexed at the interphalangeal (IP) joints with recruitment of metacarpophalangeal (MP) flexion as load increases. The thumb plays no roll in this type of grip. Power grip is a more sophisticated form of grasp but is still nonmanipulative. The thumb becomes involved by applying counter pressure over the dorsum of the flexed fingers or by acting as the post for holding of an object in the palm. The most sophisticated form of grip is precision grip, whereby an object can be manipulated by the fingers.

The bridge between nonmanipulative and precision handling is pinch. In lateral pinch, an object is held by the palmar surface of the distal phalanx of the thumb against the middle and distal phalanx of the index finger. The thumb is abducted and medially rotated while the first dorsal interosseous muscle abducts and laterally rotates the index finger. Two additional types of pinch are used during prehension grip: palmar pinch and tip pinch. In palmar pinch, an object is held between the distal pad of the thumb and the distal pad of one or two adjacent fingers. Three-point palmar pinch (3-jaw chuck) is the primary manipulative pinch used by the normal hand. Tip pinch uses the tip of the thumb opposed to the tip of an adjacent finger (usually index) to form a circle in the side view to manipulate small fine objects.

In the course of normal development, a child will maintain the hands in a flexed position and clench upon stimulation until about 2 months of age. Voluntary opening comes into play at about 2 months, and primitive power grip using the ulnar digits begins at approximately 3 months. By 7 months, thumb opposition begins and pinch begins at 10 to 12 months. Precision opposition with voluntary release is usually in place at 15 to 18 months. This development occurs bilaterally and independent of handedness, which will not become apparent until 30 to 36 months.

Incidence and Genetics

Of newborns, 1 to 2% have a congenital malformation. However, not all of these abnormalities require treatment. An abnormality of the upper extremity occurs in about 10% of these children. The cause of these limb anomalies may be genetic, secondary to exposure to environmental teratogens, or a combination of both. Genetic causes include single-gene (Mendelian), multiple-gene (polygenic), or chromosomal disorders.

Syndactyly and polydactyly are the most common congenital anomalies of the upper extremity and demonstrate a single-gene dominant inheritance pattern. However, many of the complex syndromes involve multiple genes with variable penetrance, and referral to a geneticist is required. Environmental agents include radiation and medications, such as thalidomide, which causes radial deficiencies and phocomelia. Despite an extensive evaluation, many of these upper extremity congenital anomalies occur in a sporadic fashion.

Classification of congenital malformations of the upper extremity includes seven groups. The classification is not all inclusive and cannot be applied to all abnormalities. Nonetheless, it provides the basis for understanding a complex array of anomalies (Table 40–1). Failure of formation implies an arrest of development that occurs in the transverse or longitudinal direction. In failure of differentiation, the basic units have developed, but the final form is not completed. This group can involve the soft tissue, skeletal elements, or a combination of both. Duplication can occur throughout the limb and is most common at the level of the digits (polydactyly). Overgrowth and undergrowth are separate categories that vary from minimal deformity to extensive. Congenital constriction band syndrome is a distinct group that is not genetic and is diagnosed by the presence of an amniotic ring. Generalized skeletal abnormalities include entities such as dwarfism, Madelung's deformity, and Marfan's syndrome.

This chapter will focus on the more common congenital anomalies of the upper extremity and serve as a guide to diagnosis and treatment of this diverse group of abnormalities. The anomalies will be presented in sequence defined by the general classification listed in Table 40–1.

SPECIFIC CONDITIONS, TREATMENT, AND OUTCOME

Failure of Formation

Transverse Deficiencies

Transverse deficiencies are also referred to as congenital amputations. They are defined by the last remaining bone segment and most commonly occur below the elbow (Fig.

TABLE 40–1 Classification of congenital limb anomalies

I. Failure of Formation of Parts
    A. Transverse deficiencies
    B. Longitudinal deficiencies
        1. Phocomelia
        2. Radial
        3. Central
        4. Ulnar
II. Failure of Differentiation
    A. Synostosis
    B. Radial head dislocation
    C. Symphalangism
    D. Syndactyly
    E. Contracture
        1. Soft tissue
            a. Arthrogryposis
            b. Pterygium
            c. Trigger
            d. Absent extensor tendons
            e. Hypoplastic thumb
            f. Clasped thumb
            g. Retroflexible thumb
            h. Camptodactyly
            i. Windblown hand
        2. Skeletal
            a. Clinodactyly
            b. Kirner's deformity
            c. Delta bone
III. Duplication
    A. Thumb
    B. Triphalangism / hyperphalangism
    C. Polydactyly
    D. Mirror hand
IV. Overgrowth
    A. Limb
    B. Macrodactyly
V. Undergrowth
VI. Congenital constriction band syndrome
VII. Generalized skeletal abnormalities

40–1). The stump is usually well padded and may contain rudimentary nubbins on the end. The elbow joint usually is stable and has good motion. Surgery is rarely required, and treatment is aimed toward prosthetic fitting. A passive prosthetic device is recommended as soon as the child develops sitting balance (about 6 months). This early fitting promotes bimanual activity away from the body, prevents abnormalities of posture, and encourages prosthetic acceptance. When the child demonstrates adequate motor skills (about 2 to 3 years old), an active prosthesis is provided that has a voluntary opening hook. Myoelectric devices may be used when the child is older and able to understand the complexities of such a prosthesis.

PEARL

Congenital upper extremity amputations most commonly occur just below the elbow joint. Prosthetic fitting is initiated at 6 months of age.

Phocomelia

Phocomelia represents a longitudinal failure of formation with an absent intervening segment of the extremity (intercalary aplasia) (Fig. 40–2). The missing segment can be the arm, forearm, or both, with the hand attached directly to the shoulder. This deformity is uncommon except for the marked increased incidence (60%) associated with thalidomide. Thalidomide causes phocomelia when taken during the first trimester of pregnancy. Phocomelia has also been seen in the

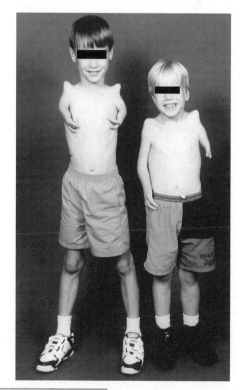

Figure 40–2 Phocomelia with a variable degree of intercalary aplasia in affected children.

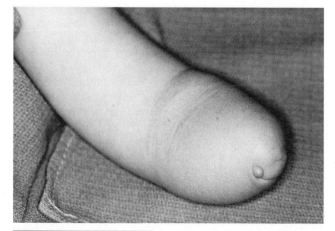

Figure 40–1 Congenital below-the-elbow amputation with rudimentary nubbins.

grandchildren of women who took thalidomide. Surgery is rarely indicated, and prosthetic fitting is beneficial, especially in bilateral cases. Prosthetic fitting can be difficult because of the extreme shortening of the limb.

Radial Clubhand

Radial clubhand is a longitudinal deficiency of the radial border of the upper extremity. The incidence varies from 1:55,000 to 1:100,000 live births. The etiology is unclear, but evidence shows that it may involve abnormal regulation of the AER. It is known to follow exposure to teratogens such as thalidomide and radiation. There is a well-known association of radial aplasia with many genetic syndromes, the most common of which include Holt-Oram (cardiac septal defects), Fanconi's anemia (aplastic), TAR (thrombocytopenia, absent radius) and VATER (vertebral, anal, tracheo-esophageal and renal abnormalities).

The musculoskeletal abnormalities associated with radial aplasia involve the entire extremity (Fig. 40–3). The humerus is shortened with deficiencies of capitellar and trochlear development. The ulna is short (60% of predicted) and bowed. Deficiencies extend distally with absence of the scaphoid and trapezium common, hypoplasia or absence of the thumb (80%), and stiffness in the radial most digits. The soft tissue abnormalities include deficiencies or aberrant insertions of all muscles that normally arise from the lateral epicondyle. The radial artery and nerve are absent with persistence of the median artery and thickening of the median nerve that supply the lateral border of the extremity distally. The classification of radial clubhand is based on the degree of absence (Table 40–2).

Treatment of radial dysplasia is initially directed toward any visceral anomalies that may be life threatening. The goal of the orthopaedic management is to provide adequate support for the carpus and hand, followed by thumb reconstruction. Contraindications to surgical treatment include, children with limited life expectancy, mild deformity with adequate support for the hand, elbow contractures that prevent the hand from reaching the mouth, and adult patients who have adjusted to their deformity. In the appropriate patient, soft tissue stretching with splinting or serial casting is the initial treatment, especially in children who require cardiac or gastrointestinal surgery, which will delay orthopaedic procedures.

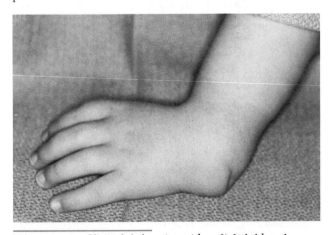

Figure 40–3 Clinical deformity with radial clubhand.

TABLE 40–2 Classification of Radial Clubhand

Type	Description	Characteristics
I	Short distal radius	Distal radial epiphysis present but delayed in appearance Radius and ulna are short without bow Adequate support for the carpus Stable elbow Thumb hypoplasia common
II	Hypoplastic radius	Both radial physes are present but defective Progressive ulnar bowing Loss of support for carpus Stable elbow
III	Partial absence	Distal and middle thirds of the radius absent or represented by an anlage without growth potential Ulna shortened, thickened, and bowed No support for the carpus and hand Elbow is usually stable
IV	Total radius	No representation of the radius Ulna shortened, thickened, and bowed No support for the carpus and hand

---

PEARL

Deficiencies in radial clubhand include the bone, muscle, tendon, nerves, and arteries. The radial sensory nerve is absent with an enlarged median nerve supplying sensation to the dorsoradial aspect of the hand.

The traditional surgical algorithm begins with passive correction followed by centralization of the carpus on the ulna. When passive correction is not possible, soft tissue release on the lateral side of the limb with Z-plasty of the skin becomes necessary. The limiting structure to centralization may be the median nerve, which is located more superficial and radial than normal. The placement of the carpus on the distal ulna with longitudinal alignment between the third ray and the long axis of the ulna is the goal of centralization. This can be accomplished by shaving the distal ulnar epiphysis to a flattened surface or by notching or resection of the lunate. Osteotomy of the ulna may be required to straighten the bow, but caution must be exercised not to excessively shorten the ulna that is already 60% of predicted length. Once the bony alignment is satisfactory, the carpus is secured by an intramedullary pin to the ulna. Soft tissue balancing is critical to a successful outcome and is accomplished by capsular reefing and extensor tendon transfer or advancement to overcome the tendency for recurrence. Postsurgical management includes full-time splinting until the child reaches school age and night splints until skeletal maturity. This regimen has inherent difficulties with patient compliance. Despite appropriate patient selection and good surgical principles, outcome studies tend to show a high rate of recurrence of the angular deformity. A recent analysis of outcomes from our institution showed a significant loss of correction in patients followed for more than 7 years. The use of thin-pin external fixation devices (Ilizarov) may be of benefit in future treatment algorithms to provide better soft tissue correction than the methods presently employed.

Central Deficiency

Cleft hand is a longitudinal deficiency of the central rays of the hand (index, long, and ring), which differentiate at a separate time from the radial and ulnar rays (thumb and small). There are two types of cleft hand (typical and atypical), possessing separate features and requiring different treatment (Table 40–3). The typical cleft hand has a "V" shaped defect with a varying degree of long ray absence. Most commonly, the phalanges are absent and the metacarpal is present (Fig.

TABLE 40–3   Comparison of Atypical and Typical Cleft Hand

Characteristic	Typical Cleft	Atypical Cleft
Inherited	Yes	No
Bilateral	Yes	No
Associated anomalies	Yes	No
Cleft foot	Yes	No
Cleft lip	Yes	No
Syndactyly	Yes	No
Several rays	No	Yes

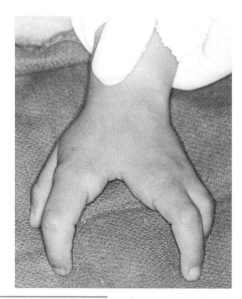

Figure 40–4   Typical cleft hand reconstructed with cleft closure and intermetacarpal ligament reconstruction.

40–4). This type is often bilateral and is usually inherited, but it may skip generations. Associated foot involvement is common, and there may be syndactyly of the thumb-index or ring-small web space that requires release prior to cleft closure.

Surgical treatment involves cleft closure to improve grasp and appearance. There is no urgency for cleft closure as development is not delayed by the presence of a cleft nor is function seriously impaired. We prefer to wait until the child is between 2 to 3 years of age, when surgical reconstruction is easier to perform. Closure of the cleft requires creation of a flap to recreate the commissure (web space), reducing the potential for scar contracture, removal of any intervening bones that block cleft narrowing, and reconstruction of the intermetacarpal ligament to prevent late splaying. Suturing the metacarpals together is insufficient to prevent metacarpal divergence. We use a surgical technique similar to Barsky (1964), with creation of a commissure from the side of an adjacent digit to the cleft, excision of any interposed metacarpal, and reapproximation of the remaining intermetacarpal ligament. More severe cases with a significant thumb adduction contracture may require transposition of the index ray to the long position to achieve thumb-index web reconstruction and cleft closure.

Atypical cleft hand is also known as symbrachydactyly and involves the central three rays. This type is usually unilateral, sporadic, and without foot involvement. Atypical cleft is more difficult to treat and requires individualized treatment. The goal is to create a good grasp with a functional pincer. Many children with atypical cleft hand demonstrate surprising proficiency. Surgery may not be required, but techniques to improve function include web deepening, rotational osteotomies, tendon transfer, or digital lengthening. Narrowing of the atypical cleft should not be performed as it may interfere with function.

Ulnar Clubhand

Ulnar clubhand is a longitudinal deficiency of the ulna border of the upper extremity. It is characterized by varying degrees of ulna absence, ulnar deviation of the hand on the forearm, and elbow instability. Digital malformation is common on the ulnar border of the hand. This deficiency occurs sporadically with no identifiable chromosomal marker. The associated anomalies are primarily of the musculoskeletal system, in contrast to radial clubhand, which has visceral abnormalities. The classification of this deficiency is based on the amount of ulna remaining and the degree of deformity (Table 40–4). The ulnar anlage is a remnant of the distal ulna made up of cartilage that has no growth potential. The anlage arises from the distal humerus or remaining proximal ulna and attaches to the ulnar carpus and/or distal radius. This structure is most commonly present in types II and IV ulnar clubhand. It may act as a tether to cause progressive bowing of the radius, ulnar tilting of the radial physis, and ulnar deviation. If progressive ulnar bowing and deviation is apparent, then early resection at approximately 6 months of age is indicated. The carpus is usually stable on the radius following anlage resection and, thus, requires no relocation procedure. The ulnar neurovascular structures are usually present and must be protected at surgery. If there is no progression of the deformity, anlage resection can be delayed. Absence of the ulna

TABLE 40–4   Classification of Ulnar Clubhand

Type	Description	Characteristics
I	Hypoplasia	Both proximal and distal ulnar physes are present Stable elbow Slight ulnar deviation of the hand Minimal bowing of the radius Usually nonprogressive
II	Partial dysplasia	Absence of the distal +/− middle third of the ulna Distal ulna anlage Stable elbow Progressive ulnar deviation and bowing common Radial head may dislocate
III	Total absence	Unstable elbow Radius relatively straight Severe deficiencies of the carpus and hand
IV	Radiohumeral synostosis	Elbow stable but fixed Ulna is represented by anlage Progressive ulnar deviation of the hand and bowing of the radius can occur

TABLE 40–5   Classification of Metacarpal Synostosis

Type	Degree of Synostosis	Characteristics
I	Fusion at the base	Divergence distally +/− abduction deformity of small digit
II	Fusion of 1/2 the metacarpal	High propensity for abduction deformity of small digit
III	Fusion of >1/2 the metacarpal	A: separate MP joint B: common MP joint

Metacarpal transverse synostosis occurs most commonly between the ring and small fingers and is frequently bilateral (up to 80%). It can be divided into three types (Table 40–5). Treatment of ring-small synostosis is indicated when small finger abduction deformity creates a functional difficulty. In these instances, the small finger cannot be brought parallel to the adjacent digits. If the digit is severely hypoplastic, amputation should be considered. If the digit is functional, lengthening osteotomy of the metacarpal can be performed with correction of the abduction deformity utilizing interposition bone graft. Soft tissue balancing of the interossei and abductor digiti quinti with extensor realignment is also necessary. Metacarpal synostosis can occur between the thumb and index fingers with subsequent significant functional difficulties. Management of thumb-index synostosis is directed toward salvage of a functional opposable digit in the thumb position utilizing the best available parts.

Carpal coalitions represent a transverse synostosis at the wrist level and is more common in the black population. Lunotriquetral is the most common, followed by capitohammate. Carpal coalitions are associated with other skeletal anomalies (i.e., tarsal coalition, Puerto Rican syndrome) but rarely require treatment.

Longitudinal synostosis at the radiohumeral joint occurs with type IV clubhand. This can be treated with correctional osteotomy if the position of the hand renders it nonfunctional. Synostosis at the elbow is most commonly transverse at the proximal radioulnar joint (Fig. 40–5). Type I is a complete synostosis. Type II is partial and is associated with radial head dislocation. Forearm rotation can be partially compensated for by intercarpal supination, but pronation

causes increased loads across the radiocapitellar joint, which may result in radial head dislocation. Surgical intervention is indicated if the radial head dislocation becomes symptomatic. If the elbow is stable with adequate proximal ulnar length, resection of the radial head is appropriate. However, with an unstable or very short proximal ulna, creation of a one bone forearm may be the treatment of choice. Osteotomy of the radius is performed proximally, translated to the proximal ulna, and secured by pins or plating. In type IV deformities, the hand may be facing backward and rest on the flank. Corrective osteotomy to better postion the hand is beneficial. The hand deficiencies of ulnar clubhand are addressed as needed, the goal being to provide opposable digits for grip and pinch.

PEARL

Ulnar clubhand is associated with musculoskeletal anomalies, whereas radial clubhand often includes visceral abnormalities.

Failure of Differentiation

Synostosis

Synostosis can occur anywhere in the upper extremity. It may be partial or complete, longitudinal or transverse. When synostosis occurs longitudinally in the digits, it is referred to as symphalangism. Transverse digital synostosis at the phalangeal level is usually part of a complex syndactyly.

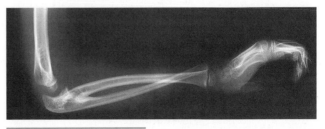

Figure 40–5   X-ray of proximal radioulnar synostosis, which inhibits forearm rotation.

deformities in excess of 45 degrees may require rotational osteotomy through the fusion mass to a more functional position. Caution must be used with severe rotational deformities to prevent neurovascular compromise. The presence of a synostosis should alert the orthopaedist to look for other skeletal anomalies. Treatment aimed at restoration of motion is universally unsuccessful and, therefore, ill advised.

PITFALL

Surgical procedures to restore motion for congenital synostosis are universally unsuccessful.

Radial Head Dislocation

Isolated radial head dislocation occurs more frequently than that associated with radioulnar synostosis. The dislocation can occur posteriorly (65%), anteriorly (18%), or posterolateral (17%). Distinguishing between true congenital dislocation and long-standing post-traumatic dislocation may be difficult in a child. Radiographic criteria include a short radius (relative to the ulna), hypoplastic capitellum with a deficient trochlea, and a dome-shaped radial head. However these findings can also develop as a result of a traumatic dislocation at an early age. Family history and bilateral involvement also infer congenital cause. In addition, any condition that results in a shortened ulna will increase force across the radiocapitellar joint and can predispose to radial head dislocation. Examples include multiple hereditary exostosis, multiple enchondromatosis, nail-patella syndrome, antecubital pterygium, and connective tissue disorders with associated joint laxity.

Congenital radial head dislocations should be followed until skeletal maturity. Indications for surgery at that time are pain along the prominence of the dislocation and/or cosmesis. Radial head excision after skeletal maturity provides pain relief and improves appearance but does not have any significant affect on forearm or elbow motion.

Symphalangism

Symphalangism is a longitudinal failure of joint differentiation that usually affects the proximal interphalangeal (PIP) joint. The child presents with a stiff, extended finger with absence of skin creases across the affected joint. Radiographs may be misleading as they appear to demonstrate a joint space. However, ossification of the connecting cartilaginous bar has yet to occur and obliteration of the joint space with bony ankylosis will appear with time (Fig. 40–6). Symphalangism is often associated with short fingers (brachydactyly) and is called symbrachydactyly. Treatment for symphalangism has been disappointing, and no reliable method exists for restoration of motion. Chondrodesis or arthrodesis can be performed to better position the finger.

Syndactyly

Syndactyly is one of the most common congenital anomalies and represents a failure of differentiation of the web space, probably from an abnormality in the AER. Syndactyly is

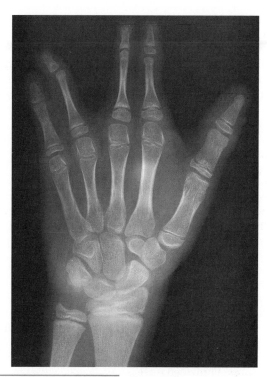

Figure 40–6 X-ray of symphalangism of the fingers with bony ankylosis of the proximal interphalangeal joint.

defined as an abnormal interconnection between adjacent digits and is described according to the magnitude and extent of the linkage. The interconnection may encompass the entire length of the adjacent digits (complete) or end proximal to the fingertip (incomplete). The syndactyly may involve only skin and fibrous tissue (simple) or may include bone (complex). Syndactyly that occurs with other anomalies (e.g., Apert's syndrome, Poland's syndrome, and macrodactyly) is referred to as complicated syndactyly. Psuedosyndactyly occurs in congenital constriction band syndrome and has an intact web space with a distal connection between digits. This is the result of intrauterine healing following an insult from the amniotic bands. This condition should be differentiated from true syndactyly. Syndactyly occurs most commonly in the third web space, followed by the fourth, second, and first. Treatment depends on the child, type of syndactyly, extent of involvement, and quality of the digits. Simple syndactyly of any significant degree will benefit from web space reconstruction. Surgery is performed between 6 and 12 months of age and requires full-thickness skin graft, usually from the groin. If multiple web spaces are affected, reconstruction should include only one side of a syndactylized digit at a time to avoid potential vascular difficulties. Therefore, staged surgery may be necessary to completely release all affected digits. It is preferable to have all releases completed before the child starts school. Priority is granted to attached digits with marked differences in their respective lengths to prevent angular deformities. For example, syndactyly of the fourth web space involves the ring and small digits which have significant length differences. Failure to separate these digits at an early age will result in a flexion and lateral deviation of the ring digit. In contrast, syndactyly of the third web space involves digits of similar lengths (long and ring), and surgery is less urgent.

Surgical goals are to create and maintain a web space of normal dimension. Therefore, flap design should avoid skin graft in the web commissure and should use zigzag incisions along the digits to limit longitudinal contracture. There are many techniques for syndactyly release and web space reconstruction. We prefer to design a dorsal flap for the commissure to replicate the normal slope of the web space. We use zigzag incisions that extend from the commissure to the midline of the connected digits. Triangular flaps are designed to interdigitate after digit separation. The dorsal flap will be placed between the separated digits to a transverse incision in the palm. The normal commissure extends approximately one third the length of the proximal phalanx. In cases of short digits with syndactyly (brachysyndactyly), we further deepen the web space for better motion and cosmesis.

Syndactyly release is performed with a tourniquet and loupe magnification. After elevating the skin flaps, the neurovascular bundles are identified along the palmar aspect of the digits prior to separation of the digits. If the bundle bifurcates distal to the proposed commissure, then microdissection of the nerve is necessary to allow web reconstruction. Ligation of a proper digital artery may be necessary and can be performed provided there is an adequate vessel from the other side. The digits are then separated by dividing the interconnecting fibrous tissue and septa, and the flaps are inset. The skin deficit is covered by full-thickness skin graft from the groin, which is harvested in an elliptical fashion to allow primary closure. Prior to skin graft application, the tourniquet is deflated and hemostasis attained to prevent skin graft failure. A No. 5-0 plain gut suture is used to avoid the need for suture removal. A large bulky compressive dressing is applied with long-arm plaster immobilization and elbow flexion greater than 90 degrees for 2 weeks.

Complex and complicated syndactyly are considerably more difficult to treat than simple syndactyly. There are often bony, tendinous, and neurovascular abnormalities. The fingertips may have a common nail which makes nail plate division and pulp reconstruction difficult. Treatment needs to be individualized with careful consideration of function. In certain instances, the hand may function better with a single conjoined digit versus two deformed stiff digits. Apert's syndrome (acrocephalosyndactyly) represents a combination of severe complex and complicated syndactyly, which usually involves all digits (Fig. 40–7). Separation of these fused digits is a formidable task, with initial attempts directed at thumb and small finger segregation and mobilization. The remaining central mass can often not be completely separated. In some cases a three-fingered hand is the best option.

PEARL

Reconstruction of any commissure should avoid skin graft or a suture line to minimize contracture.

Arthrogryposis

Arthrogryposis multiplex congenita is a syndrome of joint contractures that are present at birth and are not progressive.

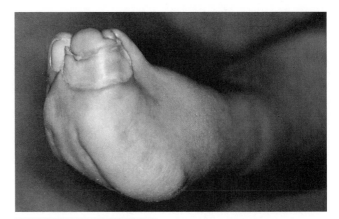

Figure 40–7 Severe syndactyly associated with Apert's syndrome.

The etiology is unclear; however, it is well recognized that the joint contractures are secondary to muscle weakness and inelasticity during development. There are two forms: neuropathic and myopathic. The neuropathic form is by far more common and is the result of degeneration of the anterior horn cells in utero. The myopathic form demonstrates inheritance patterns similar to muscular dystrophy. The degree of joint involvement may be minimal, moderate, or severe. Presentation can be divided into three groups: group I, distal hand involvement only; group II, diffuse upper extremity involvement; and group III, upper and lower extremity involvement.

The contractures are bilaterally symmetric with limitations of both active and passive motion. Clinical features include waxy skin devoid of skin creases, significant muscle wasting, and a paucity of subcutaneous tissue. Associated anomalies frequently involve the musculoskeletal system, for example, Klippel-Feil cervical anomalies, Sprengel's deformity, synostoses, and syndactyly. The typical attitude of the affected upper extremity is that of adduction and internal rotation at the shoulder, elbow extension, forearm pronation, and wrist flexion and ulnar deviation (Fig. 40–8). The digits are stiff and semiflexed, and the thumb is clenched in the palm. This creates functional difficulties with activities of daily living, especially self care.

Treatment is individualized to each childs needs; however, the traditional goals include independent function for self-feeding and peroneal care. Early and frequent passive movement of all involved joints is recommended. Internal rotation deformities of the shoulder that are severe are best managed by external rotation osteotomy, but most authors agree that shoulder surgery is rarely necessary. Most often surgical attention is directed toward elbow, wrist, and finger mobility.

Restoring elbow function requires a careful assessment of the child's total needs. The goal is to achieve one elbow capable of flexion and the other extension. However, lower extremity involvement may create the need for ambulatory assistive devices where active elbow extension is more important than elbow flexion. Passive motion that cannot be achieved by therapy may be an indication for joint release or fractional tendon lengthening. If adequate passive motion can be gained but inadequate active motion is present, tendon transfers may be considered. Unfortunately, standard elbow flexion transfers (pectoralis major, latissimus dorsi, triceps,

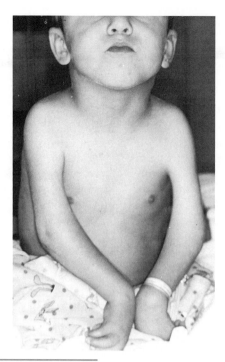

Figure 40–8 Typical upper extremity posture in arthrogryposis multiplex congenita.

Steindler flexorplasty) have been disappointing in restoring functional elbow flexion due to poor motor function of the donor muscle.

Wrist flexion contractures are similarly difficult to overcome because of inadequate active extension power. Options are wrist arthrodesis or proximal row carpectomy, if adequate wrist extension is present.

Pterygium Cubitale

Congenital webbing of the elbow is part of the pterygium syndrome, which also involves webbing of the neck, axilla, knees, and digits. It is similar in appearance to arthrogryposis, and the etiology is unknown. Associated anomalies include cardiac, genitourinary, craniofacial, and congenital hand deformities. All structures about the elbow are involved including skin, subcutaneous tissue, muscle, and bone. The elbow can usually flex across the web, but extension is severely limited and is seldom beyond 90 degrees. Brachial and antebrachial muscles are atrophic or absent. Associated skeletal deformities include radial head dislocation, radioulnar synostosis, hypoplastic or absent radius and/or ulna, and hypoplasia of the distal humerus. Thus far, most attempts to correct the deformity result in recurrence, and surgical treatment is not recommended.

Trigger Digits

Congenital trigger thumb is far more common than trigger finger. The diagnosis is often delayed because infants normally posture their thumb in a flexed position. The child presents with an inability to extend the thumb at the IP joint, and the condition can be bilateral. A vague history of trauma is not uncommon but typically not related. The etiology is secondary to a nodular thickening of the flexor pollicis longus

tendon and narrowing of the flexor sheath. This prevents the flexor tendon from entering the sheath. Palpation of the nodular thickening of the flexor tendon can be appreciated just proximal to the sheath. Passive manipulation may produce a noticeable click or pop as the thumb extends. Splinting can be used to maintain this position but has not been efficacious. Approximately one third of trigger thumbs diagnosed prior to 1 year will resolve, and a delay in surgery up to 3 years of age has no harmful effects. Therefore, a period of observation can be recommended in young children. Delayed presentation, parental decision, or failure to spontaneously resolve are indications for surgical release of the first annular pulley. Careful attention should be taken to identify and protect digital nerves, particularly the radial digital nerve of the thumb, as it traverses the sheath just beneath the thumb MP flexion crease.

> ## PEARL
>
> **Trigger thumbs have a palpable nodular thickening of the flexor pollicis longus tendon just proximal to the sheath.**

Absent Extensor Tendons

Absent extensor tendons are a rare congenital anomaly that can effect single or multiple digits. The single digit variant consists of hypoplasia or absence of the central slip with lack of PIP joint extension. The multiple digit type involves hypoplasia of the extensor digitorum communis with subluxation of the underdeveloped tendons into the valleys and loss of MP joint extension. This type is often associated with a similar flexion deformity of the thumb. The goal for either variety is to correct the flexion contracture, followed by tendon transfer to substitute for the deficiency. The contracture may be overcome by splinting, serial casting, or surgery. Tendon transfer for single digit central slip hypoplasia utilizes the flexor digitorum superficialis of the involved finger or a lateral band of an adjacent finger. Tendon transfer for multiple digits uses one or several of the flexor digitorum superficialis tendons routed to the dorsum of the hand or the extensor carpi radialis extended with a multitail tendon graft.

Hypoplastic Thumb

Thumb hypoplasia refers to an underdevelopment secondary to a failure of differentiation. Thumb hypoplasia is a different entity from partial thumb aplasia, which usually results from a transverse deficiency or congenital constriction band syndrome. Hypoplasia of the thumb can occur to variable degree and most commonly occurs as part of a radial deficiency of the upper extremity. However, a short thumb can be associated with many syndromes (e.g., de Lange's syndrome, diastrophic dwarfism, and Apert's syndrome).

The underdeveloped thumb has been classified into five types (Table 40–6). This classification is extremely helpful when contemplating treatment options. However, it can be difficult to distinguish between types II and IIIA (thumbs that can be reconstructed) and type IIIB, which is best treated with pollicization. The determining factor is the presence or

TABLE 40–6 Classification and Treatment of Thumb Hypoplasia

Type	Characteristics	Treatment
I	Minor hypoplasia Minimal shortening	None
II	Moderate hypoplasia First web contracture Instability of MP joint Hypoplastic thenars	Reconstruction
III	Severe hypoplasia Type II characteristics plus extreme thenar hypoplasia Extrinsic abnormalities Partial aplasia metacarpal A: CMC stable B: CMC unstable	Reconstruction Pollicization
IV	Pouce flottant (floating thumb) Rudimentary bony elements Narrow skin pedicle	Ablation and pollicization
V	Complete absence	Pollicization

TABLE 40–7 Joint, Tendon, and Bone Reorganization in Pollicization

Structure	Pollicization Function
Distal IP joint	IP joint
PIP joint	MP joint
MP joint	CMC joint
First palmar interosseous	Adductor pollicis
First dorsal interosseous	Abductor pollicis brevis
Extensor indicis propius	Extensor pollicis longus
Extensor digitorum	Abductor pollicis longus
Metacarpal	Trapezium

absence of a carpometacarpal (CMC) joint. A vestigial CMC joint that lacks stability requires pollicization, whereas a stable CMC joint can serve as a foundation for thumb reconstruction. Unfortunately, the trapezium and trapezoid do not ossify until 4 to 6 years of age, which further complicates the decision-making process.

Thumb reconstruction in types II and IIIA requires addressing all elements of the hypoplasia. The adducted posture of the thumb is corrected with web space deepening and reconstruction by Z-plasty or dorsal transposition flap. The MP joint instability involves the ulnar side and can be rectified by ulnar collateral ligament reconstruction or epiphyseal chondrodesis. The thenar hypoplasia is augmented by opposition transfer with the abductor digiti quinti or a flexor digitorum superficialis tendon. Type IIIA thumbs also require

transfer or rerouting to overcome the extrinsic tendon and muscle abnormalities, which can include aberrant or deficient extensor pollicis longus and/or flexor pollicis longus tendons.

Pollicization is the procedure of choice for types IIIB, IV, and V hypoplasia (Fig. 40–9). This complex procedure involves neurovascular transposition of the index digit to the thumb position with reconstruction of the intrinsic muscles of the thumb. The index digit must be rotated at least 120 degrees to attain proper orientation of the new thumb. The index must be shortened by removal of the diaphysis, and a metacarpal epiphysiodesis should be performed to prevent excessive length of the thumb. The neurovascular bundles must be carefully protected throughout the procedure. Joint and tendon reorganization is necessary for pollicization (Table 40–7). The index distal IP joint becomes the thumb IP joint, the index PIP joint becomes the thumb MP joint, and the index MP joint becomes the thumb CMC joint. The muscles are reorganized to optimize function of the created thumb. The extensor digitorum communis becomes the abductor pollicis longus, the extensor indicis proprius becomes the extensor pollicis longus, the first dorsal interosseous becomes the abductor pollicis brevis, and the first palmar interosseous becomes the adductor pollicis (Fig. 40–10).

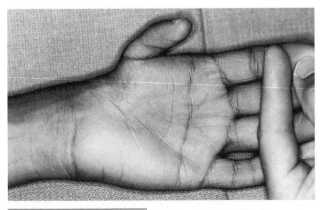

Figure 40–9 Pouce flottant (floating thumb) attached by skin bridge.

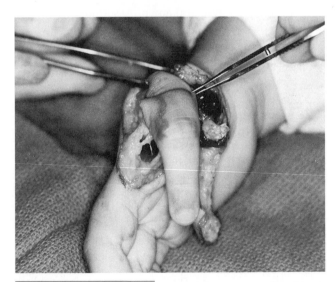

Figure 40–10 Index finger pollicization to the thumb position.

The time to perform this procedure remains controversial, with a trend toward early surgery to encourage incorporation of the pollicized digit into daily use. This avoids the development of compensatory side-to-side pinch between adjacent fingers. We prefer to perform the surgery at approximately 1 year of age, when the structures are of substantial size and prior to significant compensatory tendencies. The results of pollicization are directly related to the status of the transposed index digit and surrounding musculature. Children with radial deficiencies may have a stiff index digit that will not perform as well a mobile pollicized index. Nonetheless, pollicization is a rewarding operation that reliably improves grasp, prehension, and cosmesis in children with severe thumb hypoplasia.

PEARL

The presence or absence of a carpometacarpal (CMC) joint in thumb hypoplasia will determine whether the existing thumb can be reconstructed or amputated, followed by pollicization.

Clasped Thumb

Congenital clasped thumb is caused by hypoplasia or absence of the thumb extensors. The diagnosis is often delayed because an infant frequently holds the thumb within the palm for the first few months. The clasped thumb rests in a flexed and adducted posture. Inadequate MP extension implies extensor pollicis brevis deficiency, and lack of IP extension indicates extensor pollicis longus abnormality. Initial treatment is prolonged splinting for at least 3 months duration. Failure to achieve improved extension by 3 months implies extreme hypoplasia or absence, and tendon transfer is indicated. The extensor indicis propius appears to be the best donor tendon, but it may also be absent when the extensor pollicis longus tendon is missing. Therefore, an alternative suitable donor may be required for transfer.

Retroflexible Thumb

Retroflexible thumb is a rare congenital anomaly due to over-pull of the extensor pollicis brevis muscle. The MP joint is hyperextended, and the IP joint is flexed creating a "swan-neck" deformity. Splinting is often the initial treatment, but surgery is frequently required for correction of the deformity. The extensor pollicis brevis tendon is lengthened by Z-plasty, and a volar capsulodesis is performed to achieve equilibrium.

Camptodactyly

Derived form the Greek, meaning "bent finger," camptodactyly refers to a nontraumatic PIP flexion deformity most commonly involving the small finger. There are two types of clinical presentation, the most common appears in infancy (84% in the first year) and affects males and females equally. The second appears after the age of 10 years and more often affects females. Both types show a tendency for progression of the deformity with growth (80%), especially during normal growth spurts, and both do not progress after the age of

18. The deformity occurs bilaterally in about two thirds of the cases, and associated syndromes may be present.

The precise etiology of the deformity is unknown. Studies have implicated all structures on the volar aspect of the joint from the skin to the volar plate and joint capsule. Anomalous or absent lumbricals, aberrant ligamentous or fibrous bands, and flexor tendon abnormalities have also been identified. Treatment is directed toward prevention or correction of the deformity. However, without a consistent pathologic anatomy, the overall results of both surgical and nonsurgical treatment are unpredictable. Conservative treatment with splinting is most effective when begun early to prevent bony changes at the joint surface. Operative treatment is reserved for failed conservative management with severe deformity. Surgery should attempt to identify the pathologic anatomy followed by release or transfer of the deforming forces.

Windblown Hand (Congenital Ulnar Drift)

The windblown hand presents with ulnar deviation and flexion contractures of the fingers at the MP joint. The extensor tendons subluxate or dislocate into the valleys between the MP heads. The thumb may be involved, causing a fixed thumb-in-palm deformity. The deformities are present at birth and will progress with growth. Treatment should be undertaken before the age of 2 years. The windblown hand is associated with craniofacial deformities (e.g., whistling face syndrome or Freeman-Sheldon syndrome) and arthrogryposis. Release of the thumb web requires Z-plasty or a dorsal rotation flap to overcome the narrowing of the web space. Lengthening of the flexor pollicis longus and intrinsic release may be necessary to overcome severe contractures. Active thumb extension may require augmentation by tendon transfer extensor indicis proprius to extensor pollicis longus. The ulnar deviation and flexion contracture of the MP joints also requires an extensive release of the soft tissue contracture, and the extensor tendons hoods need to be centralized dorsally over the MP joints. If the deformity exists above the age of 5 or 6 years, the results of releases are less satisfactory. In the untreated adult, a shortening osteotomy of the metacarpals is necessary to achieve satisfactory correction.

Clinodactyly

Clinodactyly refers to an angular deformity in the coronal plane. Although it can occur in any digit, the most common is the distal IP of the small finger. It is usually inherited as a dominant trait but can occur sporadically. There is a high incidence of associated anomalies (more than 30 syndromes, most notably Down's) and a correlation with mental retardation. The critical factor in identifying clinodactyly may be in identifying the associated syndrome. Clinically, the affected digit has a short middle phalanx with an inclination shorter on the radial side. The joint surface is subsequently angulated away from the normal perpendicular orientation to the long axis of the phalanx. Treatment may consist of splinting in the very young child, and is usually more for cosmetic than functional benefit. Closing wedge osteotomy is performed in the older child (older than age 6) if the deformity is severe.

Kirner's Deformity

Kirner described a deformity of volar and radial angulation of the distal phalanx of the small finger (Carstam and Eiken, 1970). It characteristically presents as painless swelling of the digit followed by progressive deformity. The deformity does not usually begin until the age of 5 years, is more common in females, and is often bilateral. Functional difficulties are limited to specific activities such as playing a musical instrument or typing. Treatment is usually not necessary, but when symptomatic, surgical correction is by multiple wedge osteotomies to correct the angulatory deformity.

Delta Bone (Delta Phalanx)

This term applies to a tubular bone that has an abnormal proximal epiphysis. The proximal growth plate is C-shaped and at least a portion of it has a longitudinal rather than transverse orientation (Fig. 40–11). A bony bracket joins the proximal and distal epiphyses (longitudinally bracketed diaphysis). The affected bone will produce an angular deformity that progresses with growth and tends to angulate toward the midline of the hand. The phalanges are affected most often, but it can occur in the metacarpals. Associated anomalies are common and include syndactyly, polydactyly, symphalangism, triphalangeal thumb, cleft hand, ulnar dysplasia, Apert's syndrome, and Poland's syndrome. The associated hand deformity may dictate treatment. Central polydactyly and triphalangeal thumb are the most frequently associated anomalies that require surgical correction. At the time of surgery, the delta bone can be addressed in a variety of ways. In very young children, resection of the longitudinal bony bracket with fat interposition has been proposed (Vickers, 1987). Opening wedge osteotomy with interposition bone graft provides the best opportunity to restore and preserve length, longitudinal alignment, and function. Reverse wedge

osteotomy has also been described where the wedge resection is based along the longitudinal physis, and then is reversed and reinserted. These procedures are technically demanding, especially when handling the small-sized delta bone. Care must be taken to prevent injury to the remaining physis. Recurrence of the deformity during a growth spurt is common regardless of the method employed for correction. Therefore, in the isolated delta phalanx, observation until significant angulatory deformity develops will allow the best opportunity for correction with a single osteotomy. In severe cases, amputation of the involved bone or digit may be indicated to maximize function of the involved hand.

Duplication

Thumb Duplication

Duplication of the thumb can be partial or complete and has been classified into various types depending on the degree of skeletal replication (Table 40–8). In this classification, the extent of duplication is defined by whether the components are attached proximally (bifid) or completely separated (duplicated). Type IV is the most common type of thumb duplication and constitutes about 50% of the cases (Fig. 40–12).

Thumb duplication involves more than the bony elements as the parts may share common nails, tendons, ligaments, joints, and neurovascular structures. Treatment often requires using portions of each component to construct a properly aligned and functional thumb. The treatment of types I and II depends on the extent and size of each duplicated part. Asymmetric duplication can be treated by ablation of the smaller thumb with transfer of the collateral ligament and centralization of the extensor tendon. Failure to restore stability by collateral ligament relocation will lead to persistent instability. Inadequate extensor tendon centralization will cause thumb deviation. Symmetric thumb duplication can be treated by resection of the central portions of bone and nail from each component and approximation of the retained borders (Bilhaut-Cloquet procedure). This operation is difficult and nail deformity and IP joint stiffness is common.

Types III and IV duplication are treated with selection of a dominant thumb and ablation of the lesser counterpart. This decision is not always straightforward and requires careful examination. If the components are equal, we preserve the ulnar thumb to retain the ulnar collateral ligament for pinch. The soft tissue from the ablated thumb should be used to augment the retained thumb. The collateral ligament is retained with an osteoperiosteal sleeve from the deleted thumb and is

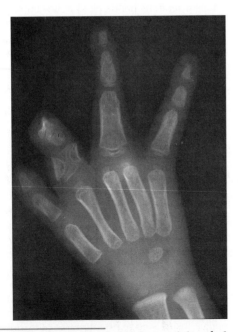

Figure 40–11 X-ray of a index finger delta phalanx with combined super digit of long and ring digits.

TABLE 40–8   Classification of thumb duplication

Type	Duplicated Elements
I	Bifid distal phalanx
II	Duplicated distal phalanx
III	Bifid proximal phalanx
IV	Duplicated proximal
V	Bifid metacarpal
VI	Duplicated metacarpal

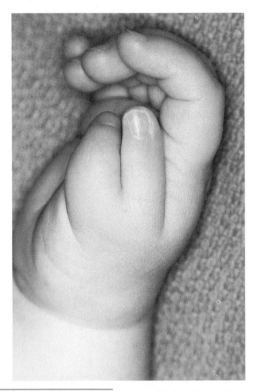

Figure 40–12   Photograph of type IV thumb duplication.

transferred to the preserved thumb. Articular surface modification and tendon realignment is necessary to optimize thumb function. Osteotomy or articular surface recontouring may be necessary to correctly align the thumb and prevent progressive angulatory deformity. The thenar intrinsic muscles require transfer from the deleted thumb to the retained thumb. The treatment of types V and VI duplication utilizes similar principles with the added complexity of additional intrinsic reconstruction.

PEARL

Surgery for thumb duplication requires collateral ligament reconstruction and tendon centralization for a good outcome.

Triphalangeal Thumb

Triphalangeal thumb can develop as an isolated anomaly or occur with thumb duplication. It can be associated with heart defects such as Holt-Oram syndrome or blood dyscrasias such as Fanconi's pancytopenia. The extra phalanx has a variable shape and will directly effect treatment. A small, wedge-shaped middle phalanx will cause deviation and requires excision with ligament reconstruction. A large, wedge-shaped extra phalanx will produce deviation and excessive length. Excision of the phalanx can be performed, but subsequent instability is common. Fusion of the abnormal phalanx with the distal or proximal phalanx along with bone removal is a better option. The bone reduction is performed to shorten and realign the thumb, and the arthrodesis eliminates the

supernumerary joint. A fully developed middle phalanx usually lies in the same plane of the fingers and represents a five-fingered hand. The preferred treatment for this type is pollicization to restore thumb prehension.

Polydactyly

Polydactyly is a common congenital anomaly that can occur as an isolated anomaly or part of a syndrome (e.g., Ellis-van Creveld syndrome). It is frequently inherited but has a variable penetrance pattern. Polydactyly is classified according to the degree of duplication (Table 40–9). Finger polydactyly usually effects the ulnar side of the hand, most commonly the small digit. Surgery should be performed early prior to the development of altered hand patterns. The treatment principles are similar to thumb duplication, with careful selection of the most functional and dominant digit. Type I polydactyly is treated by simple ablation, and complete duplication (type III) can be managed by ray resection. Partial duplication (Fig. 40–13) is more difficult to treat and requires excision of the least developed digit. Preservation of collateral ligament stability with an osteoperiosteal sleeve is required to maintain stability, and tendon transfer from the discarded digit may be necessary to maximize motion. In certain situations, the duplication is so complex and intertwined that reconstruction is not possible. Treatment options are to retain an extra digit hand or to create a three-fingered hand.

TABLE 40–9   Classification of Polydactyly

Type	Features
I	Extra soft tissue mass without skeleton
II	Some skeleton that articulates with bifid metacarpal or phalanx
III	Complete duplication with own metacarpal

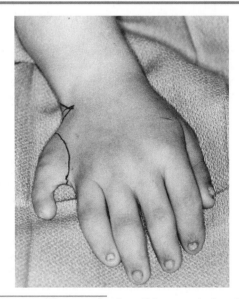

Figure 40–13   Photograph of small finger polydactyly.

Mirror Hand

Mirror hand or ulnar dimelia is rare, with two ulna, no thumbs, and duplicated digits. Treatment is difficult, and goals are to make a thumb and reduce the number of digits. Pollicization combined with deletion of adjacent digit(s) provides a thumb and first web space.

Undergrowth

Undergrowth or hypoplasia can effect the entire limb or be isolated to the hand. This anomaly can be classified as a failure of formation, failure of differentiation, or undergrowth. In addition, hypoplastic digits are common with constriction band syndrome. Thumb hypoplasia is a distinct entity and has been discussed previously.

Brachydactyly refers to a hypoplastic digit that is short but has the normal complement of bones. This shortening most commonly occurs in the middle phalanx. Asymmetric phalangeal shortening will lead to clinodactyly. Metacarpal shortening is uncommon and usually effects the ulnar digits (ring and small). This type of brachydactyly presents with absent knuckles of the ring and small digits (knuckle, knuckle, bump, bump) and is often associated with a syndrome such as pseudohypoparathyroidism or pseudo-pseudohypoparathyroidism.

The length and size discrepancy of the hypoplasia will not improve with growth, and the disparity may increase throughout childhood. Treatment depends on the degree of hypoplasia and quality of the adjacent digits. Mild hypoplasia requires no treatment, whereas severe underdevelopment may warrant amputation. In brachysyndactyly, web deepening with a more proximal placement of the commissure can be used to help compensate for shortening. Digital lengthening can be useful, and techniques include transposition of a hypoplastic digit or toe transfer to another digit. The transfer can be placed on the end of the digit (on-top-plasty) or into a metacarpal osteotomy (intercalary lengthening). Lengthening by distraction is a viable option in brachydactyly secondary to short metacarpals, but is usually not used at the phalangeal level.

PEARL

Brachydactyly is most commonly caused by shortening of the middle phalanx.

Overgrowth

Macrodactyly

Macrodactyly represents overgrowth of all structures of the involved digit and is different from an isolated enlargement of the bone (e.g., enchondroma) or vessels (e.g., hemangiomas). This disfiguring condition can effect a single digit or multiple digits, with the radial fingers more commonly effected (Fig. 40–14). The thumb is typically spared. Macrodactyly usually occurs as an isolated abnormality but can

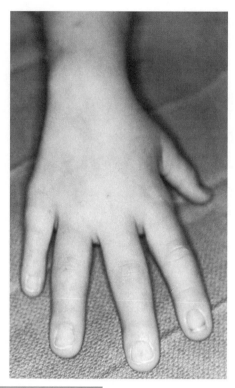

Figure 40–14   Macrodactyly of the index, long, and ring digits.

occur with neurofibromatosis or limb hypertrophy, hemangiomas, and varicose veins (Klippel-Trenaunay-Weber syndrome). The etiology remains unknown, and two forms have been described. True macrodactyly consists of an enlarged digit at birth that grows proportionately over time. Progressive macrodactyly is more common, begins in childhood, and increases in size throughout growth. Digital enlargement tends to stiffen the finger, and this progression continues until physeal closure.

Treatment of the soft tissue component involves surgery to remove excessive fat, subcutaneous tissue, and skin. Epiphysiodesis is indicated when the digit reaches the length of the sex-matched parent. Simultaneous arrest of all the phalangeal physis is often necessary for longitudinal growth inhibition, but circumferential growth control will require bone removal to narrow the width. If the enlargement is relentless and grotesque, amputation may be the only solution.

Congenital Constriction Band Syndrome

Congenital constriction band syndrome (or early amnion rupture sequence) is a condition resulting from entrapment of developing embryonal tissue by the fetal lining. It occurs in 1:15,000 live births, and there in no pattern of inheritance identified. The manifestations in the upper extremity vary, ranging from autoamputation to simple constriction rings (Fig. 40–15). It can be differentiated from failure of formation by the presence of a constriction band elsewhere on the child

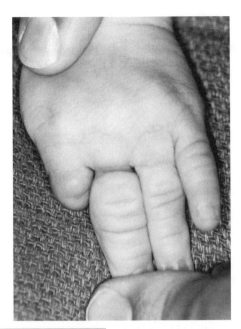

Figure 40–15 Congenital constriction band of long digit with adjacent amputation of index and thumb.

and failure of differentiation by the fact that the affected limb is normal to the point of constriction. Associated anomalies

TABLE 40–10 Classification of Constriction Band Syndrome

Type	Characteristics
I	Simple constriction
II	Constriction with deformity of distal parts
III	Constriction with fusion of distal parts (acrosyndactyly or pseudosyndactyly)
IV	Intrauterine amputation

include club foot, cleft lip and palate, syndactyly, hypoplasia, symphalangism, brachydactyly, and symbrachydactyly. The syndrome is divided into four classes (Table 40–10).

Clinical manifestations stem from the degree of involvement. Simple constriction rings may present as a cosmetic problem. Deep circumferential rings can cause vascular insufficiency with cold intolerance, neurologic compromise, and tendon dysfunction. When treatment is indicated, the standard method includes staged Z-plasty and excision of tight fibrous bands. One half of the digit is operated on at a time to prevent potential vascular compromise. Multiple digital amputations require reconstruction or augmentation by a variety of techniques including lengthening procedures or combining parts of adjacent digits. In addition, separation of the fusion of distal digits (pseudosyndactyly) may be required to improve function.

SELECTED BIBLIOGRAPHY

Embryology

BEATTY E. Upper limb tissue differentiation in the human embryo. *Hand Clin.* 1985;1:391–403.
ZALESKE DJ. Development of the upper limb. *Hand Clin.* 1985;1:383–390.

Growth and Development

FLATT AE. *The Care of Congenital Hand Anomalies.* 2d ed. St. Louis, MO: Quality Medical Publishing; 1994.

Incidence and Genetic

BIRCH-JENSEN A. *Congenital Deformities of the Upper Extremity.* Copenhagen, Denmark: Ejnar Munksgaard; 1949.
FLATT AE. *The Care of Congenital Hand Anomalies.* 2nd ed. St Louis, MO: Quality Medical Publishing; 1994.

Classification

SWANSON AB, SWANSON G deG, TADA K. A classification for congenital limb malformation. *J Hand Surg.* 1983;8:693–702.

Failure of Formation

BARSKY AJ. Cleft hand; classification, incidence, and treatment: review of the literature and report of 19 cases. *J Bone Jt Surg.* 1964;46A:1707–1720.
BAYNE LG, KLUG WS. Long-term review of the surgical treatment of radial deficiencies. *J Hand Surg.* 1987:12A:169–170.
CARROLL RE, LOUIS DS. Anomalies associated with radial dysplasia. *J Pediatr.* 1974;84:409–411.
DaMORE E, KOZIN SH, THODER J. The recurrence of deformity after surgical correction of radial clubhand. Presented at the 51st Annual Meeting of The American Society of the Hand, Nashville, September 1996.
DOBYNS JH, WOOD VE, BAYNE LG. Congenital hand deformities. In: Green DP, ed. *Operative Hand Surgery.* 3rd ed. New York, NY: Churchill Livingstone, 1993;251–548.
FLATT AE. *The Care of Congenital Hand Anomalies.* 2nd ed. St Louis, MO: Quality Medical Publishing, 1994.
MacDONELL JA. Age of fitting upper-extremity prosthesis in children. *J Bone Jt Surg.* 1958;40A:655–662.
MILLER JK, WENNER SM, KRUGER LM. Ulnar deficiency. *J Hand Surg.* 1986;11A:822–829.
SKERIK SK, FLATT AE. The anatomy of congenital radial dysplasia: its surgical and functional implications. *Clin Orthop.* 1969;66:125–143.

TAUSSIG HB. A study of the German outbreak of phocomelia: The thalidomide syndrome. *JAMA* 1962;180:1106–1114.

Failure of Differentiation

BAUER TB, TONDRA JM, TRUSLER HM. Technical modification in repair of syndactyly. *Plast Reconstr Surg.* 1986;77: 282–287.

BROWN LM, ROBSON MJ, SHARRARD WJW. The pathophysiology of arthrogryposis multiplex congenita neurologica. *J Bone Jt Surg.* 1980;62B:291–296.

BUCK-GRAMCKO D, WOOD VE. The treatment of metacarpal synostosis. *J Hand Surg.* 1993;18A:565–581.

CAMPBELL CC, WATERS PM, EMANS JB. Excision of the radial head for congenital dislocation. *J Bone Jt Surg.* 1992;74A: 726–733.

CLEARY JE, OMER GE. Congenital proximal radioulnar synostosis: natural history and functional assessment. *J Bone Jt Surg.* 1985;67A:539–545.

DINHAM DM, MEGGITT BF. Trigger thumbs in children. *J Bone Jt Surg.* 1974;56B:153–155.

DOBYNS JH, WOOD VE, BAYNE LG. Congenital hand deformities. In: Green DP, ed. *Operative Hand Surgery.* 3rd ed. New York, NY: Churchill Livingstone; 1993;251–548.

EATON CJ, LISTER GD. Syndactyly. *Hand Clin.* 1990;6:555–575.

FLATT AE. *The Care of Congenital Hand Anomalies.* 2nd ed. St Louis, MO: Quality Medical Publishing; 1994.

HOOVER GH, FLATT AE, WEISS MW. The hand and Apert's syndrome. *J Bone Jt Surg.* 1970;52A:878–895.

SHUN-SHIN M. Congenital web function. *J Bone Jt Surg.* 1954;36B:268–271.

STEEL HH, PISTON RW, CLANCY M, BETZ, RR. A syndrome of dislocated hips and radial heads, carpal coalition, and short stature in Puerto Rican children. *J Bone Jt Surg.* 1993;75A:259–267.

STEENWERCKX A, DESMET L, FABRY G. Congenital trigger thumb. *J Hand Surg.* 1996;21A:909–911.

WEEKS PM. Surgical correction of upper extremity deformities in arthrogryposis. *Plast Reconstr Surg.* 1965;36:459–465.

Thumb Hypoplasia

BUCK-GRAMCKO D. Pollicization of the index finger: methods and results in aplasia and hypoplasia of the thumb. *J Bone Jt Surg.* 1971;53A:1605–1617.

CRAWFORD HH, HORTON CE, ADAMSON JE. Congenital aplasia or hypoplasia of the thumb and finger extensor tendons. *J Bone Jt Surg.* 1966;48A:82–91.

KOZIN SH, WEISS AA, WEBBER JB, BETZ RR, CLANCY M, STEEL HH. Index finger pollicization for congenital aplasia or hypoplasia of the thumb. *J Hand Surg.* 1992;17A:880–884.

LISTER GD. Reconstruction of the hypoplastic thumb. *Clin Orthop.* 1985;195:52–65.

MANSKE PR, McCARROLL HR, JAMES M. Type III-A hypoplastic thumb. *J Hand Surg.* 1995;20A:246–253.

Camptodactyly

McFARLANE RM, CLASSEN DA, PORTE AM, BOTZ JS. The anatomy and treatment of camptodactyly of the small finger. *J Hand Surg.* 1992;17:35–44.

MIURA T, NAKAMURA R, TAMURA Y. Long-standing extended dynamic splintage and release an abnormal restraining structure in camptodactyly. *J Hand Surg.* 1992;17B:665–672.

SIEGERT JJ, COONEY WP, DOBYNS JH. Management of simple camptodactyly. *J Hand Surg.* 1990;15B:181–189.

Windblown Hand

DOBYNS JH, WOOD VE, BAYNE LG. Congenital hand deformities. In: Green DP, ed. *Operative Hand Surgery.* 3rd ed. New York, NY: Churchill Livingstone; 1993.

FLATT AE. *The Care of Congenital Hand Anomalies.* 2d ed. St. Louis, MO: Quality Medical Publishing; 1994.

FREEMAN EA, SHELDON JH. Craniocarpotarsal dystrophy: an undescribed congenital malformation. *Arch Dis Child.* 1983;13:277–283.

Clinodactyly

DOBYNS JH, WOOD VE, BAYNE LG. Congenital hand deformities. In: Green DP, ed. *Operative Hand Surgery.* 3rd ed. New York, NY: Churchill Livingstone; 1993.

FLATT AE. *The Care of Congenital Hand Anomalies.* 2d ed. St. Louis, MO: Quality Medical Publishing; 1994.

Kirner's Deformity

CARSTAM N, EIKEN O. Kirner's deformity of the little finger. *J Bone Jt Surg.* 1970;52A:1663–1665.

DOBYNS JH, WOOD VE, BAYNE LG. Congenital hand deformities. In: Green DP, ed. *Operative Hand Surgery.* 3rd ed. New York, NY: Churchill Livingstone; 1993.

Delta Phalanx

FLATT AE. *The Care of Congenital Hand Anomalies.* 2d ed. St. Louis, MO: Quality Medical Publishing; 1994.

JONES GB. Delta phalanx. *J Bone Jt Surg.* 1964;46B:226–228.

THEANDER G, CARSTAM M. Longitudinally bracketed diaphysis. *Ann Radiol.* 1974;17:355–360.

VICKERS D. Clinodactyl of the little finger: a simple operative technique for reversal of the growth abnormality. *J Hand Surg.* 1987;12B:335–345.

Thumb Duplication

FLATT AE. *The Care of Congenital Hand Anomalies.* 2nd ed. St Louis, MO: Quality Medical Publishing; 1994.

WASSEL HD. The results of surgery for polydactyly of the thumb: a review. *Clin Orthop.* 1969;64:175–193.

Polydactyly

DOBYNS JH, WOOD VE, BAYNE LG. Congenital hand deformities. In: Green DP, ed. *Operative Hand Surgery.* 3rd ed. New York, NY: Churchill Livingstone; 1993.

Macrodactyly

FLATT AE. *The Care of Congenital Hand Anomalies.* 2nd ed. St Louis, MO: Quality Medical Publishing; 1994.

Congenital Constriction Band

ASKINS G, GER E. Congenital constriction band syndrome. *J Pediatr Orthop.* 1988;8:461–466.

FOUKES GD, REINKER K. Congenital constriction band syndrome: a 70-year experience. *J Pediatr Orthop.* 1994;14: 242–248.

LIGHT TR, OGDEN JA. Congenital constriction band syndrome. *Yale J Bio Med.* 1994;66:143–155.

SAMPLE QUESTIONS

1. Radial clubhand is associated with:
   (a) heart defects
   (b) thumb hypoplasia
   (c) vertebral anomalies
   (d) thrombocytopenia
   (e) all of the above

2. Syndactyly that extends to the fingertips without bony involvement is classified as:
   (a) complete and complex
   (b) incomplete and complex
   (c) incomplete and simple
   (d) complete and simple
   (e) complex and complicated

3. The most important aspect for successful treatment of thumb duplication is ablation and:
   (a) nerve reconstruction and web deepening
   (b) artery reconstruction with transposition
   (c) nail-bed reconstruction or graft
   (d) tendon transfer to augment thenar hypoplasia
   (e) collateral reconstruction and tendon realignment

4. The most effective treatment of congenital radial head dislocation in a 5-year-old is:
   (a) prompt reduction and annular ligament reconstruction
   (b) radial head resection
   (c) observation
   (d) ulnar lengthening to promote spontaeous reduction
   (e) radial shortening

5. During upper extremity embryogenesis, what structure is critical to cell death and formation of the web spaces:
   (a) AER
   (b) somatic mesoderm
   (c) somatopleure
   (d) chondrogen
   (e) weboderm

Answers: 1) e; 2) d; 3) e; 4) c; 5) a

Chapter 41

Disorders of the Lower Extremity in Children

John J. Williams, MD

Outline

Pediatric lower extremity disorders can have grave consequences for adult function. Deformities can affect gait and joint mechanics. Seemingly minor subtle disorders can be neglected and can cause disabling degenerative joint disease in adulthood. A thorough understanding of normal and abnormal, the natural history of lower extremity disorders, and the principles of treatment facilitate the management of these often difficult problems.

ETIOLOGY

Pediatric lower extremity disorders can result from a variety of etiologies, including osteomyelitis and septic arthritis, developmental hip dislocation, Legg-Calve-Perthes Disease, a slipped capital femoral epiphysis, leg-length discrepancy, intoeing, angular knee deformities, and Blount's disease. These will be elucidated in greater detail below.

BASIC SCIENCE

Osteomyelitis and Septic Arthritis

Osteomyelitis in children is typically hematogenous and occurs in metaphyseal regions where there is an extensive vascular network to support physeal growth. High-volume, low-pressure, low-velocity flow occurs in the metaphyseal vascular network. Minor trauma may be the precipitating event. Typical sources of bacteremia include upper and lower respiratory infections and skin excoriation. The causative organisms are usually *Staphylococcus aureus* or *Haemophilus influenzae* type B. Recent *H influenzae* type B vaccination programs have decreased the incidence of osteomyelitis due to this organism. Gram negative organisms and opportunistic host organisms should be considered in immunosuppressed children.

Septic arthritis can occur primarily or can be the result of metaphyseal abscess extension through the cortex and into the nearby joint. Causative organisms include *S aureus*, group B streptococcus, and gram negative organisms in neonates. Between 18 months and 4 years of age, *S aureus*, β-hemolytic streptococcus, and *H influenzae* type B are common. Infection with *S aureus* and β-hemolytic streptococcus are common in children more than 4 years of age. *Neisseria gonorrhea* should be considered in teenagers.

Developmental Hip Dislocation

The incidence of hip dislocation in newborns is more than 1 per 1000 live births. "Loose" or subluxable hips at birth occur in almost 1 per 100 births. Hip instability is 4 to 6 times more common in females, and a large number of affected children are firstborns, often with breech presentation. Other risk factors include oligohydramnios, torticollis, and other associated positional deformities such as metatarsus adductus and calcaneovalgus feet. These observations suggest that restricted intrauterine space plays a role in the development of hip dislocation. Hormonal factors may also be involved. Circulating

Orthopaedic Surgery: The Essentials. Edited by M.E. Baratz, A.D. Watson, and J.E. Imbriglia. Thieme Medical Publishers, Inc., New York © 1999

maternal estrogens increase pelvic laxity in the mother and increase hip capsule laxity in the fetus. Postpartum positioning may also play a role, given that hip dysplasia is much more common in cultures where babies are swathed with the hips and legs extended and adducted.

Increased capsular laxity allows the femoral head to migrate superiorly and posteriorly out of the acetabulum. Secondary bone and soft tissue adaptive changes then occur that maintain the dislocated position. The adductors, hamstrings, and iliopsoas become contracted. The tight iliopsoas creates an "hourglass" constriction of the inferior joint capsule. The acetabulum becomes dysplastic and dish-shaped and fills with fatty debris called pulvinar. Pressure on the labrum causes it to enlarge and infold. The femoral head becomes flattened. The proximal femur develops an anteverted, valgus deformity.

Legg-Calve-Perthes Disease

Although much work has been done to elucidate the etiology of Legg-Calve-Perthes disease, the cause is still unknown. It is currently presumed that the damage to the femoral head is the result of avascular necrosis. There does not appear to be a genetic predisposition, and environmental factors have not clearly been shown to be related. Trauma, hematologic abnormalities, endocrine abnormalities, and synovitis have all been implicated as causative factors. The typical child with Legg-Calve-Perthes is small for his or her age, with bone age being 2 or more years less than the chronologic age. Males are affected about 4 times more frequently than females. These children are physically very active, and a significant percentage have true hyperactivity. The disease is bilateral in 10% of cases.

Disruption of the arterial circulation leads to an infarct along the anterolateral aspect of the femoral head (Fig. 41–1). Repetitive compressive and shear forces then cause a subchondral fracture. This is followed by fragmentation and collapse of the avascular femoral head. During this fragmentation period, which can last 2 to 3 years, synovitis may occur, and the hip may become stiff and painful. Radiographs will show varying degrees of femoral head involvement possibly including lateral extrusion and metaphyseal cysts (Fig. 42–1). The healing phase consists of new bone formation in the subchondral areas of the femoral head. This may last 1 to

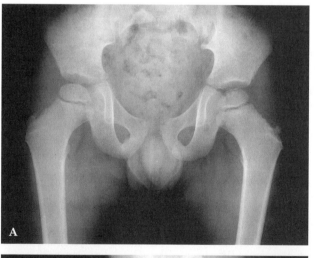
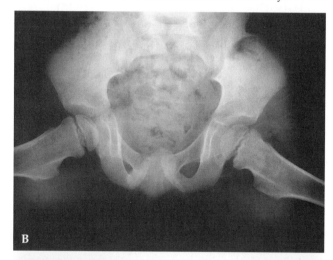
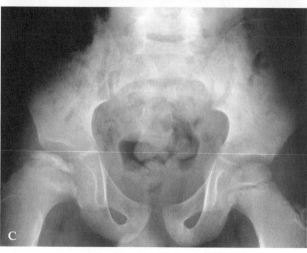
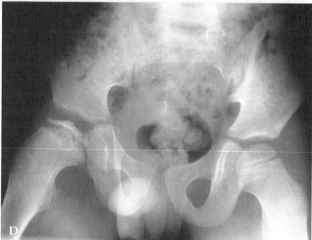

Figure 41–1 Legg-Calve-Perthes disease. (**A, B**) The only radiographic finding in early Legg-Calve-Perthes disease is a subchondral fracture seen best on the frog-lateral x-ray. The radiographic changes become more dramatic with flattening and lateral subluxation of the femoral head and with formation of metaphyseal cysts as femoral head collapse and fragmentation progress (**C, D**).

2 years during which time the pain and stiffness begin to resolve.

The healing femoral head is typically flattened, and, thus, incongruent with the acetabulum. The degree of flattening is usually related to the extent of femoral head involvement and the age of onset of the disease. Hips with more femoral head involvement usually develop more flattening. Children who have an early onset (younger than age 6) generally have a long time for remodeling to occur within the mold of the acetabulum and, therefore, have less flattening of the femoral head. Older children have less potential for remodeling and, therefore, a worse long-term prognosis.

Slipped Capital Femoral Epiphysis

Slipped capital femoral epiphysis (SCFE) is a displacement of the capital femoral epiphysis from the metaphysis through the physis. The femoral head remains in the acetabulum while the proximal femur displaces anteriorly. Radiographically, the femoral head appears to displace posteriorly and into varus. (Fig. 41–2) This is especially apparent on the frog-lateral x-ray.

The condition usually occurs just before puberty when the child is going through the adolescent growth spurt.

Affected children are often obese and have delayed skeletal maturity. It is more common in males and in blacks, and the condition is often associated with underlying metabolic disturbances such as hypothyroidism, hypogonadism, and renal osteodystrophy.

Histologically, SCFE differs from a typical physeal fracture. Displacement occurs through the hypertrophic zone of the physis, which has become widened and mechanically weakened. Normal enchondral ossification is absent, and irregular clusters of chondrocytes replace the normal columnar arrangement.

Obesity and excessive femoral retroversion combined with abnormal hormonal influences may be responsible for the weakened growth plate. Sex hormones normally increase the strength of the growth plate. Obese children with delayed onset of puberty have relative deficiency of sex hormones and increased shear forces acting on the proximal femur. Synovitis of the hip is often present and may also weaken the physis.

Leg-length Discrepancy

Causes of leg-length discrepancy include congenital deformities (Fig. 41–3) and growth plate disturbance caused by trauma, infection, or neurologic and neoplastic disorders.

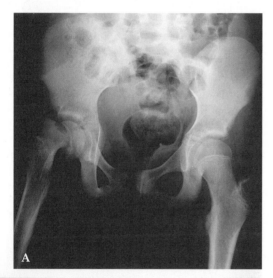

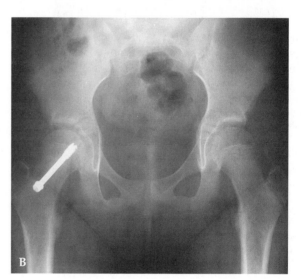

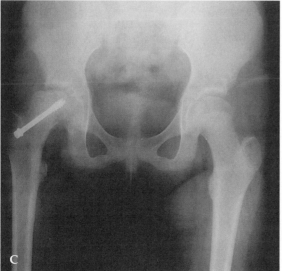

Figure 41–2 Acute slipped capital femoral epiphysis (SCFE). (**A**) A ten year-old girl fell onto her right hip, developed immediate pain, and was unable to walk. X-rays demonstrate a grade III SCFE. (**B**) She was treated with in situ pinning with a single, percutaneous cannulated screw. (**C**) Three months later, she began to develop a limp and recurrent hip pain. X-rays show the onset of avascular necrosis of the femoral head.

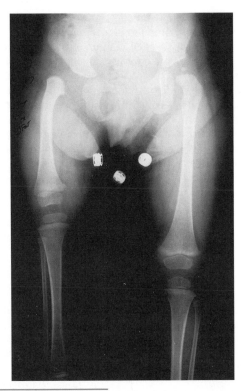

Figure 41–3 Proximal femoral focal deficiency is a congenital cause of leg-length discrepancy due to abnormal development of the proximal femoral physis. The ossification of the entire femoral head and neck is delayed, and asymmetric growth causes coxa vara. The relative shortening of the femur will be constant over time; thus, a 20% shortening at birth will become a 20% shortening at skeletal maturity.

(Fig. 41–4). Congenital deformities include proximal femoral focal deficiency, fibular hemimelia, and hemihypertrophy.

Intoeing

Intoeing is most commonly a normal variant that resolves spontaneously with growth. Three common benign causes of intoeing in children are metatarsus adductus, tibial torsion, and femoral anteversion. Metatarsus adductus is the most common cause of intoeing in children prior to walking age. It is usually caused by intrauterine positioning and can be associated with congenital hip dislocation and/or torticollis. Intoeing in the toddler is generally caused by internal tibial torsion. The inward twist of the tibia is produced in utero by the infolded position of the legs. Femoral anteversion or femoral torsion causes intoeing in children aged 3 to 5. These children are probably born with a more anteverted femoral neck, and often other family members have a similar intoed gait. Sitting in a "W" position instead of cross-legged increases the femoral anteversion. Pathologic causes of intoeing include clubfoot and neuromuscular conditions that produce equinovarus such as cerebral palsy, Charcot-Marie-Tooth, arthrogryposis, and spinal cord disorders.

Angular Knee Deformities

Genu varum (bowlegs) and genu valgum (knockknees) are typically physiologically normal. Children typically have a

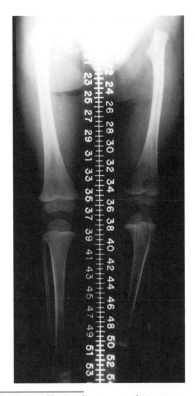

Figure 41–4 Late effects of osteomyelitis are apparent in this 5 year-old who was treated for neonatal sepsis. The diagnosis of septic arthritis of the hip and knee with proximal femoral and tibial osteomyelitis was delayed, and late surgical drainage was performed. Consequently, the patient developed severe proximal femoral and proximal tibial growth arrest. A significant leg-length discrepancy is demonstrated on scanogram.

bowlegged appearance to their gait when they begin walking. Physiologic bowing is caused by a combination of internal tibial torsion and external rotation of the hips (Fig. 41–5).

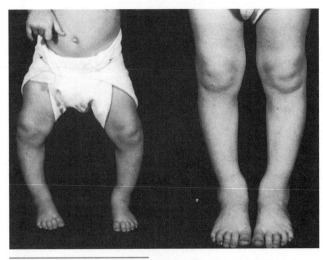

Figure 41–5 Typical clinical appearance of physiologic bowing. The hips are externally rotated, the tibiae are internally rotated, and the knee axis is laterally deviated to yield a bowed appearance **(left)**. As the child grows, the external rotation contractures of the hips resolve, the tibial torsion resolves, and the knee axis returns to normal **(right)**.

External rotation of the hips is due to normal physiologic contracture that allows children to have a wide base for their gait when they begin walking. Hip external rotation combined with internal tibial torsion rotates the knee axis laterally and causes a bowed appearance.

Genu valgum occurs most commonly between ages 3 and 6 and can recur in early adolescence. Physiologic genu varum in toddlers gradually overcorrects to physiologic genu valgum, which then corrects to normal adult alignment of 5 to 7 degrees of valgus. A radiographic study of normal children in Finland by Selenius and Vankka (1975) documented the normal progression of the tibiofemoral angle between birth and 13 years of age (Fig. 41–6).

Pathologic causes of genu varum and genu valgum include rickets (renal osteodystrophy, hypophosphatemia, nutritional) and skeletal dysplasias (spondyloepiphyseal dysplasia, multiple epiphyseal dysplasia, achondroplasia). Blount's disease causes genu varum.

Blount's Disease

Blount's disease, or tibia vara, is caused by a growth disturbance of the proximal tibial physis. Infantile tibia vara causes severe bowlegs with an onset prior to 3 years of age. Adolescent tibia vara occurs in obese children older than 8 years of age. Children with infantile tibia vara are often very large for their age and have a history of beginning ambulation very early in life. Abnormal compressive forces on the medial tibial physis in the overweight child with physiologic bowing

likely damages the physeal cartilage and retards normal growth medially.

Histologically, the physis and the cartilage medial to the epiphysis have areas of dead or severely damaged cartilage intermingled with areas of repair in infantile Blount's disease. Normal physeal growth and bone formation is delayed medially. Continued growth laterally causes varus deformity and shear forces instead of compressive forces on the medial physis. Thus, the medial physis closes prematurely to cause additional varus deformity. The histologic findings are similar but less severe in adolescent Blount's disease.

ANATOMY AND SURGICAL APPROACHES

Hip Joint

Relevant Anatomy

Nerves

The lateral femoral cutaneous nerve passes under the inguinal ligament as it leaves the pelvis between the anterior superior iliac spine and the midinguinal point. The nerve runs over the sartorius muscle and is a landmark for the interval between the sartorius and the tensor fascia lata (Fig. 41–7). The femoral nerve runs along the medial border of the iliopsoas muscle as it crosses the pelvic brim. This nerve must be protected when releasing the iliopsoas tendon via the anterior approach.

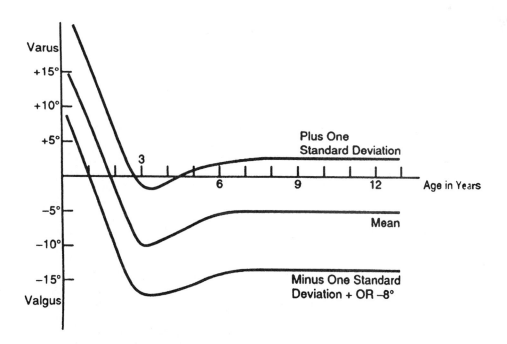

Figure 41–6 The tibiofemoral angle in children as depicted by the Salenius curve. From birth to 18 months, children have a tibiofemoral angle in varus. Between the ages of 18 months and 3 years, the varus gradually changes to valgus. By age 6 to 7 years, the valgus corrects back to the normal adult tibiofemoral angle (5–6 degrees valgus). All children go through this normal progression. Children at the extremes of the curve may have a markedly abnormal appearance during the peak periods of normal development. Reproduced with permission from Salenius P. Vankka E. The development of the tibiofemoral angle in children. *J Bone Jt Surg.* 1975;57A:260.

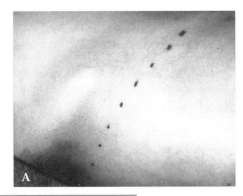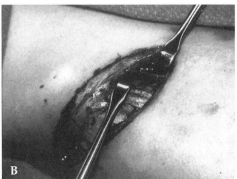

Figure 41–7 Anterior approach to the hip joint. (**A**) A transverse or oblique incision is used centered on the anterior inferior iliac spine. (**B**) The lateral femoral cutaneous nerve is in the interval between the sartorius and the tensor fascia lata.

The obturator nerve is encountered during the medial approach to the hip. The anterior branch runs deep to the adductor longus muscle on the anterior surface of the adductor brevis. The posterior branch of the obturator nerve runs on the posterior surface of the adductor brevis just above the adductor magnus. Both branches of the obturator nerve should be protected while releasing the adductor longus and brevis tendons.

Vessels

The femoral artery lies medial to the femoral nerve and is rarely at risk during routine exposures to the hip. The ascending branch of the lateral femoral circumflex artery runs through the distal end of the plane between the sartorius and tensor fascia lata and must be ligated if encountered during the anterior approach to the hip. The medial femoral circumflex artery runs deep to the iliopsoas tendon and crosses the inferior hip capsule, where it is vulnerable to injury with the medial approach.

Tendons

The iliopsoas muscle crosses the pelvic brim and forms a well-defined tendinous structure that attaches to the lesser trochanter. It can be released through either the anterior or medial approach to the hip. The rectus femorus muscle has two heads of origin. The direct head attaches to the anterior inferior iliac spine. The reflected head attaches to the anterior capsule of the hip joint and to the superior lip of the acetabulum. Both heads must be released to expose the hip capsule from the anterior approach.

The gracilis, adductor longus, adductor brevis, and adductor magnus muscles all have a tendinous origin on the pubis. Intervals can be developed between these muscles by identifying their tendinous origin.

Surgical Approaches

Anterior Approach to the Hip Joint

The anterior approach to the hip is useful for drainage of the septic hip, open reduction of a developmental hip dislocation, and pelvic osteotomies. The superior and inferior hip capsule and entire ilium can be exposed through the same incision.

The patient is positioned supine with a sandbag under the affected buttocks. A transverse or oblique incision is centered over the anterior inferior iliac spine (Fig. 41–7a). The dissection is carried through the superficial fascia to identify the lateral femoral cutaneous nerve in the interval between the sartorius and the tensor fascia lata (Fig. 41–7b). The sartorius-tensor interval is developed by blunt dissection, and the sartorius is then released from its origin on the anterior superior iliac spine.

The iliac apophysis is then sharply split, and the medial and lateral walls of the ilium are exposed by subperiosteal dissection. The tensor fascia lata and abductors are retracted laterally, and subperiosteal dissection is continued along the lateral wall of the ilium until the hip capsule is exposed. Careful hemostasis of perforating arteries is essential during exposure of the lateral wall. Subperiosteal exposure of the medial wall of the ilium permits medial retraction of the iliacus muscle. The iliopsoas tendon can be followed distally and released, if necessary, from its insertion on the lesser trochanter. The direct and reflected heads of the rectus femoris muscle are identified and released to expose the medial and inferior hip capsule.

Medial Approach to the Hip

The medial approach to the hip is used to treat a developmental hip dislocation in children who are not yet walking. The exposure is ideal for removing the obstacles to a closed reduction such as the iliopsoas tendon, ligamentum teres, or transverse acetabular ligament. Capsulorraphy cannot be performed through the medial approach, however.

The patient is positioned supine at the end of the operating table to allow the assistant to maximally abduct the affected leg. A transverse incision is made over the adductor longus tendon 1 to 2 cm distal to its origin on the pubis. The dissection is carried through the superficial fascia, and the adductor tendon is divided close to its origin on the pubis. Blunt dissection is then used to develop the interval between the adductor brevis and the pectineus. A small portion of the pectineus and adductor brevis can be released from their origins to improve exposure. Superior retraction of the pectineus muscle exposes the iliopsoas tendon as it inserts onto the lesser trochanter. The iliopsoas tendon is divided, if necessary. A deep retractor can then be placed in the interval between the pectineus and the anterior hip capsule. The medial circumflex artery is identified and protected as it crosses the inferior hip capsule. A capsulotomy can now be performed, and the ligamentum teres and transverse acetabular ligament can be released to reduce a dislocated hip.

EXAMINATION

History

It can be difficult to obtain a thorough history from a child. Parents' observations are essential. The history should include prenatal, birth, developmental, and family histories. Recent infections and past trauma should be identified. Many lower extremity conditions are age specific.

The onset and time course of symptoms are important. Acute symptoms suggest infection, trauma, or acute events such as avascular necrosis with synovitis in Legg-Calve-Perthes disease or displacement in slipped capital femoral epiphysis. Gradually progressive chronic symptoms suggest developmental and idiopathic conditions. Often, the only presenting symptom may be a limp, refusal to bear weight, or neglect of the extremity instead of pain.

Examination

The gait and station should be evaluated for limp, leg-length discrepancy, and deformity. Detailed neurologic examination is necessary when any of these are present. Leg-lengths should be measured from the anterior superior iliac spine to the tip of the medial malleolus. Deformities should be measured and compared with the contralateral leg.

The foot-progression angle is the angle subtended by the long axis of the foot with a line that defines the path of the child while walking. It is used to assess intoeing. The thigh-foot angle is also used to assess intoeing. It is measured by positioning the child prone and flexing the knees to 90 degrees. The angle is subtended by the long axis of the foot and the longitudinal axis of the thigh. It is a measure of tibial torsion. The bimalleolar axis is a theoretical line that connects the tips of the malleoli. Its position is compared to the tibial tubercle to assess tibial torsion.

Metatarsus adductus can be differentiated from clubfoot by involvement of the forefoot only. The hindfoot is in a neutral position, and there is no evidence of equinus. The forefoot is in adductus, and the great toe may be deviated medially. The thigh-foot angle and bimalleolar axis is rotated internally in internal tibial torsion. The patella points straight forward when the child is standing. Femoral anteversion causes the patella to point medially when the child is standing. Hip internal rotation is increased, and external rotation is decreased.

The point of maximal tenderness should be identified to help localize infection and trauma. Metaphyseal tenderness with painless range of motion suggests osteomyelitis. Limited or painful joint motion suggests an underlying synovitis or infection. Painless increased internal rotation of the hip with decreased external rotation suggests increased femoral anteversion. Differences in hip abduction, and especially painful, limited hip abduction, suggest hip dislocation.

Provocative signs useful for assessing developmental hip dislocation include the Ortolani and Barlow tests. The Ortolani test attempts to reduce a dislocated hip. The examiner places the child supine, abducts the hips, and manually translates the proximal femur anteriorly. A palpable "clunk" into a congruent acetabulum can be felt. The Barlow test attempts to dislocate or at least sublux an unstable hip. The examiner places the child supine, adducts and flexes the hip, and pushes the proximal femur posteriorly and laterally in an attempt to sublux or dislocate the hip. A "click" without dislocation suggests instability.

Children with hip dysplasia can present with a wide variety of clinical findings. In most cases, the hip is dislocated at birth but can easily be reduced. Teratologic hip dislocations are fixed and irreducible. Hips that are "loose" due to increased capsular laxity often improve spontaneously and "tighten up" within a few days after birth. However, some loose hips remain subluxed and develop acetabular dysplasia. Despite widespread neonatal screening, a number of children first present with hip dysplasia at walking age. These children will present with a shortened extremity due to the proximal migration of the dislocated femoral head (Fig. 41–8). They will also have limited hip abduction and asymmetric thigh folds.

PEARL

The Galleazzi sign can identify children with a developmental hip dislocation. Place the child supine with the hips and knees flexed. If the hip is dislocated, the knee will be lower on the affected side, indicating proximal migration of the femur (Fig. 41–9).

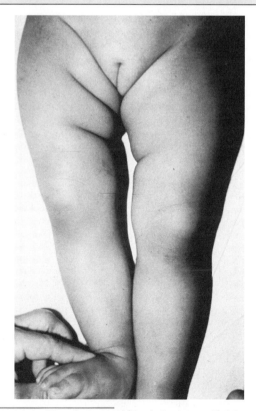

Figure 41–8 Developmental hip dislocation. Children more than 6 months old with developmental hip dislocation will present with a shortened extremity with asymmetric thigh folds.

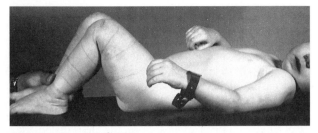

Figure 41–9   The Galleazzi sign is a clinical finding that usually indicates a developmental hip dislocation. With the hips and knees flexed, the knee on the affected side is lower due to proximal migration of the femoral head.

Children with SCFE may present with either chronic or acute onset of symptoms. A chronic slip will cause mild groin or hip pain, which is often referred to the knee. The child will have a noticeable limp with the affected leg being slightly externally rotated. Often the condition will go undiagnosed for several months until the child is finally brought to the orthopaedist because of increasing hip or knee pain.

The child with an acute slip will suddenly develop severe groin, hip, or knee pain that may occur after a minor traumatic event. The pain will be so severe that the child will not be able to walk, and any movement of the leg will elicit pain. The acute-on-chronic slip occurs in the child with chronic symptoms for several months that suddenly worsen to the point that weight-bearing is difficult.

Children with infantile tibia vara walk with a lateral thrust to the knee, and their bowlegs are severe and progressive. Early on, the deformity resembles physiologic bowing, and in fact, physiologic bowing may be a precursor to Blount's disease in overweight toddlers. Adolescent Blount's disease is commonly seen in obese black males. It is unilateral in 50% of cases, and often patients will present with knee pain.

AIDS TO DIAGNOSIS

Laboratory studies are essential for the evaluation of osteomyelitis and septic arthritis. Blood cultures, joint aspiration, and percutaneous aspiration of the metaphysis are imperative. A complete blood count (CBC), erythrocyte sedimentation rate (ESR), and C-reactive protein (CRP) can all be useful. Normal values for the CBC, ESR, and CRP do not rule out an infection. It is especially useful to follow sequential CRP values to assess the response to treatment in osteomyelitis. The ESR is almost always elevated within 48 to 72 hours of the onset of infection and returns to normal 2 to 4 weeks after eradication of the infection. The CRP may be elevated within 6 hours of infection, peaks around day 2, and returns to normal within 1 week.

Radiographs have variable utility in evaluating pediatric lower extremity problems. The bones in young children with metatarsus adductus or developmental hip dislocation are not yet fully ossified. Acute osteomyelitis may have no radiographic manifestations until 5 to 7 days after the onset of symptoms (Fig. 41–10). Increased intra-articular fluid manifested by increased joint space may be apparent in septic arthritis (Fig. 41–11). As children get older, radiographs become more useful.

Special radiographs can be useful in evaluating deformity or leg-length discrepancy. Standing x-rays of the lower extremities are essential to evaluate angular knee deformities. An anteroposterior view of the pelvis with the legs abducted and internally rotated is useful to evaluate femoral head coverage with bracing or femoral osteotomy in Legg-Calve-Perthes disease. Scanograms are essential for following a leg-length discrepancy and planning treatment.

The radiographic changes of developmental hip dislocation include a break in Shenton's line, location of the femoral head superior and lateral to the acetabulum, and increased acetabular index (Fig. 41–12). Shenton's line is a line drawn along the medial cortex of the femoral diaphysis and neck

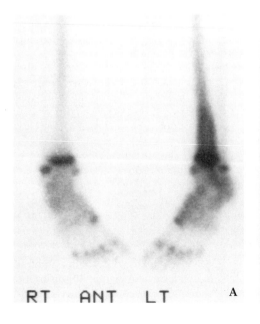

RT   ANT   LT   **A**

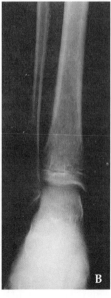

B

Figure 41–10   Acute osteomyelitis may have a normal appearance on plain radiographs, but a three-phase bone scan will demonstrate increased activity on the delayed images. (**A**) After 5 to 7 days, the plain radiographs will begin to show irregular lytic areas with periosteal reaction (**B**).

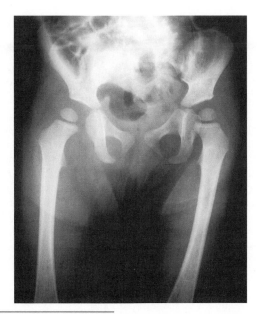

Figure 41–11 Septic arthritis will cause a joint effusion that is sometimes apparent on plain radiographs. This 1-year-old had a 48-hour history of fever with an irritable right hip. The x-ray shows a widened joint space on the right hip, suggesting the diagnosis of septic arthritis. In young children, the intra-articular pressure in a septic hip can cause the joint to dislocate, so aspiration and surgical drainage is a surgical emergency.

and continued along the inferior margin of the superior pubic ramus. A break of this line implies a nonanatomic position of the proximal femur. The acetabular index is the angle subtended by a horizontal line connecting the triradiate cartilage of each acetabulum and a second line connecting the triradiate cartilage to the lateral margin of the acetabulum.

Three radiographic classifications of Legg-Calve-Perthes disease have been proposed to predict outcome and guide treatment. Catterall's system (1971) is based on the amount of femoral head involvement. Groups I and II usually have a good prognosis and require little treatment, whereas groups III and IV have more extensive head involvement and may do better with treatment. Salter and Thompson (1984) described a classification based on the extent of the subchondral fracture line. The subchondral fracture involves less than one half of the femoral head in type A hips, and extends to the lateral margin of the femoral head in type B hips. Type A hips have a good prognosis, and type B hips have a poor prognosis. Herring's lateral pillar classification (Herring et al, 1992) evaluates the lateral pillar of the femoral head on an anteroposterior radiograph. Type A hips with a normal lateral pillar have an excellent prognosis. The prognosis worsens with progressive collapse in type B and C hips, and treatment may be indicated (Fig. 41–13).

A radiographic classification of SCFE evaluates the degree of femoral head displacement. The epiphysis is nondisplaced in a preslip, but the physis is widened. A minimal slip has epiphyseal displacement of less than one third of the diameter of the femoral neck. Epiphyseal displacement between

one third and one half the diameter of the femoral neck defines a moderate slip. A severe slip has epiphyseal displacement greater than one half the diameter of the femoral neck (Fig. 41–2).

Langenskold (1981) described and classified the radiographic changes in Blount's disease. There are six stages ranging from beaking and fragmentation of the medial metaphysis to a complete closure of the medial physis with a sharp medial slope of the articular surface. The x-ray changes of adolescent tibia vara are less severe than those of infantile tibia vara. The physis can be irregular in thickness with mild medial beaking (Fig. 41–14). Fragmentation is rare.

Ultrasonography is useful for assessing hip instability in infants. It is possible to evaluate the anatomy of the acetabulum, labrum, capsule, and femoral head. One examiner can image the hip while another attempts to sublux the hip to evaluate hip stability.

Computed tomography (CT) scanning, magnetic resonance imaging (MRI), and technetium bone scanning are rarely used. Computed tomography scanning may be necessary to evaluate reduction of a dislocated hip. Magnetic resonance imaging is useful to evaluate the spine and spinal cord when neuromuscular etiologies are suspected. Technetium bone scanning and MRI imaging may be necessary to identify osteomyelitis (Fig. 41–10).

SPECIFIC CONDITIONS, TREATMENT, AND OUTCOME

Osteomyelitis and Septic Arthritis

Diagnosis of osteomyelitis or septic arthritis can be difficult, and delay in treatment is not unusual. A good outcome of treatment depends on early diagnosis and prompt initiation of treatment. Any child with a fever and pain localized to an extremity requires thorough evaluation to rule out musculoskeletal infection. Many severe deformities are long-term sequelae of untreated bone and joint infections. These include complete joint destruction with dislocation and complete physeal destruction causing severe limb-length inequality (Fig. 41–4). The diagnosis of osteomyelitis is often imprecise, and the treatment is often empiric.

Treatment of osteomyelitis is based on a thorough knowledge of the microbiology of bone and joint infections. S aureus is the most common organism responsible for hematogenous osteomyelitis; therefore, after obtaining cultures, empiric treatment with intravenous antibiotics that "cover" S aureus should be initiated immediately. Sensitivity results from the cultures may suggest alternative antibiotics. S aureus coverage should be continued if cultures are negative. Additional empiric coverage for streptococcus and H influenzae type B may be necessary. The incidence of H influenzae type B infections is decreasing now that children are receiving immunizations for this virus.

Nafcillin, oxacillin sodium, and first- and second-generation cephalosporins are usually effective for osteomyelitis. Intravenous therapy is started in the hospital, where the patient's clinical course can be monitored. The child can be switched to oral therapy when clinically improved. Serum

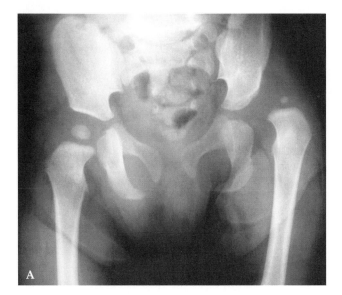

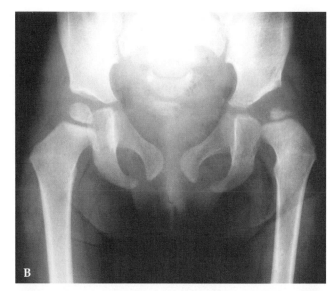

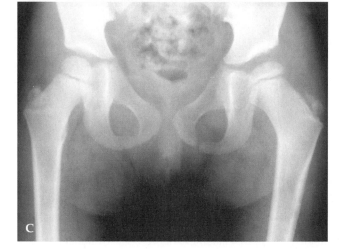

Figure 41–12   Closed reduction of developmental hip dislocation. A 16-month-old baby girl presented with a limp and leg-length inequality. (**A**) Plain radiographs demonstrate a right hip dislocation with delayed ossification of the femoral head ossific nucleus, a break in Shenton's line, and increased acetabular index. (**B**) Six months after closed reduction, the hip is reduced, Shenton's line is restored, but the acetabular index is still elevated. (**C**) Two years later, the hip is still reduced, the acetabular index has returned to normal, and the femoral head has fully ossified.

bacteriostatic and bacteriocidal levels of the antibiotic should be adequate prior to discharging the patient on oral therapy. Total treatment time for combined intravenous and oral antibiotics should be 6 weeks.

Surgical drainage is indicated for abscess or sequestrum formation in the bone, or if antibiotic therapy alone does not result in clinical improvement. Ultrasound, CT, or MRI will often demonstrate a subperiosteal or intraosseous abscess. Special consideration should be given to infections occurring in the foot after a puncture wound through a shoe. Pseudomonas is almost always present in these polymicrobial infections. Thorough surgical debridement and intravenous aminoglycoside antibiotics are necessary.

The differential diagnosis of a hot, swollen joint includes septic arthritis, toxic synovitis, juvenile rheumatoid arthritis, rheumatic fever, Henoch-Schonlein purpura, Lyme disease, and tuberculosis.

Gram stain and cultures from purulent joint fluid do not always reveal bacteria, so blood cultures should also be obtained.

Broad spectrum antibiotics should be initiated for septic arthritis once cultures have been obtained. Intravenous

---

PEARL

Joint aspiration is mandatory if septic arthritis is suspected. A joint fluid leukocyte count of greater than 50,000 to 100,000 usually indicates a septic joint, whereas a white cell count of less than 50,000 usually indicates other inflammatory disorders.

administration is necessary for initial treatment after thorough surgical drainage of the joint. Once the clinical course begins to improve, antibiotics can be switched to oral administration, if adequate serum levels of the drug can be measured. Typically, the duration for combined intravenous and oral therapy in septic arthritis is 3 to 4 weeks.

Arthrotomy, irrigation and drainage are essential in the treatment of septic arthritis. It is imperative to remove the bacteria and inflammatory products, which can destroy articular cartilage. Repeat joint aspirations are not feasible in chil-

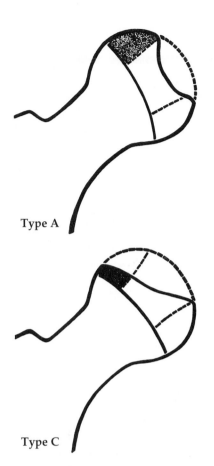

Type A

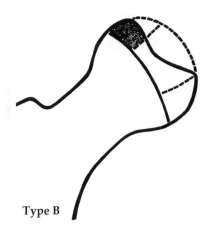

Type B

Type C

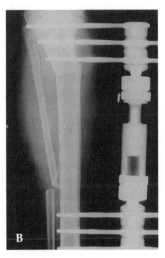

Figure 41–13   Lateral pillar classification of Legg-Calve-Perthes. The femoral head can be divided into three zones, or pillars on the anteroposterior radiograph. (**A**) The amount of collapse of the lateral pillar has prognostic significance. The hip with no collapse of the lateral pillar has an excellent prognosis. (**B**) The prognosis is variable and depends on the age of onset of the disease when there is 50 to 100% collapse of the lateral pillar. (**C**) The prognosis is poor with greater than 50% collapse of the lateral pillar. Reproduced with permission from Herring JA, Neustadt JB, Williams JJ. The lateral pillar classification of Legg-Calve-Perthes disease. *J Pediat Orthop*. 1992;12:144–148.

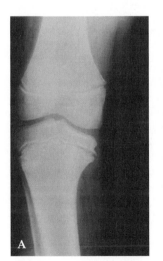

Figure 41–14   Adolescent Blount's disease. A ten-year-old girl with typical x-rays of adolescent Blount's disease. (**A**) The physis is widened, with medial beaking. (**B**) The varus deformity of the proximal tibia is corrected with tibial and fibular osteotomy with application of an Orthofix external fixator (EBI Medical Systems, Parsippany, New Jersey).

dren, and it is unlikely that antibiotics alone will prevent the destructive effects of a bacterial infection. Arthrotomy can be performed through a small incision with minimal morbidity, and a drain can be left in place for several days. In older children, septic joints can be drained and irrigated arthroscopically. The hip joint merits special attention because intra-articular pus under pressure can compromise the intracapsular vascular supply of the femoral head and cause avascular necrosis.

Developmental Hip Dislocation
Age Newborn to Six Months

Newborn screening for hip dislocation is a standard part of every pediatrician's physical exam. The Ortolani and Barlow tests are performed at birth and at every subsequent office visit until the child is of walking age. If the pediatrician notices an abnormality on the physical exam, especially in newborns, who have risk factors for hip dysplasia, the child is then referred to the orthopaedist.

The treatment for dislocated hips with a positive Ortolani test is a Pavlik harness (Fig. 41–15). The harness maintains hip abduction and flexion while allowing the baby to kick his or her legs. It is well tolerated and has a low complication rate. A total of 6 weeks full-time treatment followed by 6 weeks part-time treatment is usually all that is necessary to ensure adequate reduction. Radiographs should be obtained at the end of this 3 month period. If acetabular dysplasia persists, the Pavlik harness should be continued. After 6 months of age, abduction splinting can be achieved with a soft plastic

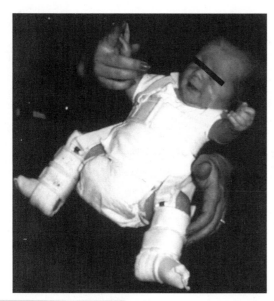

Figure 41–15 *The Pavlik harness is used to treat developmental hip dislocation in children younger than 6 months of age. The harness holds the hips in 90 degrees of flexion and no more than 60 degrees of abduction. The harness is worn full-time until the hips have become stable on clinical exam and have a normal radiographic or sonographic appearance.*

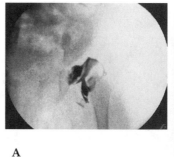
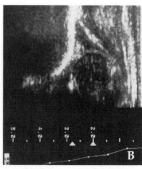

A

Figure 41–16 Hip arthrogram is performed intra-operatively under anesthesia during closed reduction of a developmental hip dislocation. (**A**) The arthrogram demonstrates superior migration of the femoral head, an infolded acetabular labrum, and a large medial dye pool. (**B**) Similar morphologic information can be obtained with a hip ultrasound in an awake child. The femoral head has migrated superior and lateral to the bony ilium, the echodense cartilaginous labrum is blunted and infolded, and there is a wide gap between the femoral head and triradiate cartilage.

brace. The few hips that fail Pavlik harness treatment are usually bilateral dislocations, hips which have delayed treatment, and hips that cannot be reduced with the Ortolani maneuver.

Hips that are not dislocated but have a click or instability can be followed with observation and serial ultrasounds (Fig. 41–16). The ultrasound can demonstrate abnormal hip morphology or abnormal motion on stress exam. If the ultrasound is normal or shows only slight capsular laxity, the child does not require treatment but should be followed with ultrasound or radiographs. The hip must have normal radiographic morphology by 4 months of age, otherwise Pavlik harness treatment should be initiated and continued until the dysplasia has resolved.

Age Six Months to Two Years

Closed or possibly open reduction is necessary for treatment. A closed reduction can be performed with or without 3 weeks of preliminary traction. A traction apparatus can be set up for home use.

Closed reduction is performed under general anesthesia and is confirmed with an arthrogram in the operating room (Fig. 41–16a). Open reduction is indicated if the hip is not adequately reduced, or if it is unstable after reduction. Adductor tenotomy may be necessary. A spica cast is applied for 18 weeks, with the legs in the "human position" of 90 degrees of hip flexion and no more than 60 degrees of hip abduction. The cast is molded to maintain pressure on the greater trochanter so the hip will stay reduced. Reduction can be evaluated with a single-cut CT scan through the hips and cast to verify that the femoral head is maintained within the acetabulum.

PITFALL
Infants should never be casted with the hips in more than 60 degrees of abduction. Abduction beyond 60 degrees can lead to avascular necrosis of the femoral head. After closed reduction, the "human position" with 90 degrees of hip flexion and only 60 degrees of abduction should be used.

Open reduction can be performed through a medial or anterior approach (Fig. 41–7). The medial approach is direct and removes the obstacles of reduction; however, the anterior branch of the medial circumflex artery is at risk. The anterior approach allows for a capsulorraphy, which is often necessary to tighten a redundant capsule in children who are of walking age. The human position is maintained in a spica cast for 6 weeks. Results of closed versus open reduction are similar. The most important complication of either closed or open reduction is avascular necrosis of the femoral head. The factor most strongly associated with avascular necrosis is excessive hip abduction in the spica cast.

Age Two Years and Older

As children get older, the secondary soft tissue and bone changes of hip dislocation make treatment more challenging. Closed reduction becomes more difficult, and acetabular dysplasia may persist even though reduction may be achieved. Contractures can cause excessive pressure on the femoral head and increase the risk of avascular necrosis. Open reduction with capsulorraphy and femoral shortening is usually necessary to achieve reduction. A pelvic osteotomy may also be necessary to increase coverage of the femoral head (Fig. 41–17).

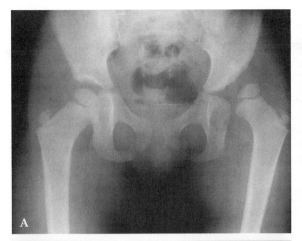

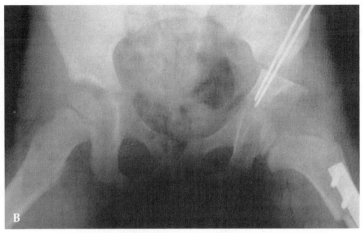

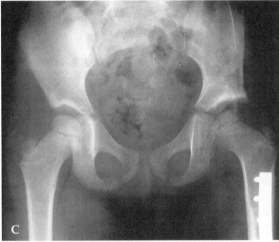

Figure 41–17 Open reduction of developmental hip dislocation. (**A**) A 3-year-old girl presented with a noticeable leg-length discrepancy, with the left leg shorter than the right. X-rays demonstrate left developmental hip dislocation. (**B**) The child underwent open reduction, capsulorraphy, femoral shortening, and Salter inominate osteotomy. (**C**) One year postoperatively, the hip is well reduced, and the acetabular dysplasia is resolving. Subtle changes in the radiographic appearance of the femoral head suggest mild avascular necrosis of the femoral head.

A pelvic osteotomy or varus femoral osteotomy may also be used to treat residual acetabular dysplasia in older children who have previously undiagnosed or persistent dysplasia despite prior treatment. Multiple pelvic osteotomies are often necessary to redirect the acetabulum in older children in whom the triradiate cartilage has closed. Salvage procedures to provide a bony shelf over the uncovered portion of the femoral head may be necessary when concentric reduction is impossible. The choice of pelvic osteotomy depends on the amount of dysplasia, the location of the acetabular deficiency, and whether or not a concentric reduction can be obtained. A CT scan of the hip with three-dimensional reconstruction can be helpful in preoperative planning.

Legg-Calve-Perthes Disease

The child with early, acute Legg-Calve-Perthes disease has intermittent pain, limping, and limited range of motion of the hip that can last for days to months. These symptoms are due to synovitis, begin at the onset of the avascular necrosis, and can last for several years until the femoral head has begun to reossify. The goals of early treatment are controlling the pain and preserving hip range of motion. Eventually, the hip pain abates as the femoral head reossifies.

Collapse of the femoral head due to subchondral fractures that occur during the fragmentation phase flattens the femoral head. The irregular shape predisposes the hip to

degenerative arthritis later in life. Thus, the ultimate treatment goal in Legg-Calve-Perthes disease is to "contain" the femoral head within the acetabulum to maintain its sphericity and hip joint congruity to prevent late, degenerative arthritis of the hip.

PEARL

Children who develop Legg-Calve-Perthes disease before age 6 and have a preserved height of the lateral pillar of the femoral head (Fig. 41–13) generally have a good prognosis with minimal late deformity and arthritis. These children rarely need more than symptomatic treatment for bouts of synovitis. Older children with whole-head involvement tend to have a worse prognosis and may benefit from containment treatment.

Children with early symptoms of Legg-Calve-Perthes disease require activity limitations, anti-inflammatory medication, and family education about the natural history. Bedrest and traction may be necessary if the synovitis and pain continue, and the hip becomes stiff and loses abduction. Buck's extension traction or "slings and springs", i.e., the patient is lying supine in bed, and legs are suspended by large springs which keep the hips flexed and abducted while still allowing hip motion, can be used in the hospital or at home. Periodic range-of-motion exercises are performed as well. Traction is discontinued after 1 to 2 weeks, when the pain and range of motion have improved. Children may go through several bouts of pain and stiffness requiring bedrest and traction before the healing phase begins. As pain diminishes, normal activities can be resumed.

Older children, and children with more extensive involvement of the lateral pillar of the femoral head may benefit from containment treatment. Theoretically, acetabular containment and coverage of the femoral head should prevent lateral subluxation and flattening of the laterally extruded femoral head. Bracing, femoral osteotomy, or inominate osteotomy can be used to achieve containment during the fragmentation and healing phases. The most commonly used brace is the Atlanta Scottish Rite orthosis, (Fillauer Orthopedic, Chattanooga, Tennessee) which maintains 45 degrees of hip abduction but still allows full ambulation. With the brace properly applied, the femoral head is completely covered while the child is weight bearing. Results of brace treatment are variable because of difficult compliance and fit.

Femoral varus osteotomies have also been moderately successful. The osteotomy increases femoral neck varus so that the lateral femoral head is contained within the acetabulum. Children often develop an abductor lurch, though, because the osteotomy shortens the abductor lever arm. The Salter inominate osteotomy also provides excellent containment of the femoral head by redirecting the acetabulum anteriorly and laterally. The best results with any form of containment have been achieved in patients with limited femoral head involvement and normal hip range of motion.

Regardless of treatment method, patients with Legg-Calve-Perthes reossify the femoral head and have a pain-free adolescence and early adulthood. The irregular contour of the femoral head eventually leads to degenerative arthritis. It is unclear whether containment treatment prevents or delays long-term degenerative changes. Any form of containment treatment theoretically improves the prognosis for degenerative arthritis of the hip. Therefore, treatment decisions should be individualized after thorough consultation with the family, considering potential risks and benefits of each treatment option.

Slipped Capital Femoral Epiphysis

The immediate goal of treatment is to stabilize the slip, prevent further displacement, and return the patient to normal ambulation. The early complications of SCFE are avascular necrosis and chondrolysis and are, in part, related to treatment. A potential long-term consequence of SCFE is degenerative arthritis of the hip. Degenerative changes are related to the severity of the slip and the proximal femur deformity. Early diagnosis and treatment of SCFE minimizes deformity of the hip and improves the long-term prognosis.

The standard treatment for SCFE is in situ pinning with a percutaneous or open technique using one or two partially threaded cannulated screws (Fig. 41–2). Avascular necrosis of the femoral head is more common when two or more screws are used. The patient should be positioned on a fracture table or a C-arm table. Reduction should not be attempted because it increases the incidence of avascular necrosis. The screw is ideally placed in the center of the femoral head. Attentive intra-operative x-ray imaging in multiple planes is essential to avoid screw penetration into the joint space. Cannulated screws are useful because a guide pin can be positioned first to ensure appropriate screw length and position. Postoperatively, patients must be kept non–weight-bearing on crutches for 6 to 12 weeks, depending on the severity of the slip.

PEARL

The femoral head is relatively posterior to the proximal femur in slipped capital femoral epiphysis (SCFE), and, therefore, the pin must enter the anterior cortex of the femoral neck to be placed perpendicular to the epiphyseal plate to enter the center of the femoral head. The more severe the slip, the more anterior the starting point must be on the femoral neck.

Acute SCFE has a high incidence of poor results. Avascular necrosis occurs in 25 to 50% of these hips despite accurate in situ pin treatment (Fig. 41–2c). It is presumed that damage to the blood supply of the femoral head occurs at the time of the acute slip. It is unclear whether emergent treatment within 6 hours or delayed treatment after several days of bedrest and traction yields a better outcome. Femoral head collapse and articular incongruity occur rapidly once avascular necrosis occurs. Minimal femoral head involvement can be managed with non–weight-bearing and activity restrictions until the avascular segment reossifies. Severe cases with more femoral head involvement may improve symptomatically with femoral and pelvic osteotomies, but hip fusion is often necessary.

The cause of chondrolysis is currently unknown. Penetration of the hip joint with the fixation screw causes chondrolysis if the screw is not replaced. Penetration of the hip joint with a guide pin likely does not cause chondrolysis, as long as the screw does not penetrate the hip joint and the guide pin is removed. Chondrolysis typically progresses to degenerative arthritis.

Severe slips result in a varus, retroverted femoral neck deformity resulting in an abnormal gait with marked external rotation of the affected extremity. Late degenerative arthritis is common in these hips. Femoral neck, intertrochanteric, or subtrochanteric osteotomies can improve the deformity but are technically difficult and can be complicated by avascular necrosis and chondrolysis.

Leg-length Discrepancy

Treatment of leg-length discrepancy depends on the cause of the discrepancy, the difference in length between the two legs, and the rate of growth of the normal and affected leg. A leg-length difference of less than 2 centimeters is usually well tolerated and can be managed with a shoe-lift. A leg-length difference of more than 2 centimeters usually produces a limp and can lead to back pain and scoliosis later in life. Therefore, surgical treatment of a leg-length discrepancy greater than 2 cm is recommended.

Physes are all functional in leg-length discrepancies due to congenital anomalies; however, the rate of growth is slower in the affected limb (Fig. 41–3). Typically, the relative shortening that is encountered is stable throughout growth. For example, a child with a 20% shortening of the leg at birth will probably end up with a 20% shortening of that extremity at skeletal maturity. On the other hand, a static loss of growth occurs in the affected limb if there is damage to a growth plate. As the child grows, the relative difference in leg lengths will increase.

Two methods are routinely used to predict the leg-length difference at skeletal maturity. The growth-remaining method uses graphs developed by Green and Anderson (1963) (Fig. 41–18) to first calculate the growth remaining of the normal leg based on the patient's age and bone length relative to his or her age. The growth of the normal and affected leg is measured over time to calculate the relative growth

inhibition of the shortened leg. The percent growth-inhibition is then multiplied by the growth remaining of the normal leg to predict the growth remaining of the shortened leg.

A simpler method has been devised by Moseley (1989) using a straight-line graph. The length of the normal leg and the length of the short leg are plotted on the graph at each visit to the physician. Over time, two diverging lines result. A vertical line is drawn from each leg-length plot to a skeletal age line. A horizontal line is then drawn from each point on the skeletal age line to a vertical skeletal maturity line. The difference between the intersection of the horizontal lines with the skeletal maturity line is the leg-length discrepancy at skeletal maturity.

Both methods require at least three measurements at different time intervals. A simple rule of thumb is that the distal femoral physis grows 1 cm per year and the proximal tibia grows 0.6 cm per year. Physes close on average at age 14 in girls and age 16 in boys. One can thus determine the timing of physeal arrest in the longer leg to correct the predicted leg-length discrepancy.

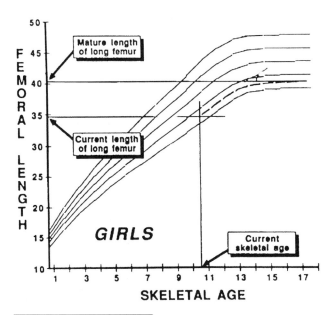

Figure 41–18   The Green-Anderson table can be used to determine the predicted leg-length discrepancy at skeletal maturity. First, the growth remaining of the normal femur or tibia is determined by plotting the skeletal age versus the bone length and following the growth line to skeletal maturity. The growth inhibition is calculated separately, over time, by dividing the growth rate of the short bone by the growth rate of the long bone. The percent growth inhibition is then multiplied by the growth remaining of the long bone to calculate the growth remaining of the short bone. This information is then used to decide if the optimal form of treatment will be a leg-lengthening or a contralateral epiphysiodesis. Reproduced with permission from Moseley CF. Assessment and prediction in leg-length discrepancy. In: Barr JS, ed. *AAOS Instructional Course Lectures.* Vol 38. St. Louis, MO: CV Mosby; 1989;38:327.

PEARL

In leg-length discrepency, for differences less than 2 centimeters, no treatment or a shoe-lift is all that is necessary. For differences of 2 to 5 cm, timed contralateral epiphysiodesis is the treatment of choice. For differences more than 5 cm, lengthening of the shortened extremity is indicated.

Epiphysiodesis has traditionally consisted of excision of the physis and fixation of the epiphysis and metaphysis with a staple. Recently, percutaneous epiphysiodesis has become a reliable procedure with low morbidity and rapid recuperation for equalizing leg lengths. Whenever the predicted leg-length difference is less than 5 cm, epiphysiodesis is preferable to lengthening due to its low complication rate and short recovery period.

Much progress has been made in the field of limb lengthening with the introduction of the Ilizarov callotasis method in this country. A small-wire, external ring fixator is applied to the shortened limb (Fig. 41–19), a metaphyseal corticotomy is performed, and the limb is gradually distracted with the external fixator at a rate of 1 mm per day. The distraction is started 5 to 7 days after surgery to allow osteogenesis to begin. By lengthening in very small increments (0.25 mm, 4 times/day) callus and regenerate bone forms in the gap created by the lengthening. The regenerate bone consolidates after the lengthening has been completed. The external fixator can be removed when the new bone is clinically strong enough to withstand normal weight-bearing stresses.

Lengthenings up to 20 cm can be performed with the Ilizarov method. Ilizarov lengthening is technically demanding and requires a cooperative patient and family who are willing to endure months of treatment and rehabilitation. The external fixator is on for 6 months to more than 1 year, depending on the amount of lengthening necessary. Complications are frequent and include pin-tract infections, joint contractures and instability, psychological disturbance, and fracture once the external fixator is removed.

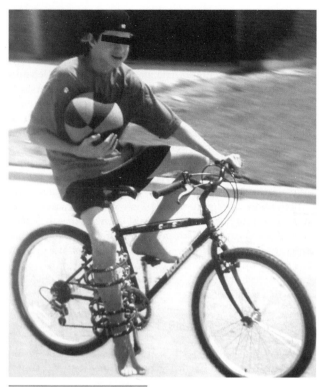

Figure 41–19 The Ilizarov technique for leg-lengthening is performed with a small-wire, ring external fixator. The external fixator is applied, a corticotomy is performed, and the rings are then slowly distracted at a rate of 1 mm per day. Regenerate bone forms in the distraction gap. The external fixator is continued until the regenerate bone has fully consolidated. Lengthenings up to 15% of the length of the bone can be successfully performed.

Intoeing

A large part of pediatric orthopaedics involves the evaluation of children with perceived gait abnormalities. Parents, grandparents, teachers, and other care-givers are often concerned with a child whose feet turn in or a child whose legs appear bowed or knockkneed during walking. In our society, a perfect appearance is of utmost priority; and therefore, any slight deviation from normal is of great parental concern. The goal of the orthopaedist is to understand the parental concern, rule out a pathologic condition, and educate families about the benign natural history of these variants of normal.

Flexible metatarsus adductus usually resolves on its own. Parents can accelerate the process by performing gentle stretching exercises several times a day. Rigid metatarsus adductus usually requires serial casting to correct the forefoot deformity. Best results are achieved when treatment starts before the child reaches 6 months of age. Other treatment modalities for metatarsus adductus include reverse last shoes or Bebax shoes (Camp International, Inc., Jackson, Mississippi), which are leather shoes with a ball joint on the plantar surface to allow gradual deformity correction. (Fig. 41–20).

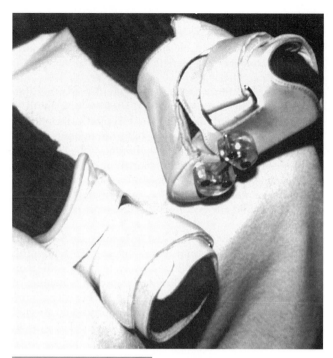

Figure 41–20 Bebax shoes are used to treat metatarsus adductus in children before walking age. The shoes have a ball joint on the plantar surface and can be adjusted to manipulate the feet into a corrected position. They are worn fulltime, and gradual correction can be achieved by adjusting the ball joints at weekly intervals.

These special shoes can be worn until the child begins walking. After ambulation begins, the forefoot deformity usually corrects on its own. Forefoot adduction may persist to school age in severe rigid cases and may require corrective metatarsal osteotomies.

Internal tibial torsion also resolves with time, usually by age 3. Reassurance and education of the family are essential. Derotational splints such as the Denis-Browne bar have been used for many years; however, there is no published evidence that they alter the natural course of gradual improvement that occurs in children with tibial torsion.

Femoral torsion lasts much longer than other causes of intoeing. Reassurance can be difficult in an older child who remains "pigeon-toed" for a few years. Femoral torsion usually resolves by age 8 or 9 or the child consciously points his or her feet straight forward when walking. Special shoes and braces have no role in the management of femoral anteversion. Often encouragement to sit in the cross-legged position or involvement in activities that point the feet straight such as skating, skiing, gymnastics, and ballet are helpful. Ultimately, the intoeing resolves before the teenage years, and femoral derotational osteotomies are rarely, if ever, required for treatment.

Angular Knee Deformities

Physiologic genu varum and genu valgum rarely require treatment other than family education and observation. Genu

---

PEARL

Intoeing after walking age rarely requires treatment. Special shoes and bracing will not alter the course of tibial torsion or femoral anteversion. The natural history is slow resolution over time. Tibial torsion usually goes away by age 3, femoral anteversion may persist to age 8 or 9.

---

varum is common in toddlers. The genu varum overcorrects to genu valgum around age 3 and then decreases to normal valgus of 5 to 7 degrees. Physiologic genu valgum in adolescence does not always correct with time. Surgical correction may be necessary when the tibiofemoral angle exceeds 15 degrees or if the valgus angulation causes a significant cosmetic deformity. Medial distal femoral physeal arrest by hemiepiphysiodesis or stapling is a simple procedure that can correct the deformity, if timed properly. A chart based on the Green-Anderson growth tables guides the timing of the operation.

Blount's Disease

Infantile tibia vara causes progressive varus deformity of the knee and degenerative arthritis. The outcome of treatment of tibia vara correlates with the Langenskold radiographic stage. Patients treated at an early stage of the disease have a much better prognosis than those treated at later stages. In children under 3 with stage I or stage II disease, complete correction can be achieved using long-leg braces that exert a valgus force and, thus, unload the medial tibial physis. Osteotomy is necessary in stage III or greater and in cases in which the deformity is not corrected after 1 year of bracing.

Corrective osteotomy of the proximal tibia in Blount's disease should over-correct the mechanical axis by 5 degrees or more to "unload" the medial physis. It should be performed before age 4 when the cartilage damage is still reversible. Fibular osteotomy is necessary for adequate realignment of the mechanical axis. Prophylactic fasciotomy is recommended to prevent compartment syndrome. Realignment osteotomy alone is not sufficient in stage IV, V, and VI deformities because of severe physeal destruction. Medial physeal resection with placement of interposition material usually must be added to realignment osteotomy. An osteotomy to elevate the entire medial plateau may be necessary in severe stage VI deformities with depression of the medial articular surface.

Untreated adolescent tibia vara also has a poor prognosis with early progressive degenerative arthritis of the knee. The goal of treatment is to restore the normal mechanical axis. A lateral proximal tibial hemiepiphysiodesis can be effective when physeal growth remains. A proximal tibial osteotomy is necessary to realign the mechanical axis in patients approaching or past skeletal maturity. Dynamic external fixation with either a unilateral or ring fixator can be used to "dial in" the correction. Fibular osteotomy and prophylactic fasciotomy are important steps in the surgical procedure (Fig. 41–14).

SUMMARY

Pediatric lower extremity disorders can usually be easily diagnosed with a thorough history and examination. Laboratory and radiographic studies facilitate both diagnosis and treatment planning. Many deformities are physiologically normal and require only reassurance and observation. Pediatric hip disorders are all at risk of evolving into adult degenerative arthritis. A thorough understanding of the natural history of each and prompt and attentive treatment can decrease this risk. Infectious disorders can be challenging and require prompt treatment to minimize the risk of long-term deformity and disability.

SELECTED BIBLIOGRAPHY

ANDERSON M, GREEN WT, MESSNER MB. Growth and prediction of growth in the lower extremities. *J Bone Jt Surg.* 1963;45A:10.

BOWEN JR, LEAHEY JL, ZHANG Z. Partial epiphysiodesis at the knee to correct angular deformity. *Clin Orthop.* 1985;198:184–190.

CANALE ST, CHRISTIAN CA. Techniques for epiphysiodesis about the knee. *Clin Orthop.* 1990;255:81–85.

CATTERALL A. The natural history of Perthes disease. *J Bone Jt Surg.* 1971;53B:37–53.

FELDMAN MD, SCHOENECKER PL. Use of the metaphyseal-diaphyseal angle in the evaluation of bowed legs. *J Bone Jt Surg.* 1993;75A:1602–1609.

GALPIN RD, ROACH JW, WENGER DR. One-stage treatment of congenital dislocation of the hip in older children, including femoral shortening. *J Bone Jt Surg.* 1989;71A:734–741.

GREEN NE, EDWARDS K. Bone and joint infections in children. *Orthop Clin North Am.* 1987;18:555–576.

HERRING JA, NEUSTADT JB, WILLIAMS JJ. The lateral pillar classification of Legg-Calve-Perthes disease. *J Pediatr Orthop.* 1992;12:143–150.

IPPOLITO E, MICKELSON MR, PONSETI IV. A histochemical study of slipped capital femoral epiphysis. *J Bone Jt Surg.* 1981;63A:1109–1113.

JOHNSTON CE. Infantile tibia vara. *Clin Orthop.* 1990;225:13–23.

KLING TF, HENSINGER, RN. Angular and torsional deformities of the lower limbs in children. *Clin Orthop.* 1983;176:136–147.

LANGENSKIOLD A. Tibia vara: osteochondrosis deformans tibiae. Blount's disease. *Clin Orthop.* 1981;158:77–82.

MEEHAN PL, ANGEL D, NELSON JM. The Scottish Rite abduction orthosis for the treatment of Legg-Perthes Disease. *J Bone Jt Surg.* 1992;74A:2–11.

Morrissy RT. *Atlas of Pediatric Orthopedics.* Philadelphia, PA: Lippincott; 1992.

Moseley CF. Assessment and prediction in leg-length discrepancy. In: Barr, JS, ed. AAOS *Instructional Course Lectures.* Vol. 38. St. Louis, MO: CV Mosby; 1989:325–330.

Nguyen D, Morrissy RT. Slipped capital femoral epiphysis: rationale for the technique of percutaneous in situ fixation. *J Pediatr Orthop* 1990;10:341–346.

Paley D. Current techniques of limb lengthening. *J Pediat Orthop.* 1988;8:73–92.

Price CT, Scott DS, Greenberg DA. Dynamic axial external fixation in the surgical treatment of tibia vara. *J Pediat Orthop.* 1995;15:236–243.

Rang M, Wenger D. *The art and practice of children's orthopaedics.* New York, NY: Raven Press;1993.

Salenius P, Vanka E. The development of the tibiofemoral angle in children. *J Bone Jt Surg.* 1975;57A:259–261.

Salter RB, Thompson GH. Legg-Calve-Perthes disease: the prognostic significance of the subchondral fracture and a two group classification of the femoral head involvement. *J Bone Jt Surg.* 1984;66:479.

Staheli LT, Corbett M, Wyss C, King H. Lower-extremity rotational problems in children: normal values to guide management. *J Bone Jt Surg.* 1985;67A:39–47.

Thompson GH, Carter JR. Late-onset tibia vara (Blount's disease). *Clin Orthop.* 1990;225:24–35.

Viere RG, Birch JG, Herring JA, Roach JW, Johnston CE. Use of the Pavlik harness in congenital dislocation of the hip. An analysis of failures of treatment. *J Bone Jt Surg.* 1990;72A:238–244.

Zionts LE, Macewen GD. Treatment of congenital dislocation of the hip in children between the ages of 1 and 3 years. *J Bone Jt Surg.* 1986;68A:829–846.

SAMPLE QUESTIONS

1. Which of the following structures may interfere with the closed reduction of a developmental hip dislocation:
   (a) the lateral femoral cutaneous nerve
   (b) the medial circumflex artery
   (c) the rectus femorus tendon
   (d) the transverse acetabular ligament
   (e) the sartorius muscle

2. Which of the following factors affects the prognosis in Legg-Calve-Perthes disease:
   (a) the age of onset of the disease
   (b) the presence of a subchondral fracture on frog-lateral x-ray
   (c) fragmentation of the femoral head on plain x-ray
   (d) decreased activity in the femoral head on bone scan
   (e) early treatment with bedrest and traction

3. What are the features of a chronic SCFE:
   (a) severe pain with inability to bear weight
   (b) anterior displacement of the femoral head
   (c) several months of mild hip pain and limping

   (d) a high incidence of developing avascular necrosis of the femoral head
   (e) displacement histologically through the resting zone of physeal cartilage

4. What is a common cause of intoeing in older children:
   (a) Blount's disease
   (b) developmental hip dislocation
   (c) proximal femoral focal deficiency
   (d) femoral anteversion
   (e) osteomyelitis

5. How is Blount's disease differentiated from physiologic bowing:
   (a) the presence of a limp
   (b) beaking of the medial proximal tibial metaphysis on plain x-ray
   (c) onset of bowing as soon as the child begins ambulation
   (d) family history of bowed legs
   (e) improvement of bowing with early brace treatment

Answers: 1) d; 2) a; 3) c; 4) d; 5) b

Chapter 42

The Pediatric Foot

Anthony A. Stans, MD, and Douglas K. Kehl, MD

Outline

Foot disorders represent the most common non-traumatic reason for pediatric patients to visit an orthopaedist. The spectrum of pathology varies greatly, from benign conditions which resolve spontaneously with no treatment, to disorders which can be treated effectively without surgery, to pathology which can only be corrected by aggressive surgery. Therefore, the most important principles for effective treatment of pediatric foot disorders are to correctly diagnose the problem, to understand the natural history of the problem, and to recognize what treatment can most favorably alter its natural history. The purpose of this chapter is to describe common pediatric foot disorders, discuss their appropriate evaluation, characterize their natural history, and review their appropriate treatment.

ETIOLOGY

Equinovarus Congenita (Clubfoot)

Postural

Teratologic

Congenital

Pes Planus

Idiopathic

Neuromuscular

Congenital vertical talus

Tarsal coalition

Miscellaneous Disorders

Metatarsus adductus

"Skew" or "Z" foot

Cavovarus deformity

BASIC SCIENCE

Problems in the pediatric foot are typically abnormalities of structure that result in subsequent abnormality in function. This implies either a pathologic special relationship of the bones relative to each other, or an abnormality in the shape of the bones themselves. One and often both situations occur in pediatric foot deformities. The etiology of pediatric foot deformity can usually be categorized into one of three groups: (1) packaging defects, (2) manufacturing defects, or (3) muscle imbalance.

Packaging Defects

An abnormal intra-uterine environment can affect foot position. Previous studies have demonstrated that an equinovarus deformity occurs in lambs born to sheep with oligohydramnios. Although a pediatric foot deformity caused by packaging defects may have an appearance similar to a deformity caused by a congenital or neuromuscular etiology, the packaging defect deformity will be associated only with abnormal relationships between normally formed bony structures. These deformities, therefore, often correct sponta-

Orthopaedic Surgery: The Essentials. Edited by M.E. Baratz, A.D. Watson, and J.E. Imbriglia. Thieme Medical Publishers, Inc., New York © 1999

neously or require only minimal nonoperative treatment. Examples of pediatric foot deformities believed to be caused by packaging defects include "postural clubfoot," calcaneovalgus in newborns, and metatarsus adductus. Although Hippocrates believed congenital equinovarus to have a postural etiology, more recent critical analysis has shown that extrinsic forces alone cannot adequately account for the pathologic anatomy present in true congenital equinovarus.

Manufacturing Defects

Manufacturing defects are thought to be the result of an error occurring during formation of an anatomic region or structure. Manufacturing defects may be associated with a genetic abnormality, may be associated with a syndrome, or may be the result of myelodysplasia. All manufacturing defects are the result of an intrinsic abnormality within the tissues of the foot and often ipsilateral leg, resulting in a more structural deformity that rarely fully corrects with nonoperative treatment alone. Manufacturing defects resulting in isolated idiopathic intrinsic foot deformities are referred to as congenital deformities. Pediatric foot abnormalities associated with identifiable syndromes or other generalized medical disorders are referred to as teratologic deformities.

A descriptive term such as equinovarus is used to label a foot deformity which may be of a postural, congenital, or teratologic origin. Postural, congenital, and teratologic etiologies for the same deformity represent a spectrum of deformity severity. Teratologic equinovarus is associated with disorders such as arthrogryposis, myelodysplasia, and diastrophic dwarfism, and it is a much more rigid and structural deformity than is encountered in the postural or idiopathic congenital clubfoot. Teratologic deformities usually require more radical surgery and have a higher recurrence rate.

Muscle Imbalance

A foot that is normal at birth, without intrinsic pathology or postural deformity, may develop deformity during growth. The most common cause of acquired foot deformity is muscular imbalance. Muscle imbalance is usually associated with an underlying neurologic abnormality and can be associated with a wide variety of causes such as a condition acquired at birth (cerebral palsy), a condition acquired through illness (polio), a condition acquired through neurologic injury (sciatic nerve laceration), or a genetic condition that becomes manifest as the child matures (Charcot-Marie-Tooth). The neuromuscular deformity may be static (cerebral palsy), or progressive (Charcot-Marie-Tooth), making successful treatment of the neuromuscular deformity challenging. An important principle in the treatment of deformity induced by muscle imbalance is that in addition to correction of the deformity, the muscular forces causing the deformity must be balanced if the foot is to remain in an acceptable position.

ANATOMY AND SURGICAL APPROACHES

A thorough knowledge of normal foot anatomy is critical for safe operative treatment of pediatric foot deformities. Making this even more important is the fact that congenital pediatric

foot deformities are often associated with neurovascular anatomic anomalies.

Medial Foot
Relevant anatomy

Bones and joints
Bones encountered on the medial border of the foot include the first metatarsal, cuneiforms, navicular, talus, and calcaneus. Between each pair of bones is a joint named for the articulating bones.

Nerves
The tibial nerve travels beneath the flexor retinaculum and divides into the medial and lateral plantar nerves at approximately the level of the subtalar joint (Fig. 42–1). The medial and lateral plantar nerves travel along the medial and lateral borders of the foot providing motor and sensory innervation.

Vessels
Paralleling the tibial nerve is the posterior tibial artery, which gives rise to the medial and lateral plantar arteries that form a plantar vascular arch. The plantar arterial arch communicates with the dorsal vessels of the foot through the deep plantar artery, which passes between the first and second metatarsals.

Muscles and tendons
Muscles and tendons that power the foot either have their origin outside the foot (extrinsic) or within the foot (intrinsic). The extrinsic muscles of the foot have their origins in the anterior, lateral, posterior, and deep posterior compartments of the leg. Extrinsic muscles of the posterior compartment, which pass medially beneath the medial malleolus as they cross the ankle, and include the flexor hallucis longus (FHL), the flexor digitorum longus (FDL), and the posterior tibialis. The anterior tibialis tendon passes beneath the extensor retinaculum to insert on to the medial aspect of the first metatarsal at its base. Similar to those in the hand, plantar intrinsic muscles are numerous and their origins and insertions complex. A muscle of particular anatomic importance to the surgeon is the abductor hallucis, which has been referred to as the "door to the cage of the foot."

Surgical approach

The medial and plantar regions of the foot are best exposed through an incision over the medial border of the foot extending from approximately the midshaft of the first metatarsal to a point posterior to the medial malleolus, adjusted in length to fit the needs of the procedure. Initial dissection is safely performed distally, where the abductor hallucis is encountered. Deep dissection proceeds posteriorly with relative safety along the dorsal border of the abductor hallucis to the anterior border of the medial malleolus. Here dissection must proceed more careful, as the posterior tibial artery and nerve come in close proximity to the origin of the abductor hallucis. The medial plantar neurovascular bundle is identified and may be followed onto the plantar surface of the foot where it runs parallel to the tendons of the FDL and the FHL through their crossing point known as Henry's knot. Further

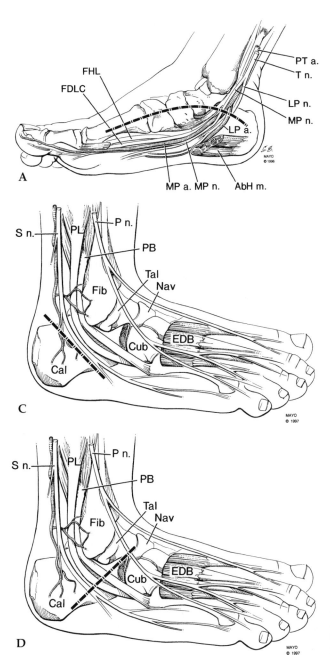

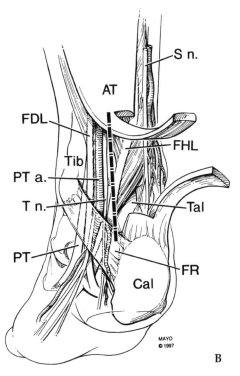

Figure 42–1 Surgical incisions and relevant anatomy of the foot. The dark dashed lines illustrate appropriate skin incision location for each approach. **(A)** The medial neurovascular bundle passes posterior to the medial malleolus, where the tibial nerve and posterior tibial artery divide to form the medial and lateral plantar nerve and artery. The plantar neurovascular bundles pass deep to the abductor hallucis onto the plantar aspect of the foot. (PTa = Posterior Tibial artery; Tn = Tibial nerve; LPn = Lateral Plantar nerve; MPn = Medial Plantar nerve; LPa = Lateral Plantar artery; MPa = Medial Plantar Artery; AbHm = Abductor Hallucis muscle, FDL = Flexor Digitorum Longus). **(B)** Approaching the foot posteriorly is usually done through an incision medial or lateral to the Achilles' tendon. A medial incision allows direct visualization of the medial neurovascular bundle as well as the posterior tibialis, flexor digitorum longus, and flexor hallucis longus muscles. AT, Achilles tendon; S n, sural nerve; FDL, flexor digitorum longus muscle; Tib, tibia; FHL, Flexor hallucis longus muscle; Tal, talus; PT a, posterior tibial artery; T n, tibial nerve; PT, posterior tibialis muscle; Cal, Calcaneus; FR, flexor retinaculum. **(C)** Calcaneal tuberosity osteotomies are performed through a posterior lateral incision, just posterior to, and paralleling, the peroneal tendons. S n, sural nerve; PL, peroneus longus muscle; PB, peroneus brevis muscle; P n, superficial peroneal nerve; Fib, fibula; Tal, talus; Nav, navicular; Cal, calcaneus; Cub, cuboid; EDB, extensor digitorum brevis. **(D)** Triple arthrodeses are performed, and calcaneonavicular coalitions are excised through an anterior lateral incision overlying the sinus tarsi. S n, sural nerve; PL, peroneus longus muscle; PB, peroneus brevis muscle; P n, superficial peroneal nerve; Fib, fibula; Tal, talus; Nav, navicular; Cal, calcaneus; Cub, cuboid; EDB, extensor digitorum brevis.

dissection posteriorly along the abductor hallucis results in exposure of the lateral plantar nerve and vessel as they course between the flexor digitorum brevis and the quadratus plantae muscles. Following either of the neurovascular bundles proximally leads to the common posterior tibial artery and tibial nerve. With the important neurovascular structures isolated and protected, all bones, joints and tendons of the medial foot are accessible.

Posterior Foot and Ankle
Relevant Anatomy

Bone and joints

The distal tibia, talus and calcaneus articulate through the ankle and subtalar joints.

Nerves

The sural nerve is located superficially just lateral to the Achilles tendon, and the tibial nerve passes beneath the flexor retinaculum on the medial aspect of the exposure

Vessels

The lesser saphenous vein accompanies the sural nerve and both cross the ankle in the subcutaneous tissues on the posterolateral aspect of the ankle. The posterior tibial artery and greater saphenous vein are located medially.

Muscles and tendons

The Achilles' tendon is located superficially and directly posterior to the ankle joint, attaching to the calcaneal tuberosity. The FHL, posterior tibialis, and FDL are located in the deep posterior compartment. Originating from the fibula, the FHL crosses from lateral to medial at the level of the ankle. The FDL and posterior tibialis originate from the posterior tibia. All three tendons pass beneath the flexor retinaculum medially. Posterolaterally, the peroneal tendons originate from the Fibula and their tendons pass laterally beneath the lateral malleolus within the peroneal sheath.

Surgical Approach

The posterior approach to the foot and ankle is used most frequently to perform Achilles' tendon lengthening, often with accompanying posterior ankle and subtalar joint release (Fig. 42–1B). The exact configuration of the incision is not important, but it is typically not made directly over the Achilles' tendon to avoid wound healing problems and adhesions between the skin and the underlying tendon. Achilles' tendon lengthening can be performed using a number of methods, the most common being the simple "Z" lengthening. Beneath the divided Achilles' tendon, a layer of fat is encountered. Incision of the fat results in exposure of the fascia of the deep posterior compartment. Dividing the fascia longitudinally exposes the FHL and its origin from the fibula and the posterior tibialis muscle originating from the tibia. The FHL is retracted medially, thus protecting the posterior tibial neurovascular bundle and the posterior ankle and subtalar joint capsule is exposed. Lateral dissection exposes the peroneal tendons and overlying sheath.

Lateral Foot
Relevant Anatomy

Bones and joints

Beneath the distal Nebula lies the talus and calcaneus. Slightly anterior to the Nebula, a fat-filled cavity forms the sinus tarsi. Further anterior is the talonavicular joint, the calcaneocuboid joint, and the variable calcaneonavicular joint.

Nerves

On the dorsal and lateral aspect of the ankle, the terminal branches of the superficial peroneal nerve enter the foot. The sural nerve passes behind the lateral malleolus toward the fifth metatarsal over the lateral border of the foot.

Vessels

In approximately 3% of patients, the terminal branch of the peroneal artery is the dominant blood supply to the dorsum of the foot.

Muscles and tendons

The peroneal tendons pass beneath the distal fibula and course towards the base of the fifth metatarsal where the peroneus brevis inserts. The more superficial peroneus longus passes into the plantar aspect of the foot just posterior to the base of the fifth metatarsal to insert on the neck of the first metatarsal. The extensor digitorum brevis has its origin on the anterior and lateral surface of the distal calcaneus.

Surgical Approach

The lateral foot can be divided into two regions: the lateral foot posterior to the fibula and the lateral foot anterior to the fibula. The posterior region is most frequently exposed for osteotomies of the calcaneus. The incision typically begins proximally and posterior extending distally while paralleling the peroneal tendons (Fig. 42–1C). The sural nerve may be encountered and should be carefully protected. With the sural nerve protected dissection proceeds directly to the bone of the calcaneus. The peroneal sheath and enclosed tendons are elevated anteriorly by subperiosteal dissection, providing adequate exposure for any desired osteotomy.

The anterior region is exposed when performing subtalar arthrodesis, triple arthrodesis, or calcaneal lengthening osteotomy. Exposure of the calcaneocuboid joint, calcaneonavicular joint, and lateral talocalcaneal (subtalar) joint is possible. The approach most frequently used to accomplish this utilizes an oblique incision in line with the skin creases that begins distal to the fibula at the peroneal tendon sheath and extends proximal and anterior to the border of the common toe extensors (Fig. 42–1D). The underlying soft tissue is divided with care to avoid dividing the terminal branches of the superficial peroneal nerve anteriorly and the sural nerve posteriorly. The extensor digitorum brevis is encountered and detached from its origin on the anterior lateral surface of the calcaneus. The sinus tarsi with its fatty tissue contents is thus exposed, and it can be excised if exposure of the subtalar joint is desired. Dissection continues directly to the bone of the calcaneus and talus. Further posterior dissection exposes the posterior facet of the subtalar joint, and more distal dissection provides access to the calcaneonavicular, talonavicular, and calcaneocuboid joints.

Dorsal Foot
Relevant Anatomy

Bones and joints

Bony architecture is subcutaneous, and the bones of the foot are easily palpable. There should be linear alignment of the talus, navicular, and first metatarsal. Deviation from this normal relationship is consistent with pathologic deformity, which is characterized by describing the pattern of abnormal anatomy of the more distal bones with respect to the more proximal bones.

Nerves

The dorsum of the foot receives innervation from 4 nerves; 3 sensory nerves and 1 nerve with both motor and sensory function. The superficial peroneal nerve provides sensory innervation to the dorsum and lateral aspect of the foot, the sural nerve has a sensory distribution over the posterior and lateral border of the foot, and the terminal branches of the saphenous nerve supply sensory innervation to the dorsum and medial aspect of the foot. The deep peroneal nerve arrives on the dorsum of the foot after passing beneath the extensor retinaculum. The deep peroneal nerve provides sensation to the first web space and motor innervation to the extensor digitorum brevis.

Vessels

The anterior tibial artery becomes the dorsalis pedis artery as it passes beneath the extensor retinaculum between the anterior tibialis and extensor hallucis longus tendons. The anterior tibialis artery consistently creates anastamosis with the plantar arterial arch through the deep plantar artery.

Muscles and tendons

Tendons from the extrinsic muscles of the foot enter the dorsum of the foot beneath the extensor retinaculum and include the anterior tibialis, extensor hallucis longus, extensor digitorum longus, and peroneus tertius. The only intrinsic muscle of the dorsal foot, the extensor digitorum brevis, has its primary origin on the anterolateral surface of the calcaneus and spans the sinus tarsi as it inserts distally on the dorsum of the toes.

Surgical Approach

Because the bones and joints of the foot are subcutaneous, a specific single intermuscular interval or internervous plane is not critical. General principles which should be employed for safe exposure include the use of longitudinal incisions and careful medial and lateral retraction of the numerous nerves, vessels and tendons that cross the exposure. This principle may be employed to expose the cuneiforms for anchoring tendon transfers, metatarsals for osteotomies, and phalanges for tendon transfer, capsular release, or arthrodesis.

EXAMINATION
History
Prenatal History

Factors such as oligohydramnios suggest a possible packaging defect.

Perinatal History

Premature birth, fetal distress, and perinatal anoxia suggest cerebral palsy as an underlying cause. The presence of a rigid deformity or an associated syndrome at birth suggests true congenital or teratologic deformity, whereas absence of deformity at birth suggests an acquired deformity.

Family History

A family history of Charcot-Marie-Tooth, Friedreich's ataxia, or other heritable disorders associated with foot deformity allows the physician to predict and characterize the potential for a future disorder. A family history positive for equinovarus congenita identifies patients at risk, as first degree relatives have a 20 to 30 times greater risk of being affected.

Present Illness

Static or progressive deformity.

Physical Examination
Appearance

Normal feet may be quite varied in appearance when suspended in mid-air, but with weight-bearing, normal feet should take on a relatively uniform shape and position. The foot should rest comfortably on the floor, with pressure and skin contact distributed evenly between the heel and the metatarsals. The hindfoot should be in neutral to 5 degrees of valgus, and the medial and lateral borders of the foot should be relatively straight.

Active Range of Motion

Active ROM is helpful to assess muscle balance and its affect on foot position and gait. A foot which can be passively placed in a plantirgrade position, but cannot actively be held in a plantargrade position may benefit from an orthotic to prevent contracture and to improve gait.

Passive Range of Motion

Assessing passive ROM is critical in determining appropriate treatment. Ankle, hindfoot, midfoot and forefoot joint ROM should be appraised. A foot which can be passively placed into a plantirgrade position may often be effectively treated with an orthosis or a tendon balancing procedure. Inability to passively correct a foot deformity implies a soft tissue contracture or abnormality of bone which requires more aggressive treatment; usually surgery of soft tissue or bone.

Flexibility

A rigid foot is unforgiving of shoe wear and orthotics, resulting in a higher incidence of skin breakdown and shoe wear problems. Rigid deformity can rarely be treated successfully by non-operative means alone.

Motor Function and Balance

Motor function can be either an essential component to normal foot function, or a deforming force causing significant deformity and disability. Normal gait requires strong, balanced, and coordinated muscle contraction. Muscle weakness can be supported with an orthosis in a foot with adequate passive ROM, such as the use of an AFO in a limb with a deep peroneal nerve palsy and foot drop. However, muscle imbalance in myelodysplasia typically results in rigid deformity which is appropriately treated by tendon excision, creating a flail foot which can effectively be braced.

Sensation

Protective sensation is essential to avoid chronic skin problems in the foot. Plantar sensation is especially critical. Highly functional patients lacking plantar sensation, such as the sacral level myelodysplasia patient, must have perfect orthotic and shoe fitting, and must be counseled on the importance of asensate foot care.

Gait

Ambulation is a culmination of all of the individual aspects of the physical exam performed to this point. While abnormal findings may be noted on static exam, the significance of these findings is often not apparent until gait is assessed. Gait involves not only muscle strength and joint motion, but also the fine coordination of these functions. In patients with cerebral palsy, normal muscle strength and normal joint motion still may result in a markedly abnormal gait due to muscles contracting out of their appropriate phase of the gait cycle. When assessing gait always provide the patient with an adequate distance to walk. This usually requires that the gait exam be performed in the hallway outside the exam room.

PEARL

In addition to assessing routine gait, have the patient walk on their toes and heels as well. "Stressing" the patient's gait by walking on the toes and heels often provides the examiner with helpful additional information regarding joint ROM, strength, and balance.

AIDS TO DIAGNOSIS

Plain Radiographs

Weight-bearing (or simulated weight-bearing anteroposterior (AP)) and lateral radiographs of the foot are utilized.

Axial "ski jump" view and oblique views are helpful in establishing the diagnosis of tarsal coalition.

Computed Tomography Scans

Computed tomography (CT) scans improve definition of the anatomy of the individual bones and joints as well as the relationship between the individual bones.

Magnetic Resonance Imaging

Magnetic resonance imaging (MRI) permits imaging of fibrous and cartilaginous coalitions.

SPECIFIC CONDITIONS, TREATMENT, AND OUTCOME

Equinovarus Congenita

The primary components of congenital equinovarus deformity include ankle equinus, hindfoot varus, medial and inferior deviation at the talar neck and head, medial subluxation of the navicular on the talar head, and forefoot adduction. Equinovarus describes a deformity that varies in severity from the flexible postural deformity from true congenital clubfoot all the way to the rigid teratologic equinovarus deformity.

Postural Equinovarus

Postural equinovarus deformities may be associated with risk factors that limit intra-uterine space such as oligohydramnios or a firstborn child. Examination demonstrates a resting equinovarus deformity that can be passively corrected to a normal anatomic position.

PEARL

In postural equinovarus, the calcaneus is palpable within the heel pad, in contrast to the "empty" heel pad often palpated in the congenital or teratologic equinovarus deformity.

The postural equinovarus deformity typically responds to gentle repetitive manipulation and retentive casting. Complete correction can usually be achieved in 2 to 4 weeks with surgery rarely being required.

Congenital Equinovarus

Congenital equinovarus represents a manufacturing defect that demonstrates all of the deformity components listed above, but in contrast to postural equinovarus, these components are structural and fixed. The calcaneus is not palpable in the heel pad. Forefoot cavus may also be present and is manifest by a deep, medial skin crease (Fig. 42–2).

Simulated weight-bearing AP and lateral radiographs of the foot should be obtained early in treatment and then repeated during treatment to confirm appropriate correction. The AP radiograph demonstrates a decrease in the normal talocalcaneal angle (angle of Kite) which is usually between

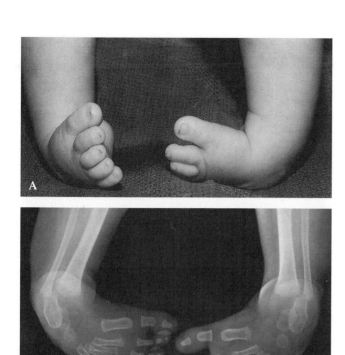

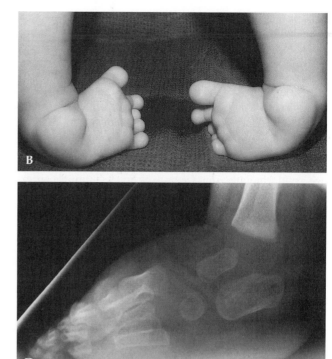

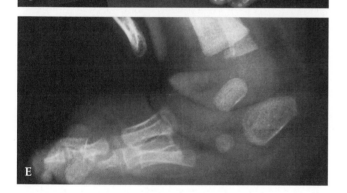

Figure 42–2 Clinical photographs and radiographs demonstrating classic features of equinovarus congenita. **(A)** Marked forefoot supination and adduction is readily apparent in this anterior photograph. **(B)** Hindfoot varus, heel crease, and medial crease are seen on this posterior view. **(C)** An anteroposterior (AP) radiograph demonstrates parallelism between talus and calcaneus (normal angle 20 to 40 degrees) and marked forefoot supination and adduction, as well as medial and posterior skin creases. **(D)** The lateral radiograph also demonstrates parallelism between talus and calcaneus (normal angle 25 to 50 degrees), equinus, and forefoot supination. **(E)** Forceful manipulation has resulted in spurious correction of equinus through the midfoot, resulting in a rocker-bottom foot deformity.

20 and 40 degrees, with the ossification center of the talus often superimposed over that of the calcaneus. The later radiograph demonstrates parallelism between the talus and calcaneus rather than a normal converging pattern. Forefoot cavus is demonstrated by plantarflexed metatarsals with respect to the axis of the talus.

The most efficacious method for treatment of true congenital equinovarus deformity remains somewhat controversial. Kite (1970), Ponseti (1996), and Lovell (1978) have been strong advocates of a nonoperative approach utilizing gentle repetitive manipulation followed by retentive casting for several months. Their reported success in achieving a corrected foot clinically and radiographically has varied from 40 to 95%. The method of manipulation and casting has been described in detail in several articles and texts. Common to each method is initial correction of the forefoot adduction and hindfoot varus. Once the subluxated talonavicular joint has

been reduced and the hindfoot varus corrected, a more concerted effort at correcting the ankle equinus contracture is undertaken.

Overzealous or premature attempts at correcting ankle equinus should be avoided for it may result in one of two common complications. A "rocker-bottom" foot may result in which the plantar structures are overstretched resulting in spurious correction of equinus through the joints of the midfoot instead of the ankle. Alternatively, a "nutcracker" effect may occur in which excessive pressure on the articular surface of the talar dome results in formation of a permanently deformed flat-top talus.

The initial treatment of congenital equinovarus continues to be manipulation and serial casting. Serial casting every 7 to 14 days continues until either full clinical and radiographic correction is achieved or until resistance to further correction is identified, at which time casting is discontinued. At present, only a small percentage of patients are able to be definitively treated by non-operative methods alone. It is unclear if this is due to loss of ability to perform the meticulous manipulation and casting techniques, due to the time constraints found in a busy office practice, poor parental acceptance of long periods of cast immobilization, or a different standard of what should be considered an acceptable correction. Whatever the reason, the majority of true congenital equinovarus deformities, by today's standards, will require some form of surgical intervention to achieve full correction. Surgical intervention typically occurs between age 5 and 8 months. This seems to be an ideal time for surgical intervention because growth has provided structures of adequate size for a safer operation, yet it is early enough for casting to be completed prior to the time the child is ready to stand and walk.

Coleman (1983) and Tachdjian (1972) have stressed the importance of correcting only those structures that are contributing to the deformity present in the foot in question.

PEARL

This selective surgical approach permits the flexibility needed to effectively address the varied severity of deformity encountered in patients with equinovarus congenita, and it reduces the risk of overcorrection, which might otherwise occur if a routine standard procedure was used for all feet.

Surgical correction of congenital equinovarus may successfully be performed through either a posteromedial or more laterally extended Cincinnati incision, as long as access is provided to structures on the medial, posterior, and posterolateral aspect of the foot and ankle.

The comprehensive equinovarus congenita release includes division of subcutaneous tissue to the level of the fascia overlying the abductor hallucis, anterior tibialis tendon, tibionavicular ligament, posterior tibial tendon, posterior tibial neurovascular bundle, and Achilles' tendon. The abductor hallucis is released from the medial border of the foot and retracted with the inferior skin flap. The posterior tibial neurovascular bundle is identified, and the sheaths of the FDL and FHL are opened. Division of the tibionavicular portion of the deltoid ligament is followed by dissection of the posterior tibialis tendon. The posterior tibialis tendon may be released from its insertion on the navicular and plantar aspect of the first metatarsal with preservation of its tendon sheath, or it may be released in a "Z" fashion at the level of the subtalar joint and ankle. The talonavicular joint capsule is then sectioned completely to include the spring ligament. If there is a significant component of cavus associated with the deformity, a plantar release is performed posterior to the neurovascular bundle. The subtalar joint is released at the talonavicular joint and extended posteriorly, taking care to preserve the remaining deep deltoid and interosseous ligaments.

With the medial release completed, the navicular should now be reducible onto the head of the talus, allowing correction of the forefoot abduction. If resistance to reduction is noted, a release of the calcaneocuboid joint may also be required. Care should be taken not to injure the tendon of the peroneus longus as it crosses the lateral side of the calcaneocuboid joint.

Release of the posterior structures begins with the Achilles' tendon. The Achilles' tendon is usually lengthened in a Z fashion. The ends of the tendon are then retracted to facilitate exposure of the posterior ankle and subtalar joints. Posterior structures typically released include the posterior talofibular ligament, the peroneal tendon sheath, the calcaneofibular ligament, the posterior ankle capsule, and the posterior and lateral subtalar joint capsule. While deformity severity determines the extent of surgical release for each foot, at the conclusion of surgery the common goal of returning the ankle and foot to a plantigrade position should be accomplished. With the foot held in a plantigrade position, the tension on the toe flexors can be assessed. If the toes cannot passively be dorsiflexed to a neutral position easily with the foot in a plantigrade position, the toe flexors should be lengthened at the level of the ankle or on the plantar aspect of the foot in the region of Henry's knot.

The use of smooth K-wires to maintain restored bony anatomy varies between surgeons. Several authors recommend that no pins be used whereas other authors suggest as many as four pins. Most surgeons recommend placement of at least one pin through the talus into the navicular, exiting through the dorsum of the foot. Intra-operative AP and Lateral radiographs should be obtained to document corrected bony alignment. The foot is then placed in an above-knee cast in a corrected position for 6 weeks. At this time, pins are removed, and a below-knee cast is applied for 6 weeks. After 3 months in casts, the correction is assessed, and a decision is made whether an orthosis or corrective shoe is indicated.

After neonatal soft tissue release, a recurrent equinovarus deformity usually indicates an incomplete primary release.

PEARL

Recurrent deformity in the face of documented, previous full correction is unusual and implies an unrecognized underlying neurologic disorder.

In the undercorrected clubfoot, it is important to radiographically document the relationship of the navicular on the talar head. If persistent medial navicular deviation is identified, correction is best achieved by a repeat soft tissue release supplemented by a lateral column shortening procedure to facilitate navicular reduction. This can be done at the calcaneocuboid joint as described by Evans (1961), or at the distal calcaneus as described by Lichtblau (1973). If the navicular is reduced on the talar head, then residual hindfoot varus is best corrected by lateral displacement calcaneal osteotomy and forefoot abduction by a closing wedge resection osteotomy of the cuboid.

An overcorrected clubfoot is always iatrogenic in origin and manifests by excessive hindfoot valgus with lateral displacement of the navicular on the talar head. Partial correction can be achieved by a medial displacement calcaneal osteotomy in the immature foot. Definitive treatment at maturity for either residual overcorrected or undercorrected deformity is best accomplished by a triple arthrodesis.

Teratologic Equinovarus

Teratologic equinovarus is resistant to all forms of treatment, tends to recur, and usually requires radical surgery to achieve adequate correction. Patients with teratologic equinovarus deformities have an associated syndrome or systemic medical condition, most commonly arthrogryposis, myelodysplasia, or diastrophic dwarfism. Controversy remains whether manipulation and retentive casting should ever be attempted because it often has no significant effect on the deformity. Initial casting may, however, allow for some stretching of the skin, which can help avoid wound healing problems following surgery.

Radical surgical release is required to achieve a plantigrade foot in teratologic equinovarus deformity. The surgical approach is similar to that used to correct congenital equinovarus deformity; however, instead of tendon lengthening, tendon segments are usually resected. Despite radical release, recurrence frequently occurs. In an attempt to achieve full correction and avoid recurrence, primary talectomy has recently been advocated. Because patients with teratologic deformities rarely function at a high level, the adverse effects of articular incongruity induced by talectomy seem to be of minimal consequence.

Pes Planus

Pes planus is a descriptive term referring to a foot with low longitudinal arch height. The appearance of a low arch may be the result of several different etiologies warranting very different treatment methods. The correct etiology and subsequent appropriate treatment are determined by a thorough knowledge of normal foot development and pertinent information gained through a complete patient history and physical exam, with the addition of selected imaging studies. All normal infants appear to have pes planus. This is due to an abundance of subcutaneous fat filling in the arch and giving a flattened appearance to the sole of the foot.

PEARL

Footprint and radiographic analysis have demonstrated that the spontaneous development of the longitudinal arch usually does not occur until later in the first decade of life.

Idiopathic Pes Planus

Knowing that the height of the longitudinal arch varies considerably in normal patients, some feet will have lower arches than others. When the longitudinal arch is significantly lower than average, this is referred to as a flatfoot (Fig. 42–3). If the patient has no associated neuromuscular disorder; has a flexible and mobile hindfoot, midfoot and forefoot; and has no identifiable iatrogenic or traumatic cause of the deformity, then it is considered to be idiopathic pes planus. In their study of Canadian military recruits, Harris and Beath (1947) reported flexible idiopathic flatfoot to be the source of little or no morbidity in adults. Despite this available information, strong parental and grandparental desire to institute some

form of treatment occasionally pushes the treating physician to prescribe benign, orthotic treatment such as corrective shoes or arch support inserts in asymptomatic idiopathic pes planus. The treating physician must remain aware that neither corrective shoes nor any arch support orthosis has ever demonstrated a significant improvement in formation of a longitudinal arch during childhood when compared to observation alone.

Rarely, the flexible flatfoot becomes painful or the deformity becomes so severe that painful callosities develop over the head of the talus. In these situations a soft custom-molded insert or a molded University of California Berkeley Labs (UCBL) orthosis may provide symptomatic relief. In the very rare patient in whom the deformity remains severe and long-standing, secondary soft tissue contractures may occur resulting in fixed deformity. In patients with persistent debilitating symptoms or fixed contracture, surgical release or lengthening of contracted soft tissues with correction of bony deformity may be indicated. In this rare situation, Achilles tendon lengthening is virtually always required and may be accompanied by medial displacement calcaneal osteotomy or by a calcaneal lengthening procedure. Rarely, triple arthrodesis may be indicated for the adult with debilitating symptoms and severe degenerative changes of the joints of the hindfoot. Although surgical intervention rarely results in complete correction of the deformity, the foot position is typically improved to significantly relieve symptoms and improve shoe wearing.

Neuromuscular Pes Planus

A history of an acquired spastic neurologic condition associated with the development of a flatfoot deformity confirms the diagnosis of neuromuscular pes planus. With triceps surae spasticity the hindfoot tends to be pulled from a balanced position into a valgus position. When a valgus hindfoot deformity occurs the forefoot typically becomes pronated to allow spurious dorsiflexion through the midfoot resulting in a flatfoot deformity. Before fixed ankle equinus develops, the foot may be held in a corrected plantigrade position using an ankle-foot orthosis. The neuromuscular flatfoot will also frequently develop secondary callus formation over the talar head. When significant equinus contracture occurs, the foot will no longer be able to be maintained in an orthosis in a plantigrade position. Surgical correction of the bone and soft tissue deformity is then indicated.

Soft tissue deformity is typically corrected through Achilles tendon and occasionally peroneal tendon lengthening. Correction of the hindfoot valgus can be performed through several operations including subtalar arthrodesis, medial displacement calcaneal slide osteotomy or calcaneal lengthening osteotomy. Subtalar arthrodesis results in permanent correction for the older child who is a household ambulator. The procedure of single screw stabilization with extra-articular arthrodesis as described by Dennyson and Fulford (1972) is preferred. Calcaneal slide and calcaneal lengthening osteotomies preserve motion but are less reliable at maintaining correction. Subtalar arthrodesis, calcaneal slide, and calcaneal lengthening are all performed through a lateral approach to the calcaneus, all require approximately 4 to 6 weeks non–weight-bearing post-operatively, and up to 8 to

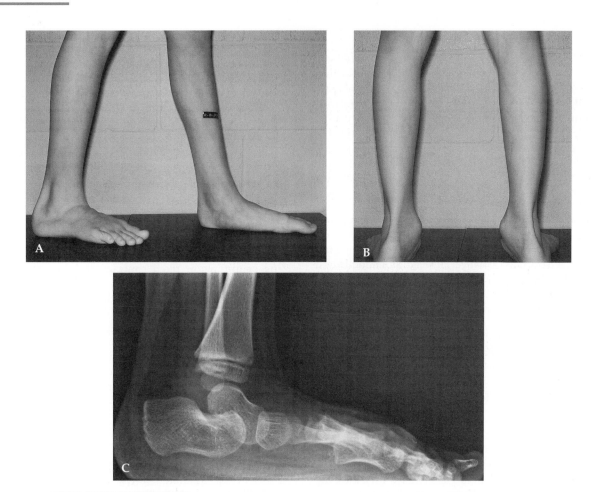

Figure 42–3   Severe idiopathic pes planus with corresponding clinical and radiographic deformity. **(A)** Clinical photographs demonstrating a convex lateral border to the right foot, complete absence of a medial arch in the right foot, with a prominent talar head and associated overlying pressure sore. **(B)** Extreme hindfoot valgus is easily seen from the posterior view. **(C)** The lateral view demonstrates excessive convergence between talus and calcaneus, a negative angle of Meary between talus and first metatarsal, with complete parallelism and overlap of the metatarsals.

12 weeks of cast immobilization. Rarely, in the older patient with longstanding severe hindfoot valgus and associated degenerative changes, corrective triple arthrodesis may be indicated.

Congenital Vertical Talus

An uncommon deformity, congenital vertical talus is the result of a manufacturing defect and has also been referred to as congenital convex pes valgus (Fig. 42–4). Unlike idiopathic pes planus or pes planus associated with a neuromuscular etiology, congenital vertical talus is a rigid deformity present at birth. The hallmark of congenital vertical talus is dorsal dislocation of the navicular from its normal articulation on the head of the talus with associated hindfoot equinus and valgus. In severe cases, the cuboid is also dorsally dislocated from its articulation with the calcaneus. The etiology of congenital vertical talus is unknown but the deformity is typically associated with other coexisting developmental neuromuscular or skeletal anomalies such as spinal dysraphism, myelodysplasia, arthrogryposis, or sacral agenesis. Isolated true congenital vertical talus without associated anomalies is rare.

Clinically, the foot exhibits a convex plantar surface with the hindfoot in fixed equinus and the forefoot held in dorsiflexion. The affected foot is frequently smaller than normal. The head of the talus can be palpated as a prominence on the sole of the foot, with a depression palpable just proximal to the tarsal navicular over the anterior aspect of the ankle. Of significance is that this depression persists when foot is plantarflexed, indicating a fixed dorsal dislocation of the talonavicular joint. In addition to weight-bearing AP and lateral radiographs of the foot, gentle stress plantar flexion and dorsiflexion lateral radiographs assist in making the proper diagnosis. In congenital vertical talus, the navicular remains dorsally dislocated on the neck of the talus in the plantarflexion radiograph, and the dorsiflexion radiograph confirms fixed hindfoot equinus. If the navicular has not yet ossified, the dislocation is manifest by the first metatarsal aligning with the neck or dome of a plantarflexed talus instead of aligning with the talar head and neck. In severe deformities, the calcaneocuboid joint also remains dislocated.

The value of nonoperative treatment by serial casting in true congenital vertical talus remains controversial. Although some stretching of soft tissues and skin on the dorsum of the foot by serial manipulation and plantarflexion casting can

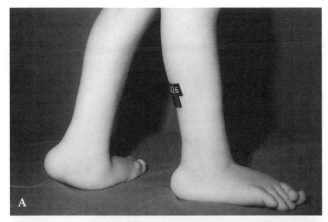
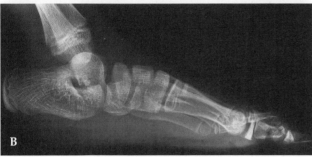

Figure 42–4   Congenital vertical talus. **(A)** Occasionally referred to as the Persian slipper foot, congenital vertical talus represents the most severe pes planus deformity. **(B)** The Lateral radiograph demonstrates complete dislocation of the navicular from the head of the talus and hindfoot equinus.

facilitate later surgery, the deformity cannot be definitively treated by manipulation and casting alone. The true congenital vertical talus deformity will require surgical correction. The key pathologic components that must be corrected include: (1) reduction of the talonavicular joint, (2) reduction of the calcaneocuboid joint, and (3) correction of hindfoot valgus and equinus. This will require access to structures on the dorsal, medial, posterior, and lateral aspects of the foot.

Although staged procedures have been advocated historically, a one-stage comprehensive release is currently preferred. Reduction of the talonavicular joint is often the first component of the deformity to be addressed. This is done through a standard posteromedial approach or a Cincinnati incision with complete talonavicular capsule release. A lengthening of the anterior tibialis tendon and long toe extensor tendons is required and is best performed above the ankle joint through a separate anterior tibial incision. Posteriorly, the Achilles tendon and, occasionally, the peroneal tendons are lengthened. A complete posterior ankle capsulotomy is required. The talonavicular joint is reduced and held in position with a smooth K-wire. The talonavicular capsule and spring ligament are repaired. The posterior tibial tendon may need to be reefed under the navicular. The lengthened tendons are then sutured at an appropriated resting tension. In an older child, a concomitant subtalar arthrodesis may be required to maintain hindfoot alignment. A well-padded cast is applied which is removed 6 weeks postoperatively, at which time the pin is extracted. At that time a decision can be made regarding the need for further casting or orthotic wear.

Congenital vertical talus deformity associated with myelodysplasia and arthrogryposis represents a more rigid deformity with an increased tendency for recurrence. This deformity may require primary talectomy to achieve adequate correction and may require prolonged bracing to maintain alignment. Less severe deformities and deformities treated before 1 year of age have a lower incidence of recurrent deformity.

Tarsal Coalition

Unlike the pediatric foot deformities discussed thus far, the patient with tarsal coalition usually does not present until adolescence (Fig. 42–5). Although tarsal coalition can be acquired by iatrogenic, traumatic, or inflammatory etiology, the vast majority of tarsal coalitions are developmental in origin and are the result of failed fetal tarsal bone separation. A strong genetic influence has been noted in several studies. Leonard (1974) studied 98 first-degree relatives of patients with tarsal coalition and found that 39% of first-degree relatives also had a coalition, compared with an estimated prevalence in the general population of less than 1%. It is important to note that very few of the first-degree relatives with tarsal coalition were symptomatic. The coalition may be fibrous, cartilaginous or bony. The coalition may involve in decreasing order of frequency, the calcaneonavicular joint, the talocalcaneal joint, the talonavicular joint, and the calcaneocuboid joint. Talonavicular and calcaneocuboid coalitions are seen most commonly in terminal limb deficiencies and are rarely found in otherwise normal limbs. The diagnosis is rarely made in infancy because patients are not symptomatic. With skeletal maturation, the coalition will progress from fibrous to cartilaginous to bony coalition, resulting in the onset of pain during adolescence in a limited number of patients.

Patients with tarsal coalition often present with a flattened longitudinal arch. The most common finding on physical examination is significant limitation in subtalar joint range of motion, which may be associated with spastic guarding of the peroneal tendons.

PEARL

Having the patient with pes planes stand on the toes should result in reconstitution of the longitudinal arch. Failure to reconstitute the arch suggests a rigid deformity and the presence of a tarsal coalition.

Suspected coalitions should be evaluated with imaging studies to obtain a diagnosis. Plain film radiographs are often able to document a coalition if the appropriate view is obtained. AP and lateral weight-bearing radiographs frequently show secondary signs of tarsal coalition which include bony traction spurs at the talonavicular joint, narrowing of the subtalar joint, and blunting of the lateral talar process. An ossified extension of the anterior calcaneus toward the navicular, the so-called anteater sign may also be seen. A calcaneonavicular coalition is usually best visualized on a 45-degree oblique projection. A middle facet talocalcaneal coalition is best demonstrated on a P-A axial ski jump

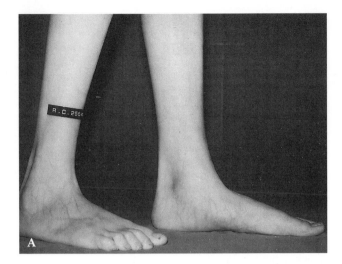

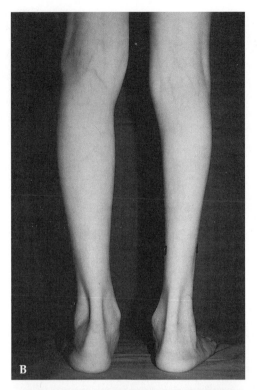

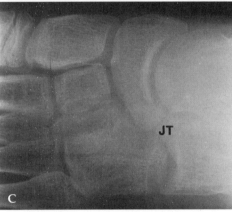

Figure 42–5 Clinical photographs and radiographs demonstrating classic features of calcaneonavicular tarsal coalition. **(A)** Decreased medial longitudinal arch is present, which does not reconstitute when standing on toes. **(B)** Slight increase in hindfoot valgus is seen. **(C)** The AP radiograph is rarely diagnostic.

view taken at 40 to 50 degrees from the horizontal (Fig. 42–6). If a coalition cannot be identified by plain radiography but is strongly suspected based on history and physical exam, a CT scan in the coronal and axial planes can be very helpful in demonstrating its presence. An MRI will assist in identifying a pure fibrous or cartilaginous coalition. The CT scan may also be used to map the size of the coalition and to demonstrate early associated hindfoot joint degeneration, which is important in determining appropriate treatment.

In patients with symptomatic tarsal coalitions, restriction of physical activity accompanied by nonsteroidal anti-inflammatory medication may result in resolution of pain. Patients not responding to this treatment regime often experience significant pain relief when temporarily placed in a below-knee cast. In patients not responding to these regimen, operative treatment may be required. Patients with calcaneonavicular coalition or with a middle facet talocalcaneal coalition of limited size and without associated degenerative changes at the

remaining hindfoot joints can be treated by complete excision of the coalition with interposition of local muscle or fat into the defect. For calcaneonavicular coalitions, the operation is performed through a lateral sinus tarsi approach. Care must be taken not to open or destabilize the talonavicular joint capsule. Middle facet talocalcaneal coalitions are best resected through a medial approach to the hindfoot. If excessive hindfoot valgus is present, a concomitant medial displacement calcaneal osteotomy should also be performed. Following coalition excision, the patient is placed in a below-knee non–weight-bearing cast for 3 to 4 weeks. The cast is then removed and active subtalar motion is initiated. Progressive weight-bearing is allowed as subtalar motion increases.

True recurrence of the coalition is rare, but inadequate excision will result in recurrence of symptoms. Medial facet talocalcaneal coalitions greater than 50% of the surface area of the posterior facet of the subtalar joint should probably not be excised. In this situation and in mature patients who

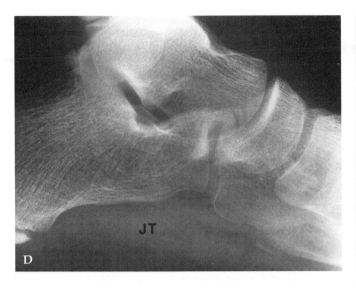

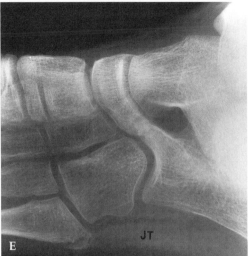

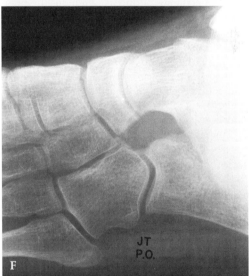

Figure 42–5D *(cont.)* **(D)** The lateral radiograph may demonstrate the "anteater sign," or prominent anterior calcaneal process, which is suggestive of calcaneonavicular coalition. **(E)** An oblique radiograph best demonstrates a calcaneonavicular coalition. **(F)** An intra-operative oblique radiograph confirms adequate resection of the coalition.

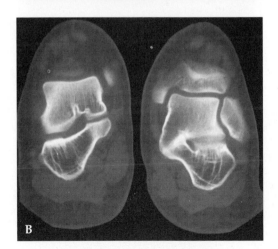

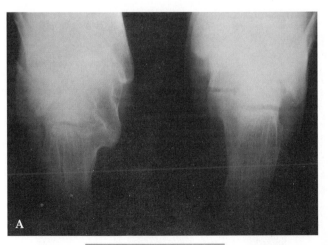

Figure 42–6 Specific imaging techniques are often required to demonstrate talocalcaneal coalition. **(A)** Posteroanterior axial ski jump view is the best plain radiographic view for imaging talocalcaneal coalition at the middle facet. The middle facet may be completely obliterated as in the left foot in this radiograph, or it may more subtly angle towards or converge with the posterior facet. The right foot represents the normal, parallel relationship between posterior and middle facets of the subtalar joint. **(B)** Computerized tomography performed in the coronal plane clearly demonstrates the talocalcaneal coalition.

have developed significant degenerative changes in the associated hindfoot joints, a triple arthrodesis remains the best treatment.

Miscellaneous Disorders

Metatarsus Adductus

Metatarsus adductus is a common foot disorder often encountered at birth and in early infancy. The disorder is differentiated from other more severe deformities by the fact that the adducted forefoot can almost always be passively corrected to a normal position. Metatarsus adductus usually resolves spontaneously during the first 2 years of life. It is unclear if stretching, manipulation, corrective shoewear, or casting actually affects the natural history of the deformity. If the deformity is passively correctable, most physicians are content to observe metatarsus adductus, often despite pressure from the family for treatment. If the deformity is not passively correctable, gentle manipulation and retentive casting for 4 to 6 weeks will usually correct the deformity. Straight-last or reverse-last shoes may also be used as a benign form of intervention, but again there is no evidence that they significantly affect the natural history of the condition. Rarely one encounters a patient older than 2 years of age with persistent, isolated, forefoot adduction that is not passively correctable. In this unusual patient, metatarsal osteotomies performed through two or three small, dorsal incisions definitively corrects the deformity. Care must be taken not to injure the physis at the base of the first metatarsal. The osteotomies are held in place with percutaneous K-wires. The foot is immobilized in a non-weight-bearing below-knee cast for 4 weeks until the pins are removed, and then in a weight-bearing cast for an additional 4 weeks. Tarsal-metatarsal joint capsulotomies have been described for persistent metatarsus adductus but can be associated with later tarsometatarsal joint abnormalities, and, therefore, are not recommended.

The "Skew" or "Z" Foot

The skewfoot, an uncommon and challenging deformity, is a foot in which fixed excessive hindfoot valgus and forefoot adduction are present (Fig. 42–7). Although the natural history of the skew foot is unknown, the deformity appears to be less likely to spontaneously correct and more likely to become symptomatic than the natural histories associated with the individual deformities of which it consists. Because patients with a skewfoot deformity rarely have symptoms during their juvenile years, the combination of significant hindfoot valgus and forefoot adduction often results in painful callosities and marked difficulty with shoewear during juvenile or early adolescent development.

The AP radiograph in skewfoot demonstrates an increased talocalcaneal angle, lateral displacement of the navicular on the head of the talar head and forefoot adduction which results in a subsequent "Z" alignment to the medial column of the foot.

Treatment for one component of the deformity risks exacerbation of the other component. Considering the condition's unknown natural history and potential for deformity exacerbation encountered with manipulation, treatment of the skewfoot is rarely instituted before age 2 or 3 years. In patients with severe deformity, gentle manipulation and retentive casting with appropriate molding to prevent worsening hindfoot valgus may be cautiously undertaken. Operative treatment is reserved for the symptomatic skewfoot in

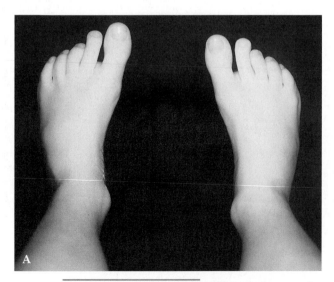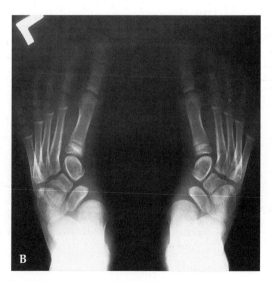

Figure 42–7   Corresponding clinical photographs and plain radiographs demonstrate bilateral skewfoot deformity. **(A)** Prominent medial malleoli due to hindfoot valgus, with forefoot adduction result in the unique appearance of the skewfoot. **(B)** Plain radiographs confirm the clinical diagnosis, demonstrating divergence of talus and calcaneus, lateral subluxation of the navicular from the head of the talus, and marked metatarsus varus.

which there is no reasonable nonoperative treatment option. Ideally, surgery is not performed until the patient is age 6 to 8 years, and it must address all major components of the deformity in the forefoot and hindfoot. Forefoot correction may be achieved through a combination of medial cuneiform opening wedge osteotomy with or without metatarsal osteotomies. A closing wedge osteotomy of the cuboid may also be required to achieve full forefoot correction. Hindfoot valgus may be corrected by calcaneal lengthening osteotomy, calcaneal slide osteotomy, or subtalar arthrodesis. A medial reefing and capsular plication of the talonavicular joint to correct the lateral navicular displacement may also be required. Frequently, there is an associated Achilles' tendon contracture that becomes apparent with correction of the hindfoot and also requires lengthening. No long-term results are available following skewfoot treatment, so prognosis is unclear.

Cavovarus deformity

Cavovarus deformity is most frequently an acquired foot abnormality associated with an underlying neurological disorder. Unilateral cavovarus deformity has been linked to spinal cord pathology and spinal dysraphism. Bilateral foot deformity is frequently seen in association with Charcot-Marie-Tooth Disease and Friedreich's ataxia (Fig. 42–8).

> ### PEARL
>
> **A thorough evaluation for an underlying neurological disorder should be undertaken in each patient prior to correction of the foot deformity.**

The exact mechanism causing a cavovarus deformity is unclear but is related to muscle imbalance of the foot. Weakness of the intrinsic muscles and the anterior tibialis with long toe extensor compensation has been proposed. As the long toe extensor muscles attempt to assist with ankle dorsiflexion, the metatarsal heads are forced into plantarflexion by the dorsiflexed proximal phalanges which results in eventual shortening and contracture of the plantar fascia and a plantarflexion deformity of the first metatarsal. The fixed plantarflexed attitude of the forefoot then forces the hindfoot into varus during weight-bearing. The hindfoot varus will initially remain flexible but with time will develop structural changes and become fixed.

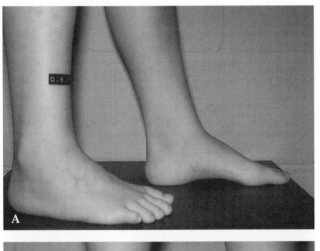
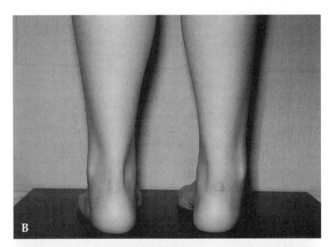
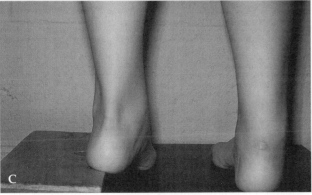
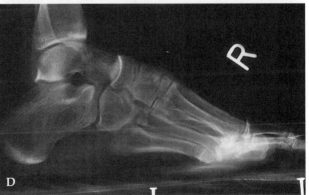

Figure 42–8   Bilateral cavovarus deformity is most commonly associated with Charcot-Marie-Tooth Disease or Friedreich's ataxia. **(A)** Significant increase in medial longitudinal arch height is apparent. **(B)** The plantarflexed first metatarsal pushes the hindfoot into varus, creating what has been referred to as the tripod effect. **(C)** The lateral (Coleman) block test neutralizes the effect of the plantar flexed first metatarsal, allowing a flexible hindfoot to assume a normal or valgus position. **(D)** The lateral radiograph demonstrates minimal overlap between talus and calcaneus, a positive angle of Meary between talus and first metatarsal, and widely converging first and fifth metatarsals, all consistent with cavovarus deformity.

Clinical presentation usually results from concern over an increased longitudinal arch height with secondary skin callosities and shoewear difficulties. A detailed history should be taken to identify possible heritable disorders. Physical examination reveals the forefoot to be pronated with excessive plantar flexion of the first metatarsal, a high longitudinal arch, and a contracted plantar fascia. The hindfoot is in varus when the position of the heel is inspected from behind the standing patient. Callosities are often present over the prominent first metatarsal head and base of the fifth metatarsal. Associated claw-toe deformities are often noted. A thorough neurologic evaluation should be performed with any motor weakness or muscle imbalance being documented. Determination of hindfoot flexibility is critical to determining appropriate treatment. This is done by performing the lateral (Coleman) block test (Fig. 42–8c). The lateral rays and the heel of the involved foot are placed on a 1-inch block with the first metatarsal hanging freely over the edge which negates its effect on the hindfoot. A flexible hindfoot will assume a neutral or slightly valgus position, which can be documented photographically or radiographically. A rigid hindfoot will remain in varus.

Weight-bearing AP and lateral radiographs of the cavovarus foot demonstrate a decrease in the talocalcaneal angle on the AP radiograph indicative of hindfoot varus. Hindfoot varus is also apparent on the lateral radiograph by visualization of the tarsal canal of the subtalar joint. Forefoot cavus is demonstrated by plantarflexion of the first metatarsal in relation to the axis of the talus—the so-called angle of Meary. A Meary angle of 5 degrees or greater indicates forefoot cavus.

Nonoperative treatment and attempts at bracing have no effect on the cavovarus deformity. Correction of the deformity can only be achieved through operative intervention. Appropriate operative treatment is individualized to each affected foot and depends upon hindfoot flexibility and the presence of muscle imbalance. In all cases of cavovarus deformity, correction of the forefoot will be required and should be performed first. The forefoot will always demonstrate a plantarflexion deformity of the first metatarsal and a contracture of the plantar fascia. This is corrected by a radical plantar release through a medial approach to the foot. The plantar fascia and origins of the quadratus plantae, abductor hallucis, flexor digitorum brevis, and abductor digiti minimi are extraperiosteally released from the calcaneus. In patients less than age 9 years, the first metatarsal can usually be corrected by casting, placing the forefoot in supination and the hindfoot in slight valgus. In older patients, the first metatarsal is usually fixed in plantar flexion and a dorsal closing wedge osteotomy performed at the base of the first metatarsal, avoiding injury to the physeal plate, is required to achieve full correction.

Attention is next directed at the hindfoot. If the hindfoot is flexible, it should return to a neutral or slightly valgus position during weight-bearing following correction of the forefoot. If the hindfoot is fixed in varus, then it also requires surgical correction. A lateral displacement calcaneal osteotomy through a posterior extension of the medial incision can be performed. In patients with more severe deformity, a triple arthrodesis may be required to achieve correction.

After correction of the forefoot and hindfoot deformities and a plantigrade foot position has been reestablished, tendon lengthenings and/or transfers may be performed to regain muscle balance about the foot. The corrected foot is immobilized in a below-knee cast for 6 weeks with weight-bearing delayed for 3 to 4 weeks.

Long-term prognosis and the risk of recurrence following surgical correction depends on the underlying neuromuscular disorder. The corrected cavovarus foot must continue to be followed for later development of muscle imbalance requiring further correction. Recent reports of long-term results in the treatment of cavovarus foot deformity demonstrate that feet requiring triple arthrodesis tend to develop accelerated degenerative arthritis in the joints of the ankle and midfoot. Current surgical treatment of cavovarus deformity is, therefore, aimed at early forefoot correction and muscle balancing in an attempt to prevent the development of hindfoot rigidity requiring correction by arthrodesis.

SELECTED BIBLIOGRAPHY

CHAMBERS RB, COOK TM, COWELL HR. Surgical reconstruction for calcaneonavicular coalition: evaluation of function and gait. *J Bone Jt Surg.* 1982;64A:829–836.

COLEMAN SS, CHESTNUT WJ. A simple test for hindfoot flexibility in the cavovarus foot. *Clin Orthop Rel Res.* 1977; 123:60–62.

COLEMAN SS. *Complex foot deformities in children.* Philadelphia, PA: Lea and Febiger; 1983:23–113.

CRAWFORD AH, MARXEN JL, OSTERFELD DL. The Cincinnati incision: a comprehensive approach for surgical procedures of the foot and ankle in childhood. *J Bone Jt Surg.* 1982;64A:1355–1358.

DENNYSON WG, FULFORD GE. Subtalar arthrodesis by cancellous grafts and metallic internal fixation in children. *J Bone Jt Surg.* 1976;58B:507–510.

DRENNAN JC, SHARRARD WJW. The pathological anatomy of convex pes valgus. *J Bone Jt Surg.* 1971;53B:455–461.

EVANS D. Relapsed club foot. *J Bone Jt Surg.* 1961;43B:722–733.

GOULD N. MORELAND M, ALVAREZ R. TREVINO S. FENWICK J. Development of the child's foot. *Arch Foot Ankle.* 1989;9:241–245.

HARRIS RI, BEATH T. *Army Foot Survey: An Investigation of Foot Ailments in Canadian Soldiers.* Vol 1. Ottawa: National Research Council of Canada; 1947.

HENRY AK. *Extensile Exposure.* Baltimore, MD: Williams & Wilkins, 1970:303.

HIPPOCRATES. *Loeb Classical Library.* Vol III. London: Heinemann; 1927.

HOLLINSHEAD WH. *Anatomy For Surgeons.* Vol III. Philadelphia, PA: Harper and Row; 1982:878.

KITE JH. The treatment of congenital clubfoot. *JAMA* 1932;99:1156.

KITE JH. Conservative treatment of the resistant recurrent clubfoot. *Clin Orthop Rel Res.* 1970;70:93–110.

LAAVEG SJ, PONSETI IV. Long-term results of treatment of congenital club foot. *J Bone Jt Surg.* 1980;62A:23–31.

LEORNARD MA. The inheritance of tarsal coalition and its relationship to spastic flatfoot. *J Bone Jt Surg.* 1974;56B: 520–526.

LICHTBLAU S. A medial and lateral release operation for club foot: a preliminary report. *J Bone Jt Surg.* 1973;55A: 1377–1384.

LOVELL WW, PRICE CT, MEEHAN PL. The foot. In: Lovell WW, Winter RB, eds. *Pediatric Orthopaedics.* Philadelphia, PA: J.B. Lippincott; 1978.

MORRISSY RT. *Atlas of Pediatric Orthopaedic Surgery.* Philadelphia, PA: J.B. Lippincott; 1992:747.

MOSCA VS. Flexible flatfoot and skewfoot. *J Bone Jt Surg.* 1995;77A:1937–1945.

PAULOS L, COLEMAN SS, SAMUELSON KM. Pes cavovarus: review of a surgical approach using selective soft-tissue procedures. *J Bone Jt Surg.* 1980;62A:942–953.

PONSETI IV. *Congenital Clubloot; Fundamentals of Treatment.* Oxford: Oxford University Press; 1996.

ROBERTS J. The inheritance of lethal muscle contracture in sheep. *Journal of Genetics* 1929;21.

STAHELI LT, CHEW DE, CORBETT M. The Longitudinal Arch. A study of eight hundred and eighty-two feet in normal children and adults. *J Bone Jt Surg.* 1987;69-A:426–428.

TACHDJIAN MO. *Pediatric Orthopedics.* Philadelphia, PA: W.B. Saunders; 1972.

TURCO VJ. Resistant congenital club foot: one-stage posteromedial release with internal fixation. A follow-up report of a fifteen-year experience. *J Bone Jt Surg.* 1979;61A:805–814.

VANDERWILDE R, STAHELI LT, CHEW DE, MALAGON V. Measurements on radiographs of the foot in normal infants and children. *J Bone Jt Surg.* 1988;70A:407–415.

WENGER DR, MAUDLIN D, SPECK G, MORGAN D, LEIBER RL. Corrective shoes and inserts as treatment for flexible flatfoot in infants and children. *J Bone Jt Surg.* 1989;71A: 800–810.

SAMPLE QUESTIONS

1. The most likely etiology for congenital equinovarus deformity (clubfoot) is:

   (a) intra-uterine posture

   (b) abnormal tendon insertions

   (c) nerve and muscle dysfunction

   (d) arrest in development

   (e) manufacturing defect

2. A 6-year-old child presents with a progressive cavovarus foot deformity secondary to a tethered cord. Hindfoot flexibility and the need for a concomitant hindfoot procedure at the time of surgical correction is best determined by:

   (a) response to shoe wear modifications

   (b) weight-bearing radiographs of the foot

   (c) lateral (Coleman) block test

   (d) computerized axial tomography

   (e) ankle arthrography

3. A 3-year-old child is seen for treatment of flatfeet. There is a family history of flatfeet, and the mother wants something done to prevent her son from having flatfeet as an adult. The patient is asymptomatic and demonstrates a low medial arch in stance without increased hindfoot valgus. A good arch is demonstrated with toe stance. The subtalar joint motion is normal. After discussion of this condition's natural history with the mother you recommend:

   (a) prophylactic arch supports

   (b) prescription shoewear

   (c) observation

   (d) exercise program

   (e) subtalar arthrodesis

4. A newborn child presents with arthrogryposis and bilateral clubfoot deformities. The deformities of the feet will most likely:

   (a) resolve spontaneously

   (b) require extensive surgical release

   (c) correct with modified shoewear

   (d) require only Achilles tendon lengthening

   (e) respond to serial casting

5. A 12-year-old male presents with a 1-year history of recurrent ankle sprains and activity related pain in the left foot. Physical examination show normal ankle motion but painful restricted subtalar motion. The hindfoot is noted to be in mild increased valgus, and the medial arch is low. The patient has tried arch supports in his shoes without relief of symptoms. Radiographs confirm an osteochondral calcaneonavicular coalition. Treatment at this time is best achieved by:

   (a) UCBL orthoses

   (b) naviculo-cuneiform fusion with posterior tibial tendon rerouting

   (c) peroneal tendon lengthening

   (d) osteochondral bar resection and muscle interposition

   (e) triple arthrodesis

Chapter 43

The Pediatric Spine

Vishwas R. Talwalkar, MD and Gregory A. Mencio, MD

Pediatric spine disorders comprise a broad spectrum of pathology including developmental and infectious diseases, deformity, and traumatic injury. Evaluation and treatment of pediatric spine disorders can be challenging and require a thorough understanding of etiology and pathomechanics. Back pain in children requires diligent evaluation because treatable pathology is often present. Spine injury is uncommon in children but requires systematic evaluation to differentiate unstable injuries that require surgical stabilization.

ETIOLOGY

Scoliosis

Scoliosis is the most common pediatric spine deformity and is defined as lateral deviation of the spine with rotation. The etiology is unknown in roughly 80% of patients. Congenital anomalies and neuromuscular disease are the etiologies in the other 20%. Idiopathic scoliosis is further subdivided by age of onset into infantile (up to 3 years), juvenile (4–10 years), and adolescent (> 10 years) types.

Infantile scoliosis occurs in children less than 3 years old and is more common in males. It is the least common type of scoliosis; however, its true incidence remains undefined. A multifactorial etiology has been proposed that includes intrauterine molding and supine postnatal positioning. Children with infantile scoliosis often have other abnormalities including inguinal hernias, developmental dysplasia of the hip, congenital heart disease, and developmental delay.

Juvenile scoliosis occurs in children between 4 and 10 years of age. The majority of juvenile curves occur in girls. The etiology is undefined, but is believed to be similar to that for adolescent idiopathic scoliosis.

Eighty percent of idiopathic scoliosis occurs in adolescents between the ages of 10 and 17. In spite of extensive research, the etiology remains elusive. It commonly occurs in families suggesting a genetic cause. Abnormalities of equilibrium reaction, serum melatonin levels, platelet calmodulin levels, and intervertebral disc collagen have been observed.

Congenital scoliosis is caused by vertebral anomalies present at birth. Progressive deformity occurs with growth. Vertebral anomalies occur early in the first trimester of pregnancy. Approximately 80% of congenital deformities are due to either failure of formation of a portion of the vertebra or failure of segmentation between vertebrae. The remainder are of either mixed or unclassifiable pathology (Fig. 43–1). The true incidence of congenital scoliosis is not known, and deformity can first present at any age. Isolated vertebral anomalies occur sporadically with no apparent inheritance pattern. There is a 5 to 10% risk of vertebral anomaly in siblings of a child with multiple vertebral anomalies and spina bifida cystica.

Intraspinal pathology is common in congenital scoliosis. Diastematomyelia is a sagittal split in the spinal cord or cauda equina caused by an osseous, fibrous, or cartilaginous process arising within the spinal canal and is present in up to 20% of patients with congenital scoliosis. Other intraspinal abnormalities include syringomyelia, teratomas, lipomas, fibrous bands, tight filum terminale, ectopic roots, and dural adhesions, which may be present and cause compression or tethering of the spinal cord. With growth, scoliosis occurs because the tethered or compressed spinal cord cannot migrate cephalad.

Orthopaedic Surgery: The Essentials. Edited by M.E. Baratz, A.D. Watson, and J.E. Imbriglia. Thieme Medical Publishers, Inc., New York © 1999

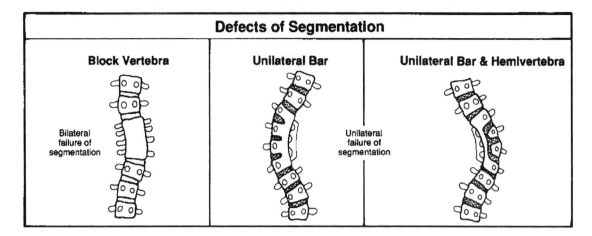

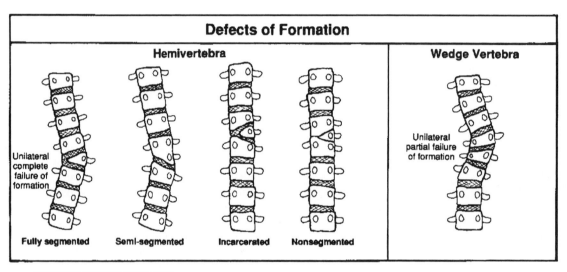

Figure 43–1   Classification of congenital scoliosis. Redrawn from McMaster MJ. Congenital scoliosis. In: Weinstein SL, ed. *The Pediatric Spine: Principles and Practice.* New York, NY: Raven Press; 1994:229.

Accompanying congenital abnormalities are frequent and include Klippel-Feil syndrome; genitourinary, cardiac, and gastrointestinal anomalies; and musculoskeletal defects such as Sprengel's deformity, longitudinal deficiencies of the appendicular skeleton, and defects in the axial skeleton. The VATER (Vertebral and Ventriculoseptal anomalies, Anal atresia, Tracheoesophageal fistula and Radial aplasia) syndrome comprises the rare, simultaneous occurrence of congenital vertebral and ventriculoseptal anomalies, anal atresia, tracheoesophageal fistula, and radial aplasia.

PEARL

Thorough evaluation for coexisting anomalies and intraspinal pathology is essential in children with congenital spine deformity.

Scoliosis may occur in neuromuscular diseases such as cerebral palsy, myelomeningocele, Duchenne's muscular dystrophy, spinal muscle atrophy, and Friedrich's ataxia. Neurologic deficit, spasticity, and muscular dystrophy associated with each of the neuromuscular diseases can result in muscle imbalance that can lead to scoliosis, especially during rapid growth spurts. Postural and balance disorders can aggravate the muscle imbalance. Children with myelomeningocele have diastematomyelia and other vertebral anomalies that contribute to scoliosis. Neuromuscular scoliosis may be neuropathic or myopathic (Table 43–1). The prevalence of spinal deformity in various neuromuscular diseases ranges from 25% in cerebral palsy to almost 100% in post-traumatic infantile quadriplegia (Table 43–2).

Scheuermann's Disease

Scheuermann's disease is a structural hyperkyphosis of the thoracic spine associated with vertebral body and intervertebral disc abnormalities. Proposed etiologies include osteopenia, growth hormone excess, repetitive trauma, osteochondrosis, and familial predisposition; however, no widely accepted etiology has been defined. The incidence is between 0.5 and 8% of healthy individuals. Males and females are affected equally. There is no defined inheritance pattern, but the deformity tends to affect multiple members of a family.

TABLE 43–1   Classification of Neuromuscular Scoliosis

Neuropathic	Myopathic
Upper motor neuron	Arthrogryposis
Cerebral palsy	Muscular dystrophy
Spinocerebellar degeneration	Duchenne
Friedreich's ataxia	Limb-girdle
Charcot-Marie-Tooth	Facioscapulohumeral
Roussy-Levy	Fiber-type disproportion
Syringomyelia	Congenital hypotonia
Spinal cord tumor	Myotonia dystrophica
Spinal cord trauma	
Lower motor neuron	
Poliomyelitis	
Other viral myelitides	
Traumatic	
Spinal muscle atrophy	
Werdnig-Hoffmann	
Kugelberg-Welander	
Dysautonomia (Riley-Day syndrome)	

Reproduced with permission from Goldstein LA, Waugh TR. Classification and terminology of scoliosis. *Clin Orthop.* 1973;93:18.

TABLE 43–2   Prevalence of Spinal Deformities in Various Neuromuscular Disorders

Diagnosis	Prevalence
Cerebral palsy	25%
Myelodysplasia	60%
Spinal muscular atrophy	67%
Friedreich's ataxia	80%
Duchenne's muscular dystrophy	90%
Traumatic paralysis (< 10 years)	100%

Reproduced with permission from Lonstein JE, Renshaw TS. Neuromuscular spine deformities. In: Griffin PP, ed. AAOS. Instructional Course Lectures. St. Louis, MO: CV Mosby; 1987:285.

Spondylolysis and Spondylolisthesis

Spondylolysis is a defect of the pars interarticularis and may be unilateral or bilateral. Isthmic spondylolysis is characterized by elongation or deficiency of the pars interarticularis. It is the most common form of spondylolysis that occurs in children and adolescents. Though not proven, it is widely believed to be a stress fracture of the pars interarticularis caused by repetitive motion and loading. Dysplastic spondylolysis is due to congenital deficiency of the facet joints. Spondylolysis due to trauma, tumor, or infection is very rare.

Isthmic spondylolysis is believed to be acquired and not congenital. The prevalence among adults in the United States is approximately 5%. Spondylolysis is more common in white males, but it is more likely to progress to symptomatic spondylolisthesis in females. The high incidence of pars interarticularis defects within families, in patients with spina bifida occulta, and in certain Eskimo tribes strongly suggests a genetic predisposition.

Spondylolisthesis is translation in any direction of one vertebral body over another. In children and adolescents, there is typically anterior translation of the spondylotic relative to a normal, more caudal vertebra. The vertebral arch of the normal vertebra can cause symptomatic nerve root or dural compression.

Spondylolisthesis occurs only in ambulatory individuals and is believed to be due to progressive displacement of a pars interarticularis stress fracture. Gymnasts, swimmers, divers, and football linemen more commonly develop symptomatic spondylolysis and spondylolisthesis. This is presumably because their sports require repetitive hyperextension and hyperlordotic motion and loading of the pars interarticularis. Forty-five percent of patients with Scheuermann's kyphosis have associated spondylolisthesis presumably because of compensatory lumbar hyperlordosis.

Cervical Spine

Torticollis is characterized by head tilt and rotation. There are both congenital and acquired causes that can be osseous or nonosseous. (Table 43–3) The most common form is congenital muscular torticollis (congenital wryneck). It is caused by contracture of the sternocleidomastoid muscle. The contracture is believed to be due to pre- or perinatal insult to the sternocleidomastoid muscle with localized compartment syndrome and fibrosis. Intra-uterine crowding has been implicated given that 20% of children with congenital muscular torticollis have developmental hip dysplasia. Other causes of torticollis include pharyngitis, gastroesophageal reflux (Sandifer's syndrome), ocular dysfunction, inflammatory disease, posterior fossa tumors, basilar impression, atlanto-occipital deformity, atlanto-axial rotatory displacement, unilateral absence of atlas, familial cervical dysplasia, and spinal neoplasms.

TABLE 43–3   Causes of Torticollis

Congenital	Acquired
Occipitocervical anomalies	Basilar impression, secondary
Basilar impression, primary	Idiopathic/inflammatory
Atlanto-occipital anomalies	Atlantoaxial rotary displacement, subluxation, fixation
Asymmetry of occipital condyles	Neurogenic
Unilateral absence of C-1 facet	Spinal cord tumors
Odontoid anomalies (aplasia, hypoplasia, os	Cerebellar tumors, posterior fossa tumors
odontoideum)	Syringomyelia
Klippel-Feil syndrome	Ocular dysfunction
Familial cervical dysplasia	Bulbar palsies
Pterygium colli	Arnold-Chiari malformation
Congenital muscular torticollis	Inflammatory
	Cervical adenitis, Grisel's syndrome, retropharyngeal
	abscess
	Juvenile rheumatoid arthritis, rheumatoid arthritis
	Disc space calcification
	Tuberculosis
	Neoplasm
	Osteoid osteoma
	Aneurysmal bone cyst
	Sandifer's syndrome

Reproduced with permission from Loder RT, Hensinger RN. Developmental abnormalities of the cervical spine. In: Weinstein SL, ed. *The Pediatric Spine: Principles and Practice.* New York, NY: Raven Press; 1994:397.

PITFALL

The differential diagnosis of torticollis is extensive. Idiopathic torticollis is, therefore, a diagnosis of exclusion.

Atlantoaxial rotatory displacement is a rotational subluxation or dislocation of the C1-2 articular facets and a common osseous cause of torticollis. The etiology is poorly understood, and likely multifactorial. The condition may occur spontaneously or following trauma, surgery, or any inflammatory condition of the neck or pharynx.

Atlanto-axial instability is due to either osseous or ligamentous insufficiency. Odontoid hypoplasia occurs when odontoid formation is defective and may be partial or complete. Failure of fusion of the odontoid to the body of C-2 is os odontoideum. An occult fracture of the odontoid process is thought to be the cause of os odontoideum.

The most common ligamentous cause of atlanto-axial instability is Down's syndrome. These children have an underlying collagen defect. Sixty percent of children with Down's syndrome have occiput-C1 instability, and 20% have C1-2 instability. However, only 2 to 3% of patients become symptomatic.

Klippel-Feil syndrome traditionally described the clinical triad of short neck, limited cervical motion, and low posterior hairline. The syndrome now refers to any congenital failure of segmentation of the cervical spine. The true incidence of Klippel-Feil syndrome is unknown, but is estimated to range from 2 to 6 per 1000 live births. Klippel-Feil syndrome is commonly associated with other well-defined syndromes including fetal alcohol syndrome, Goldenhar's syndrome, and VATER syndrome. Associated musculoskeletal anomalies include congenital scoliosis, Sprengel's deformity, cervical ribs, developmental hip dysplasia, clubfoot, and defects of the radius.

Basilar impression is an abnormality of the craniocervical junction in which the base of the skull invaginates into the cranium, which in turn "settles" caudally onto the upper cervical spine. "Crowding" within the foramen magnum may cause brainstem or vertebral artery compression or occlusion of cerebrospinal fluid flow. Primary basilar impression is a developmental defect and is often associated with craniovertebral anomalies such as occipitalization of the atlas, Klippel-Feil syndrome, odontoid defects, hypoplasia of the atlas, skeletal dysplasias such as Morquio's syndrome, spondyloepiphyseal dysplasia, and achondroplasia. Neural element abnormalities such as Chiari malformation, syringobulbia, and syringomyelia may occur.

Secondary basilar impression is an acquired deformity associated with systemic disorders that cause softening of the occipital bone. Etiologic conditions include rickets, osteomalacia, osteogenesis imperfecta, neurofibromatosis, renal osteodystrophy, rheumatoid arthritis, and trauma.

Back Pain

Infection is the most common cause of back pain in children less than 5 years old but can occur in children of any age.

Diskitis and osteomyelitis can both occur and often coexist. *Staphylococcus aureus* is the most common infecting organism.

Scheuermann's kyphosis is the most common cause of thoracic back pain in the adolescent population. Males are more commonly affected. Spondylolysis and spondylolisthesis are the most common causes of lumbar pain in the adolescent. Lumbar Scheuermann's disease is a less common source of pain.

Herniated nucleus pulposus occurs much less frequently in children and adolescents than in adults, but can cause severe low back and radicular leg pain. Apophyseal ring avulsion causes similar symptoms but occurs much less frequently than herniated nucleus pulposus. Flexion with axial compression causes avulsion of the vertebral end plate from the vertebral body. The end plate displaces into the spinal canal to cause compression. The posteroinferior rim of L-4 is the most common site. Apophyseal ring avulsion classically occurs in adolescent, male weight lifters.

Inflammatory arthropathies such as juvenile rheumatoid arthritis and ankylosing spondylitis may also cause back pain in children. Juvenile rheumatoid arthritis usually produces cervical pain but can occasionally cause low back pain. Ankylosing spondylitis causes low back and sacroiliac pain.

Certain benign and malignant neoplasms have a predilection for the spine and can cause back pain. Osteoid osteoma, osteoblastoma, and aneurysmal bone cysts occur in the posterior elements of the spine and can cause pain and neurologic compression. Eosinophilic granuloma affects the vertebral body and may be part of a systemic disease such as Hand-Schüller-Christian, Letterer-Siwe, or histiocytosis X. Leukemia, Ewing's sarcoma, osteosarcoma, and chordoma are the most common primary malignant tumors of the spine.

Neuroblastoma is the most common metastatic neoplasm, and astrocytoma is the most common spinal cord tumor.

PITFALL

Do not "write off" back pain in children and adolescents. It rarely occurs without underlying pathology.

Trauma

Spine fractures are rare in children and constitute fewer than 3% of all pediatric fractures. Blunt trauma caused by falls and motor vehicle accidents is the most common cause of injury. Other common mechanisms of spine fractures in children are sports injuries, gunshot wounds, and child abuse. Roughly half of all spine injuries occur in the cervical spine. Of patients with a spine fracture, 50% have another axial or appendicular fracture, and 20% have an associated spinal cord injury.

BASIC SCIENCE

Embryology of the Spine

The vertebral column formation begins in the fourth week of gestation and continues until the third decade of life. Its development comprises three stages (Fig. 43–2). The first is the mesenchymal stage. Mesenchymal cells derived from sclerotomes of adjacent somites arranged along the longitudinal axis of the embryo organize into three regions during the fourth week of development. The first region surrounds

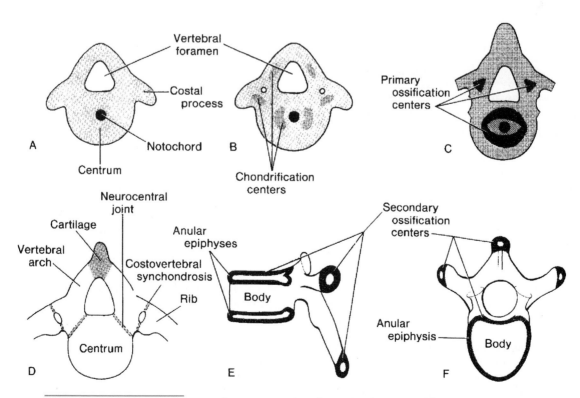

Figure 43–2 Schematic diagram illustrating embryologic development of the vertebral column.

the notochord and becomes the intervertebral discs and centra, which will become vertebral bodies. The second region is posterior to the first, surrounds the neural tube, and produces the vertebral arch. The third region develops peripherally from the first two along the body wall and becomes the ribs.

The cartilaginous stage begins during the sixth week of embryonic development. Chondrification centers develop in the centra and vertebral arches. Spinous and transverse process precursors develop from the vertebral arches. These chondral elements fuse to become a cartilaginous spinal column.

The bony stage begins near the end of the embryonic period when primary ossification centers appear in the centrum and in each half of the posterior arch of each vertebra. At birth, the typical vertebra consists of three bony parts joined by cartilage. The posterior arch elements fuse by 5 years of age, and the arch fuses with the centrum, or vertebral body, by age 8. Thus, the majority of radial growth of the spinal canal is completed by the end of the first decade. After puberty, annular apophyses appear at the vertebral endplates, and secondary ossification centers appear at the tips of the transverse and spinous processes. Completion of vertebral ossification occurs by age 25.

Development of the atlas (C-1) and axis (C-2) differs from the remainder of the spinal column (Fig. 43–3). The anterior ossification center of C-1 does not appear until approximately 9 to 12 months of age, and its three ossification centers fuse by age 6 years. Therefore, the spinal canal at this level reaches adult size at a relatively younger age than the remaining spinal canal.

Development of the odontoid process of C-2 begins with formation of the dens. The dens results from fusion of two ossification centers at approximately 3 years of age. The dens fuses to the centrum at the dentocentral synchondrosis by age 7. A secondary ossification center called the os terminale develops cephalad to the dens by age 10 years and fuses to the dens by age 13.

PEARL

The timing of the appearance and fusion of these ossification centers must be considered when evaluating the dens for hypoplasia or trauma.

The longitudinal growth rate of the spine varies throughout childhood. Growth is fairly rapid during the first 5 years of life at an average rate of 0.85 cm per segment per year. It slows to 0.05 cm per segment per year between 5 and 10 years of age. Growth accelerates to 0.11 cm per segment per year during the adolescent growth spurt. The spinal column reaches approximately 50% of adult height by age 1 and 80% by age 10 years.

ANATOMY AND SURGICAL APPROACHES

The vertebral column consists of 7 cervical, 12 thoracic, and 5 lumbar vertebra. Each vertebra consists of a cylindrical vertebral body anteriorly and a posterior bony ring that contains the spinal cord and cauda equina. The posterior bony ring is comprised of the pedicles that project posteriorly from either side of the posterior wall of the vertebral body. The pedicles are bridged posteriorly by the lamina, which complete the ring. A transverse process arises at the junction of each pedicle and lamina and projects laterally. The articular facets are located at this junction. The orientation of the articular facets varies along the vertebral column, but generally the superior articular facet faces posteriorly, cephalad, and laterally, and the inferior articular facet faces anteriorly, caudad, and medially. Each thoracic vertebra also has an articular facet for its corresponding rib on the proximal transverse process. The spinous process arises from the posterior midline junction of the laminae and projects posteriorly.

The vascular supply arises from segmental arteries that arise from the aorta anteriorly. Each segmental artery courses along the wall of its respective vertebral body and is encountered in the "valley" between intervertebral discs. The anterior spinal artery arises from the cervical vertebral arteries and provides collateral circulation to the anterior spinal cord.

Posterior Approach

The posterior approach to the spine is useful for posterior spinal fusion, deformity correction, posterior decompression, and infection or neoplasm of the posterior elements. A longitudinal skin incision is made along the line of the spinous processes so that it is in line with any deformity that is present. The spinous processes are approached through sharp dissection of the subcutaneous tissue. A cartilaginous apophysis is present on each spinous process until adolescence; therefore, sharp dissection should not be directly to bone. Each apophysis is split sharply, and the paraspinal musculature is elevated by subperiosteal dissection from the underlying spinous processes, laminae, and transverse processes. Dissection between transverse processes must be cautious to minimize blood loss from the inevitable injury to muscular branches of the paravertebral arteries.

Anterior Approach

The anterior approach to the spine is useful for anterior spinal fusion, anterior decompression, and infection or neoplasm of the vertebral body. It may also be necessary for deformity correction. Anterior approaches are less commonly used in children than in adults.

Cervical Spine

The anterior approach to the cervical spine is performed via a transverse incision on the left neck. The left recurrent laryngeal nerve is less susceptible to traction injury than the right. Blunt dissection through subcutaneous tissue is performed to approach the thin platysma muscle. The fascia is incised in line with the skin incision, and the fibers of the platysma are split longitudinally. The underlying deep cervical fascia is incised along the anterior margin of the sternocleidomastoid muscle, which is retracted posteriorly. The pretracheal fascia is incised in the interval between the trachea and the carotid sheath, which are retracted anteriorly and posteriorly, respectively, to expose the underlying longus colli muscles on either side of the anterior cervical spine. The periosteum over the vertebral bodies between the left and right longus colli is incised and elevated to expose the cervical vertebral bodies.

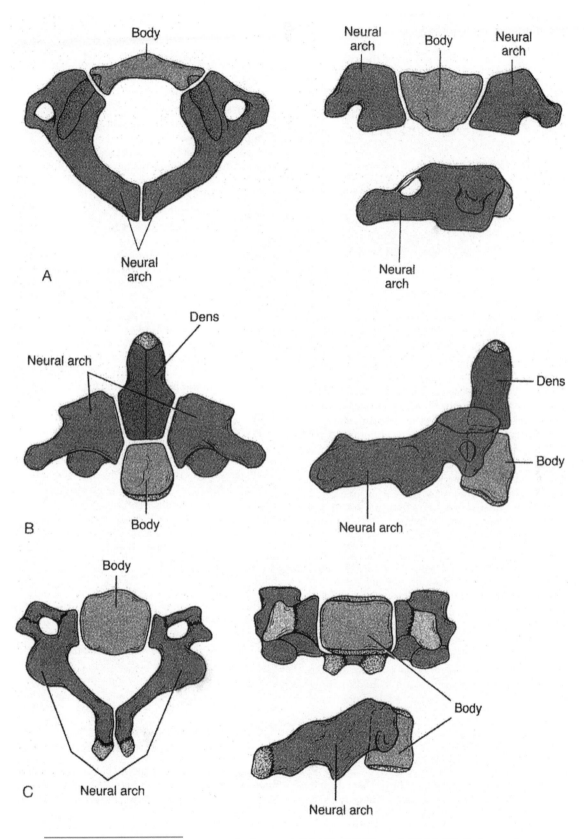

Figure 43–3   Ossification centers and physes of C-1 **(A)**, C-2 **(B)**, and C3-L5 **(C)**. Redrawn from Sullivan JA. Fractures of the Spine in Children. In: Green NE, Swiontkowski MF, eds. *Skeletal Trauma in Children.* Philadelphia, PA: WB Saunders; 1993:284.

Thoracic Spine

The anterior approach to the thoracic spine is performed with the patient in the semi-Fowler position with the arms above the head. The incision is made over the rib corresponding to the vertebral body to be approached. Sharp dissection through the subcutaneous tissue is performed to approach the lattisimus dorsi, which is incised over the rib. The underlying serratus anterior is incised over the rib. The periosteum over the rib is incised along the rib, and the superior margin of the rib is exposed by subperiosteal dissection because the neurovascular structures lie on the inferior, deep surface of the rib. The ribs are spread apart or the rib can be resected after careful subperiosteal exposure of the entire rib. The lung is deflated and retracted anteriorly. The parietal pleura is incised over the anterior vertebral column, taking care to avoid the stellate ganglia posteriorly and the vascular structures anteriorly. The segmental arteries can be ligated as necessary.

Lumbar Spine

A midline transabdominal approach or flank retroperitoneal approach can be used to expose the anterior lumbar spine. The former is better for the lower lumbar spine and the latter for the upper lumbar spine. The retroperitoneal approach can expose more of the lumbar spine, but is more difficult.

The transabdominal approach begins with a midline incision over the lower abdomen. Sharp dissection through the subcutaneous tissue exposes the rectus abdominis fascia. The midline linea alba is incised and the rectus abdominis split longitudinally to expose the peritoneum. The peritoneum is incised longitudinally and the abdominal contents retracted out of the way to expose the underlying aorta, vena cava, and their bifurcations. The bifurcations are at L-4. The periosteum over the sacral promontory is incised up to the bifurcation to expose L-5 and S-1. More cephalad exposure requires mobilization of the iliac arteries and veins.

A flank incision just inferior and parallel to the 12th rib is used for the retroperitoneal approach. The patient is positioned in semi-Fowler or lateral decubitus. Sharp dissection through the subcutaneous tissue exposes the external oblique, which is incised in line with the skin incision. The underlying internal oblique and transversalis muscle are each incised similarly to expose the peritoneum. The peritoneum is mobilized anteriorly by blunt dissection posteriorly to expose the psoas muscle and the genitofemoral nerve laterally and the aorta medially. The segmental arteries are ligated to allow mobilization of the aorta medially to expose the underlying vertebral bodies.

EXAMINATION

Important elements of the history include birth, growth, and developmental history; the presence, duration, intensity, and character of pain; factors that either worsen or relieve the pain; daily and athletic activity levels; neurologic deficits; associated musculoskeletal or neuromuscular disorders; and age of onset and manner in which the abnormality was discovered. The menstrual and pubertal history are helpful for predicting spinal deformity progression in adolescents.

A thorough general physical examination of the patient should precede focused examination of the spine to rule out associated abnormalities that would suggest a syndrome. The presence of a cutaneous lesion, hairy patch, or foot deformity may be the only sign of intraspinal pathology.

Leg lengths should be measured, and an evaluation of standing posture and gait performed. Neurologic examination should include manual motor testing, dermatomal sensation testing, and an assessment of appendicular and abdominal reflexes.

Examination of the spine begins with assessment of standing and forward-bending alignment and mobility in all planes. Elevation of the one side of the thorax relative to the other when the patient is bent forward suggests rotatory deformity of the spine and can be easily quantitated with an inclinometer. Rotation greater than 5 degrees warrants radiographic evaluation. A plumb line dropped from the C-7 spinous process while the patient is standing should fall into the gluteal cleft. Pelvic or shoulder girdle obliquity, a flank crease, arm-to-flank asymmetry, and a rib prominence all suggest curvature or rotation of the spine. Palpation of all the spinous processes may reveal a subtle deformity.

Areas of pain should be palpated for tenderness. Percussion over the spine may elicit pain when infection or tumor is present. The patient should be asked to perform any maneuvers that reproduce or exacerbate the pain. The trunk and extremities should be carefully evaluated for any evidence of trauma. Hamstring tension should be assessed because it is frequently increased in spondylolysis.

Spine trauma evaluation presents a unique challenge. Evaluation of a very young, unconscious, postconcussive, frightened, or otherwise uncooperative patient can be quite challenging. Mass reflex withdrawal movements in the infant may be indistinguishable from voluntary movements. In the cooperative, communicative individual, the mechanism of injury and of the presence of any transient or ongoing neurologic symptoms should be determined. Facial bruising, evidence of seatbelt trauma, unexplained hypotension, and a history of cardiopulmonary arrest suggest an occult injury. Palpable step-off between adjacent spinous processes, tenderness to palpation, crepitus, ecchymosis, torticollis, neck rigidity, painful range of motion, and neurologic deficit all require thorough investigation. Detailed neurologic examination including rectal exam and bulbocavernosus reflex testing should be performed initially, and frequently. Serial neurologic examinations are necessary in children without initial deficit because delayed neurologic deterioration can occur.

AIDS TO DIAGNOSIS

Radiographs of the spine should be obtained after a thorough interview and examination. Standing posteroanterior and lateral radiographs of the thoracolumbar spine are taken for spine deformity. The Cobb technique is used to measure scoliosis in the frontal plane and kyphosis and lordosis in the sagittal plane. (Fig. 43–4) A line is drawn parallel to the end plate of the most cephalad vertebra and the most caudad vertebra that define the curve. Another line is drawn perpendicular to the first line for both vertebra. The angle subtended by

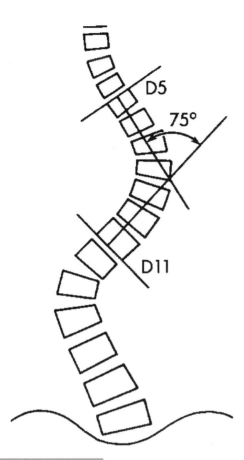

Figure 43–4 Diagram of the Cobb method for measuring frontal plane deformity (scoliosis) of the spine. The most tilted vertebral bodies at the superior and inferior ends of the curve are identified. Lines are drawn across the endplates. The angle of the intersecting perpendicular lines represent the magnitude of the curve. Redrawn from Cobb JR. Outline for the study of scoliosis. In: Edwards, JW, ed. *AAOS Instructional Course Lectures*, Vol. 5. Ann Arbor, MI: American Academy of Orthopaedic Surgeons; 1948;5:266.

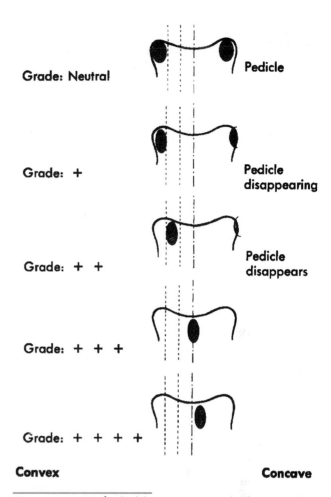

Figure 43–5 Method of determining vertebral rotation. Vertebral body is divided into segments and rotation is graded based on the location of the convex pedicle. Redrawn from Nash CL Jr, Moe JH. A study of vertebral rotation. *J Bone Jt Surg.* 1969;51A:224.

the second lines is the Cobb angle. Higher Cobb angles signify greater curvature. Two Cobb angles must be measured for double or S-shaped curves.

Vertebral rotation can be graded, but not quantitated, by the position of the pedicles (Fig. 43–5) The pedicles should appear symmetric and equidistant from the midline when there is no rotation. The pedicles appear asymmetric, and one pedicle will approach the midline of the patient as rotation of a vertebral body increases.

Anteroposterior (AP) and lateral radiographs of the affected portion of the spine should be obtained when back pain is present. Back pain in children and adolescents is almost always associated with spinal pathology.

The Risser sign describes the extent of iliac apophysis fusion to the ilium and is a radiographic indicator of skeletal maturity (Risser, 1958). Absence of formation of the iliac apophysis is Risser stage 0 and complete fusion is Risser stage 5. Risser stages 1 through 4 describe increasing formation and fusion of the iliac apophysis to the ilium.

The Technetium bone and single photon emission computed (SPECT) scans are more sensitive for bony pathology than plain radiographs. Neither is very specific, however. Computerized axial tomography offers better resolution than plain radiographs to confirm or localize osseous pathology of the spinal column. Magnetic resonance imaging (MRI) is the best imaging modality for evaluating the spinal canal, intervertebral discs, and neural elements.

Radiographic evaluation of spine trauma should include plain radiographs. Injured and poorly imaged levels require computed tomography (CT) scan evaluation. The upper cervical spine often requires a CT scan from the occiput to C-2. Magnetic resonance imaging is necessary in any child with neurologic deficit. Dynamic studies such as flexion and extension views should not be done acutely or in any child who is not completely awake and alert.

Laboratory studies may be necessary if infection or inflammatory disease is suspected. Blood cultures may be positive when osteomyelitis is present but are rarely positive in discitis. Similarly, the white blood cell count is often normal in discitis.

SPECIFIC CONDITIONS, TREATMENT, AND OUTCOME

Idiopathic Scoliosis

The Scoliosis Research Society has proposed a classification of spinal deformity that helps guide treatment (Table 43–4). Scoliosis is further classified by the level of the apical vertebrae and the direction and shape of the curve.

Infantile

Infantile scoliosis typically affects the thoracic spine and is convex to the left. Infantile scoliosis may be divided clinically into two types: resolving and progressive. Progressive curves occur in 10 to 30% of cases. The remainder are resolving. They do not progress and usually improve. Infantile scoliosis requires vigilant clinical and radiographic followup for at least 6 months following diagnosis to rule out progression.

Progression is inversely related to flexibility and directly related to curve magnitude at the time of diagnosis. Curves greater than 35 degrees or with secondary curve formation will likely progress. The rib-vertebral angle difference (RVAD) is helpful in predicting progression (Fig. 43–6). Curves with a Cobb angle greater than 35 degrees and a RVAD greater than 20 degrees are considered progressive until proven otherwise.

Resolving and flexible curves with a RVAD less than 20 degrees are followed with serial standing radiographs every 4 to 6 months until the curve resolves. A progressive curve is treated initially with casting to gain correction and then by prolonged bracing. Brace treatment must be continued until curve progression is halted or resolution occurs.

Surgical treatment is indicated when the curve progresses in spite of brace treatment. Options include spinal fusion and subcutaneous rodding. Arthrodesis with or without instrumentation must be performed anteriorly and posteriorly to minimize the risk of "crankshafting," wherein continued growth anteriorly with posterior fusion leads to recurrence of deformity. Arthrodesis effectively halts curve progression at the expense of truncal height because fusion causes cessation of vertebral growth.

Subcutaneous rodding theoretically permits some growth. Anterior arthrodesis of the apical vertebrae is combined with subcutaneous placement of an expandable rod on the concave side of the curve. This may control the curve during growth until posterior spinal arthrodesis with instrumentation can be performed at a more suitable age (> 10 years). Hooks are placed only in the most cephalad and caudal vertebrae of the curve. Arthrodesis is not performed. The curve is corrected by distracting the rod. The rod must be lengthened periodically as the child grows. Bracing is continued throughout treatment. The advantages of preserving vertebral growth and truncal proportion are offset by the protracted course and a high complication rate.

Juvenile

Juvenile scoliosis is typically characterized by a right thoracic pattern. Lumbar curves are rare and less likely to progress. The majority of thoracic juvenile scoliosis curves progress. Progression is slow until the age of 10 and greatly accelerates during the adolescent growth spurt.

The risk and rapidity of progression requires thorough neurological examination and aggressive treatment. Curves with Cobb angles less than 20 degrees can be followed with serial radiographs every 4 to 6 months until skeletal maturity. Curves between 20 and 30 degrees that have not progressed more than 10 degrees between serial radiographs should be followed at 3-month intervals. Curves greater than 20 degrees that have progressed more than 10 degrees and all curves larger than 30 degrees should be treated with a brace to prevent progression.

The effectiveness of brace treatment is followed with standing AP radiographs taken in the brace every 3 to 4 months. Part-time bracing (16 hours/day) may be considered after a year of full-time brace wear, if curve progression is halted. Brace treatment is continued until the patient reaches skeletal maturity. Occasionally, brace treatment can be discontinued prior to skeletal maturity if the curve is reduced to less than 20 degrees and remains stable. However, close clinical and radiographic followup should continue until growth ceases, and brace treatment reinstituted if progression resumes.

Surgical treatment is indicated for curve progression in the brace beyond 45 degrees. Surgery should be delayed until the patient is close to skeletal maturity to maximize truncal height and eliminate the need for anterior arthrodesis. Anterior arthrodesis is necessary in young patients to avoid deformity progression due to the crankshaft phenomenon.

Younger children with curves greater than 60 degrees may

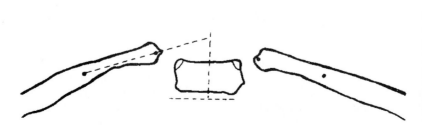

Figure 43–6 Method of determining the rib vertebral angle as described by Mehta. The difference between the rib vertebral angle measured on the convex and concave sides of the apical vertebra is the rib vertebral angle difference (RVAD); a RVAD less than 20 degrees is thought to be predictive of curve progression. Redrawn from Koop SE. Infantile and juvenile scoliosis. *Orthop Clin North Am.* 1988;19:332.

TABLE 43–4 Classification of scoliosis

Idiopathic	Neurofibromatosis
Infantile (0 to 3 years)	Mesenchymal
Resolving	Marfan's
Progressive	Homocystinuria
Juvenile (4 years to puberty onset)	Ehlers-Danlos
Adolescent (puberty onset to epiphyseal closure)	Other
Adult (epiphyses closed)	Traumatic
Neuromuscular	Fracture or dislocation (nonparalytic)
Neuropathic	Postradiation
Upper motor neuron lesion	Other
Cerebral palsy	Soft tissue contractures
Spinocerebellar degeneration: Friedreich's,	Postempyema
Charcot-Marie-Tooth, Roussy-Levy	Burns
Syringomyelia	Other
Spinal cord tumor	Osteochondrodystrophies
Spinal cord trauma	Achondroplasia
Other	Spondyloepiphyseal dysplasia
Lower motor neuron lesion	Diastrophic dwarfism
Poliomyelitis	Mucopolysaccharidoses
Traumatic	Other
Spinal muscular atrophy	Tumor
Myelomeningocele (paralytic)	Benign
Dysautonomia (Riley-Day)	Malignant
Other	Rheumatoid disease
Myopathic	Metabolic
Arthrogryposis	Rickets
Muscular dystrophy	Juvenile osteoporosis
Duchenne (pseudohypertrophic)	Osteogenesis imperfecta
Limb-girdle	Related to lumbosacral area
Facioscapulohumeral	Spondylolysis
Congenital hypotonia	Spondylolisthesis
Myotonia dystrophica	Other
Other	Thoracogenic
Congenital	Post-thoracoplasty
Failure of formation	Post-thoracotomy
Partial unilateral (wedge vertebra)	Other
Complete unilateral (hemivertebra)	Hysterical
Fully segmented	Functional
Semisegmented	Postural
Nonsegmented	Secondary to short leg
Failure of segmentation	Due to muscle spasm
Unilateral (unilateral unsegmented bar)	Other
Bilateral (bloc vertebrae)	
Mixed	
Associated with neural tissue defect	
Myelomeningocele	
Meningocele	
Spinal dysraphism	
Diastematomyelia	
Other	

Reproduced with permission from Goldstein LA, Waugh TR. Classification and terminology of scoliosis. *Clin Orthop.* 1973;93:18.

require subcutaneous rodding to control the curve until they are old enough for arthrodesis. Older children should undergo posterior spinal fusion with instrumentation combined with anterior arthrodesis or instrumented anterior spinal arthrodesis alone. Anterior arthrodesis is indicated in skeletally immature children at risk for developing crankshaft phenomenon. The risk is greatest in children less than 10 years old, those in whom the triradiate cartilage remains open, and those who have not reached the period of peak growth velocity.

Adolescent

Adolescent idiopathic scoliosis is defined as a curve greater than or equal to 10 degrees. Lesser curves are considered normal variants. The prevalence of curves less than 30 degrees is approximately 2 to 3 per 100 and is equally distributed between genders. The prevalence of curves greater than 40 degrees is much higher in females at a ratio of approximately 3 or 4:1 (Table 43–5).

School screening for adolescent idiopathic scoliosis is performed in 35 states. The efficacy and costs of of school screening programs have been challenged because fewer than 1% of the screened population eventually require treatment. The premise of screening programs is that early recognition of scoliosis results in early brace treatment to minimize progression and the need for surgery.

Progression risk is a function of curve severity, skeletal maturity, curve pattern, and gender. Curves less than 30 degrees will not progress beyond skeletal maturity. Curves measuring 30 to 40 degrees may progress, but few will require surgery. Approximately 40% of curves greater than 40 degrees will progress and require surgery.

Adult patients with adolescent idiopathic scoliosis have comparable rates of low back pain, mortality, and pregnancy complications as the general population. Clinically significant restrictive pulmonary dysfunction occurs in curves greater than 50 degrees. Pulmonary dysfunction worsens with increasing curve severity, and statistically significant increases in morbidity and mortality related to pulmonary dysfunction have been documented in curves greater than 100 degrees.

Bracing does not "correct" scoliosis but is used to prevent significant curve progression in skeletally immature children with (1) a flexible curve as measured by side-bending AP, (2) apex at T-8 or more caudad, and (3) curvature between 30 and 45 degrees. It should also be used in children with a curve between 20 and 30 degrees that has progressed 5 degrees in 6 months or 10 degrees over any length of time.

TABLE 43–5   Prevalence of Adolescent Idiopathic Scoliosis

Cobb Angle	Female/Male Ratio	Prevalence (Percent)
> 10 degrees	1.5:1	2–3%
> 20 degrees	5.4:1	0.3–0.5%
> 30 degrees	10:1	0.1–0.3%
> 40 degrees		< 0.1%

Reproduced with permission from Weinstein SL. Adolescent idiopathic scoliosis: prevalence and natural history. In: Weinstein SL, ed. *The Pediatric Spine: Principles and Practice.* New York, NY: Raven Press; 1994:463.

Brace treatment may also be initiated as a temporizing measure for curves of greater magnitude in younger adolescents to allow for trunk growth and skeletal maturation prior to spinal fusion.

Brace treatment is more likely to be effective if the curve magnitude in the brace is corrected by 50% on the initial in-brace radiograph. Daily brace wear is gradually increased to 16 hours per day, which has been shown to be as effective as full-time wear, and is more likely to foster compliance by the adolescent. Prompt attention to skin problems and poorly fitting braces will increase patient compliance. Radiographs should be performed every 3 to 4 months to rule out progression. Brace wear is continued until the patient reaches Risser stage 4.

Brace treatment is effective in 85% of compliant patients. Recent studies suggest that it is the only effective nonoperative treatment to prevent progression of curves less than 45 degrees in skeletally immature patients. Options include the Milwaukee brace, which supports the head, and the lower profile, underarm braces such as the Boston brace or TLSO (thoracolumbosacral orthosis).

Indications for surgery in adolescent idiopathic scoliosis include progression beyond 40 degrees despite adequate bracing in a skeletally immature patient, thoracic curves greater than 50 degrees, and lumbar curves greater than 45 degrees. Relative indications include truncal asymmetry, cosmetic deformity, and thoracic hypokyphosis or frank lordosis that may compromise pulmonary function. The goals of surgery are restoration of truncal balance with level shoulders centered over a level pelvis and C-7 aligned directly with the gluteal cleft, preservation of sagittal alignment, and safe correction of spinal deformity.

Posterior spinal fusion with instrumentation is performed in children with Risser stage 2 or greater. Less skeletally mature patients require combined anterior and posterior arthrodesis to prevent recurrence due to the crankshaft phenomenon. Supine side-bending AP radiographs are performed for S-shaped curves to determine which curve is more flexible because the more flexible curve can compensate its alignment after realignment of the less flexible curve. This allows the surgeon to minimize the number of levels fused and thus maximize residual spinal motion.

All of the vertebra within the curve that are rotated in the same direction as the apical vertebra should be included in the fusion, as should the stable vertebrae cephalad and caudad to the curve. The stable vertebrae are the first vertebrae cephalad and caudad to the curve that are neutrally rotated. The fusion should spare as many motion segments as possible. The fusion should not include L-5 and S-1, if at all possible.

Segmental instrumentation with a rod on either side of midline anchored to the vertebrae with hooks, pedicle screws, sublaminar wires, or spinous process wires provides powerful deformity correction, stable fixation, and usually obviates postoperative casting or bracing. Thoracoplasty may be cosmetically indicated in patients with a prominent rib hump. The resected ribs are an excellent source of autologous bone graft for arthrodesis. Somatosensory-evoked potential (SSEP) monitoring and the wake-up test are commonly used to evaluate spinal cord function intra-operatively. Hypotensive anesthesia, red blood cell retrieval systems, and acute nor-movolemic hemodilution are useful methods to minimize blood transfusions.

Congenital Spinal Deformity

Scoliosis is the most common congenital spinal deformity fol-lowed by kyphosis (Table 43–6) and then lordosis (Table 43–7). The deformity is determined by the type and location of the vertebral malformation. The risk of progression is a function of the type of anomaly, its location, and the age at diagnosis.

The prognosis for progression is worst with unilateral unsegmented bar with a contralateral hemivertebra and best

TABLE 43–6 Classification of Kyphosis

Postural
Scheuermann's disease
Congenital
Defect of segmentation
Defect of formation
Mixed
Paralytic
Poliomyelitis
Anterior horn cell
Upper motor neuron
Myelomeningocele
Post-traumatic
Acute
Chronic
Inflammatory
Tuberculosis
Other infections
Ankylosing spondylitis
Postsurgical
Postlaminectomy
Postexcision (e.g., tumor)
Postradiation
Metabolic
Osteoporosis
Senile
Juvenile
Osteogenesis imperfecta
Other
Developmental
Achondroplasia
Mucopolysaccharidoses
Other
Tumor
Benign
Malignant
Primary
Metastatic

Reproduced with permission from Goldstein LA, Waugh TR. Classification and terminology of scoliosis. *Clin Orthop.* 1973;93:18.

with a block vertebra. Congenital kyphosis due to a posterior hemivertebra has a significant risk for progression and neu-rologic deterioration. Deformity due to thoracic, thoracolum-bar, and lumbosacral vertebral anomalies have an increased risk of progression. Younger children have a worse prognosis for progression than older children, and the rate of progres-sion is highest during periods of rapid skeletal growth.

Treatment options include bracing and surgery. Bracing is rarely effective for congenital scoliosis and never effective for congenital lordosis or kyphosis. It may control compen-satory curves cephalad or caudad to the congenital curve, but surgery is usually necessary for these typically progressive deformities.

The goals of surgical therapy are to halt progression and restore balance. Surgery should be performed as soon as safely possible once progression has been documented. Pro-longed observation or bracing increases the riskiness of the usually inevitable surgery. Deformity correction procedures are difficult and neurologically risky, especially in patients with kyphotic deformities. The high incidence of associated intraspinal anomalies also increases the risk of neurologic injury. Fusion in situ is the most reliable technique.

Immediate surgery should be considered for congenital kyphosis due to a posterior hemivertebrae because of the high risk of progression and paraplegia. Immediate surgery is also indicated for congenital scoliosis due to an unsegmented bar with a contralateral hemivertebra because of the rapidly progressive nature of this deformity.

Posterior spinal fusion is sufficient in older children with scoliosis, but anterior arthrodesis should be added in young patients and in patients of any age with coexisting lordosis. Instrumentation with hooks and rods provides rigid internal fixation, obviates postoperative immobilization, and may improve the fusion rate. It should never be used for major correction of a curve because of the significant risk of neuro-logic injury.

Two other options for correction of scoliosis caused by hemivertebrae are convex anterior and posterior hemiepi-physiodesis and hemivertebra excision. Hemiepiphysiodesis is most effective in children less than 5 years old because it relies on continued growth of the concave side of the curve to provide gradual correction. Hemivertebra excision provides immediate correction but is neurologically risky, particularly in the thoracic spine. It is an excellent choice for a hemiverte-bra at L-5 causing truncal imbalance.

TABLE 43–7 Classification of Lordosis

Postural
Congenital
Paralytic
Neuropathic
Myopathic
Contracture of hip flexors
Secondary to shunts

Reproduced with permission from Goldstein LA, Waugh TR. Classification and terminology of scoliosis. *Clin Orthop.* 1973;93:18.

Posterior spinal fusion alone is usually sufficient for kyphotic curves measuring 55 degrees or less in children less than 5 years old and in older children with a curve of any magnitude. Correction should not be attempted because of the risk of neurologic injury. Combined anterior and posterior arthrodesis is necessary in younger children with curves greater than 55 degrees to prevent "bending" of the fusion mass. Anterior arthrodesis is performed for lordotic curves.

Neuromuscular Scoliosis

Children with neuromuscular scoliosis typically have many other problems that reflect the global nature of the underlying disorders responsible for the spinal deformity. The needs of these children must be prioritized and are usually best served by a multidisciplinary approach. Goals of treatment must be realistically derived and clearly communicated. Treatment priorities for patients with neuromuscular diseases are to maximize communicative ability, activities of daily living, mobility, and ambulation. Management of spinal deformity is important to maintain or restore trunk posture and stability to maximize sitting, standing, and walking.

The severity of the scoliosis and the likelihood of curve progression correlates with the severity of the underlying neuromuscular disorder. The natural history of spinal deformity in children with neuromuscular diseases is continuous progression with dramatic accelerations of progression during periods of rapid skeletal growth. Curve progression is more common in neuromuscular than in idiopathic scoliosis, the curves are more severe, and the functional consequences are often greater.

Treatment goals are to control deformity and maximize mobility and upright seating potential. Options include bracing, accommodative seating, and spinal fusion. Brace treatment rarely halts progression and at best slows curve progression and delays surgical treatment until the child reaches an appropriate age and size. A foam-padded, total contact TLSO is usually better tolerated than one made of more rigid polypropylene. Wheelchair-bound patients who are not operative candidates benefit from seating systems that accommodate the spinal deformity and any associated pelvic obliquity or lower extremity contractures.

Surgical treatment is indicated to restore truncal balance and when progression threatens truncal balance. Posterior arthrodesis with instrumentation from upper thoracic level (T-2 or T-3) to L-5 or the pelvis is performed with sublaminar wire fixation of long contoured rods. Fixation to the ilium using the Galveston technique is often necessary. Anterior spinal release and fusion may be necessary in patients with rigid pelvic obliquity and in those without posterior spinal elements. Families of children with tenuous ambulatory status must be made aware of the risks of losing the ability to walk, particularly following arthrodesis to the pelvis.

The risk of perioperative complications is significantly increased in children with neuromuscular disease. Chronic pulmonary and urinary tract infections are common and increase the chance of hematogenous bacterial seeding of the spine. Children with neuromuscular disease are often poorly nourished and immunocompromised. Pre- and postoperative hyperalimentation may be necessary if preoperative total protein, albumin, and total lymphocyte count suggest malnutri-

tion. Seizure disorders are common. Osteopenia due to antiepileptic medication may compromise fixation. Prolonged intubation, or even tracheostomy, may be necessary in patients with severe pulmonary dysfunction. Blood loss and transfusion requirements can be minimized with hypotensive anesthesia, acute normotensive hemodilution, and red blood cell retrieval systems.

Cerebral Palsy

The overall incidence of scoliosis in cerebral palsy is 25%. The incidence varies from 5% in diplegia to 65% in quadriplegia. Two curve patterns have been described (Fig. 43–7). Type I curves typically occur in ambulatory patients and are treated like idiopathic curves. Type II curves are long, sweeping curves with pelvic obliquity, which typically occur in nonambulators. Both the magnitude and the functional consequences of scoliosis are greater in nonambulators. The timing of the adolescent growth spurt is less predictable in cerebral palsy, and curves often progress during adulthood, requiring long-term observation.

Contractures of the hips and knees can disrupt truncal balance and can appear worse after correction of the spinal deformity. Nonetheless, the spinal deformity should be corrected first. Indications for surgery are loss of sitting balance and curve progression. Posterior arthrodesis is adequate for most curves that correct to less than 70 degrees on lateral-bending radiographs. Anterior spinal release may be necessary for more rigid curves. Every effort should be made to return the patient to an upright position as soon as possible to decrease the risk of aspiration and other pulmonary complications. Postoperative casting or bracing is usually not necessary.

Myelomeningocele

Spinal deformity in myelomeningocele may be congenital, paralytic, or both. Paralytic curves are long and C-shaped, whereas congenital curves are often acutely angulated. The incidence of scoliosis in myelomeningocele is about 60%. The incidence is greater at higher neurosegmental levels of involvement. Scoliosis typically appears before age 10 and progresses rather insidiously. Tethered cord, progressive hydrocephalus, and syringomyelia should be suspected whenever scoliosis progresses.

Curves less than 30 degrees can be observed, but curves greater than 30 degrees or those causing truncal imbalance are likely to progress. A total contact TLSO may effectively slow progression in a skeletally immature individual with a flexible curve and delay surgical treatment until skeletal maturity. Breakdown of insensate skin is a common complication of brace treatment.

Surgical treatment is indicated to halt progression and restore truncal balance. Caudal fixation is often complicated by the absence of the posterior elements. Anterior spinal release and arthrodesis are often necessary. Pelvic obliquity often coexists and requires arthrodesis and fixation to the pelvis (Fig. 43–8).

Congenital and/or paralytic kyphosis of the lumbar spine occurs in 10 to 15% of children with myelomeningocele. Two types of deformity have been described: a supple collapsing C-shaped kyphus and a rigid S-shaped deformity with cephalad lordosis. Both deformities are severe and progressive.

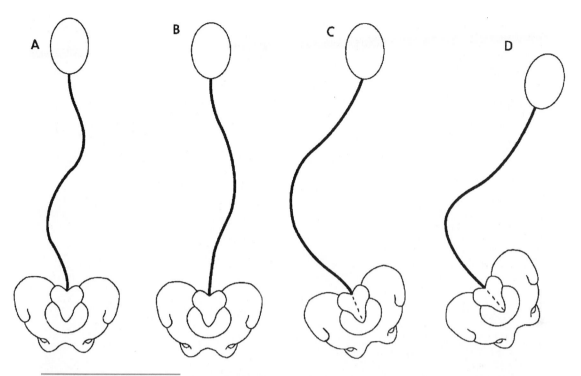

Figure 43–7   Curve patterns in cerebral palsy. Type I curves occur in ambulatory patients and do not cause pelvic obliquity **(A,B)**. Type II curves occur in more severely involved individuals and are typically associated with significant pelvic obliquity **(C,D)**. Redrawn from Lonstein JE, Akbarnia BA. Operative treatment of spinal deformity in patients with cerebral palsy or mental retardation: an analysis of 107 cases. *J Bone Jt Surg.* 1983;65A:45.

Seating problems and skin breakdown over the prominence of the deformity are common. Thoracic deformity and crowding of the abdominal viscera compromise pulmonary function, eating, and urinary drainage.

Brace treatment for kyphosis in myelomeningocele is futile. Surgical treatment fares best when it can be deferred until after age 8. The goal of surgery is to produce a flat, balanced back. Many techniques have been described that have in common shortening of the spine by way of posterior vertebrectomy, extensive bone grafting, rigid segmental instrumentation, and stable sacral or iliosacral fixation. Tension-band wiring provides sufficient fixation in children less than 1 year of age.

Wound-healing complications are common following surgery for either kyphosis or scoliosis in children with myelomeningocele because their skin is thin and insensate. Tissue expansion or myocutaneous flap coverage may be necessary. Latex allergy is very prevalent among children with myelomeningocele; therefore, all latex products should be avoided during the care of these patients.

Duchenne's Muscular Dystrophy

The incidence of scoliosis in Duchenne's muscular dystrophy is 95%. Scoliosis develops once the child becomes wheelchair-bound; typically between the ages of 11 and 13. Virtually all curves progress and compromise pulmonary function and positioning. Pulmonary function declines by 4% for every 10 degrees of scoliosis progression.

Brace treatment is contraindicated for scoliosis due to Duchenne's muscular dystrophy. Posterior spinal fusion is indicated for curves greater than 20 degrees as soon as the patient stops walking to minimize pulmonary deterioration. Surgery should be performed before the forced vital capacity decreases below 30%. The goal of surgery is to preserve trunk balance and optimal sitting posture. Arthrodesis should extend from T-2 to the pelvis if there is any pelvic obliquity; otherwise, arthrodesis from T-2 to L-5 is adequate.

Spinal Muscle Atrophy

The risk of scoliosis in patients with spinal muscular atrophy increases with the severity of neurologic involvement. Patients who never sit independently develop scoliosis by age 2. Marginal ambulators and those who are able sit but not walk typically develop scoliosis at age 7 or 8. The typical curve is long, C-shaped, and progressive.

A sitting support orthosis or a total contact TLSO may slow, but not halt curve progression. Posterior spine fusion with segmental fixation is indicated for progression beyond 40 degrees. Patients with pelvic obliquity require fusion to the pelvis. Anterior spinal release is necessary for rigid

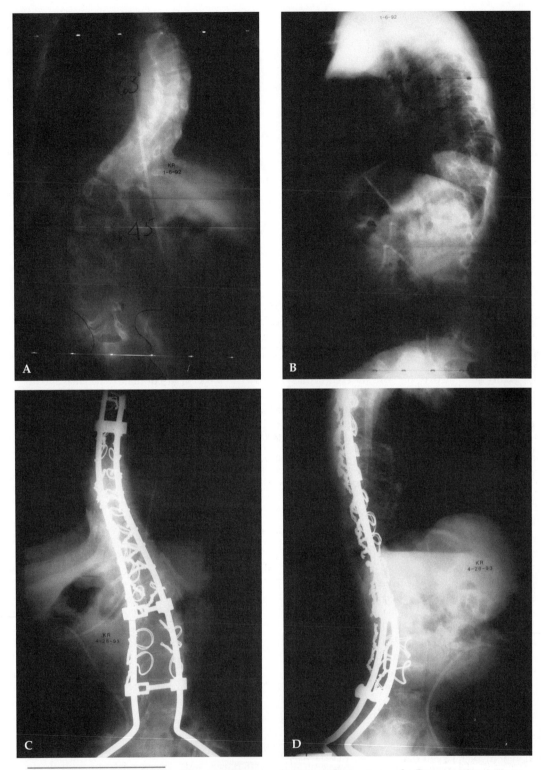

Figure 43–8 A 16-year-old with paralytic curve due to myelomeningocele. Preoperative antero-posterior and lateral radiographs **(A,B)**. Postoperative radiographs demonstrating segmental spinal instrumentation with sublaminar wires (Luque technique) and iliosacral fixation (Galveston) **(C,D)**.

curves greater than 70 degrees and fixed pelvic obliquity greater than 25 degrees. Spinal fusion should be performed before vital capacity diminishes to less than 30 percent of predicted, below which the risk of pulmonary complications and perioperative morbidity and mortality increases precipitously.

Friedreich's Ataxia

Scoliosis occurs in nearly all patients with Friedreich's ataxia. The curve patterns resemble idiopathic scoliosis. About two thirds are progressive and require surgical treatment. The risk of progression is greatest in younger children. Brace treatment does not effectively control progression. Seating devices may be helpful but have no effect on the natural history of the curve.

Posterior spinal arthrodesis with instrumentation is indicated for any curve greater than 60 degrees. Curves less than 40 degrees should be followed for progression. Treatment of curves between 40 and 60 degrees depends on evidence of progression and age of the patient.

Scheuermann's Disease

This deformity must be distinguished from postural hyperkyphosis, which is a more flexible curvature lacking struc-

---

> **PEARL**
>
> **Congenital and neuromuscular scoliosis often require surgery to halt disabling progression and maximize functional ability.**

tural abnormalities. Active spinal growth worsens the pain and progressive deformity. Symptoms often diminish after skeletal maturity. Neurologic signs are rare and should be evaluated immediately with MRI.

Scheuermann's disease is diagnosed radiographically on a standing lateral radiograph when three adjacent vertebrae have anterior wedging of at least 5 degrees (Fig. 43–9). Classic Scheuermann's disease affects the thoracic spine with an apex between T-7 and T-9 and is usually accompanied by a flexible lumbar lordosis. Thoracolumbar Scheuermann's disease with an apex between T-10 and T-12 is less prevalent,

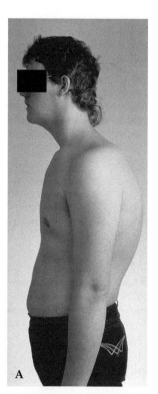

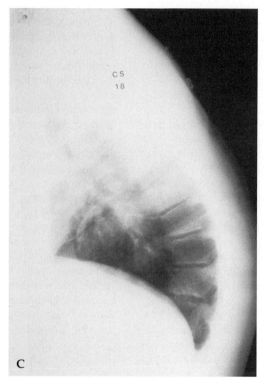

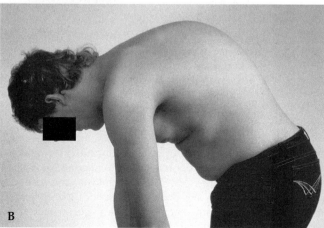

Figure 43–9   Typical appearance of Scheuermann's kyphosis in a 17-year old **(A,B)**. Lateral radiograph shows vertebral wedging and endplate irregularities **(C)**.

and may be accompanied by a compensatory thoracic lordosis. Lumbar Scheuermann's disease typically occurs in male athletes or laborers. Radiographs demonstrate vertebral endplate changes and disc space narrowing with loss or reversal of lumbar lordosis.

The natural history of classic Scheuermann's disease is benign. Eighty percent of patients with curves greater than 60 degrees may slowly progress, but few develop severe deformity. Patients have few functional limitations. Back pain tends to be more severe when the apex of the deformity is below T-8. Symptoms in lumbar Scheuermann's disease typically improve with decreased activity. Pulmonary compromise is minimal in curves less than 100 degrees. Cosmesis and self-esteem are difficult to quantify, but are important considerations.

Patients with kyphosis measuring less than 60 degrees without evidence of progression may be followed with serial radiographs every 4 to 6 months. An exercise program emphasizing hamstring and lumbar spine stretching and flexibility should be initiated. Skeletally immature patients with flexible curves between 60 and 75 degrees should undergo brace treatment. Brace treatment is more likely to succeed when initiated early after diagnosis in flexible curves. The Milwaukee brace (CTLSO [cervicothoracolumbo-sacral orthosis]) is effective, but compliance is often a problem. Curves with apices in the lower thoracic spine may be effectively treated with low profile, TLSO braces.

Surgical treatment is indicated for adolescents with curves that continue to progress beyond 75 degrees despite bracing, adults with painful or cosmetically unacceptable curves, or in patients beginning to experience pulmonary dysfunction. Staged or concurrent anterior and posterior procedures are most likely to yield maximum permanent correction. Instrumentation should include all vertebra in the curve and extend at least one level above and below the most cephalad and caudal vertebrae that are tilted toward the apex of the curve. Paraplegia following instrumentation and reduction of deformity is a rare complication attributed to thoracic disc herniation or traction injury to the anterior spinal artery. Intra-operative spinal cord monitoring or a wake-up test should be performed in all patients. If injury to the spinal cord is detected, hardware should be removed immediately to reverse correction of the deformity and to relieve tension on the anterior vasculature. If a herniated disc is identified, it should be decompressed.

Spondylolysis and Spondylolisthesis

Spondylolisthesis develops in 50% of patients with spondylolysis. A small subset will actually become symptomatic with low back pain, thigh pain, and hamstring tightness. Patients with more severe listhesis may have hyperlordosis of the lumbar spine, kyphosis with a palpable step-off at the lumbosacral junction, heart-shaped buttocks, and a waddling gait. Nerve root and cauda equina compression are rare. Radiographic severity of the listhesis is measured as the amount of displacement of the more cephalad vertebra relative to the more caudal vertebra and expressed as a percentage. Kyphosis at the lumbosacral junction is measured by the slip angle (Fig. 43–10). A radiographic classification has been described that suggests etiology (Fig. 43–11).

Nonoperative symptomatic treatment of spondylolisthesis is usually successful. Predictors of unsuccessful nonoperative treatment include dysplastic spondylolisthesis, a slip angle greater than 30 degrees, spondylolisthesis greater than 50%, female gender, and age less than 15. The slip angle is the most reliable predictor of progression in skeletally immature patients. Treatment goals include pain relief and prevention of progression. Asymptomatic skeletally mature patients do not require treatment or followup unless symptoms develop. Skeletally immature patients with an asymptomatic grade I or II spondylolisthesis should be followed until maturity. Patients with low-grade spondylolisthesis with gradual onset of symptoms can be effectively treated with activity restriction and physical therapy for hamstring and lumbar stretching and abdominal strengthening. Brace treatment with a TLSO effectively relieves pain in 60 to 80% of patients with acute or persistent symptoms. Children with grade I spondylolisthesis can safely return to sports when their symptoms abate. Those with a grade II slips should be discouraged from returning to collision sports.

Surgical treatment is indicated for patients with any degree of spondylolisthesis who remain symptomatic despite exhaustive nonoperative treatment and in those with a slip greater than 50 percent. In situ, single level (L-5–S-1) posterolateral arthrodesis is indicated for symptomatic patients with grade I or II slips. Two level (L-4–S-1) arthrodesis is recommended for listhesis greater than grade II because the significant displacement of L-5 leads to an increased incidence of pseudarthrosis. Decompression is indicated for patients with objective neurologic signs but not isolated hamstring tightness, and it should be performed in conjunction with fusion. Postoperatively, patients are placed in an ambulatory pantaloon cast or brace for 3 to 6 months.

Progression may occur after operative treatment when the preoperative slip angle is greater than 45 degrees. Therefore, internal fixation may be indicated for in situ posterolateral arthrodesis when the preoperative slip angle is greater than 45 degrees. Spinal instrumentation should not be used to reduce the anterior vertebral displacement because of an increased risk of neurologic injury. Patients with spondyloptosis may require resection of the L-5 vertebra and combined anterior and posterior arthrodesis.

Cervical Spine

Atlanto-axial Instability and Os Odontoideum

Symptoms in atlanto-axial instability can be mechanical or myelopathic. Severity of symptoms is inversely proportional to the size of the dens. Frank aplasia results in a functionally incompetent transverse ligament and C1-2 instability, whereas mild hypoplasia may go unnoticed forever.

Radiographic measurement of the atlanto-dens interval (ADI) can guide treatment. Within the ring of C-1, an equal amount of space is occupied by the odontoid process, the spinal cord, and additional space around the cord. The ADI measures the space between the anterior ring of C-1 and the odontoid process and indirectly measures the space available for the spinal cord (SAC). In children, the normal ADI is less than 4 mm, and the SAC is greater than 13 mm (Fig. 43–12). These measurements should be made on neutral, flexion, and extension lateral radiographs of the cervical spine.

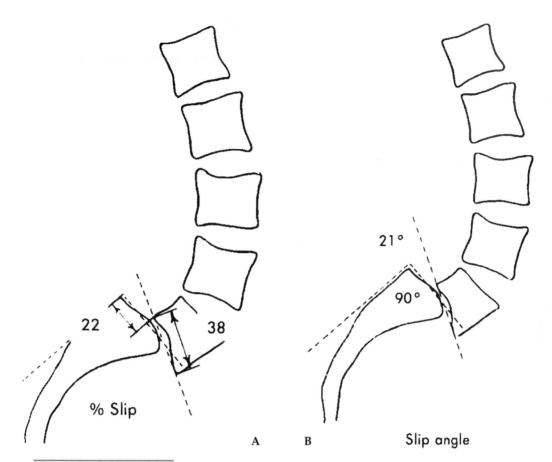

Figure 43–10   Percentage of slipping is calculated by measuring the distance between tangents drawn from the posterior sacrum and the posterior body of L-5 (in this case 22 mm) and then dividing that value by the width of the inferior body of L-5 (38 mm). In this example, slip percentage is 22/38 = 58% **(A)**. Slip angle is determined by measuring the angle subtended by a line drawn across the inferior body of L-5 and the perpendicular to the tangent of the posterior sacrum. In the example, this measures 21 degrees **(B)**. Adapted from Boxall D, Bradford DS, Winter RB. Management of severe spondylolisthesis in children and adolescents. *J Bone Jt Surg.* 1979;61A:480, 482.

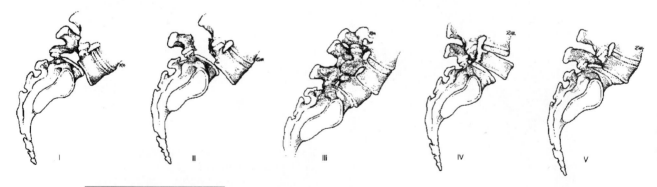

Figure 43–11   Wiltse classification of spondylolisthesis: type I, dysplastic; type II, isthmic; type III, degenerative; type IV, traumatic; type V, pathologic. Reproduced with permission from Freeman BL III. The pediatric spine. In: Canale ST, Beaty JH, eds. *Operative Pediatric Orthopaedics.* St. Louis, MO, C.V. Mosby; 1996:599.

The radiographic appearance of the os odontoideum is also prognostic. The orthotopic ossicle occurs in the usual location of the dens, and the dystopic ossicle is located just inferior to the clivus, where it may be fused to the occiput (Fig. 43–13). The atlanto-axial complex is more unstable and

likely to be associated with neurologic symptoms in the dystopic type.

Surgical stabilization with posterior C1-2 arthrodesis is indicated for *symptomatic* patients with radiographic instability characterized by an ADI greater than 4 mm on a lateral

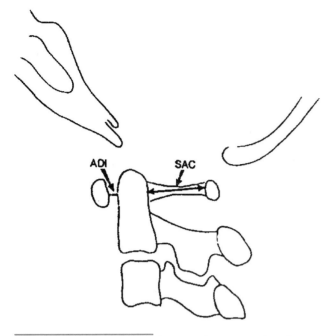

Figure 43–12 Illustration of atlanto-dens interval, and space available for the cord.

PEARL

The Committee on Sports Medicine of the American Academy of Pediatrics recommends that children with Down's syndrome who wish to participate in sports with potential for head or neck trauma should be evaluated with flexion and extension lateral radiographs of the cervical spine prior to participation. Participation should not be permitted if the ADI is greater than 4.5 mm or structural abnormalities of the odontoid are present.

extension radiograph. Periodic screening and treatment of asymptomatic patients with radiographic instability remains undefined.

Posterior cervical arthrodesis should be performed in any Down's syndrome child with neurological symptoms, regardless of the ADI, or when the ADI is greater than 10 mm, regardless of symptoms. Arthrodesis should be extended to include the occiput if craniocervical instability is present. Complications including pseudoarthrosis and neurologic compromise are common after posterior cervical arthrodesis in children with Down's syndrome.

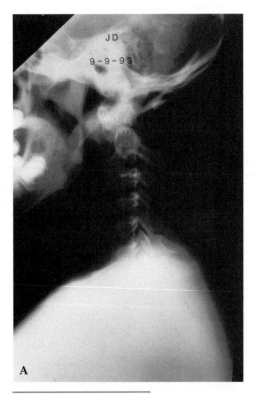

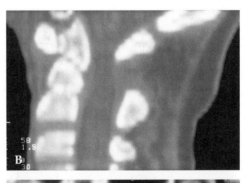

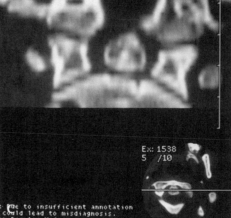

Figure 43–13 Lateral radiograph showing an orthotopic os odontoideum in a patient with transient episodes of quadriparesis **(A)**. Coronal and sagittal computed tomography reconstructions of the same patient illustrating a distinct line of separation, which is superior to the physeal scar at the base of the dens **(B,C)**.

Torticollis

Congenital muscular torticollis may progress and lead to asymmetric flattening of the skull and facial features if untreated. The sternocleidomastoid muscle contralateral to the direction the chin points is contracted. Associated deformities such as clubfoot, metatarsus adductus, and developmental hip dysplasia may be present. Thorough physical and radiographic examination and detailed neurologic and ophthalmologic examination are essential to rule out a primary etiology.

Gentle passive stretching performed by the parents and diligence to positioning for sleep often reverse the deformity. Persistent deformity with restricted range of motion at 1 year of age requires surgical release of the sternocleidomastoid muscle. Recurrence is less likely with proximal and distal release, but strength preservation is theoretically better with distal release only. Postoperatively, patients are either placed in a rigid cervical orthosis or begin physical therapy without any immobilization.

Four types of rotatory subluxation may cause torticollis (Fig. 43–14). Type I is rotatory displacement without anterior translation; type II is a rotatory displacement with anterior translation of 5 mm or less; type III is rotary displacement with anterior translation greater than 5 mm; and type IV is rotatory displacement with posterior translation. Type I is most common and usually resolves spontaneously. Types II, III, and IV have a worse prognosis. Sternocleidomastoid muscle spasm occurs on the side toward which the chin is pointed (the opposite of muscular torticollis). The deformity rarely becomes fixed; but if the deformity becomes fixed, pain will subside and range of motion will be limited. Fixed subluxation of the C1-2 facet joints is present on dynamic axial CT scan.

The duration and severity of the deformity determine treatment. Rest and a soft cervical collar are usually adequate when symptoms have been present for less than 1 week. Cervical halter traction, analgesics, and muscle relaxants are necessary if treatment fails or if symptoms have been present for more than 1 week. Reduction is clinically apparent when neck range of motion improves and is confirmed by reduction of the C1-2 facet joints on dynamic CT. Symptoms present for more than 1 month occasionally respond to 3 weeks of cervical halter traction, but reduction is unlikely. In situ posterior arthrodesis of C1-2 is recommended for symptomatic patients with persistent deformity.

Klippel-Feil Syndrome

Associated anomalies are present in 15 to 35% of patients with Klippel-Feil syndrome. Anomalies include sensorineural hearing loss, significant genitourinary and renal anomalies with unilateral renal agenesis being the most common, cardiac anomalies, central nervous system anomaly with synkinesia (involuntary paired movements of extremities), and skeletal anomalies. Thus, congenital cervical fusion should be considered when any of these anomalies are discovered. Furthermore, diagnosis of Klippel-Feil syndrome should initiate a diligent search for other associated conditions.

Presenting symptoms can be mechanical, neurogenic, or myelopathic. Only 40 to 50% of patients present with the classic triad of decreased neck range of motion, low hairline, and short neck. Decreased lateral bending and rotation is the most common complaint. The age at presentation varies widely; patients with C1-2 fusions present earlier than those with lower level fusion. Of patients who develop neurologic symptoms, 20% do so by 5 years of age and 65% by age 30.

Radiographic evaluation of the entire spine is necessary to rule out other congenital abnormalities. Instability should be assessed with flexion and extension lateral radiographs of the cervical spine. Computed tomography scan may be more useful in younger children. Magnetic resonance imaging should be performed to evaluate for the presence of spinal cord injury, intraspinal pathology, or brain stem anomaly when instability or symptoms are present.

The natural history of Klippel-Feil syndrome is unknown. Severe neurologic compromise can occur, but most patients lead active lives. Risk factors for neurologic compromise include congenital stenosis, hypermobility, and the presence of two or more fusion segments separated by an open segment. A common pattern associated with spinal cord injury is fusion of C-1 to the occiput coupled with fusion of C2-3 and an unfused C1-2.

Treatment of the symptomatic patient requires surgical stabilization with posterior cervical fusion. Neural decom-

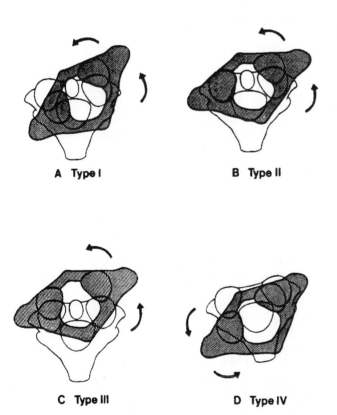

A Type I   **B Type II**

C Type III   **D Type IV**

Figure 43–14 Rotatory displacement can be divided into four types: Type I is simple rotatory displacement without a translatory shift **(A)**; Type II is rotatory displacement with anterior displacement less than or equal to 5 mm. Type III is rotatory displacement with an anterior shift greater than 5 mm. Type IV is rotatory displacement with a posterior shift. Reproduced with permission from Fielding JW, Hawkins RJ. Atlanto-axial rotatory fixation (fixed rotatory subluxation of the atlanto-axial joint). *J Bone Jt Surg.* 1977; 59A:42.

pression is rarely indicated. Treatment of the asymptomatic patient remains undefined. All patients with congenital cervical fusions should be advised to avoid collision sports or recreational activities that place them at increased risk of head and neck trauma.

Basilar Impression

Common findings include short neck, skull asymmetry, and painful range of motion of the cervical spine. Torticollis occurs in 15% of patients. Signs of brainstem compression such as hyperreflexia, ataxia, spasticity, or weakness require immediate attention. Hydrocephalus may occur if the dens compresses the aqueduct of Sylvius in the medulla oblongata.

A number of radiographic parameters have been defined to measure the relationship between the dens and the base of the skull. However, sagittal plane MRI is more useful because it can evaluate the osseous relationships and the neural elements.

Surgical decompression is indicated for neurologic compromise. Anterior neural compression is treated by transoral odontoid resection. Suboccipital decompression is performed for posterior neural compression. Following either anterior or posterior decompression, the craniocervical junction must be stabilized by a posterior arthrodesis extending from the occiput to C-2 or C-3.

Cervical Stenosis

A spinal canal diameter that measures 10 mm or less constitutes absolute stenosis, and a measurement of 10 to 13 mm is relative stenosis. Pavlov et al (1987) described a ratio of vertebral body width to canal diameter in the sagittal plane to account for anthropomorphic differences. A ratio of 0.8 or less represents stenosis. Hyperextension or hyperflexion further diminishes the spinal canal diameter.

Traumatic spinal cord injury is more common in children with cervical stenosis. Transient neurapraxia may present as burning pain, numbness, weakness, paraplegia, or complete quadriplegia. Neurologic symptoms typically resolve within 10 to 15 minutes, but may persist as long as 48 hours. Routine radiographs typically show no fracture or dislocation. Whether to allow an athlete with cervical stenosis to return to a contact sport following an episode of transient neurapraxia remains unresolved. The presence of concomitant pathology such as disc disease, spondylosis, or instability should preclude participation in contact sports.

Back Pain in Children

Back pain in children requires thorough evaluation because treatable pathology is present in 85% of cases. Factors often associated with a positive diagnosis include constant pain, radicular pain, male gender, and a short duration of symptoms.

Intermittent pain associated with activities occurs with spondylolisthesis. Constant or nocturnal pain suggests a neoplasm. Constitutional symptoms suggest a systemic process such as infection or malignancy. Radicular symptoms are due to nerve root irritation caused by a herniated disc or apophyseal ring avulsion. Back pain may also be a manifestation of pulmonary, gastrointestinal, genitourinary, or other intraabdominal or intrathoracic pathology. Abnormal spinal align-

ment or gait suggests a herniated disc, hamstring tightness is common with spondylolysis; and abnormal reflexes occur when intraspinal pathology is present.

Posteroanterior and lateral radiographs of the thoracolumbar spine should be obtained in all symptomatic children less than 5 years old and in all children with symptoms for more than 2 weeks, night pain, or constitutional symptoms. Adolescents with lumbar complaints or hamstring tightness should also have oblique radiographs of the lumbosacral spine and a standing lateral radiograph of L-5–S-1 to rule out spondylolysis or spondylolisthesis. Lytic or blastic lesions are due to either tumor or infection. Discitis is suggested by disc space narrowing and vertebral endplate irregularities. Radiographic scoliosis represents a reaction to spinal pathology. Bony lesions on radiographs require further evaluation with CT scan.

Technetium bone scan is a sensitive test for children with pain, normal radiographs, and a normal neurologic examination. The SPECT scan can localize a lesion identified on bone scan. Magnetic resonance imaging is useful when neurologic or constitutional symptoms are present. Laboratory evaluation including complete blood count with differential, erythrocyte sedimentation rate, and C-reactive protein should be performed in all young children and in any child with constitutional symptoms or night pain.

Infection

Empiric treatment with antibiotics to cover Staphylococcus species is recommended. Aspiration of the disc space or vertebra is not necessary because the low diagnostic yield with positive cultures in only 60% of cases does not justify the operative risk. Rest and brace treatment with a TLSO provide adequate symptomatic relief. Surgical debridement is necessary only for patients who develop an abscess. Tuberculosis is re-emerging as a cause of vertebral osteomyelitis and should be considered in refractory cases.

Herniated Nucleus Pulposis and Apophyseal Ring Avulsion

Severe back and leg pain occur in both groups. There may be a history of antecedent trauma. Gait and postural abnormalities and positive straight-leg raise are present. However, motor weakness, absent reflexes, and paresthesias are rarely seen. Radiographs typically are normal, MRI is usually diagnostic for herniated nucleus pulposus, and CT is useful for ring apophyseal avulsion.

Initial treatment should be nonoperative and consists of analgesics, anti-inflammatories, and activity modification for 3 to 6 weeks. Nonoperative treatment is often effective for herniated nucleus pulposus. Surgical excision is effective when nonoperative treatment fails. Surgical excision of a displaced ring apophyseal avulsion is usually required.

Neoplasms

The most common vertebral neoplasm is osteoid osteoma. The classic presentation is night pain relieved by anti-inflammatory medication. The lesion involves the posterior elements and is often difficult to see on plain radiographs. Bone scan demonstrates an isolated focus of increased uptake, and

CT scan demonstrates a lesion with a sclerotic rim and central nidus. The pain usually resolves as the patient approaches late adolescence. Nonsteroidal anti-inflammatory medications are often palliative. Failure to adequately control pain with medication is an indication for en bloc resection of the lesion.

Other neoplasms that involve the posterior elements include osteoblastoma and aneurysmal bone cyst. Both are larger than osteoid osteoma and can progress in size to cause neurologic compression. Both require surgical excision by curettage and bone grafting.

Eosinophilic granuloma is a painful neoplasm of the spine that occurs in children and involves the vertebral body. Radiographic characteristics include bony lysis and vertebra plana. Biopsy is often necessary to differentiate the lesion from infection and leukemia. Eosinophilic granuloma typically resolves spontaneously with reconstitution of the vertebrae. Neurologic symptoms may be an indication for radiation therapy, or rarely, surgical debridement and stabilization.

Spine Trauma

Spine injury should be suspected in any child who has been involved in trauma or has been found unconscious. Initial trauma management protocols should be followed with immediate and ongoing assessment of the airway, breathing, and circulation. The patient must be immobilized as soon as possible and transported carefully. A hard cervical collar is used to immobilize the cervical spine, and tape and sandbags are used to immobilize the head and torso for transport. A standard spine board should not be used for immobilization and transport because it will cause flexion of the neck due to the disproportionate head-chest circumference ratio in children. The torso must be elevated with a pad or blanket or a pediatric spine board with an occipital cutout should be used to allow the head and neck to maintain a normal relationship with the thorax. Football or hockey helmets should not be removed from an injured athlete until several trained personnel are available to immobilize the head as the helmet is spread apart and removed.

Options for cervical immobilization while intubating an unconscious patient include in-line traction, nasotracheal intubation, and fiberoptic intubation. Overdistraction of an unstable spine fracture may occur with in-line traction. Nasotracheal and fiberoptic intubation minimize manipulation but require more time and expertise.

Spinal Cord Injury
Without Radiographic Abnormality

Spinal cord injury without radiographic abnormality (SCIWORA) is unique to the pediatric population and occurs in approximately 20% of children with spinal cord injuries. It is more common in children younger than 8 years old. The cervical spine is more commonly involved than the thoracic and lumbar spine. The etiology of the syndrome is unknown, but ligamentous laxity, hypermobility of the spine, and immature spinal vasculature are believed to contribute to the pathophysiology because the elasticity of the

spinal column is much greater than of that of the spinal cord. Proposed etiologies include traction injury with cord rupture, transient disc rupture or endplate avulsion, and vascular infarction. Incomplete neurologic injuries have a good prognosis for recovery, whereas complete injuries have a dismal prognosis. The onset of symptoms is delayed from the time of injury in approximately 50% of patients. Careful radiographic and MRI evaluation are essential to identify occult apophyseal fractures, transient disc herniation, or subtle instability of the spinal column.

Cervical Spine

Spinal cord injury rarely accompanies cervical spine fracture or dislocation. The prognosis for recovery when spinal cord injury does occur in children is better than it is for adults. However, children with permanent spinal cord injury have a high risk for developing spinal deformity.

The pattern of cervical spine injury varies with age. Injury tends to occur above C-3 in children younger than 8 years old because the relatively large size of the head relative to the trunk places the fulcrum of motion in the upper cervical spine at C2-3 where the facet joint angles are relatively horizontal. The fulcrum of motion gradually moves caudally with age, and by age 12, cervical spine injuries are similar to those that typically occur in adults.

Radiographic evaluation of the cervical spine requires familiarity with the location and timing of appearance and fusion of the multiple ossification centers in the atlas and dens to differentiate normal variants from fractures. Persistent synchondroses in the ring of C-1 can be mistaken for fractures. Incomplete ossification of the tip of the odontoid can be confused with odontoid hypoplasia. "Pseudosubluxation" of up to 3 mm, particularly at C2-3, is often normal, because of the relatively horizontal facet joints and ligamentous laxity.

PEARL

Thick soft tissues anterior to C2-3 suggest traumatic subluxation. Crying, however, will cause the soft tissues to thicken.

Atlanto-occipital dislocation is usually fatal in the younger child. The injury involves ligamentous and soft tissue disruption, and, thus, may not be radiographically evident unless there is marked displacement of the occipital condyles. The Power's ratio can help make the diagnosis and is calculated by comparing the length of a line drawn from the basion to the posterior arch of atlas and dividing it by the length of a line extending from the occiput to the anterior arch of atlas (Fig. 43–15). Ratios less than 0.9 are normal, and a ratio greater than 1 diagnoses dislocation. Halo vest immobilization without distraction is applied immediately in the rare survivor, and posterior occipitocervical arthrodesis is performed once the patient is medically stable.

Neurologic injury rarely occurs in atlas and axis injuries with occipital involvement because of the large amount of space available for the spinal cord. Computed tomography scan is often necessary to evaluate atlas fractures (Jefferson

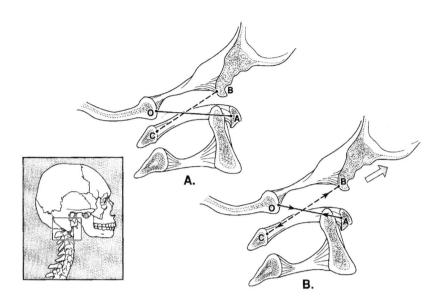

Figure 43–15 Power's ratio is determined by drawing a line from the basion (B) to the posterior arch of atlas (C), and another line from the opisthion (O) to the anterior arch of atlas (A). The length of line BC is divided by the length of line OA. A ratio greater than 1 is diagnostic of anterior occipital dislocation. Values less than 0.9 are normal. Reproduced with permission from Lebwohl NH, Eismont FJ. Cervical spine injuries in children. In: Weinstein SL, ed. *The Pediatric Spine: Principles and Practice.* New York, NY: Raven Press; 1994:729.

fractures) in children younger than 8 years old to distinguish fracture from normal synchondrosis. Cervical collar immobilization is sufficient for stable fractures, and a Minerva cast or halo vest is necessary for unstable injuries. Atlanto-axial stability should be ruled out radiographically before discontinuing immobilization.

Atlanto-axial instability can be due to rupture or avulsion of the transverse ligament, or fracture of the synchondrosis at the base of the odontoid process. An anterior dens interval (ADI) greater than 4 mm in flexion diagnoses atlanto-axial instability. Open reduction and posterior C1-2 arthrodesis is indicated when the ADI is greater than 5 mm in flexion or when neurologic deficit symptoms are present regardless of the amount of displacement. Halo vest or Minerva jacket immobilization are necessary postoperatively.

Odontoid fractures typically occur in children younger than 6 years old, and such a fracture is a Salter-Harris type I physeal separation through the synchondrosis at the base of the dens. Neurologic deficits are rare. Halo vest or Minerva cast immobilization in hyperextension to reduce displacement is sufficient. Failure to recognize this injury may lead to formation of an os odontoideum.

The hangman's fracture is a fracture through the pedicles of C-2 that can occasionally cause traumatic spondylolisthesis. Persistent synchondroses droses just anterior to the C-2 pedicles and physiologic pseudosubluxation at C2-3 are normal variants that are often misdiagnosed as a hangman's fracture. These fractures are typically stable. Fractures that are displaced less than 3 mm can be treated with a rigid cervical collar until healed. More displacement requires reduction and halo vest immobilization for 8 weeks.

Subaxial cervical spine injuries usually occur in children older than 8 years. Flexion is the most common mechanism of injury and compression fractures the most common fracture pattern. These injuries are stable unless the posterior ligaments are ruptured. Cervical collar immobilization is sufficient in stable injuries, but posterior cervical arthrodesis is necessary for unstable injuries.

Facet dislocations are uncommon in children. Unilateral dislocations are treated by traction and closed or open reduction. Bilateral facet dislocations are unstable injuries that require posterior arthrodesis following reduction. Vertebral endplate fractures may go unrecognized if the fragment spontaneously reduces. These injuries may be a cause of SCIWORA and may require stabilization. Anterior arthrodesis should be avoided in children unless an anterior surgical approach is necessary to decompress the spinal canal because progressive kyphosis due to cessation of anterior growth may occur. Deformity is also common after laminectomy.

Thoracolumbar Spine

Apophyseal endplate fractures occur mostly in the lumbar spine in adolescents and clinically resemble herniated nucleus pulposus. Displacement of the fragment into the spinal canal, neurologic deficit, and failure of rest and activity restriction to relieve symptoms are indications for surgical decompression.

The 3-column classification of thoracolumbar spine fractures described in adults can be extrapolated to pediatric spine fractures. The anterior column comprises the anterior longitudinal ligament, the anterior half of the intervertebral disc, and the anterior half of the vertebral body. The middle column includes the posterior half of the vertebral body and intervertebral disc, the posterior longitudinal ligament, and the pedicle. The posterior column comprises the facet joints, the ligamentum flavum, the posterior laminar arch, the interspinous ligaments, and the supraspinous ligament.

Spine fractures are also classified by the mechanism of injury. Flexion injuries cause anterior column failure and anterior compression fracture. Axial compression injuries produce burst fractures with failure of the anterior and middle columns, and occasionally the posterior column. Flexion-distraction injuries cause compressive failure of the anterior column and tension failure of the middle and posterior columns. High-energy combinations of flexion, axial compression, and distraction cause multiplane failure of all 3 columns and result in complex fracture-dislocations.

Thoracolumbar injury is also classified by the presence or risk of mechanical and/or neurologic compromise. First-degree instability implies deformity or risk of deformity. Neurologic deficit without deformity defines second-degree instability. Third-degree instability is present when both deformity and neurologic deficit occur. Acute instability is apparent at the time injury, and chronic instability becomes evident during followup.

Compression fractures are due to flexion, are the most common fracture type, and are usually mechanically stable. Neurologic deficits are rare. Mild compression deformity can be treated symptomatically, but more significant deformity requires cast or brace treatment. Residual deformity is usually clinically insignificant.

Burst fractures are more severe injuries caused by flexion and axial loading. Mechanical instability and neurologic injury are more likely. Important determinants of treatment are the number of columns involved, the magnitude of kyphosis, the amount of canal compromise, and the loss of vertebral height. Bracing with a TLSO is appropriate in two-column injuries without kyphosis, canal compromise, and neurologic deficit. Open reduction and instrumented fusion with or without decompression is necessary when there is mechanical instability and/or canal compromise.

Flexion-distraction injuries, also known as seatbelt injuries or Chance fractures are caused by a flexion of the spine with a fulcrum anterior to the patient. A common mechanism occurs in automobile accidents wherein the seat belt acts a fulcrum for forceful flexion of the spine following sudden deceleration of the motor vehicle. Children are particularly susceptible to this fracture mechanism because their size and body habitus does not allow them to sit in an automobile seat with the lap belt in proper position across the pelvis. The seatbelt rests across the lower abdomen and is the axis of rotation.

Mechanical failure of the spine can occur either through the bony elements or the soft tissues. Bony injuries are amenable to postural reduction and hyperextension casting. Injuries with predominantly soft tissue involvement, unreducible fractures, and late instability following closed treatment require open reduction, stabilization with a simple dual compression rod construct or interspinous wire, and posterior arthrodesis.

Fracture dislocations are complex, high energy injuries that typically occur at the thoracolumbar junction and are associated with spinal cord or cauda equina injury. These injuries are always unstable and require operative reduction and arthrodesis with instrumentation.

Seemingly benign fractures of the spinous and transverse processes typically do not require any treatment but should raise the index of suspicion for an intra-abdominal or intrathoracic injury because of the blunt trauma typically incurred to cause fracture.

The long-term consequences of spine and spinal cord injuries can be devastating. Joint contractures, pulmonary insufficiency, pressure sores, autonomic dysreflexia, sphincter dysfunction, and spasticity are common problems. Children less than 10 years of age develop progressive scoliosis below the level of injury, which often requires surgical stabilization.

SUMMARY

The natural history and treatment of idiopathic scoliosis varies with age. Juvenile idiopathic scoliosis requires more aggressive treatment because of the risk of prognosis. The risk of progression of adolescent idiopathic scoliosis decreases with increasing skeletal maturity. Congenital and neuromuscular spinal deformity require early, aggressive treatment to maximize mobility and function.

Scheuermann's disease, spondylolysis, and spondylolisthesis can cause mechanical back pain but rarely require operative treatment. Other causes of back pain in children include infection, neoplasm, herniated nucleus pulposus, and apophyseal ring avulsion. Back pain in children warrants thorough evaluation because "idiopathic" back pain is rare.

Cervical spine disorders are rare in children but can have important implications. Congenital torticollis has infectious, mechanical, ophthalmologic, and neurologic etiologies, but it is most commonly due to sternocleidomastoid fibrosis caused by intra-uterine crowding. Klippel-Feil syndrome is highly correlated with other anomalies with significant long-term implications.

Spine trauma is rare in children and is associated with spinal cord injury in 20% of cases. Spinal cord injury without radiographic abnormality is unique to the pediatric population. Systematic clinical and radiographic evaluation is essential to determine appropriate treatment to minimize long-term neurologic and mechanical compromise.

SELECTED BIBLIOGRAPHY

CANALE ST, GRIFFIN DW, HUBBARD CN. Congenital muscular torticollis: a long-term followup. *J Bone Jt Surg.* 1982;64A: 810–816.

CEBALLOS T, FERRER-TORELLES M, CASTILLO F, FERNANDEZ-PAREDES E. Prognosis in infantile idiopathic scoliosis. *J Bone Jt Surg.* 1980;62A:863–875.

FIELDING JW, HENSINGER RN, HAWKINS RJ. Os odontoideum. *J Bone Jt Surg.* 1980;62A:376–383.

FIGUEIREDO UM, JAMES JI. Juvenile idiopathic scoliosis. *J Bone Jt Surg.* 1981;63B:61–66.

GINSBURG GM, BASSETT GS. Back pain in children and adolescents: evaluation and differential diagnosis. *J Am Acad Orthop Surg.* 1997;5:67–78.

GREEN NE. Part-time bracing of adolescent idiopathic scoliosis. *J Bone Jt Surg.* 1986;68A:738–742.

HENSINGER RN. Spondylolysis and spondylolisthesis in children and adolescents. *J Bone Jt Surg.* 1989;71A:1098–1107.

KING HA, MOE JH, BRADFORD DS, WINTER RB. The selection of fusion levels in thoracic idiopathic scoliosis. *J Bone Jt Surg.* 1983;65A:1302–1313.

LONSTEIN JE, CARLSON JM. The prediction of curve progression in untreated idiopathic scoliosis during growth. *J Bone Jt Surg.* 1984;66A:1061–1071.

MCMASTER MJ, OHTSUKA K. The natural history of congenital scoliosis: a study of 251 patients. *J Bone Jt Surg.* 1882; 64A:1128–1147.

MURRAY PM, WEINSTEIN SL, SPRATT KF. The natural history and long-term followup of Scheuermann's kyphosis. *J Bone Jt Surg.* 1993;75A:236–248.

NACHEMSON AL, PETERSON LE. Effectiveness of treatment with a brace in girls who have adolescent idiopathic scoliosis: a prospective, controlled study based on data from the Brace Study of the Scoliosis Research Society. *J Bone Jt Surg.* 1995;77A:815–822.

PAVLOV H, TORA JS, ROBIE B, JAHRE C. Cervical spinal stenosis: determination with vertebral body ratio method. *Radiol.* 1987;164:771–775.

PHILLIPS WA, HENSINGER RN. The management of rotatory atlanto-axial subluxation in children. *J Bone Jt Surg.* 1989;71A:664–668.

RING D, JOHNSTON CE II, WENGER DR. Pyogenic infectious spondylitis in children: the convergence of discitis and vertebral osteomyelitis. *J Pediatr Orthop.* 1995;15:652–660.

RISSER J. The iliac apophysis: an invaluable sign in the management of scoliosis. *Clin Orthop.* 1958;11:111–119.

SANDERS JO, LITTLE DG, RICHARDS BS. Prediction of the crankshaft phenomenon by growth height velocity. *Spine.* 1997;33:1352–1357.

TREDWELL SJ, NEWMAN DE, LOCKITCH G. Instability of the upper cervical spine in Down's syndrome. *J Pediatr Orthop.* 1990;10:602–606.

WINTER S. Preoperative assessment of the child with neuromuscular scoliosis. *Orthop Clin North Am.* 1994;25:239–245.

SAMPLE QUESTIONS

1. The most appropriate treatment for a 14-year-old girl with a 37-degree right thoracic scoliosis that corrects to 23 degrees with lateral bending and is Risser stage 4 would be:
   - (a) posterior spinal fusion to L-4
   - (b) posterior spinal fusion with instrumentation to L-4
   - (c) posterior spinal fusion with instrumentation to the pelvis
   - (d) 16-hour/day TLSO brace treatment
   - (e) physical therapy

2. Predictors of slip progression in spondylolisthesis include:
   - (a) slip angle less than 30 degrees
   - (b) skeletal maturity
   - (c) dysplastic spondylolysis
   - (d) male gender
   - (e) grade II or less

3. Atlanto-axial rotatory subluxation is characterized by which of the following:
   - (a) requires open reduction
   - (b) presents with torticollis
   - (c) sternocleidomastoid muscle spasm on opposite side from direction chin is pointed
   - (d) b and c
   - (e) a, b, and c

4. The most appropriate next step in the evaluation and management of a 7-year-old boy with a 3-week history of back pain, fatigue, no fever, and L3-4 disc space narrowing on lateral radiographs is:
   - (a) open vertebral and intervertebral biopsy
   - (b) radiographically (flouroscopy or CT) guided needle aspiration of the vertebrae and intervertebral disc
   - (c) MRI of the lumbar spine
   - (d) technetium bone scan
   - (e) TLSO brace and rest

5. A 5-year-old boy presents to the emergency department after an unwitnessed fall from a swingset. The child is hysterical and cannot state whether he has pain. The cervical spine is difficult to examine but is nontender. Neurologic examination is grossly normal. Cervical spine radiographs are normal. Supervised flexion and extension radiographs demonstrate 3 mm of anterior subluxation at C2-3 with flexion. The most appropriate treatment is:
   - (a) halo vest immobilization
   - (b) observation and serial neurologic examination
   - (c) open reduction and posterior C2-3 arthrodesis
   - (d) hard cervical collar immobilization
   - (e) cervical halter traction

Answers: 1) d; 2) c; 3) b; 4) c; 5) b

Chapter 44

Neuromuscular Disorders in Children

Stephanie L. Schneck-Jacob, MD and Mark J. Sangimino, MD

Outline

Neuromuscular disorders in children are complex disorders. Musculoskeletal deformity, gait disturbance, and disability are common and are typically due to distruption of the fine balance between the muscles that move each joint. Neuromuscular disorders in children can have profound long-term consequences. These disorders share the basic etiology of a primary derangement that alters the delicate balance between the neurologic, muscular, and skeletal systems, and, thus, compromises function. Normal growth and development in the presence of neuromuscular imbalance may cause progressive deformity.

ETIOLOGY

Common neuromuscular disorders with orthopaedic manifestations include cerebral palsy, myelomeningocele, Duchenne's muscular dystrophy, and arthrogryposis. Cerebral palsy is not progressive, myelomeningocele and arthrogryposis can be progressive, and Duchenne's muscular dystrophy is fatally progressive.

BASIC SCIENCE

Cerebral Palsy

Cerebral palsy is a nonprogressive neurological disorder. It is due to maldevelopment of or injury to the immature brain. Cerebral palsy affects movement and posture and can cause sensory, cognitive, emotional, or communicative dysfunction. Perinatal and postnatal causes have been theorized, but prenatal developmental disturbance is the likely etiology in at least 80% of cases. A history of prematurity and low birth weight is common.

Spasticity is the most common cause of movement and posture problems, but athetosis, ataxia, dystonia, or chorea may be present. Spasticity has been defined as a motor disorder characterized as a velocity-dependent increase in tone resulting from hyperexcitability of stretch reflexes as a component of an upper motor neuron syndrome. Increased tone and asynchrony of motor control make it difficult or even impossible for the afflicted child to initiate or maintain normal motion and posture.

Increased tone in an extremity may cause muscle force imbalance and a non-neutral resting joint position. Over time, musculotendinous units may shorten because of the altered resting joint position, become contracted, and thus maintain the pathologic joint posture. The pathologic joint posture compounds the muscle force imbalance across the joint and the corresponding physes. Bony deformity, dysplasia, and/or joint malalignment often result.

Myelomeningocele

Spina bifida encompasses a wide range of neural tube defects. Spina bifida occulta is a benign, localized defect of the vertebral arch that occurs in 10% of normal adults. Spina bifida cystica comprises vertebral arch defects with meningeal, and possibly, neural element involvement. A meningocele involves only the meninges. Abnormal neural elements are present in a myelomeningocele, which is the most common neural tube defect (Fig. 44–1).

Most neural tube defects result from failure of neural tube closure at 3 to 4 weeks of gestation. The cause is unknown and believed to be multifactorial. Recent studies have demonstrated that preconception dietary supplementation

Orthopaedic Surgery: The Essentials. Edited by M.E. Baratz, A.D. Watson, and J.E. Imbriglia. Thieme Medical Publishers, Inc., New York © 1999

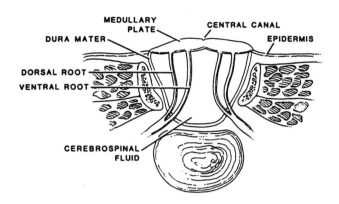

Figure 44–1 Cross section of myelomeningocele with the abnormal neural elements elevated out of the spinal canal. Reproduced with permission from Lindseth RE. Myelomeningocele. In: Morrissy RT, Weinstein SL, eds. *Lovell and Winter's Pediatric Orthopaedics*. Philadelphia, PA: Lippincott-Raven; 1996:504.

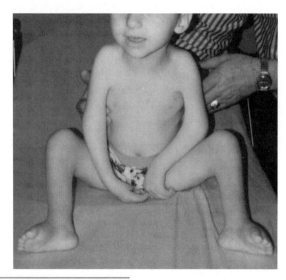

Figure 44–2 Typical limb contractures seen in arthrogryposis multiplex congenita.

with 400 mg of folic acid per day can reduce the risk of spina bifida cystica.

Muscle imbalance, postural contracture in utero, or pathologic posture due to muscle weakness may lead to skeletal deformity. Muscle imbalance can result from normal muscles overpowering weak or flaccid antagonists or from spastic muscles overpowering normal, weak, or flaccid antagonists. The imbalance may cause joint malposition and contracture of the shortened anatagonist. As in cerebral palsy, pathologically aligned joint and/or physis forces may cause progressive deformity with growth.

Growth can indirectly cause neurologic deterioration, increased spasticity, scoliosis, and worsening urologic function because scarring at the site of the myelomeningocele closure may tether the spinal cord and restrict caudad migration of the spinal cord with longitudinal vertebral growth. Hydrocephalus and hydromyelia are commonly present and may also lead to neurologic deterioration.

Duchenne's Muscular Dystrophy

Duchenne's muscular dystrophy is the third most common neuromuscular disease after cerebral palsy and myelomeningocele. It is typically hereditary with an X-linked recessive inheritance pattern, but one third of cases are new mutations. It is believed that individuals with Duchenne's muscular dystrophy lack the gene that codes for the protein dystrophin. This gene is located on the X chromosome. The absence of dystrophin appears to impair neuromuscular transmission at the muscle fiber sarcoplasmic reticulum. Progressive weakness develops in selected muscle groups. Compensatory gait abnormalities develop, which in turn lead to contractures and secondary skeletal deformities.

Arthrogryposis Multiplex Congenita

Arthrogryposis comprises a group of approximately 150 syndromes characterized by joint contractures present at birth. Ninety percent of patients with congenital joint contractures have classic arthrogryposis multiplex congenita or amyoplasia. It is believed that patients with arthrogryposis multiplex

congenita have a decreased number of anterior horn cells in the spinal cord. This results in myofibrosis and limited active intra-uterine motion. Featureless, fusiform limbs that lack skin creases develop (Fig. 44–2).

ANATOMY AND SURGICAL APPROACHES

Hip

The anterior approach is useful for access to the hip flexors, the hip joint, and the ilium. The lateral femoral cutaneous nerve crosses the interval between the sartorius and the tensor fascia lata, but its course may vary. The ascending branch of lateral femoral circumflex artery is encountered in the interval between the gluteus medius and the rectus femoris. The internervous plane is between the gluteus medius, which is innervated by the superior gluteal nerve and the rectus femoris, which is innervated by the femoral nerve.

Surgical Approach

A slightly oblique "bikini" incision is made just below the anterior iliac crest. The lateral femoral cutaneous nerve is identified and retracted medially, and blunt dissection proceeds through the interval between the sartorius and tensor fascia lata (Fig. 44–3). The ascending branch of the lateral femoral circumflex artery is identified between the gluteus medius and rectus femoris and is ligated. Blunt dissection continues between the gluteus medius and rectus femoris. The straight and reflected origins of the rectus femoris are detached from the anterior inferior iliac spine and anterior hip capsule, respectively. Inferomedial to the hip capsule, the iliopsoas tendon can be identified as it courses to its insertion onto the lesser trochanter.

The medial approach is used for access to the hip adductors, iliopsoas, and hamstrings. The anterior division of the obturator nerve courses over the upper portion of the adductor brevis muscle. The posterior division of the obturator nerve courses over the adductor magnus in the interval

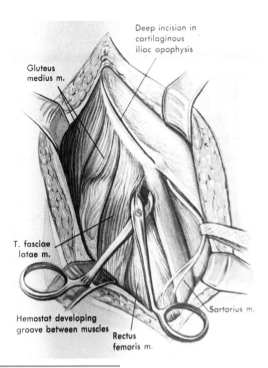

Figure 44–3 In the anterior approach to the hip, dissection proceeds in the internervous plane superficially between the sartorius and tensor fascia lata muscles and more deeply between the rectus femoris and gluteus medius muscles. Reproduced with permission from Tachdjian MO. *Pediatric Orthopedics*. Philadelphia, PA: WB Saunders; 1990:381.

between it and the adductor brevis. The medial femoral circumflex artery lies along the inferior hip capsule.

The patient is positioned supine with the hip flexed and abducted. Either a transverse incision 1 cm distal to the groin crease or a longitudinal incision centered over the adductor longus tendon is used. The sheath of the adductor longus is incised longitudinally, and the muscle is divided transversely close to its origin on the pelvis. The adductor brevis is encountered and can be identified by the presence of the anterior branch of the obturator nerve overlying it. The gracilis is posterior to the adductor brevis and may require division for further exposure. The iliopsoas tendon is identified by retracting the pectineus anteriorly and palpating the lesser trochanter (Fig. 44–4). The large posterior muscle is the adductor magnus, over which the posterior branch of the

oburator nerve courses. The origins of the hamstring tendons are further posterior and can be divided using this approach in the nonambulatory cerebral palsy patient, if indicated. The sciatic nerve, which lies anterior and slightly lateral to the hamstrings, should be palpated and pushed laterally prior to hamstring release.

Knee

The posterior approach is used for access to the knee flexors and posterior capsule. The medial sural cutaneous nerve lies superficial to the fascia and lateral to the small saphenous vein. The sciatic nerve divides into the tibial and common peroneal nerves proximal to the knee joint. Both branches are the most lateral structures in the popliteal fossa. The small saphenous vein is superficial to the posterior fascia. The popliteal vein and artery are medial to the tibial nerve and deep to the fascia.

The hamstring muscles insert onto the tibia and fibula, and the gastrocnemius muscle originates from the femoral condyles. The muscle borders form a diamond-shaped fossa within which lie the major vessels and nerves to the leg. The medial hamstring tendons include the semitendinosus, semimembranosus, gracilis, and sartorius (Fig. 44–5). The biceps femoris tendon is the lateral hamstring.

When muscle lengthening without posterior capsulotomy is necessary, longitudinal incisions over the medial and lateral hamstrings suffice. A transverse incision approximately 1 cm proximal to the knee flexion crease is necessary when posterior capsulotomy is necessary. The transverse incision must be made through the skin only with blunt dissection of the subcutaneous tissue to avoid injuring the small saphenous vein and medial sural cutaneous nerve. It may be necessary to release the medial and lateral origin of the gastrocnemius from the femoral condyles and to expose the posterior knee capsule (see Fig. 44–5). A moist sponge may be used to develop this plane deep to the neurovascular bundle so that these structures can be safely retracted posteriorly. Additional posterior release can be achieved by dividing the posterior cruciate ligament, medial and lateral collateral ligaments, and iliotibial band.

EXAMINATION

The evaluation should begin with the prenatal, birth, growth, developmental, and family history. The timing of develop-

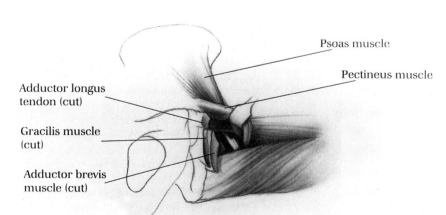

Figure 44–4 The iliopsoas is visualized by retracting the pectineus muscle superiorly. Reproduced with permission from Morrissy RT. *Atlas of Pediatric Orthopaedic Surgery*. Philadelphia, PA: Lippincott-Raven; 1996:378. Bernie Kida, illustrator.

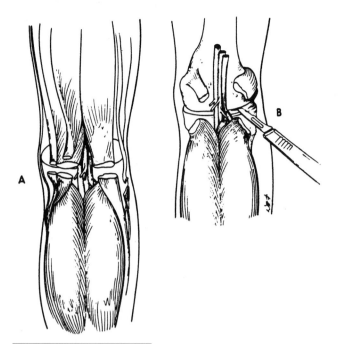

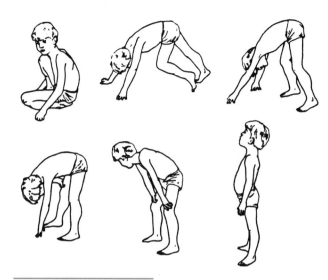

Figure 44–6 Gower's sign. Reproduced with permission from Seigel IM. *The Clinical Management of Muscle Disease.* Philadelphia, PA: Lippincott-Raven; 1977;1:13.

Figure 44–5 Posterior approach to the knee. **(A)** In myelomeningocele patients, all the hamstring tendons are divided and resected for a length of 2 cm. **(B)** The gastrocnemius is divided from its origins medially and laterally, and the posterior capsule is incised. Reproduced with permission from Beaty JH. Paralytic disorders. In: Crenshaw AH, ed. *Campbell's Operative Orthopaedics.* St. Louis, MO: Mosby Year Book; 1992:2443.

PEARL

In patients with asensate limbs from spina bifida or in noncommunicative patients with cerebral palsy, apply well-molded postoperative casts by making a hybrid of plaster followed by fiberglass, for added strength. In addition, pad all bony prominences with pieces of one-eighth inch felt, in addition to the usual cotton cast padding. Common areas for breakdown include the heel, plantar foot, patella, greater trochanter, anterior and posterior iliac crests, and sacrum.

---

mental milestones should receive special attention. Patients with cerebral palsy may initially appear normal, and the first indication of pathology may be delayed standing or walking. Myelomeningocele is usually obvious at birth, but rare patients with sacral or even low lumbar involvement may not manifest symptoms until they begin ambulating. Duchenne's muscular dystrophy typically does not become evident until 18 to 36 months of age.

An evaluation of the child's functional ability including sitting, crawling, standing, walking, and eating is useful for prognosis and treatment planning. Urologic function should be assessed as well. It is imperative to observe an ambulatory child's gait to effectively plan treatment. Although detailed

gait analysis can assist or even direct treatment planning, much useful information can be gained from simple observation. Subtle hemiplegia can be elicited in a normal appearing child with cerebral palsy by having the child run.

Detailed neurological examination is imperative. The examination should be repeated at each visit in children with spina bifida and Duchenne's muscular dystrophy. Subtle, progressive deficits in spina bifida suggest tethered cord, uncompensated hydrocephalus, and hydromyelia. Progressive weakness that starts with the proximal muscle groups is characteristic of Duchenne's muscular dystrophy. Gower's sign (Fig. 44–6) is useful in demonstrating this proximal weakness in a young child.

Periodic range-of-motion examination is essential in all neuromuscular diseases. The Thomas test (Fig. 44–7) measures hip flexion contracture. The popliteal angle (Fig. 44–8) measures knee flexion contracture. Heelcord contracture should be evaluated with the foot inverted and the knee in full extension. These measurements can help elucidate the causes of a gait abnormality. Examination of the spine for both scoliosis and sagittal deformities is also important.

AIDS TO DIAGNOSIS

Plain radiographs are usually all that is necessary for characterizing deformity. Specialized views such as abduction-internal rotation views of the hips to determine concentricity of reduction or weight-bearing views of the feet are often indicated. Spine films should be performed in the sitting or standing positions whenever possible.

Magnetic resonance imaging (MRI) of the brain and spinal cord is indicated whenever the neurologic status worsens or scoliosis progresses in a patient with spina bifida. This will help rule out worsening hydrocephalus, tethered cord, or hydromyelia. Detailed gait analysis is useful for planning brace or surgical treatment.

Laboratory studies are of little use in cerebral palsy, spina bifida, and arthrogryposis. Creatine phosphokinase (CPK) is

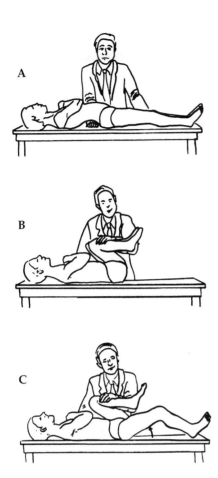

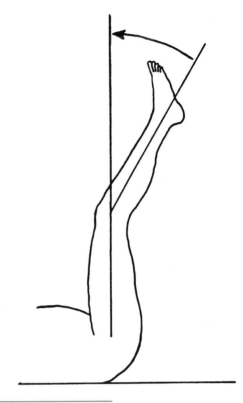

Figure 44–8 The popliteal angle.

Figure 44–7 Thomas test. **(A)** A fixed flexion contracture results in compensatory increased lumbar lordosis when the patient attempts to lie supine. **(B)** In testing for hip flexion contracture, first flex both hips as far as possible to stabilize the pelvis and flatten the lumbar lordosis. **(C)** Allow one limb to extend as far as possible. The angle between the table and the longitudinal axis of the patient's right femur is the magnitude of hip flexion contracture. Adapted from Hoppenfeld S. *Physical Examination of the Spine and Extremities.* Old Tappan, NJ; Appleton-Century-Crofts; 1976:156.

markedly elevated in early Duchenne's muscular dystrophy. Muscle biopsy in Duchenne's muscular dystrophy reveals degeneration, muscle fiber heterogeneity, connective tissue proliferation, and fibrofatty replacement of muscle tissue. The fibrofatty replacement is manifested clinically by pseudohypertrophy of the calf. Chromosome analysis is replacing muscle biopsy for diagnosis of Duchenne's muscular dystrophy.

Electromyography (EMG) is occasionally useful, especially in the differential diagnosis of Duchenne's muscular dystrophy. Low amplitude polyphasic action potentials of short duration are characteristic of Duchenne's muscular dystrophy. Fibrillation potentials are present in arthrogryposis. Dynamic EMG during gait analysis can illustrate the timing of asynchronous muscle activity in cerebral palsy, and, thus, help determine whether tendon transfers may be useful. It can also be used in myelomeningocele to determine which muscles are active during gait; however, there is no asynchrony in myelomeningocele, and manual motor testing may be sufficient.

SPECIFIC CONDITIONS, TREATMENT, AND OUTCOME

Cerebral Palsy

Geographic and neurologic classification of cerebral palsy is useful for prognosis and treatment. Hemiplegia describes involvement of the upper and lower extremity on one side. Diplegia is bilateral lower extremity involvement. Tetraplegia, formerly quadriplegia, is involvement of all four extremities. Total involvement includes severe cognitive impairment with tetraplegia. Adult function is best with hemiplegia and worst with total involvement. Neurologic types include spastic, flaccid, athetotic, and ataxic. Adult function is best with spastic involvement, which is the most common type. Therefore, spastic hemiplegia has the best prognosis for adult function, followed by spastic diplegia. These two forms are the most common. Ambulation, perineal function, and cognitive function are impaired in more severe forms of involvement.

The goal for the child with cerebral palsy is to maximize function and ambulatory efficiency. The primary cerebral abnormality or insult is usually irreversible, and therefore, the treatment team must deal with the secondary hypertonicity and deformities. Early, aggressive multidisciplinary management includes physical therapy, electrical stimulation, positioning and casting, pharmacologic agents, peripheral nerve blocks, tendon transfer, and rhizotomy.

Diligent physical therapy is the mainstay of treatment for cerebral palsy. Stretching of hypertonic muscle groups, splinting, and postural training are essential to maintain function and prevent progressive contracture and deformity.

Baclofen is an effective muscle relaxant that can be administered orally or by way of an implanted pump that delivers the medication directly into the intrathecal space. Baclofen inhibits monosynaptic and polysynaptic reflexes at the spinal cord level to reduce hypertonicity.

Selective dorsal rhizotomy can reduce hypertonicity in spastic patients that are not athetotic. This procedure can delay or even prevent orthopaedic procedures in select patients. Laminectomy is performed between L-1 and L-5 and the dorsal rootlets are electrically stimulated. Rootlets in which incremental, clonic, and multiphasic potentials are generated are divided. Usually, 60 to 70 rootlets are stimulated, and 25 to 50% are divided. Complications include loss of postural control, trunk asymmetry, and weakness of the lower extremities.

Muscle or tendon lengthening may be necessary when tone management fails to prevent contracture. Realignment osteotomies may be necessary when longstanding contracture causes dysplasia.

Progressive Hip Subluxation and Dislocation

The incidence of progressive hip subluxation and dislocation in patients with cerebral palsy is between 18 and 28%. Patients with spastic quadriplegia are at highest risk. The incidence in patients with spastic diplegia is much lower, and it is rare in spastic hemiplegia.

Spastic hip flexors and adductors overpower the extensors and abductors and sublux or even dislocate the hip. Contracture of the shortenened flexors and adductors subsequently develop. Limited abduction occurs early; lumbar lordosis, hip instability, and a crouched or scissor gait occur later. Hip pain may result from the femoral head resting against the ilium.

Soft tissue releases are necessary to balance the forces across the hip when nonoperative management of spasticity fails. Flexion contractures greater than 25 degrees can be treated with release or lengthening of the rectus femoris, tensor fascia lata, and the iliopsoas as it traverses the pelvic brim. Adduction contractures allowing less than 40 degrees of abduction should be treated with adductor tenotomy or transfer. Adductor transfer is preferred in ambulatory patients because it results in better hip motion and stability and minimizes the risk of recurrence.

Patients under the age of 4 with hip subluxation and at least 50% acetabular coverage of the femoral head require soft tissue release and tendon lengthening or transfer as previously described to improve hip stability and prevent dysplasia. Tight hamstrings may also require release. Intertrochanteric varus rotation osteotomy should supplement soft tissue surgery in patients older than 4 years with less than 50% femoral head coverage. Bony deformity may recur in younger patients. Pelvic osteotomy may be necessary in an older child or young adult when acetabular dysplasia is present.

Windswept Hips

A "windswept" deformity occurs when flexion-adduction contracture of one hip coexists with flexion-abduction contracture of the contralateral hip. Dislocation may occur on the side of the flexion-adduction contracture and may lead to pelvic obliquity and scoliosis. Perineal care and seating of children with windswept hips can be very difficult. Muscle releases need to be performed early and combined with realignment osteotomies. The abduction contracture must be corrected to prevent recurrence of the contralateral flexion-adduction contracture.

Chronic Painful Hip Dislocation

Inadequately treated children with flexion-adduction contracture eventually develop hip dislocation, which becomes painful even if they are nonambulatory. Unfortunately, there is no uniformly reliable treatment option. Proximal femur resection may result in proximal migration of the femoral shaft, leg-length discrepancy, and soft tissue complications. Interposition arthroplasty may improve the results of resection arthroplasty, if the technique is meticulously performed. Hip fusion can effectively relieve pain, but pseudoarthrosis is common in the neurologically impaired child. Total hip replacement is a viable option in very selected individuals. Aggressive, well-timed, prophylactic nonoperative and operative treatment is essential to avoid hip dislocation.

Crouched Gait

Crouched gait is common in patients with spastic diplegia. It may be due to any combination of hip flexion contracture, knee flexion contracture, or pescalcaneus deformity. The patient appears to be crouching while walking.

Treatment must be directed at all contractures that may be present, and the effects of lengthening muscles that cross two joints must be considered. For example, hamstring lengthening will improve knee extension but may result in increased hip flexion, anterior pelvic tilt, and compensatory lumbar hyperlordosis if hip flexion contracture is not corrected. Equinus contracture may, in rare instances, develop postoperatively because knee extension tightens the gastrocnemius. Cylinder casts are applied postoperatively, and the child is allowed to ambulate.

Stiff Knee Gait

Reduced knee flexion during swing phase and a decreased arc of knee motion characterizes stiff knee gait. Out-of-phase activity of the rectus femoris during swing phase is often identified during EMG gait analysis.

Treatment options consist of proximal or distal release of the rectus femoris or distal transfer of the rectus femoris to the sartorius muscle. Recent gait analysis studies have demonstrated better peak knee flexion with transfer.

Equinovarus Foot Deformity

Equinovarus foot deformity occurs most often in patients with spastic hemiplegia or diplegia. The deformity is due to posterior tibialis muscle spasticity and peroneal muscle weakness. Plantigrade weight-bearing and shoe wearing are difficult or even impossible.

Nonoperative treatment includes accomodative shoewear, orthotics, and brace management. Surgical treatment is indicated when nonoperative treatment fails. Flexibility of the deformity determines the appropriate surgical treatment. The Coleman block test is used to assess hindfoot and midfoot flexibility. The patient stands with the heel and lateral rays on a one half-inch block and allows the medial ray to fall towards the floor. The hindfoot and midfoot are deemed flexible if the hindfoot corrects from varus to neutral or valgus. Gait analysis is also useful preoperatively to determine which muscles are spastic and during which phase of gait.

Tendon transfer attempts to balance tendon forces across the foot and ankle to correct flexible deformity. Split posterior tibial tendon transfer weakens a spastic posterior tibialis muscle, maintains plantar flexion strength, and augments weak peroneal muscles. Three incisions are used. One incision is made over the navicular insertion of the posterior tibial tendon to release and split the plantar half of the tendon. A second incision is made proximal to the tarsal tunnel to continue splitting the tendon proximally to the musculotendinous junction and to pass the tendon transfer posterolaterally. The third incision is placed laterally to retrieve the tendon transfer and to weave it into the peroneus brevis.

Split anterior tibial tendon transfer to the cuboid is combined with lengthening of the posterior tibial tendon when the anterior tibialis is spastic in stance and swing phase. A dorsal incision is made over the navicular insertion of the anterior tibialis tendon to release and split the lateral half of the tendon. A second incision is made proximal to the ankle to continue splitting the tendon proximally to the musculotendinous junction. The tendon transfer is passed subcutaneously towards the dorsal cuboid bone, where it is retrieved through a third longitudinal incision. The tendon transfer is anchored to the periosteum of the cuboid or through a drill hole. After tendon transfer, corrective casts are applied and changed biweekly for 6 weeks. Weight-bearing is initiated 2 weeks after surgery.

Rigid deformity requires realignment triple arthrodesis to correct and maintain alignment. Degenerative joint disease of the ankle occurs 40 years after triple arthrodesis in nearly three quarters of patients. An extended sinus tarsi approach is used to fuse the subtalar and calcaneocuboid joints, and a medial longitudinal incision over the talonavicular joint is used to fuse it. Correction is easier to obtain by shortening the lateral foot at the calcaneocuboid joint than by lengthening the medial foot at the talonavicular joint. The talonavicular joint should be positioned and fixed first to correct the deformity, followed by the subtalar joint and the calcaneocuboid joint. It is imperative to remove all cartilage from the joint surfaces. A short-leg cast is applied postoperatively and changed every 4 weeks until solid arthrodesis occurs. Weight-bearing may begin 6 weeks postoperatively if there is radiographic evidence of progressive healing.

Equinovalgus Foot Deformity

Equinovalgus foot deformity is commonly caused by heelcord contracture and most often occurs in children with spastic diplegia. The deformity occurs because the ankle cannot dorsiflex normally during gait because of the tight heelcord. Midfoot dorsiflexion and hindfoot eversion occur to allow the tibia to progress over the foot during stance phase of gait. Eventually equinovalgus deformity develops.

Nonoperative treatment options include accomodative shoes and bracing. Surgical treatment for failed nonoperative treatment includes heelcord lengthening and lateral calcaneal

lengthening with a bone block. Percutaneous heelcord lengthening is often sufficient for mild contracture. Stab wounds are made just proximal to the insertion, just distal to the musculotendinous junction, and midway between the first two incisions. The medial half of the tendon is divided in the distal and proximal wounds, and the lateral half is divided in the center wound. Manual ankle dorsiflexion force is applied until a "snap" is heard. Ten to fifteen degrees of passive dorsiflexion should be possible.

Severe equinus contracture due to gastrocnemius and soleus contracture requires a Z-lengthening of the Achilles' tendon. It is important to remember that the Achilles' tendon fibers internally rotate as they approach the calcaneal insertion. The posterior fibers insert onto the calcaneus laterally.

Severe equinus due to isolated gastrocnemius contracture is treated with step-cut lengthening at the musculotendinous junction via a posteromedial or posterolateral incision. Only the tendinous and fascial fibers are divided, and the underlying muscle is left intact. Manual ankle dorsiflexion force is applied to stretch the muscle and distract the step-cut.

Calcaneal lengthening is performed via a lateral longitudinal incision over the anterior calcaneus and calcaneocuboid joint. A coronal osteotomy is made in the anterior calcaneus 1.5 cm proximal to the calcaneocuboid joint. The osteotomy is distracted, and a tricortical iliac crest bone block approximately 1 cm wide is placed in the osteotomy. A smooth or threaded Kirschner wire (K-wire) is used for fixation. A short-leg cast is used for 6 to 12 weeks postoperatively. Weight-bearing may begin 4 to 6 weeks postoperatively, if there is radiographic evidence of progressive healing.

The Grice extra-articular subtalar arthrodesis, conventional subtalar arthrodesis, or Crawford staple arthroeresis can be used to correct hindfoot valgus. Crawford's procedure is more useful in children less than 4 years old. Neither corrects the planus or forefoot abductus deformities as well as the calcaneal lengthening. The Grice procedure consists of removing a core of bone from the lateral talus and calcaneus at the posterior facet of the subtalar joint and packing cancellous bone graft. The hindfoot is realigned, and staples or a cast can be used to maintain position. Arthroeresis is not performed in Crawford's staple arthroeresis; instead, the hindfoot position is corrected and fixed with staples.

Conventional subtalar arthrodesis is reliable. It is performed via a sinus tarsi approach. Cartilage and subchondral bone is removed from the talar and calcaneal articular surfaces of the subtalar joint. The hindfoot position is corrected. Fixation is with threaded K-wires or staples. A short-leg cast is applied postoperatively after subtalar arthrodesis or arthroeresis, and weight-bearing is permitted 4 to 6 weeks postoperatively. Casting is continued for 6 to 10 weeks postoperatively.

Myelomeningocele

Children with myelomeningocele are classified according to the lowest nerve root functioning with antigravity strength (Fig. 44–9). This classification helps determine prognosis and guides treatment planning.

IgE-mediated hypersensitivity to latex is very prevalent among patients with myelomeningocele. It is believed to be due to repetitive latex exposure from frequent urethral catheterization and surgical procedures. Reactions can range from skin rash and bronchospasm to anaphylaxis and death.

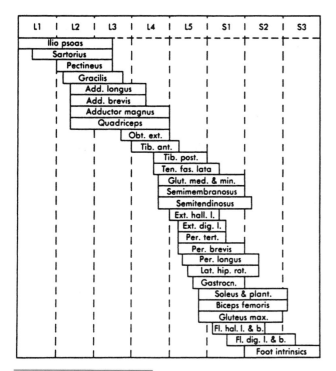

	L1	L2	L3	L4	L5	S1	S2	S3
	Ilio psoas							
	Sartorius							
		Pectineus						
		Gracilis						
		Add. longus						
		Add. brevis						
		Adductor magnus						
		Quadriceps						
			Obt. ext.					
			Tib. ant.					
			Tib. post.					
			Ten. fas. lata					
			Glut. med. & min.					
			Semimembranosus					
			Semitendinosus					
			Ext. hall. l.					
			Ext. dig. l.					
			Per. tert.					
			Per. brevis					
			Per. longus					
			Lat. hip. rot.					
			Gastrocn.					
				Soleus & plant.			
				Biceps femoris			
				Gluteus max.			
				Fl. hal. l. & b.			
				Fl. dig. l. & b.			
					Foot intrinsics		

Figure 44–9 Neurosegmental innervation of muscles of lower limb. Reproduced with permission from Sharrard WJW. Posterior iliopsoas transplantation in the treatment of paralytic dislocation of the hip. *J Bone Jt Surg.* 1964;46B:427.

Strict latex precautions are necessary when caring for a patient with myelomeningocele.

Ambulation

The most important treatment goal for the orthopaedic surgeon is to maximize the myelomeningocele patient's mobility. This requires a plantigrade foot, adequate trunk balance, and functional lower extremity alignment. Nearly all children will ambulate in early childhood with the aid of orthoses. The neurologic level determines the prognosis for ambulation beyond adolescence. Patients with an L3-4 level or lower have a much better prognosis for adult ambulation because they have sufficient knee extension strength and do not require above-the-knee orthoses. Scoliosis and pelvic obliquity due to either lower extremity deformity or scoliosis compromise trunk balance and may limit ambulation. Surprisingly, hip dislocation does not preclude ambulation.

Spinal Deformity

Scoliosis

Scoliosis may be paralytic, congenital, or neurogenic. The initial presentation of scoliosis or progression of scoliosis requires evaluation for tethered cord, hydrocephalus, or hydromyelia. Nearly 100% of thoracic-level patients will have scoliosis, as opposed to 50% of lumbar-level and 5% of sacral-level patients.

Paralytic curves can usually be controlled by bracing until age 9 or 10. Progression occurs with the adolescent growth spurt and requires anterior and posterior spinal fusion with segmental instrumentation; fusion to the pelvis is recommended only if the child is not a reciprocal walker. Posterior fusion requires anterior supplementation because of the deficient posterior elements available for fusion.

Neurogenic curves may stabilize or even improve if the underlying cause is treated. Congenital curves should be treated with short in situ fusion in early childhood with extension of the arthrodesis at maturity.

PITFALL

Examine patients with myelomeningocele for infrapelvic contractures prior to surgical spine fusion. Hip flexion contractures greater than 20 degrees require release, or it will be difficult to position the patient prone on the operating table without exaggerating lumbar lordosis. Severe flexion contractures will stress lumbosacral spinal instrumentation and increase the risk of pseudoarthrosis and instrumentation failure.

Kyphosis

Sagittal deformity occurs most often in thoracic or high lumbar myelomenigocele. Paralytic kyphosis is C-shaped, and congenital kyphosis is an S-shaped curve. Bracing controls paralytic curves until fusion becomes necessary for progression during the adolescent growth spurt. Congenital kyphosis is often rigid, may approach 180 degrees, and resists bracing because of frequent skin ulceration. Surgical correction requires resection of the vertebrae of the rigid segment proximal to the apex of the deformity (Fig. 44–10) and segmental instrumention from the upper thoracic spine to the sacrum.

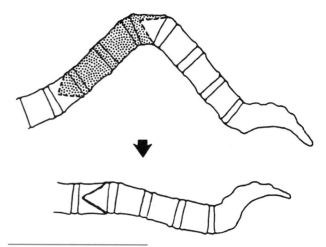

Figure 44–10 In the congenital S-shaped kyphosis, the stippled area of rigid lordosis proximal to the apex of the kyphosis is the area to be resected. Reproduced with permission from Lindseth RE. Myelomeningocele. In: Morrissy RT, Weinstein SL, eds. *Lovell and Winter's Pediatric Orthopaedics.* Philadelphia, PA: Lippincott-Raven; 1996:520.

Hip

Contractures

Flexion contractures are most common in high lumbar or thoracic-level myelomeningocele patients. Surgical release is indicated when contractures are greater than 20 degrees and interfere with walking or bracing. A complete release of sartorius, tensor fascia lata, rectus femoris, iliopsoas, and anterior hip capsule is necessary.

Flexion-abduction–external rotation contractures occur in thoracic level patients. Flaccid limbs assume this posture in the supine patient and become contracted. Nonoperative treatment includes night splints and daytime stretching. Surgical release of the tensor fascia lata fascia proximally and the iliotibial band distally is indicated if bracing fails to control deformity.

Subluxation and Dislocation

Hip instability usually occurs before age three in L3-4 level patients who have intact hip flexors and adductors and weak hip extensors. Surgical treatment is indicated only if the patient has sufficient quadriceps strength to ambulate in below-knee orthoses. The goals of surgery are concentric reduction and muscle balance. Open reduction, release of contractures, and muscle transfer are usually necessary. Longstanding hip instability with secondary bone deformity often requires femoral and/or pelvic osteotomies.

Knee

Flexion contractures are common in thoracic or high-lumbar-level patients because of prolonged wheelchair sitting. Night splints and physical therapy are often effective, but hamstring release and posterior capsulotomy are necessary when flexion contracture greater than 20 degrees mitigates successful bracing.

Extension contractures occur in patients with an L3-4 level who have strong quadriceps and weak hamstrings. V-Y advancement of the suprapatellar portion of the quadriceps tendon can release the contracture while maintaining sufficient quadriceps strength.

Ankle and Foot

Valgus ankle deformity occurs in L4-5 level patients because of gastrocnemius-soleus weakness. Skin breakdown may occur over the medial malleolus. Weight-bearing radiographs of the feet and ankles are useful for differentiating ankle valgus from hindfoot valgus. Nonoperative treatment includes accomodative shoewear and judicious bracing. Surgical treatment includes Achilles' tendon tenodesis to the fibula in the young child, hemiepiphysiodesis of the distal medial tibia in the older child, and supramalleolar osteotomy in adolescents with little or no growth remaining.

Foot deformities are present in 90% of children with spina bifida. Nonoperative treatment includes accomodative shoewear, bracing, and diligent physical therapy. Bracing must be done carefully because of insensate skin. Surgical treatment is indicated when nonoperative measures fail to adequately control deformity or impending or actual skin ulceration occurs.

Flexible deformities are often amenable to soft tissue surgery. The tendons of spastic or flaccid muscles should be excised. Tendons under adequate volitional control should then be transferred to balance the foot. The result is a flail but braceable foot with little chance of recurrence. Stiff or rigid deformities may require realignment osteotomies. Arthrodesis should be avoided in patients with myelomeningocele.

Talipes equinovarus is the most common foot deformity in myelomeningocele and is treated surgically with complete subtalar release and radical excision of all tendons. Congenital vertical talus occurs in 10% of patients with myelomeningocele. Nonoperative treatment is rarely successful. Complete subtalar release and tendon excision are usually necessary.

Equinus deformity is easily preventable, but may require Achilles' tendon lengthening as previously described when nonoperative treatment fails. Calcaneus deformity is due to active ankle dorsiflexors and paralyzed plantar flexors. Anterior tibial tendon transfer to the posterior calcaneus is recommended in younger children, and a proximal displacement osteotomy of the calcaneus may be necessary in older children.

Valgus hindfoot deformity can easily cause skin breakdown over the head of the talus. Calcaneal lengthening as described previously can improve the valgus hindfoot and reconstitute the longitudinal arch. Cavovarus deformity and clawfoot occur in children with sacral-level myelomeningocele because of intrinsic muscle and gastrocnemius-soleus muscle paralysis. Split transfer of either the posterior tibialis tendon or the anterior tibialis tendon to the midfoot may balance the foot and correct a flexible deformity. A lateral closing wedge osteotomy of the calcaneus may be necessary if the Coleman block test demonstrates that the hindfoot and midfoot are not flexible. Radical plantar release and/or midfoot osteotomy may also be necessary to correct a rigid cavovarus foot deformity.

Rotational Deformities

Out-toeing gait may be due to either external femoral or tibial torsion (Fig. 44–11). External femoral torsion occurs in the thoracic- or L-5-level patient. Bracing can be used to control out-toeing, but subtrochanteric rotational osteotomy may be necessary. External tibial torsion is usually associated with valgus ankle deformity. Surgical treatment is indicated when gait is compromised by the deformity and consists of a derotation varus closing-wedge supramalleolar osteotomy.

In toeing gait (Fig. 44–11) occurs in L4-5 level patients who have active medial hamstrings but inactive lateral hamstrings. Transfer of the semitendinosus tendon to the head of the fibula will balance tibial rotation if significant bony deformity is absent. Internal tibial torsion greater than 10 degrees requires a rotational osteotomy in addition to the semitendinosus tendon transfer.

Fractures

Patients with myelomeningocele typically sustain neuropathic fractures in insensate limbs with minimal trauma. Predisposing factors include osteopenia, poor proprioception, and fixed contractures. The fractures are painless and present only with erythema, warmth, swelling, and fever. Fractures are often misdiagnosed as cellulitis or osteomyelitis, and,

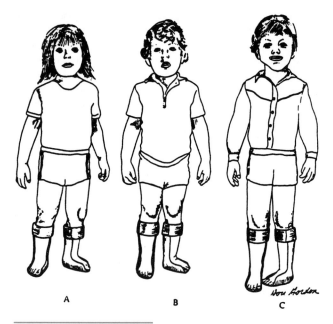

Figure 44–11 Common torsional deformities in myelomeningocele. **(A)** Out-toeing gait secondary to left external femoral torsion. **(B)** Out-toeing gait due to external tibial torsion on the left. **(C)** Left internal tibial torsion causing intoeing gait. Reproduced with permission from Dias LS, Jasty MJ, Collins P. Rotational deformities of the lower limb in myelomeningocele. *J Bone Jt Surg.* 1984; 66A:216.

fractures are usually undisplaced and may only be apparent on stress radiographs. Physeal fractures have a more guarded prognosis and may require cast immobilization for 4 to 6 weeks.

PEARL
A red, hot, swollen limb in a paralytic patient is a fracture until proven otherwise.

Duchenne's Muscular Dystrophy

The goal of treatment is to preserve ambulation for as long as possible. Patients are usually wheelchair bound by adolescence and succumb to respiratory failure in their early 20s. Physical therapy is initiated early in the course of disease to preserve muscle strength and limit contractures. Surgical release of hip, knee, or ankle contractures may be necessary for pain relief or if ambulation is impaired. Progressive scoliosis occurs in 95% of patients and is treated by posterior spinal fusion from the upper thoracic spine to the pelvis when the curve exceeds 20 degrees.

Arthrogryposis Multiplex Congenita

Physical therapy beginning during the neonatal period is essential to maximize range of motion. Passive, but not active, range of motion can improve with therapy. Soft tissue releases may be necessary before age 2 to align the limbs for standing or ambulating in orthoses. After age 2, soft tissue releases are unsuccessful because of progressive joint incongruity. Osteotomies are then necessary for realignment.

Unilateral hip dislocation in infancy should be treated surgically, but bilateral dislocated hips are best left alone. Resistant clubfoot is characteristic of arthrogryposis and requires radical soft tissue release. Primary talectomy should also be considered because of the high incidence of failed soft tissue surgery. Scoliosis occurs in one third of patients and is treated as in other neuromuscular diseases.

therefore, should be suspected and ruled out with radiographs of the affected extremity.

Fracture healing in children with myelomeningocele is exuberant and nonunion is rare. Metaphyseal and diaphyseal fractures are treated with immobilization for 2 to 4 weeks in a well-padded, well-molded cast, followed by treatment in a brace as soon as callus is radiographically apparent. Physeal

SELECTED BIBLIOGRAPHY

ASHER M, OLSON J. Factors affecting the ambulatory status of patients with spina bifida cystica. *J Bone Jt Surg.* 1983;65A: 350–356.

DIAS LS. Hip deformities in myelomeningocele. In: Tullos HS, ed. *AAOS Instructional Course Lectures.* Park Ridge, IL: American Academy of Orthopaedic Surgeons; 1991:4: 273–279.

DIAS LS, JASTY MJ, COLLINS P. Rotational deformities of the lower limb in myelomeningocele: evaluation and treatment. *J Bone Jt Surg.* 1984;66A:215–223.

DRENNAN JC. Foot deformities in myelomeningocele. In: Tullos HS, ed. *AAOS Instructional Course Lectures.* Vol. 4. Park Ridge, IL: American Academy of Orthopaedic Surgeons; 1991;4:287–291.

EMANS JB. Allergy to latex in patients who have myelodysplasia: relevance for the orthopaedic surgeon. *J Bone Jt Surg.* 1992;74A:1103–1109.

GAGE JR. Distal hamstring lengthening/release and rectus transfer. In: Sussman MD, ed. *The Diplegic Child.* Rosemont, IL: American Academy of Orthopaedic Surgeons; 1992:317–336.

GALASKI CSB, DELANEY C, MORRIS P. Spinal stabilization in Duchenne's muscular dystrophy. *J Bone Jt Surg.* 1992;74B: 210–214.

LINDSETH RE. Spine deformity in myelomeningocele. In: Tullos HS, ed. *AAOS Instructional Course Lectures.* Park Ridge, IL: American Academy of Orthopaedic Surgeons; 1991;4:273–279.

LOCK TR, ARONSON DD. Fractures in patients who have myelomeningocele. *J Bone Jt Surg.* 1989;71A:1153–1157.

MOSCA VS. Calcaneal lengthening for valgus deformity of the hindfoot: results in children who had severe symptomatic flatfoot and skewfoot. *J Bone Jt Surg.* 1995;77A:500–512.

RENSHAW TS, GREEN NE, GRIFFIN PP, ROOT L. Cerebral palsy: orthopaedic management. *J Bone Jt Surg.* 1995;77A:1590–1606.

ROOT L, LAPLAZA FJ, BROURMAN SN, ANGEL DH. The severely unstable hip in cerebral palsy: treatment with open reduction, pelvic osteotomy, and femoral osteotomy with shortening. *J Bone Jt Surg.* 1995;77A:703–712.

SARWARK JF, MACEWEN GD, SCOTT CI. Amyoplasia: a common form of arthrogryposis. *J Bone Jt Surg.* 1990;72A:465–469.

SCHOPLER SA, MENELAUS MB. Significance of the strength of the quadriceps muscle in children with myelomeningocele. *J Pediatr Orthop.* 1987;7:507–512.

SHAPIRO F, SPECHT L. The diagnosis and orthopaedic treatment of childhood spinal muscular atrophy, peripheral neuropathy, Friedrich ataxia, and arthrogryposis. *J Bone Jt Surg.* 1993;75A:1699–1714.

SAMPLE QUESTIONS

1. A 6-year-old ambulatory child with spastic diplegic cerebral palsy and without any athetosis has developed increased intoeing and a scissoring gait. Physical exam reveals increased tone in her lower extremities. Hip abduction is greater than 45 degrees bilaterally, and she has no significant hip, knee, or ankle contractures. She has no significant femoral anteversion or tibial torsion and no hip instability. The recommended intervention is:

   (a) release of hip adductors and flexors bilaterally

   (b) release of hip adductors bilaterally

   (c) selective dorsal rhizotomy

   (d) release of hip adductors with varus rotation osteotomy

   (e) release of hip flexors, adductors, hamstrings, and heelcords bilaterally

2. A 7-year-old child with right-sided spastic hemiplegic cerebral palsy ambulates with a stiff knee gait. On the right, he has areas of toe irritation from striking the ground during swing phase. He has greater than 45 degrees of passive abduction of the hip and no hip, knee, or heelcord contractures. Electromyographic analysis during gait demonstrates continuous activity of the rectus femoris during stance and swing phase. The recommended intervention is:

   (a) right rectus femoris transfer to the sartorius

   (b) right rectus femoris release

   (c) right iliopsoas recession

   (d) right heelcord lengthening

   (e) right adductor transfer

3. A 2-year-old girl with myelomeningocele and an L-2 motor level has a left hip dislocation and no pelvic obliquity. She has good sitting balance, bilateral hip flexion contractures of 10 degrees, and no other significant contractures. Recommended treatment would be:

   (a) placement in standing brace

   (b) release of hip flexion contractures and placement in standing brace

   (c) release of hip flexors and adductors and placement in standing brace

   (d) open reduction of left hip and placement in hip spica cast

   (e) open reduction of left hip, proximal femur varus osteotomy, and muscle transfers to balance the hip

4. A 7-year-old myelomeningocele patient has an L-4 motor level and a thoracic scoliosis that has increased from 22 to 32 degrees. The next step would be:

   (a) wheelchair modification

   (b) MRI of the brain

   (c) MRI of the brain and spinal cord

   (d) anterior spinal fusion

   (e) anterior-posterior spinal fusion

5. A 14-year-old boy with Duchenne's muscular dystrophy has difficulty sitting in his wheelchair and a 30-degree scoliosis that includes the pelvis. Recommended treatment is:

   (a) wheelchair modification

   (b) Boston overlap brace

   (c) custom-molded Thoraco-Lumbo Sacral Orthotic (TLSO) brace

   (d) posterior spinal fusion to the pelvis with segmental instrumentation

   (e) anterior spinal fusion with instrumentation

Answers: 1) c; 2) a; 3) a; 4) c; 5) d

Nerve Injuries

Chapter 45

Acute Injuries to Peripheral Nerves

Greg P. Watchmaker, MD and Susan E. Mackinnon, MD

Acute upper and lower extremity nerve injuries require the attention of a surgeon skilled in the technique of microsurgical repair. More importantly, however, nerve injuries require a detailed preoperative assessment to determine the grade and extent of injury in order to correctly time exploration and repair. Some nerve deficits are best treated expectantly with serial electrodiagnostic testing. This chapter highlights nerve injury classifications and their potential for regeneration, in addition to surgical timing and technique.

ETIOLOGY

Penetrating Trauma

Acute peripheral nerve injury may result from penetrating trauma, fractures, dislocations, iatrogenic damage during surgery, injections or venipuncture. Penetrating trauma accounts for the vast majority of these injuries especially in the upper extremity.

Frazier et al (1978) reported that upper extremity injuries account for one third of all surgical emergency department visits. Penetrating injuries of the hand and wrist are twice as common as fractures, infections, and burns combined. Following deep laceration of the hand, nerves are injured 27% of

the time. Iconomou et al (1993) pointed out that the diagnosis may be missed in a child or in a patient who is intoxicated.

Penetrating trauma may be divided into high and low velocity injuries. Low velocity injuries with a knife, glass, or metal edge typically have a small zone of injury surrounding the path of the glass or metal. If the patient complains of numbness or tingling distal to the level of a low velocity injury, there is a high likelihood that a nerve is partially or completely transected. Sensory and motor examination is important to confirm the diagnosis but should not outweigh the patient's subjective complaints when deciding to explore the wound. In a partial nerve injury, the sensory exam may be normal due to sensory overlap. A near-normal motor exam may also be observed due to compensatory motor actions. On occasion, bleeding or swelling from a low velocity injury may cause a neural deficit secondary to compression and not laceration. It is better to err on the side of exploration with these injuries.

High velocity injuries typically have a large zone of injury surrounding the path of the projectile. Nerve dysfunction may occur due to direct nerve injury or may occur indirectly from the concussive effect of the passing projectile. In the authors' experience, gunshot wounds commonly result in a neurapraxia or axonotmesis. Unless exploration is planned for associated vascular or bony injuries, observation and serial nerve studies constitute the best treatment as many nerve injuries resulting from gunshot wounds will recover spontaneously (Fig. 45–1).

PEARL

Knives and glass cut. Bullets bruise.

Fractures, Dislocations, and Sprains

Nerve injuries are associated with fractures and dislocations for several reasons. First, the high impact necessary to cause the fracture may cause direct, blunt nerve trauma. This is especially true where nerves travel in a subcutaneous position, as does the common peroneal nerve around the head of the fibula or the ulnar nerve about the medial epicondyle. Second, the fracture or dislocation may cause stretching of nerves if displacement is significant such as in posterior knee dislocations and anterior shoulder dislocations. Third, post-traumatic swelling and bleeding may cause direct compression of nerves, as in acute carpal tunnel syndrome following

751

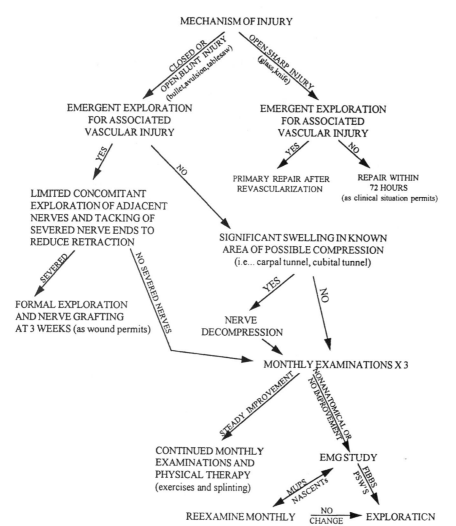

MECHANISM OF INJURY

CLOSED OR OPEN BLUNT INJURY (bullet, avulsion, tablesaw)

OPEN SHARP INJURY (glass, knife)

EMERGENT EXPLORATION FOR ASSOCIATED VASCULAR INJURY

YES

NO

EMERGENT EXPLORATION FOR ASSOCIATED VASCULAR INJURY

YES

NO

PRIMARY REPAIR AFTER REVASCULARIZATION

REPAIR WITHIN 72 HOURS (as clinical situation permits)

LIMITED CONCOMITANT EXPLORATION OF ADJACENT NERVES AND TACKING OF SEVERED NERVE ENDS TO REDUCE RETRACTION

SEVERED

NO SEVERED NERVES

SIGNIFICANT SWELLING IN KNOWN AREA OF POSSIBLE COMPRESSION (i.e... carpal tunnel, cubital tunnel)

YES

NO

FORMAL EXPLORATION AND NERVE GRAFTING AT 3 WEEKS (as wound permits)

NERVE DECOMPRESSION

MONTHLY EXAMINATIONS X 3

STEADY IMPROVEMENT

NONANATOMICAL OR NO IMPROVEMENT

CONTINUED MONTHLY EXAMINATIONS AND PHYSICAL THERAPY (exercises and splinting)

EMG STUDY

MUPS NASCENTS

FIBBS PSW'S

REEXAMINE MONTHLY

NO CHANGE

EXPLORATION

Figure 45–1 Algorithm for management of nerve injuries. Reproduced with permission from Peimer C, Watchmaker GP, MacKinnon SE. Nerve injury and repair. In: Peimer C, ed. *Surgery of the Hand and Upper Extremity*. New York, NY: Mc Graw-Hill; 1996:1260.

a distal radius fracture. Lastly, the fracture fragments themselves may cause direct neural injury, as in radial nerve injuries following humerus fracture.

Iatrogenic

Unintended nerve injuries can occur with almost any surgical approach. Common mechanisms include traction, laceration, or compression from swelling or hematoma.

Knowledge of anatomy is the best defense against iatrogenic nerve injury. Equally important is a complete preoperative nerve exam. When evaluating fractures, it is tempting to perform a cursory sensory or motor examination due to the patient's discomfort or bandages. However, the trauma that caused the fracture may have traumatized nearby nerves, a condition that is best discovered preoperatively.

Once a nerve deficit is identified, the course of action depends on the surgeon's intraoperative visualization of the affected nerve. If the nerve was identified and protected during the surgical procedure and is not functioning postoperatively, the best course of action is usually observation. If the nerve was not visualized as in an endoscopic approach, immediate exploration is the safest action. Neither patient nor surgeon will be satisfied in the long run observing such a deficit.

Several iatrogenic injuries are regularly reported includ-

ing ulnar neuropathy following open treatment of a distal humerus fracture, sciatic neuropathy following total hip arthroplasty, and radial nerve injury following surgical treatment of a humeral shaft fracture.

BASIC SCIENCE

Embryologically, nerves develop from primitive neural crest cells that send axonal projections into the developing limb buds. By day 38 of development, the median, radial, and ulnar nerves have entered the hand plate. During development, large motor and sensory axons become ensheathed in myelin containing Schwann cells. The insulating layers of myelin with periodic interruptions at the nodes of Ranvier are responsible for rapid (saltatory) conduction (Fig. 45–2). Loss or degradation of the myelin sheath results in slowed conduction or even conduction block.

Each group of nerves and associated Schwann cells are enclosed by a collagen layer referred to as endoneurium. Groups of endoneurial tubes form discrete bundles within the nerve, referred to as fascicles (or funincles). Fascicles are in turn wrapped by tightly connecting cells in a layer called perineurium (Fig. 45–3). Finally, groups of fascicles are held together by the epineurium, which is also predominantly

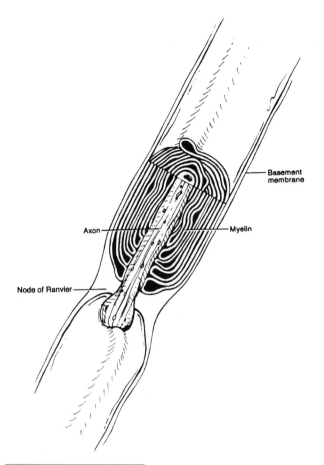

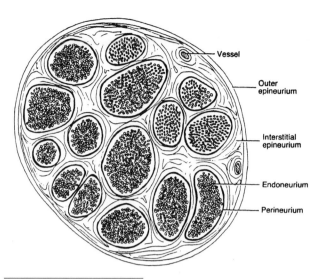

Figure 45–3   Cross-sectional view of nerve. Reproduced with permission from Peimer C, Watchmaker GP, MacKinnon SE. Nerve injury and repair. In: Peimer C, ed. *Surgery of the Hand and Upper Extremity*. New York, NY: McGraw-Hill; 1996:1255.

Figure 45–2   Schematic view of axon with its layers of myelin and the node of Ranvier. Reproduced with permission from Peimer C, Watchmaker GP, MacKinnon SE. Nerve injury and repair. In: Peimer C, ed. *Surgery of the Hand and Upper Extremity*. New York, NY: McGraw-Hill; 1996:1255.

composed of collagen. Clinically, the nerve is handled by the outer epineurium with longitudinal fascicles visible beneath. On the cut end, healthy fascicles often pouch 1 to 2 mm beyond the end of the nerve.

When a nerve fiber is traumatized, compressed, or crushed but not divided, there is local swelling associated with degradation of the Schwann cell lamina (focal demyelination). The patient experiences the resulting slowed or blocked conduction as numbness or weakness. If not severe, conduction is usually restored within several weeks.

When a nerve fiber is completely divided the result is much more profound and quickly apparent along the entire length of the nerve cell. The cell body swells and begins producing RNA, lipids, and proteins that are important for cell repair. The distal segment of nerve begins a process of irreversible degeneration referred to as Wallerian degeneration. No technique in humans has been able to functionally reconnect the severed ends and halt this process of degeneration. Recovery of nerve function, therefore, depends on outgrowth of new nerve endings at the level of injury.

To predict an individual's nerve recovery as well as to compare results among investigators, several classification schemes have evolved to characterize the severity of nerve injuries. Two schemes are commonly used to evaluate

nerve injuries. Seddon (1943) popularized three terms; neurapraxia, axonotmesis, and neurotmesis. In his words:

> Neurapraxia is used to describe those cases in which paralysis occurs in the absence of peripheral degeneration. It is more accurate than transient block in that the paralysis is often of considerable duration, though recovery always occurs in a shorter time than would be required after complete Wallerian degeneration; it is invariably complete.

> Axonotmesis—here the essential lesion is damage to the nerve fibers of such severity that complete peripheral degeneration follows; and yet the epineurium and more intimate supporting structures of the nerve have been so little disturbed that the internal architecture is fairly well preserved. Recovery is spontaneous, and of good quality, because the regeneration fibers are guided into their proper paths by their intact sheaths.

> Neurotmesis describes the state of a nerve in which all essential structures have been sundered. There is not necessarily an obvious anatomical gap in the nerve; indeed, the epineurial sheath may appear to be in continuity, although the rest of the nerve at the site of damage has been completely replaced by fibrous tissue. In both the effect is the same as if anatomical continuity had been lost. Neurotmesis is, therefore, of wider applicability than division.

PEARL

Seddon's classification of nerve injury comprises neurapraxia: nerve fiber intact, local block to conduction; axonotmesis: nerve fiber degenerated, overall nerve structure preserved; and neurotmesis: nerve fiber and all supporting structures injured or divided.

These terms provide greater clarity than terms such as concussion, contusion, and physiologic disruption. An even more detailed classification scheme involving five degrees of injury was proposed by Sunderland (1951):

First degree injury: Conduction is blocked at the site of injury but the continuity of all components comprising the nerve trunk, including the axon is preserved.... The fundamental basis of this injury is therefore interruption of conduction with preservation of anatomical continuity.

Second degree injury: Disintegration of the axon and all the associated changes collectively referred to as Wallerian degeneration occur below the site of the injury and perhaps for a short distance above it. The general arrangement of the axon sheaths and the remaining structures comprising the nerve is preserved and at no time is the integrity of the endoneurial tube threatened.... Because recovery depends on the regrowth of the axon, structures recover in the order in which they were innervated. Owing to the preservation of the endoneurial tubes, this regeneration results in the complete restoration of the original pattern of innervation.

Third degree injury: The internal structure of the funiculi (fasciculi) are disorganized though the bundles (fascicles) remain in continuity and show little, if any, deformation of their outlines. In addition to axonal disintegration and Wallerian degeneration, continuity of the endoneurial tubes is also destroyed.... The fundamental basis of a third degree injury is the disorganization of the contents of the funiculi so that the continuity of endoneurial tubes is destroyed and the chances of erroneous cross-shunting of regenerating axons are introduced.

Fourth degree injury: The funiculi are breached and disorganized so that they are no longer sharply demarcated from the epineurium in which they are embedded. Continuity of the nerve trunk is preserved; however, the involved segment being ultimately converted into a strand of tissue composed of a tangled mass of connective tissue, Schwann cells, and regenerating axons, which may become enlarged to form a neuroma. The fundamental basis of a fourth degree injury is complete disorganization of the internal structure of the nerve with preservation of continuity.

Fifth degree injury: The fundamental basis of a fifth degree injury is severance of the nerve trunk.

Sixth degree injury: Mackinnon (1989) has coined the term sixth degree injury to describe the concept of a mixed injury. In this type of injury there may be some fascicles that are perfectly normal adjacent to fascicles that demonstrate varying degrees of injury.

Both systems of classification have proven their clinical utility. Using either system, nerve injuries may be divided into those that will get better without intervention versus those that will require surgery. Clinically, Sunderland grade I (neurapraxia) and grade II (axonotmesis) will spontaneously improve and are best observed. Sunderland grades IV and V (neurotmesis) will not.

Grade I lesions (neurapraxia) will improve rapidly (weeks to months). Grade II lesions (axonotmesis) will improve

slowly at the rate of 1 to 2 mm per day. Because the endoneurial tubes remain intact, the prospects for near normal recovery exist for distal injuries. We educate our patients in this grading system and give an estimate of where their injuries belong. As more information from serial exams or electromyograms (EMGs) becomes available, the patient is given a revised estimate of the grade of the injury and expected recovery rate. In this way, the patient stays informed and interested in what can be a protracted recovery.

ANATOMY AND SURGICAL APPROACHES

The surgical approach to peripheral nerves for exploration, repair, grafting, or neurolysis follows several basic tenants independent of the specific nerve involved: Make incisions generous to allow ample exposure of the nerve proximal and distal to the zone of injury. Use a tourniquet for a bloodless field when possible, but limit tourniquet time to 30 minutes or less so that intra-operative nerve stimulation may be performed. Resist unnecessary dissection and handling of the nerve, which may lead to future scarring to surrounding structures. Use microsurgical technique with magnification and appropriate sutures and instruments. Perform repairs without tension, and utilize nerve grafts when nerve retraction or deficit indicates (Fig. 45–4).

EXAMINATION

The Upper Extremity

Prior to examining the injured extremity, its overall appearance yields significant information about innervation and function, especially in the subacute injury. Well-innervated skin will have a dull surface with occasional sweat beads. Shiny and atrophic skin with loss of joint creases indicates long-standing dysfunction or disuse. Calluses, on the other hand, are a good indication of function and use of the hand. Evidence of machine oil or grease embedded in the patient's palmar creases is also a good clue of the patient's ability to carry out tasks with the involved extremity. A dense paresthesia or complete anesthesia with loss of protective sensation is usually apparent by observation alone. Unless the patient is exceedingly careful, the numb part will be subjected to small burns and cuts, which often go untended. Patients who smoke cigarettes are at especially high risk of recurrent, fingertip burns.

Sudomotor function provides additional objective information regarding dennervation. Following dennervation, the involved skin becomes dry and smooth. The Ninhydrin test will demonstrate where there has been loss of sweat production. Dennervated skin will also not wrinkle normally when immersed in warm water. Bathing the extremity in 40°C water for half an hour will induce fingertip wrinkling in normally innervated areas. Although neither of these tests provide quantitative nor precise enough information on which to base surgery, they may be useful when following the recovery of an established nerve injury.

Active examination of the extremity may be done in a proximal to distal manner or in a nerve by nerve manner. The

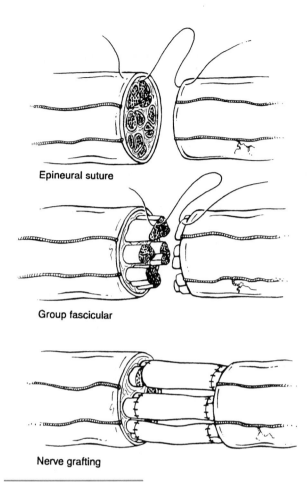

Epineural suture

Group fascicular

Nerve grafting

Figure 45–4 Schematic of epineurial nerve repair without tension and nerve grafting when there is a nerve gap. Reproduced with permission from Peimer C, Watchmaker GP, MacKinnon SE. Nerve injury and repair. In: Peimer C, ed. *Surgery of the Hand and Upper Extremity*. New York, NY: McGraw-Hill; 1996:1261.

order of the examination is not as important as the completeness and reproducibility of the testing. The authors prefer to follow a proximal to distal exam, skipping examination of the injured area until the end. It is difficult to gain useful information once the patient has retracted the extremity in discomfort. Important sensory areas to test in the upper extremity are (Fig. 45–5):

- dorsal first web space (radial nerve)
- small finger pad (ulnar nerve)
- index finger pad (median nerve)
- lateral aspect forearm (lateral antebrachial cutaneous [LABC] branch of musculocutaneous)
- skin overlying deltoid insertion (axillary nerve)

PEARL

Numbness in the thumb may occur from injury to any of three nerves: the median nerve, radial sensory nerve, or lateral antebrachial cutaneous (LABC) nerve.

Sensory testing may include testing light-touch versus pin-prick sensation using a broken wooden cotton swab. Light touch sensation may be quantitized using Semmes-Weinstein filaments. Two-point discrimination finger pad testing may be performed using a device with two tips calibrated with seperations of 1 to 20 mm.

Important upper extremity motor testing includes:

- metacarpophalangeal (MCP) extension (radial nerve)
- index finger abduction while palpating the first dorsal interosseous muscle (ulnar nerve)
- thumb opposition (median nerve)

PEARL

Posterior interosseous nerve injuries may be easily missed because wrist extension is preserved. Be sure to test metacarpophalangeal (MCP) extension.

Systematic examination of the upper extremity may be confounded by one of several commonly occurring innervation variations. The best know anomaly is a motor branch arising from the median nerve high in the forearm that joins the ulnar nerve more distally. This anomaly, referred to as a Martin-Gruber anastomosis, occurs in 10 to 20% of individuals. The most common pattern involves motor fibers crossing

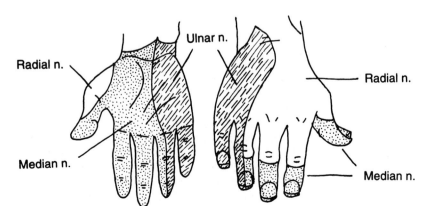

Radial n.

Ulnar n.

Radial n.

Median n.

Median n.

Figure 45–5 Zones of sensory innervation of the hand. Larson Langschwager, illustrator.

from median to ulnar nerve to innervate "normally median" muscles in the hand. Sensory fibers are not involved.

The Lower Extremity

Examination of the lower extremity is similar to that of the upper extremity. Examination should include muscles in each compartment of the leg. Sensory testing of the foot will yield significant information regarding nerve injury if the examiner understands its innervation pattern (Fig. 45–6).

Additional testing may include percussion along the course of the nerve to elicit a Tinel's sign. This sign is characterized by tingling or shocklike sensations in the sensory distribution of the nerve. This should not be confused with pain or other sensations felt at the site of the injury. Within several days of nerve fiber transection, the regenerating nerve endings from the proximal stump begin their distal growth. Tapping on these bare nerve endings elicits the classic Tinel's sign. This sign is, therefore, while not always useful acutely (<48°), can be very useful in older injuries or to monitor regeneration following repair. Because nerve fiber continuity is not lost in a neurapraxia grade injury, this sign is absent.

Examination of nerve injuries associated with significant bleeding or distal ischemia can be challenging. A limb with a deep laceration producing arterial bleeding and distal limb ischemia provides little information on examination and is best explored at the time of vascular repair. If the limb remains perfused, time should be spent preoperatively performing a neurologic examination. This examination not only helps direct operative incisions and exploration but also avoids discovery of unsuspected injuries postoperatively.

Often, the limb is hypoperfused secondary to the vascular injury in addition to the pressure applied to control bleeding.

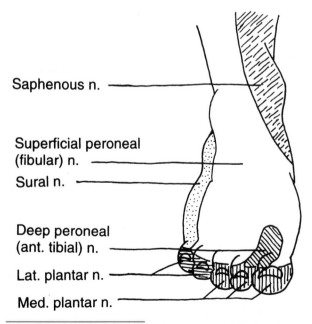

Saphenous n.

Superficial peroneal (fibular) n.

Sural n.

Deep peroneal (ant. tibial) n.

Lat. plantar n.

Med. plantar n.

Figure 45–6   Zones of sensory innervation of the foot. Larson Langschwager, illustrator.

The physician should personally apply direct pressure to the bleeding while attempting to allow as much collateral circulation to the limb as possible. After 10 minutes, a neurologic examination may yield important information regarding injured and uninjured nerves. This period of perfusion preoperatively is also important if a tourniquet has been applied in the field or emergency department because tourniquet ischemia during surgery will be necessary to perform repairs.

AIDS TO DIAGNOSIS

The nature and extent of acute nerve injuries can be straightforward in low velocity penetrating injuries (i.e., knife, glass injuries), but confusing and difficult in high velocity injuries, crush injuries, and stretch injuries. Several aids to diagnosis have been detailed previously including the sweat test, two point discrimination testing, and examination of skin character. Additional testing including radiographs and electromyography are also useful.

Radiographs or the injured extremity are useful for:

1. identifyng any embedded glass or metal (including bullets) in proximity to nerves
2. characterizing underlying fractures or dislocations and their likelihood of injuring neighboring nerves
3. identifyng fixation pins or plates postoperatively that may be irritating or entrapping nearby nerves

Electromylograms (EMGs) and nerve conduction studies (NCTs) provide concise and detailed information that sometimes cannot be attained by clinical examination. In the setting of a low velocity injury with identifiable nerve deficit, EMGs are unnecessary as wound exploration and nerve repair should proceed without delay. In the case of high velocity injuries, crush, or compression injuries, serial EMGs and NCTs along with the clinical exam guide decision making.

An EMG study details the health of the muscle being needled and, indirectly, the nerve supply to that muscle. Several terms need to be understood to interpret the results of an EMG.

Fibrillations (fibs) indicate spontaneous electrical activity (depolarizations) of muscle fibers while at rest. A normal muscle is electrically silent when not being stimulated by its supplying nerve. After a muscle has been dennervated for several weeks, it begins to have minute spontaneous depolarizations. These depolarizations are recorded as very low amplitude fibrillations. This spontaneous activity is important in differentiating a neurapraxia from a higher-grade injury because fibrillations do not occur unless the axon has been divided. Fibrillations are different from fasciculations, which are depolarizations of entire motor units. Fasciculations are higher in amplitude, and a small number occur at rest in healthy muscles.

Insertional activity is the amount of electrical activity that occurs immediately on insertion of the EMG needle into the muscle. Normal muscle that is well innervated has a small amount of insertional activity, whereas a muscle that has been dennervated for several weeks to months has a high insertional activity.

Motor unit potentials (MUPs) represent the electrical activity caused by depolarization of muscle motor units when a muscle is stimulated by its supplying nerve. Motor unit potentials are brief and high in amplitude in a healthy muscle, similar to the narrow QRS complex seen on a normal electrocardiogram. When conduction in the nerve supplying the muscle is slowed (as in neurapraxia) or collateral sprouting has occurred, the MUPs may be few, wide, and of low amplitude. Motor unit potentials are an important indicator of innervation because they may be detectable months before clinical evidence of muscle contraction is seen.

PEARL

Remember that fibrillations (fibs) indicate denervation of the muscle and motor unit potentials (MUPs) indicate innervation of the muscle.

The NCT provides additional information as to the health of the nerve. Because major motor and sensory axons transmit their impulses via saltatory (jumping) conduction, propagation velocities of 50 meters per second or more are typical in the extremities. Following complete division of the nerve (neurotmesis) or axons (axonotmesis), no conduction will be elicited across the site of division. Distal conduction will persist for several days before Wallerian degeneration consumes the axons. Following a neurapraxia injury, conduction may be slowed. In more severe neurapraxia injuries, no conduction may be elicited across the level of injury. Serial NCTs at monthly intervals will allow the clinician to follow conduction velocity improvements as a marker of recovery of neurapraxia.

SPECIFIC CONDITIONS, TREATMENT, AND OUTCOME

Although penetrating trauma may involve any nerve of the upper or lower extremity, several nerves are especially vulnerable given their location and anatomy.

The common peroneal nerve is vulnerable due to its subcutaneous location around the head of the fibula and to tethering by its branches, which may lead to traction injury. The most common mechanism is blunt trauma (e.g., from a hockey puck or soccer kick) that pins the nerve against the unyielding fibula. This often results in a neurapraxia requiring hours to weeks to resolve. Traction injuries that may be incurred with lower leg injuries can be more severe (e.g., axonotmesis). Meals (1977) has demonstrated that 15% of all grade II and grade III lateral ankle sprains have evidence of damage to the peroneal nerve as documented by EMG. Peroneal nerve injuries caused by nonpenetrating trauma should be treated conservatively with serial exam and EMG. Fitting of a foot drop splint until dorsiflexion motion returns is recommended. Exploration, if necessary, should include intra-operative nerve stimulation and nerve-to-nerve testing to isolate the nonconducting segment for grafting.

Nerve Injuries About the Elbow

Elbow dislocations and supracondylar fractures of the humerus may be complicated by acute injuries of the median, ulnar, or radial nerves. Injuries to the radial nerve are seen in conjuction with humeral shaft fractures. The anterior interosseous branch of the median nerve is frequently injured in pediatric supracondylar humerus fractures. The ulnar nerve is often contused in intra-articular fractures of the distal humerus. The posterior interosseous portion of the radial nerve can be injured in Monteggia fractures; fractures of the proximal humerus with dislocation of the radial head. Incomplete recovery is more often associated with ulnar nerve lesions; however, as in radial nerve palsy following distal humeral shaft fracture, spontaneous resolution is the norm. Occasionally, the nerve may become entrapped in scar tissue or hypertrophic bone leading to a traction neuritis. Neurolysis and placement of the nerve in a padded bed of muscle can alleviate this problem.

Radial Nerve Injuries

The axillary nerve is also vulnerable to injury by direct trauma as well as stretching from an anterior shoulder dislocation. The injury is relatively common in football, wrestling, and rugby, with presenting symptoms including weakness in shoulder abduction and decreased sensation on the lateral aspect of the upper arm. Mild or subclinical injury is common. Electromyographic study of patients following anterior dislocation has demonstrated a 45 to 65% incidence of nerve damage. As is true of all such closed injuries, observation and EMG study are indicated.

Axillary Nerve Injuries

The radial nerve is protected in the arm by its deep position with overlying muscle and fat. Humerus fractures, however, can result in radial nerve injury from stretching, swelling, or direct impailment. A short, oblique fracture at the junction of the middle and distal thirds of the humerus is referred to as Holstein-Lewis fracture and is important for its association with radial nerve injury (Fig. 45–7). The literature remains divided on the appropriate management of closed injuries where the underlying fracture does not require open fixation because return to near-normal function occurs in up to 95% of patients. Open injuries, however, have a high association with nerve laceration and interposition between bone fragments. If closed fracture treatment is elected, an EMG should be performed monthly if objective clinical improvement is not seen. Waiting 4 or 5 months before performing the first EMG study risks losing valuable baseline information from which future studies may be compared. The median and ulnar nerves at the wrist are vulnerable due to their superficial location. Impact of the wrist against plate glass when the wrist is extended may injure either nerve. The

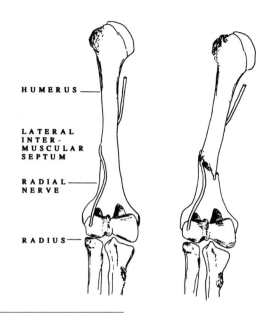

HUMERUS

LATERAL INTER-MUSCULAR SEPTUM

RADIAL NERVE

RADIUS

Figure 45–7 Schematic of the Holstein-Lewis fracture with the mechanism by which the radial nerve is trapped in the fracture. Larson Langschwager, illustrator.

patient often relates a history of hurrying to leave a home or garage, pushing on the glass of the door, and breaking the glass. Most local building codes now require the use of tempered or safety glass on doors due to the frequency of this injury. The approach to this injury is straightforward as emergent exploration is usually indicated. Epineurial repair should be performed using fascicular pattern and longitudinal epineurial vessels for orientation.

Distal Median Nerve Injuries

Results from distal median nerve injuries were reported by Novak (1992) in a study of 14 patients at an average of 4 years after median nerve grafting. Of the 14 patients, 10 had suffered a laceration injury. Two patients achieved 2-point discrimination of 2 to 3 mm, and three patients achieved 2-point discrimination of 4 to 7 mm. These results are superior to those previously reported and are likely due to an aggressive sensory re-education program.

The median nerve is also vulnerable to iatrogenic injury during a palmaris longus tendon harvest. By appearance alone, these two structures appear surprisingly similar, especially through a small incision. This mistake can be avoided by preoperative examination of the forearm to confirm a palmaris tendon is indeed present. In addition, the median nerve is deep to the palmar forearm fascia, whereas the palmaris longus is superficial.

SELECTED BIBLIOGRAPHY

BATEMAN JE. Nerve injuries about the shoulder in sports. *J Bone Jt Surg.* 1967;49A:785–792.

BERRY H, BRIL V. Axillary nerve palsy following blunt trauma to the shoulder region: a clinical and electrophysiological review. *J Neurol Neurosurg Psychiatry.* 1982;45:1027–1032.

BROWN IC, ZINAR DM. Traumatic and iatrogenic neurological complications after supracondylar humerus fractures in children. *J Pediatr Orthop.* 1995;15:440–443.

DELAAT EA, VISSER CP, COENE LN, PAHPLATZ PV, TAVY DL. Nerve lesions in primary shoulder dislocations and humeral neck fractures: a prospective clinical and EMG study. *J Bone Jt Surg.* 1994;76B:381–383.

FOSTER RJ, SWIONTKOWSKI ME, ALLAN W, SACK IT. Radial nerve palsy caused by open humeral shaft fractures. *J Hand Surg.* 1993;18A:121–124.

FRAZIER WH, MILLER M, FOX RS, BRAND D, FINSETH F. Hand injuries: incidence and epidemiology in an emergency service. *JACEP.* 1978;7:265–268.

FRYKMAN GK. Peripheral nerve injuries in children. *Orthop Clin North Am.* 1976;7:701–716.

GALBRAITH KA, MCCULLOUGH CJ. Acute nerve injury as a complication of closed fractures or dislocations of the elbow. *Injury.* 1979;11:159–164.

GUSE TR, OSTRUM RF. The surgical anatomy of the radial nerve around the humerus. *Clin Orthop Rel Res.* 1995;320:149–153.

HOLMLUND T. Electrodiagnosis and neurologic evaluation. In: Peimer C, ed. *Surgery of the Hand and Upper Extremity.* New York, NY: McGraw Hill; 1996:1277–1290.

HOLSTEIN A, LEWIS G. Fractures of the humerus with radial nerve paralysis. *J Bone Jt Surg.* 1963;45A:1382–1388.

ICONOMOU TG, ZUKER RM, MICHELOW BJ. Management of major penetrating glass injuries to the upper extremities in children and adolescents. *Microsurgery.* 1993;14:91–96.

JOHANSON NA, PELLICCI PM, TSAIRIS P, SALVATI EA. Nerve injury in total hip arthroplasty. *Clin Orthop Rel Res.* 1983;179:214–222.

LIEBERMAN AR. The axon reaction: a review of the principle features of perikaryal responses to axon injury. *Int Rev Neurobiol.* 1971;14:49–124.

LOREI MP, HERSHMAN EB. Peripheral nerve injuries in athletes: treatment and prevention. *Sports Med.* 1993;16:130–147.

MACKINNON SE. New directions in peripheral nerve surgery. *Ann Surg.* 1989;22:257–273.

MANNERFELT L. Studies on the hand in ulnar nerve paralysis: a clinical-experimental investigation in normal and anomalous innervation. *Acta Orthop Scand.* 1966;(suppl 87):1.

MCILVEEN SJ, DURALDE XA, D'ALESSANDRO DF, BIGLIANI LU. Isolated nerve injuries about the shoulder. *Clin Orthop Rel Res.* 1994;306:54–63.

MEALS RA. Peroneal nerve palsy complicating ankle sprain. *J Bone Jt Surg.* 1977;59A:966–968.

NOVAK CB, KELLY L, MACKINNON SE. Sensory recovery after median nerve grafting. *J Hand Surg.* 1992;17A:59–68.

O'RIAIN S. New and simple test of nerve function in hand. *Br Med.* 1973;3:615–616.

POLLOCK FH, DRAKE D, BOVILL KG, DAY L, TRAFTON PG. Treatment of radial neuropathy associated with fractures of the humerus. *J Bone Jt Surg.* 1981;63A:239–243.

RICHARDS RR, HUDSON AR, BERTOIA JT, URBANIAK JR, WADDELL JP. Injury to the brachial plexus during Putti Platt and Bristow procedures: a report of 8 cases. *Am J Sports Med.* 1987;15:374–380.

SCHMALZRIED TP, AMSTUTZ HC, DOREY FJ. Nerve palsy associated with total hip replacement. Risk factors and prognosis. *J Bone Jt Surg.* 1991;73A:1074–1080.

SEDDON HJ. Three types of nerve injury. *Brain.* 1943;66:238–287.

SEDDON HJ, MEDAWAR PB, SMITH H. Rate of regeneration of peripheral nerves in man. *J Physiol.* 1943;102:191–215.

SHAH JJ, BHATTI NA. Radial nerve paralysis associated with fractures of the humerus: a review of 62 cases. *Clin Orthop Rel Res.* 1983;172:171–176.

STROMBERG WB, MCFARLANE RM, BELL LL. Injury of the median and ulnar nerves. *J Bone Jt Surg.* 1961;43A:717–730.

SUNDERLAND S. A classification of peripheral nerve injuries producing loss of function. *Brain.* 1951;74:491–516.

TOOLANEN G, HILDINGSSON C, HEDLUND T, KNIBESTOL M, OBERG L. Early complications after anterior dislocation of the shoulder in patients over 40 years: an ultrasonographic and electromyographic study. *Acta Orthop Scand.* 1993;64:549–552.

WALLER A. Experiments on the section of the glossopharyngeal and hypoglossal nerves of the frog, and observations of the alterations produced thereby in the structure of their primitive fibres. *Philos Trans Royal Soc London.* 1850;140:423–429.

SAMPLE QUESTIONS

1. Clinical evidence of nerve regeneration following a complete nerve laceration and repair proceeds distally at approximately:
   (a) 1 inch per day
   (b) 1 mm per day
   (c) 1 mm per month
   (d) neural regeneration rarely occurs following repair

2. A dennervated muscle is receptive to reinnervation:
   (a) for about 3 months
   (b) for several years optimally and up to 10 years total
   (c) for up to a year with best results before 6 months
   (d) seldom. If the nerve is completely cut, the muscle usually cannot be reinnervated.

3. Muscle fibrillations seen on EMG study are important because they:
   (a) indicate the muscle has been at least partially dennervated
   (b) indicate evidence of muscle recovery and reinnervation
   (c) are normal in most people at rest, and indicate injury if absent
   (d) can be seen on EMG within hours of nerve injury, making them useful in assessing acute nerve injuries

4. Thumb sensation is supplied by all of the following nerves except the:
   (a) radial nerve
   (b) digital nerves derived from the median nerve
   (c) LABC
   (d) palmar cutaneous branch of the median nerve

5. Neurapraxia (first degree injury):
   (a) is associated with fibrillation on EMG
   (b) improves at a rate of 1 inch per month
   (c) includes injuries where the axon is severed but the nerve itself remains in continuity
   (d) is a local block to impulse conduction in an otherwise intact nerve and is best treated conservatively.

Answers: 1) b; 2) c; 3) a; 4) c; 5) d

Chapter 46

Chronic Nerve Injuries and Neuropathies

Thomas W. Wright, MD

Chronic nerve injuries and compressive neuropathies can be a source of substantial morbidity. The key to effective treatment is accurate diagnosis. This chapter will review the most common forms of chronic nerve injuries along with an approach to diagnosis and treatment.

ETIOLOGY

Chronic neuropathies may be caused by multiple factors, both local and host. The causes essentially can be divided into two main groups: mechanical and medical. Of the mechanical causes, the primary culprit is believed to be compression.

Other possible factors include traction, strain, friction, and repetitive low-grade trauma. Compression is the most extensively studied of the mechanical causes of chronic neuropathy. Direct pressure on a nerve causes a decrease in nerve function by two possible means: direct effect of pressure on nerve axoplasmic flow or direct effect of pressure on nerve blood flow. The exact contribution of each of these to deteriorating nerve function has not been clearly delineated and is somewhat controversial.

Not all nerve fibers respond to compression in a similar manner. Large myelinated sensory fibers are the most susceptible to compression; whereas, nonmyelinated fibers are resistant to even high levels of compression.

Compression at a proximal site to a nerve makes the nerve more susceptible to a lower grade compression at a second, more distal location. This phenomena is referred to as the double crush syndrome. The most common explanation for the double crush syndrome is decreased axoplasmic flow occurring at the first site of compression, making a distal site more susceptible to a second but lower level of compression.

Traction, repetitive strain, friction, and repetitive trauma all contribute to a mechanical neuropathy. These factors, (although not as significant as compression) may act in synergy with compression in the pathomechanism of a mechanical compressive neuropathy.

Medical causes of chronic neuropathy can be divided into three main groups: (1) metabolic, (2) inherited disorders, and (3) toxins. Metabolic causes of peripheral neuropathy include diabetes, hypothyroidism, and some vitamin deficiencies. One theory for the cause of diabetic neuropathy is that an accumulation of sorbitol, a metabolite of glucose, causes endoneural edema. The edema results in decreased axoplasmic flow in the peripheral nerves and, therefore, more susceptiblity to a second compressive injury. This is similar to the double crush model as mentioned earlier. Another possible reason for diabetic neuropathy may be peripheral microvascular lesions. Hypothyroidism and B_6 and B_{12} deficiencies have all been associated with chronic peripheral neuropathies.

Charcot-Marie-Tooth disease, a mixed motor and sensory neuropathy that affects the feet and hands is an example of a heritable cause of chronic peripheral neuropathy. Finally, toxic causes of neuropathies are numerous, including heavy metals, chemotherapy (vincristine), and long-term effects of radiation therapy.

Orthopaedic Surgery: The Essentials. Edited by M.E. Baratz, A.D. Watson, and J.E. Imbriglia. Thieme Medical Publishers, Inc., New York © 1999

BASIC SCIENCE

Compression is felt to be the primary component of mechanical peripheral neuropathy. A pressure of 30 mm Hg has been shown to significantly retard blood flow in neural venules (Rydevik et al, 1981; Ogata and Naito, 1986). With increases of pressure to 60 to 80 mm Hg, complete blood flow is arrested to the nerve. The critical threshold for blocking axoplasmic flow has been shown to be 30 mm Hg. With pressure of longer duration, a pressure as low as 20 mm Hg may produce the same effect. Pressure decreases axoplasmic flow in both a proximal and distal direction. This pressure and its effect on axoplasmic flow has significant implications on the double crush syndrome mentioned earlier. Compression has its greatest effects at the actual compression gradient, or the edge. This has been referred to as the edge effect. Long-term compression (chronic neuropathy) results histologically in what has been called a tadpole lesion: an area of retraction of myelin at the compressed area and an accumulation of myelin at the internodal areas outside of the compressed area (Neary and Eames, 1975).

Another potential cause of chronic neuropathy is traction. Peripheral nerves require significant excursion to accommodate extremity motion. The further a nerve is from the center of rotation of a joint as it crosses that joint, the greater the amount of nerve excursion necessary to accommodate motion of that joint. If this ability to move with limb motion is impeded, the nerve will see significant increase in strain. It appears that this may also be responsible for mechanical injury to nerve; although it has not been well elucidated. It is possible that traction in synergy with compression may add to a mechanical chronic neuropathy.

ANATOMY AND SURGICAL APPROACHES

The anatomy of and surgical approaches to the most common sites of compressive neuropathy will be discussed in this section. For the median nerve, the most common compression sites include the carpal tunnel and pronator teres region at the elbow. The ulnar nerve, or its origin nerve, can be compressed at the cubital tunnel at the elbow, Guyon's canal at the wrist, and the thoracic outlet area. The radial nerve can be compressed at or about the radial tunnel. The posterior tibial nerve can be compressed in the tarsal tunnel.

Median Nerve at the Wrist: Carpal Tunnel Syndrome

The carpal tunnel is a confined space bordered by the carpal bones dorsally, the carpal trapezium radially, the hook of the hamate on the ulnar side, and volarly by a thick ligamentous structure called the transverse carpal ligament. In this confined space run nine tendons and the median nerve (Fig. 46–1). Occasionally, a persistent median artery will also run in the confines of the carpal tunnel. The tendons are surrounded by tenosynovium, which at times may become thickened and take up more room in the already restricted and unyielding confines of the carpal tunnel. This in turn places increased pressure on the median nerve. The median nerve, prior to entering the carpal tunnel, gives a branch called the palmar cutaneous nerve, which pierces the antebrachial fascia proximal to the carpal tunnel and supplies sensation to the skin over the thenar eminence. The median nerve proceeds through the carpal tunnel and gives off a motor branch, which normally occurs at the end of the carpal tunnel (Fig. 46–2). There is significant anatomic variation concerning the median motor branch that may, in some cases, actually traverse the ligament. At or near the end of the carpal tunnel, the median nerve begins branching into the common digital nerves. The median nerve as previously discussed is responsible for sensation to the thumb, index, long, and radial one half of the ring finger.

The surgical approach to the carpal tunnel involves two basic methods, both of which are directed at release of the transverse carpal ligament. One is an open incision through the palm, palmar fascia, and the transverse carpal ligament. This incision is started just distal to the distal wrist flexion

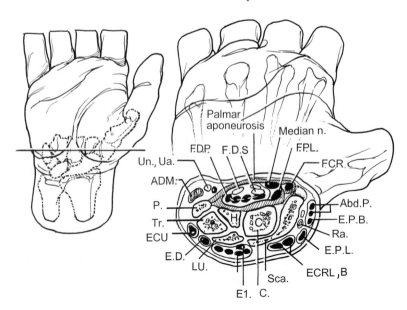

Figure 46–1 Cross section anatomy of the carpal tunnel.

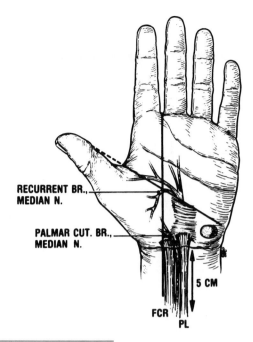

Figure 46–2 Anatomy of the branches of the median nerve at the level of the carpal tunnel. (Reproduced with permission from Elizabeth Roselius, *Operative Nerve Repair and Reconstruction*. Richard H. Gelberman. Philadelphia, PA: Lippincott; 1991:903.)

PITFALL

Placing the carpal tunnel incision too radial will place the palmar cutaneous and median motor nerves at increased risk of injury. It will also leave no retinaculum over the median nerve, promoting scarring between the median nerve and the overlying skin.

---

crease and extends distally in line with the midaxial line of the ring finger for 2.5 cm (Fig. 46–3).

Over the last few years a somewhat controversial approach to carpal tunnel release has been performed using an endoscope, whereby the transverse carpal ligament is cut from the inside of the carpal tunnel. This is done through either one or two incisions with an endoscope leaving the skin intact over the carpal tunnel itself (Figs. 46–4 and 46–5). Potential advantages of this technique are earlier rehabilitation and less pain. Potential disadvantages are an increased risk of nerve or tendon injury. This is an area of an intense controversy at present and cannot be comprehensively discussed in this text. However, the standard operation for carpal tunnel syndrome is the open technique using the incision discussed above.

Median Nerve at the Elbow

The median nerve at the elbow may be compressed, although this is far less common than carpal tunnel syndrome. The

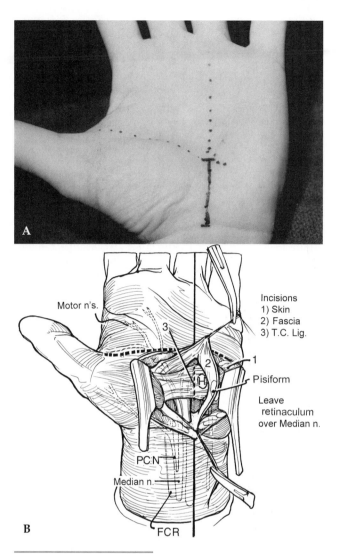

Figure 46–3 **(A)** Drawing of planned carpal tunnel incision. Incision runs distal from the distal wrist flexion crease in the midaxial line of the ring finger. Distal transverse line marks Kaplan's cardinal line which runs from the base of the first web space to the hook of the hamate. This marks the approximate level of the superficial palmar arch. **(B)** Schematic illustrating exposure of the transverse carpal ligament.

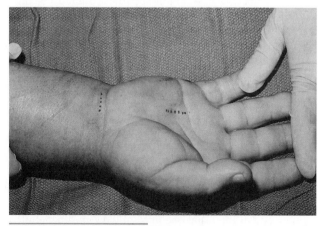

Figure 46–4 Planned incision for the two-incision endoscopic carpal tunnel release technique.

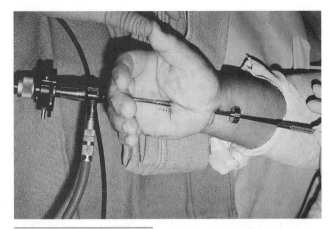

Figure 46–5   Two-incision endoscopic carpal tunnel release. The endoscope is distal, and the cutting knife is proximal.

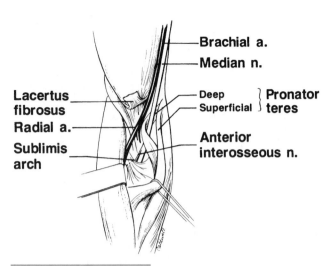

Figure 46–6   Drawing of the median nerve at the elbow. Reproduced with permission from Richard H. Gelberman. *Operative Nerve Repair and Reconstruction.* Philadelphia, PA: Lippincott; 1991:991.

median nerve proximal to the elbow is contained in the anterior compartment of the arm and is just medial to the brachial artery. It then passes under the lacertus fibrosis just proximal to the elbow flexion crease, penetrates the two heads of the pronator teres, and finally traverses through the flexor digitorum superficialis (Fig. 46–6). Proximal to the superficialis, the median nerve gives off an anterior interosseous nerve branch, which is responsible for motor function of the flexor pollicis longus, flexor digitorum profundus to the index and long finger, and the pronator quadratus. There is considerable anatomic variation when considering the anatomy of the median nerve as it traverses the pronator teres. The median nerve at the elbow may be compressed at a number of sites: the ligament of Struthers (if a humeral supracondylar process is present), lacertus fibrosis, pronator teres, or the superficialis origin (Fig. 46–7).

To release the median nerve at the elbow, a 12-cm skin incision is made starting along the medial border of the biceps and curving obliquely across the elbow flexion crease. This is carried on down through fascia. The median nerve is encountered proximally along the medial border of the brachialis. At this level, if a ligament of Struthers is present, then it is released. The nerve is then dissected distal to the lacertus fibrosis, which is released. The median nerve is followed as it penetrates the pronator teres. The lateral antebrachial cutaneous nerve is more superficial but must be protected at this level. Just proximal to this level, the anterior interosseous nerve branches off dorsally. The anterior interosseous nerve is released over its course to the interosseous membrane. Further release of the median nerve proper is done by spreading through the pronator and then the flexor digitorum superficialis. Avoid transecting the superficial head of the pronator, if possible.

Ulnar Nerve at the Elbow: Cubital Tunnel Syndrome

The ulnar nerve is formed by the medial cord of the brachial plexus. It passes through the upper two thirds of the arm along the anterior medial portion of the medial intermuscular septum, and at the distal one third of the arm it penetrates the septum to course distally along the anterior medial portion of the triceps (Fig. 46–8). At the medial epicondyle the

nerve passes into the cubital tunnel, which is formed posteriorly by the aponeurotic arcuate ligament (Osborne's fascia) anteriorly and medially by the medial epicondyle, and distally and laterally by the medial collateral ligament. There is significant anatomic variation in the arcuate ligament, sometimes called the cubital tunnel retinaculum. This variation has been demonstrated by O'Driscoll et al (1991). The cubital tunnel retinaculum may be significantly thickened by an atavistic muscle called the anconeus epitrochlearis. The nerve is closely accompanied throughout its course by a longitudinal vascular bundle, which supplies the nerve in a segmental fashion. There are no significant branches of the ulnar nerve in the upper arm. The first branch of significance is a branch to the flexor carpi ulnaris. Compressive sites of the ulnar

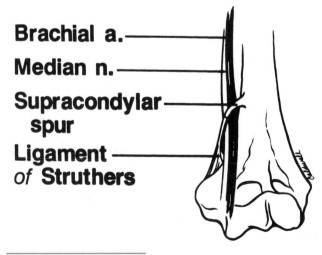

Figure 46–7   Drawing of the ligament of Struthers. Reproduced with permission from Richard H. Gelberman. *Operative Nerve Repair and Reconstruction.* Philadelphia, PA: Lippincott; 1991:999.

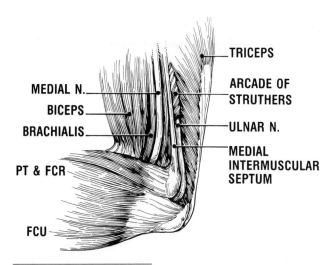

MEDIAL N.
BICEPS
BRACHIALIS
PT & FCR
FCU

TRICEPS
ARCADE OF STRUTHERS
ULNAR N.
MEDIAL INTERMUSCULAR SEPTUM

Figure 46–8 Ulnar nerve in the distal arm. Reproduced with permission from Richard H. Gelberman. *Operative Nerve Repair and Reconstruction*. Philadelphia, PA: Lippincott; 1991:1058.

nerve from proximal to distal include the arcade of Struthers, the medial intermuscular septum, the medial epicondyle, the cubital tunnel retinaculum, a hypertrophied ossified medial collateral ligament, and the flexor carpi ulnaris (Fig. 46–9).

Surgical approaches to cubital tunnel syndrome are numerous. The least complex approach to ulnar nerve compression at the elbow is a simple release, which has been advocated by some authors for mild cubital tunnel syndrome. Another approach, medial epicondylectomy, requires a small 3-cm incision placed over the posterior medial portion of the medial epicondyle. The nerve is protected, the medial epicondyle is exposed subperiosteal, and the epicondyle medial to the insertion of the ulnar collateral ligament is removed. The overlying soft tissue is then repaired, and the nerve is left in situ. Medial epicondylectomy has been advocated for patients with subluxation of the ulnar nerve and milder forms of cubital tunnel syndrome. For more severe forms of cubital tunnel syndrome, transposition of the ulnar nerve is indicated. Transposition of the ulnar nerve may be submuscular, intramuscular, or subcutaneous. To perform an ulnar nerve transposition, a 15-cm posterior incision is made.

The ulnar nerve is found anterior to the medial border of the triceps. The longitudinal blood vessel is protected with the ulnar nerve to maintain some blood flow to the nerve over the dissection area. The nerve is then circumferentially dissected from where it penetrates the medial intermuscular fascia at the arcade of Struthers to the branches to the flexor carpi ulnaris. It is then transposed anterior to the medial epicondyle. The terminal portion of the medial intramuscular septum is excised, and several large blood vessels in the area are cauterized so as to not kink the nerve at this site. If the nerve is left subcutaneously, a small fascial sling is created to keep the nerve from subluxating posterior. If it is placed intramuscularly, an incision is made in the flexor pronator mass. If it is placed submuscularly, the flexor pronator mass is elevated, and the nerve is then placed under the flexor pronator mass. The flexor pronator mass is loosely repaired or Z-lengthened and repaired.

Ulnar Nerve at the Wrist

The ulnar nerve passes from the forearm into the palm, through Guyon's canal. In this area it runs with the ulnar artery. The nerve gives off a motor branch, which supplies the intrinsic muscles of the hand, including the hypothenar muscles, dorsal interossei, the palmar interossei, the ulnar

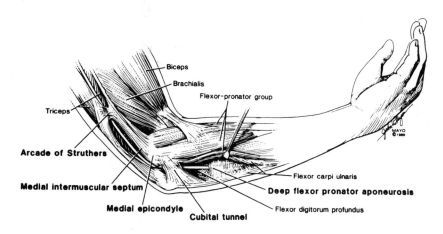

Biceps
Brachialis
Flexor-pronator group
Triceps
Arcade of Struthers
Medial intermuscular septum
Medial epicondyle
Cubital tunnel
Flexor carpi ulnaris
Deep flexor pronator aponeurosis
Flexor digitorum profundus

Figure 46–9 Drawing of the potential compression sites of the ulnar nerve at the elbow. Reproduced with permission from the Mayo Foundation. *Operative Nerve Repair and Reconstruction*. Philadelphia, PA: Lippincott; 1991:1111.

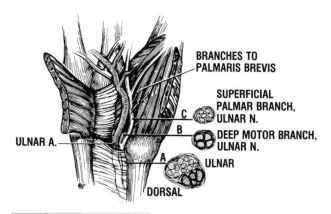

Figure 46–10 Drawing of the ulnar nerve at the level of Guyon's canal. Reproduced with permission from Elizabeth Roselius. *Operative Nerve Repair and Reconstruction*. Philadelphia, PA: Lippincott Co; 1991:1132.

two lumbricals, as well as the adductor pollicis. It finally terminates in the deep head of the flexor pollicis brevis. The motor branch of the ulnar nerve may be injured by a fracture of the hook of the hamate in its course along the base of the hook. Guyon's canal is created dorsally by the transverse carpal ligament, the pisohamate ligament, and pisometacarpal ligaments. Volarly, it consists of palmar fascia, fat, and palmaris brevis. The ulnar nerve lies medial to the ulnar artery throughout this course. The sensory portion of the ulnar nerve passes through Guyon's canal and supplies sensation to the small finger and ulnar half of the ring finger (Fig. 46–10). The ulnar artery runs with the ulnar sensory nerve and terminates in the superficial palmar arch. A branch of the ulnar artery that runs with the ulnar motor branch contributes to the deep palmar arch. This deep branch of the ulnar artery may primarily supply local muscle.

The operative approach to Guyon's canal consists of a 2-cm skin incision made from the distal wrist flexion crease and extending distally in line with the ulnar border of the ring finger. This is deepened through the subcutaneous tissue, palmaris brevis, and palmar fascia. The ulnar nerve and artery are then exposed. The ulnar motor branch is exposed,

taking off from the ulnar nerve proximal to the hook of the hamate and proceeding deep in a radial direction toward the midpalm.

Thoracic Outlet Syndrome

Thoracic outlet syndrome (TOS) is relatively common, but rarely requires surgical management. Thoracic outlet syndrome is caused by compression of the lower trunk or medial cord of the brachial plexus. The sites of compression are numerous and may include compression between the anterior and medial scalene muscles, compression by a cervical, or first rib, or compression by the clavicle or pectoralis minor.

Surgical approaches for TOS are very complex, varied, and rarely necessary. They are beyond the scope of this text for discussion.

Radial Nerve at the Elbow

The radial nerve enters the distal one third of the arm as it penetrates the lateral intermuscular septum. It then runs between the brachioradialis and brachialis. The radial nerve gives motor branches to the brachioradialis and extensor carpi radialis longus before dividing proximal to the elbow into the radial sensory and the posterior interosseous nerves. The radial sensory nerve sometimes provides a motor branch to the extensor carpi radialis brevis (ECRB) before extending along the deep surface of the brachioradialis to the distal forearm, where it provides sensation to the dorsal radial aspect of the hand. The radial sensory nerve is rarely compressed, although it can be irritated where it penetrates the fascia in the distal one third of the forearm. The posterior interosseous nerve (PIN) penetrates the supinator muscle, and at the end of the supinator it branches extensively to supply motor function to the extensor pollicis longus, abductor pollicis longus, extensor pollicis brevis, extensor indicis proprius, extensor digitorum communis, extensor digiti minimi, and extensor carpi ulnaris. The PIN may be compressed at a number of sites from proximal to distal: the leading edge of the ECRB fascia, vascular leash of Henry, the arcade of Frohse (the proximal leading edge of the supinator), and finally the supinator proper (Fig. 46–11).

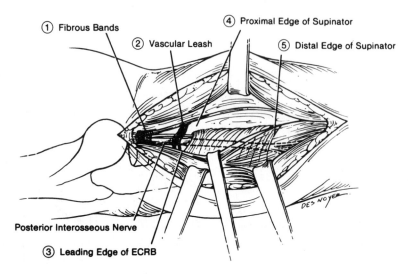

Figure 46–11 Schematic of radial tunnel nerve compression sites. Reproduced with permission from Richard H. Gelberman. *Operative Nerve Repair and Reconstruction*. Philadelphia, PA: Lippincott; 1991:1007.

Surgery for the radial nerve at the elbow is less common than for compressive lesions of the ulnar and median nerves. The results of surgical release for this nerve are not as consistent as release of several of the other nerves. The PIN may be approached anteriorly, posteriorly, or through the brachioradialis. Anteriorly, an incision is made beginning at the elbow flexion crease along the medial border of the brachial radialis. The dissection is carried down along the medial border of the brachioradialis. The interval between the pronator and brachioradialis is developed. This brings the dissection down onto the supinator. The PIN is encountered penetrating the supinator. At this point, the arcade of Frohse and the entire supinator may be released, as well as any more proximal lesions. The trans brachioradialis approach is performed through a 10-cm longitudinal incision starting at the lateral epicondyle and extending distally over the brachioradialis. The brachioradialis is then split in line with its muscle fibers. The dissection is carried down onto the supinator, which can be released as previously described. The dorsal approach of Thompson can be made through a 10-cm incision made between the ECRB and the extensor digitorum communis starting at the lateral epicondyle. This interval is then split longitudinally all the way up to the lateral epicondyle. This brings the dissection down onto the supinator, which again can be released as previously described.

Tarsal Tunnel Syndrome

Tarsal tunnel syndrome occurs from compression of the posterior tibial nerve by either the flexor retinaculum behind the medial malleolus or by the membranous origin of the abductor hallucis muscle. The posterior tibial nerve enters the ankle area through the deep posterior compartment of the leg. It passes behind the medial malleolus in conjunction with the flexor hallucis longus, the tibialis posterior, the flexor digitorum, as well as the posterior tibial artery. The compartment is confined by a thick flexor retinaculum. The nerve then continues on towards the plantar aspect of the foot, where it branches into a lateral or medial plantar branches. This area may be compressed by the membranous origin of the abductor hallucis. The nerve also gives off a calcaneal branch just proximal to branching into the plantar nerves. Release of the tarsal tunnel is made by a 6-cm curved incision starting just proximal to the medial malleolus and coursing distally behind the medial malleolus. Release of the flexor retinaculum and the fibrous origin of the abductor hallucis is then performed.

Morton's Neuroma

Morton's neuroma occurs in the third webbed space of the foot. This is thought to be secondary to perineural fibrosis of the common digital nerve of this web space. It is caused by friction between the two metatarsal heads.

Surgical approach to this is through a 2-cm dorsal incision between the third and fourth metacarpal heads. The neuroma is then excised.

EXAMINATION

Most chronic peripheral neuropathies will have a slow onset. The majority will not have a single initiating event. Patients will often complain of a general aching sensation sometimes associated with numbness and tingling in the anatomic distribution of the affected nerve. The symptoms are worse at night. The symptoms may then progress from a rare intermittent process to a more persistent process, to finally constant pain and numbness. Individuals will also report some weakness, and occasionally in advanced cases, some loss of muscle mass.

Physical examination consists of observation, which may reveal abnormal posturing, particularly of individuals' shoulders, wrist or elbow. Wasting of both the musculature and skin is also obvious with observation.

PEARL

A gross objective test of sensation is the absence of sweat on the involved digit. The absence of sweat is consistent with a significant sensory deficit. The absence of wrinkling of skin after prolonged emersion in water is another good objective test of a significant sensory neuropathy.

The Tinel's test, when positive, is an excellent test to use when looking for the site of peripheral nerve pathology. The Tinel's test is performed by tapping over the affected nerve, which causes an electrical sensation and discomfort projecting into the anatomic distribution of the nerve. In severe neuropathies that are recovering, the presence of a Tinel's sign that is advancing from proximal to distal over time, is positive evidence of nerve recovery. Digital compression over the nerve with numbness in the appropriate anatomic distribution also is an excellent sensitive test for compressive neuropathy.

Concerning the median nerve at the wrist, a Phalen's test performed with the wrist held in flexion resulting in numbness in the appropriate distribution is indicative of carpal tunnel syndrome. Wasting of the abductor pollicis brevis and inability to oppose the thumb is indicative of a severe carpal tunnel syndrome (Fig. 46–12).

Anterior interosseous neuropathy results in weakness or paralysis of flexion of the interphalangeal joint of the thumb and distal interphalangeal joints of the index and long fingers.

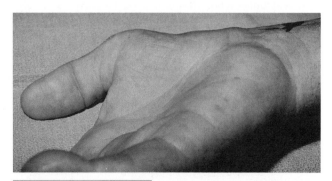

Figure 46–12 Atrophy of the abductor pollicis brevis consistent with a severe long-standing median neuropathy.

Pronator syndrome will have tenderness over the median nerve at the elbow, and resisted supination or pronation may make the symptoms worse.

A provocative test for cubital tunnel syndrome is the elbow flexion test. It is performed by flexing the elbow to 130 degrees, and if positive, will result in numbness in the ulnar nerve distribution. Other signs of a significant ulnar motor neuropathy include: clawing of the hand, a Wartenberg sign (abduction stance of the little finger), Froment's sign (flexion of the interphalangeal joint of the thumb when pinching), weakness of grip, weakness of pinch, wasting of the interossei, and wasting of the hypothenar muscles.

Thoracic outlet symptoms may be reproduced by abducting and externally rotating the shoulder rotating the neck, to the opposite side. The symptoms maybe also be reproduced by reaching overhead and exercising the hand by repetitively making a fist.

Posterior interosseous nerve syndrome will have significant weakness or paralysis of the finger and thumb extensors in the presence of intact wrist extension.

PITFALL

Patients will be able to extend the metacarpophalangeal (MP) joints of their hand with the wrist in flexion even if the posterior interosseous nerve (PIN) is not functioning secondary to the tenodesis effect.

PEARL

To determine if a patient cannot extend the MP joints of the hand secondary to incompetent tendons or to a PIN injury, the tenodesis effect can be used. With the wrist in full flexion the extensor tendons of the fingers have increased tone secondary to stretching and can extend the fingers at the MP joint level. If the wrist is extended the finger extensors are relaxed and the MP joints fall into flexion.

Radial tunnel syndrome presents with tenderness over the course of the PIN in the supinator and may be made worse with resisted supination. Loading of the long finger extensor may also exacerbate the symptoms.

Morton's neuroma patients will have exquisite tenderness between the third and fourth metatarsal heads. Squeezing the metatarsal heads together will exacerbate the symptoms.

Other modalities that can help with delineation of the sensory deficits include vibrometer, two-point discrimination both moving and static, and Semmes-Weinstein monofilaments. Motor evaluation can be determined by manual muscle testing, grip strength measurements, and pinch strength measurements.

AIDS TO DIAGNOSIS

There are a number of tests that will help delineate the degree of sensory dysfunction. One shortcoming of these tests, however, is that they all require some subjective interpretation by the patient and are subsequently prone to manipulation in some patients. Vibrometer testing is performed by touching a vibrometer of different frequencies to the skin. Normals have been well established, and this appears to be a good test for a compressive neuropathy. Semmes-Weinstein monofilament testing is performed by touching monofilaments of different thicknesses to the skin. Normals have been well established. Two-point testing is performed by having the patient note the difference between contact with one and two-points and measuring the distance between the two points. The two point test may be performed by using moving two-point or static two-point. Normal in the hand in someone without heavy callouses is 4 mm.

Electrodiagnostic testing is an important adjunct to the workup of a chronic peripheral neuropathy. Nerve conduction velocities are sensitive and specific for the presence of a number of neurocompressive lesions. A delay in the distal sensory latency of the median nerve at the wrist is consistent with a carpal tunnel syndrome. These must be interpreted in light of clinical findings. A small percentage of patients with normal nerve conduction velocities will still have carpal tunnel syndrome. For the ulnar nerve, a significant number of patients will have normal nerve conduction velocities when they have mild cubital tunnel syndrome. In other words, the electrodiagnostic studies are not sensitive enough to pick up all patients with carpal tunnel or cubital tunnel syndrome.

Electromyography (EMG) is performed by placing small, wire electrodes into the muscle proper that record electrical activity of the muscle. The presence of fibrillation potentials is indicative of a significant neuropathy. Nerve conduction velocities and EMGs are good objective tests for peripheral neuropathy. Injections about peripheral nerves can be an excellent adjunct to determine the exact peripheral nerve injury. This is particularly helpful when there are overlapping nerves. Injection also has a role in treatment.

PEARL

If an injection of the carpal tunnel results in temporary improvement in a patient with carpal tunnel syndrome, it is an excellent predictor of a good result if the carpal tunnel is released. This test is particularly helpful in the patient who has symptoms of carpal tunnel syndrome but a normal nerve conduction velocity.

X-ray examination when indicated can be a valuable adjunct to the workup of compressive neuropathies. X-rays of the elbow might reveal a supracondylar process with its associated ligament of Struthers responsible for a pronator teres syndrome. A cubital tunnel X-ray may also show heterotopic ossification about the cubital tunnel. X-rays of the wrist in a patient who has had a distal radius fracture may reveal a significant malunion of the distal radius, which can be responsible for significant mechanical compression of the median nerve at the carpal tunnel. Carpal-tunnel view X-rays may reveal a fracture of the hook of the hamate responsible for injury to the ulnar motor nerve. X-rays of the ankle in a patient with tarsal tunnel syndrome may reveal ossifications in the area of the tarsal tunnel.

SPECIFIC CONDITIONS, TREATMENT, AND OUTCOME

Carpal Tunnel Syndrome

Carpal tunnel syndrome is a compressive neuropathy caused by pressure on the median nerve in the constrained carpal tunnel. This is caused by a relative space mismatch between the flexor tendons, flexor tenosynovium, and median nerve in the confines of the carpal tunnel. Pressure rises in the carpal tunnel, and the median nerve is the structure most sensitive to pressure in the carpal tunnel.

Nonoperative treatment includes rest, splinting of the wrist in neutral, anti-inflammatory medication, and modification of work activities. Metabolic abnormalities, such as thyroid dysfunction or vitamin B_6 or B_{12} deficiencies, should be corrected. In carpal tunnel syndrome secondary to pregnancy, nonoperative treatment should be aggressively pursued, with the exception of medications, until the woman has delivered. When the patient is post partum, the carpal tunnel symptoms will slowly subside.

When carpal tunnel syndrome has failed to respond to this nonoperative management, then carpal tunnel release is indicated. Two basic approaches for the surgical treatment of carpal tunnel syndrome are available. A significant controversy exists between the choices of endoscopic versus open release of the carpal tunnel. Both surgical approaches were previously discussed.

PITFALL

In endoscopic carpal tunnel surgery, failure to clearly identify the transverse orientation of the fibers of the transverse carpal ligament prior to cutting can result in either an unreleased transverse carpal ligament or injury to the median nerve.

Postoperatively, the wound is dressed in a soft, compressive dressing for 7 to 10 days, and finger and wrist motion is begun immediately. Some physicians still splint the wrist for a short period of time postoperatively.

Carpal tunnel release is one of the most common operative procedures performed in the United States today. The expected outcome is excellent with 90% of patients noting significant pain relief. Some individuals, however, will have significant scar sensitivity and pain along the ulnar and radial pillars of the transverse carpal ligament. This incidence

---

PEARL

It is imperative that finger motion and, preferably, wrist motion begin immediately after carpal tunnel release to promote nerve gliding. It has been shown that with finger motion, the median nerve alone glides significantly. This movement is more than doubled once wrist motion is added. If the fingers and wrist are not moved, the median nerve will become encased in nonyielding scar with resulting tethering of the median nerve.

---

appears to be higher with the open carpal tunnel release than with the endoscopic carpal tunnel release in the early postoperative course. Complications include reflex sympathetic dystrophy (rare), persistent pain in the incision area, persistent numbness and tingling (occurs in cases of severe neuropathy), and neurologic injury (rare).

Incidence of neurologic injury is extremely low when surgery is performed by an experienced hand surgeon. The incidence of neurologic injury or tendon or vascular injury is higher with the endoscopic technique. The value of the endoscopic carpal tunnel technique is decreased postoperative pain during the first 90 days of resuming work. Recurrence of carpal tunnel syndrome is uncommon but can occur in individuals who return to a work activity that places very high demand on their hands such as prolonged exposure to vibrational tools. The majority of workers will be able to return to their previous occupation.

In cases of severe median neuropathy with thenar atrophy, carpal tunnel release is less predictable. These patients will often regain some sensation, although very rarely will regain normal sensation. Motor function return is unpredictable. In these cases, a Camitz transfer is performed at the time of the carpal tunnel release. The Camitz procedure is a tendon transfer using the palmaris longus elongated with a strip of palmar fascia to restore abduction (Fig. 46–13). There

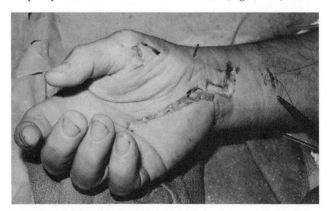

Figure 46–13 Postoperative photograph of a Camitz transfer for a long-standing severe median neuropathy. The direction of pull of the palmaris transfer is shown by the arrow. Note the positioning of the thumb.

are numerous other opponensplasties that have been described in the literature. These include transfer of the flexor digitorum superficialis of the ring finger or the transfer of the extensor indicis proprius.

Anterior Interosseous Neuropathy

Anterior interosseous neuropathy (AIN) is a neuropathy of the anterior interosseous nerve, which is the motor nerve to the flexor pollicis longus, the flexor digitorum profundus to the index and long fingers, and the pronator quadratus.

Treatment options include nonoperative methods: rest, anti-inflammatory medication, occasional long-arm splinting in neutral rotation, modification of work activities, and time. If the nerve has not returned in 4 to 6 months, then operative intervention should be performed. The operative approach is the same as the one described previously for the pronator teres release.

Postoperative care includes early active and passive range of motion of the elbow after suture removal. A significant number of AIN neuropathies will spontaneously resolve without surgical intervention. Anterior interosseus neuropathy secondary to a stretch injury, as one would see with supracondylar fractures, almost always resolves with nonoperative management. Anterior interosseus neuropathy that does not spontaneously resolve has a reasonable outcome with surgery, resulting in more than 50% of patients obtaining near-normal function. Patients that do not have return of function of the AIN despite operative management are then candidates for a tendon transfer. The recommended tendon transfers are the transfer of the brachioradialis to the flexor pollicis longus and suturing the tendons of the profundus of the index and long fingers side to side to the profundus of the ring and small fingers.

A recurrence of AIN neuropathy has not been reported to the author's knowledge. Complications of surgery include hypertrophic scar in the antecubital fossa, injury to the lateral antebrachial cutaneous nerve, and failure of recovery of the AIN.

Pronator Syndrome

Pronator syndrome is a compressive neuropathy of the median nerve at the elbow. Pronator syndrome presents with proximal forearm pain and subjective numbness in the hand. Objective numbness in the median nerve distribution of the hand is not a feature of pronator syndrome. Pronator syndrome usually occurs alone but may occur in conjunction with a carpal tunnel syndrome more distally.

Nonoperative management includes rest, modification of activities, anti-inflammatory medication, long-arm splinting (usually in neutral rotation), and, occasionally, corticosteroid injection. If such treatment should fail and nerve conduction studies are positive, then surgical treatment is indicated. The surgical approach has been described previously. It is critical that the following potential compressive lesions be released from proximal to distal: ligament of Struthers, lacertus fibrosis, pronator fascia, and fascial arcade of the superficialis. Postoperative management includes splint immobilization until the skin is healed and then early active and passive range of motion of the elbow. Expected outcome of surgical treatment for pronator syndrome is good, if the diagnosis is correct. The biggest problem with pronator syndrome is the lack of good objective tests to confirm the diagnosis. Studies of the results of operative management of pronator syndrome have reported from 80 to 90% good results (Johnson et al, 1979: Hartz et al, 1981). Complications of pronator release include misdiagnosis, hypertrophic scar, and injury to the lateral antebrachial cutaneous nerve from retraction.

Cubital Tunnel Syndrome

Cubital tunnel syndrome is the most common cause of ulnar nerve neuropathy. Cubital tunnel syndrome is a compressive neuropathy occurring at the elbow. The ulnar nerve may be injured by a direct blow at the cubital tunnel level, by compression in the confined space of the cubital tunnel, by a traction on the nerve during elbow flexion. The nerve can also be injured by subluxation around the medial epicondyle in individuals who have a poorly formed cubital tunnel retinaculum.

Treatment of mild, cubital tunnel syndrome includes night splinting the elbow in extension, an elbow pad for protection of the nerve, anti-inflammatory medication, rest, and modification of work activities. Operative intervention varies somewhat depending on the severity of the ulnar neuropathy and its underlying cause.

Multiple operative options are available to the surgeon. In mild grades of ulnar neuropathy associated with subjective numbness and/or objective numbness without motor weakness, a medial epicondylectomy, previously described, may be performed. Medial epicondylectomy is also a good choice for subluxation of the ulnar nerve. Other surgical techniques used for mild grades of cubital tunnel syndrome include simple in situ release and ulnar nerve transposition. Ulnar nerve transposition is also used for more severe grades (muscle weakness and wasting) of cubital tunnel syndrome. There is no clear evidence that one type of ulnar nerve transposition is superior to another. The choices are subcutaneous, intramuscular, and submuscular. The operative technique has been previously discussed.

Postoperative care involves immediate active and passive range of motion of the elbow. Resistive activities are avoided for 6 weeks. The need for splinting the elbow to protect the flexor pronator mass after epicondylectomy or submuscular transposition is not necessary because the flexor pronator mass has an extensive ulna origin and will not retract significantly.

Outcome of cubital tunnel surgery is primarily related to the severity of cubital tunnel syndrome noted preoperatively. In other words, patients with mild ulnar neuropathy, Dellon or McGowan stage I (mild sensory only), can predictably obtain 90% good relief with any operative procedure mentioned (Dellon et al, 1989). Patients with more severe ulnar neuropathy, Dellon stage II (mild weakness) or stage III (significant weakness and atrophy), in which motor involvement is a prominent feature, have a less predictable result. Kleinman and Bishop have reported 87% excellent and good results for all stages of cubital tunnel syndrome with intramuscular transposition of the ulnar nerve (Kleineman and Bishop, 1989).

<table>
<tr><td>

PITFALL

Incomplete release of the ulnar nerve from the arcade of Struthers to the flexor carpi ulnaris branch may result in an acute turn and kinking of the transposed nerve. If the distal medial intermuscular septum is not resected, the transposed nerve may be compressed by the septum.

</td></tr>
</table>

Complications of failed ulnar nerve surgery are uncommon but may be severe. These include reflex sympathetic dystrophy, neuroma of the medial brachial or medial antebrachial cutaneous nerves, and persistent or increased ulnar nerve symptoms. Treatment of these complications may be difficult and includes injections, transcutaneous electrical stimulation (TENS), antidepressant medication, and, in some cases, the use of an implantable electrical stimulator directly on the nerve. Operative management of ulnar motor neuropathy with significant weakness that has not improved with a transposition involves tendon transfers. There are numerous described tendon transfers for ulnar neuropathy. Tendon transfers that have been described to correct clawing of the ring and small fingers include flexor digitorum superficialis of the ring finger transferred to the A2 pulley of the ring and small fingers (low ulnar nerve palsy), extensor carpi radialis longus transfer with plantaris tendon graft elongation to the proximal phalanx of the ring and small fingers (high or low ulnar neuropathy), and flexor carpi radialis tendon with plantaris tendon graft elongation to either the A2 pulley or proximal phalanx of the ring and small fingers.

Ulnar Nerve Compression in Guyon's Canal

The ulnar nerve may be compressed in Guyon's canal at the wrist. This site of ulnar nerve compression is not as common as cubital tunnel syndrome. The nerve may be compressed by an aneurysm of the ulnar artery, a ganglion in Guyon's canal, or by direct injury. Nonoperative management of the ulnar nerve in Guyon's canal includes splinting, rest, use of padding or heavy glove in individuals who perform heavy work, and modification of work activities. If this should fail, a workup with magnetic resonance imaging (MRI) is indicated to evaluate for a mass lesion. If the ulnar nerve has not responded to conservative nonoperative management or if a mass lesion has been identified, then operative intervention is indicated. Operative intervention includes direct release of the ulnar nerve at the wrist as previously described. If compression is due to an aneurysm, the aneurysm is excised, and the ulnar artery is reconstructed with a vein graft. If a ganglion is present, it is excised. Postoperative management is dependent on the intra-operative findings. If a vascular reconstruction was performed, immobilization is indicated for 3 weeks. If no reconstruction was performed, then a soft, padded dressing and immediate motion is indicated. The expected outcome for release of the ulnar nerve in Guyon's canal is excellent, particularly in cases of early neuropathy associated with a compressive mass. Recurrence is rare. Complications include persistence of neuropathy in severe cases and hypertrophic painful scar. If no neurologic return should

occur, then tendon transfers can optimize the hand function. These transfers are the same as mentioned for low ulnar nerve palsy under the cubital tunnel section.

An isolated low ulnar motor neuropathy can occur with normal sensory findings. This occurs most commonly with fractures of the hook of the hamate, which should be suspected in anyone who plays racquet sports, golf, or baseball and who has tenderness over the hook of the hamate. This diagnosis can be confirmed by a carpal-tunnel view x-ray, 30-degree supinated x-ray, or computed tomography scan. Treatment consists of excision of the hook of the hamate. Results of ulnar motor neuropathy secondary to a hook of the hamate nonunion are excellent. Complications of excision of the hook of the hamate are injury to the motor branch of the ulnar nerve that runs intimately around the base of the hamate and, in rare exceptions, subluxation of ulnar flexor tendons.

Thoracic Outlet Syndrome

Thoracic outlet syndrome is caused by compression of the lower trunk and/or medial cord of the brachial plexus. It presents with pain and numbness in the ulnar nerve distribution, particularly with overhead-type activities. Treatment involves physical therapy with particular emphasis on postural training, stretching, mobilization of the neck and shoulder girdle area, and general muscle strengthening of the shoulder girdle muscles. This is very effective in the majority of patients. In a very small group of patients that do not respond at all to this treatment and who have severe symptoms, further anatomic causes of the TOS should be evaluated. Surgical treatment is rarely indicated and only in recalcitrant cases with severe symptoms. Surgical treatment is varied. It may include a first-rib resection, a scalenotomy, or a pectoralis minor tenotomy. The results of nonoperative treatment for TOS are good, with the majority of patients responding to a significant degree to an exercise and postural training program. In the recalcitrant stages, surgical management in the hands of a very experienced surgeon may also give good results. A significant problem is the lack of objective evidence for TOS. Nerve conduction velocities and EMG are almost invariably normal, and the diagnosis is dependent on history and the presence of nonspecific provocative tests. Surgical complications include pneumothorax, persistence of symptoms, brachial plexus injury, injury to the long thoracic nerve, and vascular injury. Because of the significant severe-complication rate, surgery for TOS should be deferred to a surgeon very experienced in this area.

Posterior Interosseous Neuropathy

Posterior interosseous neuropathy is a compressive neuropathy of the PIN at or slightly proximal to the supinator that results in weakness or inability to extend the fingers at the MP joint level, inability to extend the thumb, and some weakness in wrist extension. Posterior interosseus neuropathy can be caused by direct trauma, a traction phenomenon (as one would see with a supracondylar humerus fracture), or a mass effect (as one might see from a ganglion or synovitis) (Fig. 46–14). Treatment for PIN neuropathy secondary to traction is nonoperative with expectation of return of function of the nerve. Treatment of PIN neuropathy secondary

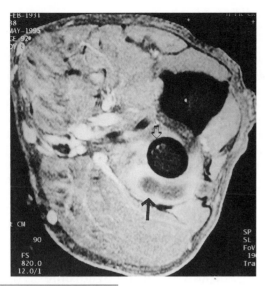

Figure 46–14   Magnetic resonance imaging of the elbow showing a large ganglion at the level of the radial head (solid arrow). The nonsolid, short arrow is pointing to the anterior portion of the radial head.

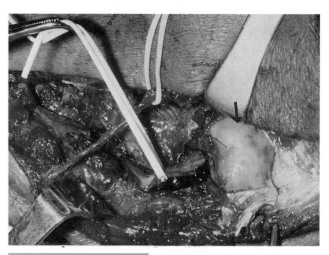

Figure 46–15   Intra-operative photograph of the posterior interosseous nerve (PIN) proximal to the supinator. The solid arrow is pointing to the large ganglion from the radial capitellar joint. Vessel loop with arrow on it is around the PIN. To the right is proximal.

to a mass lesion as one would see with a ganglion or synovitis of the radiocapitellar joint in patients with rheumatoid arthritis is decompression of the PIN with resection of the mass (Fig. 46–15). Treatment of spontaneous PIN neuropathy without a mass lesion (ruled out by MRI) is treated with rest, anti-inflammatory medication, and splinting in a supination long-arm splint. Modification of work activities also plays a role. If this should fail with no improvement in 3 months, then operative intervention is indicated. Operative intervention can precede through any of the three basic surgical approaches previously described, depending on the need for resection of a mass, if present. In cases of mass lesions such as a ganglion, the surgical approach is determined by the location of the mass, and excision of the ganglion is indicated. In rheumatoid synovitis, a synovectomy of the elbow with probable radial head excision is indicated. Release of the PIN from proximal to distal must include release of the leading edge of the ECRB; release of the vascular leash of Henry; release of the arcade of Frohse; and as some authors would recommend, release of the entire body of the supinator. Postoperative care may include splinting until the skin is healed, followed by active and passive motion. The wrist is splinted in neutral until it obtains adequate strength with neurologic recovery. This is sometimes not necessary depending on whether the ECRB is innervated by the PIN or a branch more proximal off the radial nerve. Expected outcome of PIN neuropathy is highly dependent on the cause. Fractures resulting in a traction injury to the PIN will recover with excellent function in 3 to 4 months. Where a mass lesion has been identified and treated early, functional recovery is usually good.

Complications of PIN neuropathy surgery include persistence of the neuropathy, injury to the lateral antebrachial cutaneous nerve (anterior approach), and hypertrophic scar (anterior approach). Late treatment of PIN palsy includes ten-

don transfers. The most common set of tendon transfers used for PIN palsy is the pronator teres transferred to the ECRB (if the ECRB is not working) for wrist extension, palmaris longus to the rerouted extensor pollicis longus for thumb extension, and flexor carpi radialis or flexor carpi ulnaris to the finger extensors for finger extension.

Radial Tunnel Syndrome

Radial tunnel syndrome is thought to represent a compressive neuropathy of the PIN about the elbow. It is distinguished from PIN neuropathy because of the lack of motor weakness. Patients with radial tunnel syndrome will complain of significant pain over the course of the PIN in the dorsal radial aspect of the forearm. There are no good objective tests. Nerve conduction velocities, and EMGs are routinely normal. Treatment of radial tunnel syndrome involves rest, anti-inflammatory medication, placement in a long-arm supination-type splint with the elbow in flexion, and work modification. If there is a lateral epicondylitis associated with the radial tunnel syndrome, which is common, the lateral epicondylitis should be aggressively treated. Often with resolution of the lateral epicondylitis the radial tunnel syndrome will resolve as well. Release of the radial tunnel is uncommonly indicated. Surgical treatment involves an approach to the PIN through any of the three approaches previously discussed: anterior, lateral, or dorsal. The structures that need to be released from proximal to distal are the leading edge of the ECRB, the vascular leash of Henry, the arcade of Frohse, and the supinator muscle itself. Outcome of radial tunnel syndrome is generally good with nonoperative management. Recurrence can occur, particularly if the original inciting event is returned to on a frequent basis. Results of surgical treatment of radial tunnel syndrome are unpredictable, with persistence of pain in a significant number of patients. Surgical complications include missed diagnosis and persistence or increased radial tunnel pain. No transfers are necessary because this is not a motor neuropathy.

Radial Sensory Neuritis

The radial sensory nerve can be injured resulting in a severely painful sensory neuritis. This occurs where the radial nerve protrudes from under the brachioradialis at the distal one third of the forearm. This neuritis is typified by a severe pain or numbness in the dorsal radial aspect of the distal forearm that radiates to the dorsal radial aspect of the hand. Radial sensory neuritis may occur spontaneously, be secondary to trauma, or be caused iatrogenically (usually by the use of external fixator pins). It also may be seen in association with DeQuervain's tenosynovitis. Treatment of radial sensory neuritis includes splinting, anti-inflammatory medication, occasional corticosteroid injection, and a TENS unit. Treatment also includes treatment of the DeQuervain's tenosynovitis, if present. If nonoperative management is not successful and the symptoms are severe, surgical intervention is indicated. Surgery is performed through a longitudinal skin incision at the level of the Tinel's sign. The dissection is then carried down to the radial sensory nerve. If a neuroma is encountered, which is common in iatrogenic causes of radial sensory neuritis, the neuroma is excised. The defect in the nerve is grafted. Postoperative care involves splinting of the wrist for 3 weeks, then active and passive range of motion is started. Expected outcome in mild cases of radial sensory neuritis treated nonoperatively is good with resolution. In severe cases, particularly in cases of neuroma from iatrogenic causes, the treatment is very unpredictable. Complications include further symptomatic neuroma formation and severe causalgia. Treatment of severe causalgia and recurrent neuroma formation is to dissect the nerve further proximally and place the nerve in a more silent muscle bed versus continued splinting, and a TENS unit. In occasional extreme circumstances, an implantable nerve stimulator is placed. No tendon transfers are necessary because this is a sensory nerve only.

Tarsal Tunnel Syndrome

Tarsal tunnel syndrome is caused by compression of the terminal portion of the posterior tibial nerve at the ankle. It also may be caused by compression of one of its terminal branches, the medial or lateral plantar nerves. Patients with tarsal tunnel will complain of pain and numbness in the plantar aspect of the feet that is exacerbated by standing. Treatment of tarsal tunnel is predominantly nonoperative. Surgery should be reserved only for patients who have significant symptoms and who have not responded to nonoperative management. Nonoperative modalities include avoidance of high heels and poor-fitting shoes, anti-inflammatory medication, and, sometimes, steroid injection. Treatment of a significant hindfoot valgus deformity with a custom orthoses may be of value. Modification of work activities including prolonged standing is important. Surgery is reserved for the small group of patients who have not responded to a nonoperative treatment regimen and in whom the diagnosis is secure. The surgical approach has previously been described. Postoperatively, patients are treated in a compressive dressing and early motion of the ankle is initiated. Weight bearing may be added as tolerated. Expected outcome for nonoperative patients is generally good. The outcome of surgical treatment of tarsal tunnel syndrome is somewhat unpredictable. Complications include missed diagnosis, a localized causalgia, neuroma formation, and persistent pain.

Hereditary Neuropathies

There are a number of rare hereditary peripheral neuropathies. Only Charcot-Marie-Tooth disease will be discussed in any detail as it is the most common of this group. A complete listing of the genetically determined peripheral neuropathies include (1) peroneal muscular atrophy (Charcot-Marie-Tooth disease); (2) progressive hypertrophic polyneuropathy (Dejerine-Sottas disease); (3) hereditary sensory neuropathy; (4) chronic polyneuropathy with ichthyosis, deafness, and retinitis pigmentosa (Refsum's disease); (5) abetalipoproteinemia; (6) Tangier disease; and (7) metachromatic leukodystrophy.

Charcot-Marie-Tooth disease is the most common hereditary peripheral neuropathy. It is a dominant heritable disease that may present in the adolescent or adult years. It is a mixed sensory motor neuropathy involving the most distal axons of the peripheral nerves. It begins in the feet and progresses proximally to as high as the midthigh. The patient will present with an equinovarus-type foot deformity. At a much later stage, it may progress to involve the intrinsic muscles of the hand. The patient may respond to orthoses or tendon transfers for the intrinsic minus foot with absence of evertors of the ankle. The hand is much less commonly involved but may benefit from tendon transfers used for treatment of the intrinsic minus hand.

Acquired Peripheral Neuropathies

There is a long list of medical causes of peripheral neuropathy, which will only be listed. Diabetic neuropathy, the most common form of peripheral neuropathy, will be discussed in more detail.

1. Poisons:
   metals: arsenic, lead, mercury, antimony, and thallium
   drugs: nitrofurantoin, isoniazid, thalidomide, vincristine, diphenylhydantoin
   organic substances: carbon monoxide
   solvents: organophosphate compounds
2. Deficiency states and metabolic disorders:
   alcoholism, berry-berry, pellagra, pregnancy and chronic gastro-intestinal disease, carcinoma of the lung, diabetes, porphyria, amyloidosis, multiple myeloma, macroglobulinemia, uremia, hypoglycemia, systemic lupus erythematosus, and hypothyroidism

3. specific inflammatory states and infections:
   acute idiopathic polyneuritis (Guillain-Barre syndrome), diphtheria, sarcoid, infectious mononucleosis, leprosy, and herpes zoster
4. vascular disease:
   includes polyarteritis nodosum, diabetes, and rheumatoid arthritis

Diabetes

Diabetes is the most common cause of peripheral neuropathy. The exact pathomechanism by which diabetes effects the peripheral nerves has not been fully elucidated. In the past, it was felt that diabetes causes changes in the microvascular circulation that in turn effect the peripheral nerves. It appears now that microvascular changes only play a minor role in diabetic peripheral neuropathy. Diabetic neuropathy may act in a similar manner as the double crush model previously discussed. Accumulation of sorbitol, which is a metabolic product of glucose in the nerve, may cause endoneural edema. This endoneural edema results in decreased axoplasmic flow and makes the nerve more susceptible to a secondary compressive injury. This may explain the high incidence of associated compressive neuropathy in addition to diabetic peripheral neuropathy.

The most common presentation of diabetic peripheral neuropathy is in the feet. The second most common site is a carpal-tunnel–like scenario. This results from a combination of a diabetic peripheral neuropathy with an associated compressive neuropathy. Treatment begins with wrist splinting, anti-inflammatory medication, modification of activities, and corticosteroid injection. Injection with temporary relief may give some indication of the what may be expected from a carpal tunnel release. Nerve conduction velocities and EMGs will give some idea of an overlying compressive neuropathy in addition to the peripheral neuropathy. Releasing the carpal tunnel will only effect the compressive component of the neuropathy and will have no effect on the peripheral neuropathy itself. Results of surgery on diabetics with a compressive neuropathy overlying a peripheral neuropathy are good but not as predictable as in patients who has a compressive neuropathy only. If a compressive neuropathy is present that has not responded to nonoperative treatment, then a carpal tunnel release should be performed because it is the only significant treatment available for the diabetic with a compressive and peripheral neuropathy. Peripheral neuropathy alone is difficult to treat, but it appears that good long-term control of diabetes may slow its progression. There are a number of antidepressant and anticonvulsant medications that may help with the dysethesias associated with a diabetic neuropathy.

Complications of carpal tunnel surgery in diabetics include infection, persistence of numbness and tingling secondary to the peripheral neuropathy, and, occasionally, causalgia.

SELECTED BIBLIOGRAPHY

Carpal Tunnel Syndrome

LEWIS DA. Cumulative trauma disorders. *J Hand Surg.* 1987;12A:823–825.

LUNDBORG G. MYERS R. POWELL H. Nerve compression injury and increase in endoneural fluid pressure: a miniature compartment syndrome. *J Neurol Neurosurg Psychiatry.* 1983;46:1119–1124.

OSTERMAN AL. The double crush syndrome. *Orthop Clin North Am.* 1988;19:147–155.

SZABO RM, CHIDGEY LK. Stress carpal tunnel pressures in patients with carpal tunnel syndrome and normal patients. *J Hand Surg.* 1989;14A:624–627.

SZABO RM, GELBERMAN RH. Peripheral nerve compression: etiology, critical pressure threshold and clinical assessment. *Orthop.* 1984;7:1461–1466.

Anterior Interosseous Nerve

FARBER JS, BRYAN RS. The anterior interosseous nerve syndrome. *J Bone Jt Surg.* 1968;50A:521–523.

JONES ET, LEWIS DS. Median nerve injuries associated with supracondylar fractures of the humerus in children. *Clin Orthop.* 1980;150:181–186.

Pronator Syndrome

HARTZ CR, LINSCHEID RL, GRAMSE RR, DAUBE JR. The pronator teres syndrome: compressive neuropathy of the median nerve. *J Bone Jt Surg.* 1981;63A:885–890.

JOHNSON RK, SPINNER M, SHREWSBURY MM. Median nerve entrapment syndrome in the proximal forearm. *J Hand Surg.* 1979;4:48–51.

Posterior Interosseous Neuropathy

SPINNER M. The arcade of Frohse and its relationship to the posterior interosseous nerve paralysis. *J Bone Jt Surg.* 1968;50B:809–812.

WHITE SH, GOODFELLOW JW, MOWAT A. Posterior interosseous nerve palsy in rheumatoid arthritis. *J Bone Jt Surg.* 1988;70B:468–471.

Radial Tunnel Syndrome

LISTER GO, BELSOLE RB, KLEINERT HE. The radial tunnel syndrome. *J Hand Surg.* 1979;4:52–59.

Radial Sensory Nerve Entrapment

DELLON AL, MACKINNON SE. Radial sensory nerve entrapment in the forearm. *J Hand Surg.* 1986;11A:199–205.

Ulnar Nerve

ADELAAR RS, FOSTER WC, MCDOWELL C. The treatment of cubital tunnel syndrome. *J Hand Surg.* 1984;9A:90–95.

CHILDRESS HM. Recurrent ulnar nerve dislocation at the elbow. *Clin Orthop.* 1975;108:168–173.

DELLON AL. Review of treatment results for ulnar nerve entrapment at the elbow. *J Hand Surg.* 1989;14A:688–699.

EATON RG, CROWE JF, PARKES JC III. Anterior transposition of the ulnar nerve with a noncompressing fasciodermal sling. *J Bone Jt Surg.* 1980;62A:820–825.

HEITHOFF SJ, MILLENDER LH. Medial epicondylectomy for treatment of ulnar nerve compression at the elbow. *J Hand Surg.* 1990;15A:22–29.

KLEINMAN WB, Bishop AT. Anterior intramuscular transposition of the ulnar nerve. *J Hand Surg.* 1989;14:972–979.

LEVY DM, APFELBERG DB. Results of anterior transposition for the ulnar neuropathy at the elbow. *Amer J Surg.* 1972;123:304–308.

O'DRISCOLL SW, HORI E, CARMICHAEL SW, MORREY BF. The cubital tunnel and ulnar neuropathy. *J Bone Jt Surg.* 1991;73B:613–617.

OGATA K, MANSKE PR, LESKER PA. The effect of surgical dissection on regional blood flow to the ulnar nerve in the cubital tunnel. *Clin Orthop.* 1985;193:195–198.

Ulnar Nerve at the Wrist

BRAND RW. Tendon transfers for median and ulnar nerve paralysis. *Orthop Clin North Amer.* 1970;1:447–454.

KUSCHNER S. GELBERMAN RH. Ulnar nerve compression at the wrist. *J Hand Surg.* 1988;13A:577–580.

Basic Science

NEARY D, EAMES RA. The pathology of ulnar nerve compression in man. *Neuropathol Appl Neurobiol.* 1975;1:69–88.

OGATA K, NAITO M. Blood flow to the peripheral nerve: effects of dissection, stretching, and compression. *J Hand Surg.* 1986;11B:10–14.

RYDEVIK B, LUNDBORG G, BAGGE U. Effects of graded compression on intraneural blood flow. *J Hand Surg.* 1981;6:3–12.

WRIGHT TW, GLOWCZEWSKIE F, WHEELER D, MILLER G. COWIN D. Median nerve excursion and strain. *J Bone Jt Surg.* In press.

SAMPLE QUESTIONS

1. Aching sensation in the proximal volar forearm with subjective numbness and tingling in the radial three and one half digits that is exacerbated with work activities are symptoms of:
   - (a) cubital tunnel syndrome
   - (b) TOS
   - (c) carpal tunnel syndrome
   - (d) posterior interosseous neuropathy
   - (e) pronator syndrome

2. A 43-year-old patient presents with acute onset of pain for several days in the proximal volar forearm followed by resolution of this pain. The patient now complains of inability to pinch. He has no subjective sensory complaints. This patient likely has:
   - (a) PIN syndrome
   - (b) carpal tunnel syndrome
   - (c) AIN syndrome
   - (d) TOS
   - (e) none of the above

3. Severe cubital tunnel syndrome will result in weakness and atrophy of all of the following muscles except:
   - (a) first dorsal interosseous
   - (b) abductor digiti minimae
   - (c) abductor pollicis brevis

   - (d) ulnar two lumbricales
   - (e) palmar interossei

4. A 43-year-old patient with a long history of rheumatoid arthritis presents with an onset of weakness of wrist extension and finger extension over a 2-week period. On physical examination, the patient can extend the wrist very weakly in radial deviation and has no ability to extend the MP joints with the wrist extended or the IP joint of the thumb. The likely site of a lesion is:
   - (a) ulnar nerve at the elbow
   - (b) carpal tunnel
   - (c) radial nerve proximal to the elbow
   - (d) radial sensory nerve at the elbow
   - (e) PIN at the elbow

5. Carpal tunnel syndrome is characterized by all of these findings except:
   - (a) nocturnal pain in the hand
   - (b) decreased subjective sensation or numbness in the radial three and one half digits of the hand
   - (c) positive Tinel's sign at the wrist
   - (d) atrophy of the abductor pollicis brevis
   - (e) inability to flex the IP joint of the thumb

Sports Medicine and Rehabilitation

Section XIV

Chapter 47

Principles of Rehabilitation

Joseph E. Tomaro, MS, PT, ATC

Many orthopaedic ailments are curable with a period of rest followed by rehabilitation. Appropriate therapy is also essential to maximize the effectiveness of surgery. This chapter will review the principles of rehabilitation including flexibility, strengthening, and proprioception along with the methods by which these characteristics are restored.

BASIC SCIENCE

Influence of the Inflammatory Process on Rehabilitation

Understanding the inflammatory process is essential in determining appropriate rehabilitation following an injury. The extent of the inflammatory process depends on the type of tissue injured and the degree of injury. Although the inflammatory process occurs with injuries to all tissues, the following sections will concentrate on the effects of injury on connective tissue.

Inflammation

The inflammatory process can be subdivided into inflammation and tissue repair. *Inflammation* comprises vascular, hemostatic, and immune responses. The primary signs of inflammation are due to changes that occur in the vascular system at the site of injury. Chemical mediators including histamine, bradykinin, and prostaglandins that cause vasodilation of the capillaries are released at the area of the injury. Increased hydrostatic pressure occurs in the capillary which causes a release of fluid into the interstitial space. The resultant edema creates increased pressure on the mechanoreceptors in the region producing *mechanical pain*. In addition, the increased fluid in the interstitial spaces causes hypoxia of the surrounding tissues leading to *chemical pain*. An elevation in tissue temperature occurs due to increased metabolism at the site of the injury. The events that occur during the vascular response lead to a loss of function of the injured area. In the later stages of inflammation, the hemostatic response begins, which allows for localized clotting at the area of injury to control blood loss.

The primary goal of treatment during inflammation is to control the vascular response through the use of cold, compression, and elevation. The reduction in vasodilation and edema will decrease pain, expediting the return to normal function. It is also important to protect the injured area from further damage. During this period, an understanding of both the inflammatory process and joint biomechanics is important in determining the appropriate amount of protection. For example, in a grade I lateral ankle sprain, the goal is to prevent excessive stress on the injured lateral ankle ligaments. Therefore, only control of the frontal plane motion of inversion is necessary while still allowing for normal sagittal plane movement of dorsiflexion and plantarflexion. Appropriate active range-of-motion exercises can be performed that will create a muscle pumping mechanism to decrease swelling. The gentle oscillatory movements also help to stimulate the mechanoreceptors that may assist in pain reduction.

Proliferation

The next phase of the inflammatory process is tissue repair, which is commonly subdivided into the proliferative and remodeling phases. One of the primary events that occurs in the *proliferative phase* is the re-initiation of the blood supply to the injured area by an ingrowth of capillary buds. Fibroblasts also begin to migrate to the area of injury and initiate the synthesis of collagen. A connective tissue matrix is re-established but lacks sufficient tensile strength due to the random arrangement of the collagen fibers.

The primary goal of rehabilitation during the proliferative phase is to allow for the re-establishment of the connective tissue matrix while preventing the deleterious effects that occur with prolonged immobilization. The adverse effects of immobilization include decreased ground substance, decreased lubrication between collagen fibers, and increased

779

cross linking of collagen fibers leading to thickening of the collagen fibers and a loss of proper orientation. These changes can result in a loss of normal motion and decreased tensile strength of the connective tissue. For example, in the rehabilitation of a grade II medial collateral ligament sprain of the knee, controlled range-of-motion exercises place tension on the medial collateral ligament preventing the adverse effects of immobilization while still allowing for re-establishment of the connective tissue matrix.

Remodeling

The final stage of the inflammatory process is tissue remodeling, which is characterized by maturation of the connective tissue matrix. Initially, the connective tissue matrix is fragile and randomly oriented leading to decreased tensile strength. During the remodeling phase, there is a reorientation of the collagen fibers based on the stress that is placed across the injured tissue.

The goal of rehabilitation during the remodeling phase is to provide controlled stress to the healing tissue to allow for re-establishment of optimal collagen alignment and strength. Graded and progressive range-of-motion and strengthening exercises will gradually increase the tension on the connective tissue leading to improved healing. In addition, the steady progression of functional activity will further enhance tissue remodeling.

PRINCIPLES OF REHABILITATION

Flexibility

Flexibility is the ability to move a joint or a series of joints through a full, unrestricted range of motion. The length of the antagonist muscle is typically the cause for inadequate range of motion about a joint. The most common muscle groups that have flexibility deficits are the bi-articular muscles. Inadequate flexibility may be a causative factor in muscle strains that typically occur during ballistic activities, such as a hamstring strain during sprinting. Rapid hip flexion and knee extension occur during the swing phase of running. If there is inadequate flexibility of the hamstrings, there may be increased susceptibility to muscular strain during sprinting. Poor flexibility may also be one cause of overuse injuries. For example, decreased flexibility of the iliotibial band may increase friction between the iliotibial band and the greater trochanter, possibly leading to trochanteric bursitis.

Achieving adequate flexibility through stretching exercises is an important part of the warm-up process. Flexibility exercises should ideally be performed following a period of light cardiovascular exercise. This increases blood flow and tissue temperature leading to increased extensibility of the connective tissue elements of skeletal muscle. The purpose of performing stretching exercises is to prevent injuries, provide adequate warm-up, and enhance performance by increasing movement capabilities.

Specific recommendations for flexibility exercises are based upon individual assessments, activity level, and injury. Stretching exercises can be static, ballistic, or make use of proprioceptive neuromuscular facilitation principles.

Static stretching is the most commonly recommended type of stretching exercise and consists of placing a muscle in a lengthened position and holding for an extended period of time at the moment of stretch. The static stretch should be held for 10 to 60 seconds with no definitive recommendations based on the results of research. During stretching, there is increased activity of the muscle spindle in the muscle being stretched, which causes a reflex contraction of the muscle through the monosynaptic stretch reflex.

> ### PEARL
>
> **If the stretch is held for a longer than 6 seconds, the golgi tendon organs will begin to be facilitated leading to an inhibition of the muscle being stretched and improved flexibility.**

Gentle, prolonged stretching is one of the most effective ways of increasing connective tissue extensibility and avoiding injury.

Ballistic stretching involves lengthening the muscle to the point of stretch and performing short magnitude, high speed, bouncing movements. The theorized, beneficial effect of ballistic stretching is that it may be more functional because most sporting activities involve ballistic movements. However, there are concerns about the safety of ballistic stretching and the increased potential for injury due to uncontrolled lengthening of the muscle. It is also been theorized that ballistic stretching will cause continual firing of the muscle spindle leading to a reflex contraction of the muscle and, therefore, prevention of adequate gains in flexibility.

Proprioceptive neuromuscular facilitation (PNF) is a group of techniques designed to use various types of input to assist in facilitation or inhibition of certain muscle groups. This type of stretching requires a skilled partner to provide appropriate resistance and stabilization. Gains in hamstring flexibility have been reported with the use of hold-relax and contract-relax stretching techniques. In contract-relax stretching, the antagonist muscle is passively moved through the range of motion until resistance is met. An isotonic contraction of the antagonist muscle is then performed followed by further passive stretching (Fig. 47–1). Hold-relax stretching tech-

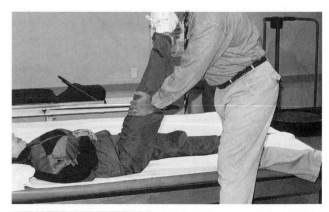

Figure 47–1   Example of contract-relax stretching. The hamstring is passively moved until resistence is met. Following isotonic contraction of the hamstring, further passive stretching is attempted.

niques involve passively stretching the antagonist muscle until resistance is met. An isometric contraction of the antagonist muscle is then performed followed by an isotonic contraction of the agonist and additional passive stretching of the antagonist.

Joint Mobilization

Osteokinematics describes the movement of the bone during joint motion. During shoulder abduction, the shaft of the humerus swings in a superior direction. Accessory joint movements also occur during joint motion and are described by *arthrokinematics*. As the humerus is swinging superiorly during shoulder abduction, the humeral head is gliding inferiorly in the glenoid fossa. When a convex surface moves on a concave surface, the swing of the bone and the glide of the joint surface are in opposite directions. When a concave surface moves on a convex surface, the swing of the bone and the glide of the joint surface are in same direction. *Joint mobilization* is the use of manual techniques to restore the accessory movements or joint gliding that occurs during motion.

There may be significant limitations in joint motion following periods of immobilization, especially following fractures. The initial goal of rehabilitation is to restore normal passive range-of-motion. In many cases, the limitations in passive range of motion are due to restrictions that have developed in the joint capsule due to the prolonged period of immobilization. In addition to performing passive range of motion exercises, joint mobilization techniques can be used to improve the accessory movements of the joint to assist in gaining motion. For example, shoulder abduction may be decreased because of joint capsule tightness limiting the normal inferior glide of the humerus in the glenoid. A joint mobilization technique of inferior gliding can be performed to restore normal arthrokinematics (Fig. 47–2). Joint mobilization techniques are graded based on the magnitude and amplitude of the stretch. There are various theories and classifications of joint mobilization techniques. It is important to have an understanding of both the osteokinematics and arthrokinematics of the joint when using joint mobilization techniques.

Spinal traction is a specific joint mobilization technique that is often used in the treatment of injuries to the lumbar and cervical spine. *Spinal traction* is the separation of the joint articular surfaces due to forces that are perpendicular to the joint surfaces. The proposed benefits of spinal traction include greater stretching of the facet joint capsules, increased superior-inferior dimensions of the intervertebral foramen, elongation of the posterior soft tissue structures, and alterations of interdiscal pressures. Lumbar or cervical traction may be beneficial in the treatment of spinal nerve root impingement secondary to degenerative disc disease, spinal nerve root impingement due to spinal stenosis, and general hypomobility of the spine. Caution should be used when applying spinal traction; begin with low amplitude movements while constantly monitoring the patient's signs and symptoms. Spinal traction is contraindicated in patients with hypermobility of the spine.

Strengthening

Strength is the ability of a muscle to generate force against resistance and plays an integral role in rehabilitation. The primary purpose of performing strengthening exercises is to return muscles to their pre-injury status following a period of immobilization or inactivity. Muscle strengthening is also important in providing dynamic joint stability and in helping to correct muscle imbalances that may lead to overuse injuries. Muscle can be divided into fast-twitch and slow-twitch fiber types based on the characteristics of the motor unit (Table 47–1). Many detrimental effects occur in muscle with inactivity or immobilization including atrophy of primarily the fast-twitch fibers. The ability to increase force production is based upon two factors: changes within the muscle fiber and improved activation of the muscle by the motor unit. Resistance training has been shown to increase the cross-sectional area of skeletal muscle. Strengthening exercises have the greatest effects on fast-twitch muscle fibers, creating hypertrophy due to an increased synthesis of myofibrillar proteins (actin and myosin). Resistance training has been shown to cause minimal changes in the number of mitochondria or capillary density within muscle. During initial resistance training, there is usually a rapid increase in muscle force production due to improvement of the efficiency of the neuromuscular system. There is an increase in the number of

TABLE 47–1   Characteristics of Motor Units

Tonic	Phasic
Type I	Type II
Small alpha motor neuron	Large alpha motor neuron
Small axon	Large axon
Slow-twitch fibers	Fast-twitch fibers
Muscle fibers (red)	Muscle fibers (white)
Aerobic oxidative enzymes	Anaerobic glycolytic enzymes
Small quantities of glycogen	Large quantities of glycogen
Rich in myoglobin	Poor in myoglobin
Longer contraction time	Shorter contraction time
More mitochondria	Fewer mitochondria
Lower muscle tension	Higher muscle tension
High oxygen consumption	Low oxygen consumption
Low fatigability	Pronounced fatigability

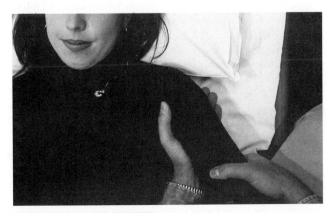

Figure 47–2   Mobilization of the shoulder using the technique of inferior gliding.

motor units recruited, increased firing of the motor units, and more synchronized firing of the motor unit.

PEARL

Strength is the ability of a muscle to generate force against resistance and plays an integral role in rehabilitation.

Muscle strengthening can be achieved through isometric, isotonic, or isokinetic exercise. *Isometric* exercise is the contraction of a muscle where tension is produced without joint movement. The primary advantages of isometric exercise is that the contraction can be performed with little or no equipment and can be used in an attempt to maintain muscle strength when joint movement is contraindicated. Therefore, isometric exercises are generally used early in the rehabilitation process to prevent the effects of immobilization while protecting the injured area. The disadvantages of isometric exercise are that the rate of strength gains are limited, and the strength gains only occur at the joint angle ($+/-$15 degrees) at which the contraction is performed.

Isotonic exercise is the contraction of a muscle through the range of motion against a constant resistance. Isotonics are the most common form of resistance exercises used in rehabilitation. The advantages of isotonic exercise are greater strength gains than isometrics and strengthening throughout the range-of-motion. Isotonic exercises are usually performed later in rehabilitation when joint movement is permitted. Due to the length-tension properties of muscle, there is a portion in the range-of-motion where a muscle produces the greatest amount of force. The length at which maximal force production occurs is the point of optimal overlap of actin and myosin. When a muscle is lengthened or shortened, there is less optimal positioning of the actin and myosin and decreased ability to generate force. During isotonic exercises, the resistance that can be used is limited by the weakest portions of the length tension curve, which limits the ability to develop maximum force through the entire range of motion. Many weight-lifting machines use variable resistance throughout the range of motion to accommodate to the length-tension curve and improve the ability to generate maximal force throughout the entire range-of-motion.

Isotonic exercises can be performed through either concentric or eccentric contractions. A *concentric* contraction is the shortening of a muscle as joint movement occurs whereas an *eccentric* contraction is the lengthening of a muscle during joint movement. Muscle can generate greater force during an eccentric contraction due to increased tension in the connective tissue elements of the muscle. Eccentric strengthening may be considered to be more functional because many movements that occur during activity require eccentric muscle contractions to control movements that occur due to gravity and ground reaction forces.

Isokinetic exercise is the performance of movement at a constant speed against variable and accommodating resistance. The advantages of isokinetic exercise are an accommodation to the length-tension curve and maximum force output at each point in the range-of-motion. Isokinetic exercise can be performed at a variety of contraction speeds that approach the velocity of joint movement that occurs during activities of daily living. However, even at faster contraction speeds, the movement does not approach the velocity of motion that occurs during sports activities. Other disadvantages of isokinetic exercise include increased joint compression and increased shear forces at low contraction velocities. These increased forces may be especially harmful following surgical procedures that are designed to provide joint stability. When properly used, isokinetic exercise can be an effective means of improving muscle strength.

Many isokinetic machines can also be used to measure force production of various muscle groups and to compare the force production of injured with uninjured extremities or agonists with antagonists. Force production during an isokinetic contraction depends on both the ability of the muscle to generate force and the status of the joint. Comparison of isokinetic force production requires interpretation and should be used as only one component in the overall evaluation of a patient's status.

Strengthening exercises can either be performed during open or closed kinetic chain movements. *Open kinetic chain* movements are movements in which the distal limb of a joint is not fixed and is free to move. An example of an open kinetic chain strengthening exercise for the quadriceps is seated knee extension. Strengthening exercises can also be performed in a *closed kinetic chain*, in which the distal segment is fixed. Examples of closed kinetic chain exercises for the quadriceps are the leg press or the squat (Fig. 47–3). During closed kinetic chain exercises, there is increased joint compression that may be beneficial depending on the injury. Closed kinetic chain exercises have also been shown to provide increased muscle co-contraction, which provides further joint stability. Closed kinetic chain exercises can be advantageous during rehabilitation because they often mimic functional movements.

The initiation and progression of strengthening exercises is based on the results of an evaluation to determine specific deficits. The goal of strengthening following a ligamentous injury is to provide dynamic stability by strengthening the muscles that span the joint. Understanding the joint biomechanics and the injury are critical in determining the specific exercises to be performed. For example, following an anterior cruciate ligament reconstruction, open kinetic chain knee extension is contraindicated during the early phases of rehabilitation. The quadriceps create a significant anterior shearing force during seated knee extension from 60 degrees of knee flexion to full extension. Therefore, during the early stages following the anterior cruciate ligament reconstruction, closed kinetic chain exercises are advocated due to the decreased anterior shear force of the quadriceps, improved joint compression, and increased co-contraction of other muscles about the knee.

Strengthening exercises can also be performed to correct muscle imbalances that may cause overuse injuries. A common muscle imbalance is weakness of the rotator cuff when compared with the larger prime movers of the shoulder. The purpose of the rotator cuff is to provide stability and positioning of the glenohumeral joint. If the rotator cuff is not properly functioning due to weakness, the prime movers of

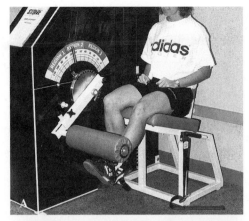

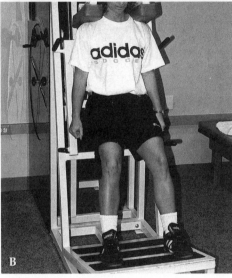

Figure 47–3 **(A)** Open kinetic chain strengthening of the quadriceps (knee extension). **(B)** Closed kinetic chain strengthening of the quadriceps (partial squats).

the shoulder will cause increased translation of the glenohumeral joint possibly leading to an overuse injury. This imbalance is particularly harmful during activities when the arm is away from the side or in an overhead position. The goal of rehabilitation is to improve the strength of the rotator cuff muscles and to improve the dynamic stability and positioning of the glenohumeral joint to decrease suprahumeral irritation. Large resistance to the rotator cuff is not required because the purpose of the rotator cuff is to provide stability over a repeated number of repetitions. Strengthening of the rotator cuff is usually accomplished through low resistance exercises with higher repetitions.

Proprioception and Functional Retraining

Obtaining normal strength, flexibility, and range of motion are the early goals of rehabilitation. However, the determinant to successful rehabilitation is often the transition of the patient back to functional activities. These functional goals may range from performance of everyday activities to return to sports activities. Once the component parts of strength,

motion, and flexibility are obtained, proprioception and functional retraining are important in gradually progressing the patient to achieve desired goals.

Mechanoreceptors are found within joint structures and ligaments and provide proprioceptive feedback concerning sensations of joint movement and joint position. Disruption of these joint receptors can occur following injury leading to a decrease in proprioception. When a ligament injury occurs, mechanical instability may occur due to loss of ligamentous integrity. Further loss of joint stability may also be due to a loss of neuromuscular reaction due to injury of the mechanoreceptors.

Studies have shown that there is a decrease in joint movement sense at the knee following anterior cruciate ligament disruption. The decreased proprioception is primarily at the end range of motion where the maximum response of joint mechanoreceptors usually occur. The loss of proprioception about the knee has been demonstrated, even following an anterior cruciate ligament reconstruction. The patient may still be at risk for further injury unless adequate proprioceptive re-training occurs, in spite of the fact that mechanical stability about the joint has been restored.

Proprioception may also be important in the treatment of shoulder instability. Several studies have found a decrease in both joint position and joint movement sense in individuals with traumatic shoulder instability. Repetitive stretching of the joint capsule may lead to a loss of shoulder stability and further mechanoreceptor injury, which may decrease neuromuscular response time. The result will be further joint instability, possibly leading to secondary impingement in individuals that perform repetitive overhead ballistic activities such as throwing, swimming, or racquet sports.

Proprioceptive exercises include activities that stimulate the joint mechanoreceptors to enhance function. These exercises are usually performed in a closed kinetic chain throughout various joint positions to allow for maximal mechanoreceptor response. Proprioceptive re-training usually corresponds with the functional progression of the patient's activities.

Functional re-training is a combination of neuromuscular coordination and agility exercises to provide a gradual return to higher-level activities. The initial step in designing a functional rehabilitation program is to understand the demands of the activity that the patient desires to perform. For example, tennis involves quick lateral movements, periods of rapid acceleration and deceleration, and pivoting motions. The current status of the patient's injury and limitations must also be examined to determine what deficits exist that are preventing the individual from performing the desired activities. Each component of the sports activity can then be divided into smaller components to allow each element to be addressed. Functional re-training is most important in individuals desiring to return to higher-level sports activities.

Functional re-training gradually progresses the individual from activities of daily living to full participation in sports activities through a gradual improvement in endurance, strength, and coordination. Following an injury, an athlete may be apprehensive about returning to full participation. Functional re-training assists in gradually decreasing the athlete's apprehension and improves his or her confidence in returning to the sport.

High-level sports activities usually involve movements that utilize the stretch-shortening cycle of a muscle. An example of this occurs in running when the quadriceps eccentrically contracts to control knee flexion at foot strike and then quickly concentrically contracts during propulsion. *Plyometrics* is a form of functional training that involves quick, powerful movements that prestretch the muscle and utilize the stretch-shortening cycle to produce a stronger, concentric contraction. During a rapid eccentric contraction, the connective tissue elements of the muscle are under tension leading to increased force production. The total contraction force during an eccentric contraction is a combination of the force of the contractile component and connective tissue elements. Increased concentric force production has been noted following an eccentric contraction. It is believed that the energy stored in the connective tissue elements during the eccentric contraction is used to enhance the concentric contraction. Plyometric activities can be an important component of functional re-training to gain strength and allow for a gradual return to sports activities.

Determination of when an individual can return to full participation is an important decision that must be made during rehabilitation. Many factors are involved including the type and extent of injury, the sport, and the level of participation. Clinical testing may indicate normal strength, flexibility, and range of motion, but these tests may not be the best determinants of the individual's ability to return to full participation. *Functional testing* such as sprinting, shuttle runs, lateral movements, and jump tests for height and distance can also be used to more effectively determine an individual's ability to return to sports.

The return of a soccer player to full participation following a grade II inversion ankle sprain can be used to demonstrate the principles of proprioceptive training and functional progression. During the early portion of rehabilitation, closed kinetic chain proprioceptive exercises can be performed in a sitting position. This may involve utilizing a wobble board or a Biomechanical Ankle Platform system (CAMP, Jackson MI) board to perform movements initially in dorsi-flexion and plantar-flexion, progressing to inversion, eversion, and rotational movements. These activities will begin to re-train the muscles that span the ankle joint throughout the range of motion in a closed chain position, which will enhance mechanoreceptor output. As healing progresses, the same type of exercises can be performed with the patient weight-bearing in unilateral stance. The sport of soccer involves quick bursts of movement with periods of rapid deceleration. There is also a high demand for pivoting movements and coordinated foot skills. Functional re-training in a soccer player will require a gradual progression from straight ahead running to re-training the rapid acceleration and deceleration movements through activities such as a shuttle run. Lateral movements can be initiated without impact forces through the use of a slide board. As the healing progresses, the athlete can then be progressed to resisted activities against elastic resistance by performing lateral movements and crossover steps (Fig. 47–4). In addition, ballistic jumping activities, through the use of plyometrics, can be performed to further enhance strength and proprioceptive re-training about the ankle. The athlete then begins participation in sports-specific drills involving passing and ball control. Evaluation of the

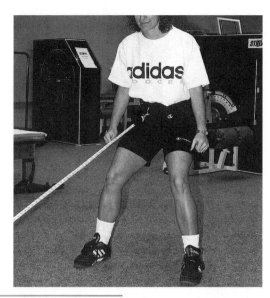

Figure 47–4   Rehabilitation of the legs with elastic resistance.

individual's performance at each phase of the functional progression will allow for a controlled resumption of sports activities while decreasing the risk of re-injury.

Modalities

Various physical agents can be used to enhance the rehabilitation process. The primary emphasis of rehabilitation should be on the components noted previously. However, modalities can be effective adjuncts to treatment in rehabilitation.

The most common physical agents used in rehabilitation are superficial heat and cold. The primary purpose of superficial *heat* is to increase blood flow and nutrients in the area of injury to enhance the healing process. Superficial heat is usually used later in the rehabilitation process, once the initial signs of inflammation have decreased. The physiological effects of superficial heat are described in Table 47–2. Heat

TABLE 47–2   Effects of Heat and Cold.

Effects	Heat	Cold
Vascular	Vasodilation	Vasoconstriction
Blood flow	Increased	Decreased
Capillary perfusion	Increased	Decreased
Metabolic activity	Increased	Decreased
Nerve conduction velocity	Increased	Decreased
Connective tissue elasticity	Increased	Decreased
Pain	Decreased	Decreased

can also be used in the warm-up process prior to beginning an exercise program. However, a disadvantage of superficial heat is its inability to penetrate to deeper muscle and connective tissue. In most cases, active movements are more effective than superficial heat at increasing blood flow to deeper structures during the warm-up process. Superficial heat is contraindicated in the initial stages following an injury when further increases in blood flow to the area of injury may be harmful.

The use of *cold* is important in the rehabilitation process to control the initial vascular changes that occur following injury. Cold modalities have a greater depth of penetration than superficial heat and will cause a decrease in temperature in muscle and connective tissue. The physiological effects of cold are summarized in Table 47–2. Cryotherapy is generally used throughout the entire rehabilitation process following exercise to decrease any inflammatory response that may occur.

Ultrasound is a form of deep heat that uses sound waves to penetrate through the superficial tissues to provide thermal effects at greater depths. Within the ultrasound head is a crystal that is vibrated at a frequency of 1 MHz or 3 MHz. The 1 MHz frequency of ultrasound has a deeper penetration than does the 3 MHz. Ultrasound produces thermal effects similar to that of superficial heat but at a depth of penetration at which important connective tissue and muscle can be targeted. Ultrasound also has nonthermal effects that are thought to assist in increasing motion by increasing the elasticity of connective tissue. Ultrasound can be used during *phonophoresis*, which is the superficial administration of medications with the use of sound waves. Further research is needed to determine the effectiveness of phonophoresis and whether the medication is reaching the target tissue. The most common use of phonophoresis is the use of hydrocortisone cream as an anti-inflammatory agent.

Electrical stimulation is another modality often used in the rehabilitation of orthopaedic injuries. The most common objective of electrical stimulation is to facilitate a muscle contraction to enhance strengthening and prevent disuse atrophy. The most common types of electrical stimulation to facilitate a muscle contraction are pulsed biphasic current and time-modulated alternating current ("Russian" current). Both of these forms of electrical stimulation use a frequency of between 35 and 50 Hz, which will elicit a tetanic muscle contraction. There is a debate as to whether electrical stimulation can truly increase muscle strength. The benefits may be increased synchronization of the motor units to provide a more efficient contraction. During volitional muscle contraction, the slow-twitch fibers are activated initially with recruitment of the fast-twitch fibers as the intensity of the contraction increases. During electrical stimulation, the fast-twitch fibers are initially recruited in a synchronous manner with increased recruitment of the slow-twitch fibers as the intensity of the electrical stimulation increases. Some studies have shown atrophy of primarily the fast-twitch fibers following periods of immobilization or disuse. Therefore, electrical stimulation may be beneficial to enhance the specific contraction of the fast-twitch fibers to assist in gaining strength following a period of immobilization.

Electrical stimulation with pulsed biphasic current has also been used to provide pain relief. This is typically achieved through sensory level stimulation, which produces a cutaneous paresthesia. Motor level stimulation can also be utilized through the use of low frequency pulses producing twitch contractions of the muscles in the area of injury. The effectiveness of pain management with electrical stimulation is controversial. The potential mechanisms of pain relief through the use of electrical stimulation include modifications of the interneuron firing pattern in the dorsal horn of the spinal cord or stimulus-produced analgesic effects from higher centers.

Recently there has been an increase in use of electrical stimulation for swelling relief. This form of electrical stimulation uses high-volt pulsed current with the cathode placed over the site of injury. The proposed mechanism is that the cathodal stimulation may repel edema from the injury site. Further study is needed to determine the effectiveness of electrical stimulation in the treatment of swelling.

Electrical current can also be used to drive medication into deeper tissues through the use of iontophoresis. *Iontophoresis* uses direct current to drive the chemical ions into the superficial body tissues. Chemical substances with a positive charge are introduced through the skin with the positive electrode, and substances with a negative charge are introduced through the negative electrode. The most common use of iontophoresis is the administration of dexamethasone as an anti-inflammatory agent. Iontophoresis with local anesthetics and salicylates has also been performed. Further study of iontophoresis is needed to determine the effectiveness of ion transfer to the target tissues.

TREATMENT GUIDELINES

Several treatment principles can be followed in the rehabilitation of orthopaedic injuries (Table 47–3). The first principle is the progression of simple to complex concepts in rehabilitation. The initial focus of rehabilitation should be on normalizing strength, motion, and flexibility. As healing progresses, the complexity of rehabilitation increases based on each individual's deficits and goals of rehabilitation. In the case of an individual with an ankle sprain desiring to return to activities of daily living, the functional rehabilitation is simplified as compared with an individual who wants to return to athletic activity. A similar guideline is the *SAID principle* (specific adaptation to imposed demands). It is important to understand the specific demands of the individual's activities to customize rehabilitation to meet the desired goals.

TABLE 47–3 Treatment Guidelines

Simple to complex
Specific adaptation to imposed demands (SAID)
Create independence, not dependence
Individualized evaluation and treatment plan
Macrotrauma vs. microtrauma

It is important for the rehabilitation process to allow an individual to gain independence. The patient must become actively involved in the rehabilitation process and must assume a large amount of responsibility through the performance of the exercise program. In the era of managed care and cost containment, the number of physical therapy visits and the length of approved rehabilitation continues to decrease. It is also important that the patient understand the appropriate guidelines for injury prevention. This is especially true with low back injury in which there is a high incidence of recurrence of symptoms. It is important during the rehabilitation process to constantly reevaluate the patient for progression of the treatment program. Treatment protocols should not be used as generic instructions but as guidelines to individually progress the patient.

Macro-trauma injuries are due to one specific event leading to an injury. The goals of rehabilitation following macro-trauma are to control the inflammatory process and to restore the individual's motion, strength, and flexibility to pre-injury status. Microtrauma injuries are due to repetitive overuse and present a challenge during rehabilitation. The characteristics of microtraumatic overuse injuries are summarized in Table 47–4.

The most important objectives in the treatment of overuse injuries is to identify and correct the cause of the injury. One of the most common areas of overuse injuries is in the lower extremities in individuals who perform repetitive running and jumping activities. Potential causes of lower extremity overuse injuries are listed in Table 47–5.

Training errors are a common cause of overuse injuries that are often overlooked. Connective tissue and muscles have the ability to adapt to the stress placed upon them. The key to injury prevention is a gradual increase in activity. An example of a training error would be when an individual who had previously been running 10 to 15 miles per week increased to 35 to 40 miles per week in a 2-week time period. The overuse symptoms that may occur with this training error are due to the inability of the body to adapt to the increased stress over a short time. The treatment of this individual would involve decreasing the inflammatory process; but more importantly the patient would need to be educated in

the appropriate progression of training activities. Other types of training prone to errors include specialized programs such as hill running, interval training, or plyometric activities. All of these activities are good training methods to enhance performance but must be gradually initiated to prevent injury.

Flexibility deficits can also contribute to overuse injuries. During running and jumping activities, knee flexion and ankle dorsi flexion occur at impact. If there is inadequate flexibility of the gastrocnemius and soleus, there may be increased susceptibility to overuse injuries such as Achilles' tendinitis and plantar fasciitis.

Strength deficits are also a potential cause of overuse injuries. During running and jumping activities, the quadriceps eccentrically contract to control the amount of knee flexion at impact. If there is quadriceps weakness, there may be increased susceptibility to overuse injuries in the patellofemoral region including quadriceps tendinitis, patellar tendinitis, and retropatellar symptoms.

Foot and ankle biomechanics have also been implicated as a major cause of lower extremity overuse injuries. Upon impact, the subtalar joint normally pronates, which decreases the osseous stability of the foot providing shock absorption and adaptation to the ground. During the later portion of stance, the subtalar joint begins to supinate to increase osseous stability to provide an effective lever for propulsion. If an individual excessively pronates, there is decreased osseous stability that may increase stress to other muscle or connective tissue structures leading to an overuse injury (Fig. 47–5). If an individual has a foot with a high arch and remains in a supinated position throughout the gait cycle, there may be a lack of shock absorption and increased lateral weight bearing that could also lead to an overuse injury. The evaluation and possible change in foot biomechanics with the use of orthotics is an important treatment component in individuals with lower extremity overuse injuries.

PITFALL

Treatment of lower extremity biomechanics with foot orthotics should not be done until a thorough evaluation is performed to determine the appropriate type and amount of correction.

TABLE 47–4 Characteristics of Microtrauma

Repetitive overuse injuries
Gradual, insidious onset
No history of trauma
Usually no indication of major inflammatory process
Must determine and correct cause of injury

TABLE 47–5 Causes of Overuse Injuries

Training errors
Flexibility deficits
Strength deficits
Biomechanical considerations
Shoes and equipment

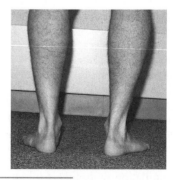

Figure 47–5 Excessive subtalar joint pronation.

Shoe assessment is another area of evaluation in individuals with overuse injuries. Running shoes are designed to provide various amounts of shock absorption and stability. It is important to match the properties of the shoe with the individual's foot biomechanics. In an individual with increased pronation, there is a loss of osseous stability. The appropriate running shoe for this individual would provide more stability features. In an individual with a foot with a high arch, there is decreased shock absorbing capabilities within the foot. Therefore, the appropriate running shoe would provide increased shock absorption to assist with the patient's biomechanical deficits. In this way, running shoes can be used as a form of biomechanical correction of an individual's foot mechanics.

SELECTED BIBLIOGRAPHY

BANDY WD, LOVELACE-CHANDLER V, MCKICTRICK-BANDY B. Adaptation of skeletal muscle to resistance training. *J Orthop Sports Phys Ther*. 1990;12:248–256.

BROTZMAN SB. *Clinical Orthopedic Rehabilitation*. St Louis, MO: CV Mosby; 1996.

KAMKAR A, IRRGANG JJ, WHITNEY SL. Nonoperative management of secondary shoulder impingement syndrome. *J Orthop Sports Phys Ther*. 1993;17:212–239.

MALONE TR, MCPOIL TG, NITZ AJ. *Orthopedic and Sports Physical Therapy*. St Louis, MO: CV Mosby; 1997.

MCPOIL TG, HUNT GC. Evaluation and management of foot and ankle disorders: present problems and future directions. *J Orthop Sports Phys Ther*. 1995;21:381–388.

MICHLOVITZ SL. *Thermal Agents in Rehabilitation*. Philadelphia, PA: FA Davis; 1990.

NORKIN CC, LEVANGIE PK. *Joint Structure and Function: A Comprehensive Analysis*. Philadelphia, PA: FA Davis; 1992.

PRENTICE WE. *Rehabilitation Techniques in Sports Medicine*. St Louis, MO: CV Mosby; 1994.

PRENTICE WE. *Therapeutic Modalities in Sports Medicine*. St Louis, MO: CV Mosby; 1994.

ROBINSON AJ, SNYDER-MACKLER L. *Clinical Electrophysiology: Electrotherapy and Electrotherapeutic Testing*. Baltimore, MD: Williams and Wilkins; 1995.

SAUNDERS HD, SAUNDERS R. *Evaluation, Treatment, and Prevention of Musculoskeletal Disorders*. Vol 1. Chaska, MI: The Saunders Group; 1993.

SODERBERG GL. *Kinesiology: Application to Pathological Motion*. Baltimore, MD: Williams and Wilkins; 1986.

WILK KE, ANDREWS JR. Current concepts in the treatment of anterior cruciate ligament disruption. *J Orthop Sports Phys Ther*. 1992;15:179–293.

ZACHAZEWSKI JE, MAGEE DJ, QUILLEN WS. *Athletic Injuries and Rehabilitation*. Philidelphia, PA: WB Saunders; 1996.

SAMPLE QUESTIONS

1. The advantages of closed kinetic chain exercises include the following:

   (a) increased co-contraction of the muscles surrounding the joint

   (b) increased joint compression forces

   (c) the distal segment is not fixed

   (d) a and b

   (e) all of the above

2. Proprioceptive exercises:

   (a) stimulate joint mechanoreceptors to enhance function

   (b) are especially important following ligamentous injuries

   (c) are used to increase joint movement and position sense

   (d) b and c

   (e) all of the above

3. The physiological effects of cold include:

   (a) decreased vascular response

   (b) increased elasticity of connective tissue

   (c) increased nerve conduction velocity

   (d) a and b

   (e) none of the above

4. The characteristics of a type I motor unit include:

   (a) large alpha motor neuron

   (b) increased mitochondria

   (c) decreased muscle tension

   (d) a and b

   (e) b and c

5. Adverse effects of immobilization include:

   (a) increased ground substance formation

   (b) increased collagen cross-linking

   (c) loss of collagen orientation

   (d) b and c

   (e) all of the above

Answers: 1) d; 2) e; 3) a; 4) e; 5) d

Chapter 48

Lower Extremity Amputations and Prostheses

Richard L. Ray, MD and Jon P. Leimkuehler, CPO

Outline

During the 20th Century, as wound care improved and antibiotics were developed, amputation was no longer the first choice of treatment or even the expected consequence of severe wounds or fractures. At the same time, the discovery of insulin and modern treatment of heart disease have resulted in a more normal life span for persons with diabetes mellitus and atherosclerosis. Lower extremity complications of these two conditions, which often co-exist, include gangrene, ischemic pain, chronic infection, and neuropathic deformity. These complications are the most common indications for amputation in the United States today. Other less common indications for amputation are neoplastic disease, intractable foot pain, nonresolvable chronic osteomyelitis, and severe fixed deformity.

INDICATIONS FOR AMPUTATION

Amputation of part of an extremity is surely one of the oldest procedures performed by surgeons. Until this century, the majority of amputations were performed for traumatic conditions. During the 18th Century, more modern weaponry resulted in increased tissue destruction in wounds and dramatically increased the number of amputations performed. Having lost his leg above the knee at the Battle of Waterloo, the Marquis of Angelsea commissioned the Royal Engineers to design the first known articulated prosthesis. During the American Civil War, an estimated 50,000 amputations were performed. This epidemic of amputations stimulated the development of modern prosthesis technology.

BASIC SCIENCE AND EVALUATION FOR LEVEL OF AMPUTATION

When amputation is considered as a treatment for a diseased or dysfunctional extremity, the surgeon must decide what is the most appropriate level at which to perform the amputation. The goals are not only to remove all of the diseased portion of the extremity but to also reconstruct the remaining extremity to provide optimal prosthetic fitting. In general, patients will wish to preserve as much as possible of their own bodies but will also desire to avoid going through more than one surgical procedure. In reasonably healthy patients, performing multiple procedures to attempt to preserve a more functional limb are justified. In severely ill or debilitated persons, additional procedures may result in unacceptable risks for questionable functional gains.

Skin that has enough circulation to remain viable may have insufficient circulation to survive the stress of surgery or to heal. Several methods have been performed successfully to evaluate the limb for appropriate level of amputation:

1. physical examination: skin temperature and appearance, capillary refill
2. Doppler assessment
3. transcutaneous oxygen pressure measurement
4. skin temperature measurement
5. laser Doppler skin perfusion pressure measurement

Each of these measures emphasizes skin circulation and can reliably, but not infallibly, predict the success of amputation at a given anatomic level. Angiographic findings and the presence/absence of pulses may be misleading as collateral circulation may provide adequate circulation for healing, even when pulses are absent or poor distal runoff is observed. Clinical examination has been estimated to have an approximately 80% success rate in predicting whether below-knee amputations will heal.

Doppler segmental pressure measurement is the simplest and most readily available objective measure beyond clinical examination. Nearly all patients with a calf Doppler systolic pressure greater than 50 mm Hg will heal a below-knee amputation (BKA), but many with lower calf pressures will

Orthopaedic Surgery: The Essentials. Edited by M.E. Baratz, A.D. Watson, and J.E. Imbriglia. Thieme Medical Publishers, Inc., New York © 1999

also heal a BKA. Ankle Doppler systolic pressure below 50 mm Hg or ankle-brachial index less than 0.4 have been associated with nonhealing of foot and ankle level amputations. Larsson et al (1993) found that a systolic toe pressure of less than 15 mm Hg was associated with 6% healing of minor amputations in the foot, whereas greater than 15 mm Hg was associated with 51% healing. In general, Doppler segmental pressure measurement is more reliable in predicting success of healing than in determining what procedures will fail at the below knee and above knee level. In the foot, the predictive value is more limited.

Objective testing that assesses skin blood flow would potentially be more accurate in predicting success of amputations in the foot. Moore (1981) has published on the Xenon-133 clearance technique for measuring skin blood flow, reporting over 95% accuracy. Unfortunately, this technique requires a highly skilled technician, and the Xenon-133 isotope is not readily available. Therefore, it is not widely used. Transcutaneous oxygen pressure ($PTCO_2$) measurement is a technique that is widely available. Transcutaneous oxygen sensors are placed at the proposed amputation site. Measurements of $PTCO_2$ at 35 to 40 mm Hg or greater reliably predict healing at the above knee or below knee level, but some individuals with lower $PTCO_2$ have healed satisfactorily. Less data is available for the foot, but generally measurements of 40 mm Hg or below are associated with failure of healing in the foot. Skin temperature measurement using a thermistor has similar prognostic value to transcutaneous oximetry. Skin temperatures of 5°C greater than ambient temperature are associated with primary healing. Accurately predicting whether a minor amputation in the foot will fail is not provided by these techniques.

Adera et al (1995) have reported on laser Doppler skin perfusion pressure (LD-SPP) measurement using a laser Doppler flow sensor within the blood pressure cuff. Several cuff sizes were available including a toe cuff. Using a LD-SPP measurement of 30 mm Hg for analysis, patients undergoing BKA or above knee amputation (AKA) healed 100% of the time at levels greater than 30 mm Hg and failed 83% of the time at levels less than 30 mm Hg. Accuracy of prediction was less in the foot where 75% of toe amputation healed when LD-SPP was greater than 30 mm Hg and 67% failed when it was less than 30 mm Hg. Further evaluation of this technique may result in the ability to predict failure of minor foot amputations with greater assurance.

In general, patients faced with an amputation, especially a below-knee amputation, will wish to know that the loss of the foot is absolutely necessary or whether some lesser amputation may be successful. Often, they will not consent to a below-knee amputation unless a lesser amputation that saves part of the foot has been attempted first. Ultimately, the surgeon's clinical judgement will come to play in making the final decision. Through careful physical examination and the use of objective measures, the patient can be reassured that the surgeon's recommendation was determined thoughtfully and not impulsively or simply for the surgeon's convenience. Unfortunately, objective testing does not tell us when an amputation at a lower level should be considered.

Several other general considerations deserve comment. Nonhealing of a toe amputation is most likely to occur at the base of the adjacent toe. Each common digital artery divides into two digital arteries at the level of the metatarsophalangeal joint. Skin circulation is usually much better at the level of the metatarsophalangeal joint and at the level of the metatarsal heads, and, therefore, transmetatarsal amputation may be successful when toe amputation has failed. Resection of the first or fifth ray can heal successfully but intercalary second, third, or fourth ray resection in the dysvascular foot may be expected to fail because of disruption of the arterial plantar arch. Midfoot, hindfoot, and through-ankle (Symes) amputations cannot be expected to heal in patients with peripheral vascular disease, although they are successful in diabetic patients with otherwise good blood flow. The extensive surgical dissection, the rotation of the skin flap, and the length of the heel flap exceed the ability of the atherosclerotic vessels to adapt.

Arterial blood supply to the skin is a much more important factor than is the presence of diabetes or infection in successful healing of amputations. Diabetic patients with good blood flow will heal well. Amputations through infected, cellulitic skin will heal if the infection is treated with appropriate antibiotics. Amputation through an area of osteomyelitis may be expected to result in continued infection problems unless the bone infection has resolved.

Deciding whether to risk failure with a BKA or to do the "sure thing" with an AKA is a frequent dilemma for the surgeon. Whenever reasonable, a BKA should be attempted. The increased energy demanded for an amputee using a BKA prosthesis is 15 to 40% whereas for an amputee using an AKA prosthesis it is 60 to 80%. When cardiopulmonary disease is present, BKA versus AKA may mean the difference between functional ambulation or wheelchair dependence. Even a short BKA, just below the level of the tibial tubercle, is usually more functional than an AKA. When severe flexion contracture is present, AKA is usually the best choice. A through-knee amputation offers little mechanical advantage over an AKA and is a more difficult prosthetic fitting. Through-knee amputation is primarily indicated in certain childhood conditions because it preserves the distal growth plate of the femur and avoids bony overgrowth at the end of the stump.

> ### PEARL
>
> **Symes amputation is rarely, if ever, successful in the dysvascular patient.**

ANATOMY AND SURGICAL APPROACHES

Anatomy

Understanding the vascular supply to the leg is essential to planning and performing an appropriate amputation. Long-standing peripheral vascular disease may lead to alteration in blood flow and, in particular, increased collateral sources of flow to the skin of the calf and foot. The femoral artery leaves the adductor canal just proximal to the medial epicondyle of the femur and passes posteriorly and laterally into the popliteal space where it becomes the popliteal artery. The popliteal artery gives off five genicular arteries that anastomose with the descending branch of the lateral circumflex artery and descending genicular artery providing collateral flow from higher in the thigh. Arterial branches of this anastomosis provide blood flow to the skin of the calf and gastrocnemius muscles. Because of the collateral flow, circulation to the skin of the posterior calf and gastrocnemius muscle is generally better than the circulation to the more anterior muscles and skin. Indeed, when necrosis of skin flaps occurs after BKA, it is most often on the anterior flap.

The popliteal artery exits the popliteal space deep to the soleus muscle; the popliteal artery divides into the anterior tibial artery and posterior tibial artery. The anterior tibial artery passes around the upper edge of the interosseous membrane into the anterior compartment. About 2 cm further distally, the posterior tibial artery gives off a peroneal branch. The level of this trifurcation may vary considerably and, therefore, it is essential that the surgeon inspect the BKA site carefully for all large arteries so that they may be ligated. The veins that accompany the posterior tibial artery are usually multiple rather than a single large vein.

The posterior tibial artery passes posterior to the medial malleolus of the ankle and then divides into the medial and lateral plantar arteries. These vessels are the primary source of circulation to the skin of the heel, which is rotated forward to cover the end of the Symes amputation. The lateral plantar artery is the largest vessel contributing to the deep plantar arch, which traverses the foot on the plantar aspect of the base of the second through fifth metatarsals. The plantar arch gives off four common digital arteries, each of which divides into proper digital arteries at the level of the metatarsal heads.

The sciatic nerve is composed of the tibial and common peroneal nerves, which separate from each other just proximal to the popliteal fossa. The sciatic nerve has a small artery that courses with it that must be ligated when the nerve is transected. The common peroneal nerve passes lateral and distal to the fibular head where it divides into the superficial and deep branches that pass through the anterior compartment to the foot. The tibial nerve courses with the posterior tibial artery on its superficial aspect and should be identified and resected proximally before ligating the artery. The sural nerve branches from the tibial nerve in the popliteal space and then passes through the crural fascia about midcalf. The sural nerve is located about midline in the posterior skin flap of a BKA adjacent to the saphenous vein, just superficial to the fascia. Each major nerve is resected as proximal as possible to avoid amputation neuromata close to the surface or in pressure-bearing areas. However, nerves are not pulled distally to resect them so as to avoid traction neuritis.

Surgical Approaches

The technique of BKA will be discussed in detail. Certain general principles apply to all lower extremity amputations. Skin flaps should be carefully planned and drawn out to have equal lengths. The skin should be handled carefully, avoiding grasping it with instruments or retractors as much as possible. Large arteries are identified and doubly ligated with nonabsorbable sutures. The distal suture ligature is passed through the artery and tied around either side to make sure it will not be pushed off by the pulsation. A second more proximal free ligature will prevent leaking of blood around the

suture that was placed through the artery. Finding and doubly ligating the major arteries is particularly important in traumatic amputations where the vessels may have retracted and may be in spasm so that bleeding is not evident. A tourniquet is placed around the thigh, whenever appropriate, and may be inflated if bleeding is a problem. A tourniquet is not used if severe peripheral vascular disease is present or if a previous vascular graft has been performed. Whenever a tourniquet is used, it is inflated the minimal length of time to complete hemostasis, then it is deflated and the wound thoroughly inspected before closing.

Below-knee amputation is the most commonly performed major leg amputation. A variety of techniques have been described, but for reasons that have been noted above, the authors believe the long posterior flap technique provides the best chance for successful healing as well as for soft tissue coverage over the end of the bone. Although a prosthetist may be able to fit some type of below-knee prosthesis at any level below the tibial tubercle, optimal prosthetic fit is probably achieved with a tibial length of 13 to 15 cm or even longer in taller individuals. The authors prefer to measure from the tibial tubercle, which is 3 cm below the joint line. A line is marked on the skin over the tibial crest, 12 cm below the tibial tubercle and 2 cm distal to the planned tibial bone cut (Fig. 48–1). The anterior skin flap extends directly laterally one third of the calf circumference and medially one third of the circumference (Fig. 48–2). The anterior flap comprises two thirds of the calf circumference with the remaining one third as the base of the posterior flap (Fig. 48–3). A parabolic pos-

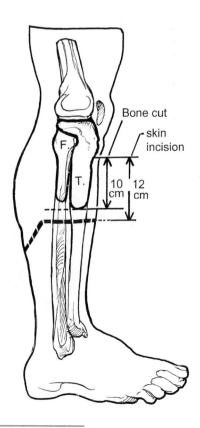

Figure 48–1 Levels of skin incision and bone cuts for below-knee amputations (BKAs).

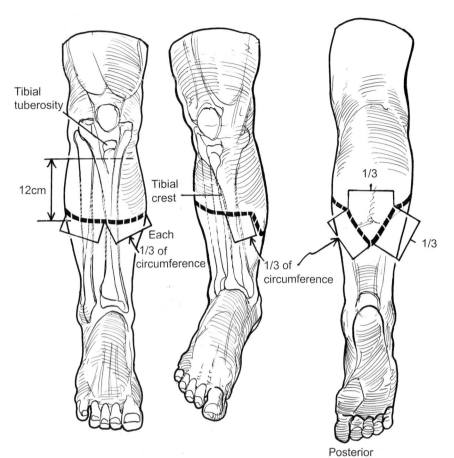

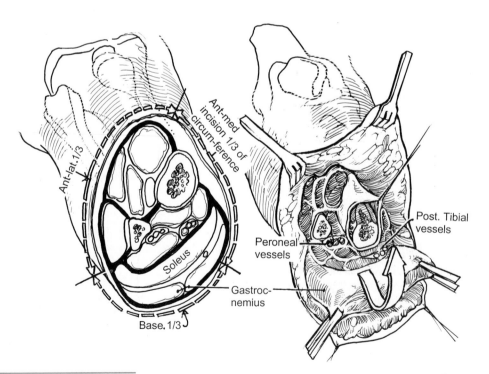

Figure 48–2 Design of the skin flaps for BKAs.

Figure 48–3 Cross-sectional view of the lower leg illustrating relative proportions for the design of skin flaps for BKAs.

terior flap is drawn out on the posterior skin with the goal of creating a skin-edge length around the parabola equal to skin-edge length of the anterior flap (i.e., two thirds of the calf circumference). To make sure the skin edges of both anterior and posterior flaps are equal, lay a hernia tape along each flap. Unequal skin flaps may result in "dog ears" at the corners of the incision. The skin is incised through the level of the fascia so that the muscle is visible and the skin edges are well separated. Both anterior and posterior flaps are completed before proceeding.

The muscles of the anterior compartment of the calf are incised to expose the lateral aspect of the tibia and the fibula. The tibia is cut with a reciprocating saw, 2 cm proximal to the skin incision, and an anterior bevel is placed on the tibia to avoid an anterior bony prominence (Fig. 48–1). The fibula is cut 1 cm proximal to the tibial cut. The amputation is completed by using a large amputation knife to cut the posterior compartment muscles and to create a flap of gastrocnemius muscle 10 to 12 cm long. The flap is accomplished by having an assistant provide distal traction on the ankle, making the muscle taught, and by cutting distal and posterior with the knife at about a 30-degree angle to the horizontal. A flap that is too thick or long will produce redundant tissue, whereas a flap that is too thin or short will not provide adequate soft tissue coverage at the end of the tibia.

Once the amputation is completed, the large vessels are identified and doubly ligated. Each vascular bundle, artery, and surrounding veins are ligated as a unit because separating the many veins from the arteries results in venous bleeding that is difficult to control. The tibial, peroneal, and sural nerves are cut proximally. The bone ends are smoothed with a power rasp. At this point, if a tourniquet has been used it should be released and further hemostasis secured with electrocautery. Any nonviable muscle tissue should be excised at this time. The gastrocnemius muscle flap is now brought over the end of the tibia, and the muscle fascia is sutured to the periosteum of the tibia (Fig. 48–4). The skin is closed with staples beginning at the axilla of the incision on each side and moving toward the midline (Fig. 48–5). By beginning at the corners, small discrepancies in flap length can be compensated for gradually, and dog ears at the corners are avoided.

In performing an AKA, skin flaps of equal length (the so-called fish mouth incision) or a slightly longer anterior flap will provide satisfactory healing. The optimal level is about 8 to 10 cm above the joint line to provide for the appropriate position of the prosthetic knee hinge. A transmetatarsal amputation should have a slightly longer plantar skin flap, if possible, so that the tougher more well-padded plantar skin can be used to cover the ends of the metatarsals. A Symes amputation presents some problems in closure because of the relatively long plantar skin flap and frequently a second procedure is needed to revise the redundant skin or dog ears. It is also important to trim the malleoli back severely; for, if the end of the Symes stump is too wide, it will be difficult to fit into the prosthesis. The tibial nerve is quite superficial as it crosses the ankle and, therefore, it should be trimmed back well proximally, or it will develop a neuroma that will be painful in the prosthesis.

Whenever reasonable, patients undergoing BKA or Symes amputation should be placed in a cast postoperatively. The cast provides a rigid dressing that limits swelling and prevents the development of knee flexion contracture. Further,

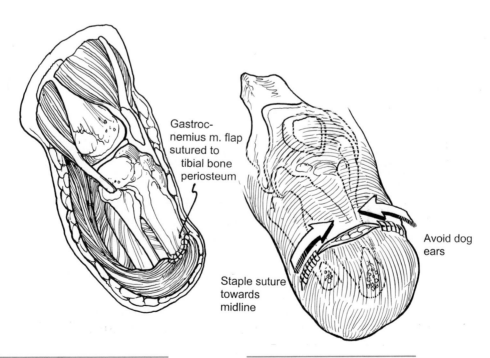

Gastroc-
nemius m. flap
sutured to
tibial bone
periosteum

Staple suture
towards
midline

Avoid dog
ears

Figure 48–4   Technique for covering tibial stump with flap of gastrocnemius muscle.

Figure 48–5   Technique for skin closure during BKA. Careful closure by starting at edges and working toward the center will minimize the creation of "dog ears."

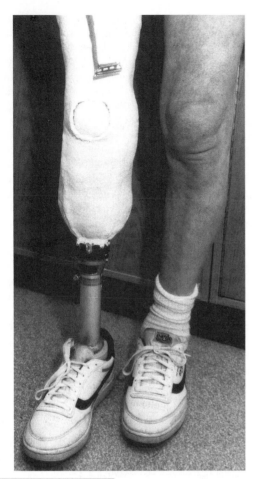

Figure 48–6   An immediate postoperative prosthesis.

the cast will protect the end of the stump in the event that the patient falls (a frequent problem). Patients with dementia, serious comorbidity, or problematic healing are not good candidates for casting. The cast is changed at 4 to 5 days postoperatively. Early or immediate postoperative prosthesis (IPOP) should be considered in healthier patients (Fig. 48–6). Not only does the amputee benefit psychologically from never being without a foot, but functionally, the amputee is able to do more and the entire process of rehabilitation is expedited.

PROSTHESIS SELECTION AND DESIGN

Functional Level

Lower limb amputees are categorized in terms of their projected functional level, which is a critical element of prosthetic selection and design (Table 48–1).

High-strength, light-weight components made from titanium and carbon fiber are combined with thermoplastic or acrylic resin sockets fabricated to be as light in weight as possible yet with sufficient strength for the amputee's weight and lifestyle requirements.

Wearing a shrinker sock, rigid dressing, or elastic bandaging helps considerably in preparing the amputee to be fit with a prosthesis. A preparatory or temporary prosthetic socket can be used to help shrink the residual limb, as well as to protect it from inadvertent falls. Prosthetic socks (covering the residual limb) of varying plies are used for adjusting the fit of the socket. Change in size (shrinking) is a major concern of the new amputee. A new amputee's residual limb frequently shrinks in size and a new socket or prosthesis is then required.

Five basic types of lower limb amputations are defined for prosthetic fitting:

1. transtibial or below-knee (BK)
2. transfemoral or above-knee (AK)

TABLE 48–1   Categories of Functional Level

Level	Functional level	Description
0	Nonambulator	Patient does not have the ability or potential to ambulate or transfer without assistance.
1	Household ambulator	Patient has the ability or potential to use prosthesis for transfers or ambulation on level surfaces.
2	Limited community ambulator	Patient has the ability or potential to traverse low level barriers such as curbs, stairs, etc.
3	Community ambulator	Patient has the ability or potential to ambulate with variable cadence; has the ability to traverse most environmental barriers; may have activity level that demands prosthetic utilization beyond simple locomotion.
4	Child, active adult, or athlete	Patient has the ability or potential for prosthetic ambulation that exceeds basic ambulation, exhibiting high impact, stress, or energy levels.

3. partial foot

4. Symes-type

5. hip disarticulations and hemipelvectomies

Transtibial Below-knee Prosthesis

The most common type of amputation is the transtibial (BK). A typical BK prosthesis comprises a socket, a method of suspension, a pylon or shin section, and a foot (Figs. 48–7 and Fig. 48–8).

A socket is made from an impression taken of the patient's residual limb, modified to achieve an intimate, total-contact fit over the entire surface of the residual limb. Upon fitting the prosthesis, the prosthetist adjusts the alignment and length of the prosthesis for optimum gait.

Suspension Systems

The most commonly used suspension systems are:

1. supracondylar cuff suspension strap: a Velcro or leather strap attached to the prosthesis that encircles the knee proximal to the femoral condyles;

2. wedge suspension: a wedge, often inserted into the flexible liner of a socket that encompasses the adductor tubercle. It fits snugly over the patella and each side of the residual limb just above the knee;

3. silicone suction socket: a silicone insert rolled on directly over the skin.

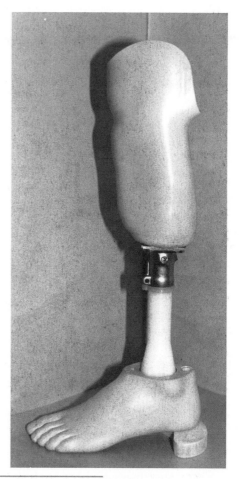

Figure 48–8 A typical BK prosthesis.

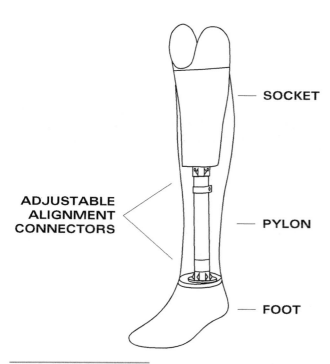

Figure 48–7 Schematic illustration of the components of a below-knee (BK) prosthesis.

Prosthetic Feet

For all levels of lower extremity amputees there are three types of feet:

1. solid-ankle cushion heel foot (functional level 1): allows flexion of the toe and compression of the heel. The basic design, most commonly used;

2. multi-axial (functional level 2 or higher): a foot that permits ankle movement or rotation in several different planes;

3. energy-storing foot (functional level 3 or higher): a prosthetic foot for the active amputee. It provides a spring or push off after weight bearing.

Above-knee Prosthesis

A typical AK prosthesis comprises a socket, a method of suspension, a knee, a pylon or shin section, and a foot (Fig. 48–9).

There are two basic methods of suspension:

1. suction suspension: where the socket is directly against the skin;

2. belt suspension: A sock is worn over the residual limb and a pelvic belt is attached to the prosthesis to hold it on.

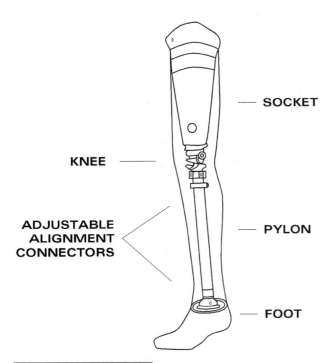

Figure 48–9 Schematic illustration of the components of an above-knee prosthesis.

Knee Mechanism

There are three basic categories of knees:

1. manual locking knee (functional Level 1 or higher): a knee design that locks straight upon full extension and can be unlocked for sitting. Suitable for unstable or weak amputees;
2. stance control knee (functional level 1 or higher): a knee that is designed with a brake to prevent buckling that is engaged when weight is placed on the prosthesis. Suitable for amputees with fair strength and balance;
3. hydraulic or pneumatic variable cadence knee (functional level 3 or higher): a design that uses pneumatic or hydraulic units to control the knee during the swing phase of walking, automatically adjusting to provide variable cadence.

Symes or Boyd Amputation Prosthesis

The Symes or Boyd level of amputation is very functional because of limb-end weight bearing on the remaining heel pad. This prosthesis is not cosmetically acceptable to many amputees (Fig. 48–10).

Hip Disarticulation and Hemipelvectomy Prosthesis

Hip disarticulation and hemipelvectomy amputees can be successfully fit with a prosthesis if they have normal strength and balance and are motivated to use a prosthesis. The socket encompasses the entire pelvis. Use of the prosthesis requires a very high energy expenditure because the hip joint as well as the knee is involved.

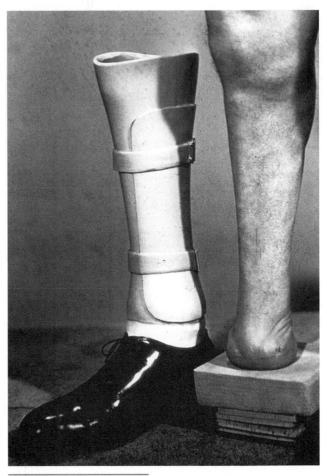

Figure 48–10 A prosthesis for a Symes or Boyd level amputation.

For more information, consult the Selected Bibliography.

PEARL
Protect the residual limb with a removable cast or a preparatory prosthesis. Many new amputees hold the leg out to catch themselves in a fall.

PEARL
Have a prosthetist help in determining the type of prosthesis. New products and designs are developed each year, so rely on a prosthetist to keep up to date.

POSTAMPUTATION RECOVERY

Following successful healing of the amputation and prosthetic fitting, all amputees will go through a period of recovery that involves acceptance of their loss, learning to use the prosthesis, and functional adaptation. The time it takes to recover will vary with each person, as will the goals and expectations of recovery. Physical therapy is begun as soon after surgery as reasonable. In the early postoperative period, the emphasis is on overcoming the effects of deconditioning that often exist preoperatively and on achieving safe ambulation.

With an AKA, particular attention is given to preventing a hip flexion contracture that can rapidly develop when a patient spends long periods in a wheelchair. Once the cast is removed from a BKA, the amputee begins exercises to regain knee motion and strength. The therapist instructs the patient in stump wrapping and in the use of a stump shrinker. Without this early physical therapy, the patient is likely to show up at the amputee clinic with a swollen stump and a hip or knee flexion contracture, delaying the prosthetic fitting and recovery.

Once the prosthesis has been fitted and completed, the amputee is admitted to a rehabilitation facility for gait training for a period of 1 or 2 weeks. This admission is particularly important for the elderly and those patients with healing concerns. Getting the amputee up and safe as quickly as possible is essential to avoiding dangerous falls and skin problems. The therapist helps the amputee develop strength, balance, and confidence while monitoring the condition of the skin over the stump. The prosthetist can make timely changes and adjustments that will prevent areas of irritation from becoming blisters or serious ulcers. During this period, the stump may begin to shrink in size rather rapidly before the amputee has learned how to adapt to these changes.

Physical therapy continues after discharge from the rehabilitation center. The amputee will have an increased energy demand in walking with a prosthesis. The increased demand will be directly proportional to the level of amputation. The older vascular amputee will tend to slow his or her gait to compensate for the increased demand. The BK amputee will have an increased energy demand of 15 to 40% as compared with normal whereas the AK amputee's energy demand will be 60 to 80% higher. The bilateral BK amputee will a have somewhat lower energy demand than a unilateral AK amputee. It is not unusual for an amputee to require a year or more to achieve maximum recovery.

Phantom pain and phantom sensation may be quite severe in the first weeks and months following amputation. All adult amputees will experience some phantom sensations throughout their lives. When the peripheral nerve is cut it will make an abortive attempt to heal, resulting in an amputation neuroma. The neuroma is sensitive to pressure or traction producing burning, tingling, or painful sensations of the amputated part of the extremity. The phantom sensations tend to become less bothersome as time passes but never completely go away. Patients with severe pain preoperatively tend to have the most severe pain after surgery. Narcotic analgesics may be necessary to control their pain. The use of various psychoactive medications, such as nortriptyline hydrochloride, may also be helpful. Successful prosthetic fitting will significantly ameliorate phantom sensations. Painful neuromata that are a problem for prosthetic fitting may need to be excised surgically. The freshly cut end of the nerve should be buried in the muscle tissue away from any pressure areas as a new neuroma may be expected to form.

Child amputees do not generally experience phantom sensation or require neuroma excision. As the child grows, appositional bone growth will occur in the diaphyseal area producing bony exostoses that may even penetrate the skin. These bony overgrowths will need to be periodically excised. Scar revision may also be necessary for tethering bands.

The psychologic impact of amputation is recognized by all those who work or live with the amputee. The visible loss of a part of one's body has been compared with the loss of a loved family member. A period of mourning the loss of the limb should be expected as a normal part of recovery. Lighthearted attempts to cheer up the patient by predicting that he or she will be "as good as new" or the "bionic man" only serve to trivialize the deeply felt loss. When the process of mourning the loss of the limb is deferred or delayed, it may be associated with severe depression at a later time. Psychiatric consultation can be helpful at any point in preventing or treating severe depression.

The orthopaedic surgeon as a member of the "amputation team" is in a unique position to guide the patient through the trauma of surgery and the recovery process. The amputation itself is thought of not simply as a resection of the diseased part but as a reconstruction of the leg to fit a prosthesis. The surgeon will have the earliest opportunity to discuss with the patient and the family the future course of recovery. The confidence of the surgeon in the other members of the team—the nurse, physical therapist, prosthetist, and psychiatrist—will be passed on to the amputee. Those patients who have gone through the trauma of an amputation are grateful for the care and consideration of those who have helped them during a time of great stress and pain.

SELECTED BIBLIOGRAPHY

ADERA HM, JAMES K, CASTRONUOVO Jr. JJ, BYRNE M, DESHMUKH R, LOHR J. Prediction of amputation wound healing with skin perfusion pressure. *J Vasc Surg.* 1995;21:823–829.

BOWKER JH, MICHAEL JW. *The American Academy of Orthopaedic Surgeons Atlas of Limb Prosthetics: Surgical, Prosthetic, and Rehabilitation Principles.* 2nd ed. St. louis, MO: CV Mosby; 1992.

BURGESS EM, ROMANO RL, ZETTL JH, SCHROCK Jr. RD. Amputations of the leg for peripheral vascular insufficiency. *J Bone Jt Surg.* 1971;53A:814–890.

DWARS BJ, VAN DEN BROEK TA, RAUWERDA JA, BAKKER FC. Criteria for reliable selection of the lowest level of amputation in peripheral vascular disease. *J Vasc Surg.* 1992; 15:536–542.

HOLLINSHED WH. *Anatomy for Surgeons. Vol 3: The Back and Limbs.* New York, NY: Harper and Row; 1969.

LARSSON J, APELQVIST J, CASTENFORS, J, AGARDH CD, STENSTROM A. Distal blood pressure as a predictor for the level of amputation in diabetic patients with foot ulcer. *Foot Ankle.* 1993;14:247–253.

MOORE WS, HENRY RE, MALONNE JM, DALY MJ, PATTON D, CHILDERS SJ. Prospective use of Xenon 133 clearance for amputation level selection. *Arch Surg*. 1981;116:86.

MOORE WS, MALONE JM. *Lower extremity amputation*. Philadelphia, PA: WB Saunders; 1989.

SAMPLE QUESTIONS

1. A 67-year-old man who underwent a BK amputation 2 months ago is admitted to the rehabilitation unit for gait training. He complains of intermittent burning pain and paresthesias in his absent toes. You should:

   (a) order an MRI scan of his stump

   (b) tell him that the sensations will go away soon

   (c) tell him that the sensations will become less severe as time passes

   (d) schedule him for neuroma excision

   (e) postpone gait training until the sensations are less severe

2. Piston action of the residual limb in a transtibial prosthesis during swing phase is most commonly caused by:

   (a) volume fluctuation of the residual limb

   (b) a prosthesis that is too long

   (c) a prosthesis that is too short

   (d) an ineffective suspension system

   (e) the SACH heel cushion is too soft

3. True or false: A hydraulic variable cadence knee prosthesis controls the knee during swing phase of walking to provide a variable cadence to gait. It can be used to raise the functional level of a household ambulator to a community ambulator.

   (a) true

   (b) false

4. True or false: A SACH foot is recommended for the amputee with a functional level of 1 (household ambulator). The SACH foot allows flexion of the toe and compression of the heel.

   (a) true

   (b) false

5. Which of the following statements regarding functional level is incorrect:

   (a) It is a method to estimate the ability of lower limb amputees to ambulate under various environmental conditions.

   (b) Functional level helps with selection of the appropriate prosthesis for a lower limb amputee.

   (c) A community ambulator can walk with a variable cadence.

   (d) A household ambulator can traverse low-level barriers such as curbs and stairs.

   (e) None of the above

Answers: 1) c; 2) d; 3) b; 4) a; 5) d

Oncology

Section

XV

Chapter 49

The Principles of Biopsy and Staging of Bone Tumors

Norbert J. Lindner, MD, and Mark T. Scarborough, MD

Outline

The evaluation and treatment of musculoskeletal tumors is an involved process due to their rarity and variety. This chapter reviews some of the fundamentals of musculoskeletal tumors: staging, surgical margins, and biopsy. Musculoskeletal tumors have different clinical behaviors depending on the histologic type and grade, the anatomic location, and extent. Staging of musculoskeletal tumors provides a common nomenclature and allows comparison of patients across multiple institutions with differing treatment protocols. The current staging system was developed by the American Musculoskeletal Tumor Society and has been accepted as the worldwide standard. This staging system is simple, reproducible, directly relates to prognosis, and facilitates treatment decisions. Definitions of surgical margins have also been developed to correlate with the staging system. Finally, types of biopsy and the associated pitfalls will be discussed.

EVALUATION

As in any other disease, a thorough evaluation of the history of the patient and physical examination are the basis for determining the correct diagnosis and therapy.

A plain radiograph in two planes is the first step in imaging bone and soft-tissue tumors. If the radiographs reveal a lesion that has a potential for malignancy or do not confirm a specific diagnosis, further staging studies are indicated. A magnetic resonance image (MRI) or computed tomography (CT) scan will serve as the best imaging to determine the exact localization of the lesion. Computed tomography best demonstrates bone destruction and mineralization, whereas MRI imaging demonstrates the soft tissue anatomy and intramedullary extension. A complete body radionuclide bone scan will give information about the biological activity of the lesion and can reveal other lesions within the skeletal system. Angiography can be performed to examine the relationship of the vascular structures to the tumor and can provide preoperative embolization to minimize blood loss. A chest radiograph and possibly a chest CT should be performed to exclude pulmonary metastases.

PEARL

When a radiograph of a patient shows a lesion that is potentially malignant, further staging studies (local magnetic resonance imaging [MRI] or computed tomography [CT], full-body radionuclide bone scan, chest radiograph or chest CT) should be performed.

From the history, physical exam, and imaging studies, an impression is formed whether the process is obviously benign or has equivocal or malignant features. Benign processes can then be managed as clinically indicated, often with clinical observation if asymptomatic. Intracapsular or marginal excision may be necessary for precise classification and staging.

CLASSIFICATION

Primary, secondary, and tumorlike lesions of the musculoskeletal system must be distinguished from one another before they are classified. Primary bone and soft-tissue tumors are those lesions that arise directly from mesenchymal cells. Secondary lesions arise in the setting of another abnormality. These include metastases from carcinomas, bone tumors secondary to radiation therapy, or malignancies arising from an underlying bone disease, such as osteosarcoma in Paget´s disease or malignant fibrous histiocytoma from bone infarcts. Tumorlike lesions mimic tumors, but are in fact of dysplastic or hyperplastic origin, often with an unknown etiology. Benign and malignant bone and soft-tissue tumors are usually characterized according to the clinical course of the disease.

Tumors of the musculoskeletal system are classified based on their cell of origin. A tumor composed of fibroblasts or fibrocytes and collagen is a fibroma or fibrosarcoma, whereas a tumor made of chondroblasts or chondrocytes and cartilage is an enchondroma or chondrosarcoma. A tumor consisting

Orthopaedic Surgery: The Essentials. Edited by M.E. Baratz, A.D. Watson, and J.E. Imbriglia. Thieme Medical Publishers, Inc., New York © 1999

of osteoblasts or osteocytes and osteoid can be an osteoid osteoma, osteoblastoma, or osteosarcoma.

The histological distinction among different lesions is simpler for benign tumors but can be difficult in malignant lesions with a mixed cell pattern. For further classification, the pathologist uses immunohistochemical stains, cytogenetics, electron microscopy, and other sophisticated techniques. An overview of the benign and malignant bone tumors is given in Tables 49–1 and 49–2, whereas Table 49–3 lists tumorlike lesions.

STAGING OF BONE AND SOFT-TISSUE TUMORS

The surgical staging system for musculoskeletal neoplasms was devised based on analysis of data compiled from various neoplasms seen between 1960 and 1975. The system was field-tested by the Musculoskeletal Tumor Society from 1976 to 1978. It was then adopted by the Society for use in interinstitutional protocols and was published in 1980. In 1985, it was adopted by the American Joint Commission on Staging and End-Result Studies (AJC) and, in 1990, by the International Union Against Cancer (UICC).

Tumor staging is based on the natural history of neoplasms arising from the connective tissues that make up the musculoskeletal system and is applicable to lesions arising both from bone and the somatic soft tissues. This system utilizes radiographic, clinical, and histological data to assign a stage. Treatment, planning, and comparison of outcomes are possible using this framework. The staging is not used for metastatic carcinomas and lesions arising from the bone marrow (lymphoma, myeloma, leukemia, etc.), which have their own separate staging systems.

The stage of a neoplasm is an indication of the biological aggressiveness and potential for distant metastases. It is based on three factors: histological grade (G), the anatomic site or extent (T), and the presence or absence of metastases (M). Benign tumors can be classified as stage 1 (latent), stage 2 (active), or stage 3 (aggressive). Malignant tumors are classified as stage I (low-grade malignant), stage II (high-grade malignant) or stage III (metastatic). Stage III includes both

TABLE 49–1   Bone Tumors

Histogenesis	Benign	Low-grade Malignant	High-grade Malignant
Fibrous and histiocytic	Histiocytic fibroma Benign fibrous histiocytoma Giant-cell tumor Desmoplatic fibroma	Grade 1 and 2 fibrosarcoma and malignant fibrous histiocytoma	Grade 3 and 4 fibrosarcoma and malignant fibrous histiocytoma
Cartilaginous	Exostosis Enchondroma Periostel chondroma Chondroblastoma Chondromyxoidfibroma	Grade 1 and 2 central chondrosarcoma Peripheral chondrosarcoma Periosteal chondrosarcoma Clear-cell chondrosarcoma Mesenchymoma	Grade 3 central chondrosarcoma Mesenchymal chondrosarcoma
Osseous	Osteoma Osteoid osteoma Osteoblastoma Fibrous dysplasia Osteofibrous dysplasia	Parosteal osteosarcoma Periosteal osteosarcoma Low-grade central osteosarcoma Surface osteosarcoma	Classic osteosarcoma hemorraghic osteosarcoma Small-cell osteosarcoma Osteosarcomatosis High-grade central osteosarcoma Surface osteosarcoma
Emopoietic			Lymphoma Multiple myeloma Ewing's sarcoma
Vascular	Hemangioma Lymphangioma	Low-grade hemangioendothelioma Hemangiopericytoma	High-grade hemangioendothelioma Hemangiopericytoma
Neurogenic	Neurilemoma Neurofibroma		Primitive neuroectodermal tumor (PNET)
Fatty	Lipoma		Liposarcoma
Mixed		Adamantinoma	Malignant mesenchymoma
Notochordal		Chordoma	

TABLE 49–2 Soft-Tissue Tumors

Histogenesis	Benign	Low-grade Malignant	High-grade Malignant
Fibrous	Fibromatosis Aggressive fibromatosis	Grade 1 and 2 fibrosarcoma	Grade 3 and 4 fibrosarcoma
Fibrohistiocytotic	Benign fibrous histiocytoma	Dermatofibrosarcoma protuberans Atypical fibroxanthoma	Malignant fibrous histiocytoma
Fatty	Atypical Lipoma Lipoma	Liposarcoma (well-differentiated)	Liposarcoma (dedifferentiated)
Smooth muscle	Leiomyoma	Grade 1 and 2 leiomyosarcoma	Grade 3 and 4 leiomyosarcoma

Vascular	Angioma
	Angiodysplasia
	Glomus tumor
	Hemangioma
	Hemangiopericytoma
		Low-grade
		  hemangioendothelioma
		Kaposi's sarcoma
		Hemangiopericytoma
			High-grade
			  hemangioendothelioma
			Kaposi's sarcoma
			Hemangiopericytoma

Synovial			Synovial sarcoma
Neurogenic	Neurinoma Neurofibroma		Malignant neurofibrosarcoma Peripheral neuroepithelioma
Cartilaginous		Myxoid chondrosarcoma Synovial chondrosarcoma	Mesenchymal chondrosarcoma
Osseous			Osteosarcoma
Unknown	Intramuscular myxoma Granular-cell tumor		Malignant granular-cell tumor Ewing's sarcoma Alueolar sarcoma Epitheloid sarcoma Clear-cell sarcoma

TABLE 49–3 Tumorlike Lesions

In Bone	In Soft Tissue
Simple bone cyst Aneurysmal bone cyst Intraosseous ganglion Progressive osteolysis Eosinophilic granuloma Brown tumor Solid aneurysmal bone cyst Periostitis	Palmar and plantar fibromatosis Nodular fasciitis Ganglion Elastofibroma Xanthoma Juvenile xanthogranuloma Proliferative fasciitis and myositis Synovial chondromatosis Neuroma Heterotopic ossification (Myositis ossificans) Pigmented villonodular synovitis Tumorous calcinosis

low- and high-grade tumors that have metastasized. Stage I and stage II tumors are subdivided into A or B groups based on whether the tumor is intracompartmental (A) or extracompartmental (B). These factors are summarized in Table 49–4.

Tumor grade (G) is a histopathological assessment based on the cell type of tumor and the degree of cellular atypia. The grade reflects the predicted behavior of the lesion, including the risk of developing satellite, skip, regional, and distant metastases. Categories of grade include G0 (benign), G1 (low-grade malignant), and G2 (high-grade malignant).

Benign lesions (G0) have variable local aggressiveness and rare metastases. Low-grade malignant lesions (G1) tend to

TABLE 49–4   Stages of Benign and Malignant Lesions

Stage (benign)	1 (latent)	2 (active)	3 (aggressive)
Grade	G0	G0	G_0
Localization	T0	T0	T_1
Metastases	M0	M0	M_0 or M_1

Stage (malignant)	IA low-grade	IB low-grade	IIA high-grade	IIB	IIIA	IIIB
Grade	G_1	G_1	G_2	G_2	G_1 or G_2	G_1 or G_2
Localization	T_1	T_2	T_1	T_2	T_1 or T_2	T_1 or T_2
Metastases	M_0	M_0	M_0	M_0	M_1	M_1

have limited local spread with few satellite nodules or skip metastases and a low rate of local recurrence. In contrast, high-grade malignant lesions (G2) have a wide reactive zone containing satellite nodules and a higher incidence of skip, regional, and distant metastases. Consequently, G2 lesions require more aggressive surgery and radiotherapy for local control, sometimes with adjuvant chemotherapy .

The site (T) of a lesion is determined by its location and extent. This is important when deciding on the margin that is necessary for local control of the tumor. The site (T) of a lesion is described as: intracapsular and intracompartmental (T0), extracapsular yet intracompartmental (T1), or extracapsular and extracompartmental (T2). Certain well-defined compartments such as the thigh, leg, arm, forearm, or within a bone itself provide a natural barrier to tumor extension. When a lesion occurs in these locations, it is considered intracompartmental. In contrast, other areas such as the popliteal fossa and the groin are poor barriers to tumor extension and are considered extracompartmental. Table 49–5 explains the system used to determine site in tumor staging.

TABLE 49–5   Anatomical Sites

Intracompartmental (T0–1), extracompartmental (T2)
Intraosseous
Intra-articular
Skin subcutaneous
Parosseous
Intracompartmental soft tissue

Intracompartmental by Origin	Extracompartmental by Origin
Ray of hand or foot	Midhand, dorsal or plantar
Posterior calf	Mid- or hindfoot
Anterolateral leg	Popliteal fossa
Anterior thigh	Peri-articular knee
Medial thigh	Femoral triangle
Posterior thigh	Obturator foramen, pelvis
Buttocks	Sciatic notch, intrapelvic
Volar forearm	Antecubital fossa
Posterior forearm	Peri-articular elbow
Anterior arm	Axilla
Posterior arm	Periclavicular
Periscapular-extraosseous extension	Paraspinal
Extra-articular extension	Head and neck
Deep extension	
Extension into bone or soft tissue	
Extracompartmental soft tissue	

The presence or absence of metastases (M0 or M1), determines the third factor in the staging system. All metastases are considered M1, regardless of whether to the lungs, bone, nodes, or other location. Metastases are almost always due to malignant tumors. Rarely, a histologically benign tumor such as a giant-cell tumor or chondroblastoma may develop pulmonary metastases. Skip metastases are defined as nodules of tumor within bone separated from the primary lesion by an intervening zone of normal, nonreactive tissue. They differ from the satellite nodules that form in the reactive zone immediately about the primary lesion. Skip metastases are almost always found within the compartment of origin of the primary lesion, although they are occasionally located across a joint in an adjacent bone. Skip metastases confer the same poor prognosis as do distant metastases, and are classified as M1. Regional metastases occur within the regional lymph nodes. Distant metastases are typically found in the lungs, but may develop in any organ or bone.

Tumors can change stage during the course of the disease. Benign tumors may undergo malignant transformation or may spontaneously involute. Malignant tumors develop worsening histological features, spread locally, and metastasize. Certain clinical situations may be associated with changes in tumor stage. Cytogenetic aberrations have been implicated in the transition of multiple familial exostoses to chondrosarcoma. Cessation of skeletal growth is clearly related to the involution of stage II, benign lesions to stage I.

Repeated local recurrences following inadequate primary resection are associated with transformation of sarcomas from grade 1 to 2. Pathological fracture, inappropriate biopsy techniques, and traumatic events are associated with progression from an intracompartmental to an extracompartmental site. Repeated manipulations are known to be associated with showers of cells in the systemic circulation and may cause metastases.

SURGICAL MARGINS

A precise definition and classification of surgical margins are useful for evaluation, planning, and treatment in the care of musculoskeletal tumors. Bone and soft-tissue tumors behave in a similar manner, and common principles are used to assess their margins. Surrounding any musculoskeletal neoplasm there is usually a capsule (or pseudocapsule) for soft-tissue tumors or a rim of reactive bone in bone tumors (Fig. 49–1).

Inside the capsule is the tumor, and on the outer surface is the reactive zone. The reactive zone is of variable thickness and can be identified best on MRI studies as a rim of increased signal intensity surrounding the lesion. Within the reactive zone is a variable amount of microscopic tumor extension. Just beyond the reactive zone is normal tissue. High-grade tumors may have neither a capsule nor reactive rim of bone.

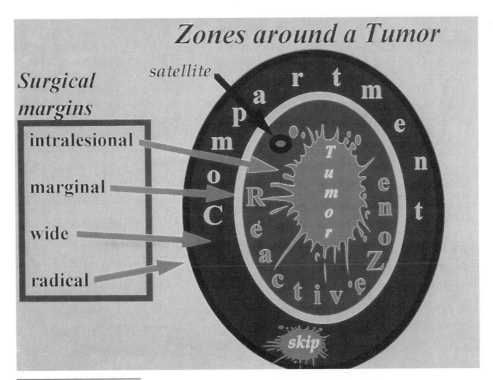

Figure 49–1 A scheme describing the zones around tumors.

TABLE 49–6   Definition of Surgical Margins

Surgical Margin	Limb Salvage	Amputation	Histology
Intralesional	Curettage, piecemeal resection within lesion	Through tumor	Tumor at margin
Marginal	Marginal en bloc excision through reactive tissue	Along reactive tissue	Reactive tissue +/− satellites
Wide	Wide en bloc excision through normal surrounding tissue	Through normal tissue in compartment	Normal tissue +/− skip lesions
Radical	Radical en bloc resection with entire compartment	Extracompartmental amputation or disarticulation	Normal tissue

Four types of surgical margins of resection have been defined: intralesional (or intracapsular), marginal, wide, and radical. Table 49–6 summarizes the surgical margins with their microscopic appearance and oncologic procedures.

Intralesional or intracapsular resection margins occur when the plane of dissection is through the lesion. By definition, microscopic residual tumor remains. The margin of resection is defined as marginal when the plane of dissection is through the reactive zone. In a soft-tissue tumor, this usually happens when the tumor is "shelled out" by means of dissection outside of the tumor capsule. With a wide resection, the plane of dissection occurs through normal tissue. There is no set distance that determines a wide margin, rather it is the quality of tissue that makes a margin wide. For instance, fat is a poor barrier to tumor extension, and several centimeters of intervening normal fat may be necessary to obtain a wide margin. In contrast, a single millimeter margin of unaffected cortical bone or fascia is considered wide. A radical margin is attained if the entire compartment in which the tumor originated is removed. With a bone tumor this means removing the entire bone. In soft-tissue masses, the entire compartment from muscle origin to insertion must be removed to achieve a radical resection.

Because certain soft tissues are poor barriers to tumor extension, they are by definition considered extracompartmental. In these instances, amputation is avoided because the importance of limb salvage supercedes that of the margin of resection (Table 49–5). For example, the popliteal fossa, axilla, and antecubital fossa are considered extracompartmental, whereas the anterior, medial and posterior portions of the thigh are intracompartmental. The margins of resection for amputations are classified with the same scheme as those of other resections. Intralesional is an amputation that extends through the tumor; marginal extends through the reactive zone, wide extends through normal tissue, and a radical amputation extends outside of the compartment of origin. The surgical stage is articulated with the surgical margin for local control of the tumor. Table 49–7 summarizes the different correlations for surgical planning.

TABLE 49–7a.   Articulation of Benign Lesions with Surgical Margins

Stage	Site	Metastasis	Margin for Control
I	T0	M0	Intralesional
II	T0	M0	Marginal or Intralesional plus effective adjuvant
III	T1–2	M0–1	Wide or marginal plus effective adjuvant

Therapeutic measures may be capable of downstaging tumors. The encapsulating-host response to neoadjuvant chemotherapy about a stage IIB osteosarcoma may produce transition to a stage IIA lesion. In a similar fashion, a soft-tissue sarcoma after preoperative radiation therapy may be downstaged from a stage IIB to a stage IIA lesion. Successful chemotherapy, when it obliterates micrometastases, downstages stage III to stage II.

BIOPSY OF BONE AND SOFT-TISSUE TUMORS

Choice of biopsy techniques in bone and soft-tissue tumors is a vital step in patient management. Errors in diagnosis or an inappropriate biopsy can have an adverse impact on the chances of limb salvage and even survival. Thus, the biopsy should be performed following completion of the radiographic staging and preoperative consultation with the radiologist, pathologist, and surgeon. Obtaining the imaging studies prior to biopsy is essential because the biopsy can

TABLE 49–7b. Articulation of Malignant Lesions with Surgical Margins

Stage	Grade	Site	Metastases	Margin for Control
IA	G1	T1	M0	Wide excision
IB	G1	T2	M0	Wide excision
IIA	G2	T1	M0	Radical resection or wide excision plus effective adjuvant therapy
IIB	G2	T2	M0	Radical exarticulation or wide amputation plus effective adjuvant therapy
IIIB	G2–1	T1	M1	Thoracotomy plus radical exarticulation or palliative procedure

alter the staging studies. The radiographs can also locate other lesions that may be more amenable to biopsy than the presenting lesion. After the staging studies are completed, a differential diagnosis should be prepared. The best method of biopsy can then be chosen.

The best biopsy method for a musculoskeletal neoplasm depends on the differential diagnosis, the location of the neoplasm, and the ability of the pathologist to make a diagnosis on a small sample of tissue. In general, needle biopsies are preferred when the diagnosis can be made on a small tissue sample, when the diagnostic possibilities are limited, or when the tumor tissue is so homogeneous that there is little potential for a sampling error. Myeloma and metastatic carcinoma, for example, are often easily diagnosed on needle biopsy. Soft tissue sarcomas may also sometimes be diagnosed with a needle biopsy. The advantages of a needle biopsy are that the procedure is quick, safe, inexpensive, and easily done with local anesthesia. The disadvantages are due to the small volume of tissue obtained from a needle biopsy. Limited tissue samples not only introduce the possibility of a sampling error but also may not provide enough tissue to do special studies such as immunohistochemistry, electron microscopy, flow cytometry, or cytogenetics.

Open incisional biopsies involve taking a sample of tumor. Open biopsy provides more tissue and improves the accuracy of diagnosis compared with needle biopsies. When an open biopsy is performed, a frozen section analysis should be performed to confirm the adequacy of the specimen. If necrotic tissue is obtained, further samples should be taken.

The frozen section assures that the sample chosen is viable tumor with sufficient cells for histological examination. In selected cases, a definitive procedure can be performed immediately following the frozen section. For example, prophylactic internal fixation of an impending pathologic fracture can be carried out following a frozen section that proves the lesion is caused by metastatic carcinoma. The biopsy of musculoskeletal neoplasms is an important procedure that should be thoroughly planned.

PEARL

Every musculoskeletal tumor has the potential to be a sarcoma and should be approached as such. Because sarcomas are implantable, proper biopsy technique is essential to avoid contamination of uninvolved structures.

Longitudinal incisions should always be used in the extremities. The most direct route from the skin to the tumor is preferred. However, the biopsy should always go through muscle rather than through intermuscular planes to avoid spread of tumor cells along these planes. The neurovascular bundle or joint should not be exposed or opened during a biopsy. If a pathologic fracture is present, the fracture callus should be avoided because the pathologist may have difficulty distinguishing this from the tumor bone seen in osteosarcoma.

It is important to be aware of the approaches made for limb salvage procedures, as well as the standard flaps used in amputations.

PEARL

If autograft bone is to be used, the donor site must not be contaminated. Either a second team separately gowned and gloved and using separate instruments should obtain the donor bone, or the surgeon should change gown, gloves, and instruments prior to harvesting the bone graft.

Once a sample is obtained and the frozen section confirms the tissue to be of adequate diagnostic quality, the wound is closed. Hematomas can be prevented by strict hemostasis and surgical drains to avoid the potential of wound contamination.

If the diagnosis is certain based on the imaging studies (e.g., a classic osteochondroma), then an incisional biopsy is not necessary.

Complete excision of a suspected benign lesion can be done if the excision does not compromise the ability to achieve a wide surgical margin should the lesion proves to

PEARL

In selected cases, an excisional biopsy can be performed, during which the entire specimen is removed and submitted to the pathologist.

be malignant. For example, a small, soft-tissue lesion (< 5 cm) in the subcutaneous tissue of the anterior thigh could be marginally excised as an excisional biopsy, without a frozen section. If the lesion is proven to be malignant then re-excision of the tumor bed could be done without difficulty. In contrast, removal of a tumor greater than 5 cm that is deep to the fascia would contaminate a large amount of normal tissue and make subsequent resection difficult.

The most common errors associated with biopsy of musculoskeletal tumors are an inadequate preoperative evaluation, transverse incisions, exposure of a joint or neurovascu-

lar bundle, a postoperative hematoma or infection, or inadequate tumor sampling. Arthroscopic biopsy will contaminate the joint and, thus, should not be done for any potentially malignant tumor. Such errors result in an increased risk of amputation and lower rates of survival. The risk is increased when the biopsy of a presumed sarcoma is done outside of a hospital that treats sarcomas. Thus, it is preferable to refer any potential sarcoma to a tertiary treatment center prior to biopsy.

PEARL

It is recommended that all soft-tissue lesions greater than 5 cm or deep to the fascia and all potentially primary bone lesions associated with pain, cortical destruction, or bone formation be referred prior to biopsy.

SELECTED BIBLIOGRAPHY

ENNEKING WF. A system of staging musculoskeletal neoplasm. *Clin Orthop Rel Res.* 1986;204:9–24.

ENNEKING WF. *A System of Staging Musculoskeletal Neoplasms.* Gainesville, FL: University, of Florida Press; 1990.

ENNEKING WF, SPANIER SS, GOODMAN MA. A system for the surgical staging of musculoskeletal sarcoma. *Clin Orthop Rel Res.* 1980;153:106–120.

GUSTAFSON P. Soft tissue sarcoma: epidemiology and progress in 508 patients. *Acta Orthop Scand.* 1994;65:1–31 (supp 259).

HEARE TC, ENNEKING WF, HEARE MM. Staging techniques and biopsy of bone tumors. *Orthop Clin North Am.* 1989; 20:273–285.

JOYCE MJ, MANKIN HJ. Caveat arthroscopos: extra-articular lesions of bone simulating intra-articular pathology of the knee. *J Bone Jt Surg.* 1983;65A:289–292.

MANKIN HJ, LANGE TA, SPANIER SS. The hazards of biopsy in patients with malignant primary bone and soft-tissue tumors. *J Bone Jt Surg.* 1982;64A:1121–1127.

MANKIN HJ, MANKIN CJ, SIMON MA. The hazards of biopsy, revisited. *J Bone Jt Surg.* 1996;78A:656–663.

PEABODY TD, SIMON MA. Principles of staging of soft-tissue sarcomas. *Clin Orthop Rel Res.* 1993;289:19–31.

SIMON MA. Biopsy of musculoskeletal tumors. *J Bone Jt Surg.* 1982;64A:1253–1257.

WUISMAN P, ENNEKING WF. Prognosis for patients who have osteosarcoma with skip metastasis. *J Bone Jt Surg Am.* 1990;72A:60–68.

SAMPLE QUESTIONS

1. An 18 year-old female presented with a distal femoral lesion. Staging studies showed the lesion to arise from the femur with soft-tissue extension into the anterior compartment of the thigh. The bone scan and chest CT showed no evidence of distant disease. An incisional biopsy revealed a high-grade osteosarcoma. The stage is:

   (a) I-A
   (b) I-B
   (c) II-A
   (d) II-B
   (e) III-B

2. An above knee amputation was done for an extensive soft-tissue sarcoma of the leg that involved the popliteal neurovascular bundle. The tissue at the amputation margin was noted to be somewhat edematous. The margins were

reported as "free of tumor". The surgical margin achieved is best described as:

   (a) intralesional
   (b) marginal
   (c) wide
   (d) radical
   (e) en-bloc

3. A 32 year-old male was found to have a lesion of the distal femur. An incisional biopsy revealed a benign giant cell tumor. There was no evidence of regional or distant spread based on the bone scan and chest radiographs. A thorough curettage procedure was done and the defect was packed with bone cement. The surgical margin is:

   (a) intralesional
   (b) marginal

(c) wide

(d) radical

(e) en-bloc

4. The most common errors associated with biopsy of musculoskeletal tumors include all of the following except:

(a) transverse incision

(b) joint exposure

(c) arthroscopic biopsy

(d) early referral

(e) inadequate evaluation

5. A 13 year-old male presented with knee pain. Radiographs revealed a lesion within the epiphysis of the distal femur. A MRI showed a lesion within the epiphyseal portion of the distal femur without cortical breakthough or a soft-tissue mass. There was significant edema within the distal femur and adjacent soft-tissue. The bone scan and chest radiographs revealed no distant disease. An incisional biopsy was consistent with a chondroblastoma. The stage is:

(a) 1

(b) 2

(c) 3

(d) I-A

(e) I-B

Chapter 50

Benign Lesions of the Musculoskeletal System

Don C. Beringer, MD, Mark S. Meyer, MD, and Mark T. Scarborough, MD

Outline

Benign lesions of bone and soft tissue range from the most innocuous curiosities noted on imaging to very aggressive processes that threaten limb or even life. A continuum exists that renders a strict definition of benign versus malignant, at times, artificial. For example, few would consider myositis ossificans anything but a benign entity, yet how is myositis ossificans progressiva, a non-neoplastic yet potentially life-threatening condition, defined? Despite its limitation, we distinguish benign from malignant processes to provide a conceptual framework for diagnosis, staging, and treatment. Benign musculoskeletal lesions usually result from a disorder in the normal processes that control the growth and differentiation of musculoskeletal tissues. However, the process, whether dysplastic, hyperplastic, or neoplastic is of limited biologic aggressiveness; it tends to remain within or in close proximity to its compartment of origin and rarely metastasizes. Developing a system for the clinical and radiographic evaluation of a musculoskeletal lesion is imperative. These principles have been discussed in Chapter 49. In this chapter, the focus is on the identifying features of each benign lesion. The most important of these are patient age at occurrence, anatomic location, clinical presentation, special imaging characteristics, and histopathology. This chapter includes benign conditions commonly encountered in orthopaedic practice and those of most relevance to the orthopaedist in training. The lesions are grouped by their most common location (bone or soft tissue) and, when possible, by their predominant histogenetic origin. Finally, several non-neoplastic but clearly benign entities in bone and soft tissue that are often confused with tumors are included for discussion.

SPECIFIC CONDITIONS, TREATMENT, AND OUTCOME

Benign Lesions in Bone

Osteogenic

Included in this group are osteoid osteoma and osteoblastoma. Despite their similarities in age distribution and histopathologic appearance, they are quite distinctive with respect to size, anatomic distribution, radiographic appearance, and clinical behavior. In addition, there are subtle differences in their histopathologies. Therefore, they have been accepted as separate entities.

Osteoid osteoma is a common lesion that constitutes 13% of all benign bone tumors. With more than 50% occurring between the ages of 10 and 20, this is a neoplasm affecting predominantly young persons. Seventy-six percent occur between the ages of 5 and 24. Males are affected more commonly by a margin of 3:1. The proximal femur is the single most common site of involvement and more than half are found in either the femur or the tibia. Other common locations include the vertebrae (where the posterior arch is involved almost exclusively), the phalanges of the hand, and the tarsal bones, especially the talar neck. Patients report throbbing pain unrelated to activity, which is worse at night and is improved by aspirin or other nonsteroidal anti-inflammatory agents. These medications work because of their ability to inhibit prostaglandins that are in high concentration in the lesion. Patients can usually localize the pain so well that they can help direct appropriate radiographic views to identify the lesion. Despite this classic presentation, approximately one-third of patients will either have no pain or lack this constellation of findings. Superficial locations are associated with swelling. The occasional lesion in the epiphysis may present with a joint effusion. Vertebral involvement can cause scoliosis due to muscle spasm. Important distinctions between this and idiopathic scoliosis is the lack of rotational deformity, absence of posterior rib hump, and the presence of pain. Although osteoid osteoma is a neoplasm, it is a self-limited process that is usually of concern to the patient more for the pain and irritation than for any danger it presents.

Although the clinical presentation varies, the radiographic features are consistent. The lesion is an intra- or paracortical

Orthopaedic Surgery: The Essentials. Edited by M.E. Baratz, A.D. Watson, and J.E. Imbriglia. Thieme Medical Publishers, Inc., New York © 1999

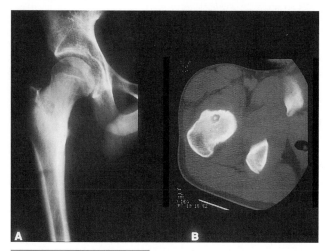

Figure 50–1 Osteoid osteoma. Lesion in the base of the femoral neck on the anteroposterior (AP) radiograph **(A)** is localized to the anterior cortex on the computed tomography (CT) scan **(B)**. Note the radiolucency surrounding the nidus within the reactive bone.

nidus that has a radiodense center and a radiolucent rim (Fig. 50–1). Most are less than 1 cm in diameter and virtually never greater than 2 cm. A striking feature that may obscure the lesion itself is the abundant, dense surrounding reactive cortical bone that appears out of proportion compared with the small nidus. In a large series of biopsy-proven osteoid osteomas, plain radiographs were diagnostic in 75% and at least suggestive of the lesion in more than 90%. Bone scans always show increased uptake in the reactive portion of the lesion that is usually more intense in the nidus itself. The value of a bone scan is questionable unless the patient with a typical presentation has normal radiographs. When a lesion is visible and the diagnosis is still in question or the surgeon needs to localize the lesion for treatment, computed tomography (CT) has been helpful and is superior to standard tomography. Owing to the abundant blood supply to an osteoid osteoma, contrast-enhanced CT can be used to confirm the diagnosis.

The nidus of an osteoid osteoma appears as irregular spicules of immmature, mineralized bone or osteoid lined with osteoblasts and occasional osteoclasts. The mesenchymal background stroma has numerous capillaries. The lesion is separated from the reactive bone surrounding it by a narrow region of fibrovascular stroma devoid of osseous tissue (Fig. 50–2).

Use of aspirin or nonsteroidal anti-inflammatory medication relieves symptoms in a significant number of patients. However, the natural history of the process, pain over several years duration, is unaltered by these medications. In addition, there are risks to the chronic use of anti-inflammatotry agents, and patients occasionally experience intolerable side effects. The surgical treatment of osteoid osteoma has changed in recent years. Historically, with plain radiographs only, the nidus was excised en bloc, taking a margin of reactive bone. Although this technique adequately removes the nidus, it involves a standard surgical exposure and its attendant morbidity and it weakens the bone, requiring protected weight bearing with the potential of a pathologic fracture. Shaving the cortex over the nidus before removing it has become an accepted alternative to en bloc resection. This is

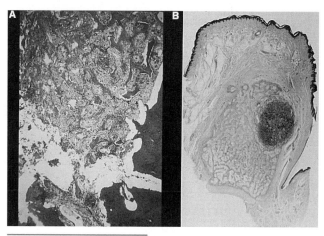

Figure 50–2 Osteoid osteoma. Photomicrograph (40×) of the nidus consisting of bony trabeculae and well vascularized mesenchymal tissue surrounded by reactive bone **(A)**. Macrosection of lesion in distal phalanx **(B)**. Note the lesion bounded by dense reactive bone.

more effective when combined with CT-guided localization. Although tetracycline labeling and intra-operative nuclear scanning have been used, CT remains the best alternative for localization. The most recent surgical advance involves techniques of percutaneous CT-guided ablation using drills and radiofrequency probes.

Osteoblastoma is an uncommon lesion, accounting for less than 3% of all benign bone tumors and approximately 1% of all primary bone tumors. Males are affected more frequently by a margin of 3:1. Most cases occur in the second and third decade and 90% present before the age of 40. The anatomic distribution is wide, with a predilection for the spine and sacrum. Like osteoid osteoma, it arises in the posterior elements and may extend into the adjacent tissues and to the vertebral body (Fig. 50–3). The femur, tibia, and mandible (so called cementoblastoma at the root of a tooth) are also common sites.

The radiographic features described for osteoblastomas are protean. However, there are a few distinguishing characteristics. Osteoblastomas tend to be ovoid and range in size from 2 to 11 cm with an average size of 3 cm. Most are either intracortical or intramedullary, can be lucent or blastic, and frequently cause expansile remodelling of bone (Fig. 50–4).

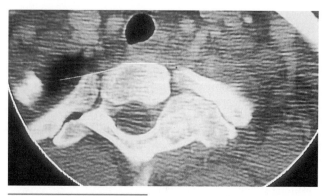

Figure 50–3 Osteoblastoma involving the posterior elements of the seventh cervical vertebrae.

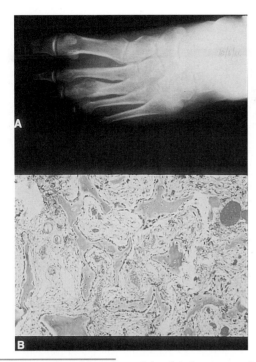

Figure 50–4 Osteoblastoma of the third metatarsal. Plain radiograph **(A)**. Photomicrograph (100×) **(B)** shows well formed trabeculae with prominent osteoblastic rimming and a vascularized fibrous stroma.

These lesions are usually confined within the bone, but an "aggressive osteoblastoma" commonly extends beyond the cortical border and may have a soft tissue component. Secondary aneurysmal bone cysts are frequently seen.

The clinical behavior of this tumor varies widely. Most patients have gradually increasing pain that is not relieved with nonsteroidal anti-inflammatories. Treatment requires biopsy and excision. Curettage is recommended when the entire lesion can be resected with minimal morbidity. In expendable bones, aggressive-appearing lesions, and some vertebral lesions, should be resected en bloc. The reconstruction depends on the site, but most defects require bone grafting. Recurrence is uncommon.

Another lesion composed of bone is the *enostosis* or "bone islands." These bone islands are totally asymptomatic, incidental radiographic densities that can be located in any bone. Although an enostosis never causes pain, it may be a source of confusion when images obtained for another reason show this lesion. It is a focal radiodensity reaching up to 2 cm in size. Located within the intramedullary space, the edges of the lesion blend with the trabeculations of the surrounding cancellous bone giving it a somewhat hazy border. Histologically, it consists entirely of compact bone. The differential diagnoses include metastatic carcinoma and low-grade osteogenic sarcoma. Osteomas are exceedingly rare outside of the skull, are larger, and have slightly different radiographic characteristics. Metastatic carcinoma, even if osteoblastic, will likely be larger, has associated bone destruction, occurs in the appropriate age group, and has a consistent history. Likewise, osteogenic sarcoma must be considered only in an appropriately aged individual with some of the radiographic characteristics of this entity. Certainly,

biopsy will conclusively distinguish all of these possibilities, but is necessary only on rare occasions.

Chondrogenic

Osteochondroma, periosteal chondroma, and enchondroma constitute this group of benign bone lesions.

Osteochondroma (also known as osteocartilaginous exostosis or exostosis) is the most common bone tumor, estimated to constitute 44% of all benign bone tumors. Most are seen in children and young adults: males more commonly than females. Exostoses usually occur as solitary lesions but can occur in multiple locations as an autosomal dominant condition known as multiple hereditary exostoses (MHE). The lesions occur in the metaphyses of the distal femur, proximal tibia, and proximal humerus but are also found in any of the long bones and in the axial skeleton. They result from a developmental abnormality in the epiphyseal mechanism, are found on the metaphyseal side of the physis as a raised lesion on the cortex, and consist of an osseous base and a cartilage cap. An osteochondroma is confluent with the cortex, can be sessile or pedunculated, and has a marrow cavity continuous with the intramedullary canal of the native bone. The pedunculated type have a stalk that is directed away from the physeal plate from which it originated. The cartilage cap is thicker in childhood (1-2 cm), becomes thinner in adults, and is similar to the physis on its deep side. Growth parallels that of the normal skeleton. Secondary chondrosarcomas rarely occur. In MHE, risk factors associated with the development of a secondary chondrosarcoma include an excessive number of lesions and a central location.

The presentation and radiographic features for any given lesion are identical in either solitary or multiple exostoses. Owing to the natural growth pattern, a certain proportion of lesions become symptomatic during the growing years. A mechanical cause for the pain includes tendon impingement, nerve compression, interference with normal joint motion, fracture of the base, or, rarely, pseudoaneurysm formation. In addition, an exostosis may interfere with physeal growth causing skeletal malalignment or limb-length discrepancy. Short stature or degenerative changes of the weight-bearing joints may occur and is seen more commonly in MHE. Lesions that are large, centrally located, or in a patient with MHE deserve surveillance for malignant transformation with serial radiographs. After skeletal maturity, new onset of pain in a previously quiescent lesion, nonmechanical pain, or noticeable enlargement are reasons for concern and further study.

The radiographic features are so distinctive that only plain radiographs are required for diagnosis and routine surveillance (Figs. 50–5 and 50–6). In the adult, a suspicious radiographic appearance would include a significant change in size, an apparently thick (greater than 1cm) cartilage cap, cortical destruction, or a soft tissue mass. Both CT and magnetic resonance imaging (MRI) are acceptable methods of evaluating a suspicious lesion. Magnetic resonance imaging is more reliable for estimating the thickness of the cartilage cap. Computed tomography provides better visualization of cortical bone and can adequately reveal adjacent soft tissue masses (Fig. 50–7).

Parosteal osteosarcoma and secondary chondrosarcoma need to be differentiated from osteochondroma. A parosteal

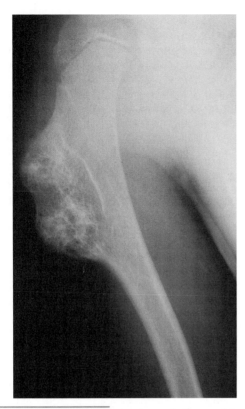

Figure 50–5   Osteochondroma. A sessile humeral lesion.

osteosarcoma can be distinguished on imaging from a sessile osteochondroma by its lack of intramedullary continuity, characteristic location, and distinctive histologic appearance. If the clinical findings are suspicious and the radiographs show change in size or calcification pattern, subtle cortical expansion or destruction, or evidence of soft tissue mass, then a secondary chondrosarcoma is likely.

Indications for removal of exostoses include pain, progressive skeletal malalignment, or limb-length discrepancy and cosmetic problems. In these cases, the entire exostosis must be resected with care to remove the cartilaginous cap to prevent recurrence. Any lesion that remains suspicious following appropriate staging should be resected.

Chondroblastoma is a rare neoplasm accounting for 1% of all benign bone tumors. Most occur in adolescents or young adults, and 90% occur between the ages of 10 and 25. Males are affected with a higher frequency than females. It occurs primarily in the epiphysis of the growing skeleton. The most common sites are the proximal humerus, proximal and distal femur, and proximal tibia. Unusual sites of occurrence include the talus, lumbar spine, and innominate bone, where it is seen in older individuals.

The patient typically presents with a several month history of gradually increasing dull, aching pain made worse with activity. Swelling, effusion, and limited motion are typical when chondroblastoma occurs around the knee. Tenderness with palpation is characteristic regardless of the site. There are rare instances of so-called malignant chondroblastoma with an an especially aggressive course and distant spread.

The secondary ossification center is the primary location in most cases (Fig. 50–8). However, extension to the physis or

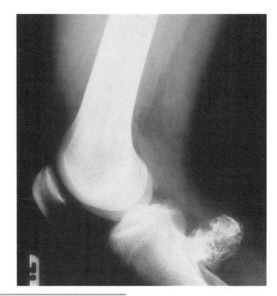

Figure 50–6   Osteochondroma. A pedunculated proximal tibial lesion.

metaphysis occurs. Radiographically, chondroblastomas present as stage II active lesions with a well-marginated border, though many are stage III aggressive lesions with cortical or subchondral perforation and associated soft tissue mass. The CT scan is superior for observing cortical penetration, periosteal reaction, and associated soft tisssue masses. The bone scan shows increased uptake, which extends slightly beyond the radiographically apparent lesion into the reactive zone. Although MRI is more useful for evaluating the size and extent rather than for diagnosis, it is useful for resolving the occasional diagnostic dilemma. On T2-weighted imaging, the lesion has a lobular appearance with a heterogenous low,

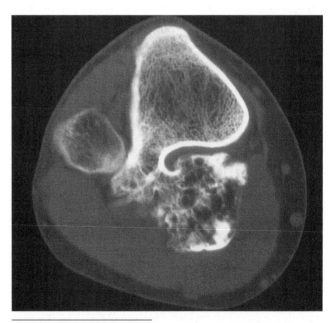

Figure 50–7   Computed tomography scan of the pedunculated osteochondroma of the proximal, posterior tibia seen in Figure 6. Note the continuity between the intramedullary canal of the tibia and the lesion.

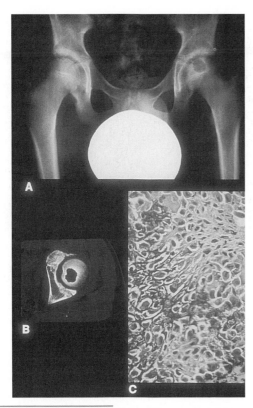

Figure 50–8   Chondroblastoma of the proximal femoral epiphysis. Plain radiograph **(A)** and CT scan **(B)** showing intact subchondral bone. Photomicrograph (100×) **(C)** demonstrates characteristic immature chondroblasts, chondroid matrix and foci of chicken-wire calcification.

intermediate, and high signal. The surrounding marrow and periosteum have a high signal intensity even in radiographically well-marginated lesions.

Consideration of typical age of occurrence, location, findings on clinical exam, and imaging will usually distinguish chondroblastoma from other possibilities. Although giant-cell tumor can extend to the epiphysis, it is rare before skeletal maturity and these lesions have no calcification.

On histology, chondroblastomas have islands of mature chondroblasts with primitive cartilage matrix, multinucleated giant cells, and lacelike or "chicken-wire" calcification (Fig. 50–8).

Chondroblastoma, owing to its close proximity to the articular surface, has the potential to damage the joint and create a poor outcome if unrecognized or untreated. Prompt diagnosis and appropriate treatment is critical. Intralesional curettage with bone grafting can be done for stage II and some stage III lesions, whereas resection is necessary for locally aggressive recurrence or neglected lesions.

Chondromyxoid fibromas (CMFs) are, rare benign neoplasms accounting for less than 0.5% of all primary bone tumors. They have features resembling chondroblastoma and have been mistaken for a myxoid chondrosarcoma. However, this lesion is clearly a benign process and is a distinct clinicopathologic entity. Most occur in the second and third decade of life but can present in all ages. The proximal tibia is the most common site. Half of all cases occur around the

knee, and 75% are in the lower extremity. Approximately 25% occur in the flat bones, especially the ilium. Although most patients have pain, the severity is variable. The duration of symptoms ranges from months to years. Local swelling and tenderness occur, but associated joint effusions are not characteristic.

The imaging and pathologic findings are more revealing than the clinical exam. Plain radiographs show a well-localized, eccentric, oval, radiolucent lesion located primarily in the metaphysis of a long bone. A radiodense or scalloped margin is usually present, suggesting a benign process and resembling nonossifying fibroma. Extension into the epiphysis after skeletal maturity may occur, but crossing an open physis is rare. Expansion or bubbling of the cortex may occur and is more characteristic of small or flat bone involvement. There are no distinguishing intralesional densities. Most lesions are 5 cm or less. Chondromyxoid fibroma presents as a stage II lesion in most cases and only on occasion has characteristics of a more aggressive process. The bone scan is not particularly helpful and tends to show increased uptake differentially about the margins of the lesion. Computed tomography and or MRI outline the extent of the lesion and are more helpful in planning treatment.

The name chondromyxoid fibroma accurately describes the microscopic appearance of the tissue. Islands of pink, chondroid matrix with large, round cells are distinguished from the fibromyxoid elements. Hyaline cartilage is distinctly unusual. Within the chondroid component, mild cellular atypia and pleomorphism are occasionally seen. The more abundant myxoid element is composed of stellate cells with inconspicuous septae, which can be differentiated histologically from a myxoid chondrosarcoma.

A CMF can be distinguished from a myxoid chondrosarcoma by the lack of permeation into the surrounding bone and the paucity of hyaline cartilage. The radiographic appearance of nonossifying fibroma and fibrous dysplasia is similar to a CMF, but neither expand the cortex and the latter shows a more radiodense, intralesional "ground glass" appearance. Chondromyxoid fibroma is usually treated with intralesional curettage and bone grafting. The recurrence rate of curettage is significant, and there is a tendency for recurrent tumor to behave more aggressively. For this reason, a marginal or wide resection (with an appropriate reconstruction) may be a preferable initial approach. Although CMF can be locally destructive, it is a benign process, even when it recurs, and malignant transformation is virtually unknown.

Enchondromas are hamartomatous collections of cartilage within bone. They are more common than all other benign lesions except exostoses and nonossifying fibromas, accounting for between 13 and 25% of benign bone tumors. They arise from a focal defect in ossification of the primary spongiosa of the physeal plate. More than half occur in the small tubular bones, and the vast majority of these are in the hands, in which it is the most common tumor (Fig. 50–9). Other common sites include the femur and humerus. They originate in the metadiaphysis and become more diaphyseal with skeletal growth.

Solitary enchondromas are distinguished from the multiple lesions of enchondromatosis or Ollier's disease. In the solitary form, it is most commonly discovered in the second through fourth decades, often as an incidental finding. There

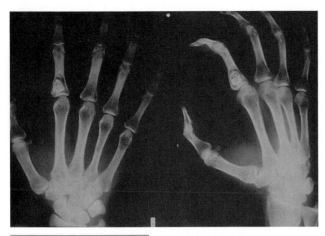

Figure 50–9 Enchondroma of the index finger proximal phalanx.

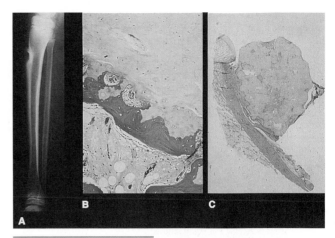

Figure 50–10 Periosteal chondroma of the proximal tibia. Lateral radiograph (**A**) and photomicrograph (40×) of this lesion (**B**) demonstrates the cartilaginous tissue against the underlying reactive cortical bone. A macrosection (**C**) of a distal femoral lesion shows the characteristic lobule of cartilage, the underlying dense cortical bone, and a remnant of periosteal covering.

is no sex predilection. Secondary chondrosarcomas develop in less than 1%, of enchondromas, occurring more commonly in centrally located lesions. The multiple lesions of Ollier's disease may present at an earlier age as a result of the associated problems with skeletal growth and alignment. In this setting, the incidence of secondary chondrosarcoma is approximately 25%. It is even higher in Maffucci's syndrome, characterized by enchondromatosis and soft tissue hemangiomas.

Enchondromas are usually found incidentally. In adults, a painful lesion requires evaluation as it may result from a pathologic fracture or, on rare occasion, an associated chondrosarcoma. A pathologic fracture is most common in enchondromas of the hand. However, in this location secondary malignancy is extremely rare.

Periosteal chondroma is a rare, benign cartilage tumor arising on the external surface of cortical bone deep to the periosteum. It occurs in the metaphyseal region of long bones and the short tubular bones of the hands and feet. Patients commonly present in the third and fourth decade, although it occurs in both children and adults. There is a male-to-female ratio of 2:1.

The clinical presentation includes a firm mass, tenderness, and pain that may have persisted for months to several years. A mass, if present, may slowly progress in size even after skeletal maturity. Radiographically, periosteal chondromas show a characteristic saucerized erosion in the metaphyseal cortex with a reactive rim of bone and, possibly, intralesional calcifications (Fig. 50–10). They rarely exceed beyond 3 to 4 cm in size.

Histologically, a periosteal chondroma consists of benign cartilaginous lobules of proliferating chondrocytes and occasional foci of calcification or osteoid. Despite the hypercellularity of the lesion, there is minimal cellular atypia, and mitoses are rare. It is bounded on its deep side by reactive cortical bone and superficially by mature fibrous periosteum.

The differential diagnostic possibilities include chondrosarcoma and exostosis. In contrast to chondrosarcoma, a periosteal chondroma usually is smaller, tends to present at a younger age, has a characteristic radiographic appearance, and usually lacks malignant histological features. Osteochondromas have some continuity with the intramedullary

canal and have features on plain radiographs or CT scan that easily distinguish it from periosteal chondroma.

Periosteal chondromas are treated surgically by wide or marginal resection. Bone grafting the defect may be indicated. Recurrence is uncommon even for marginal resections. Observation with serial radiographs is acceptable for small, asymptomatic lesions.

Fibrous

The fibrous lesions of bone are represented by several entities, not all neoplastic, that have widely different clinicopathologic characteristics. These include nonossifying fibroma, fibrous dysplasia, desmoplastic fibroma, and periosteal desmoid.

Nonossifying fibroma (NOF) is a benign proliferation of fibroblastlike mesenchymal tissue that is more likely a hamartomatous process than a true neoplasm. It is usually a stage I latent lesion and is an incidental finding in the vast majority of cases. It is one of most common benign bone lesions. Owing to its harmless course and its classic radiographic appearance, few are biopsied and, consequently, account for only 2% of all benign bone biopsies. It occurs at a young age; more than 80% present before the age of 20. It is located in the metaphysis or metadiaphysis and can occur almost anywhere in the appendicular skeleton (Fig. 50–11). However, it is most common in the long bones, especially the distal femur and the tibia.

Although most are incidental findings, NOFs can present as a stage II active process with either pain, a stress fracture or, less commonly, an outright pathologic fracture. Growth abnormalities and articular involvement are uncommon. Following skeletal maturity, NOFs enter a regressive phase whereby they are gradually replaced by reactive bone and leave only a remnant of their previous existence. Most regress by the time patients reach 30 years of age.

The classic radiographic appearance is an eccentric metaphyseal lesion, always involving the medullary canal, with a

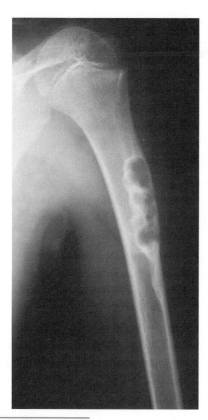

Figure 50–11 Nonossifying fibroma in the proximal humerus. Note the eccentric, metaphyseal location and loculated appearance. The lesion is typically well marginated with thinning but no destruction of the cortex.

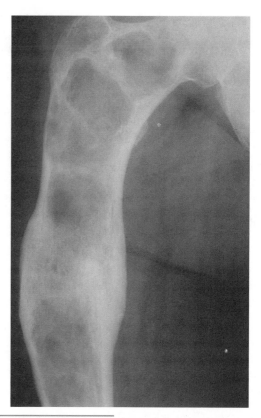

Figure 50–12 Fibrous dysplasia of the proximal femur in a patient with polyostotic disease ("shepherd's crook" deformity).

loculated appearance and a radiodense rim. Aside from the septations, it has no intralesional density. The cortex may undergo remodeling. A CT scan is occasionally indicated to evaluate the risk of pathologic fracture.

The histologic appearance depends on whether the lesion is in an early or incipient phase during skeletal growth or in a regressive phase later in adulthood. Early, the lesion is extremely cellular, consisting of fibroblastic spindle cells with plump nuclei. Mitoses can be seen but are not common, and the overall appearance is quite monotonous. Giant cells are a prominent feature, are evenly distributed, and have nuclei that are different from those in the matrix. As the lesion matures, the collagen content increases, lipid rich macrophages appear, and hemosiderin deposits are seen. Finally, reactive bone, initially from the periphery, is increasingly seen.

Differential diagnosis includes giant-cell tumor, brown tumor of hyperparathyroidism, desmoplastic fibroma, fibrous dysplasia, and fibrosarcoma.

Fibrous dysplasia is a non-neoplastic condition of aberrant bone development resulting in localized fibro-osseous metaplasia. More commonly, skeletal involvement is limited to a single location in monostotic disease, but up to 25% of individuals may have multiple sites of involvement that tend to predominate on one side of the body. Brown patches of skin pigmentation with irregular borders (café au lait) may be an associated finding in either form. Albright's syndrome, the combination of polyostotic fibrous dysplasia, café au lait skin

patches, and precocious puberty, occur rarely and more often in females. The incidence of this disease, especially the monostotic form, is difficult to estimate because many patients are asymptomatic. Females are affected slightly more often than males. The most common extremity location is the proximal femur followed by the tibia, although any bone may be involved. In the axial skeleton, head (skull and jaw) and rib lesions are most common. The disease is usually in an active phase of growth in childhood, and adolescents and most symptomatic patients are diagnosed by early adulthood.

The clinical presentation varies depending on the number of lesions, the specific location, and the extent of bone involvement. If a lesion is incidentally discovered, it usually is solitary, small, and in a low-stress region of the skeleton such as a rib. Typically, pain results from fatigue-related microfractures or pathologic fracture through a lesion. The subtrochanteric region of the femur is the most frequent site but this can occur in any weight-bearing portion of the skeleton (Fig. 50–12). Although fractures through the lesions heal at a normal rate, they do so with dysplastic bone, which is as likely to fracture again. Less commonly, a painful mass presents in a small bone such as a rib or metacarpal. In older patients, deformity or limb-length discrepancy may follow repeated cycles of fracture and repair. Despite the tendency of the lesion itself to stop growing and enter a latent phase in adulthood, fractures can still occur and any deformity may worsen and subsequently cause fracture. Fibrous dysplasia occurs in the skull or mandible in between one-third and one-half of cases. The potential clinical problems, including facial disfigurement and cranial nerve dysfunction, can be severe and of great concern to the patient. On rare occasion, a lesion may degenerate into a sarcoma, usually a fibrosarcoma or malignant fibrous histiocytoma. These high-grade lesions tend to have a similar response to treatment as primary sarcomas of the same histogenetic origin.

Radiographically, fibrous dysplasia is usually metaphyseal, oval, with a radiolucent but ground glass appearance within the lesion. The small, rather evenly dispersed trabeculae of dysplastic bone against a fibrous background stroma account for this appearance. Although the lesion may cause cortical expansion, it grows rather slowly as seen by the surrounding radiodense rim (Fig. 50–13). Occasionally, secondary aneurysmal bone cysts or large cystic areas can develop within the lesions, thus, altering the characteristics of the radiograph. Clinical exam and plain radiographs are usually sufficient for making the diagnosis, but additional imaging may be required. On the bone scan, uptake within the lesion is usually intense. The CT scan shows an homogenous intramedullary soft tissue density that contrasts with the surrounding bone. Computed tomography is more useful in evaluating extent of cortical involvement. In an adult, significant radiographic change, rapid enlargement of the lesion, or cortical destruction are worrisome and require an appropriate workup to rule out malignant degeneration.

The most notable pathologic feature in fibrous dysplasia is the immature, woven bone trabeculae within a background stroma of collagen-rich tissue. The small dysplastic bone particles resemble Chinese letters. The dysplastic bone appears to arise in a haphazard fashion from the stroma (Fig. 50–13). There is no appreciable osteoblastic rimming about the bone as seen in osteofibrous dysplasia and osteoblastoma. The tissue is well vascularized with abundant capillaries, which accounts for the intense bone scan activity.

The differential diagnsosis includes mostly benign entities. Osteoblastoma, giant-cell tumor, aneurysmal bone cyst, osteofibrous dysplasia (when the lesion occurs in the tibia), and brown tumor are included.

Simple observation is adequate treatment in most cases. When a lesion is very large or enlarging, in a high-stress location, or has become symptomatic, a minimum of serial radiographs and counseling to modify activities is indicated. The indications for surgical treatment depend on the lesion's location, its extent, and the presence of pathologic fracture or deformity. Active disease in a growing child mandates different treatment considerations than disease in its quiescent phase in adulthood. Similar to the pattern of fracture healing in fibrous dysplasia, curettage of these lesions results in healing with dysplastic, mechanically deficient bone regardless of whether cancellous graft is used. Therefore, the goals of surgical treatment, when indicated, are clearly different from other benign active or aggressive lesions. Rather than resect the lesional tissue, the goals are to stabilize the bone, prevent or correct deformity, and relieve pain. Recommendations for stabilizing dysplastic long bones, especially the proximal femur, include cortical bone grafts such as fibular strut (Fig. 50–14). Cortical bone, especially allograft, is very useful because of its limited ability to incorporate that parallels its lower rate of resorption. In deformity or pathologic fracture, internal fixation may be required but is more successful in adults than children.

Reticuloendothelial

Eosinophilic granuloma (EG) is a focally destructive bone lesion that may occur as a solitary finding or within the spectrum of related disorders known collectively as histiocytosis X (Langerhans cell histiocytosis). When EG is associated with exopthalmos and diabetes insipidus it is called Hand-Schuller-Christian disease. Onset at a very young age with disseminated lesions in multiple organs carries a poor prog-

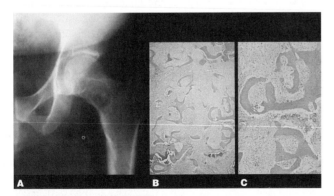

Figure 50–13 Fibrous dysplasia. Anteroposterior radiograph **(A)** showing the lesion in the base of the femoral neck. Low-power photomicrograph (100×) **(B)** demonstrates immature bone in "Chinese letters" pattern in a sea of fibrous connective tissue. In the high power photomicrograph **(C)** note the lack of rimming osteoblasts about the dysplastic trabeculae in contrast to osteoblastoma.

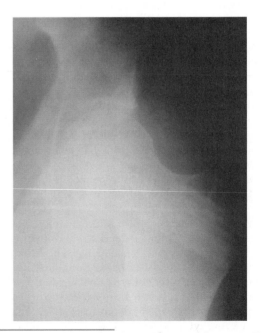

Figure 50–14 Fibrous dysplasia. The same lesion in Figure 12 stabilized with fibular cortical strut graft.

nosis and is known as Letterer-Siwe disease. In each of these entities, the lesion is composed of abnormally proliferating histiocytes that derive from a dendritic histiocytic precursor. It presents in both children and adults of all ages but occurs most commonly between ages 1 and 3. More than 90% occur before the age of 15. Although the incidence of histiocytosis is underestimated (by the number of patients with asymptomatic lesions), it is rare and has a frequency of approximately 4 per 1,000,000. It has a distinct male predilection. Eosiniphilic granuloma has a wide distribution, but 70% of lesions present in the axial skeleton, most commonly in the skull, vertebral body, ribs, and pelvis. The other 30% occur in the long bones, especially the tibia and femur.

The clinical presentation varies with the stage and size of the lesion and whether a single or multiple sites are involved. Most eosinophilic granulomas present as solitary stage 2 active lesions. Although their behavior is variable, these lesions tend to regress and enter a latent phase with skeletal maturity. When symptomatic, dull aching and swelling are common complaints. A soft tissue mass may coexist with the lesion and, if close to the skin, is palpable. Pathologic fracture occurs infrequently in the long bones, and vertebral involvement may result in collapse and subsequent neurological compromise. Elevated erythrocyte sedimentation rate, leukocytosis, and fever occur but are not diagnostic.

The radiographic appearance of EG varies widely with the stage of the lesion and its location. It may appear similar to a large number of benign and malignant processes and is appropriately referred to as the "great mimicker." It ranges from a focal, well-marginated radiolucency to a permeative appearance with periosteal elevation, "onionskinning" of the cortex and an associated soft tissue mass (Fig. 50–15).

Histologically, eosinophilic granuloma and the soft tissue lesions of histiocytosis X appear similar. Sheets of lipid-laden histiocytes on a backround of inflammatory cells with variable numbers of eosinophils constitute this lesion (Fig. 50–15). Birbeck granules, tennis racket-shaped cytoplasmic structures

identified only by electron microscopy, are found within the histiocytes and are pathognomic.

In view of the protean radiographic and clinical manifestations of EG, a biopsy may be required to rule out malignancy and curettage may be performed concurrently. However, spontaneous resolution occurs in months to years in the localized form of the disease. Nonoperative treatment includes activity modification, weight-bearing restrictions, and occasional bracing for vertebral lesions. Surgical alternatives include curettage and bone grafting, and corticosteroid injections. Only on rare occasions is radiation appropriate for localized disease.

Giant-cell tumor (GCT) of bone is relatively common, accounting for 22% of biopsy-proven primary bone tumors. This neoplasm appears to arise from monocytic precursor cells. Eighty percent of GCTs occur after the second decade, thus this tumor occurs primarily after skeletal maturity. The typical location is the metaepiphyseal end of the long bones. The most common site is the distal femur, and half occur around the knee in either the femur or tibia. Other common locations include the distal radius, proximal humerus, and the sacrum. Only 2% occur in the small bones of the hands and feet. Vertebral involvement above the sacrum occurs on occasion.

The clinical presentation varies from incidental discovery to pathologic fracture, but more than 80% of patients are symptomatic. Most cases of giant-cell tumor are stage 2 active or stage 3 aggressive, benign lesions. Pain, swelling, joint effusion, loss of motion, and a mass are common findings. Vertebral (or sacral) lesions can result in neurologic compromise owing to either instability or an impinging soft tissue mass. Although GCT has little tendency for distant spread, lung metastases are noted in approximately 3%. Lung metastases from GCT usually behave indolently, with few patients dying of these lesions. An extremely rare variant of GCT is the "multicentric" GCT, which accounts for approximately 1% of all cases. Malignant transformation of a completely benign GCT in the absence of previous radiation is also very rare.

The radiographic appearance of GCT in the long bones is classic in most cases. It is a well-localized metaepiphyseal radiolucent lesion with minimal reactive bone about the margin. GCTs often approach or violate the subchondral bone and even the articular cartilage (Fig. 50–16). There are no radiodensities seen within the lesion except for occasional septations representing incomplete cortical destruction (Fig. 50–17). The CT scan shows cortical and subchondral bone destruction and can identify fluid-fluid levels of commonly associated secondary aneurysmal bone cysts. The MRI shows an homogenous, low signal intensity on T1- and a high signal on T2-weighted images, extra-osseous soft tissue masses if present, and occasionally fluid-fluid levels.

The histopathology of GCT is characterized by homogenous sea of cells devoid of matrix with evenly distributed multinucleated giant cells. The cells have oval to spindle-shaped nuclei with abundant pink cytoplasm but an indistinct border between them. The multinucleated giant cells have scores of nuclei that appear identical to those of the stroma (Fig. 50–17). Occasional foci of necrosis are seen. Mitoses are common and do not predict the behavior of the lesion.

The most common form of treatment is intralesional curettage, usually with an adjuvant such as phenol, methacrylate,

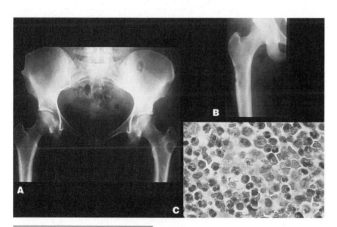

Figure 50–15 Eosinophilic granuloma. The radiographic presentation varies widely. This small, well-marginated radiolucency in the lateral trochanteric region **(A)** contrasts with this destructive appearing subtrochanteric lesion **(B)**. The photomicrograph (400×) **(C)** demonstrates the typical pale staining histiocytes admixed with variable numbers of smaller eosinophils with bilobed nuclei and dark, granular cytoplasm.

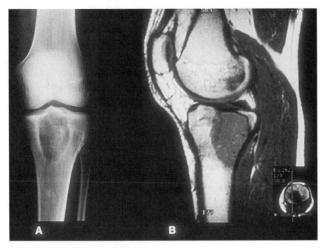

Figure 50–16 Giant-cell tumor of the proximal tibia. The characteristic radiolucent, meta-epiphyseal lesion is seen on the AP radiograph **(A)**. The T1-weighted magnetic resonance imaging (MRI) scan typically has an homogenous signal abnormality corresponding to the radiolucency and delineates soft tissue extension if present **(B)**.

PEARL

In giant-cell tumors (GCTs), the nuclei in the giant cells appear identical to those of the stroma. There are several lesions with a similar pathologic appearance, yet they have a markedly different clinical behavior and response to treatment. The most important distinction is between GCT and a number of malignant processes. "Giant-cell rich" variants of osteosarcoma, fibrosarcoma, and malignant fibrous histiocytoma occur uncommonly and so-called malignant GCT is rare. Benign lesions masquerading as a GCT include aneurysmal bone cyst and a brown tumor of hyperthyroidism.

---

and/or liquid nitrogen. Unroofing the lesion through the most accessible or weakest cortex, curetting out all macroscopic disease, and burring the margins are critical to minimizing local recurrence. The rate of local recurrence ranges from approximately 10 to 50% and is dependent on the stage of the tumor, surgical technique, and appropriate use of adjuvant therapies. The defect is usually filled with methacrylate. Local recurrence may be recognized earlier with methacrylate in the defect rather than bone graft. However, the mechanical properties of methacrylate differ so markedly from bone that its use in subchondral locations is likely to result in accelerated degenerative changes in the articular cartilage. Solutions to this problem are currently being explored.

Indications for a wide resection and reconstruction include stage 3 aggressive lesions with cortical or articular destruction, some cases with pathologic fracture, and when local recurrence severely limits the chance of success with repeat curettage. Radiation therapy has proven beneficial in achieving local control in surgically inaccessible sites or when unacceptable morbidity is expected with surgical resection. How-

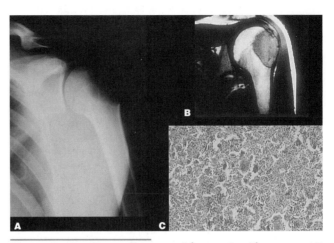

Figure 50–17 Giant-cell tumor of the proximal humerus. AP radiograph **(A)** and T1-weighted MRI **(B)** with homogenous signal abnormality corresponding to the lucency seen in the radiograph. Photomicrograph (-100×) **(C)** of the lesion demonstrates a sea of multinucleated giant cells, which appear to arise from the background stromal cells.

ever, evidence for occasional malignant transformation of GCT treated with radiation is growing and should be considered in determining the best treatment approach.

Uncertain Origin

Aneurysmal bone cysts (ABCs) account for 1 to 2% of all benign bone lesions. The ABC has a distinctive place in the study of benign bone tumors for a number of reasons. This non-neoplastic entity may be radiographically similar to many benign as well as malignant processes within bone. ABCs may behave in a very aggressive fashion, causing significant bone destruction. They occur in association with many benign and malignant processes as "secondary ABCs" in up to 30% of cases. One third occur in association with giant-cell tumor. A wide range of other associated benign and malignant lesions are found including osteogenic sarcoma (especially telangiectatic osteosarcoma), nonossifying fibroma, chondroblastoma, fibrous dysplasia, and previous trauma. The etiology is not known, although they appear to be a reactive process. This is a disease of the growing skeleton with more than 80% of cases occurring in the first two decades. Males and females are affected equally. Fifty percent of ABCs present in the long bones, and the vast majority occur in either the long bones, spine, or pelvis. An ABC typically occurs in the knee region with the distal femur and proximal tibia the most common of all sites. In the extremities, lesions most commonly are found eccentrically in the metaphysis followed, much less commonly, by diaphyseal lesions. Epiphyseal lesions are rare and may be associated with a chondroblastoma or giant-cell tumor. More than 20% involve the vertebrae. The posterior elements are the primary site of involvement, although they frequently extend into the body.

Pain and swelling are the common symptoms at the time of presentation. Limitations in range of motion are common, and 20% will present with a pathologic fracture. In the spine, additional neurologic problems include nerve root impingement and associated pain, sensory disturbance or, less commonly, motor deficits (Fig. 50–18).

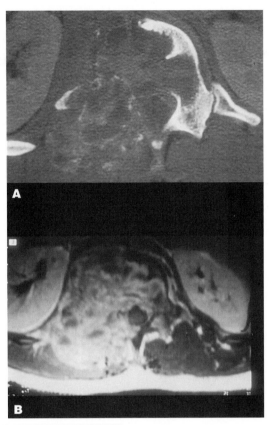

Figure 50–18 Aneurysmal bone cyst of the 12th thoracic vertebrae. Computed tomography scan **(A)** and MRI **(B)** show destruction of the posterior elements with extension to the body and a soft tissue mass encroaching on the vertebral canal.

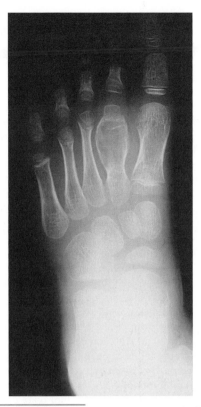

Figure 50–19 Aneurysmal bone cyst of the second metatarsal. Anteroposterior radiograph showing cortical expansile remodeling.

PEARL

If you see an aneurysmal bone cyst (ABC), consider a coexisting primary bone lesion.

The radiographic picture varies significantly, depending on the location and the stage of the lesion. ABCs occur subperiosteally, intracortically, within the medullary cavity, or in conjunction with other lesions. An ABC usually shows expansile remodeling (Fig. 50–19). The bone scan often shows an area of intense uptake, with less uptake in the central portion of the lesion. The CT scan and MRI are extremely helpful in distinguishing ABCs from other benign and malignant processes. Both of these imaging modalities are capable of showing the characteristic fluid-fluid interface that represents differential layering of hemoglobin-containing and serum components of the blood within the lesion.

An ABC represents a reactive vascular process within a dense connective tissue (i.e., bone). The histological features consist of hemorrhagic spaces bounded by fibrous stroma of variable thickness apparent on low power. On higher power, plump spindle cells in a collagen matrix constitute the stroma. There is no endothelial lining about the vascular space. Interspersed among the spindle cell stroma are multinucleated giant cells and small wisps of osteoid or chondroid (Fig. 50–20).

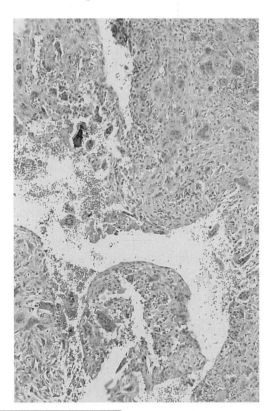

Figure 50–20 Biopsy of the lesion seen in Figure 19 illustrates the characteristic cellular mesynchymal stroma, occasional giant cells, and cystic, hemorrhagic areas devoid of endothelial lining.

Given the frequency of secondary ABCs, the differential diagnoses must always be given consideration. Distinguishing osteosarcoma with an ABC component or telangiectatic osteosarcoma from a primary ABC can be extremely challenging. Careful review of the clinical information, all imaging, and the biopsy material with close communication among surgeon, pathologist, and radiologist are imperative. Although the fibrous stroma in ABC can be very cellular with mitoses present, there is little pleomorphism. The occasional osteoid in an ABC occurs as wisps of reactive tissue, which can be distinguished from tumor osteoid by an experienced pathologist. Large intramedullary radiolucencies can resemble unicameral bone cysts. However, their typical locations differ, and imaging characteristics on CT and MRI can distinguish these entities as well. Giant-cell tumor must be considered in an adult with epiphyseal extension of the lesion. In ABCs, the nuclei of giant cells have a different appearance than their stromal counterparts. This pattern is different than the giant-cell tumor in which the nuclei of the giant cells arise from the surrounding stromal cells. A chondroblastoma should be considered in any epiphyseal lesion occuring in a growing child. Distinguishing a vertebral osteoblastoma from an ABC can be difficult. Impressive cortical expanile remodeling of the posterior vertebral elements is usually seen with ABC's while osteoblastoma usually involves the vertebral body.

The usual treatment for aneurysmal bone cysts is curettage and bone grafting. Making a large cortical window to adequately remove all portions of the tumor followed by burring the entire cavity are key aspects of the procedure, as the recurrence rate can reach 20%. In an expendable bone such as the fibula, an en bloc resection may be preferable. Radiation therapy has been associated with late malignant transformation, so this should be considered only when resection carries a very high risk of complications or morbidity.

Unicameral bone cyst (simple cyst) is a benign tumorlike process consisting of a fluid-filled cavitary defect in bone. It arises on the metaphyseal side of the growth plate and is displaced toward the diaphysis with skeletal growth. It occurs most frequently in young children and adolescents, with a peak between 5 and 15 years of age. The pathogenesis of unicameral bone cysts (UBCs) remains unclear, but favored theories include hemodynamic alterations, trauma-related defects in enchondral bone formation, and the presence of local factors causing bone resorption such as prostaglandins. The UBC has a predilection for males by a 2:1 margin. The most common locations are the proximal humerus, proximal femur, and calcaneus. However, it has a wide distribution including the spine and flat bones.

The classic radiographic appearance is a central metaphyseal radiolucency surrounded by a very thin rim of overlying cortical bone (Fig. 50–21). The entire cavity may be loculated by septations, and a pathognomonic fragment of cortical bone ("fallen leaf"), may be seen within the lesion. Otherwise there are no intralesional densities. It may slightly expand the cortex, but periosteal reaction is uncommon in the absence of fracture. A CT scan is occasionally indicated to evaluate the risk for pathologic fracture or to show its relationship with the physeal plate. The bone scan shows an area of increased uptake corresponding to the reactive margin of the lesion and less than background uptake in the cystic portion.

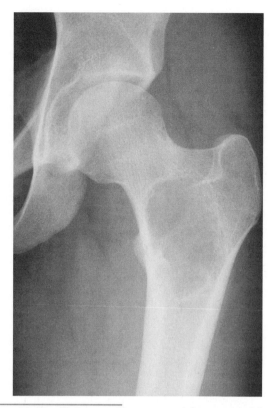

Figure 50–21   Unicameral bone cyst of the proximal femur.

Histologically, a fluid-filled space is bounded by a thin rim of fibrous tissue with interspersed multinucleated giant cells and hemosiderin deposits. Beneath this membrane lies a thin vascularized zone of areolar tissue, and osteoclasts can be seen resorbing the cortical surface in active lesions. The fluid within the cyst resembles synovial fluid, although hemorrhage occurs with fracture.

The most common differential possibilities include fibrous dysplasia and ABC, which can usually be distinguished on clinical exam and imaging studies. Both CT and MRI can be helpful in distinguishing fluid from soft tissue within the lesion or in identifying a fluid-fluid level. Occasionally, a needle biopsy will be useful to distinguish these entities.

A UBC tends to enlarge with skeletal growth as an active (stage 2) lesion in younger children and, consequently, may present with pain or a pathologic fracture. After skeletal maturity the lesion returns to a latent phase (stage 1), ceases growing, is resorbed, and is replaced by normal bone. For small lesions at low to moderate risk of fracture, observation and activity restriction may be all that is necessary. Treatment is directed at lesions with pathologic fracture or those at high risk for fracture or deformity. In most cases, a pathologic fracture should be treated nonoperatively until it heals before embarking on further treatment. Often this results in resolution of the lesion, especially in older adolescents or adults. Surgical treatment options include curettage with bone grafting and flouroscopically guided percutaneous corticosteroid injection. Regardless of the approach, the recurrence rate is very high in patients younger than 10 years of age with active lesions; the lesion approximates the growth plate and shows signs of expansion on serial radiographs. In active lesions, treatment should be delayed, if possible, until the cyst has reached a latent stage.

Benign Lesions in Soft Tissue
Synovial

In addition to rheumatoid arthritis and nonspecific synovitis, there are two other diseases of synovial tissue that appear to have a common pathogenesis and are distinguished only by the anatomic localization. These entities are pigmented villonodular synovitis and GCT of tendon sheath. Whether these are genuinely neoplasms or inflammatory processes is currently under debate. Recent evidence, including cytogenetic studies, supports a neoplastic etiology.

Pigmented villonodular synovitis (PVSN) is a proliferative process that is usually monoarticular and involves a major joint. In more than 25% of cases the knee is involved; the most frequent site of occurrence. Other common sites include the hip, wrist, ankle, and shoulder. There is no clear sex predilection. The initial presentation is typically in young adulthood but can range from adolescence through the fourth decade. An "apple-core lesion" on radiographs is characteristic. Bone about the neck of the femur or humerus is eroded, resembling bites around the circumference of an apple.

Fibrous

Aggressive fibromatosis, also commonly referred to as extra-abdominal desmoid, is a benign but aggressive form of fibrous tissue proliferation. It typically arises from the connective tissue of muscle or its overlying fascia. The biologic activity is, in general, between that of other benign fibrous lesions and fibrosarcoma, but it does not have the ability to metastasize. These lesions tend to be poorly encapsulated and infiltrate surrounding tissues leading to high local recurrence rates following marginal excision. Although fibromatosis has the potential to arise from the fascial compartments or connective tissue of any anatomic site, data from the Armed Forces Institute of Pathology (1983) shows that extra-abdominal fibromatosis has a predilection for the shoulder girdle (22%), chest wall and back (17%), thigh (12%), neck (8%), and pelvic girdle (6%). Muscle groups commonly involved include the deltoid, gluteal muscles, and quadriceps. Multicentric lesions have been reported, but are rare. The hands (Dupuytren's disease) and feet (Ledderhose's disease) are commonly involved with superficial forms of fibromatosis, but their clinical course does not follow the infiltrative pattern of aggressive fibromatosis. Fibromatosis is primarily a disease of adolescence and young adulthood, with a peak in the third decade of life.

The clinical presentation of fibromatosis is usually of a deep seated, slowly enlarging mass that typically causes little or no pain. Paresthesias, hypesthesia, and motor weakness are occasionally seen as the lesion infiltrates or encases neural structures.

As with many soft tissue lesions, fibromatosis is best visualized with MRI. The radiographic appearance on plain films is unremarkable. The exception is if the lesion has reached such a size that a soft tissue density mass is appreciated or if there is erosion of the underlying bone. Computed tomography will help to localize the lesion in relation to normal anatomic structures, but the similar radiodensity of the mass to the surrounding muscle and connective tissues does not allow for differentiation of the mass from other soft tissue neoplasms. The classic description of the MRI signal characteristics of fibromatosis is of low signal intensity on both T1- and T2-weighted images. However, more recent reports have shown variability in the MRI signal characteristics that are probably related to the degree of cellularity within the lesion. More cellular lesions will demonstrate low signal intensity on T1-weighted images and a heterogeneous signal on T2-weighted images with the majority of the lesion having a signal intensity greater than that of surrounding muscle. Those lesions that are histologically more hypocellular are more likely to show low signal intensity on both sequences. Administration of gadolinium will typically demonstrate moderate enhancement, corresponding to the areas of increased cellularity.

Unless the lesion shows the classic low signal intensity on both T1- and T2-weighted MRI, the differential diagnosis is large, including soft tissue sarcomas.

On macroscopic examination, the cut surface of the tumor reveals a firm white to tan tissue resembling dense scar tissue. Microscopically, the lesion consists of bland spindle-shaped cells with little pleomorphism within an abundant collagen matrix. The matrix typically assumes a fascicular or whorling pattern of bundles of collagen. Examination of the spindle cells can show varying amounts of cellularity, but nuclear atypia or hyperchromatism is absent. (Fig. 50–22) Infiltration of surrounding skeletal muscle is common.

The primary treatment of aggressive fibromatosis is surgical excision. Because of its infiltrative nature, tumor boundaries are often difficult to assess and a large cuff of normal tissue may have to be sacrificed where surgically feasible to decrease the risk of local recurrence. Local recurrence rates are high (up to 90% of marginally excised lesions). In those cases in which pathological evaluation of the resected specimen reveals less than wide (marginal or intralesional) margins, postoperative radiation therapy has been shown to provide local control in 83% of cases at a radiation dose averaging 55 Gy. Radiation therapy has also been successful for recurrent and surgically inaccessible lesions.

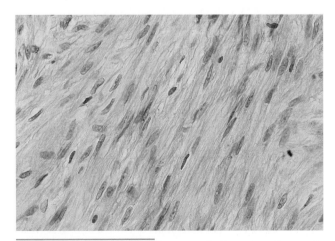

Figure 50–22 Aggressive fibromatosis demonstrating moderate hypercellularity and occasional mitoses. Note the lack of pleomorphism and nuclear atypia (400✕).

Neurogenic

Neurolemmoma and *neurofibroma* are the most common benign tumors of peripheral nerves. Both arise from benign proliferation of periaxonal Schwann cells that embryologically arise from the neural crest. Although the primary function of Schwann cells is to produce and maintain myelin, it has been shown that they also have the potential to produce collagen. This accounts for the collagen matrix seen in both neurolemmoma and neurofibroma. Although they share a common cell of origin, the clinical and morphologic findings separate the two as distinctly separate entities.

Neurolemmomas can be seen in patients of all ages, but they are most often found in young adults in the third to fifth decades of life. In the extremities, they are most commonly found on the flexor surfaces and have a predilection for the peroneal and ulnar nerves. The vast majority are solitary lesions, but rare cases of multiple neurolemmomas have been reported.

The clinical presentation is usually an asymptomatic mass that slowly enlarges over a period of months to years. Although they arise from the nerve sheath, neurological symptoms are unusual until they become so large that they compress the underlying nerve. On physical examination, a positive Tinel's sign with percussion over the mass is not uncommon.

The characteristics of neurolemmomas on MRI are a mass of low or intermediate signal intensity on T1-weighted images and highly intense signal on T2-weighted images. The neurolemmoma is usually located in intramuscular planes, sometimes associated with a large peripheral nerve. Occasionally, a heterogeneous signal can be seen on T2-weighted images corresponding to the variable cellularity between cellular (Antoni A) and myxoid (Antoni B) areas. Plain radiographs are generally not helpful in establishing a diagnosis. The exception is when there is gross foraminal widening of an intervertebral space, suggesting a peripheral nerve sheath tumor.

The differential diagnosis includes neurofibroma, reactive lymph nodes, GCT of tendon sheath, PVNS, and soft tissue sarcoma.

Macroscopically, neurolemmomas are truly encapsulated by the epineurium overlying the lesion and nerve fibers. They are typically fusiform in shape and eccentric in relation to the underlying nerve. Although fascicles of nerve fibers may be splayed over the lesion, infiltration of the nerve is not typical, and the lesion can usually be marginally "shelled out" of the nerve after the epineurium is incised. The cut surface of the lesion is white to yellow in color, and areas of cystic degeneration may be seen in large neurolemmomas. Microscopically, the classic finding in neurolemmomas is a biphasic pattern of alternating Antoni A and Antoni B areas (Fig. 50–23). The Antoni A areas are characterized by compact cellular areas of spindle cells arranged in pallisading or whorling patterns. Verocay bodies are commonly formed in Antoni A areas by the parallel alignment of rows of nuclei with cytoplasmic streaming between the rows of nuclei. Antoni B areas are characterized by hypocellular areas of spindle cells within an unorganized, loosely arranged collagen and myxoid matrix.

Treatment of neurolemmomas consists of marginal surgical excision. Overlying nerve fibers can usually easily be

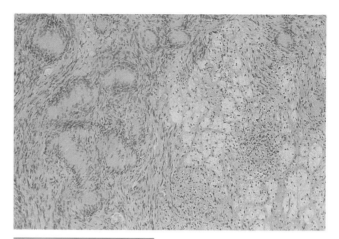

Figure 50–23 Biphasic pattern of cellular (Antoni A) and myxoid (Antoni B) areas typical of neurolemmoma. Verocay bodies can be seen in the Antoni A areas (100×).

mobilized and preserved as the lesion is marginally shelled out. Recurrence following marginal excision is rare.

Neurofibroma, like neurolemmoma, usually presents during young adulthood and peaks in incidence during the third and fourth decades. In contrast to neurolemmomas, the majority of neurofibromas arise within the subcutaneous tissue, are most commonly found within cutaneous sensory nerves, and are equally distributed over flexor and extensor surfaces. They may present as solitary lesions or as multiple lesions in association with neurofibromatosis (von Recklinghausen's disease), but the majority are solitary. The clinical findings are similar to those seen with many other benign soft tissue lesions; that is, an asymptomatic mass. In the case of neurofibromatosis, the usual subcutaneous location along with other easily visible manifestations of the disease such as café-au-lait spots, axillary freckling, or Lisch nodules in the iris of the eye.

Like other benign peripheral nerve sheath tumors, neurofibromas typically manifest as low to intermediate signal lesions on T1-weighted images. A characteristic "target" appearance has been described on T2-weighted images with a peripheral high signal intensity area surrounding a central low signal intensity core. This appearance has also been described for neurolemmomas, to a lesser degree. This zoning phenomenon correlates histologically with a more myxoid stroma peripherally and a more cellular, fibrous center. Administration of gadolinium will typically result in enhancement of the central area on T2-weighted images.

The differential diagnosis is similar to that of neurolemmoma and includes reactive lymph nodes, GCT of tendon sheath, PVNS, and soft tissue sarcoma.

Macroscopically, the typical neurofibroma presents as a centrally located fusiform mass within a peripheral nerve. In contrast to the usual eccentric location of neurolemmomas, in neurofibromas the nerve typically appears to enter and exit the lesion. Infiltration of the tumor around individual nerve fascicles is more common than with neurolemmoma, making excision with preservation of nerve fascicles more difficult. Plexiform neurofibromas, a subtype of neurofibroma usually

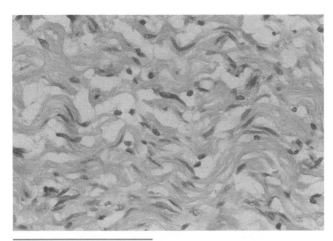

Figure 50–24 Neurofibroma demonstrating the typical pattern of loosely arranged wavy collagen, myxoid stroma, and wavy nuclei (400×).

seen in association with neurofibromatosis, appear as irregularly shaped, wormian masses that extend over large segments of a nerve. Microscopically, neurofibromas consist of spindle cells with elongated wavy nuclei within a loosely arranged, wavy collagen and myxoid stroma (Fig. 50–24). They can occasionally appear quite cellular but can be differentiated from neurolemmoma by their lack of the biphasic Antoni A and B areas classically seen with that lesion.

As with neurolemmoma, the treatment of neurofibroma is by marginal surgical excision. However, because of the more infiltrative nature of the lesion, it is often more difficult to free the tumor from the intertwined nerve fascicles. The risk of malignant transformation of neurolemmomas or solitary neurofibromas is exceedingly rare. In contrast, malignant transformation of neurofibromas in the face of neurofibromatosis is well documented. Most reports estimate the risk of malignant transformation in the range of 10% of patients with neurofibromatosis, but according to data collected by Enzinger and Weiss (1995) this estimate is more likely to be around 2%. Clinical symptoms leading to suspicion of malignant transformation include rapid enlargement of a neurofibroma and pain, along with a history of longstanding disease. Five-year survival in this setting has been estimated at 20% or less.

Lipogenic

Lipomas and other benign lipomatous tumors are the most common soft tissue neoplasms. They commonly present during middle age, and most studies report a slight male predominance. Superficial lipomas are commonly located on the trunk, shoulder girdle, and thigh. Deep and intramuscular lipomas are far less common. They are typically much larger than superficial lipomas at initial presentation due to their subfascial location. Deep lipomas are also sometimes referred to as atypical lipomas.

Most lipomas begin as a painless, slow growing mass. Neurologic symptoms may be present if nerve compression occurs. An example is a radial nerve palsy (the posterior interosseous portion) resulting from a deep lipoma around the neck of the proximal radius. Lipomas generally have a soft consistency on palpation, although deep lipomas may feel more firm as they increase volume within a fascial space.

PEARL

Deep (atypical) lipomas in the proximal forearm may present as a soft tissue mass with a posterior interosseous nerve palsy.

As opposed to most soft tissue neoplasms, radiographs of lipomas can often confirm the diagnosis. Plain radiographs will often reveal a mass with the same radiodensity as subcutaneous fat. This is more easily appreciated in the case of intramuscular lipomas, in which the radiodensity of the surrounding muscle contrasts with that of the lipoma. This isodensity with the subcutaneous fat is easily seen on CT. Similarly, MRI will show a homogenous signal with the same intensity as subcutaneous fat; that is, high signal intensity on T1-weighted images and intermediate signal on T2-weighted images (Fig. 50–25). Any heterogeneity of the MRI signal within the lesion should alert the clinician of the potential of malignancy. There is negligible enhancement following administration of gadolinium.

With adequate imaging, the differential diagnosis is usually limited to benign lipogenic tumors.

Macroscopically, lipomas present as a multilobular, soft, encapsulated mass with a yellow or tan color. Microscopically, they are made of mature adipocytes with small, uniform nuclei (Fig. 50–25c). A delicate vascular network runs between the adipocytes in the interstitial spaces.

Treatment of both superficial and deep lipomas should be individualized. Asymptomatic lesions confirmed by CT or MRI to be lipomas may be observed clinically. For large intramuscular lipomas, symptomatic lesions, or those cosmetically unacceptable to the patient marginal excision is the treatment

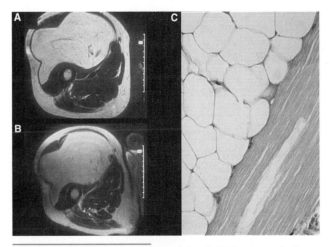

Figure 50–25 T1 **(A)** and T2-weighted **(B)** images of a large lipoma of the thigh. Note the identical signal intensity as the subcutaneous fat in both sequences. **(C)** Mature fat cells encasing skeletal muscle fibers within the lipoma (400×).

of choice. Recurrence rates have been reported to be 5% or less for superficial lesions and up to 15% for large intramuscular lipomas. Heterogeneity of the density or signal intensity on CT or MRI, respectively, can be due to hemorrhage, calcification, central necrosis, entrapped muscle fibers, or may indicate malignancy. If the etiology of the heterogenous signal remains in question, these lesions should be biopsied, resected, or watched very carefully.

Angiolipoma is an uncommon benign lipomatous neoplasm. In contrast to the middle-age presentation of typical lipomas, patients with angiolipomas usually present in early adulthood. Angiolipomas also have an unusual predilection for the forearm and are commonly multicentric.

The clinical presentation is usually dominated by complaints of pain that seem out of proportion to the limited findings on physical examination. The mass is usually small (less than a few centimeters) and may be exquisitely tender to palpation.

Macroscopically, the angiolipoma appears similar to the typical lipoma with the exception of an occasional reddish tint. Microscopically, the lesion consists of mature adipocytes mixed with areas of cellular, thin vascular channels. The vascular network is much more prominent than that seen in the typical benign lipoma. In addition, multiple thrombi can often be seen within the vascular channels.

The cause of the pain seen with angiolipomas is unknown. However, symptoms are usually relieved following surgical excision. Marginal excision is the treatment of choice.

Vascular

Hemangiomas are one of the most common benign soft tissue tumors. They account for 7% of vascular lesions. Hemangiomas are characterized by increased numbers of both normal and abnormal blood vessels. They have been classified into capillary and cavernous types among others, but because of their common cell origin and microscopic appearance they fall into the broad definition of hemangioma. Lesions are most commonly found superficially on the head and neck but may be seen anywhere. The peak in incidence is during the first decade of life, most commonly at birth or early infancy.

Superficial hemangiomas are red/purple masses present at birth or, more commonly, shortly thereafter. They enlarge quickly over a period of several months before tending toward slow resolution. Of more interest to the orthopaedic surgeon is the deep or intramuscular hemangiomas. Much less common than superficial lesions, intramuscular hemangiomas tend to be incidentally noticed during childhood as an asymptomatic mass or one associated with dull, intermittent pain. In postmenarchal females, the pain may vary in intensity in relation to the menstrual cycle. On palpation they have a soft, doughy consistency. When suspected, a useful diagnostic test is to assess changes in the size of the lesion with the limb elevated and in a dependent position.

Radiographically, phleboliths are commonly seen and help to establish the diagnosis. (Fig. 50–26). In the past, angiography was a useful, albeit invasive imaging technique revealing the highly vascular nature of the lesion. Magnetic resonance imaging has become a more favorable means of evaluation. On T1-weighted images, the lesion has a low to

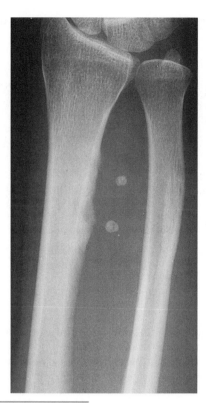

Figure 50–26   Hemangioma of the distal forearm. Note the cortical irregularity of the distal radius and the phleboliths in the soft tissue.

intermediate signal intensity often similar to the surrounding muscle. On T2-weighted images, they appear as areas of very high intensity signal. This is due to pools of slowly flowing blood with a signal intensity of muscle or fat.

The differential diagnosis includes the more rare but malignant forms of vascular tumors such as hemangioendothelioma, hemangiopericytoma, and angiosarcoma.

Microscopically, hemangiomas consist of masses of capillary-sized vascular channels (capillary hemangioma) or a mixture of capillary and larger-sized vessels (cavernous hemangioma). They are often mixed with striated muscle fibers and can contain a variable amount of fat.

The treatment of deep or intramuscular hemangiomas should be individualized. Because of the high rate of local recurrence, up to 50% in some studies, hemangiomas should be followed. For symptomatic lesions refractory to conservative treatment, surgical excision may be attempted in spite of the high risk of local recurrence.

Glomus tumor is a rare, benign perivascular tumor with predilection for the subungual regions of the fingers. The normal glomus body assists in thermoregulation by limiting blood flow through arteriovenous anastamoses in the dermis via modified smooth muscle cells. Glomus bodies are commonly found in the digits and palms. After subungual lesions, other sites affected by glomus tumors include elsewhere on the digits, palm, forearm, and foot. They represent less than 2% of all soft tissue lesions.

Glomus tumors present with severe, episodic pain exacerbated by tactile stimulation and cold. Once the tumor is located, the complaints seem out of proportion to the appearance of the lesion. The lesions are usually quite small (millimeters) and are red or blue in color. When located subungually, a nail deformity may be present.

The value of radiographic imaging is limited. Plain radiographs may show scalloping of the dorsal cortex of the distal phalanx if the tumor is beneath the nail bed (subungual). Magnetic resonance imaging is nonspecific but may show a lesion high signal intensity on T2-weighted images.

The differential diagnosis is limited to other subungual lesions such as malignant melanoma and subungual hematoma. History and examination are usually pathognomonic for the tumor.

Microscopically, the glomus tumor appears as a well circumscribed collection of capillaries encased by glomus cells. The glomus cells are characterized by their plump, rounded shape and round, central nuclei surrounded by eosinophilic cytoplasm.

Glomus tumors are treated with wide or marginal excision. Recurrence rates are 10% or less, and the resolution of symptoms is usually dramatic and immediate.

Pseudotumorous Conditions

Synovial chondromatosis is a rare benign cartilaginous lesion of large joints. Controversy exists as to whether this is a true neoplasm or an aberrant expression of normal, pleuripotent mesenchymal cells. It tends to be monoarticular and commonly affects the knee. Other large joints such as the hip, shoulder, and elbow may be involved. The process is not limited to large joints as evidenced by reports of synovial chondromatosis of the hand and tenosynovium. The condition is most commonly seen in young adults in the third and fourth decades of life. The etiology of the condition appears to be aberrant differentiation of mesenchymal cells within the synovial lining into chondroblasts. As they grow beneath the synovial lining of the joint, they protrude into the joint, connected by a thin synovial stalk. They may detach from the synovium to form loose bodies. The loose bodies continue to grow, obtaining nutrition from the surrounding synovial fluid. When they reach a sufficiently large size, the central chondrocytes lose access to the synovial fluid by diffusion and become necrotic. The necrotic cartilage calcifies. It is at this point that the loose bodies become visible on plain radiographs. Those lesions that become vascularized within the synovium may undergo enchondral ossification. Malignant degeneration of synovial chondromatosis into chondrosarcoma has been reported but is extremely rare.

The clinical presentation consists of intermittent "locking" or "catching" of the joint, pain, and loss of motion.

Radiographs obtained early in the course of the process may be entirely normal. Arthrography obtained at that time may reveal multiple filling defects in the areas of the uncalcified cartilage nodules. Once the nodules calcify or ossify they become readily apparent on plain radiographs. Spur formation and joint-space narrowing may be apparent illustrating associated degenerative joint disease. Magnetic resonance imaging can be quite nonspecific until loose bodies detach from the synovium.

The differential diagnosis includes multiple osteocartilaginous loose bodies. With adequate imaging and clinical history the diagnosis is seldom in question.

Microscopically, nests of moderately hypercellular but benign cartilage of various sizes can be seen within the synovial lining. Loose bodies also have the appearance of active cartilage with varying amounts of central calcification.

Treatment of synovial chondromatosis is directed toward removal of the existing nodules and loose bodies as well as their source, the synovium. Recurrence rates are low, and when it does occur it is easily managed. Arthroplasty is indicated when there is advanced joint degeneration.

Ganglion cysts are among the most common pseudotumorous lesion. The most common location is the dorsum of the wrist overlying the scapholunate joint. The second most common location is the palmar aspect of the wrist, just ulnar to the radial artery. Ganglion cysts are most commonly noted in early adulthood. The etiology of the lesion is mucoid degeneration of connective tissue or mucin production by surrounding fibroblasts.

Ganglion cysts present as a mass that may or may not be tender. The pain associated with dorsal ganglions has been attributed to compression of the terminal branches of the posterior interosseous nerve. The size of the lesion fluctuates. On examination, ganglion cysts may feel boggy or firm and transilluminate light.

Magnetic resonance imaging is usually unnecessary for superficial cysts. For deep lesions that cannot be diagnosed on examination, MRI will show a low signal intensity on T1-weighted images and homogenous hyperintensity on T2-weighted images.

Microscopically, the lesion is a thick-walled, cystic space containing myxoid debris. Mucin may be found outside the confines of the cyst wall.

Treatment of ganglion cysts is directed toward aspirating or excising the symptomatic lesion. Surgical aspiration with or without injection of corticosteroids has been reported to have varying success. In general, the recurrence rate is high. Open excision reduces the recurrence rate significantly. "Unroofing" the capsule or tendon sheath under the lesion is recommended to fully remove the nidus of mucoid production.

Myositis ossificans is a common pseudotumorous condition often related to trauma. Atraumatic forms, sometimes referred to as "pseudomalignant" myositis ossificans, can also occur. The condition most often affects adolescents and young adults, with a male predominance. The most common location for myositis ossificans in the lower extremity is the quadriceps muscle. In the upper extremity the brachialis muscle is most commonly affected.

The clinical presentation is related to a specific traumatic event in most cases. The pain associated with the initial injury is followed by swelling in the area. Within several weeks the swollen area becomes discreet and firm or indurated. The mass slowly hardens over the next several weeks; often to a distinct, hard mass.

Initial radiographs obtained after injury may show no abnormality. Serial radiographs taken as the condition develops will show faint areas of soft tissue ossification progressing to mature trabecular bone. This may occur over the span of weeks to months. The ossification proceeds from the periphery of the lesion towards the center. This "zoning phenomenon" can also be appreciated histologically. Computed tomography will help define the peripheral zone of ossification as the lesion matures (Fig. 50–27). Magnetic resonance imaging of early (preossification) lesions will show a heterogenous, intermediate to high signal intensity lesion with surrounding soft tissue edema. This appearance is also consistent with many soft tissue sarcomas for which myositis ossificans can be mistaken early in its development.

The differential diagnosis of myositis ossificans includes extraskeletal osteosarcoma. The radiographs, MRI, and histologic appearance of myositis ossificans may look remarkably similar to extraskeletal osteosarcoma early in the course of the condition. With maturation of the lesion, however, the typical peripherally mature zoning phenomenon becomes evident. In contrast, extraskeletal osteosarcoma typically presents with a reversal of the zoning phenomenon, with more mature areas located centrally and more immature areas peripherally.

Microscopically, the zoning phenomenon of myositis ossificans is clearly evident. The ossification at the periphery of the lesion is mature trabecular bone. The interior of the lesion contains immature mesenchymal cells and fibroblasts, often with moderate pleomorphism and frequent mitoses. This can be easily mistaken for a sarcoma.

The most important aspect of the treatment of myositis ossificans is to recognize the lesion and question the patient carefully about any history of trauma. Once the diagnosis is suspected, serial radiographs or CT will usually reveal the zoning phenomenon of ossification. Biopsy of the lesion early in its development or of its central portion may lead to the erroneous diagnosis of a soft tissue sarcoma because of its immature histologic appearance. If the patient continues to be symptomatic (pain, restricted range of motion) from the lesion after its maturation, surgical excision may be performed. Surgical intervention prior to maturation of the lesion will lead to high recurrence rates.

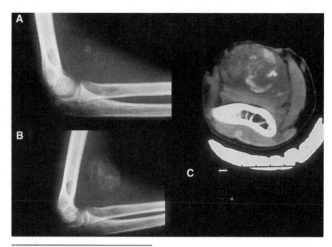

Figure 50–27   Initial radiograph **(A)** and radiograph taken 5 days later **(B)** show the rapid ossification often seen in myositis ossificans. **(C)** CT scan of the lesion seen. Note the peripheral ossification pattern.

PEARL

Myositis ossificans is characterized by mature bone on the periphery and immature bone in the center. An extra-osseous osteosarcoma has the opposite appearance.

PITFALL

Do not rule out myositis ossificans if ossification is not seen on plain radiographs. Early lesions may not show ossification until maturity.

Tumoral calcinosis is an unusual pseudotumorous condition of soft tissue calcification. Affected individuals are usually children or young adults. The disorder is often associated with mild hyperphosphatemia. Calcium levels, however, are normal. The soft tissue calcification usually occurs in the periarticular regions of the shoulder, hip, and elbow.

Tumoral calcinosis usually presents with painless, firm masses that occur around large joints and are firmly attached to the underlying soft tissues.

Radiographically, tumoral calcinosis appears as heavily calcified round or amorphous masses around large joints.

The differential diagnosis includes other diseases associated with soft tissue calcification such as chronic renal disease, hyperparathyroidism, hypervitaminosis D, and milk-alkali syndrome.

SELECTED BIBLIOGRAPHY

Bone

Osteogenic Lesions

HEALEY JH, GHELMAN B. Osteoid osteoma and osteoblastoma: current concepts and recent advances. *Clin Orth.* 1986;204: 76–85.

UNNI KK. Benign Osteoblastoma. In: *Dahlin's Bone Tumors: General Aspects and Data on 11,087 Cases.* Philadelphia, PA: Lippincott-Raven; 1996:131–143.

Chondrogenic Lesions

BORIANI S, BACCHINI P, BERTONI F, CAMPANACCI M. Periosteal chondroma: A review of 20 cases. *J Bone Jt Surg* .1983;65A: 205–212.

RAHIMI A, BEABOUT JW, IVINS JC, DAHLIN DC. Chondromyxoid fibroma: a clinicopathologic study of 76 cases. *Cancer.* 1972;30:726–736.

ROCKWELL MA, SAITER ET, ENNEKING WF. Periosteal chondroma. *J Bone Jt Surg.* 1972;54A:102–108.

SCARBOROUGH MT, MOREAU G. Benign cartilage tumors. *Orthop Clin North Am.* 1996;27:583–589.

SPRINGFIELD DS, CAPANNA R, GHERLINZONI F, PICCI P, CAMPANACCI M. Chondroblastoma: a review of 70 cases. *J Bone Jt Surg.* 1995;67A:748–755.

WEATHERALL PT, MAALE GE, MENDELSOHN DB, SHERRY CS, ERDMAN WE, PASCOE HR. Chondroblastoma: classic and confusing appearance at MR imaging. *Radiology.* 1994;190: 467–474.

ZILLMER DA, DORFMAN HD. Chondrmyxoid fibroma of bone: 36 cases with clinicopathologic correlation. *Human Pathology.* 1989;20:952–964.

Eosinophilic Granuloma

BROADBENT V, EGELER RM, NESBIT ME Jr. Langerhans cell histiocytosis: clinical and epidemiologic aspects. *Br J Cancer.* 1994;23:S11-6.

MIRRA JM, PICCI P, GOLD RH. Histiocytoses. In: *Bone Tumors.* Philadelphia, PA: Lea and Febiger; 1989:1023–1060.

Lesions of Uncertain Origin

BERTONI F, BACCHINI R, CAPANNA R, RUGGIERI P, BIAGINI R, FERRUZZI A, et al. Solid variant of aneurysmal bone cyst. *Cancer.* 1993;71:729–734.

BIESECKER JL, MARCOVE RC, HUVOS AG, MIKE V. Aneurysmal bone cyst: a clinicopathologic study of 66 cases. *Cancer.* 1970;26:615–625.

CAPANNA R, CAMPANACCI DA, MANFRINI M. Unicameral and aneurysmal bone cysts. *Orthop Clin North Am.* 1996;27: 605–614.

DAGHER AP, MAGID D, JOHNSON CA, MCCARTHY EF Jr, FISHMAN EK. Aneurysmal bone cyst developing after anterior cruciate ligament injury and repair. *AJR.* 1992;158:1289–1291.

ENNEKING WF. Lesions of uncertain origin originating in bone. In: *Musculoskeletal Tumor Surgery.* New York, NY: Churchill Livingstone; 1983:1494–1512.

JAFFE HL, LICHTENSTEIN L. Solitary unicameral bone cyst with emphasis on the roentgen picture, the pathologic appearance, and the pathogenesis. *Arch Surg.* 1992;44:1004–1025.

LEVY WM, MILLER AS, BONAKDARPOUR A, AGEGERTER E. Aneurysmal bone cyst secondary to other lesions: report of 57 cases. *Am J Clin Pathol.* 1975;63:1–8.

LICHTENSTEIN L. Aneurysmal bone cyst: observations on 50 cases. *J Bone Jt Surg* 1957;39A:873–882.

RUITER DJ, VAN RIJSSEL T, VAN DER VELDE E. Aneurysmal bone cyst: a clinicopathologic study of 105 cases. *Cancer.* 1977;39:2231.

SZENDROI M, CSER I, et al. Aneurysmal bone cyst: a review of 52 primary and 16 secondary cases. *Arch Orthop Trauma Surg.* 1992;116:318–322.

WILLIAMS RR, DAHLIN DC, GHORMLEY RK. Giant cell tumor of bone. *Cancer.* 1954;7:764–773.

Soft Tissue
Fibromatoses

BARBER HM, GALASKO CSB, WOODS CG. Multicentric extra-abdominal desmoid tumors: report of 2 cases. *J Bone Jt Surg.* 1973;55B:858–863.

ENZINGER FM, WEISS SW. Fibromatoses. In: *Soft Tissue Tumors.* St. Louis, MO: CV Mosby; 1995:201–229.

HARTMANN WH, COWAN WR. Tumors of the soft tissues, lattes, raffaele. *AFIP: Atlas of Tumor Pathology.* Armed Forces Institute of Pathology; 1982.

HAWNAUR JM, JENKINS JPR, ISHERWOOD, I. Magnetic resonance imaging of musculoaponeurotic fibromatosis. *Skeletal Radiol.* 1990;19:509–514.

MCCOLLOUGH WM, PARSONS JT, VAN DER GRIEND R, ENNEKING WF. Radiation therapy for aggressive fibromatosis. *J Bone Jt Surg.* 1991;73A:717–725.

ROCK MG, PRITCHARD DJ, REIMAN HM, SOULE EH, BREWSTER RC. Extra-abdominal desmoid tumors. *J Bone Jt Surg.* 1984;66A:1369–1374.

SUNDARAM M, DUFFRIN H, MCGUIRE MH, VAS W. Synchronous multicentric desmoid tumors (aggressive fibromatosis) of the extremities. *Skeletal Radiol.* 1988;17:16–19.

SUNDARAM M, MCGUIRE MH, SCHAJOWICZ F. Soft tissue masses: histologic basis for decreased signal (short T2) on T2-weighted MRI images. *AJR.* 1987;148:1247–1250.

Benign Neurogenic Tumors

ASBURY AK, JOHNSON PC. Pathology of peripheral nerve. In: *Major Problems in Pathology.* Philadelphia, PA: WB Saunders; 1978:22–23.

CEROFOLINI E, LANDI A, DESANTIS G, MAIORANA A, CANOSSI G, ROMAGNOLI R. MR of benign peripheral nerve sheath tumors. *J Comput Assist Tomogr.* 1991;15:593–597.

CHURCH RL, TANZER M, PFEIFFER SE. Collagen and procollagen production by a clonal line of Schwann cells. *Proc Natl Acad Sci USA.* 1973;70:1943–1946.

ENZINGER FM, WEISS SW. Benign tumors of peripheral nerves. In: *Soft Tissue Tumors.* St. Louis, MO: CV Mosby; 1995: 821–888.

GUCCION JG, ENZINGER FM. Malignant schwannoma associated with von Recklinghausen's neurofibromatosis. *Virchows Arch A, Pathological Anatomy and Histology.* 1979; 383:43–57.

PURCELL SM, DIXON SL. Schwannomatosis: an unusual variant of neurofibromatosis or a distinct clinical entity? *Arch Dermatol.* 1989;125:390–393.

SUH JS, ABENOZA P, GALLOWAY HR, EVERSON LI, GRIFFITHS HJ. Peripheral (extracranial) nerve tumors: correlation of MR imaging and histologic findings. *Radiology.* 1992;183: 341–346.

Benign Lipogenic Tumors

ADAIR FE, PACK GT, FARRIER JH. Lipomas. *Am J Cancer*. 1932;16:1104–1120.

DOOMS GC, HRICAK H, SOLLITTO RA, HIGGINS CB. Lipomatous tumors and tumors with fatty components: MR imaging potential and comparison of MR and CT results. *Radiology*. 1985;157:479–483.

ENZINGER FM. Benign lipomatous tumors simulating a sarcoma. In: *Management of Primary Bone and Soft Tissue Tumors*. St. Louis, MO: CV Mosby; 1977:11–24.

ENZINGER FM, WEISS SW. Benign lipomatous tumors. In: *Soft Tissue Tumors*. St. Louis, MO: CV Mosby; 1995:381–430.

RYDHOLM A, BERG NO. Size, site, and clinical incidence of lipoma: factors in differential diagnosis of lipoma and sarcoma. *Acta Orthop Scand*. 1983;54:929–934.

Benign Vascular Tumors

BEHAM A, FLETCHER CDM. Intramuscular angioma: a clinicopathologic analysis of 74 cases. *Histopathology*. 1991; 18:53–59.

ENZINGER FM, WEISS SW. Benign tumors and tumorlike lesions of blood vessels. In: *Soft Tissue Tumors*. St. Louis, MO: CV Mosby; 1995:579–626.

ENZINGER FM, WEISS SW. Perivascular tumors. In: *Soft Tissue Tumors*. St. Louis, MO: CV Mosby; 1995:701–733.

GREENSPAN A, McGAHAN JP, VOGELSANG P, SZABO RM. Imaging strategies in the evaluation of soft-tissue hemangiomas of the extremities: correlation of finding on plain radiography, CT, MRI, and ultrasonography in 12 histologically proven cases. *Skeletal Radiol*. 1992;21:11–18.

SHUGART RR, SOULE EH, JOHNSON EW. Glomus tumor. *Surg Gynecol Obstet*. 1963;117:334–340.

TSUNEYOSHI M, ENJOJI M. Glomus tumor: a clinicopathologic and electron microscopic study. *Cancer*. 1982;50:1601–1607.

Pseudotumorous Lesions

BERTONI F, UNNI KK, BEABOUT JW. Chondrosarcomas of the synovium. *Cancer*. 1991;67:155–162.

CAMPANACCI M. Synovial chondromatosis. In: *Bone and Soft Tissue Tumors*. New York, NY: Springer-Verlag; 1990: 1087–1097.

ENZINGER FM, WEISS SW. Benign soft tissue tumors of uncertain type. In: *Soft Tissue Tumors*. St. Louis, MO: CV Mosby; 1995:1039–1093.

ENZINGER FM, WEISS SW. Osseous soft tissue tumors. In: *Soft Tissue Tumors*. St. Louis, MO: CV Mosby; 1995:1013–1037.

MINSINGER WE, BALOGH K, MILLENDER LH. Tenosynovial osteochondroma of the hand: a case report and brief review. *Clin Orthop*. 1985;196:248–252.

SAMPLE QUESTIONS

1. Osteoid osteoma is characterized by all of the following except:
   (a) pain at rest
   (b) radiodense nidus with radiolucent rim
   (c) osteoid lined with osteoclasts and osteoblasts
   (d) persistant symptoms without surgical intervention
   (e) vascular stroma

2. Which of the following are characteristic of chondroblastoma:
   (a) epiphyseal lesion
   (b) multinucleated giant cells
   (c) "chicken-wire" calcification
   (d) a and c
   (e) a, b, and c

3. Multinucleated giant cells are found in which of the following lesions:
   (a) aneurysmal bone cyst
   (b) GCT
   (c) nonossifying fibroma
   (d) a and b
   (e) a, b, and c

4. Which of the following are associated with fibrous dysplasia:
   (a) brown skin patches
   (b) central lucent lesion with ground glass appearance
   (c) immature woven bone in collagen-rich stroma
   (d) pathological fractures
   (e) all of the above

5. Which of the following are capable of malignant degeneration:
   (a) neurofibromas in patient with neurofibromatosis
   (b) GCT of tendon sheath
   (c) multiple hereditary exostoses
   (d) a and c
   (e) all of the above

Chapter 51

Malignant Lesions of the Musculoskeletal System

Richard Lackman, MD

Outline

Etiology

Basic Science
Histology of Malignant Lesions of Bone and Soft Tissue

Anatomy and Surgical Approaches
Tumor Anatomy
Patterns of Metastasis
Surgical Approaches

Evaluation

Aids to Diagnosis
Plain Radiographs
Nuclear Medicine Scans
Computed Tomography Scans
Magnetic Resonance Imaging
Biopsy Techniques

Specific Conditions, Treatment, and Outcome
Osteosarcoma
Ewing's Sarcoma
Chondrosarcoma
Multiple Myeloma
Soft Tissue Sarcoma

Selected Bibliography

Sample Questions

Malignant tumors of soft tissue and bone are unusual. Accurate diagnosis is facilitated by the ability to recognize patterns of clinical presentation, radiographic features, and histology. Incisional biopsy through a longitudinal incision is the standard of care for most lesions. Recent chemotherapy protocols have permitted the use of limb salvage techniques where previously the only option was amputation.

ETIOLOGY

The cause of malignant musculoskeletal tumors remains a mystery. Hereditary tumors such as neurofibromatosis exist, but most tumors of connective tissue have no inherited genetic basis. Environmental factors are difficult to implicate and have never been clearly demonstrated as a cause of these lesions. Following the experience of the United States Military during the Vietnam War, Agent Orange was investigated as a possible link to the onset of soft tissue tumors in exposed soldiers, but no clear relationship was established.

Radiation, whether environmental or iatrogenic is a known cause of sarcoma formation including an association with osteosarcoma in bone and malignant fibrous histiocytoma in soft tissues.

BASIC SCIENCE

Histology of Malignant Lesions of Bone and Soft Tissue

Histological recognition of bone and soft tissue tumors is less complex than commonly thought and is facilitated by an understanding of the patterns that help define histological classification.

Bone

In bone forming lesions, it is important to understand that the presence of rimming osteoblasts on woven bone indicates that the woven bone is reactive such as seen in myositis ossificans (Fig. 51–1). The presence of woven bone in a lesion with no osteoblastic rimming indicates a neoplasm. Among neoplasms, it is the nature of the cells that constitute the fibrous

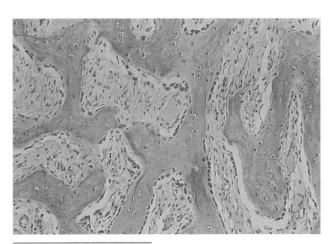

Figure 51–1 Osteoblastic rimming of the trabeculae of woven bone signifies a reactive lesion such as fracture callus or myositis ossificans.

831

Orthopaedic Surgery: The Essentials. Edited by M.E. Baratz, A.D. Watson, and J.E. Imbriglia. Thieme Medical Publishers, Inc., New York © 1999

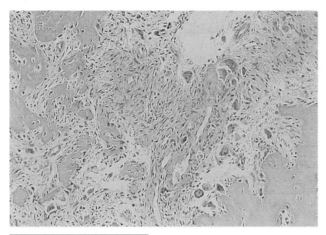

Figure 51–2 Woven bone with a benign, spindle cell stroma indicates a benign bone forming neoplasm such as osteoid osteoma, osteoblastoma, or fibrous dysplasia.

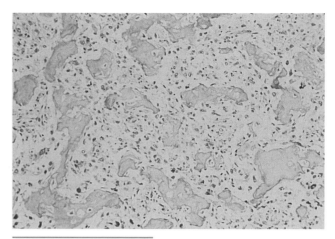

Figure 51–3 Osteosarcoma is defined by the presence of a malignant, spindle cell stroma that produces woven bone.

stroma that separates benign from malignant lesions. Benign osseous neoplasms, such as fibrous dysplasia, osteoid osteoma, and osteoblastoma, have a benign-appearing population of stromal cells. Benign stromal cells are homogeneous in size, shape, and staining, with an absence of mitoses and necrosis (Fig. 51–2). Malignant lesions such as osteosarcoma have stromal cells with heterogeneous size, shape, and staining, as well as the presence of mitoses and necrosis (Fig. 51–3).

PEARL

Osteoblasts rimming woven bone is characteristic of reactive bone. Woven bone without osteoblasts rimming is characteristic of neoplasms.

Cartilage

Cartilage tumors show three distinct patterns. The first is the spectrum of histological change from benign enchondroma to high-grade chondrosarcoma. Enchondromas are painless lesions with cartilaginous calcification but no cortical or intramedullary erosion on plain radiographs. Chondrosarcomas are painful and have intralesional lysis, endosteal scalloping, and cortical thinning or expansion on radiographs. The classification of cartilage as benign or malignant depends on the appearance of the two components of cartilage, cells, and matrix. Benign cartilage has few cells situated 1 cell per lacuna with small, eccentric nuclei and abundant, uniform matrix.

The changes associated with low-grade malignant cartilage include increased cellularity, large plump cell nuclei, and occasional binucleate cells. In addition, there may be more than one cell in many lacunar spaces, as well as cells lying outside of lacunae (Fig. 51–4). As these changes progress, the matrix typically becomes less uniform and more irregular. All of these changes are more exaggerated in progressively higher grade chondrosarcomas (Fig. 51–5).

The second pattern of cartilage lesions is that seen in chondroblastoma. These lesions have polygonal "cobble-stone"

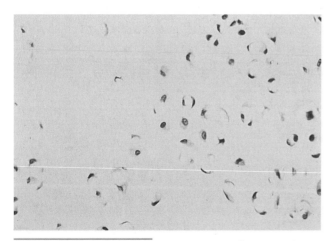

Figure 51–4 The upper left quadrant of this slide shows benign appearing cartilage with rare picnotic cells and abundant chondroid matrix. The other three quadrants of this slide show the hallmarks of low-grade malignant cartilage that include plump cells, binucleate cells, cells outside lacunar spaces, and lacunae with more than one cell.

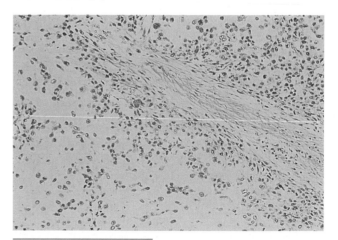

Figure 51–5 High grade of chondrosarcoma show increased cellularity with less and less normal chondroid matrix.

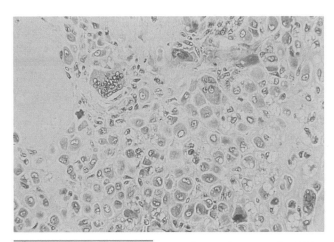

Figure 51–6 Chondroblastoma shows the typical cobblestone cells associated with chondroid matrix.

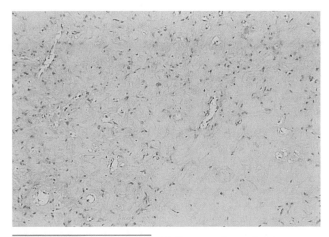

Figure 51–7 Chondromyxoid fibroma shows benign, spindle cells intermixed with areas of immature chondroid matrix.

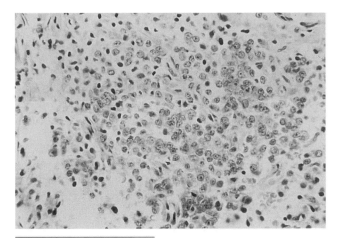

Figure 51–8 Ewing's sarcoma shows the presence of uniform, round cells with indistinct cell borders.

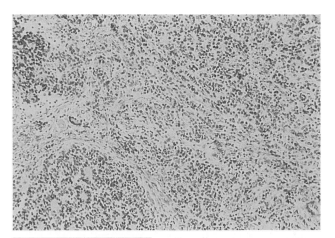

Figure 51–9 Neuroblastoma shows cells that look similar to those seen in Ewing's sarcoma but also contains rings of these cells about pink amorphous material called "pseudo-rosettes."

cells with "chicken-wire" calcification and chondroid matrix (Fig. 51–6).

The third is that pattern, seen in chondromyxoid fibroma which contains fibroblastic stromal cells with varying areas of chondroid matrix and loosely arranged myxoid regions (Fig. 51–7).

Round Cell Tumors

Round cell lesions are another distinct group of primary bone lesions. Each time a round cell infiltrate is noted, the differential diagnosis includes infection, inflammatory condition, Langerhan's cell histiocytosis, primary round cell tumor and small round cell metastatic carcinoma. Bacterial infections are typically associated with the presence of polymorphonucleocytes, as well as a mixed infiltrate of lymphocytes and plasma cells. Langerhan's cell histiocytosis is diagnosed by the presence of histiocytes in combination with variable numbers of eosinophils. Eosinophils are recognized by their bilobed nuclei and abundant red cytoplasm.

Primary round cell tumors of bone include mainly Ewing's sarcoma (Fig. 51–8) and neuroblastoma (Fig. 51–9) in children and plasmacytoma (Fig. 51–10) and lymphoma

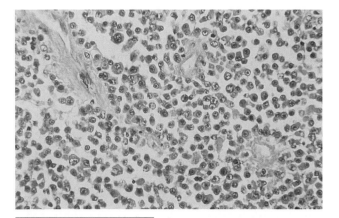

Figure 51–10 Plasmacytoma (myeloma) lesions demonstrate uniform sheets of plasma cells, which are indentified by their large dark nucleus and eccentric red cytoplasm.

(Fig. 51–11) in adults. Small round cell metastatic carcinomas must also be considered whenever lymphoma is suspected.

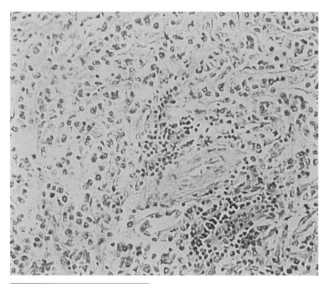

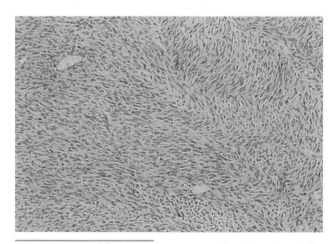

Figure 51–11 Any round cell tumor in an adult that does not appear to be a plasmacytoma is probably either a lymphoma, as in this slide, or a small, round cell metastatic carcinoma.

Figure 51–13 A herringbone pattern of malignant spindle cells indicates a fibrosarcoma.

Immunohistological testing may be required to differentiate between these lesions.

Soft Tissue Tumors

The most common soft tissue tumors are malignant fibrous histiocytoma, liposarcoma, synovial sarcoma, and fibrosarcoma. Histologially, these lesions are usually easy to distinguish. Liposarcomas (Fig. 51–12) are recognized by the presence of lipoblasts, "signet ring" appearing cells with eccentric nuclei and abundant cytoplasm, and by the presence of malignant fat cells. Fibrosarcomas (Fig. 51–13) are characterized by malignant spindle cells in a "herringbone" pattern, whereas synovial sarcoma (Fig. 51–14) shows a villonodular pattern of epithelial components and mesenchymal stromal cells. Malignant fibrous histiocytoma (Fig. 51–15) is a diagnosis of exclusion. It is seen in malignant lesions with none of

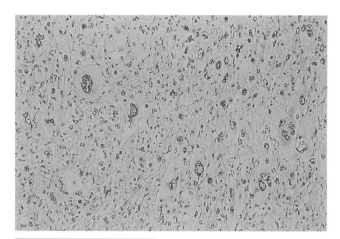

Figure 51–12 Liposarcoma is identified by the presence of lipoblasts and malignant fat cells.

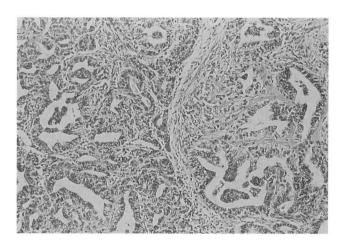

Figure 51–14 Synovial sarcoma is typically biphasic tumor containing a villonodular pattern of mesenchymal spindle cells and columnar epithelium.

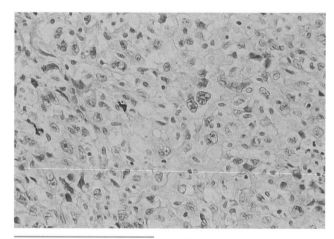

Figure 51–15 Malignant fibrous histiocytoma is a diagnosis of exclusion.

the above patterns or with none of the other patterns of more obscure soft tissue neoplasms.

ANATOMY AND SURGICAL APPROACHES

Tumor Anatomy

The major consideration for bone lesions is whether the tumor is confined within the bone. In low-grade malignancies, smaller tumors are frequently contained by the cortex. Even in these cases, resections are safer when done in an extraperiosteal plane to insure an adequate wide margin. High-grade primary bone malignancies are rarely confined to the intra-osseous compartment. These tumors can rarely be resected in this state and require preoperative chemotherapy to kill the lesion and facilitate wide resection.

Malignant soft tissue tumors are also difficult for the body to contain. Although most soft tissue sarcomas appear encapsulated, all have, by definition, cells that have escaped beyond the limits of their pseudo capsule to the surrounding zone of reactive tissue. As such, it is virtually never appropriate to "shell out" a malignant soft tissue tumor, even if the lesion appears encapsulated.

Patterns of Metastasis

The majority of patients treated for primary bone and soft tissue malignancies never develop clinically apparent metastasis. Among those who do, the lung is the most common site. Bone lesions represent a distant second in terms of metastatic frequency. Rarely, patients have metastases to the lymphatics, viscera, connective tissues, and skin.

Surgical Approaches

Surgical approaches for tumor surgery generally differ little from those utilized for open fracture treatment. Surgery for both conditions is performed along tissue planes, which provides for the protection of neurovascular structures.

Lesions of the neck and body of the scapula are normally approached posteriorly. Large resections of the scapula require access to the medial margin as well as laterally for the neurovascular structures and joint capsule. This is usually accomplished via a curvilinear incision, which may be connected to the perpendicular arm of a "T" if needed for adequate exposure.

For tumors of the proximal humerus, the delta-pectoral incision is still the most useful and forgiving. This approach can be extended proximally or distally. Lateral longitudinal incisions through the deltoid are to be avoided, as they are impossible to extend without injury to the axillary nerve. The humeral shaft area and the middle of the upper arm may be approached medially, laterally, or posteriorly, depending on the location of the lesion in question. Approaches to the elbow and forearm are either anterior or posterior.

For tumors about the hip, the posterior approach is the most extensile and can easily be connected to a "Y" approach if more anterior exposure is necessary. The femoral shaft may be exposed from the anterolateral or anteromedial approach, with the latter being more flexible and also providing a much easier dissection and exposure of the femoral vessels. The lower leg can be approached anteriorly or posteriorly as needed depending on the location of the lesion.

EVALUATION

The history in patients with a musculoskeletal tumor is rarely surprising. However, several misconceptions should be mentioned. It is important for the physician to realize that many patients with musculoskeletal neoplasms will relate the lesion to recent trauma. It is imperative that the physician maintain a high index of suspicion relative to traumatic etiologies of musculoskeletal masses and to proceed with imaging studies or biopsy if there is any deviation from the expected courses of recovery. Likewise, the history provided by a patient regarding the duration of a mass or symptoms can also be deceiving. It is not that unusual for the biopsy of a mass that the patient claims has been present for a prolonged period (i.e., months to years) to yield malignant pathology.

The physical examination focuses on the area of interest relative to the presence of a mass or pain. Localized masses, tenderness, erythema, or adenopathy should be noted as well as the range of motion of adjacent joints.

AIDS TO DIAGNOSIS

Plain Radiographs

Radiographs are the best preliminary study for any patient with a suspected tumor of the musculoskeletal system. Radiographs distinguish bone from soft tissue masses and can support the diagnosis of a particular lesion. Hemangiomas, for example, frequently contain phleboliths, which appear on radiographs as smooth, round calcified masses. Diffuse calcification in a soft tissue mass with no perceptible pattern may be seen with synovial sarcoma, which is the most frequently calcifying primary soft tissue malignancy. Myositis ossificans demonstrates a typical pattern of "eggshell" calcification in which the lesion is more calcified at the periphery than at the center. This radiographic appearance goes along with the histological tendency of peripheral maturation seen with this lesion.

In bone lesions, important radiographic parameters include lytic change, matrix calcification, type of tumor margin (i.e., geographic, moth-eaten or permeative), cortical destruction, periosteal elevation, and soft tissue extension. All of these factors give clues to the nature of the lesion.

Nuclear Medicine Scans

Nuclear medicine scans frequently aid in the evaluation of skeletal lesions. Although technicium bone scans are sensitive, they are nonspecific and will be positive due to a wide variety of causes including tumor, trauma, infection, and inflammation. The best use of a bone scan is to screen for metastatic lesions.

Computed Tomography Scans

The computed tomography (CT) scan is a tremendous aid in the delineation and characterization of bone lesions. It is the best imaging study to look at the effects of lesions on cortical bone or for characterizing lytic changes in the medullary canal. Computed tomography scans are also useful for

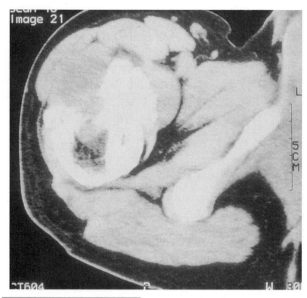

Figure 51–16 This computed tomography scan readily shows the cortical erosion as well as the calcified matrix produced by this surface osteosarcoma.

detecting metastatic lesions to the lung. Spiral CT technology detects lesions as small as 2 to 3 mm in diameter.

Magnetic Resonance Imaging

Magnetic resonance imaging (MRI) scanning is not as good as CT scanning for looking at cortical erosions (Fig. 51–16), but it is much superior to CT scanning when assessing marrow replacement and extra-osseous extension of bone lesions (Fig. 51–17). Magnetic resonance imaging scans are the gold standard for delineation of all masses in soft tissue (Fig. 51–18).

PEARL

MRI scans are used to assess the extension of a tumor within the marrow and into the soft tissues.

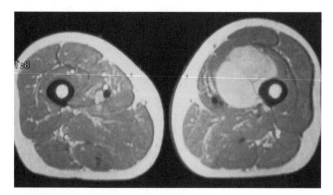

Figure 51–18 Magnetic resonance imaging scans are the best study to delineate the extent of soft tissue masses such as this malignant fibrous histiocytoma of the anteromedial thigh.

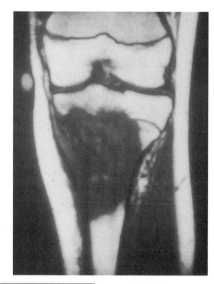

Figure 51–17 The extent of marrow involvement by this osteosarcoma of the proximal tibia is easily demonstrated by the magnetic resonance imaging (MRI) scan.

Biopsy Techniques

The most important aspect of extremity tumor surgery is the biopsy. For most cases, the safest and most effective option is a well-planned and well-executed open incisional biopsy. These are typically associated with minimal morbidity and give enough specimen to minimize the effects of sampling error. Table 51–1 outlines the rules to be followed when performing an incisional open biopsy.

TABLE 51–1   Rules of Open Biopsy

1. Use as small an incision as possible.
2. Always use longitudinal incisions on the extremities (transverse incision is acceptable about the pelvis where the major resection incisions are parallel to the superior bony margin of the pelvis).
3. Always make a small incision in the capsule of the tumor to make it easy to close and to avoid excessive blood loss.
4. Never directly contaminate a neurovascular bundle.
5. Avoid unnecessary damage to major flap structures (e.g., gluteus maximus) or functionally important structures (e.g., rectus femoris).
6. Use minimal retraction to facilitate later resection.
7. Keep within one structure if possible rather than going between two.
8. Always get a frozen section to verify that adequate diagnostic material is obtained.
9. Drains are rarely necessary for a biopsy, if one is used it should be brought out through the skin just proximal or distal to the tip of the incision.
10. All biopsies require careful closure in multiple layers.

Needle biopsy techniques are also available. These yield small specimens that may be difficult for pathology analysis unless the institution has significant experience with these procedures. The one area where needle biopsies are commonly the best choice is in spine lesions for which the CT control facilitates obtaining tissue from areas that are otherwise difficult to reach via a small surgical procedure. Most adult patients undergoing CT-directed needle biopsies of spine lesions will ultimately be found to have either metastasis or infection. Both of these are readily diagnosed via needle biopsy specimens.

SPECIFIC CONDITIONS, TREATMENT, AND OUTCOME

Osteosarcoma

Osteosarcoma (Fig. 51–19) is the most common primary sarcoma of bone. It occurs primarily in adolescents, with a second peak in the elderly in which it is associated with Paget's disease. The tumor is composed of a malignant spindle cell stroma that produces woven bone. Prior to the onset of effective systemic chemotherapy, the only other treatment was an amputation. The cure rate was roughly 15%. During the past 15 years, chemotherapy protocols have increased the cure rate to approximately 70%. As preoperative chemotherapy has increased in popularity, the amputation rate has dropped to less than 10% in most studies. The vast majority of patients with osteosarcoma are eligible for limb salvage resections and reconstruction. The two most common forms of reconstruction after segmental bone resections includes segmental replacement prostheses and allografts.

Two subtypes of osteosarcoma appear as lesions primarily on the surface of the bone. Periosteal osteosarcoma is a high-grade, condroblastic lesion on the surface of the bone. This is an aggressive lesion that may invade the medullary canal. Parosteal osteosarcoma is a low-grade lesions that is frequently located on the posterior aspect of the distal femur. This lesion crawls along the surface of the bone and usually grows to a large size before penetrating the cortex to reach

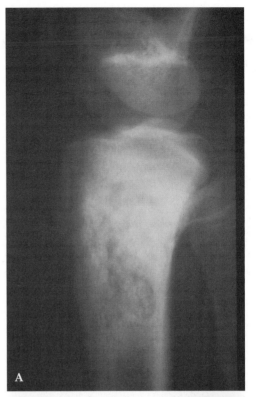

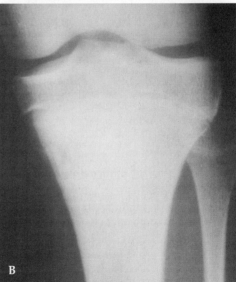

Figure 51–19   These anteroposterior **(A)** and lateral **(B)** x-rays of the proximal tibia demonstrate a typical osteosarcoma (MRI seen in Fig. 51–17).

the medullary canal. Periosteal osteosarcomas are treated the same as high-grade central lesions, whereas parosteal lesions, because of their low-grade nature, are treated with a wide resection.

The most frequent site of distant metastasis in patients with osteosarcoma is the lung. Fortunately, few patients present with multiple pulmonary lesions at diagnosis. Although those patients that do will have a grim prognosis. The prognosis for patients who develop pulmonary nodules in the course of their treatment is good, especially if the number of

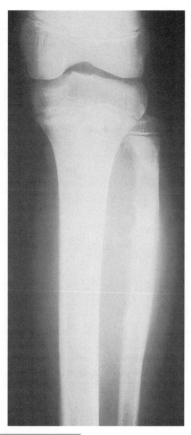

Figure 51–20 A typical Ewing's sarcoma appearing as a diaphyseal lesion of the fibula with permeative margins and soft tissue extension in a 16-year-old male.

lung lesions is small. In these patients, all pulmonary nodules should be removed.

Ewing's Sarcoma

Ewing's sarcoma (Fig. 51–20) is a round cell lesion of uncertain histogenesis that occasionally appears primarily in soft tissues but most frequently occurs in bone. It is an aggressive lesion usually found in a metadiaphyseal location associated with "onionskin" periosteal reaction and a large amount of extra-osseous extension. Occasionally, Ewing's sarcoma mimics bacterial osteomyelitis by producing an acute illness associated with fevers, chills, and a high sedimentation rate. Histologically, this lesion shows a monotonous array of round cells that stain positive for periodic acid—schiff. Electron microscopic study often reveals the presence of starch granules in the cytoplasm of these neoplastic cells.

Ewing's sarcoma is an aggressive lesion requiring local and systemic treatment. Multidrug chemotherapy is usually the first part of an integrated treatment program. Following chemotherapy, the two local options are wide resection surgery or radiation. Following the local treatment, aggressive adjuvant chemotherapy is again given in a fashion similar to that used for osteosarcoma.

There are three major complications following radiation for Ewing's sarcoma that have caused wide resection surgery to become the most popular option. These radiation-induced complications include local tissue fibrosis, increased risk for pathologic fracture, and late malignant transformation. Few patients with Ewing's sarcoma ever require an amputation. The prognosis for curing patients presenting with localized disease is currently 60% at 5 years.

Chondrosarcoma

Unlike osteosarcoma and Ewing's sarcoma, the majority of chondrosarcomas are low-grade lesions. Because they are resistant to treatment with chemotherapy and radiation, the only available treatment is wide resection. High-grade lesions are rare, accounting for only about 15% of chondrosarcomas. These are treated in a fashion similar to osteosarcoma. Although most chondrosarcomas arise as new lesions in bone, it is not uncommon for this tumor to develop following malignant transformation of a previously benign cartilage tumor such as an osteochondroma or enchondroma. Whereas enchondromas are painless lesions with calcification that blends into the surrounding medullary bone, chondrosarcomas typically show a more aggressive appearance. The hallmarks of a chondrosarcoma include intralesional lysis, endosteal scalloping, and cortical thinning or expansion (Fig. 51–21).

Multiple Myeloma

Multiple myeloma is a tumor of plasma cells characterized by multiple skeletal lytic lesions and the presence of immunoglobulin (Ig) molecules or light chains in serum or urine. Anemia, hypercalcemia, renal failure, and an increased

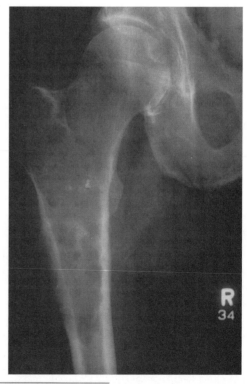

Figure 51–21 A chondrosarcoma of the proximal femur showing a calcified matrix with intralesional lysis and endosteal scallopping.

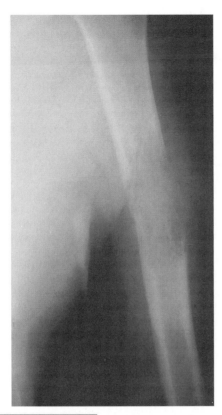

Figure 51–22 Myeloma typically appears as a lytic lesion with geographic margins and no surrounding sclerosis.

risk of infection are associated with this disease and may dominate presenting symptoms or late complications.

The bone lesions or myeloma are typically "punched-out" lytic areas (Fig. 51–22) with no surrounding reaction and a sharply defined margin. Diffuse osteoporosis is a less common presentation but may disguise the underlying disease. Serum and urine protein electrophoresis should be performed in all patients in whom myeloma enters the differential diagnosis and constitutes the most direct noninvasive method of suggesting the disorder. Treatment of this disease involves chemotherapy and radiation.

Soft Tissue Sarcoma

Soft tissue sarcomas are a group of malignant tumors occurring primarily in adults. These lesions are seen frequently in or between muscles. The most common histologic tumor types include malignant fibrous histiocytoma, liposarcoma, synovial sarcoma, and fibrosarcoma.

The biological potential of soft tissue sarcomas depends on the size and histologic grade of the tumor rather than the specific histologic type. Large high-grade lesions have a greater tendency for metastatic spread.

The local treatment for these lesions combines wide margin surgery and radiation therapy. The radiation is equally effective whether given pre- or postoperatively.

Smaller lesions that are easily removed surgically can be treated with an initial wide resection and postoperative radiation. Those tumors that are difficult to resect can be made easier to resect by the administration of preoperative radiation therapy. This tends to shrink the tumors making them firmer and less vascular.

The most common site of metastasis of soft tissue sarcomas is the lung. Despite recent advances in chemotherapy, present data suggests that this treatment modality cannot prevent the occurrence of pulmonary metastases. Chemotherapy is not routinely given to patients with soft tissue sarcomas who have no sign of metastatic spread. If pulmonary metastases are present, most patients are entered into chemotherapy clinical trials.

SELECTED BIBLIOGRAPHY

Biopsy Techniques

AYALA AG, ZOMOSA J. Primary bone tumors: percutaneous needle biopsy: radiographic-pathologic study of 222 biopsies. *Radiology.* 1983;149:675–679.

PEADBODY TD, SIMON MA. Making the diagnosis: keys to a successful biopsy in children with bone and soft tissue tumors. *Orthop Clin North Am.* 1996;27:453–459.

SHIVES TC. Biopsy of soft tissue tumors. *Clin Orthop.* 1993;289: 32–35.

Osteosarcoma

HUDSON M, JAFFEE MR, AYALA A et al. Pediatric osteosarcoma: therapeutic stratagies, results and prognostic factors derived from a 10-year experience. *J Clin Oncol.* 1990;8:1988–1997.

RUGGIERI P, DE CRISTOFARO R, PICCI P et al. Complications and surgical indications in 144 cases of non-metastatic osteosarcoma of the extremities treated with neoadjuvant chemotherapy. *Clin Orthop.* 1993;295:26–238.

Ewing's Sarcoma

BEN-ARUSH M, KUTER A, PEREZ M, COHEN Y, BIDIK V. Results of multimodal therapy in Ewing's sarcoma. *J Surg Oncol.* 1991;48:51–55.

CARA JA, CARRADELL J. Limb salvage for malignant bone tumors in young children. *Journal of Pediatric Orthopedics.* 1994;14:112–118.

Chondrosarcoma

SPRINGFIELD DS, GEBHARDT MC, MCGUIRE MH. Chondrosarcoma: a review. *Instruct Course Lec.* 1996;45:417–424.

Soft Tissue Sarcomas

CHENG EY, DUSENBERY KE, WINTERS MR, THOMPSON RC. Soft tissue sarcomas: Preoperative versus postoperative radiotherapy. *J Surg Oncol.* 1996;61:90–99.

SUIT HD, MANKIN HJ, WOOD WC, PROPPE KH. Preoperative intraoperative and postoperative radiation in the treatment of primary soft tissue sarcoma. *Cancer.* 1985;55: 2659–2667.

SAMPLE QUESTIONS

1. The presence of osteoblastic rimming of trabeculae of woven bone signifies:
   (a) a malignant lesion
   (b) a reactive lesion
   (c) a benign neoplastic lesion
   (d) infection
   (e) none of the above

2. The histologic changes that occur in low-grade malignant cartilage tumors include:
   (a) increased cellularity
   (b) cells with plump nuclei
   (c) binucleate cells
   (d) cells outside of lacunar spaces
   (e) all of the above

3. The most sensitive test for the presence of pulmonary metastases is the:
   (a) bone scan
   (b) Magnetic resonance imaging scan
   (c) spiral CT scan
   (d) anteriogram
   (e) chest x-ray

4. Which of the following are true concerning biopsy techniques for extremity tumors:
   (a) Long incisions should be performed for adequate exposure.
   (b) Longitudinal incisions should be used on the extremities.
   (c) Drains should be brought out adjacent to the middle of the incision.
   (d) Frozen section is rarely indicated.
   (e) Excisional biopsy is preferred over incisional biopsy.

5. The proper treatment for a non-metastatic soft tissue sarcoma of the anterior thigh that is 6 cm in diameter includes:
   (a) a radical resection and radiation
   (b) radiation and chemotherapy
   (c) wide resection and radiation
   (d) radical resection and chemotherapy
   (e) none of the above

Answers: 1) b; 2) e; 3) c; 4) b; 5) c

Metastatic Lesions to Bone

Scott C. Wilson, MD

DIFFERENTIAL DIAGNOSIS

Metastatic Carcinoma

(Breast, Prostate, Lung, Kidney, Thyroid, and Gastrointestinal)

Other Malignancies Involving Bone

Multiple myeloma

Leukemia

Lymphoma

Primary Bone Sarcoma

Other Lesions

Langerhans cell granulomatosis (eosinophilic granuloma)

Giant-cell tumor

Hyperparathyroidism

Chondroblastoma

Paget's disease

Infection

The goals of contemporary orthopaedic management of patients with metastatic bone disease are to provide pain control and improved functionality. This is often done with palliative operations designed to prevent pending pathological fractures and to treat pathological fractures that have occurred. However it is an oversimplification to assume that pathological lesions should be managed in the same fashion as traumatic fractures. Issues regarding the diagnosis of the lesion, reduced life expectancy, concomitant illness, the possibility of further progression of local disease after surgical stabilization, and the roles of radiation therapy and chemotherapy must be addressed in order to orchestrate an appropriate treatment plan. The following text will discuss these issues and outline selected treatment outcomes by anatomic location. Most of the chapter will deal with metastatic carcinoma and multiple myeloma. Other lesions that may present with metastatic or multifocal disease including eosinophilic granuloma, giant cell tumor, and chondroblastoma will be discussed.

BASIC SCIENCE

Mechanisms of Tumor Metastases

Because bone has no lymphatic system, metastases to bone spread by the venous system. A cancer cell's entry into bone may be facilitated by large gaps found in the endothelial lining of the sinusoidal system of red marrow. Batson's paravertebral venous plexus is located along the spinal column and connects with the superior vena cava and the inferior vena cava thus bypassing the pulmonary and portal circulation. Because there are no one-way valves in this plexus, an increase in intra-abdominal pressure can cause venous blood to preferentially flow throughout Batson's plexus connecting the paravertebral region to the head, neck, shoulder girdle, pelvis, and hip region. This may explain the presence of skeletal metastases in the absence of pulmonary metastases, and may explain the rarity of metastases distal to the humerus and femur.

Once a cancer cell has gained access to the bone, it must establish its own vascular supply. The cell accomplishes this using angiogenic factors such as prostaglandins, fibroblast growth factor, and epidermal growth factor. Tumor cells may destroy bone directly or indirectly by the recruitment and activation of osteoclasts and the production of collagenase. Factors that may be involved in this process include

Orthopaedic Surgery: The Essentials. Edited by M.E. Baratz, A.D. Watson, and J.E. Imbriglia. Thieme Medical Publishers, Inc., New York © 1999

parathyroid hormone-related protein, prostaglandins, and cytokines, including interleukins, transforming growth factors, tumor necrosis factors, and osteoclast activating factor (produced by myeloma and lymphoma cells).

EXAMINATION

When confronted with a bone tumor, the orthopaedist must work to distinguish a primary lesion from a metastatic lesion. This is especially true in the adult population, in which metastatic and multifocal cancers involving bone are 25 times more common than primary bone sarcomas.

A history helps to determine the diagnosis and to establish the tempo of the disease. The age of the patient will help to prioritize the differential diagnosis. For example, osteosarcoma, Ewing's sarcoma, chondroblastoma and eosiniphilic granuloma usually present in children and adults under the age of 30. Hyperparathyroidism and giant cell tumor tend to occur in adults 30 to 50 years of age, while carcinoma, lymphoma, multiple myeloma, and Paget's disease affect adults over the age of 50 (Table 52–1). Symptoms of metastatic cancer include unexplained weight loss, pain that is worse at night, and decreased energy level. Fevers, chills, and night sweats suggest infection but can occur in Ewing's sarcoma, Hodgkin's disease, and acute leukemia.

The lesion may or may not be tender to palpation. Tenderness suggests weakness of the bone, periosteal reaction due to the tumor, or soft tissue extension of the tumor. Auscultation of a bruit or pulsations indicates a very vascular tumor such as a renal cell carcinoma. A sudden jarring force on the spine, generated when a patient quickly drops from a toe-standing position to a foot-flat position, causes pain in

TABLE 52–2 Appearance of bony metastases on plain radiograph

	Lytic	Mixed	Blastic
Prostate			3/4
Breast	3/6	2/6	1/6
Lung	3/4		
Kidney	most		
Thyroid	most		
Multiple myeloma	most		
GI, other	+	+	rare
Lymphoma	variable		
Leukemia	variable		

patients with pathological fractures of the vertebral bodies. Physical examination of the breasts, prostate, rectum, abdomen, thyroid, and uterus may identify the primary focus of metastatic carcinoma. Enlarged lymph nodes may occur with carcinoma, lymphoma, or leukemia but rarely with primary bone sarcomas (approximately 3%).

AIDS TO DIAGNOSIS

Plain radiographs are the most expedient way to visualize a suspected bone metastasis. Radiographs of the entire bone are necessary to identify multiple lesions (Fig. 52–1). Lesions can be lytic (lung, kidney, thyroid and multiple myeloma), blastic (prostate), or contain both elements (lymphoma, leukemia,

TABLE 52–1 Age range for metastatic or multifocal diseases

Characteristic Age Range				
< 10	10–30	> 30	Usual Age	Unlikely Age
Neuroblastoma			< 3	
Eosinophlic granuloma			5–15	> 30
Chondroblastoma			10–20	> 30
OS*			10–20+	< 10
ES**			10–20+	> 30
Giant cell			20–50	< 16
Carcinoma			50+	
Lymphoma			50+	
Multiple myeloma			60+	
Paget's disease			60+	< 50
Hyperparathyroidism			30–50	
Wide age range				
Infection				
Chondrosarcoma			rare < 10	
Acute myelogenous leukemia			rare < 20	
Acute lymphocytic leukemia			17% < 20	

*OS: Osteogenic sarcoma

**ES: Ewing's sarcoma

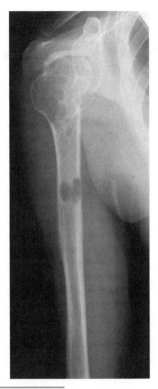

Figure 52–1   Multiple myeloma of the humerus with lesions in the head and shaft. Complete skeletal survey is necessary to identify all metastatic involvement, and stabilization of the entire humerus is necessary.

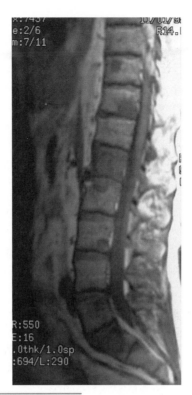

Figure 52–2   Sagittal, T-1 weighted magnetic resonance image of the spine showing multiple metastases in the vertebral bodies that were not apparent on plain radiograph.

and gastrointestinal). Some lesions like breast cancer can present with either a blastic, lytic or mixed appearance (Table 52–2). However, radiographs can fail to detect early metastases.

PITFALL

Lytic lesions that destroy up to half of the bone's mineral mass may remain undetected.

A total body technetium bone scan will identify roughly half of all metastases that are not apparent on plain radiographs. As such, the bone scan is preferable to a skeletal survey as a screening tool. A bone scan can successfully identify the most easily accessible metastasis for biopsy, and serial bone scans can be used to monitor the effects of treatment of bone metastasis. Although the sensitivity of a bone scan is greater than plain radiographs, it is less specific. False positive results can occur due to non-neoplastic lesions including trauma, arthritis, Paget's disease, and infection. Purely lytic lesions can be falsely negative because there are no areas of active mineral deposition for binding of the technetium pyrophosphate. In particular, Langerhans' cell granulomatosis and multiple myeloma generate purely lytic lesions, which may be negative on bone scan. A skeletal survey is required for patients with these or other tumors where the bone lesions are purely lytic.

Computed tomography (CT) scans are used primarily to examine the lungs, abdomen, and pelvis. In one study, CT

PITFALL

Bone scans may be negative in patients with multiple myeloma.

scans of these three regions enabled identification of the occult primary carcinoma in 75% of patients presenting with bone metastases. Since metastatic diseases are often focused in the marrow, magnetic resonance imaging (MRI) of skeletal metastases is superior in delineating the extent of marrow involvement (Fig. 52–2). MRI also is preferable in characterizing the tumor's extension into the soft tissues. Laboratory tests and other imaging tests can help to identify the type of cancer and the location of the primary lesion (Table 52–3).

An incisional biopsy should be performed promptly. Cultures of the lesion should be taken routinely unless the frozen section provides a definitive diagnosis. Computed tomography-guided needle biopsy may be used for lesions in the spine and pelvis that are difficult to access. This technique has limited success with blastic lesions, which are harder to penetrate and have a lower volume of diagnostic cells.

PEARL

Never assume a lesion is metastatic without a tissue diagnosis.

TABLE 52–3   Useful laboratory tests and radiology studies in workup of a bony lesion.

Laboratory Tests	
CBC differential	WBC > 25,000 in one third of leukemia patients.
Peripheral Smear	Blast cells present in 90% of leukemia patients
ESR	< 30 (Westergren method) in primary benign or malignant tumors of bone; however, can be elevated in metastatic carcinoma and infection.
Alkaline Phosphatase	Elevated in two thirds of patients with metastatic carcinoma. Also elevated in Paget's disease and osteogenic sarcoma.
Ca/PO$_4$	Hypercalcemia is common in multiple myeloma. If Ca is elevated and PO^4 depressed, consider hyperparathyroidism.
Liver function	Enzymes elevated with significant tumor burden in liver
SPEP/UPEP	Together, 99% diagnostic of multiple myeloma
PSA	Generally superior to prostate specific acid phosphatase
UA	60% of renal cell carcinomas have hematuria
Fecal occult blood	High false negative and false positive rate
Thyroid function	Thyroid scan or needle biopsy may also be useful
Radiology Studies	
CXR	Useful for initial evaluation
Mammogram	Useful when correlated with physical exam
CT chest	25% of lung cancers not seen on chest radiograph
CT abdomen/pelvis with contrast	Particularly helpful for kidney and bladder carcinoma

The value of a biopsy to finalize the diagnosis prior to definitive surgical treatment cannot be overstated because palliative stabilization procedures are vastly different from curative procedures. An untimely open reduction and internal fixation of a presumed metastatic carcinoma may forfeit the opportunity of a limb-sparing resection in a patient who actually has a primary bone sarcoma.

SPECIFIC CONDITIONS, TREATMENT, AND OUTCOME

Pain from a bone metastasis is caused by the direct biological effects of the tumor on the surrounding tissues and by the mechanical instability that the lesion causes in the bone. Treatment of bone metastases with surgery, radiation therapy, or chemotherapy is primarily palliative. The range of medications to treat metastases is vast and includes standard antineoplastic agents, anti-estrogen and anti-androgen agents for breast and prostate cancer, bisphosphonates, anti-inflammatory agents, and narcotics. The goal of operative treatment is to control pain by removing the tumor and to restore function by stabilizing the affected bone.

Metastatic lesions may progress after operative stabilization and may re-appear in other areas of the same bone. Bone healing is compromised by the presence of tumor. Gainor and Buchert (1983) found that 74% of 129 pathological fractures

required more than 6 months of cast treatment for healing to occur. Rates of healing included: 67% in multiple myeloma, 44% in renal cell cancer, 37% in breast cancer, and 0% in lung cancer. If the construct used to stabilize a pathological fracture fails, a more difficult revision operation may be necessary. Therefore, the entire bone should be stabilized even if the disease process currently affects only one area. Immediate stability should be provided to maximize pain relief, restore mechanical strength, and facilitate ambulation. The construct should be strong enough to outlive the patient even in the absence of bone healing. Patients with a pathological fracture should have a life expectancy of at least one month and those with pending fractures should have a life expectancy of at least 3 months.

Immediate and durable stability can be achieved using methacrylate cement to fill defects left by the tumor and to augment the stability of metal constructs. In the majority of cases the lesion is directly accessed and removed by curettage prior to stabilization. Long-stem cemented endoprostheses are preferred in proximal humeral and proximal femoral lesions adjacent to the articular surface. In long bones with mid-diaphyseal lesions, locked intramedullary rods augmented with cement may be used. Anterior spinal decompression should be followed by reconstruction of the space in the vertebra previously occupied by the tumor. Bone cement reinforced with pins, or plates and screws, has been used successfully. Radiation therapy in the range of 30–40 Gy should be used after an intralesional resection to control

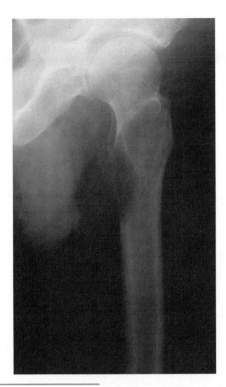

Figure 52–3 This radiograph shows a lytic lesion at the lesser trochanter of the femur that is at high risk for pathological fracture.

residual microscopic disease. Radiation treatments should be delayed until the surgical wounds are well healed to minimize the risk of infection or wound dehiscence. The radiation portal should include the entire bone and adjacent soft tissues encountered during surgery.

Occasionally, wide excision with the hope of a cure is indicated as is the case with metastatic sarcoma or indolent renal cell carcinoma. Amputation may be the most expedient way to control intractable pain. This may be indicated for aggressive metastases to the digits or for lesions that have received maximal radiation and have eroded the skin.

Prophylactic stabilization of a metastatic lesion to prevent fracture must take into account the location of the lesion, the amount of bone lost, the amount of pain, and whether radiation has been used. Lesions found in weight-bearing bones and those eroding 50% of the diameter of the bone or one inch in the axial plane are at significant risk for fracture (Fig. 52–3).

> **PEARL**
>
> Prophylactic stabilization should be considered for any lesion in the intertrochanteric region of the proximal femur.

Also, lesions causing unremitting pain, especially after a full course of radiation therapy, may benefit from surgical stabilization. Any lesion in the intertrochanteric region of the proximal femur is at risk of causing fracture and should be considered for prophylatic stabilization. Mirels (1989) described a useful scoring system to determine the likelihood of a metastatic lesion causing a fracture. Four parameters (location, pain, radiographic appearance, and portion of the diameter involved) were graded using a 3-point scale. A score of 9 indicates a 33% chance of fracture, and prophylactic fixation is recommended (Table 52–4).

> **PEARL**
>
> Postoperative radiation after intralesional surgery is necessary to control residual local disease.

Preoperative embolization should be considered in patients with renal and thyroid lesions and any purely lytic lesion, especially in proximal locations where a tourniquet cannot be used. Greater blood loss should be expected due to bleeding from the tumor.

Acetabulum

Metastatic lesions about the hip are the most common site of pathological fractures. Acetabular lesions can be classified into four groups according to Harrington (1981). In class I lesions the acetabulum is intact in the lateral, superior, and medial areas and can be reconstructed with a standard acetabular component. Class II lesions have deficiency of the medial wall requiring reconstruction with a protrusio ring. Class III lesions have deficiency in the lateral and superior walls. Reconstruction utilizes cement to replace lost bone and reinforcing rods, placed along the anterior and posterior columns of the pelvis, to transmit load to the intact portions

TABLE 52–4 Pathological fracture prediction according to Mirels

Score	1	2	3
Location	Upper extremity	Lower extremity	Peritrochanteric
Pain intensity	Mild	Moderate	Severe
X-ray appearance	Blastic	Mixed	Lytic
Diameter involved	< 1/3	1/3–2/3	> 2/3
Score (% fracture rate)	7 (4%)	9 (33%)	11 (96%)

Reproduced with permission from Mirels H. Metastatic Disease in Long bones. A proposed scoring system for diagnosing impending pathological fractures. *Clin Orthop Rel Res.* 1989;249:258.

of the ilium. These rods can be inserted retrograde through the acetabulum or antegrade through the iliac crest using a separate incision. This foundation is used to cement an acetabular component into place. The component may be secured with screws through the component and into bone or the cement mantle. Class IV lesions have complete peri-acetabular deficiency and require resection. Reasonable options for reconstruction include a "saddle" prosthesis, which has a U-shaped component that contains the cut end of the ilium, or a "girdlestone" arthroplasty (resection of the femoral head and neck). Of 58 patients in Harrington's study, 67% had good or excellent pain relief and 80% were ambulatory 6 months postoperatively. At 2 years, slightly less than half had good pain control and were still able to ambulate. Prosthesis loosening occurred in 5 patients (9%), and there were 2 operative deaths.

Femur

Long-stem (300 to 350 mm) bipolar devices are best used if the head, neck, or intertrochanteric region of the femur is involved. In a study of 101 long-stem cemented bipolar endoprostheses, Lane and associates (1980) reported 87% of patients were ambulatory postoperatively with good to excellent pain control. Average survival of these patients was 9 months. Of the patients in the study, 3% developed deep venous thromboses and 1 patient developed a nonfatal pulmonary embolism; 3% developed a wound infection. Hypotension developed and death occured during or after cementation of the prosthesis in 4% of patients in this series. To avoid this complication, a vent hole in the diaphysis of the femur is made prior to cementing the intramedullary stem. A history of pulmonary radiation or an arterial oxygen pressure (paO$_2$) of less than 70m Hg are contraindications to cementing long stems. In this setting, a noncemented prosthesis or a girdlestone arthroplasty are more appropriate options. Compression hip screws are not recommended for lesions in this area because fracture healing is not expected, and these devices do not stabilize the whole bone (Fig. 52–4). Proximally and distally locked intramedullary rods augmented with cement may also be used in subtrochanteric and diaphyseal lesions.

PEARL

Bony stabilization should follow the dictum: one bone, one operation.

Spine

Spine metastases have been classified by Harrington into five classes:

I: no major neurological impairment
II: bone involvement that is mechanically stable
III: major neurological impairment with stable bone
IV: unstable, fractured, or collapsed bone without major neurological impairment
V: both unstable bone and major neurological impairment

Patients with class I to III lesions should initially be treated with radiation and steroids if there is significant neurological

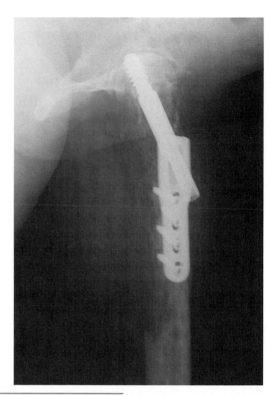

Figure 52–4 Progression of disease has caused failure of the hip screw. The entire bone should have been stabilized during the initial operation using a long-stem bipolar endoprosthesis.

involvement. Unstable spines should be considered for surgical stabilization. Harrington reported on his results of 77 patients who underwent anterior decompression and stabilization with distraction rods and cement. Of those, 66 patients had class V lesions, 62 had significant neurological involvement (Frankel A in 15, B in 20, C in 17, and D in 10), and 69 had lesions in the cervical or thoracic spine. Following treatment, 72 patients had relief of back pain. There were 4 postoperative deaths not attributed to malignancy, 5 failures of fixation, and 1 deep infection due to esophageal perforation and 3 due to reoperation. Fifty-two of 62 patients with neurological involvement improved. Sixty-five patients were alive at 6 months and 35 were alive at 2 years.

Miscellaneous Lesions
Eosinophilic Granuloma

Eosinophilic granuloma is known by many names: Hand-Schüller-Christian disease (multifocal bone involvement, especially of the skull; sometimes with exophthalmos, or diabetes insipidus); Letterer-Siwe disease (a lethal disease of children usually less than 3 years of age involving the spleen, liver, lymph nodes, and skin; and associated with infection, anemia, and hemorrhage); and histiocytosis X (a name encompassing all varieties). Langerhans' cell granulomatosis is a name used more commonly these days, in part because the Langerhans' cells, not the eosinophils, establish the histological diagnosis.

A skeletal survey is recommended to identify multifocal lesions. Because the skull and femur are the most commonly affected locations, plain radiographs of both areas should be included in the survey. A bone scan is less reliable and may be falsely negative in patients with purely lytic lesions. A chest x-ray should be performed to look for pulmonary involvement. Urinalysis is obtained to check for low specific gravity, which is an indication of diabetes insipidus.

Multifocal disease, which is found in 10 to 20% of patients, is treated with chemotherapy. The lesions are radiosensitive and low doses of radiation less than 1 Gy are useful especially in the spine, ilium, and weight-bearing bones. Surgical intervention is reserved for spinal cord compression or imminent pathological fracture. One year after successful treatment of a solitary lesion, there is little risk that multifocal involvement will subsequently occur.

Giant-cell Tumor

Both malignant and benign giant-cell tumors can produce metastases that are generally found in the lungs. Malignant giant-cell tumors are sarcomatous tumors that either arise within a benign giant-cell tumor or at the site of a prior giant-cell tumor or arise after radiation therapy. Their incidence is 5 to 7% of all giant-cell tumors. Pulmonary metastases associated with these lesions herald an aggressive neoplasm and a poor prognosis.

Benign giant-cell tumors may also have "'benign pulmonary metastases," which are recognized by their calcifications on plain x-rays. These are thought to be produced by iatrogenic seeding during forceful curettage and occur in 1 to 2% of all benign giant-cell tumors. Surgical resection of the pulmonary lesions is advised and is associated with long-term survival. If unresectable, chemotherapy is recommended because, in rare instances, these lesions can grow large enough to be fatal. Most metastases occur within 3 years of diagnosis, although some have been reported 7 years or more after treatment. Also, "benign" metastases in the soft tissues and lymph nodes have occasionally been seen.

Multicentric bone lesions have also been described but are exceedingly rare. It is much more likely that multiple giant-cell-rich tumors are brown tumors of hyperparathyroidism. These tumors radiologically and histologically mimic giant-cell tumors. An elevated serum calcium and a depressed serum phosphate indicate hyperparathyroidism.

Chondroblastoma

Like giant-cell tumor, chondroblastoma can produce benign metastases in approximately 1% of cases. These metastases are thought to be caused by vigorous curettage, venous transport, and pulmonary seeding. Usually these metastases are not progressive, developing 5 months to more than 30 years after diagnosis. However, several examples of "malignant chondroblastomas" have been described, exhibiting progressive growth and spread of the pulmonary metastases resulting in death. Patients with chondroblastoma or giant-cell tumor should be followed with serial chest x-rays to identify pulmonary lesions.

Hypercalcemia

Hypercalcemia of malignancy is the most common and potentially lethal metabolic disorder associated with cancer and occurs in 10 to 20% of patients. Hypercalcemia can be found in hematologic malignancies (especially multiple myeloma), in metastatic carcinomas (especially breast, lung, and kidney), lymphoma, and tumors without bone metastases (especially squamous cell carcinoma). Initial symptoms are vague and can be confused with the terminal stages of the underlying cancer. Patients may have bone pain, polyuria/polydipsia, GI symptoms (including abdominal pain, nausea, constipation, dehydration, and anorexia), and neurological symptoms ranging from lethargy to coma. Because hypercalcemia can cause death from cardiac arrhythmia, central nervous system depression, or renal failure, the surgeon must check for hypercalcemia during the preoperative evaluation. Calcium levels must be corrected for albumin binding using the equation:

$$\text{corrected [Ca] (mg/dl)} = \text{measured [Ca](mg/dl)} - [\text{albumin}](\text{g/dl}) + 4.$$

PEARL
Always check the calcium level preoperatively.

Elevations in serum calcium may occur due to the activity of osteoclast activating factors secreted at the sites of bone metastases. Inactivity due to enforced bed rest and dehydration can also contribute to hypercalcemia; therefore, prophylactic measures include ambulation and adequate hydration. Acute treatment of hypercalcemia consists of intravenous hydration and antiresorptive agents such as bisphosphonates, calcitonin, or gallium nitrate. If the cancer can be arrested by appropriate therapy, further hypercalcemia can be prevented.

SELECTED BIBLIOGRAPHY

GAINOR BJ, BUCHERT P. Fracture healing in metastatic bone disease. *Clin Orthop.* 1983;178:297–302.

HARRINGTON KD. The management of acetabular insufficiency secondary to metastatic malignant disease. *J Bone Jt Surg.* 1981;63A:653–664.

HARRINGTON KD. Anterior decompression and stabilization of the spine as a treatment for vertebral collapse and spinal cord compression metatatic malignancy. *Clin Orthop.* 1988;233:177–197.

LANE JM, SCULCO TP, ZOLAN S. Treatment of pathological fractures of the hip by endoprosthetic replacement. *J Bone Jt Surg.* 1980;62A:954–959.

MIRELS H. Metastatic disease in long bones: a proposed scoring system for diagnosing impending pathologic fractures. *Clin Orthop.* 1989;249:256–264.

NIELSEN OS, MUNRO AJ, TANNOCK IF. Bone metastases: pathophysiology and management policy. *J Clin Oncol.* 1991; 9:509–524.

ROUGRAFF BT, KNEISL JS, SIMON MA. Skeletal metastases of unknown origin: a prospective study of a diagnostic strategy. *J Bone Jt Surg.* 1993;75American:1276–1281.

WARRELL RP Jr. Metabolic emergencies. In: DeVita VT Jr, Hellman S, Rosenberg SA, eds. *Cancer: Principles and Practice of Oncology.* Philadelphia, PA: Lippincott; 1993:2128–2134.

SAMPLE QUESTIONS

1. A patient has pain at the lesser trochanter due to a lytic breast metastasis. The size of the lesion is less than one third the diameter of the femur. The most appropriate management is:
   - (a) operative stabilization
   - (b) antiresorptive medications
   - (c) non-weight bearing with crutches
   - (d) bed rest
   - (e) observation

2. A patient presents with a pathological hip fracture due to an unknown lesion in the proximal femur. The best initial course of treatment is:
   - (a) open reduction and internal fixation
   - (b) incisional biopsy
   - (c) wide excision and proximal femoral replacement
   - (d) hip spica cast
   - (e) an exhaustive search for the primary lesion

3. Goals of operative stabilization of metastatic bone lesions include all of the following except:
   - (a) prevent local progression of disease
   - (b) stabilize only the portion of the bone affected by tumor
   - (c) provide immediate stability because bone healing may not occur
   - (d) alleviate bone pain
   - (e) facilitate mobility

4. Essential workup in a patient suspected of having multiple myeloma includes all of the following except:
   - (a) skeletal survey
   - (b) complete blood count
   - (c) serum protein electrophoresis
   - (d) serum calcium
   - (e) total body technitium bone scan

5. Symptoms associated with hypercalcemia include all of the following except:
   - (a) lethargy
   - (b) bone pain
   - (c) spasticity
   - (d) nausea
   - (e) polyuria

Answers: 1) a; 2) b; 3) b; 4) e; 5) c

Infections

Chapter 53

Infections: Overview and Management

David C. Rehak, MD

Outline

Musculoskeletal infections are extremely common and are included in the differential diagnosis of extremity and spinal disorders treated by many different medical specialists. These infections often require urgent, if not emergency, treatment. Therefore, all physicians should be familiar with their diagnosis and management. Musculoskeletal infections can involve many different tissues including skin, subcutaneous tissue, fascia, muscle, tendon, joints, bursae, and bone. These infections range from superficial cellulitis to chronic osteomyelitis. The three most important aspects of treating musculoskeletal infections are accurate organism identification, appropriate selection and administration of antibiotics, and thorough drainage and debridement when indicated.

ETIOLOGY

To result in infection, a microorganism must first be introduced into tissue. The mechanisms by which this occurs include hematogenous spread, direct inoculation (penetrating trauma including surgery), and spread of an adjacent focus of infection. Conditions that increase susceptibility to an acute infection include vascular insufficiency, immunosuppression, rheumatoid arthritis, diabetes mellitus, sickle cell anemia, local and distant sites of infection, and devitalized tissue. The vascular status of the patient is particularly important as it helps determine if an introduced microorganism will cause an infection, as well as the effectiveness with which it can be eradicated. Individuals with small vessel insufficiency to the digits often develop ischemia followed by ulceration, cellulitis, and osteomyelitis. This problem is seen in the toes of patients who have diabetes and in the fingertips of patients who have scleroderma. Necrotic tissue provides an ideal medium for the growth of microorganisms. The inadequate blood supply prevents host defense mechanisms and antibiotics from confronting the infection.

BASIC SCIENCE

Orthopaedic Implants

The development of orthopaedic implants has greatly facilitated the management of musculoskeletal disease. However, prosthetic implants increase the risk of infection. The host considers the implant a foreign body and reacts by coating it with ionic and glycoproteinaceous constituents. The coating may attract bacteria, which prefer to attach to surfaces. Many bacterial species have the ability to produce exopolysaccharides known as glycocalyx. Production of glycocalyx creates a biofilm that is important for bacterial colonization and subsequent infection of implants. The bacteria replicate and form microcolonies within the biofilm matrix. Bacteria in biofilms are resistant to host defense mechanisms and antibiotic therapy. Consequently, the effects of implants must be considered when treating musculoskeletal infections.

Septic Arthritis and Lysosomal Enzymes

During bacterial septic arthritis, destruction of articular cartilage is caused by the release of lysosomal enzymes into the joint. Cartilage softening and fissuring secondary to glycosaminoglycan depletion occur within 7 days of infection. Erosion of the joint capsule can occur within 3 weeks of infection. Removal of leukocytes and their destructive enzymes should prevent additional damage to articular cartilage.

Orthopaedic Surgery: The Essentials. Edited by M.E. Baratz, A.D. Watson, and J.E. Imbriglia. Thieme Medical Publishers, Inc., New York © 1999

Nutrition and Its Relationship to Orthopaedic Infections

Nutritional deficiencies can complicate the treatment of musculoskeletal infections. Protein malnutrition decreases the immune response of the patient. In addition, tissue edema can occur. These events can profoundly affect wound healing and sepsis. The clinician can identify patients who have malnutrition with the serum albumin level and total lymphocyte count. Correction of malnutrition can prevent unnecessary complications in the patient who has a musculoskeletal infection.

GENERAL CONCEPTS IN MUSCULOSKELETAL INFECTIONS

Evaluation

The presenting features of musculoskeletal infection vary depending on the following factors: type of infection (e.g., soft tissue, bone, joint), site of infection, infecting organism, delay in diagnosis (acute vs. chronic), and host factors including immune status and concurrent disease. Localized symptoms include pain, tenderness, swelling, warmth, and erythema. Systemic symptoms include fever, chills, and malaise; most often present during acute infections. The clinician should find out if the patient has a history of penetrating trauma and local or distant sites of infection. Relevant history includes concurrent disease and immune status. Plain radiographs should always be taken when a musculoskeletal infection is considered. Findings vary from soft tissue swelling and loss of soft tissue planes to erosive osteolytic changes. Aspirated pus from any site confirms the diagnosis. A complete blood cell count with differential and erythrocyte sedimentation rate should be obtained. Blood cultures should be obtained for acute infections and in patients who have systemic symptoms of fever, chills, and malaise. Cultures from local (skin ulcer or nearby abscess) or distant (respiratory and genitourinary tracts) sites should also be obtained. Technetium-99, gallium, and indium-111-labeled leukocyte scans can be extremely helpful. The definitive diagnosis of any musculoskeletal infection lies in the identification of a microorganism.

Organism Identification

No infection can be adequately treated without accurate identification of the infecting microorganism. Accurate cultures enable the clinician to identify the infecting organism(s) and help dictate treatment. For example, if anaerobic organisms are identified in patients who have musculoskeletal infections, the wounds should never be closed. If *Mycobacterium tuberculosis* is identified, it should be treated with multiple drugs. The single most important factor in deciding which antibiotics should be used is antibiotic sensitivities of the isolated microorganisms.

Cultures should always be taken from as deep within infected tissue as possible. Culturing sinus tracts and superficial wounds should be avoided because they are often colonized by multiple organisms that have not caused the infection. Obtaining actual tissue samples for cultures is preferable

to swabbing a wound. Tissue obtained during debridement provides the most accurate culture. Cultures obtained by sterile aspiration may also be very helpful. It is extremely important to obtain culture material in the absence of systemic antibiotics. If antibiotic administration has already begun, it should be discontinued (as long as a life- or limb-threatening situation does not exist) far enough in advance of obtaining culture material so the cultures are not adversely affected. If culture material has been obtained in the presence of antibiotics, the microbiology laboratory should be informed, and the clinician should use this information when interpreting culture results.

The clinician must always be aware of the possibility of multiple organisms.

PEARL

Never begin antibiotic therapy until adequate specimens have been obtained for culture, unless there is a life- or limb-threatening situation.

Antibiotics

The clinician must carefully consider the administration of antibiotics to treat musculoskeletal infections. Antibiotics should never be given before obtaining adequate culture material unless a life- or limb-threatening situation exists. After material has been obtained for culture, empirical selection of broad-spectrum antibiotics is based on gram stain (or other organism-specific stains), knowledge of common pathogens, clinical picture, concurrent disease, immune status of the host, and local and distant sites of infection.

The clinician must obtain antibiotic sensitivities of the infecting organisms. Once sensitivity results are known, antibiotics can be selected based on serum bactericidal titer, toxicity, route of administration, dosing frequency, and cost. The serum bactericidal titer is used as an indicator of effectiveness. The minimal inhibitory concentration and the minimal bactericidal concentration are used to determine if a given antibiotic has bactericidal activity.

Most musculoskeletal infections require urgent, if not emergency, care including debridement and high serum antibiotic levels. Consequently, inpatient intravenous antibiotic therapy is often initiated. Based on culture and sensitivity results, the clinical response of the patient, and the antibiotic chosen, the clinician can decide whether to continue administering intravenous antibiotics or to switch to oral therapy. Local administration (topical or intra-articular) of antibiotics has little or no role in the treatment of musculoskeletal infections. One exception is in the treatment of prosthetic joint infections and chronic osteomyelitis, for which antibiotic-impregnated cement is commonly used.

The duration of antibiotic therapy depends on many factors including location of infection, infecting organism, delay in diagnosis, host immune status, and response to treatment. In general, osteomyelitis and septic arthritis should be treated for a minimum of 6 weeks, and soft tissue infections must be treated for 2 weeks. The duration of antibiotic treatment increases with coexisting disease, immunosuppression, age of the host, delay in diagnosis, and the specific microorganism. Antibiotics cannot penetrate necrotic tissue and abscesses. Therefore, in addition to the administration of antibiotics, adequate surgical debridement to remove necrotic, nonviable tissue and subsequent management of the wound are absolute necessities for the care of musculoskeletal infections.

Parenteral Prophylactic Antibiotics

Parenteral prophylactic antibiotics have been shown to reduce the infection rate after orthopaedic operations. The chosen antibiotic should be directed against a specific pathogen, which is most commonly staphylococci in postoperative infections. Cefazolin is an ideal parenteral prophylactic antibiotic because of its activity against staphylococci, its route of administration, and its half life. Alternatives include erythromycin and vancomycin hydrochloride. The drug should be administered at least 10 minutes before the tourniquet is inflated or the skin is incised. This amount of time has been shown to produce antibiotic tissue levels greater than the minimal bactericidal concentration for *Staphylococcus aureus*. Antibiotic therapy for 24 hours after surgery may also be indicated.

Incision, Drainage, and Debridement

Incision, drainage, and debridement are indispensable in the treatment of musculoskeletal infections. Infection can produce necrotic tissue that has no blood supply. Consequently, host defense mechanisms and antibiotics cannot penetrate the infected area, resulting in an ideal culture medium. Therefore, it is essential that all necrotic tissue be debrided when treating musculoskeletal infections. It cannot be overemphasized that cultured material must be obtained during debridement and before beginning antibiotic therapy.

Not all musculoskeletal infections require operative treatment; however, the clinician should always consider this option and should not hesitate to recommend operative intervention when indicated. There are many indications for incision and debridement. The presence of an abscess, purulent fluid (pus), or necrotic tissue is usually an absolute indication for debridement. When the diagnosis of infection is uncertain, debridement can help establish the diagnosis from the gross appearance of the tissues, microscopic evaluation, organism-specific stains, and cultures. Culture and biopsy specimens should always be obtained.

Preoperative antibiotics are withheld if possible. Elevation should be used to exsanguinate the extremity. Avoid using an esmarch. After cultures have been obtained, intravenous antibiotics are given. When the gross purulent material and obviously necrotic tissue have been removed, the tourniquet can be deflated and the tissues can be further assessed for viability. The most practical method to determine tissue viability is to check for bleeding with the deflated tourniquet. If there is doubt as to the viability of tissue, it is often best to delay further debridement and reassess the area during a second-look operation. This technique prevents unnecessary loss of tissue volume, which can create dead space, coverage problems, and structural instability (bone).

Copious amounts of antibiotic-containing irrigation should be used. If the patient has a soft tissue infection or osteomyelitis, wounds are often initially left open. However,

---

PITFALL

Aggressive debridement of infected but viable tissue can create a large dead space, which may complicate later reconstruction.

---

exposed bone and implants should be covered by soft tissue. The clinician should not hesitate to perform a second-look operation and additional debridement if there is inadequate clinical response, persistent drainage, or the possibility of additional necrotic tissue.

PEARL

The cornerstone of treating musculoskeletal infection lies in the adequate removal of the organism, its by-products, and necrotic tissue, as well as in the acquisition of appropriate material for culture.

After surgery, an adequate pathway must be provided for drainage. This can be accomplished either by leaving the wound open or by closing the wound over drains. In the case of septic arthritis, the joint capsule is usually closed over large suction drains. Wounds that have an abscess with necrotic, nonviable tissue and wounds that are infected with an anaerobic organism should always be left open. If a wound can be adequately debrided and converted to a clean wound, it may be closed over drainage tubes. When drains are used to close wounds, they should be removed in 48 to 72 hours. If drainage persists, the surgeon should consider debriding the wound again. Any infected wound that is closed must be closely monitored for signs of recurrent infection.

Debrided wounds that are left open should be packed and kept moist. Subsequent wound care includes daily dressing changes, whirlpools, and limited bedside debridement.

The purpose of leaving a wound open is to allow it to drain. Overpacking a wound can prevent drainage, create dead space, and prevent the skin edges from re-approximating during healing by secondary intention. Therefore, a wound should be gently packed with the least amount of material possible to prevent the depths of the wound, as well as the overlying skin, from closing prematurely. It is best to use the wick packing technique.

PITFALL

Overpacking wounds can prevent drainage, create dead space, and prevent wounds from healing by secondary intention.

With proper debridement and antibiotic administration, the wound should appear healthy with clean, granulating tissue and no evidence of infection. If additional necrotic tissue or pus forms, the wound should be debrided again. Wounds left open can be closed by secondary intention, delayed primary closure, or tissue transfer. These techniques require the wound to be healthy, clean, and granulating, by repeated debridement if necessary. Wounds considered for delayed primary closure can be evaluated for persistent infection by gram stain, tissue white cell count, or quantitative tissue cultures. A positive gram stain, a white cell count of more than 5 polymorphonuclear cells per high-powered field, or a quantitative tissue culture count of more than 10^{-5} organisms indicates persistent infection; these wounds should never be closed. At the time of delayed primary closure, the surgeon should again debride the wound to remove granulating tissue, which should be considered to be colonized by bacteria but not infected.

PEARL

If there is any doubt whether an infected wound should be left open or closed, it is always safest to leave the wound open.

Musculoskeletal Infections in an Immunocompromised Host

Musculoskeletal infections occur more often in patients who are immunocompromised. In addition to normal pathogens, there is a propensity to develop infection from opportunistic microorganisms that do not normally cause infection. The infection may go undiagnosed because the immunocompromised patient cannot develop a normal inflammatory response. Both congenital and acquired conditions can be associated with an immunocompromised state. Congenital conditions include chronic granulomatous disease, hemophilia, hypogammaglobulinemia, sickle cell hemoglobinopathy, and terminal complement deficiency. Acquired conditions include hematological malignancy, human immunodeficiency virus (HIV), pharmacological immunosuppression, and uremia. In addition, age can be a contributing factor.

The signs and symptoms of infection are often blunted secondary to the immune deficiency. Consequently, the clinician must suspect infection in any patient who has musculoskeletal symptoms and who is also immunocompromised. This is especially true for the nonbacterial organisms that frequently infect this patient population but do not provoke a dramatic inflammatory response. This less dramatic response often significantly delays the diagnosis and treatment of these musculoskeletal infections and leads to chronic infection. Infectious arthritis is the most common musculoskeletal infection seen in immunocompromised patients.

Diagnosis and Management

Suspecting that any musculoskeletal complaint may be an infectious process is the first step to correctly diagnosing and managing a musculoskeletal infection in an immunocompromised host. Much of the care when dealing with an immunocompromised host is similar to that for normal hosts; however, the clinician must anticipate the possibility of opportunistic infections. Stains for mycobacteria and fungi

should be requested in addition to a gram stain. Cultures should be sent to a laboratory not only for aerobic and anaerobic organisms, but also for fungal, mycobacterial, viral, and mycoplasmal organisms. Antibiotic administration is determined using the same criteria as for normal patients. Prolonged antimicrobial therapy is often required. More patients require surgical debridement because their defense system cannot adequately respond to infection.

PEARL

Musculoskeletal infections in immunocompromised hosts do not always produce the typical dramatic inflammatory response. Consequently, infection must always be ruled out in any immunocompromised patient with musculoskeletal symptoms.

SPECIFIC CONDITIONS, TREATMENT, AND OUTCOME

Osteomyelitis

Osteomyelitis is classified as acute or chronic. Acute hematogenous osteomyelitis most commonly occurs in children under the age of 16 years. It can, however, occur in adults. Osteomyelitis secondary to a contiguous focus of infection usually occurs in patients who are more than 50 years of age. Bone infection frequently develops after trauma or surgery. Osteomyelitis associated with vascular insufficiency occurs most commonly in patients who are more than 50 years old and who have diabetes or atherosclerosis.

Acute Osteomyelitis

Diagnosis

The symptoms of acute osteomyelitis include localized pain, warmth, swelling, and erythema. Systemic symptoms include fever, chills, and malaise. These features are often less dramatic in adults. In adults, the diaphyses of long bones and the lumbar and thoracic vertebrae are most frequently involved. In children, acute osteomyelitis is usually found in the metaphyseal region of long bones. Radiographic evidence of acute osteomyelitis may not be present for 1 to 2 weeks after the onset of infection. Radiographic changes include soft tissue swelling, demineralization by 10 to 14 days, and sequestra (dead bone with surrounding reactive bone). Bone scans may be positive as early as 48 hours after the onset of infection. Technetium-99, gallium, and indium-111-labeled leukocyte scans can be helpful in cases that are difficult to diagnose. Magnetic resonance imaging (MRI) may reveal a decreased signal intensity in marrow spaces before change is detectable in plain films. Blood cultures should be obtained in all cases of acute osteomyelitis and are positive in approximately 50% of cases. The area of maximum tenderness should be aspirated and sent for appropriate stains, culture, sensitivity, microscopic evaluation, cell count, and differential. If no material is obtained from aspiration, an open biopsy with subsequent debridement may be necessary. If there is a joint effusion or joint pain, the joint should also be aspirated.

Treatment

If osteomyelitis is diagnosed early (within 48 hours), an abscess with sequestrum may not yet be present. Consequently, patients who have acute osteomyelitis that is diagnosed early and who rapidly respond to the administration of systemic antibiotics may not need debridement. If debridement is performed, parenteral antibiotics are given as soon as specimens are obtained. The issues concerning the selection of an antibiotic are similar to those for all musculoskeletal infections. A minimum of 6 weeks of treatment is required. Intravenous administration is recommended for at least the first 2 weeks while adequate debridement is accomplished and culture and sensitivity results are obtained. Once the organism has been identified and sensitivities have been determined, oral administration of antibiotics may be acceptable. As with all musculoskeletal infections, antibiotic therapy is an adjunct to surgical management when necrotic tissue exists.

Chronic Osteomyelitis

Chronic osteomyelitis often occurs in patients who are elderly, immunosuppressed, diabetic, or intravenous drug abusers. Chronic drainage and sinus tract formation are common. Systemic symptoms of fever, chills, and malaise are rarely present. If the osteomyelitis has been present for a number of years malignancy should be ruled out, particularly squamous cell carcinoma.

Plain radiographs of chronic osteomyelitis demonstrate erosive osteolytic lesions and sclerotic bone with or without sequestrum. Indium-111-labeled white blood cell scans are helpful if the diagnosis has not been established. Computed tomography and MRI can be used to determine the extent of bone involvement. The erythrocyte sedimentation rate is often elevated; however, the blood cell count is usually normal. Blood cultures are rarely helpful. Exact organism identification is no less important in chronic osteomyelitis. This is further emphasized by the fact that many of these cases may have been misdiagnosed or inappropriately treated. Chronic osteomyelitis is not an emergency. Careful planning and execution of treatment are required for optimal results (Fig. 53–1). Culture material should always be obtained without the presence of antibiotics. Consequently, all antibiotic administration should be discontinued far enough in advance of obtaining culture material so that cultures are not affected. Cultures can be sent to a laboratory at the time of initial debridement, then antibiotics can be selected based on routine considerations as well as previous culture results. The duration of antibiotic therapy varies from a minimum of 6 weeks to suppressive oral therapy for life.

Debridement

The cornerstone of treating chronic osteomyelitis is adequate debridement of necrotic bone, soft tissue, and sinus tracts followed by skeletal stabilization and eradication of the infection. This treatment can then be followed by reconstruction including tissue transfer, bone grafting, or distraction osteogenesis as needed.

It is important that soft tissue and bony defects be eliminated to prevent continued infection and restore stability and function. Skin and subcutaneous tissue, muscle, bone, and cutaneous and osteocutaneous flaps can be transferred to reconstruct these defects. Because of its superficial, subcutaneous location, the tibia often requires coverage. In general, the gastrocnemius muscle is used to cover defects of the proximal third of the tibia, the soleus muscle is used to cover the middle third, and free-tissue transfer is used to cover the distal third. For defects up to 6 cm involving any bone, autogenous cancellous bone grafting can be performed. Bone grafting is usually performed 6 weeks or more after initiation of treatment for osteomyelitis. Because bone graft is nonviable, nonvascularized tissue, the infection must be totally eradicated before performing a bone graft. Free vascularized bone graft or bone transport (distraction osteogenesis) is indicated to compensate for defects larger than 6 cm.

Fractures Complicated by Osteomyelitis

Osteomyelitis can arise secondary to the trauma of an open fracture or from surgery for a closed fracture. Infection can lead to nonunion by producing necrotic avascular bone, loss of fixation, and gaps at the fracture site through osteolysis and debridement. When deciding how to treat an infected fracture, the clinician must consider two separate but related issues: the treatment of the fracture and the treatment of the infection. Open fractures must be adequately stabilized. This accomplishes two objectives; it allows the bone to unite, and it affords stability to the soft tissues, allowing them to heal. Healthy, vascularized tissue is crucial for eradication of infection. The relationship between bone and soft tissue is symbiotic. As the bone heals, it provides additional stability to the soft tissues. As the soft tissues heal, they provide a vascular supply to the bone, which further contributes to union.

Bacteria in the biofilms around implants are isolated from host defense mechanisms and antibiotics. Consequently, the surgeon must decide whether to remove these implants when treating infection. Stability is mandatory. If the internal fixation is required to stabilize a fracture and it is providing that stability, then it should be retained, and the infection should be treated accordingly with debridement and antibiotics. On the other hand, if fixation is inadequate and the fracture is unstable, it should be either revised or replaced with an external fixator. If osteomyelitis develops near a healed fracture with retained metal, the implant should be removed because it is not necessary for stability.

Septic Arthritis

Septic arthritis is most commonly caused by joint invasion secondary to bacteremia from distant sites. Acute hematogenous septic arthritis most commonly involves infants and children. *Haemophilus influenzae* is the most common organism in children who are less than 5 years of age, and staphylococcus is the most common organism in children who are more than 5 years of age. Common sources for hematogenous seeding include urinary tract infections, pneumonia, and bacterial endocarditis. Contiguous spread of soft tissue infections, such as cellulitis, bursitis, or local abscess formation can also result in septic arthritis. Direct inoculation through a penetrating injury can introduce bacteria directly into the joint space. Common causes include trauma, arthrocentesis, arthroscopy, and arthrotomy. The risk of inoculating a joint through injection can be minimized if strict aseptic technique is employed.

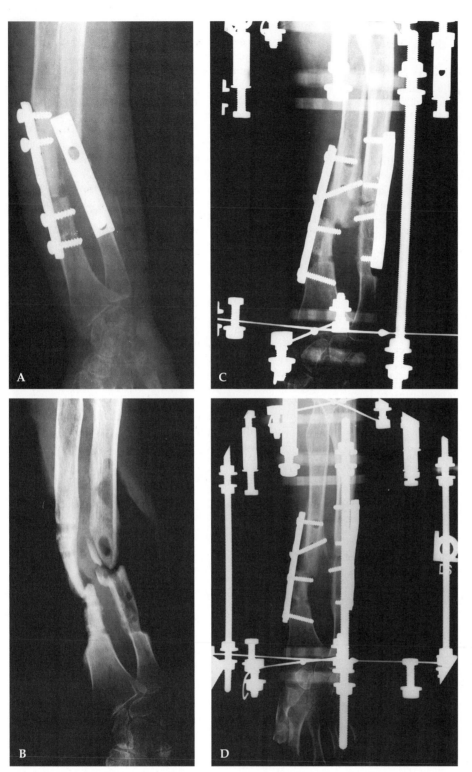

Figure 53–1 **(A)** A 37-year-old woman with a chronic, infected, nonunion of a forearm fracture with loss of fixation, exposed metal, and a draining sinus tract. **(B)** The patient underwent metal removal and extensive debridement. Deep cultures were obtained. Intravenous antibiotics were begun and modified when the culture and sensitivities were known. A central indwelling intravenous catheter was placed during a separate procedure in anticipation of long-term intravenous antibiotic administration. **(C)** One week after initial debridement and antibiotic administration, the patient had a second-look operation. All tissues appeared healthy. Consequently, internal fixation was applied and supplemented with an external fixator. The patient was treated with intravenous antibiotics for a total of 6 weeks. **(D)** Ten weeks after internal fixation, the soft tissues had completely healed with no evidence of infection. The radius and ulna were uniting. The fixator was removed. The fracture went on to heal uneventfully.

Medical conditions that increase the risk of developing septic arthritis include rheumatoid arthritis or any condition that causes chronic inflammation and joint damage. Rheumatoid arthritis is thought to be one of the most significant predisposing factors in adult septic arthritis. One problem in patients who have rheumatoid arthritis is the difficulty of distinguishing a rheumatoid flare from an acute infection.

Poor prognostic indicators for septic arthritis also include polyarticular involvement and delay in diagnosis. The most common organisms involved in adult septic arthritis are *S aureus* and *Neisseria gonorrhoeae*. The most commonly involved joints are the knee, hip, shoulder, elbow, ankle, and wrist.

Diagnosis

One of the most important prognostic factors in septic arthritis is the time of diagnosis. A delay in diagnosis puts the patient at risk for a poor outcome and is seen in patients who are elderly, are immunocompromised, have established joint disease, or have involvement of large joints, such as the hip and shoulder. Common clinical features of septic arthritis include joint pain, tenderness, swelling, heat, erythema, and limited, painful range-of-motion. Other symptoms include fever and chills. Limited, painful motion is the most helpful symptom in establishing the diagnosis of bacterial septic arthritis. A patient who can comfortably move a joint through a normal range of motion most likely does not have bacterial septic arthritis unless he or she is immunocompromised.

Plain radiographs show soft tissue swelling and are used to rule out other diagnoses (e.g., trauma). A whole-body technetium bone scan followed by an indium-111-labeled white blood cell scan can be helpful in diagnosing septic arthritis when routine methods fail. The most important step in the diagnosis of septic arthritis is aspiration of the joint fluid. Aspiration should always be performed before antibiotics are administered. The joint should not be entered through an area of skin or soft tissue that is suspected to be infected. The fluid should be sent to the laboratory for cell count, differential, microscopic evaluation (including crystals), gram stain, and other organism-specific stains if indicated. Cultures should be obtained for aerobes and, if indicated, for anaerobes, fungi, and mycobacteria.

Septic arthritis is diagnosed by demonstrating a positive synovial fluid culture or organisms. Joint fluid cultures are positive in more than 85% of cases of septic arthritis not caused by gonococcus but are positive in only 25% of infections caused by gonococcus. Gram stain of joint fluid demonstrates bacteria in 50 to 75% of the patients who have nongonococcal septic arthritis but demonstrates bacteria in less than 25% of the patients who have gonococcal septic arthritis.

PEARL

Cultures and gram stains of patients with gonococcal septic arthritis are positive in 25% or fewer of cases.

Urinary tract cultures can be extremely helpful for diagnosing gonococcal septic arthritis whereas cultures from other sources are not. Additionally, patients who have gonococcal septic arthritis often have polyarticular involvement. Blood cultures are indicated if systemic symptoms exist or if an immunocompromised state exists. Blood cultures are positive in approximately 50% of patients who have nongonococcal arthritis but are positive only in 10% of patients who have gonococcal arthritis. The differential diagnosis includes inflammatory arthritis (e.g., rheumatoid, crystal induced), trauma, and overlying soft tissue infection (e.g., cellulitis, bursitis).

Joint Aspiration

Synovial fluid has been classified as normal, noninflammatory, inflammatory, septic, and hemorrhagic. These groups have limited diagnostic value because fluids from a single disease may fall into any group. In general, normal and noninflammatory fluids are transparent, straw, or yellow in color. Inflammatory fluid is usually translucent or opaque. However, there is no discrete, gross appearance that separates infected from noninfected fluid. The white blood cell count indicates the severity of inflammation present and suggests the likelihood of bacterial infection. Fluids with a white blood cell count of less than 2000 mm^3 are traditionally considered noninflammatory. Fluids with a cell count of more than 100,000 mm^3 should be considered septic until proven otherwise. Synovial fluid with a white blood cell count between 50,000 mm^3 and 100,000 mm^3 is more difficult to evaluate. In this range, septic arthritis is certainly a possibility, particularly with tuberculosis, fungus, gonococcal, and partially treated infections. In addition, infected synovial fluid in the immunocompromised host can present in this range and even below 50,000 mm^3. Nonseptic inflammatory arthritis (e.g., crystal-induced arthritis, rheumatoid arthritis, and Reiter's syndrome) can have white cell counts in this range. The differential leukocyte count can be used to help establish a diagnosis. A noninflammatory fluid generally has considerably fewer than 50% neutrophils, whereas inflammatory fluids usually have a higher percentage. Infected synovial fluid generally has more than 95% neutrophils, but rheumatoid fluids usually have fewer than 90%.

All fluids should be examined with routine microscopy, including polarizing light. However, even the demonstration of crystals in a highly inflammatory fluid does not rule out coexisting infection. The presence of organisms on gram stain or other appropriate stains establishes the diagnosis of infection (Fig. 53–2).

Treatment

Joint debridement and antibiotic administration are required to treat septic arthritis. The initial decompression of the joint can be accomplished at the time of aspiration, and the clinician should remove as much fluid as possible at that time. The ideal technique for further decompression of the joint is controversial. The three most popular methods are repeated needle aspiration, arthroscopic irrigation, and arthrotomy. In general, if an uncomplicated infection is diagnosed and treatment is initiated within 72 hours, repeated aspiration or arthroscopic irrigation are acceptable techniques in healthy patients. Arthroscopic irrigation or arthrotomy is indicated if the diagnosis and treatment have been delayed for more than 72 hours, if a large amount of purulent material exists within the joint, or if the patient is immunocompromised. Arthrotomy should be performed in an infected hip. When in doubt,

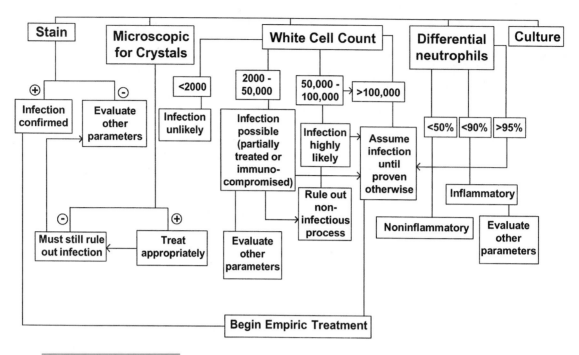

Figure 53–2   Synovial fluid analysis.

the clinician should not hesitate to perform arthrotomy, irrigation, and debridement and to repeat it as necessary.

Antibiotic selection is similar to that for all musculoskeletal infections. Usually a penicillinase-resistant, antistaphylococcal antibiotic is chosen and modified based on the clinical circumstances. Patients who have gonococcal infection may receive intravenous penicillin G. Antibiotics should never be injected directly into the joint because such treatment can result in a chemical synovitis. As long as serum bactericidal levels can be achieved, either intravenous or oral routes can be used. A minimum of 6 weeks of antibiotic administration is indicated to treat nongonococcal bacterial septic arthritis. Only 2 weeks of antibiotic administration is necessary to treat gonococcal arthritis.

Musculoskeletal Manifestations of Lyme Disease

Lyme disease is caused by the spirochete *Borrelia burgdorferi* and is transmitted by the *Ixodes dammini* tick. Lyme disease is endemic in the northeastern coastal, northern midwestern, and western United States. Early diagnosis is difficult because the tick bite may not be noticed, and the classical clinical cutaneous manifestations may not be present. Consequently, the clinician must anticipate and be familiar with the orthopaedic manifestations of the disease. The differential diagnosis includes juvenile rheumatoid arthritis and septic arthritis. Lyme disease should be considered in the differential diagnosis of unexplained joint inflammation regardless of evidence of tick bite or rash. The clinical course of Lyme disease

is described in three stages (Table 53–1). The most common joint affected is the knee.

Clinical diagnosis of Lyme disease is challenging. Enzyme-linked immunosorbent assay (ELISA) is the preferred test for serologic diagnosis. This test is extremely sensitive and specific during later stages of the disease but much less helpful during stage 1. Consequently, early diagnosis requires the clinician to know the clinical characteristics of Lyme disease.

To treat stage 1 Lyme disease, the patient must take tetracycline, doxycycline, or penicillin orally for 10 to 14 days. Administration of intravenous antibiotics is recommended for stage 3 in which the patient has established arthritis.

Spinal Infections

Osteomyelitis of the vertebral end plates can secondarily invade the disc space. Hematogenous spread is the most common mechanism of infection. Symptoms include localized back pain and tenderness with spasm and painful, decreased range of motion. Neurological deficits occur with abscess formation. Plain radiographic findings include disc space narrowing or destruction and end-plate erosion. Bone scan and MRI are the diagnostic tests of choice. Cultures from blood or aspirate are required. Antibiotics can be used without debridement in patients who do not have severe kyphosis, neurological deficit, or abscess formation. Anterior debridement and structural bone grafting are required for patients who have abscess formation, neurological deficit, extensive

TABLE 53–1   The three stages of Lyme disease

	Stage 1 Early infection	Stage 2 Disseminated infection	Stage 3 Late infection
Chronology	3 to 30 days after initial infection	Weeks to months after initial infection	Months to years after initial infection
Cutaneous manifestations	Erythema chronicum migrans (fades within 3 to 4 weeks)	Secondary skin lesions resembling erythema chronicum migrans	
Musculoskeletal symptoms	Arthralgia	Asymmetric oligoarticular arthritis and musculoskeletal pain in bursae, tendons, muscles, and bones	Chronic or intermittent arthritis
Other symptoms	Fatigue, malaise, and fever	Fatigue and malaise	

bony destruction, or marked deformity and for patients who are not responding to antibiotic administration.

Mycobacterial and Fungal Infections of Bone and Joints

Mycobacterial and fungal organisms can infect the musculoskeletal system. The diagnosis is often delayed because infection with these organisms follows an indolent clinical course. Additionally, these organisms often infect immunocompromised hosts who cannot mount a typical inflammatory defense with its subsequent clinical indicators of infections. If mycobacteria and fungi are not included in the differential diagnosis of inflammatory arthritis and tenosynovitis, delayed or inappropriate treatment can result. An injection of corticosteroids can be mistakenly used, further masking the symptoms of the disease and leading to additional delays in diagnosis. The diagnosis of these infections ultimately is made because the clinician suspects that the infection is present.

PEARL

Musculoskeletal infections caused by mycobacterial or fungal organisms do not present with the acute, dramatic inflammatory response seen in bacterial infections.

Tuberculosis

Musculoskeletal tuberculosis is most often found in the spine and weight-bearing joints. However, it can affect any bone, joint, tendon, or bursa. Tuberculosis should be considered in the differential diagnosis in patients who have chronic undiagnosed musculoskeletal symptoms. Skeletal involvement occurs in 1 to 3% of patients who have tuberculosis; however, a history of tuberculosis infection does not always exist. Musculoskeletal involvement of tuberculosis is caused by hematogenous dissemination. The characteristic pathological response to the infection by mycobacteria is the formation of

tubercles. Central caseating necrosis also occurs. The synovium develops an inflammatory reaction and formation of granulation tissue occurs. Unlike bacterial septic arthritis, tuberculosis infection does not produce lytic enzymes. Cartilage and bone are slowly destroyed from the erosion caused by the proliferation of the pannus. A positive tuberculin skin test supports the diagnosis. However, a negative result does not rule out the diagnosis; false negatives do exist. The definitive diagnosis of musculoskeletal tuberculosis relies on the demonstration of *Mycobacterium tuberculosis* in affected tissue by acid-fast stain or by culture. Synovial or bone biopsies may be necessary to obtain adequate material for culture.

The cornerstone of treatment of musculoskeletal tuberculosis is combination chemotherapy. Surgery, however, is indicated when a large abscess or proliferative synovial pannus is present. Multiple-drug-resistant tuberculosis isolates that are resistant to at least isoniazid and rifampin are increasing in prevalence. The clinician must anticipate that drug resistance exists. The recommended duration of treatment varies from a minimum of 6 months for uncomplicated cases in immunocompetent patients to more than 12 months for systemic cases in immunocompromised patients. The clinician must determine the drug susceptibility of all isolates. Antituberculosis chemotherapy should be initiated when *M tuberculosis* is present in another site or when clinical evidence supports this diagnosis. The most common musculoskeletal location of tuberculosis is the spine. Spinal tuberculosis can cause destruction of several contiguous levels or result in skip lesions or abscess formation. Anterior debridement and strut grafting are indicated in patients who have neurological deficit, abscess formation, or severe kyphosis. Chemotherapy should be started 10 days before debridement.

Nontuberculosis Mycobacteria

Musculoskeletal infections caused by nontuberculosis mycobacteria are similar to those caused by tuberculosis. These infections most commonly occur after penetrating injuries. Nontuberculous mycobacteria typically involve tenosynovium around the hand or wrist. This synovium is often thick and similar to that seen in patients who have rheumatoid arthritis. A specific history of exposure can often aid in the diagnosis. *Mycobacterium marinum* infections are often associated with aquatic exposure, and *Mycobacterium terrae* infections are often associated with farm work. The demonstration of granuloma or acid-fast bacilli aids in the diagnosis. Proliferative synovium is often an indication for surgical debridement, with extensive tenosynovectomy providing a source for culture and microscopic examination.

Fungal Infections and Mycoses

Fungi are not a common cause of musculoskeletal infection. However, the number of musculoskeletal infections from these organisms has increased because of the increase in the number of immunosuppressed patients (e.g., HIV, transplant, chemotherapy, drug abuse, intravenous antibiotics, parenteral nutrition). Musculoskeletal fungal infections have well-documented demographics that assist in early diagnosis. *Coccidioides immitis, Histoplasma capsulatum, Blastomyces dermatitidis,* and *Sporothrix schenckii* are the organisms that most frequently cause musculoskeletal fungal infections in healthy hosts. Common fungi that cause musculoskeletal infection in immunocompromised patients are *Candida, Aspergillus, Cryptococcus,* and *Histoplasma.* Hematogenous seeding is the most common mechanism of infection, but infections can also develop by direct inoculation. The vertebrae and discs are commonly affected in adults. Treatment includes debridement, if indicated, and pharmacological agents such as fluconazole, ketoconazole, itraconazole, and amphotericin B.

Soft Tissue Infections

Septic Bursitis

Septic bursitis is a common musculoskeletal infection. The superficial (subcutaneous) bursae are most commonly involved. The anatomic locations typically include the olecranon, prepatellar, and superficial infrapatellar bursae. Direct percutaneous penetration of bacteria into the bursa is the most common cause of septic bursitis. Secondary spread of primary cellulitis can also result in septic bursitis.

Septic bursitis should be placed in the differential diagnosis of a painful, swollen joint. A history of trauma often exists. Physical findings include bursal swelling, tenderness, warmth, and erythema. Joint motion is usually preserved, which helps distinguish septic bursitis from septic arthritis. Cellulitis commonly exists and may obscure the underlying bursar findings. Remember that infection can involve the bursa and its neighboring joint simultaneously. If septic arthritis is suspected, then the joint must be aspirated.

The diagnosis of septic bursitis is made by the aspiration of fluid from the bursa. As with septic arthritis, the aspirate should be sent to a laboratory for appropriate cultures and stains, cell count and differential, and microscopic evaluation (including crystals). Gram-positive organisms, especially *S aureus,* are the most common causes of septic bursitis.

The treatment of septic bursitis must include both bursal drainage and antibiotic therapy. Direct intrabursal injection of antibiotics should be avoided. Needle aspiration of the bursa is acceptable if adequate drainage can be accomplished.

Otherwise, incision and drainage are indicated. As a general rule, the wounds should always be left open.

Musculoskeletal Infections that Require Emergency Care

Almost all acute musculoskeletal infections require urgent, if not emergency, care. Delays in treatment can lead to local and distant spread of infection including sepsis, to severe dysfunction, and to the need for lengthy medical care. The following musculoskeletal infections require emergency care: necrotizing fasciitis, flexor tendon sheath infection, acute bacterial septic arthritis, acute hematogenous osteomyelitis, and human bite injuries.

Necrotizing Fasciitis

Necrotizing fasciitis is a soft tissue infection that spreads rapidly along fascial planes. Overlying cellulitis may or may not be present. This infection is often caused by a single organism (e.g., streptococcus) or by a combination of organisms that may include aerobic and anaerobic bacteria. Necrotizing fasciitis may develop after any trauma to the skin and in any anatomic location. However, the extremities are most often affected. This condition most commonly occurs in patients who have diabetes or use intravenous drugs. Necrotizing fasciitis can be distinguished from simple cellulitis by the presence of edema beyond the area of erythema, rapid development of bullae and ecchymosis, gangrenous skin, fluctuance, crepitus, and severe pain.

Patients who have necrotizing fasciitis will not improve with antibiotic therapy alone. Early extensive debridement of all involved skin and fascia is mandatory. Antibiotic therapy without debridement leads to a significant risk of mortality. High doses of antibiotics that are active against streptococci, anaerobes, and aerobic gram-negative bacilli should be started immediately. Careful postoperative monitoring is necessary, and patients who are not improving should have a second-look operation with repeat debridement. Skin grafts are usually required after the infection has been controlled.

Flexor Tendon Sheath Infection

Bacterial infection within the tendon sheaths can lead to rapid destruction of the gliding mechanism and to rapid spread of infection. These infections are most commonly caused by penetrating injury. Kanavel described the classical findings of flexor tendon sheath infection: flexed posture of the finger, swelling, tenderness over the flexor sheath, and severe pain with passive finger extension. Pain with passive finger extension is the most consistent and reliable finding. If diagnosed within the first 48 hours after infection, intravenous antibiotics can be given alone. However, patients who do not have an obvious response to antibiotics or who are diagnosed after 48 hours should have drainage and irrigation of the entire involved portion of the flexor sheath immediately. The wounds can be left open or closed over drains. Within 48 hours of surgery, patients should begin active range of motion and wound care.

Acute Bacterial Septic Arthritis and Hematogenous Osteomyelitis

Acute bacterial septic arthritis is without question an orthopaedic emergency. The production of lytic enzymes, which can lead to the rapid destruction of articular cartilage and subsequent dysfunction, necessitates rapid diagnosis and treatment of any intra-articular bacterial infection.

Acute hematogenous osteomyelitis also requires emergency care. Patients should be admitted to the hospital immediately, and appropriate cultures should be obtained through aspiration or surgical debridement. Intravenous antibiotics should be started as soon as possible.

Human Bite Injuries

Human bite injuries can cause serious infections and require immediate treatment. The most common organism is *S aureus*; however, Eikenella is also common. If a joint or bone has possibly been penetrated, formal incision and debridement are mandatory. These wounds should always be left open. Antibiotic administration of penicillin or amoxicillin and clavulanate potassium (Augmentin) is recommended.

SELECTED BIBLIOGRAPHY

Basic Science
Nutrition and its relationship to orthopaedic infections

SMITH TK. Nutrition: its relationship to orthopedic infections. *Orthop Clin North Am*. 1991;22:373–377.

General Concepts in Musculoskeletal Infections
Antibiotics

OISHI CS, CARRION WV, HOAGLUND FT. Use of parenteral prophylactic antibiotics in clean orthopaedic surgery: a review of the literature. *Clin Orthop*. 1993;296:249–255.

Musculoskeletal Infections in an Immunocompromised Host

BRENNAN PI, DEGIROLAMO MP. Musculoskeletal infections in immunocompromised hosts. *Orthop Clin North Am*. 1991;22:389–399.

Specific Conditions, Treatment, and Outcome
Osteomyelitis

DICKIE AS. Current concepts in the management of infections in bones and joints. *Drugs*. 1986;32:458–475.
DIRSCHL DR, ALMEKINDERS LC. Osteomyelitis: common causes and treatment recommendations. *Drugs*. 1993;45:29–43.
KHARDORI N, YASSIEN M. Biofilms in device-related infections. *J Indust Med*. 1995;15:141–147.

Septic Arthritis

ESTERHAI JL Jr, GELB I. Adult septic arthritis. *Orthop Clin North Am*. 1991;22:503–514.
GRISTINA AG, NAYLOR PT, MYRVIK QN. Mechanisms of musculoskeletal sepsis. *Orthop Clin North Am*. 1991;22:363–371.

Musculoskeletal Manifestations of Lyme Disease

JOUBEN LM, STEELE RJ, BONO JV. Orthopaedic manifestations of Lyme disease. *Orthop Rev*. 1994;23:395–400.

Mycobacterial and Fungal Infections of Bone and Joints

MEIER JL, BEEKMANN SE. Mycobacterial and fungal infections of bone and joints. *Curr Opin Rheum*. 1995;7:329–336.

Tuberculosis

YAO DC, SARTORIS DJ. Musculoskeletal tuberculosis. *Radiol Clin North Am*. 1995;33:679–689.

Fungal Infections and Mycoses

CUÉLLAR ML, SILVEIRA LH, CITERA G, CABRERA GE, VALLE R. Other fungal arthritides. *Rheum Dis Clin North Am*. 1993;19:439–455.

Soft Tissue Infections

ZIMMERMANN B III, MIKOLICH DJ, HO G Jr. Septic bursitis. *Sem Arth Rheum*. 1995;24:391–410.

Musculoskeletal Infections That Require Emergency Care

BISNO AL, STEVENS DL. Streptococcal infections of skin and soft tissues. *New Engl J Med*. 1996;334:240–245.
GANNON T. Dermatologic emergencies: when early recognition can be lifesaving. *Postgrad Med*. 1994;96:67–82.
KANAVEL AB. *Infections of the hand. A Guide to the Surgical Treatment of Acute and Chronic Suppurative Processes in the Fingers, Hand, and Forearm*. 7th ed. Lea & Febiger, Philadelphia, 1973.

SAMPLE QUESTIONS

1. Common routes by which musculoskeletal tissue is infected include all of the following except:

   (a) hematogenous

   (b) penetrating trauma

   (c) surgery

   (d) spread of adjacent infection

   (e) aspiration

2. Musculoskeletal infections in the presence of implants are difficult to treat because:

   (a) the implants cannot be removed

   (b) removal of the implants spreads the infection

   (c) the implants often are coated with a biofilm that protects the bacteria

   (d) the implants obscure the radiographic findings characteristic of infection

3. Acute bacterial septic arthritis is a surgical emergency for the following reason:

   (a) the fluid collection within the knee can cause severe, agonizing pain

   (b) the infection can spread to nearby bone

   (c) lysosomal enzymes cause rapid destruction of articular cartilage

   (d) fever and chills can develop rapidly

4. Antibiotics should never be given before obtaining culture material because they will:

   (a) treat the infection and make subsequent debridement unnecessary

   (b) adversely affect the culture and sensitivity results

   (c) increase the likelihood of fungal or mycobacterial infection

   (d) prevent wound healing

5. Musculoskeletal infections in immunocompromised hosts are more difficult to diagnose because:

   (a) the patients are often taking multiple medications

   (b) the patients wait too long before seeking medical attention

   (c) the typical inflammatory response is not produced

   (d) the patients do not respond to antibiotic administration

Orthopaedic Issues in Aging

Chapter 54

Orthopaedic Issues in Aging

Edward Snell, MD and Michael Scarpone, MD

Common musculoskeletal problems with orthopaedic implications in the elderly include osteoporosis and arthritis. Osteoporosis is a metabolic bone disease characterized by a diffuse reduction in the bone mass. There is no abnormality of matrix composition or mineralization. Osteoporotic bones are susceptible to fracture. Arthritis is a progressively disabling condition regardless of its etiology. Pain and limitation of motion can make activities of daily living difficult for elderly individuals. Both osteoporosis and arthritis are amenable to medical management.

ETIOLOGY

Osteoporosis

Osteoporosis occurs when bone formation is decreased, bone resorption is increased, or a combination of both occurs. Causes of osteoporosis include aging, menopause, endocrine disorders, metabolic disorders, malnutrition, malabsorption, and malignancy. Menopause and aging are the most common causes of osteoporosis. Endocrine, metabolic, and nutritional disorders are more likely to cause osteomalacia, which radiographically resembles osteoporosis but is metabolically and clinically different from osteoporosis.

After age 40, men lose 25% of their peak bone mass, and women lose approximately 50% of their peak bone mass. The difference between men and women is due to menopause. The severity of osteoporosis in a given individual is therefore a function of the individual's peak bone mass.

Several factors influence peak bone mass in young adulthood. These factors include nutrition, calcium intake, age of menarche, intensity of athletic activity, skeletal frame size (especially in women), and race. Poor nutrition and calcium intake strongly affect peak bone mass. Delayed ovarian function with late menarchal age may predispose young females to early osteoporosis. Athletic activity improves peak bone mass, but intensely athletic females may be amennorheic with decreased ovarian function and may develop osteoporosis at a young age. Small-framed and caucasian women have a higher risk of osteoporosis.

Loss of bone mass accelerates when estrogen production and ovarian function decrease. Decreased ovarian function can be due to normally occuring menopause or surgically induced menopause. Significant bone mass is lost during the first year of menopause. Postmenopausal osteoporosis preferentially affects trabecular bone.

The relationship between osteoporosis and decreased estrogen is not known. Recent studies have demonstrated estrogen receptors on osteoblasts. It is believed that these receptors enhance sensitivity to parathyroid hormone or some other mediator of bone metabolism.

Age-related loss of bone mass that is independent of hormonal influences occurs in both men and women after the age of 75. Both cortical and trabecular bone are affected. Long-term calcium deficiency is believed to be causative.

Arthritis

Causes of osteoarthritis include degenerative joint disease, ochronosis, and familial chondrodysplasia. Degenerative joint disease is the most common etiology and can be due to post-traumatic or congenital malalignment, instability, or repetitive loading and cumulative microtrauma. Common to all etiologies is failure of an entire diarthrodial joint due to abnormal joint mechanics, wear, and inadequate repair.

Malalignment can be intra- or extra-articular. Intra-articular incongruity causes load and contact maldistribution. Certain areas of the articular surface receive excessive load, whereas other areas atrophy because of insufficient load. Extra-articular malalignment may maldistribute load by redirecting joint reaction force vectors through articular surfaces not designed to accomodate them. Instability leads to abnormal joint motion, which in turn, redistributes load and pathologically increases shear stresses.

Orthopaedic Surgery: The Essentials. Edited by M.E. Baratz, A.D. Watson, and J.E. Imbriglia. Thieme Medical Publishers, Inc., New York © 1999

Ochronosis is due to accumulation within the cartilage of homogentisic acid polymers that stiffen the articular cartilage. Familial chondral dysplasia is due to a mutation in the cDNA coding for type II collagen. Both diseases alter the wear and load-bearing characteristics of articular cartilage.

Repetitive loading and cumulative microtrauma cause mechanical wear of articular cartilage. Biochemical changes also occur that contribute to deterioration. Articular cartilage has poor repair mechanisms and eventually degenerative arthritis develops. Repetitive loading within normal ranges can cause early degenerative arthritis in "at risk" joints such as a developmentally dysplastic hip or an avascular talus.

Rheumatoid arthritis is a systemic autoimmune disorder of unknown etiology. The association of rheumatoid arthritis with the HLA-DR4 antigen suggests a genetic component to the etiology. Environmental factors, such as neuroendocrine hormones and infectious agents, are thought to contribute to the risk of developing rheumatoid arthritis. Joint pain and destruction are due to hypertrophic synovial proliferation known as pannus. The event or factor that incites pannus formation has not been identified.

The crystalline arthropathies include gout and chondrocalcinosis (or pseudogout). Gout occurs when hyperuricemia leads to urate crystal deposition in oversaturated joint tissues. Hyperuricemia can be caused by uric acid overproduction or undersecretion. Undersecretion is much more common and can be due to renal insufficiency, dehydration, lactic acidosis, diuretic use, low dose salicylate use, and cyclosporine use. Causes of overproduction include excessive dietary purine (e.g., red meat) intake, increased nucleotide turnover as in myeloproliferative disorders, cancer, hemolytic diseases, or idiopathic uric acid overproduction. Pseudogout is caused by the deposition of calcium pyrophosphate crystals in cartilage, tendons, ligaments, articular capsules, and synovium.

The seronegative spondyloarthrophathies, including ankylosing spondylitis, psoriatic arthritis, and Reiter's syndrome, constitute a group of multisystem inflammatory disorders that are genetically associated with the HLA-B27 gene. The pathophysiology of the seronegative spondyloarthropathies is not known.

BASIC SCIENCE

Osteoarthritis begins with hypertrophic repair of the articular cartilage manifested by increased cartilage water content and increased proteoglycan synthesis by chondrocytes. With time, proteoglycan content begins to decrease to below-normal levels. The proteoglycan chains also become smaller. Consequently, cartilage loses its elasticity and wears more rapidly. Eventually, there is progressive loss of articular cartilage. Appositional new bone formation in the subchondral trabeculae and formation of new cartilage and bone at the joint margins occur to redistribute load no longer borne by the articular cartilage. Erosive synovitis of peripheral joints begins with microvascular endothelial cell changes and is followed by the appearance of mononuclear cells. Pannus, or hypertrophic inflammatory synovium, forms a highly proliferative and invasive granulation tissue that actively invades and destroys bone and cartilage. This process begins at the joint margins

where synovium attaches to bone. The pannus continues to hypertrophy and to invade and destroy the remaining articular surface.

Rheumatoid factor is an immunoglobulin that binds with the Fc portion of IgG molecules. It is commonly found in rheumatoid arthritis, and it is believed to amplify the inflammatory process. It does not appear to be a primary triggering factor.

AIDS TO DIAGNOSIS

Osteoporosis

Radiographs demonstrate diffuse osteopenia. It must be remembered that osteopenia is not radiographically evident until 30 to 50% of bone mass has been lost.

The vertebral body end plates stand out because of trabecular bone loss. Vertical trabeculae predominate because of preferential loss of horizontal trabeculae. A Schmorl's nodule may be apparent, wherein the intervertebral disc ruptures through the weak end plate into the vertebral body. Compression fractures with anterior vertebral wedging and loss of vertebral height may be present.

Radiographs of the proximal femur demonstrate loss of the normal trabecular pattern. The secondary compressive and tensile trabeculae are the first to diminish, followed by the principal tensile trabeculae and, finally, the principal compressive trabeculae.

Laboratory studies are performed to rule out other causes of osteopenia. Osteomalacia is the most common osteopenic condition and can be due to hyperparathyroidism, vitamin D deficiency, and renal failure. Screening studies to differentiate osteomalacia from osteoporosis include serum calcium, serum phosphorous, serum 1,25-dihydroxy-vitamin D, urine calcium, and alkaline phosphatase. Serum parathyroid hormone, thyroid function tests, and protein immunoelectorphoresis may also be indicated. Alkaline phosphatase may be decreased and serum calcium increased in osteoporosis, but laboratory studies are usually normal in osteoporosis. High urine hydroxyproline occurs in high-turnover osteoporosis.

Bone mineral density 2 standard deviations less than normal confirms the diagnosis of osteoporosis. Several tests are available to measure bone mineral density and include single or dual energy x-ray absorptiometry (SXA or DEXA) and quantitative computed tomography (QCT) scanning. Dual energy x-ray absorptiometry is the most precise and requires less radiation and time than does QCT, but bone mineral density can be falsely elevated if the area studied has significant osteoarthritis. Bone biopsy may be necessary to rule out osteomalacia and / or accurately determine bone mineral density.

Arthritis

Radiographs of the affected joint can differentiate arthritides. Osteoarthritis is characterized by joint space narrowing, subchondral sclerosis, osteophytes, and subchondral bone cysts. Articular erosions and periarticular cysts accompany joint space narrowing in rheumatoid arthritis. Disuse osteopenia is frequently present.

Radiographs are often normal in acute gout, but a joint affected by chronic gout may radiographically resemble osteoarthritis. Soft tissue calcifications are gouty tophi. Pseudogout is characterized by calcifications within the joint space that represent calcification of cartilage and fibrocartilage.

Sacroiliac joint space narrowing, subchondral sclerosis, and joint fusion are apparent in ankylosing spondylitis. The "bamboo spine" comprises anterior vertebral ankylosis at the intervertebral disc and syndesmophytes. It is pathognomonic for ankylosing spondylitis. Psoriatic arthritis and Reiter's syndrome are characterized by joint space narrowing and extra-articular erosions at the sites of ligamentous attachment. The "pencil-in-cup" appearance of the distal interphalangeal joints of the fingers and toes wherein the base of the distal phalanx forms a cup around the head of the middle phalanx is common in psoriatic arthritis and Reiter's syndrome.

PEARL

Erosion at the margin of a joint or at the locations of ligamentous attachment suggests inflammatory arthritis. Subchondral sclerosis and osteophytes suggest osteoarthritis.

Laboratory analysis of synovial fluid may be helpful. The white blood cell count is typically between 50,000 and 100,000 in inflammatory arthritis. It can be as high in osteoarthritis or crystal arthritis but is typically between 25,000 and 50,000. There is a slight predominance of lymphocytes. Monosodium urate crystals of gout are typically needle-shaped, strongly negatively birefringent, and bright yellow on compensated polarized light microscopy. Calcium pyrophosphate dihydrate crystals of pseudogout are short blunt rods, rhomboids, and cuboids that are weakly positive birefringent under compensated polarized light.

Serology has poor positive predictive value but may be useful. Rheumatoid factor may or may not be positive. A negative rheumatoid factor does not rule out rheumatoid arthritis. A positive, low-titer rheumatoid factor can occur in 5 to 42% of healthy older individuals without rheumatoid arthritis. HLA-B27 may be positive in seronegative spondyloarthropathies, but again, it may be positive in healthy individuals without seronegative spondyloarthropathy.

Hyperuricemia defined as serum urate concentrations greater than 7.0 mg/dl in males and 6.0 mg/dl in females frequently accompanies gout; however, as many as 10% of patients with acute gouty arthritis will have a normal urate level during the attack. No blood chemistry abnormalities accompany pseudogout.

PEARL

The definitive diagnosis of gout is made by joint aspiration with identification of intracellular, negatively birefringent needle-shaped crystals. (Remember gout = negative needles).

SPECIFIC CONDITIONS, TREATMENT, AND OUTCOME

Osteoporosis

Osteoporosis is typically asymptomatic until a fracture occurs. Fractures in the elderly are most common in the vertebral body, hip, pelvis, humerus, and distal radius fractures. Generalized bone pain is uncommon in osteoporosis and suggests osteomalacia.

PITFALL

Osteoporosis is clinically silent until fracture occurs or incidental radiographs suggest it. Symptomatic osteopenia is likely due to osteomalacia and warrants thorough medical evaluation.

Vertebral fractures usually manifest as a sudden onset of back pain. The patient may not recall any specific trauma. Local muscle spasm is frequently present, and an ileus may develop. Neurologic compromise rarely occurs. Occasionally, nonspecific back pain is present before the vertebral fractures occur. Progressive fracture and vertebral body collapse or multiple episodes of vertebral body fracture can result in thoracic kyphosis with compensatory cervical lordosis. This deformity is often referred to as the "dowager's hump."

Appendicular fractures are associated with trauma. Proximal and distal humerus fractures and distal radius fractures are typically due to a fall on an outstretched hand. Hip fractures are commonly due to tripping. Elderly individuals with osteoporosis may have balance disturbances or subtle neurologic disorders that predispose them to falling. Syncope should also be considered in elderly individuals who present with a fracture due to a fall.

Treatment of osteoporosis should begin before bone mass declines. Young adults require 500 mg of dietary calcium per day. Pregnant females require 1500 mg, and lactating females require 2000 mg. All patients with osteoporosis or at risk for osteoporosis should receive 1500 mg of dietary calcium per day and vitamin D supplementation. Weight-bearing exercise such as walking is essential for developing and maintaining adequate bone mass.

Type I, or postmenopausal, osteoporosis responds to estrogen replacement therapy. Women on estrogen replacement should also receive progesterone if they have not undergone hysterectomy. Estrogen replacement should be avoided in patients with known breast or uterine cancer. Testosterone replacement is useful in males with decreased serum testosterone.

Allendronate is a bisphosphonate that is useful in type II, or age-related, osteoporosis, and when estrogen is contraindicated or insufficient alone. Bisphosphonates bind to bone surfaces and prevent osteoclast resorption. Gastrointestinal upset is the most common side effect and can be minimized by gradually building up the dose to therapeutic levels.

Calcitonin directly inhibits osteoclasts and is useful in high turnover osteoporosis. It is administered either nasally or by injection. Antibodies to salmon-derived calcitonin may develop but do not appear to affect its efficacy. Nasal irritation is the most common side effect.

Calcium and vitamin D supplementation have been shown to decrease the incidence of hip fractures in the elderly by 30 to 40%. Estrogen replacement has been shown to retard or even halt the progression of osteoporosis. Controlled studies that evaluated allendronate demonstrated 50% decrease in hip and spine fractures. Allendronate arrests bone mass loss and may even increase bone mass slightly.

Arthritis

Symptoms universal to all types of arthritis include diffuse joint pain, swelling, stiffness, erythema, and limitation of motion. The onset is typically insidious and the symptoms are progressive.

Osteoarthritis

Osteoarthritis commonly involves the knees, hips, cervical and lumbar spine, proximal and distal interphalangeal joints of the fingers, and the first carpometacarpal and metatarsophalangeal joints. Onset may initially be unilateral, but symmetric involvement is typical. Pain worsens with activity and is relieved or at least improved by rest. The pain becomes persistent and more severe as the disease progresses. Stiffness after periods of inactivity is common. Inflammation of the joint manifested by redness, tenderness, and local heat may characterize the initial onset of osteoarthritis.

Physical examination of involved joints may reveal diffuse tenderness, crepitus, deformities, subluxation, swelling, bony overgrowths, and limitation of motion. Heberden's nodes are painless bony swellings of the distal interphalangeal joints of the fingers, and Bouchard's nodes are similar enlargements at the proximal interphalangeal joints of the fingers.

The goals of treatment of arthritis are to relieve pain, prevent deformity, and maintain mobility. Physical therapy and medical management often provide sufficient relief until progression requires surgical intervention.

Patients should be encouraged to judiciously participate in exercise programs that emphasize comfortable range of motion and conditioning such as pool exercise and walking. Rest should be prescribed carefully because contractures, disuse atrophy of muscles, and osteoporosis may develop.

Medications should be used carefully in the elderly popultaion because of several age-related changes in renal and hepatic function. Analgesics such as acetaminophen, nonsteroidal anti-inflammatory drugs (NSAIDs), and centrally acting opioid receptor agonists are useful for pain relief. To minimize the increased risk of toxicity in the elderly population, NSAIDs should be iniated at low doses and increased gradually to the lowest efficacious dose. Opioid receptor agonists such as codeine and propoxyphene should be used cautiously to avoid respiratory depression, drowsiness, constipation, and addiction behavior. The hepatic toxicity of acetaminophen must be considered when it is used alone or when it is combined with an opioid receptor agonists. Elderly individuals are frequently on multiple medications for other comorbidities that may enhance the toxicity of analgesics.

Rheumatoid Arthritis

Morning stiffness that lasts 30 minutes or more is a hallmark of rheumatoid arthritis. Systemic symptoms such as fatigue, malaise, low-grade fever, weight loss, and rash are common. Joint involvement is typically symmetric. Any appendicular joint can be involved, but sparing of the distal interphalangeal joints of the fingers and toes is common. Spine involvement is usually limited to the cervical spine but can produce instability and neurologic compromise. Pannus formation within the cervical spine can cause spinal cord compression.

The involved joints are typically swollen and warm. Typical deformities of the hand include ulnar deviation of the fingers, boutonniere or "swan neck" deformities, and dorsal dislocation of the distal ulna. Extensor tendon ruptures of the hand are common. Typical foot deformities include pes planovalgus, hallux valgus, and dislocated hammertoes. Table 54–1 outlines the diagnostic criteria proposed by the American Rheumatism Association.

Rheumatoid nodules, or Haygarth's nodes, are fusiform periarticular masses that usually involve the metatarsophalangeal joints. They are often painful, especially on the plantar surface of the foot, and can be tender, warm, or erythematous.

The natural history of rheumatoid arthritis can be influenced by several disease-modifying medications when NSAIDs become ineffective or toxic. Sulfasalazine combines sulfonamide and salicylate, which inhibit folate absorption and prostaglandin synthesis. Side effects include nausea and vomiting. Corticosteroids are powerful medications that provide dose-dependent suppression of inflammation. Common side effects include adrenal gland suppression, osteoporosis, immunosuppression, and cataracts. Rebound exacerbation of disease often occurs with abrupt withdrawal or rapid tapering of corticosteroids.

Methotrexate inhibits DNA synthesis and thus inhibits inflammatory cell division and proliferation. Toxicity results from its action on all cells. Bone marrow suppression, diarrhea, and cirrhosis may occur. Azathioprine inhibits DNA synthesis and transcription. Leukopenia and chemical hepatitis are common adverse effects. The anti-inflammatory mechanism of gold salts has not been established. Adverse effects include pruritic rashes, proteinuria, and hematologic toxicity. Urine protein and a complete blood count should be obtained before each gold salt injection.

The toxicity associated with the second-line disease-modifying medications requires monitoring during treatment. Thorough physical examination is imperative, and laboratory studies should include a complete blood count and serum and urine chemistry. Liver function tests and urine protein measurement may also be necessary.

Crystalline Arthropathies

Gout and pseudogout both present as an acute monoarthritis. Gout tends to affect peripheral joints such as the first metatarsophalangeal joint because it is cool relative to more proximal joints, thus decreasing the local solubility of urate. Pseudogout tends to affect the knees or other large joints. Both cause acute, extreme pain, swelling, tenderness, erythema, and occasionally fever, and thus may be confused

TABLE 54–1   Diagnostic criteria for rheumatoid arthritis. Diagnosis requires presence of at least 5 of the 7 criteria

1. Morning stiffness	Joint stiffness in the morning upon awakening that lasts at least 1 hour before maximal improvment.
2. Arthritis of three or more joints	Simultaneous soft tissue swelling or effusion (not bony overgrowth) in at least three joints observed by a physician. Areas of possible involvement include proximal interphalangeal (PIP), metacarpophalangeal (MCP), wrist, elbow, knee, ankle, and metatarsophalangeal (MTP) joints.
3. Arthritis of hand joint(s)	At least one area swollen in PIP, MCP, or wrist joint(s), as defined in criterion 2 above.
4. Symmetric arthritis	Simultaneous involvement of same joint bilaterally, as described in criterion 2 above. Asymmetric bilateral involvement of PIP, MCP, or MTP joints is acceptable without absolute symmetry.
5. Rheumatoid nodules	Subcutaneous nodule over bony prominence(s), extensor surface(s) of a joint, or juxta-articular region(s).
6. Serum rheumatoid factor	Abnormally increased titer of serum rheumatoid factor by any laboratory method for which the result is positive in < 5% of normal control subjects.
7. Radiographic changes	Typical radiographic changes on posteroanterior hand and wrist radiographs including erosions and unequivocal bony decalcification localized to or most marked adjacent to involved joint(s).

Adapted with permission from Schumacher H, eds. *Primer on the Rheumatic Diseases*. 10th ed. Atlanta, GA: The Arthritis Foundation; 1993.

with cellulitis or septic arthritis. Gouty tophi are hard deposits of crystalline urate in the skin, cartilage, or joints that are usually seen in patients with chronic gout. History of previous monoarticular joint arthritis and gouty tophi may be the only clues that suggest acute gouty arthritis on history and physical examination.

Sacroiliitis manifested by posterior pain in the sacroiliac joint is the hallmark of ankylosing spondylitis. It occurs less frequently in Reiter's syndrome and psoriatic arthropathy. Low-back pain and stiffness is common in ankylosing spondylitis. Ankylosing spondylitis affects males more often than females. The typical age of onset for the seronegative spondyloarthropathies is the 30s and 40s.

Maneuvers that confirm sacroiliac joint involvement include palpation of the sacroiliac joints, lateral compression of the pelvis with the patient lying on the side, or anteroposterior compression of the anterior iliac crests with the patient lying supine. The Patrick's test and Gaenslen's test isolate the sacroiliac joint. The Patrick's test is performed in a supine patient by placing the hip in maximal flexion, abduction, and external rotation with flexion of the ipsilateral knee. The examiner pushes the ipsilateral knee towards the examining table while stabilizing the pelvis. The Gaenslen's test is performed in a supine patient flexing the knee and hip on the affected side while the examiner hyperextends the unaffected hip by allowing it to "fall" over the side of the table. Both tests are positive if sacroiliac joint pain is reproduced.

Enthesopathic pain in the appendicular skeleton is more likely to occur with Reiter's syndrome and psoriatic arthropathy. Both also tend to involve the small joints of the fingers and toes. Reiter's syndrome includes arthritis, nongonococcal urethritis, and conjunctivitis. Typical infectious organisms include *Chlamydia trachomatis*, *Salmonella*, *Shigella*, *Yersinia*, or

Campylobacter. Arthritis appears within 1 to 3 weeks after the inciting infection. Psoriatic arthritis may appear before the typical scaly, erythematous rash on the extensor surfaces of joints, but definitive diagnosis cannot be made without evidence of skin or nail changes.

Indomethacin and colchicine are useful for acute gouty attacks. Aspirin, especially in lower doses, will exacerbate the attack by decreasing renal excretion of uric acid. In the hospitalized patient, a single dose of intravenous colchicine can dramatically eliminate the symptoms of an acute attack. Patients presenting to the office can be treated with 200 mg of indomethacin, followed by 50 mg 3 times a day until the symptoms abate. Oral steroids are an alternative for those patients who cannot take nonsteroidal anti-inflammatories.

After acute gout resolves, medical treatment is directed to decreasing serum uric acid levels. Methods include lifestyle and dietary changes, uricosuric medication (probenicid), or xanthine oxidase inhibitor medication (allopurinol). Probenecid or allopurinol are used in patients with recurrent gouty attacks, urinary stones, tophi, or dramatically elevated uric acid level. Gastrointestinal upset and hypersensitivity rash are the most common adverse effects of probenicid. Allopurinol inhibits conversion of hypoxanthine and xanthine, products of purine metabolism, to uric acid. Its toxicity includes hypersensitivity reaction characterized by fever and eosinophilia, hepatocellular injury, and renal insufficiency.

Medical management of seronegative spondyloarthropathies is less effective than it is for rheumatoid arthritis. Corticosteroids may be necessary, especially for controlling psoriatic arthritis. Control of psoriatic skin disease often relieves psoriatic arthritis. Recent evidence suggests a prolonged course of antibiotics improves Reiter's syndrome with evidence of Chlamydia infection.

Surgical treatment of arthritis is indicated when medical management fails to relieve pain and function can be improved.

SUMMARY

The orthopaedic implications of the growing elderly population are profoundly influenced by osteoporosis and arthritis.

Recognition, prevention, and medical treatment of osteoporosis decreases the incidence of debilitating fractures in the elderly. Appropriate medical management of arthritis likewise may maximize function among the elderly and delay surgical reconstruction. However, the pathophysiology of all forms of arthritis remains undetermined, and progression is inevitable.

SELECTED BIBLIOGRAPHY

BRAUNWALD E, eds. *Harrison's Principles of Internal Medicine.* 11th ed. New York, NY: McGraw-Hill; 1987.

DIEPPE P et al. *Atlas of Clinical Rheumatology.* London, England: Gower Medical; 1986.

NESHER G, MOORE T. Clinical presentation and treatment of arthritis in the aged. *Clin Geriatr Med.* 1994;10:659–675.

SCHUMACHER H, RALPH, KLIPPEL, JOHN H. KOOPMAN, WILLIAM J. (eds). *Primer on the Rheumatic Diseases.* 10th ed. Atlanta, GA: The Arthritis Foundation; 1993.

SAMPLE QUESTIONS

1. Type I osteoporosis is characterized by which of the following:
   (a) postmenopausal
   (b) equal incidence in men and women
   (c) vertebral fractures predominate
   (d) recalcitrant to calcitonin
   (e) a and c

2. Medical treatment of osteoporosis in a 67-year-old female with a history of cervical dysplasia should include:
   (a) estrogen
   (b) calcium and vitamin D
   (c) estrogen and progesterone
   (d) allendronate
   (e) b and d

3. A 37-year-old male develops heel pain that resolves over 3 months. He then develops pain of the second and third metatarsophalangeal joints. Rheumatoid factor is negative. Joint aspiration is notable for 82,000 white blood cells with a lymphocytic predominance. No crystals are identified. The most likely diagnosis is:
   (a) ankylosing spondylitis
   (b) rheumatoid arthritis
   (c) Reiter's syndrome

   (d) gout
   (e) degenerative osteoarthritis

4. The most appropriate initial and follow-up treatment of a first-time acute gout attack of the first metatarsophalangeal joint is:
   (a) aspirin and colchicine until the attack subsides, then initiate long-term probenicid
   (b) aspirin and colchicine until the attack subsides, then initiate long-term allopurinol
   (c) indomethacin and colchicine until the attack subsides, then initiate long-term probenecid
   (d) indomethacin and colchicine until the attack subsides, then initiate long-term probenecid and 6 months of colchicine
   (e) indomethacin and colchicine until the attack subsides, then initiate long-term allopurinol and 6 months of colchicine

5. Routine followup for a patient with rheumatoid arthritis on prednisone and methotrexate should include:
   (a) ophthalmologic examination
   (b) urine protein
   (c) complete blood count
   (d) a, b, and c
   (e) a and c

Answers: 1) e; **2)** e; **3)** e; **4)** c; **5)** e

Ethics

Chapter 55

Ethics in Orthopaedic Surgery

David C. Napoli, MD and Joseph E. Imbriglia, MD

Outline

Throughout the past century, the medical profession has been held in a position of high esteem, in large part because of the high ethical standards it has maintained. Indeed, society has come to expect that physicians maintain a standard of ethics and a level of altruism far above that of other professions. According to the American College of Physicians (1992), "Although the physician deserves fair compensation for services rendered, professionalism and a sense of duty to the patient and to society should take precedence over concern about compensation; the physician's primary commitment is to the patient." The health care environment has been undergoing many changes including the trend toward managed care, as well as a change in philosophy from the paternalistic role that physicians traditionally played to the concept of increased patient autonomy and self-determination. If our profession is to maintain the level of respect it has earned, it will become more and more imperative to take and keep the moral high road, and to live it by example. Only then will public support be maintained. Indeed, according to Baldwin et al (1996) there is evidence that "high levels of moral reasoning may provide a protective element against malpractice claims."

If ethical standards are not set by physicians, they may be set by others, or worse, by no one at all. In an effort to maintain such standards, the American Academy of Orthopaedic Surgeons (AAOS) has developed the Principles of Medical

Ethics in Orthopaedic Surgery (Table 55–1) as well as the Code of Ethics for Orthopaedic Surgeons. It has also published a series of Opinions on Ethics dealing in detail with specific issues such as the relationship of orthopaedic surgeons with industry, physician advertising, continuing medical education, the managed care setting, research, sexual harassment, patents, reporting of abuse, second opinions/referrals, and sexual misconduct in the physician-patient relationship. The purpose of this chapter is to familiarize the reader with some of the ethical issues of today and to review some of the published and more prevailing opinions on these issues.

PEARL

The AAOS has developed both a code and a series of opinions on ethics to help guide orthopaedists in their relationships with patients, industry, and their colleagues.

PRINCIPLES IN MEDICAL ETHICS

Principles in medical ethics can be grouped under three basic concepts: beneficence/nonmaleficence (doing good/not doing harm), justice, and respect for persons (Thompson, 1987). When ethical decisions arise, the physician must consider each situation individually and apply his or her best judgment. Moral and legal obligations may or may not coincide. If such conflicts arise, legal counsel is recommended. Ethical issues can arise in any of the following three relationships: the physician and the patient, the physician and other physicians, or the physician and society. The guiding theme in the first and second groups is to maintain the patient's welfare and treat the patient with compassion and respect. The theme in the third group is not as clear cut; the physician's obligations to society and to the individual patient may conflict, in particular when it comes to resource allocation. It is important to understand that many of these issues do not have obvious answers. As Allen (1984) points out, "a person relating to you from a different frame of reference may hold a different ethical opinion than yours and not necessarily be unethical." An interesting study by Novack et al (1989) surveyed physician opinion on the use of deception to resolve ethical dilemmas. Their work "suggests that the majority of our physician-respondents are willing to use deception in at least some

873

TABLE 55–1   Principles of medical ethics in orthopaedic surgery

The following Principles of Medical Ethics have been adopted by the American Academy of Orthopaedic Surgeons. They are not laws, but rather standards of conduct that define the essentials of honorable behavior for the orthopaedic surgeon.

I. The orthopaedic profession exists for the primary purpose of caring for the patient. The physician-patient relationship is the central focus of all ethical concerns. The orthopaedic surgeon should be dedicated to providing competent medical service with compassion and respect.

II. The orthopedic surgeon should maintain a reputation for truth and honesty with patients and colleagues and should strive to expose, through the appropriate review process, those physicians who are deficient in character or competence or who engage in fraud or deception.

III. The orthopaedic surgeon must respect the law, uphold the dignity and honor of the profession, and accept its self-imposed discipline. The orthopaedic surgeon also has a responsibility to seek changes in legal requirements that are contrary to the best interest of the patient.

IV. The practice of medicine inherently presents potential conflicts of interest. Wherever a conflict of interest arises, it must be resolved in the best interest of the patient and, if it cannot be resolved, the orthopaedic surgeon must withdraw from the care of the patient.

V. The orthopaedic surgeon must respect the rights of patients, of colleagues, and of other health-care professionals and safeguard patient confidences within the constraints of the law.

VI. The orthopaedic surgeon must continually strive to maintain and improve medical knowledge and make relevant information available to patients, colleagues, and the public.

VII. The primary bond among physicians, nurses, and other health-care professionals is a mutual concern for the patient. The orthopaedic surgeon should promote the development of an expert health-care team that will work together harmoniously to result in optimum patient care.

VIII. The fees for orthopaedic services should be commensurate to the services rendered without exploiting patients or others who pay for the services. Orthopaedic surgeons should deliver high-quality care to all regardless of race, color, gender, religion, national origin, or any basis that would constitute illegal discrimination, and regardless of ability to pay.

IX. The orthopaedic surgeon should not publicize himself or herself through any medium or form of public communication in an untruthful, misleading, or deceptive manner.

X. The orthopedic surgeon has a responsibility to the individual patient, to colleagues and orthopaedic surgeons-in-training, and to society. Activities that have the purpose of improving both the health and well-being of the individual and community deserve the interest, support, and participation of the orthopaedic surgeon.

Source: Hensinger, 1992.

situations when confronted by conflicting moral values. They evaluate the consequences of their decisions and appear to place a higher value on their patients' welfare and keeping patients' confidences than on truth-telling for its own sake."

addition, one would like to think that the standards of medical ethics would be more stringent than those of the law. The leadership in ethical practice must come from within the medical community (Todd, 1992)

THE ROLE OF GOVERNMENT AND LAW IN ETHICS

There is precedent for a government role in the determination of ethically acceptable medical practices with the creation in 1978 of the President's Commission for the Study of Ethical Problems in Medicine and Biomedical and Behavioral Research. Prior to this, ethical issues were addressed in private. Although there are certain issues, such as allocation of resources and distribution of care, which by their nature are of general public concern, the prospect of relying on the federal government as a moral lighthouse is disconcerting. Ethical principles are difficult if not impossible to legislate. In

COST CONTROL AND RATIONING

In the debate over health-care reform, the issue as to whether health care is a right or a privilege was raised. According to Dougherty (1992), "Society is obligated only to provide basic care, not everything that medicine can offer." Cost control is a virtue, both because it allows more people to receive basic care, and because it allows more of the nation's GNP to go to nonhealthcare related issues (e.g., education, housing, etc.). The AAOS has stated that "it is ethical for the orthopaedic surgeon to consider costs as one factor in determining the appropriateness of care." Sulmasy (1992) condemns bedside rationing decisions as morally problematic. He discusses the concept of a dual role for the physician; one as a citizen, answering to society and helping to determine macroallocation of resources, and the second as a physician, acting as the individual patient's advocate. He notes that, if the two roles are kept separate, then "no excessive moral burdens should occur." Although not the solution to problems of access to health care, charitable care of the indigent can help reduce their overall suffering. The Council on Ethical and Judicial Affairs of the AMA (1993) states that "the American Medical Association has long recognized an ethical obligation of physicians to assume some individual responsibility for making health care available to the needy. Caring for the poor is not a practice reserved for those who lack the skills to be more gainfully employed, but is reflective of the purpose of the healing arts." The Council has summarized their views with the recommendations in Table 55–2.

ETHICS CONSULTATION

Ethics consultation is an emerging clinical specialty, the role of which is still evolving. The role, for instance, of such a service in emergency medical situations has been debated. Detractors fear costly and harmful delays if physicians are expected to contact an ethics consultant in emergencies, even in situations in which the ethicist is available on a 24-hour basis.

Their role of ethics consultation in nonemergency situations is also a topic of much discussion. Although proponents feel that such properly trained experts in moral decision-making can be a valuable part of the health-care team, others express concerns over how this moral expertise is acquired, its applicability to clinical situations, the potential transfer of decision-making responsibility from physicians to those without medical expertise, and the cost of supporting such a service (particularly in an increasingly cost-conscious society).

CARING FOR FAMILY AND FRIENDS

The American College of Physicians states, (1992) "Physicians should be discouraged from treating close friends or members of their own families," listing concerns of impaired objectivity due to emotional ties and abbreviated history taking and physical examination. Perhaps it is wise to adopt such a stance as a general policy. Situations may arise, however, in which such treatment is not ethically unacceptable. These would include cases in which the above concerns can be controlled, or in which it becomes necessary to treat one's own friends and family for optimal care.

HEALTH MAINTENANCE ORGANIZATIONS

The rise of health maintenance organizations (HMOs) has raised certain ethical issues. Factors cited as advantages of HMOs include the following: HMOs control cost, thereby theoretically increasing access to health care for the public; they emphasize and encourage preventive care; and they lack incentives to overtreat. On the other hand, the typical HMO model provides an incentive to undertreat. In addition, there has been recent publicity regarding pressure on physicians to withhold information regarding all treatment options. Naturally, the orthopaedic surgeon has an ethical obligation to keep the patient informed of such options. The AAOS (1994) has published an Opinion on Ethics on the topic of managed care that states that "it is unethical for the physician to enter into an agreement with the MCO (managed care organization) that prohibits the provision of medically necessary care." The managed care environment has also led to difficulties with continuity of care; the AAOS has stated that the

TABLE 55–2   Recommendations of the Council on Ethical and Judicial Affairs of the AMA on caring for the indigent

1. Each physician has an obligation to share in providing care to the indigent. The measure of what constitutes an appropriate contribution may vary with circumstances such as community characteristics, geographic location, the nature of the physician's practice and specialty, and other conditions. All physicians should work to ensure that the needs of the poor in their communities are met. Caring for the poor should be a normal part of the physician's overall service to patients.

   In the poorest communities, it may not be possible to meet the needs of the indigent for physicians' services by relying solely on local physicians. The local physicians should be able to turn for assistance to their colleagues in prosperous communities, particularly those in close proximity.

   Physicians are meeting their obligation, and are encouraged to continue to do so, in a number of ways such as seeing indigent patients in their offices at no cost or at reduced cost, serving at freestanding or hospital clinics that treat the poor, and participating in government programs that provide health care to the poor. Physicians can also volunteer their services at weekend clinics for the poor and at shelters for battered women or the homeless.

   In addition to meeting their obligation to care for the indigent, physicians can devote their energy, knowledge, and prestige to designing and lobbying at all levels for better programs to provide care for the poor.

2. State, local, and specialty medical societies should help physicians meet their obligations to provide care to the indigent. By working together through their professional organizations, physicians can provide more effective services and reach more patients. Many societies have developed innovative programs and clinics to coordinate care for the indigent by physicians. These efforts can serve as a model for other societies as they assist their members in responding to the needs of the poor.

Source: Council on Ethical and Judicial Affairs, 1993.

orthopaedic surgeon has a continuing "obligation to provide medically necessary care … for the initial followup period" to a patient whose enrollment in the program is terminated if there is no provision for alternative care.

SELF-REFERRAL

The issue of self-referral, that is, referring patients to a facility in which the referring physician has ownership interests, raises the prospect of conflict of interest. It is estimated that approximately 10% of physicians in this country have such ownership interests in a healthcare facility of some type, a typical example being an orthopaedic surgeon owning all or part of a rehabilitation facility to which he refers his patients. Although such physician ownership has its potential advantages regarding patient care, the disadvantages, including the potential for overutilization, are of concern. The matter has been further complicated by an increasing and often inconsistent government role that tends to treat physicians more as business people and entrepreneurs rather than professionals. In the words of the Council on Ethical and Judicial Affairs of the AMA (1993), "Physicians are more than a special class of business professionals or entrepreneurs; they must continue to embrace elemental moral objectives if they are to maintain the mantle of professional integrity." For physicians to be able to "police" their own ethics, the incentives and forces driving them towards a business-minded approach may need to be lifted; an increasingly accepting view of shrewd and/or cut-throat business practices tends to erode at the moral fabric of the profession.

In an effort to guide the medical community through this issue, the Council on Ethical and Judicial Affairs of the AMA has provided a series of recommendations (Table 55–3).

SEXUAL MISCONDUCT

Sexual misconduct in the physician-patient relationship is condemned by current ethical thought. Even in instances in which the patient consents to such a relationship, the validity of that consent is questionable in light of the fact that patients often seek medical care when they are vulnerable, either physically or emotionally, or both. The physician who engages in sexual relations with a patient is at serious risk for compromising the patient's welfare.

If a physician and a patient find themselves mutually attracted to each other to the point where the physician's judgment may be compromised, the physician is ethically obligated to terminate the professional relationship in an appropriate fashion. According to the AAOS, (1993) sexual contact with a former patient is also considered unethical if it "occurred as a result of the use or exploitation of trust, knowledge, influence or emotions derived from the former professional relationship." The conclusions of the December, 1990 report by the Council on Ethical and Judicial Affairs of the AMA are summarized in Table 55–4.

RESEARCH

There are several aspects of research that lend themselves to ethical consideration. The AAOS (1994) Opinion on Ethics on this topic is quite extensive. It discusses issues regarding the purpose of the research: "Health research should be designed and conducted to develop new or confirmatory knowledge that promotes health, prevents diseases and injuries and improves diagnosis and treatment of diseases and injuries," financial support, the use of animals, the use of human subjects, the nature and content of the research, and credit for the work.

RELATIONSHIP WITH INDUSTRY

There is a potential in the dealings of the orthopaedic surgeon with industry for ethical dilemmas, particularly regarding the possibility of financial incentive to use a particular commercial product. Such incentives may be quite powerful, and it is incumbent on the physician to remain aware of such situations. Naturally, decisions in treatment should be based on the benefit to the patient and overall cost to society. The AAOS has published a series of recommendations regarding these matters (Table 55–5).

ETHICS IN SPORTS MEDICINE

Sports medicine differs from traditional medicine in several ways. First, the setting is different, often occurring on the sidelines or a health club, versus a more traditional institutional setting (e.g., a hospital). Second, the injury is generally caused by, and has a direct effect on, the individual's pursuit. Third, athletes as a class of patients are generally more in tune to their injuries and their physical well-being. Lastly, the patients are generally healthy.

These differences lead to conflicts that are common in sports medicine. For instance, there is the conflict between the goals of immediate performance enhancement and long-term well-being, as exemplified by anabolic steroid use. Generally speaking, the physician or trainer is in the best position to make the decision to return to play for two reasons. First, he or she is better qualified from a medical standpoint to make such a decision. Second, the physician or trainer has less of a conflict of duty than does the coach. The sports physician however may also be placed in a conflict of duty to the team versus duty to the individual player/patient; for example, if the physician is asked to give a pain-killing injection to allow an injured player to continue to play, risking further injury. The physician's contractual obligation is pitted against his or her professional obligation. The physician's primary obligation is to the patient.

ETHICS AND CHILD AND ELDER ABUSE

The physician has a duty to report child abuse and elder abuse to the appropriate authorities when it is diagnosed. This is in keeping with the ethical principles of beneficence, nonmaleficence, and justice through the fostering of self-respect (Jecker, 1993). The AMA has cited the following as reasons for failing to report and treat such abuse: lack of

TABLE 55–3   Recommendations of the Council on Ethical and Judicial Affairs of the AMA on physician ownership of medical facilities

---

Recommendation 1

Physician investment in health-care facilities can provide important benefits for patient care. However, when physicians refer patients to facilities in which they have an ownership interest, a potential for conflict of interest exists. In general, physicians should not refer patients to a health-care facility outside their office practice at which they do not directly provide care or services when they have an investment interest in the facility.

Recommendation 2

Physicians may invest in and refer to an outside facility, whether or not they provide direct care or services at the facility, if there is a demonstrated need in the community for the facility and alternative financing is not available. There may be situations in which a needed facility would not be built if referring physicians were prohibited from investing in the facility. Need might exist when there is no facility of reasonable quality in the community or when use of existing facilities is onerous for patients. In such cases, the following requirements should also be met:

a. Individuals who are not in a position to refer patents to the facility should be given a bona fide opportunity to invest in the facility, and they should be able to invest on the same terms that are offered to referring physicians. The terms on which investment interests are offered to physicians should not be related to the past or expected volume of referrals or other business from the physicians.

b. There should be no requirement that any physician investor make referrals to the entity or otherwise generate business as a condition for remaining an investor.

c. The entity should not market or furnish its items or services to referring physician investors differently than to other investors.

d. The entity should not loan funds or guarantee a loan for physicians in a position to refer to the entity.

e. The return on the physician's investment should be tied to the physician's equity in the facility rather than to the volume of referrals.

f. Investment contracts should not include "noncompetition clauses" that prevent physicians from investing in other facilities.

g. Physicians should disclose their investment interest to their patients when making a referral. Patients should be given a list of effective alternative facilities if any such facilities become reasonably available, informed that they have the option to use one of the alternative facilities, and assured that they will not be treated differently by the physician if they do not choose the physician-owned facility. These disclosure requirements also apply to physician investors who directly provide care or services for their patients in facilities outside their office practice.

h. The physician's ownership interest should be disclosed, when requested, to third-party payers.

i. An internal utilization review program should be established to ensure that investing physicians do not exploit their patients in any way, as by inappropriate or unnecessary utilization.

j. When a physician's financial interest conflicts so greatly with the patient's interest as to be incompatible, the physician should make alternative arrangements for the care of the patient.

Recommendation 3

With regard to physicians who invested in facilities under the Council's prior opinion, it is recommended that they reevaluate their activity in accordance with this report and comply with the guidelines in this report to the fullest extent possible. If compliance with the need and alternative investor criteria is not practical, it is essential that the identification of reasonably available alternative facilities be provided.

Source: Council on Ethical and Judicial Affairs, Conflicts of Interest, 1992.

knowledge, societal misconceptions, and lack of resources for victims of abuse. Both the accused abuser and the victim may plead to keep the matter from being reported, and the physician may feel reluctant to violate patient confidentiality.

Despite this dilemma, there is a strong consensus that physicians should report abuse because there is strong evidence that failure to report is often followed by further abuse and even death.

TABLE 55–4 Conclusions of the report on sexual misconduct prepared by the Council on Ethical and Judicial Affairs of the AMA

1. A physician's sexual contact or romantic relationship with a current patient is unethical.

2. A physician's sexual contact or romantic relationship with a former patient is unethical if the physician uses or exploits trust, knowledge, emotions or influence derived from the previous professional relationship.

3. Medical training should include education on the issue of sexual attraction to patients and sexual misconduct at all levels.

4. Disciplinary bodies must be structured to deal effectively with physician sexual misconduct.

5. Physicians who learn of sexual misconduct by a colleague must report the misconduct to the local medical society, the state licensing board, or other appropriate authorities. Exceptions to reporting may be made in order to protect patient welfare or the physician-patient privilege.

6. Many states have legal prohibitions against relationships between physicians and current or former patients.

Source: American Academy of Orthopaedic Surgeons, Sexual misconduct in the physician-patient relationship, 1993.

TABLE 55–5 AAOS guidelines for relationship with industry

To avoid acceptance of inappropriate gifts, the American Academy of Orthopaedic Surgeons recommends that orthopedic surgeons observe the following guidelines:

1. Any gifts accepted by orthopaedic surgeons individually should primarily entail a benefit to patients and should not be of substantial value (e.g., $100.00 or more). Accordingly, textbooks, modest meals, and other gifts are appropriate if they serve a genuine educational function. Cash payments should not be accepted under any circumstances. For example, the attendance at journal clubs sponsored by orthopaedic manufacturers would be acceptable so long as there was no substantial financial benefit to the orthopaedist-in-training involved.

2. Individual gifts of minimal value are permissible as long as the gifts are related to the orthopaedic surgeon's work. For example, it is acceptable for an orthopaedic surgeon to accept small pharmaceutical samples or pens and notepads from orthopaedic manufacturers.

3. Subsidies to underwrite the costs of continuing medical education conferences or professional meetings can contribute to the improvement of patient care and, therefore, are acceptable. A subsidy given directly to an orthopaedic surgeon by a company's sales representative creates a relationship that could be perceived to influence the orthopaedic surgeon's use of the company's products and should be avoided. Any corporate subsidy should be received by the conference's sponsor, which in turn can use the money to reduce the conference's registration fee. This is appropriate and acceptable so long as the curriculum of the conference or meeting is determined solely by the organization sponsoring the educational course, not the orthopaedic manufacturer. Orthopaedic surgeons should not accept direct payments from a company to defray the cost of attending an educational conference.

4. Orthopaedic surgeons should not accept subsidies, directly or indirectly, from orthopaedic manufacturers to pay for or defray the costs of travel, lodging, or other personal expenses of attending conferences or meetings, nor should they accept subsidies to compensate for their time. In addition, orthopaedic surgeons should not accept subsidies for hospitality outside of modest meals or social events held as part of a conference or meeting.

   It is appropriate for faculty at conferences or meetings to accept reasonable honoraria and to accept reimbursement for reasonable travel, lodging, and meal expenses. It is also appropriate for consultants who provide genuine services to receive reasonable compensation and to accept reimbursement for reasonable travel, lodging, and meal expenses. Token consulting or advisory arrangements cannot be used to justify compensating orthopaedic surgeons for their time, travel, lodging, or other out-of-pocket expenses.

5. Scholarships or other special funds to permit orthopaedic surgeons-in-training to attend carefully selected educational conferences may be permissible as long as the selection of students, residents, or fellows who will receive the funds is made by the orthopaedist-in-training's institution or by the program sponsor.

6. Orthopaedic surgeons should not accept gifts with strings attached. For example, orthopaedic surgeons should not accept gifts if they are given in relation to a physician's surgical practice. In addition, when companies underwrite medical conferences or lectures other than their own, responsibility for and control over the selection of content, faculty, educational methods, and materials should rest with the organizers of the conferences or lectures.

Source: American Academy of Orthopaedic Surgeons, Gifts and the orthopaedic surgeon's relationship with industry, 1992.

SELECTED BIBLIOGRAPHY

American Academy of Orthopaedic Surgeons. *Code of Ethics for Orthopaedic Surgeons.* American Academy of Orthopaedic Surgeons; 1991.

American Academy of Orthopaedic Surgeons. *Opinion on Ethics.* Gifts and the orthopaedic surgeon's relationship with industry. February, 1992.

American Academy of Orthopaedic Surgeons. Advertising by orthopaedic surgeons. *Opinion on Ethics.* December, 1992.

American Academy of Orthopaedic Surgeons. Sexual harassment and exploitation. *Opinion on Ethics.* February, 1993.

American Academy of Orthopaedic Surgeons. Reporting of suspected abuse or neglect of children, disabled adults or the elderly. *Opinion on Ethics.* October, 1993.

American Academy of Orthopaedic Surgeons. Sexual misconduct in the physician-patient relationship. *Opinion on Ethics.* October, 1993.

American Academy of Orthopaedic Surgeons. Ethics in health research in orthopaedic surgery. *Opinion on Ethics.* October, 1994.

American Academy of Orthopaedic Surgeons. The orthopaedic surgeon in the managed care setting. *Opinion on Ethics.* October, 1994.

American Academy of Orthopaedic Surgeons. Medical and surgical procedure patents. *Opinion on Ethics.* August, 1995.

American College of Physicians Ethics Manual. Part II: Research, Other Ethical Issues, Recommended Reading. *Ann Intern Med.* 1984;101:263–274.

American College of Physicians Ethics Manual. *Ann Intern Med.* 1992;117:947–960.

BALDWIN DC et al. Moral reasoning and malpractice: a pilot study of orthopaedic surgeons. *Amer J Orthop.* 1996; 481–484.

Council on Ethical and Judicial Affairs, American Medical Association. Conflicts of interest: physician ownership of medical facilities. *JAMA.* 1992;267:2366–2369.

Council on Ethical and Judicial Affairs, American Medical Association. Physicians and domestic violence: ethical considerations. *JAMA.* 1992;267:3190–3195.

Council on Ethical and Judicial Affairs, American Medical Association. Caring for the poor. *JAMA.* 1993;269:2533–2537.

DOUGHERTY CJ. Ethical values at stake in health care reform. *JAMA.* 1992;268:2409–2412.

Ethical emergencies. *Lancet.* 1992;339:399. Editorial.

FLINT FA, WEISS MR. Returning injured athletes to competition: a role and ethical dilemma. *Can J Sports Sci.* 1992;17: 34–40.

JECKER NS. Privacy beliefs and the violent family: extending the ethical argument for physician intervention. *JAMA.* 1993;269:776–780.

NOVACK DH et al. Physicians' attitudes toward using deception to resolve difficult ethical problems. *JAMA.* 1989;261:2980–2985.

SULMASY DP. Physicians, cost control, and ethics. *Ann Intern Med.* 1992;116:920–926.

THOMPSON IE. Fundamental ethical principles in health care. *Br Med J.* 1987;295:1461–1465.

TODD JS. Must the law assure ethical behavior? *JAMA.* 1992;268:98.

ALLEN BL. Ethical issues at the interface between orthopaedics and bioengineering. *Journal of Investigative Surgery.* 1992;5:191–199.

American College of Physicians Ethics Manual. *Annals of Internal Medicine.* 1992;117:947–960.

HENSINGER R. The principles of medical ethics in orthopaedic surgery. *J Bone Jt Surg.* 1992;74A:1439–1440.

SAMPLE QUESTIONS

1. Your community is considering building a physical therapy center. It is considered appropriate to invest in and refer patients to this center if:

   (a) you provide care at this facility

   (b) there is a need for this center and alternate financing is not available

   (c) physicians who aren't in a position to refer to the center are given a opportunity to invest

   (d) patients are given a list of alternative facilities

   (e) all of the above

2. It is considered unethical to accept the following gift(s) from product representatives or the orthopaedic manufacturing industry:

   (a) a textbook valued at $50.00

   (b) a meal at a journal club

   (c) a subsidy to defray the cost of a continuing education conference if you are the conference sponsor

   (d) a subsidy to defray the cost of travel and lodging to attend a conference

   (e) compensation for consulting services

3. A paper on tibial fractures is being prepared. The following individuals should be included as authors:

   (a) all surgeons who have provided cases for the study

   (b) the individuals who have planned and implemented the study and who have provided significant input to the preparation of the manuscript

   (c) the department chairperson

   (d) all of the above

4. True or False: There are many areas of potential ethical impropriety when a physician becomes romantically involved with a current or former patient.

   (a) true

   (b) false

5. A patient who you have recently operated on changes medical insurance to an HMO in which you are not a participating physician. The appropriate course is to:

    (a) arrange followup with a qualified surgeon in the HMO

    (b) continue to provide care if a qualified surgeon cannot be identified

    (c) allow the HMO to arrange appropriate followup

    (d) all of the above

    (e) a and b

Economic, Legal, and Political Issues in Orthopaedics

Chapter 56

Economic Realities of Orthopedic Practice

The Practical and Ethical Aspects of Changing Healthcare Reimbursement Systems

Dennis B. Phelps, MD, FACS

The vast majority of orthopaedic surgeons are astute clinicians, talented technicians, and highly motivated and competitive individuals who hold their patients' welfare foremost in their practices. They deserve to be reasonably compensated for their professional efforts—particularly in light of the lengthy and demanding training that is required of them and the importance of the care that is provided to the life and livelihoods of patients with musculoskeletal problems.

This chapter examines in depth how physicians are compensated in a rapidly changing medical environment and how the method of compensation may affect medical practice. Included are an examination of historical payment methods, the evolution of health care insurance and third party payers, the effect of governmental involvement in payment and regulation, the recent and dramatic changes resulting from the emergence of managed care and the multifaceted entities called health maintenance organizations (HMOs), the evolution of a significantly different reimbursement system called capitation, and the effect of changing reimbursement systems on the practice of medicine.

Orthopaedic surgeons may have very different opinions about reimbursement depending on the nature of their practices, the length of time they have been in practice, their experience with different payers or payment systems, and a variety of other factors. In a free-market economy, the optimal medical reimbursement system would create economic incentives for the physician to see a patient as quickly as possible and to resolve the patient's problem in the most time-efficient and cost-efficient manner. There would be no financial incentives to provide unnecessary services, and there would be penalties for failure to provide appropriate care or to achieve satisfactory outcomes. Unfortunately, there is no ideal medical reimbursement system. Each system has inherent advantages for patients and/or physicians, and each system has very real disadvantages, dangers, and potential abuses. In the rapidly changing health-care environment of the '90s, a variety of reimbursement programs exist, and there is extensive experimentation attempting to align economic incentives with appropriate care.

It is hoped that the reader will gain a useful perspective about the complexity of compensation for medical services, an understanding of the ethical issues that attend different reimbursement systems, and an appreciation for the true meaning of the "medical profession."

HISTORICAL PERSPECTIVE: THE EVOLUTION OF PHYSICIAN REIMBURSEMENT IN AMERICA AND THE FALL OF FEE FOR SERVICE

The image of the country doctor, transported by buggy to an ailing neighbor's home and embodied by more art than science—exchanging a "house call" for a hot meal and a bushel of the latest harvest—recalls a wonderful time in American medicine. Doctors and patients traded goods for services in a simple, barterlike manner quite different from the sophisticated transactions of our current high-tech world. But the exchange was well intentioned, honest, and there was no complicated intermediary requiring pre-authorization and demanding "continuing quality improvement" or "utilization review."

The introduction of third party payers, indemnity health care coverage, governmental payment and regulation, and, more recently, Wall Street and big business have dramatically altered the practice of medicine in America. All intermediary payers provide "insurance" that a defined set of benefits will be provided in whole or in part to those who are "covered"

Orthopaedic Surgery: The Essentials. Edited by M.E. Baratz, A.D. Watson, and J.E. Imbriglia. Thieme Medical Publishers, Inc., New York © 1999

through the payment of a premium or tax. Under entitlement programs, the government may be a third party payer for individuals who could not contribute through payment to an indemnity plan such as Social Security.

The concept of insurance is neither new nor complicated. Risk can be shared by those who are at risk; the unfortunate can escape financial devastation through protection from a monetary pool funded by all who are at risk. In an ideal insurance world, catastrophic events occur randomly, but the likelihood and magnitude of such events is relatively predictable. Actuaries can calculate the contributions required from those at risk to allow any specific type of insurance to provide reasonable financial protection to the insured—and reasonable profit to the insurer for assuming that risk.

At first glance the use of insurance to protect individuals and families against the financial consequences of disease, injury, aging, or a myriad of other health risks appears reasonable and logical. No one knows in advance that misfortune will strike, risk appears to be equally distributed, and the financial burden for each insured can be shared equitably. Unfortunately, there are many fallacies in this concept. While the risk of theft, fire, earthquake, or other events may be random, the risk of injury, illness, or other health problems vary widely among the population. Obesity, smoking, high blood pressure, alcoholism, high risk behaviors, or a family history of illness may make one individual much more likely to consume health insurance resources than another. Ironically, high risk individuals tend to be those least able to pay for insurance. One "solution" to this inequity of risk factors has been higher premium costs for higher risk individuals or denial of insurance altogether. Because the elderly become increasingly greater health care risks, private insurance becomes increasingly costly and, for most, unaffordable. This led to governmental intervention into the provision of health care benefits to individuals over age 65, resulting in the massive entitlement program we know as Medicare.

Another economic anomaly exists in the nature of American indemnity health insurance. In virtually all other types of insurance, untoward events resulting in financial losses are uncontrolled. In health care, the demand for services, particularly costly services, is controlled to a large degree by the insured (the patient) and the doctor. This sets the stage for wide variation in utilization of services and abuses. Imagine an automobile insurance policy that would permit an automobile owner to visit a mechanic, whenever the owner desired, to determine what work needed to be done, and that allowed the work to be paid for by the insurance company rather than by the owner. This would create incentives for the owner to get more (and perhaps unimportant) repairs or maintenance done and would create even greater incentives for the mechanic to discover problems that would incur costly repair bills.

Patients who demand excess services or unnecessary technology drive up the cost of health care and health care insurance as do physicians who practice "expensive" or inefficient medicine. Unfortunately, there are also physicians who perform income-generating procedures without proper indications. The term unnecessary surgery, to the discredit of the medical profession, refers to a very real and substantial problem.

Thus, indemnity insurance is a well-intentioned but flawed concept in traditional American fee-for-service health care. Lack of controls and exploding technology escalated the cost of health care for more than a quarter of a century beginning in the 1960s. The emergence of computer systems and information management, however, allowed insurance companies to quickly compile enormous data banks relative to fees, costs, geographic variances, and a host of other parameters. This created the opportunity for a revolutionary change in physician reimbursement. Physicians had historically defined the usual and customary charge for the services that they provided. Patients were responsible for any co-payment or deductible not covered by their policies. If a physician charged reasonably and did not raise fees greater than inflation, there would be a reasonable relationship between the uncovered portion and the total fee. Physicians could even raise fees more than inflation required, "write off" a portion of the patient's responsibility, and still expect the carrier to cover the increased costs. As a consequence, third party payers experienced quantum leaps in medical expenses during the '70s and '80s. Carriers found it increasingly difficult to increase premiums and pass on the rising costs to subscribers. With extensive data firmly in hand, they soon refused to pay more than a "reasonable" or "allowed" charge, which was now defined by the insurance industry. A patient would receive an explanation of benefits (EOB) as a claim was processed. This letter would state that the doctor's fee exceeded the usual and customary charge for a given service or procedure. Health insurance language evolved to state that coverage applied only to "allowable" charges rather than "usual and customary" charges. This was the beginning of many mechanisms employed to control spiraling health-care costs. Physicians, who had previously controlled their own reimbursements, lost that control to the third party payer.

American medicine must shoulder some of the blame for its own economic demise. Medical practices and hospitals have historically been inefficient businesses but have been able to pass on costs to patients and third party payers. This lack of responsibility, combined with an American appetite for costly technology and failure of the profession to identify, monitor, and control the problem resulted in health-care costs rising at an enormous rate relative to inflation. American medicine rapidly became much too expensive.

The movement to control the costs of medical care escalated in the '90s. Managed care exploded as individuals and employers sought less costly solutions to health-care needs. Contracting became commonplace for physicians, who were forced to accept "discounted" fee for service in exchange for access to patient populations. Physicians began to accept reimbursements that were substantially less than they had previously hoped to receive. Prevented by antitrust legislation and an inability to agree on matters of mutual self-interest, physician ranks were broken and reimbursement quickly tumbled—particularly in locations with an oversupply of physicians and specialists.

The most recent and dramatic change in reimbursement has been the move to capitation. This will be discussed in greater depth in the final section of the chapter. In general, capitation is prepayment to a doctor or group of doctors to provide a defined set of services for a specific time interval to a given patient population for a predetermined amount—no matter how much or how little care is required. This is conceptually the economic and philosophic opposite of fee for service.

Fee-for-service medical reimbursement in America has undergone radical surgery. The horse and buggy doctor has entered a far less friendly 21st century and is now forced to practice not only better quality, but more efficient and cost-effective, medicine.

GOVERNMENT AS PAYER AND REGULATOR: ESCALATION OF LEGISLATION, REGULATION, AND ECONOMIC CONTROLS

The federal and state governments are enormously important payers and players in the health-care arena. Historically, the federal government had a somewhat limited role in funding and controlling health-care services until the passage of public law 89-97, the Social Security Amendments of 1965. This important legislation established a hospital insurance program for the elderly (Medicare Part A), a voluntary supplemental medical insurance program (Medicare Part B), as well as state grants for medical assistance programs (Medicaid). Though opposed initially by the medical profession, these programs have grown enormously and constitute a major source of physician reimbursement.

Over the following three decades health care legislation proliferated. The Health Maintenance Organization Act of 1973 assisted in the establishment and expansion of HMOs and the Health Maintenance Organization Amendments of 1976 relaxed requirements for HMOs to qualify for federal support. In 1977, the Medicare-Medicaid Anti-Fraud and Abuse Amendments tightened requirements for reporting financial data and increased penalties for fraud under Medicare-Medicaid. The Omnibus Reconciliation Act of 1986 included no less than 58 Medicare-Medicaid reimbursement provisions. In 1982, the Tax Equity and Fiscal Responsibility Act eliminated reimbursement for assistants at surgery if a training program existed at the hospital in the specialty providing the service. It also established "utilization and quality control peer review organizations."

The Social Security Amendments of 1983 established prospectively determined Medicare reimbursement rates for hospital inpatient services for each of 467 diagnosis-related groups (DRGs). The Deficit Reduction Act the following year placed a freeze on physician fees for 15 months and established the Medicare "participating physician" program. The freeze was extended in 1985 under the Emergency Extension Act and again in 1986 under the Consolidated Omnibus Budget Reconciliation Act. The latter legislation also initiated the development of the "resource-based" relative value scale (RBRVS) for physician reimbursement and tightened regulations regarding fees.

The National Practitioner Data Bank—the clearing house for information on physician malpractice and incompetence—was established in 1986 under the Health Care Quality Improvement Act. This attempted to provide some protection for physicians who participate in peer review.

The Omnibus Budget Reconciliation Act (OBRA) of 1987 further extended cuts in Medicare reimbursement and targeted 12 "overpriced" procedures that included carpal tunnel release, knee arthroscopy, total hip replacement, and total knee replacement. The OBRA of 1989, however, was an even more aggressive Medicare cost-containment legislation, implementing the RBRVS, establishing the Medicare volume performance standards (MVPSs), banning patient referrals to laboratories in which physicians had financial interest, and enacting numerous other cost controls and medical practice standards. The 1990 OBRA version reduced or eliminated many surgical assistant's fees and further reduced surgical reimbursement while raising primary care reimbursement. The OBRA of 1993 updated physician fees but redefined calculations for MVPS and practice expense calculations. This was followed by a mandated resource-based practice expense study under the Social Security Act Amendments of 1994, which was incorporated into the fee schedule in January of 1996.

The history of federal legislation in health care is concisely chronicled in the *Socio-Economic Factbook for Surgery* published by the American College of Surgeons (see Selected Bibliography). In 1995, it appeared that sweeping "health-care reform" legislation might be enacted, but the aggressive proposals under consideration did not survive the political process. The focus shifted to making health insurance coverage more available, particularly to individuals who might lose their jobs or become ill. The Health Insurance Portability and Accountability Act of 1996 provided protection for individuals with preexisting conditions or who were changing insurance and—perhaps more importantly—created several fraud and abuse control programs that establish or extend substantial penalties to deter medical fraud. The legislation created incentives for whistle-blowers to report fraudulent providers and also extended penalties and data collection for fraud and abuse under Medicare, as well as certain private-sector activities. The effect of this portion of the Act is uncertain, but there are enormous implications to the medical profession if this legislation is liberally interpreted and aggressively enforced.

Another important feature of this legislation was the establishment of a pilot program for medical savings accounts (MSAs), which are available to a limited population of approximately 750,000 for a period of 4 years beginning on January 1, 1997. This is a relatively new form of health insurance that allows employees and employers to deposit pretax dollars into a special account to be used for medical expenses up to a certain level, beyond which coverage is provided by a catastrophic policy. The first dollars contributed purchase the catastrophic coverage, and the remaining dollars are used against the actual medical expenses incurred during the year. Unused dollars can be carried forward in the tax-free account to the next year. Thus, the unused dollars can grow without being taxed, unless they are withdrawn for nonmedical purposes, at which time they are taxable.

The important anticipated feature of MSAs is a self-imposed control of expenditures by the individual, whose own money is used to pay for necessary medical care. Presumably that individual has incentives to spend that money wisely. There is debate over the desirability of MSAs. Ongoing study will probably show that they are appropriate health coverage vehicles for some but not all individuals.

At the time of this writing, the federal government has extended its power into the medical decision-making process, including hospital lengths of stay and indications for medical/surgical procedures. It appears that further intrusion into medical practice will occur.

MANAGED CARE: HOW PHYSICIANS LOST CONTROL OF THE HEALTH CARE SYSTEM

The term managed care is deceptively simple. It implies the subtle imposition of rational, cost-conscious control on the delivery of health care. This is, at first glance, an attractive improvement for a health-care system that became unaffordable for individuals, employers, and government. The key concept, however, relates to the nature of the controls imposed. These controls extend far beyond efficient management techniques, effective business decision making, and elimination of unnecessary services. Before we examine this further, we need to understand more about the nature of this new direction in health care.

What is managed care? This term describes a number of medical practice and reimbursement models that have the following characteristics:

- a management organization (managed care organization [MCO] or management service organization [MSO]) that markets the insurance plan, manages the administration of services, negotiates contracts, and pays expenses. Although the MCO or MSO is usually a business entity separate from the physician providers, the independent practice association (IPA) model may bring administrative and compensation functions into an alliance of physician providers.

- a continual focus on control and containment of the costs of providing care and services to the insured patient population

- a service and reimbursement model designed to keep the cost of physician services as low and as predictable as possible—usually with the creation of financial incentives to control utilization and deter expensive procedures or services

- a shift of risk from the management organization to the provider whenever possible

The management organization may be an insurance company or other business entity such as a hospital, group of physicians, or even an alliance or partnership between such entities. Physician providers may be independent contractors (as individuals or physician groups) in competition with other providers or they may have an exclusive provider relationship with the MCO. In some cases, physician providers may be employees. Physicians who are not employed (salaried) by the MCO are usually reimbursed under discounted fee-for-service or capitation contracts.

In many managed care plans the patient is tightly controlled by the primary care physician/provider (PCP), who acts as a "gatekeeper" for patient referrals—particularly those that may result in expensive diagnostic studies, surgical intervention, or other costly specialty care. If the PCP is reimbursed under a capitation agreement, the cost of referral services may be deducted from the PCPs capitation payment. This creates a financial disincentive for the PCP to make those referrals. So-called point-of-service plans allow the insured individual to seek specialty care without the approval of the PCP for a higher premium and often with penalties. Unfortunately, many individuals and employers simply do not understand the rapidly changing and increasingly complex world of managed care and are unable to make appropriate choices as they attempt to select a satisfactory plan.

Managed care is filled with a confusing lexicon of terminology and a rapidly expanding set of acronyms to describe organizational models, activities, relationships and functions. The reader is referred to the excellent text *Health Care Reform and Managed Care* published by the American Academy of Orthopaedic Surgeons for an extensive study of the multifaceted nature of managed care (see Selected Bibliography).

Managed care has proliferated rapidly. In some locations, the majority of patients are covered under some type of managed care plan. The evolution and structure of managed care in different communities will vary depending on a number of factors. A community with a surplus of physicians and/or specialists will evolve differently from one with a limited supply. Urban areas will progress differently—and probably faster—than rural or remote locations. Communities that currently have a significant percentage of managed care patients already face a different set of problems and uncertainties than those communities that will enter managed care at some time in the future. Individual state laws, insurance regulation, federal antitrust legislation, and other factors are also likely to impact the evolution of managed care.

Let us return to the issue of control in managed care. Historically, physicians dictated the treatment given to patients and did not require approval or preauthorization to do what they felt was in the best interest of their patients. With the advent of the gatekeeper, control shifted from specialists to primary care providers. As managed care became increasingly more competitive, MCOs saw an increasing need to reduce costs by influencing the medical decision-making process. Physicians awakened to the harsh reality that they needed to get permission to obtain certain diagnostic studies, perform surgical procedures, order therapy, or provide countless other services. That permission was often delayed or withheld, and denial was often determined by a nonphysician. Control of many aspects of patient care was taken from the medical profession by managed care organizations. The control of payment became the control of the patient.

How did doctors lose control of the health-care system? Physicians have long held themselves "above" the business of medicine, shunning most administrative functions and choosing only to provide traditional medical care for patients. Physicians have had no incentives to control costs and are even prevented by antitrust law from attempting to manage rising fees (the Federal Trade Commission, under the Sherman Anti-Trust Act, may prosecute physicians who interfere with the free and open marketplace in determining medical fees). Physicians were generally unaware and apathetic about the magnitude and velocity of the changes taking place until it was too late to be proactive. Many were convinced that managed care was a momentary fad. Despite a rather obvious reality, there are still physicians who remain convinced that managed care will be destroyed by unhappy patients and unsatisfactory outcomes. This can best be described as terminal denial.

American medicine has changed. The eventual format remains uncertain, but never again will the health-care dollar be controlled only by doctor and patient.

CAPITATION: DOCTORS NOW TAKE THE RISK—FOR LESS

Although capitation may appear to be a new and radically different reimbursement system, the concept of prepayment for health care services has been operational for more than 60 years. In the 1930s, prepaid plans were developed by hospital associations in Washington and Oregon. At the same time, industrialist Henry J. Kaiser and Dr. Sidney R. Garfield, a surgeon, pioneered prepaid, comprehensive plans in California and Arizona. Some of the early programs, such as the Kaiser Permanente plans, survive today but must compete against corporate giants in a highly competitive and cost conscious health-care environment. These corporations have taken business and management techniques to a new level in the health care arena.

Capitation is a payment method in which the providers receive a contracted monthly payment to provide a defined group of services to a defined patient population. Under capitation, the providers receive payment on a per member per month (PMPM) basis. For example, a contract might define a payment of $2.00 PMPM and 50,000 "covered lives" might be enrolled for particular month, resulting in a payment to the providers of $100,000—no matter how much or how little care is actually provided.

Beyond the obvious conceptual differences between capitation and fee for service, there are some enormously important economic and practice implications when orthopaedists enter into this potentially dangerous arrangement. Under fee for service, the provider assumes no financial risks relative to the quantity or costliness of the services that are provided to the insured population. This is the risk of the third party payer. If more services are rendered than anticipated, more money will be spent. This means lower profits or even losses for the third party payer. Under capitation, the third party payer has predictable costs each month that are fixed for each enrollee. There is no risk that costs will increase if unanticipated services are required. Where has that risk gone? The risk is now borne by the providers. If unusually high numbers of patients incur illness or injury, or if more patients come into the office than were expected, the providers must provide more care without additional income. Conversely, if the need or demand for care is less, the providers still receive the full capitation payment, but do not need to work as hard.

Capitation differs markedly from fee-for-service medicine. Incentives for patients and doctors are radically altered. Ideally, the manner of reimbursement is irrelevant to the care delivered. In the "real world", however, economic incentives may influence practice patterns and have, in fact, been shown to do so. It is easy to see that under fee for service economic incentives may encourage providers to see more patients and provide more services. Under capitation, economic incentives may encourage providers to see fewer patients and to withhold or delay the provision of services. The result may be a blatant change in the ability of a patient to see a doctor or receive the care desired or a more subtle change such as a revision of indications for an elective surgical procedure. The implications of this will be discussed further in the section on ethics.

Another important facet of capitation concerns the effect this reimbursement system may have on the day-to-day operations of an orthopaedic practice and on the individual physicians in that practice. Fee for service is relatively forgiving to a medical practice. Cash flow, budgeting, identification of productive activities, tracking of desirable payers and calculation of the "bottom line" is not difficult. Each service or procedure, device or implant, medication, etc., has a known cost or value, and profitability of various practice activities is reasonably obvious. Under capitation, these business and management activities become much more difficult to identify, quantify, and evaluate. Unfortunately, they are also much more important to the medical practice with capitation contracts, in which a knowledge of costs, resource utilizations, and many other parameters is essential. The capitated practice needs to know the cost of taking care of each patient and the work performed in that process to know if providing that care is profitable or not. This requires sophisticated information management systems, which many practices do not possess. Without these essential tools, a practice may struggle or fail. This has occurred and is likely to continue as the capitation reimbursement system becomes better understood.

Another potential problem involves the method by which a medical group may distribute their monthly capitation payment to its physicians. Most groups have divided income and shared overhead using a formula. Each physician's contribution or productivity is easy to evaluate. Generally, productivity relates to the nature and volume of services or procedures each physician provides. Though a group could choose to share all income equally between the physicians, this tends to punish the hardest working doctors and reward the least productive members of the group. More commonly the income distribution (combined with overhead allocation) is designed to create incentives for hard work and penalties for poor production. Under a capitation reimbursement, system the group must determine how to distribute the lump sum payment each month. If this is done on the basis of what each individual physician would have billed (if fee-for-service charges had been submitted), there is a financial incentive for the physicians to do more and bill more. This is counter-productive in the capitation model, which is most successful when the practice efficiently provides only those services which are required and necessary. If one physician has different indications for a total knee arthroplasty than does an associate, there will be a difference in their "billings." If fee-for-service productivity determines each surgeon's share of the capitation payment, the more conservative surgeon will be penalized when, in fact, that surgeon should be rewarded in the capitation model. In addition, orthopaedic subspecialties are not equally valued in the fee-for-service system. Procedures requiring 2 hours of operating time may be reimbursed very differently, depending on the exact procedure performed. The value of 2 hours is the same to each of the surgeons, but the reward may be different if fee-for-service productivity is used to distribute the capitation payment. This inequity is meaningless in a fee-for-service reimbursement system, but it is very important in a capitation setting, where each member of the group is competing for a share of the capitation payment. This can be a source of discord and may lead to a very unhealthy type of peer review. The ideal income distribution method under the capitation model will reward the provider for seeing new patients and solving their orthopedic problems in the most efficient manner. It will not provide incentives for practicing aggressive or procedure-oriented orthopedics. It will very likely create financial incentives to achieve a high level of patient satisfaction.

The capitation model controls and reduces costs. It also shifts the risk from the third party payer to the physician but may not reward the physician for assuming that risk. Provider groups who practice high quality, but efficient and conservative orthopaedics can be financially successful under the capitation model. The structure and function of this reimbursement model is evolving. Orthopedists must be very cautious as they become involved in capitation contracts.

ETHICAL CONSIDERATIONS OF CHANGING REIMBURSEMENT PATTERNS: HOW ECONOMIC INCENTIVES MAY ERODE THE QUALITY OF MEDICAL PRACTICE

Having practiced medicine for more than a quarter of a century, the author has seen some of the best of American medicine … and unfortunately some that is not so praise worthy. To deny that economic incentives influence patient care is to deny that physicians are human and that there are bad apples in the noblest of all professions. To be truly professional a physician is to always do what is best for the patient without regard for reimbursement or any other factor. Most physicians know this, and many live by this ethic. Why then is there ever greater need for the medical profession and government to regulate the actions of physicians and protect the quality of medical care?

In the beginning of this chapter we noted that there is no ideal reimbursement system. Let us now examine this in greater depth. Under fee for service, physicians are compensated for what they do. A physician is paid for seeing a patient in the office for an initial visit and for follow-up visits. If the patient is seen every week, instead of some appropriate longer interval, the physician is "busier" and receives greater compensation. A surgeon is paid more for performing surgery than for recommending nonoperative treatment. This economic incentive encourages operative intervention, relaxation of indications, "staging" of procedures, and rewards poor surgical technique that may require re-operation or "revision." There are many other examples of abuses that may be encouraged by the fee-for-service reimbursement format. Only the highest personal ethics prevent physicians from falling for the subtle seduction of payment-driven medical decision making.

Managed care has attempted to remove the incentives to "do too much" through the capitation reimbursement model. As we have already seen, however, the incentives under capitation are to withhold care—permitting the physician to be reimbursed better for spending less time or effort providing care or for shifting the burden of care to a lower paid assistant or employee. The capitated orthopaedist may have a longer "waiting list" for procedures.

There are other abuses and unethical behaviors that may occur in an attempt to maximize reimbursement. "Unbundling" is an unethical (and now illegal) billing practice that is characterized by submitting a charge for a surgical procedure (or other types of services) with the submission of additional charges for integral components of that procedure. An example might be the submission of a separate charge for "neurolysis" of a nerve that is merely exposed and protected during the exposure routinely required for the performance of a procedure. Another unethical billing practice is called "upcoding" and is characterized by charging for a similar, but more complex and higher-paying procedure than the procedure actually performed. Other examples of fraudulent or abusive behaviors can relate to the use of surgical assistants, charges for facilities or equipment, and many other activities that occur in medical practice.

Medicine is going through a difficult evolution. Economic pressures on physicians, particularly young physicians who may have substantial debts following training, will continue to rise. In the struggle to maintain or establish lifestyle, there is danger in not recognizing that erosion of objectivity and personal ethics can harm patients and the medical profession.

DOCTORS ARE IN BUSINESS—LIKE IT OR NOT: HOW AND WHY TO COMMUNICATE WITH YOUR ACCOUNTANT, ATTORNEY, OFFICE MANAGER, AND FINANCIAL ADVISOR

The traditional preparation for the practice of medicine focuses—appropriately—on medicine and does not prepare young physicians for entry into a practice world that is complex, confusing, chaotic, and consuming. Medicine has attempted to remain above the financial, managerial, and operational aspects of the business of medical practice. As we have already seen, the abdication of the control of these essential components of the practice of medicine merely permits this control to be seized by others.

Many physicians want minimal involvement in day-to-day operations and decision making. Some choose to become employed by a multispecialty clinic or large institution, receive a salary, and concentrate their efforts on patient care. This is becoming more common and is a rational choice for many individuals. If that is your choice you must realize that you give up a degree of autonomy in these settings. No physician, however, is immune from the need to develop business acumen to be as successful as possible—regardless of the practice setting that is chosen. The more an individual desires to have control of his or her medical practice, the more business expertise becomes mandatory.

One important lesson that physicians must learn about the business of medicine is that it is common knowledge in the business community that physicians are notoriously bad business people. The reason for this is not that physicians lack intelligence or formal business education, but rather that physicians (and particularly surgeons) generally believe that they know everything and have the same level of expertise in other areas that they have in medicine. This intellectual arrogance leads to costly errors in medical practice, personal investments, retirement and estate planning, and many other endeavors. With this in mind, the sage physician seeks out the best advisors and establishes long-term relationships with those advisors, just as chief executives with MBA degrees do in their business and personal lives. Accountants, bankers, lawyers, financial advisors, and many other experts are resources to physicians and should be utilized the same way specialists and subspecialists are used in medical practice. More importantly, there is wide variation in the quality and expertise of these individuals, and the physician must research and evaluate the credentials and performance of these individuals to select the very finest advisors.

Returning to the acquisition of business acumen, one of the most important skills for physicians to acquire is a working level of knowledge in accounting. The ability to read an income statement and balance sheet is fundamental. Understanding the difference between cash accounting and accrual accounting is necessary to understand why reimbursement methods, accounts receivable, and expenses may create false impressions about the financial health of a practice. The ability to create a budget and a pro forma plan for a practice is critical, particularly if multiple reimbursement systems are involved. Accounting is the language of business and finance. It is a language worth learning, and it allows the physician to receive and understand financial advice.

Despite the distrust that many physicians feel toward the legal profession, there are many excellent lawyers, and more importantly, there are legal experts in contracting, capitation, medical mergers, malpractice, and many other specialty areas of health-care law. The physician is well advised to gain a working knowledge of contracts, torts, recent health-care legislation, workers compensation, informed consent, etc., to feel comfortable that the practice is performing properly and well within the boundaries defined by law.

Most practices have a nonphysician who administrates or manages daily activities. The physician must understand that medical practices are governed by the same federal and state labor laws, discrimination policies, health and safety requirements, and a myriad of other rules and regulations that apply to all other businesses. A medical practice may run into substantial difficulties if the expertise of the practice manager is insufficient or if the physician is unaware of the importance of these issues.

Physicians usually find that a solid banking relationship is essential to efficient medical practice as well as to personal financial management. The ability to contact a banker who can give solid advice and who can represent the best interests of the physician is another resource of great value. These relationships are far more important than the interest paid on a checking account or whether the bank has an attractive advertising campaign.

Lastly, physicians must understand that successful business people approach decisions and problems in a logical and detailed fashion. The term "due diligence" is a fundamental concept in the business world, but is often ignored by physicians in their practices and in their personal financial lives. To be successful, it is critical to get all of the pertinent information, to get the very best advice, to refuse to be pressured or hurried to make important decisions, and to fully understand the immediate and long-term implications of all decisions.

THE FUTURE: KEYS TO SUCCESS

Young physicians have been admonished for decades that their success is determined by the "three As": ability, affability, and availability. This remains conceptually, although now only partially, correct. The changes and complexities of the American health-care system will require physicians to be aware of many additional determinants of long-term medical practice success.

Although there is no simplistic recipe to ensure happiness and prosperity in the medical practice of the future, certain observations and suggestions may prove helpful:

1. The most important mission of the physician is to maximize the happiness and quality of life of his or her patient. Range-of-motion measurements, radiographic assessments, and all of the other tools of the orthopaedic trade are merely means to accomplish this goal. It is far more important to help a patient achieve a satisfactory and realistic outcome to an orthopaedic problem than it is to merely improve the radiographic appearance of that problem. The change to outcomes research will result in a far greater emphasis on patient satisfaction with treatment than has existed in the past. Formerly, the doctor defined the parameters that determined whether the final result of treatment was satisfactory or not. In the future, the assessment of the patient will be much more important. As a consequence, physicians will need to communicate effectively with patients throughout the course of treatment. It will be important to prevent patients from having unrealistic expectations. The understanding and compassion of the physician and the entire office staff will become more, not less, important in the future.

2. Understand and accept reality. Physicians may desire to be paid more than professional athletes or entertainers, but that is currently not the case. Many may wish to return to prior times of medical practice prosperity. Unfortunately, time marches only forward. Unrealistic expectations about the financial rewards of medical practice may entice a naive orthopedist entering practice to commit to a lifestyle that cannot be supported. Expensive homes, private schools, exotic cars, and vacations are aging symbols of success and do not equate with personal happiness or professional achievement. Material possessions may be a source of pleasure but can never be more important than the proper care of a patient.

3. Successful businesses are continually assessing the nature of their customer bases, interacting with their customers, and seeking new and better ways to serve their customers. This is termed being "close to the customer." In medical practice, it is becoming increasingly more difficult to identify the actual customer. Is the patient the customer or is the true customer the third party payer? Certainly the satisfaction of the payer is important or the payer will select other physician providers. Similarly referring physicians,

attorneys, and other patient sources must remain satisfied "customers" of a successful practice.

4. Physicians often assume that the product or service that they "sell" is the knowledge and technical skill that they possess. In reality, physicians, like most professionals, are paid for their time. A physician who works inefficiently in the office or in the operating room is paid less than an efficient colleague. This is true for any reimbursement system. Medical practice efficiency begins with the physician, but must also include support personnel, office systems, and over-all practice management.

5. Although advertising by the medical profession has become much more aggressive, patients and third party payers remain skeptical of flashy self-promotion by doctors. It is possible to remain professional during the process of building a practice. Successful surgeons are active and visible in their communities. They participate in educational programs and community service. They are active in professional societies and serve on hospital committees. They take leadership positions, and they expand the scope of their activities far beyond the field of medicine.

6. Throughout a physician's career, an important but intangible element characterizes his or her professional activities. Reputation is the collective judgment of the medical profession and the lay community about the quality of our work. A superior reputation may not guarantee a successful practice, but a tarnished reputation will almost certainly prevent the achievement of success to some degree. The highest standards of professional and ethical conduct are the building blocks of a superior reputation.

SUMMARY

An understanding of reimbursement systems and economic incentives is important for all physicians. The acquisition of business expertise is now a mandatory education for successful physicians, who must find a way to regain control of those components of the health-care system that are essential to the proper treatment of patients. The medical profession must be aggressive and proactive to recover its leadership role in American medicine.

SELECTED BIBLIOGRAPHY

American Academy of Orthopaedic Surgeons. *Health Care Reform and Managed Care*. Rosemont, IL: American Academy of Orthopaedic Surgeons; 1994.

American Academy of Orthopaedic Surgeons. *Capitation and Other Managed Care Payment Systems for Orthopaedic Surgeons*. Rosemont, IL: American Academy of Orthopaedic Surgeons; 1996.

American College of Surgeons. *Socio-Economic Factbook for Surgery*. Chicago, IL: American College of Surgeons; 1996–1997.

GALLAGHER C. What surgeons should know about … medical savings accounts. *Bulletin of the American College of Surgeons*. 1997;82:8–11.

HANSEN JR, FREDERIK C. What does your future hold: capitation or decapitation? *Bulletin of the American College of Surgeons*. 1996;81:12–23.

KRIEGER LM. Young surgeons at managed care's ground zero. *Bulletin of the American College of Surgeons*. 1996;81:18–22.

Chapter 57

Critical Pathways in Orthopaedics

Thomas A. Mutschler, MD, MS

Outline

HISTORY

Throughout the 1970s and 1980s, the United States experienced improvement in the quality of medical care and a marked increase in the available treatment options. These factors coupled with a rapid expansion of the delivery system led to unchecked inflation in the cost of medical care. Congress, with the Omnibus Budget Reconciliation Act of 1989, created the Agency for Health Care Policy and Research (AHCPR). One responsibility of the agency was the promotion, development, and dissemination of *clinical practice guidelines*. The AHCPR looked to the Institute of Medicine (IOM) and received the assistance of a 12-member committee of physicians, doctorates, and nurses. The IOM has been instrumental in setting priorities for the development of guidelines. Although the initiation of clinical guidelines has come about through governmental prompting, since inception their development has been under the leadership of the medical community.

DEFINITION

Clinical practice guidelines are known by a number of different terms, for example, clinical algorithms, clinical guidelines, clinical pathways, and *critical pathways*. However, there are differences in the meanings of these terms that follow a logical progression of increasing complexity but also increasing usefulness.

Many disease states can be placed into categories such as the diagnostic related groupings (DRGs). *Clinical practice guidelines* are systematically developed statements designed to assist in the formulation of treatment plans for these specific clinical groupings. These statements can be placed into an algorithm or flowchart for ease of representation. This generates a *clinical pathway*.

Clinical pathways include all of the elements of care regardless of their effect on the clinical outcome. The clinical pathway can include elements that are "good to do" or "won't do any harm" but whose impact may be minimal or unknown.

Clinical pathways can be honed to a *critical pathway*, which is a treatment plan that includes only the vital elements that are proven to positively affect patient outcomes and that are delivered in a timely fashion.

The term critical pathway is not indigenous to medicine. This term originated in industry and is used as a process management tool. These pathways are used in manufacturing to identify areas that can bottleneck production. They are strictly monitored and are modified to achieve the goals of the pathway such as timely production and decreased cost.

Most health-care workers use the terms clinical pathway and critical pathway interchangeably. The intent, regardless of usage, should be to create a pathway that is monitored, can be modified, and that continually focuses on the improvement in the pathway's ability to achieve its goals, such as improved patient outcomes or satisfaction. The term critical pathway more accurately describes these traits and will be used here.

DEVELOPMENT AND IMPLEMENTATION

At present, business is concerned with the cost of medical care. Physicians are concerned about the quality of care. Both parties agree that cost and quality are interrelated. However, high cost does not always equate to high quality and a good patient outcome. Conversely, low cost does not necessarily denote low quality or a poor outcome. The challenge in medicine for the 1990s has been to control or decrease the cost of care while maintaining or improving the quality. Critical pathways are essential to this endeavor as they provide, as in industry, the process management tool needed to control unwanted variability.

The development of a critical pathway usually begins with the need to improve the competitive position of a health-care delivery entity. It is clear that in the current climate of competition among insurers, hospitals, and physician groups for declining health-care dollars, inefficiencies in the delivery and quality of care can lead to the financial collapse of the

891

health-care entity. A critical pathway that is properly developed and implemented can produce a rapid decline of unwanted variability in the delivery of care. This variability is costly, not only in fiscal terms but also in patient outcome.

PEARL

Involve everyone who delivers patient care in the development of the critical pathway.

The key to pathway development is to elicit the support of the whole of the health-care institution. Representatives from each facet of care should be present at development meetings. As can be seen in Table 57–1, the representatives encompass the whole of the care delivery process. The critical pathway built by consensus will empower those involved in the care process with the management of the process. Involving all will invest all and ensure that the critical pathway will succeed. Each representative should be on an equal par with the other with the traditional barriers between them discarded. Information for pathway development can be exchanged at meetings or gathered via questionnaire. A team leader, usually a physician, is needed to coordinate the meetings of the representatives. It is extremely important that the team leader moderates, not dominates, these meetings.

PITFALL

Rather than seek consensus, the team leader attempts to dictate the development of the critical pathway.

Critical pathways are affected by both global and local environments. As such, a pathway cannot readily be imported from another institution without modification to accommodate local factors. In addition, attempts to initiate an imported critical pathway will likely lead to resistance within the health-care institution. This, in turn, will result in the failure or disuse of the pathway.

The critical pathway can and should be benchmarked against the global environment to determine if it has been honed to its maximum efficiency. The global environment also serves as a resource for new ideas or for the experience of an institution that underwent changes being contemplated by the local institution. Benchmarking also serves as a prime motivator for the development of critical pathways and is the logical place to begin. Comparison between health-care institutions identifies discrepancies in care and drives the health-care team's desire to develop pathways to decrease these discrepancies.

Once the need for pathways is acknowledged, a review of the present methods of delivering care is conducted. This

TABLE 57–1 Critical Pathway Development Team

Hospital administration	Physical therapy
Anesthesiology	Occupational therapy
Orthopaedic surgeons	Pyschiatry
Operating room personnel	Admission personnel
Unit nursing	Social service
Recovery room	Home care

PEARL

Compare present methods of care at your institution to global practices to determine the direction for the pathway.

---

review identifies variables in each team member's area. The review should be extensive. This allows it to uncover the most variables and presents the best opportunities for process control.

The next step is the most difficult and involves multidisciplinary collaboration to find more efficient methods for delivering care. Compromise is necessary, but individuals need not lose their identity. The orthopaedic surgeons, for example, may decide collectively to use a standard preoperative antibiotic prophylaxis given at a set time but still continue to perform an operation according to individual perferences.

The outcome to the patient of some of the treatments currently rendered has little or no support in the medical literature. The efficacy of such treatments should be challenged. If the efficacy is in doubt and a compromise cannot be reached, the treatment can be included in the pathway and the outcome monitored. If the positive benefit to the patient is not realized, then the pathway can be modified to eliminate the treatment.

Once consensus has been reached, the critical pathway is constructed on a tracking document (Fig. 57–1). The tracking document is the process control document. It usually is constructed on a per-day basis and details the events that should occur that day. It assures that care is delivered in a timely fashion.

Typically for orthopaedics, the pathway is implemented in the operating room. The tracking document initiates there and is accompanied by a postoperative standard order set (Fig. 57–2), for a given surgical procedure, for example, total hip arthroplasty (THA). The order set should detail the entire length of stay.

The critical pathway is a dynamic process that must be monitored. Patient outcomes in terms of complications and satisfaction are recorded. Variances from the pathway are also recorded. Variances can positively or negatively affect the patient outcome.

The critical pathway team is required to meet on a periodic basis to review the outcome and variance reports (Fig. 57–3). Positive variances are reinforced, and negative variances are obliterated through modifications to the tracking document. Again, multidisciplinary collaboration is necessary to affect these modifications. This will focus the pathway to its maximum efficiency and maintain the goals for which the pathway was constructed, for example, decrease length of stay. Note that a critical pathway that becomes static and is not monitored will revert to a clinical pathway, and the gains accomplished by the pathway will erode. A summary of these development and implementation steps is given in Table 57–2.

PITFALL

Not monitoring variances will produce a static pathway that will deteriorate.

PRIMARY TOTAL HIP ARTHROPLASTY   Pg. __1__
☐ With Diabetes   ☐ Without Diabetes

Allegheny General Hospital
320 East North Avenue
Pittsburgh, PA 15212-4772   *AGH*
                                ALLEGHENY GENERAL HOSPITAL

Code ____THA.1____   DRG# ___209___

Expected LOS _____5 days_____

Service _____ORTHO_____

Outcomes ___Discharge in 5 days without complications___

IMPRINT PATIENT'S PLATE HERE

UNIT(s)	Pre-Op				OR			
Day		INITIALS			Day of Surgery	INITIALS		
Date		D	E	N		D	E	N
Assessment	Critical Pathway THA Pre-Admission Evaluation				Time in room Time of incision Time of closure Time out of room			
Consults	As necessary				Anesthesia General Spinal			
Labs	As per anesthesia				Blood Glucose as ordered			
Tests								
Meds					Antibiotic Ancef Vancomycin			
IV					IV Fluids			

Treatments					Abductor splint applied
					Name of Manufacturer
					   Cemented _____
					   Cementless_____
					   Hybrid _____
					Hemovac in place			

Activity	PT: Home Evaluation							
Nutrition	NPO				NPO			
Teaching	Pre-Op							
Discharge	Administrative Case Manager: Begin D/C plan							
Intermediate Outcomes	To OR without delay							
Initial Signature Title								

The Critical Pathway is only a guideline and may be modified at the discretion of the physician or care giver, based on patient responses.
301-468 4/96

A

Figure 57–1   (A–G). Tracking document

PRIMARY TOTAL HIP ARTHROPLASTY
☐ With Diabetes ☐ Without Diabetes

Pg. __2__

Allegheny General Hospital
320 East North Avenue
Pittsburgh, PA 15212-4772

AGH™
ALLEGHENY GENERAL HOSPITAL

Code ___THA.1___ DRG# ___209___
Expected LOS ___5 days___
Service ___ORTHO___
Outcomes ___Discharge in 5 days without complications___

IMPRINT PATIENT'S PLATE HERE

UNIT(s)	RECOVERY ROOM				10C			
Day	Day of Surgery	INITIALS			Day of Surgery	INITIALS		
Date		D	E	N		D	E	N
Assessment	Neurovascular checks Hemovac emptied cc				V.S. q4° x 24° Hemovac emptied Neurovascular checks Adjust insulin as orders q2hr x 24 hr as indicated			
Consults	Diabetic Practitioner if applicable				PT OT Social Service Home Care Diabetes educator/dietician			
Labs	H & H 2 hr Post Op Blood glucose as ordered							
Tests	X-ray obtained							
Meds	PRN				Pain meds IM/IV/POEPI Compazine IM 10 mg Anticoagulant as ordered q6 hrx24 hr prn N&V Ancef 1 gm IV q 8 hrs x Colace 100 mg PO bid 6 doses; if allergic Oral hypoglycemic/ Vancomycin 500 mg insulin as ordered IV q 6 hrs x 8 doses			
IV	IV Fluids				IV Fluids I & O q8 hrs			
Treatments	Elastic stockings				Straight cath q6 hrs if necessary Reinforce Dsg.			
Activity	Bedrest				Bedrest			
Nutrition	NPO				Clear diet, adv. as tolerated or ADA			
Teaching	Cough & deep breath q 2 hr W/A				Cough & deep breath q 2 hrs W/A			
Discharge								
Intermediate Outcomes	Stable to 10C				Free of any neuro-vascular complicatons & hip dislocation BS within 100-200 mg/dl if applicable Self administration of insulin if applicable			
Initial Signature Title								

The Critical Pathway is only a guidline and may be modified at the discretion of the physician or caregiver.
301-468 4/96

B

Figure 57–1 *(cont.)*

PRIMARY TOTAL HIP ARTHROPLASTY   Pg. __3__
☐ With Diabetes   ☐ Without Diabetes

Allegheny General Hospital
320 East North Avenue
Pittsburgh, PA 15212-4772   **ALLEGHENY GENERAL HOSPITAL**

Code _____ **THA.1** _____   DRG# ___ **209** ___
Expected LOS _____ **5 days** _____
Service _____ **ORTHO** _____
Outcomes ___ **Discharge in 5 days without complications** ___

IMPRINT PATIENT'S PLATE HERE

UNIT(s)	10C			
Day	POD1		INITIALS	
Date		D	E	N
Assessment	V.S. q 4 hrs. x 24 hrs. Hemovac emptied Neurovascular checks q 4 hrs. Adjust hypoglycemic therapy as ordered			
Consults				
Labs	H & H in am Pro-Time in am BS premeal _____ hs _____ as ordered			
Tests				
Meds	Pain meds IM/IV/POEPI Compazine IM 10 mg Anticoagulant as ordered q 6 hrs x24 hr prn N&V Ancef 1 gm IV q 8 hrs x Colace 100 mg 6 doses; if allergic PO BID Vancomycin 500 mg Oral hypoglycemic/insulin as ordered IV q 6 hrs x 8 doses then D/C			
IV	D/C IV Fluids I & O q 8 hrs.			
Treatments	Indwelling cath if unable to void after 3 straight caths. Abductor splint change to pillow and send urinalysis Reinforce dsg prn Abductor pillow			
Activity	PT as tolerated Review THA precautions OT: Evaluation			
Nutrition	Advance as tolerated or ADA diet			
Teaching	Cough & deep breath q 2 hrs. W/A Nursing: Review and do above exercises with patient Review diabetic survival skills if applicable			
Discharge	Administrative Case Manager: Consult SS if necessary			
Intermediate Outcomes	Comfortable with pain management (Scale 1-5) free of hip dislocation BS within 100-200 mg/dl if applicable Self administration of insulin if applicable			
Initial Signature Title				

The Critical Pathway is only a guideline and may be modified at the discretion of the physician or care giver, based on patient responses.
301-468   4/96

C

Figure 57–1 *(cont.)*

PRIMARY TOTAL HIP ARTHROPLASTY   Pg. __4__
☐ With Diabetes   ☐ Without Diabetes

Allegheny General Hospital
320 East North Avenue
Pittsburgh, PA 15212-4772   **ALLEGHENY GENERAL HOSPITAL**

Code ___THA.1_____   DRG# ___209_____

Expected LOS _____5 days_____

Service _____ORTHO_____

Outcomes ___Discharge in 5 days without complications_____

IMPRINT PATIENT'S PLATE HERE

UNIT(s)	10C			
Day	POD2	INITIALS		
Date		D	E	N
Assessment	V.S. q shift Assess bladder function Neurovascular checks q 4 hrs. Notify MD if foley in place Assess bowel function Hemovac removed			
Consults				
Labs	Pro-Time in am H & H today BS premeal ____ hs ____ as ordered			
Tests				
Meds	Pain meds IM/IV/PO Colace 100 mg PO BID Anticoagulant as ordered Oral hypoglycemics/insulin as ordered MOM 30 cc PO BID prn			
IV	D/C I & O's			
Treatments	Premed for PT Dsg. change BID			
Activity	PT BID Review THA precautions OT: ADL's functional mobility/transfers			
Nutrition	Advance as tolerated or ADA diet			
Teaching	Cough & deep breath q 2 hrs. Reinforce & do above exercises with patient Review diabetic survival skills if applicable			
Discharge	Administrative Case Manager: Consult Gwen Bronson if necessary			
Intermediate Outcomes	Free of urinary complication and hip dislocation BS within 100-200 mg/dl if applicable Self administration of insulin if applicable			
Initial Signature Title				

The Critical Pathway is only a guideline and may be modified at the discretion of the physician or care giver, based on patient responses.
301-468 4/96

D

Figure 57–1 *(cont.)*

PRIMARY TOTAL HIP ARTHROPLASTY   Pg. __5__
☐ With Diabetes   ☐ Without Diabetes

Allegheny General Hospital
320 East North Avenue
Pittsburgh, PA 15212-4772   **AGH.**
ALLEGHENY GENERAL HOSPITAL

Code ____THA.1____   DRG# ____209____

Expected LOS ____5 days____

Service ____ORTHO____

Outcomes ___Discharge in 5 days without complications___

IMPRINT PATIENT'S PLATE HERE

UNIT(s)	10C			
Day	POD3	INITIALS		
Date		D	E	N
Assessment	V.S. q shift Assess bladder function Neurovascular checks q 4 hrs. Notify MD if foley in place Assess bowel function			
Consults				
Labs	H & H today Pro-Time in am BS premeal _____ hs _____ as ordered			
Tests				
Meds	D/C IM/IV pain med Colace 100 mg PO BID Pain med PO Anticoagulation as ordered Fleet enema prn Oral hypoglycemics/insulin as ordered			
IV				
Treatments	Premed for PT Dsg. change BID			
Activity	PT BID OT: Functional mobility/transfers Review THA precautions ADL's			
Nutrition	Regular or ADA diet			
Teaching	Nursing: Review & do above exercises with patient Diabetes education as if applicable			
Discharge	Administrative Case Manager: Discharge plan in place			
Intermediate Outcomes	Free of any signs/symptoms of hip dislocation Contact Spot/Spot for functional mobility transfers OT: Independent with ADL's Discharged to CCC/Rehab/Home Independent with diabetes care if applicable BS within 100-200 mg/dl if applicable			
Initial Signature Title				

The Critical Pathway is only a guideline and may be modified at the discretion of the physician or care giver, based on patient responses.
301-468   4/96

E

Figure 57–1 *(cont.)*

PRIMARY TOTAL HIP ARTHROPLASTY   Pg. __6__
☐ With Diabetes   ☐ Without Diabetes

Allegheny General Hospital
320 East North Avenue
Pittsburgh, PA 15212-4772   **AGH**™
                              ALLEGHENY GENERAL HOSPITAL

Code ____THA.1_____   DRG# ___209_____

Expected LOS ____5 days_____

Service _____ORTHO_____

Outcomes ___Discharge in 5 days without complications_____

IMPRINT PATIENT'S PLATE HERE

UNIT(s)	10C			
Day	POD4	INITIALS		
Date		D	E	N
Assessment	Neurovascular checks q 4 hrs VS q shift Assess bowel function			
Consults				
Labs	Pro-Time in AM H&H in am BS premeal _____ hs _____ as ordered			
Tests				
Meds	Stepdown pain med Oral hypoglycemics/insulin as ordered Anticoagulation as ordered Colace 100 mg PO BID Fleet enema prn			
IV				
Treatments	Premed for PT Dsg. change BID			
Activity	PT BID OT: ADL's THA exercises: Functional mobility/transfers			
Nutrition	Regular or ADA diet			
Teaching	Nursing: Review & do above exercises with patient Diabetes Education if applicable			
Discharge	Administrative Case manager: To order equipment and Home Care if necessary			
Intermediate Outcomes	OT: Independent with ADL's and use of equipment for D/C Contact Spot/Spot for functional mobility transfers Free of infection and hip dislocation Independent wiht diabetes care if applicable Discharged to CCC/Rehab/home BS within 100-200 mg/dl if applicable			
Initial Signature Title				

The Critical Pathway is only a guideline and may be modified at the discretion of the physician or care giver, based on patient responses.
301-468   4/96

F

Figure 57–1   *(cont.)*

PRIMARY TOTAL HIP ARTHROPLASTY   Pg. __7__
☐ With Diabetes   ☐ Without Diabetes

Allegheny General Hospital
320 East North Avenue
Pittsburgh, PA 15212-4772   **AGH**
                                  ALLEGHENY GENERAL HOSPITAL

Code ____THA.1____   DRG# ___209___
Expected LOS ____5 days____
Service ____ORTHO____
Outcomes __Discharge in 5 days without complications__

IMPRINT PATIENT'S PLATE HERE

UNIT(s)	10C			
Day	POD5	INITIALS		
Date		D	E	N
Assessment	Neurovascular checks q 4 hrs VS q shift Assess bowel function			
Consults				
Labs	PT in AM H&H in AM BS premeal _____ hs _____ as ordered			
Tests				
Meds	Stepdown pain med Oral hypoglycemics/insulin as ordered Anticoagulation as desired Colace 100 mg PO BID Fleet enema prn			
IV				
Treatments	D/C Premed for PT Dsg. change BID			
Activity	PT BID OT: ADL's THA exercises: Functional mobility/transfers			
Nutrition	Regular or ADA diet			
Teaching	Nursing: Review & do above exercises with patient			
Discharge	Administrative Case Manager: To order equipment and Home Care if necessary			
Intermediate Outcomes	Independent with transfers Contact Spot/Spot for functional mobility transfers Free of infection and hip dislocation Independent with diabetes care if applicable Discharged to rehab/home/CCC BS within 100-200 mg/dl if applicable			
Initial Signature Title				

The Critical Pathway is only a guideline and may be modified at the discretion of the physician or care giver, based on patient responses.
301-468 4/96

G

Figure 57–1   *(cont.)*

ALLEGHENY GENERAL HOSPITAL

Pittsburgh, Pennsylvania 15212

PHYSICIAN'S ORDER SHEET
Unless Specified

"This Brand Only", The Generic Equivalent
or
Therapeutic Alternative Will be Dispensed

USE BALL-POINT PEN ONLY

Form DC 470-06A Rev/ 6/88

IMPRINT PATIENT'S PLATE HERE

Time Noted By Nurse		Ordered		DIET MEDICATION TREATMENT WITH DOCTORS SIGNATURE
Hour	Name	Date	Hour	
				COMPLETE ALLERGY INFORMATION AT TIME OF ADMISSION
				ALLERGIES:
				CLINICAL PATHWAY PRE-ADMISSION ORDERS FOR TOTAL, REVISION
				AND BIPOLAR HIP ARTHROPLASTY
				☐ with Diabetes Mellitus ☐ without Diabetes Mellitus
				Pre-op Testing Guidelines: (√) *Check mark which tests are appropriate*
				MALES: ____ EKG if over 40
				____ EKG, CBC, Surgical Profile if over 60
				____ EKG, CBC, Surgical Profile and CXR if over 74
				____ U/A
				____ Type & Screen
				FEMALES: ____ CBC if under 50
				____ CBC, EKG if over 50
				____ CBC, EKG, Surgical Profile if over 60
				____ CBC, EKG, Surgical Profile, CXR if over 74
				____ U/A
				____ Type & Screen
				OPTIONAL: ____ PT/PTT ____ BUN ____ PLTS
				____ Creatinine ____ Hemoglobin A_1C ____ Fasting Blood Glucose
				☐ Hold Metformin (Glucophage) 48 hrs pre-procedure
				☐ Day of surgery: Hold oral hypoglycemic
				☐ _____ insulin _____ units sq at ____ am
				Same Day Admission Orders for Total Knee Arthroplasty
				☐ with diabetes mellitus ☐ without diabetes mellitus
				☐ Type & Screen (if not drawn in Pre-admission Testing)

Initiator _____ Department Chair *[signature]*

ECMS Date Approved ___6-18-96___ Cntrl # ___864___ (Assigned by Staff Office)

A

Figure 57–2 (A–C). Standard order set

ALLEGHENY GENERAL HOSPITAL

Pittsburgh, Pennsylvania 15212

PHYSICIAN'S ORDER SHEET
Unless Specified

"This Brand Only", The Generic Equivalent
or
Therapeutic Alternative Will be Dispensed

USE BALL-POINT PEN ONLY

IMPRINT PATIENT'S PLATE HERE

Form DC 470-06A Rev/ 6/88

Time Noted By Nurse		Ordered		DIET MEDICATION TREATMENT WITH DOCTORS SIGNATURE
Hour	Name	Date	Hour	
				COMPLETE ALLERGY INFORMATION AT TIME OF ADMISSION
				ALLERGIES:
				PRIMARY TOTAL HIP ARTHROPLASTY CLINICAL PATHWAY ORDERS (Page 1 of 2)
				☐ with Diabetes Mellitus ☐ without Diabetes Mellitus
				Admit to RR s/p _____ THA
				Condition:
				VS: q 4 hours x 24 hrs then q shift
				Neurovascular check q 2 hrs x 8 hrs
				Activities: Bed rest in bilateral thigh high ted hose or toe-to-thigh ace wraps DOS
				POD #1 until discharged OOB to gym bid
				Nursing: I & O's, Hemovac drainage
				Reinforce dressing prn
				Cough and deep breathe
				Straight cath q 6 hrs prn UTV if 3 straight caths in 24 hrs, insert indwelling
				catheter and send a urinalysis.
				If the R & M WBC count return at > 50, send C & S and notify MD
				☐ Review DM skills knowledge
				Diet: ☐ Clear diet, advance as tolerated to ADA _____ calories
				☐ Clear diet, advance to regular
				IVF:
				D/C IVF when taking PO well
				Labs: H/H 2 hrs post-op then H/H, PT q AM x 3 then PT q AM only
				☐ Blood glucose by meter in RR then ac & hs. Call MD if < _____ or > _____
				☐ Give subcut. _____ insulin: _____ units q am 30 min ac
				☐ Give subcut. _____ insulin: _____ units q pm 30 min ac
				☐ Oral hypoglycemic agent: _____ , _____ mg po q _____

Initiator _____   Department Chair _____

ECMS Date Approved _____6-18-96_____   Control # _____870_____ (Assigned by Staff Office)

142

B

Figure 57–2   *(cont.)*

Pittsburgh, Pennsylvania 15212

PHYSICIAN'S ORDER SHEET
Unless Specified

"This Brand Only", The Generic Equivalent
or
Therapeutic Alternative Will be Dispensed

USE BALL-POINT PEN ONLY   IMPRINT PATIENT'S PLATE HERE

Form DC 470-06A Rev/ 6/88

Time Noted By Nurse		Ordered		DIET MEDICATION TREATMENT WITH DOCTORS SIGNATURE
Hour	Name	Date	Hour	
				COMPLETE ALLERGY INFORMATION AT TIME OF ADMISSION
				ALLERGIES:
				PRIMARY TOTAL HIP ARTHROPLASTY CLINICAL PATHWAY ORDERS **(Page 2 of 2)**
				☐ with Diabetes Mellitus ☐ without Diabetes Mellitus
				Pain Meds:
				Acetaminophen (Tylenol) 1000 mg by mouth every 6 hrs prn pain
				Docusate (Colace) 100 mg by mouth twice daily
				Prochlorperazine (Compazine) 10 mg IM q 6 hrs x 24 hrs prn nausea/vomiting
				Milk of Magnesia 30 ml by mouth twice daily prn constipation
				Zolpidem (Ambien) _____ mg by mouth at bedtime prn sleep
				RECOMMENDED INITIAL DOSE IN ELDERLY/DEBILITATED PATIENTS IS 5 mg.
				OTHERS MAY RECEIVE 10 mg
				Antibiotics:
				☐ Cefazolin (Ancef-Kefzol) 1 gm IV q 8 hrs x 48 hrs
				IF PENICILLIN-ALLERGIC, give ☐ Vancomycin 500 mg IV q 6 hrs x 48 hrs
				Anticoagulants:
				☐ Warfarin (Coumadin) 5 mg by mouth on evening of surgery,:
				then per following schedule
				PT < 13 give Warfarin (Coumadin) 5 mg by mouth in AM
				PT = 13-15 give Warfarin (Coumadin) 2.5 mg by mouth in AM
				PT > 15 NO AM Warfarin (Coumadin)
				☐ Other DVT Prophylaxis:
				☐ X-Ray _____ hip in Recovery Room
				Consult Social Service
				Consult Physical Therapy
				Consult Occupational Therapy
				Consult Home Care
				☐ Consult: _____ for diabetes management
				☐ Consult Diabetes educator/dietitian

Initiator _____   Department Chair _____

ECMS Date Approved ____6-18-96____   Control # ____870____ (Assigned by Staff Office)

Page 2 of 2

C

Figure 57–2   *(cont.)*

17774

Medical Record
Number

ADDRESSOGRAPH

TOTAL HIP and REVISION HIP ARTHROPLASTY
VARIANCE FORM
Please use only black ink pen

Admission Date ☐☐ / ☐☐ / ☐☐

Discharge Date ☐☐ / ☐☐ / ☐☐

Please circle the appropriate pathway.
Only ONE choice permitted.

○ Total Hip Arthroplasty(tha)
○ Revison Hip Arthroplasty(rtha)

Does patient have diabetes mellitus?   Yes No
　　　　　　　　　　　　　　　　　　　① ②

Unit ☐☐☐☐   Shade circles like this: ●   Not like this: ⊗ ✓   Date ☐☐ / ☐☐ / ☐☐

Day of Surgery:

	True	False	Source P S C	Comments	Initials
Patient went to OR without delay	①	②	○ ○ ○		
No evidence of hip dislocation	①	②	○ ○ ○		
Diabetes clearance per MD	①	②	○ ○ ○		

Unit ☐☐☐☐   Date ☐☐ / ☐☐ / ☐☐

POD 1:

	True	False	Source P S C	Comments	Initials
No evidence of hip dislocation	①	②	○ ○ ○		
OOB to chair	①	②	○ ○ ○		
Physical therapy BID	①	②	○ ○ ○		
Consults diabetes educator/dietitian	①	②	○ ○ ○		

THIS FORM MUST ACCOMPANY PATIENT WHEN TRANSFERRED TO ANOTHER UNIT

THIS FORM IS NOT PART OF THE PERMANENT CHART. COMPLETED FORMS SHOULD BE RETURNED TO CLINICAL PRACTICE SPECIALIST(CPS) COORDINATING THIS CRITICAL PATHWAY.

CPS ==>Sue Leininger   p2655 x8197

Developed by OUTCOMES MEASUREMENT GROUP
rtha1xx.qes 7/11/96,2/7/96,7/11/95

A

Figure 57–3   (A,B). Variance and outcomes report

17774

Medical Record
Number

If you initial this form please print your name in the box below

Initials	Please PRINT name	Initials	Please PRINT name

Unit [ ][ ][ ][ ]

Shade circles like this: ●
Not like this: ⊗ ✓

Date [ ][ ] / [ ][ ] / [ ][ ]

POD 2:

	True	False	Source P S C	Comments	Initials
Patient is voiding on own	①	②	○ ○ ○		
Physical therapy twice a day	①	②	○ ○ ○		
Patient education done re: hypoglycemic agent hypoglycemia hyperglycemia	①	②	○ ○ ○		

Unit [ ][ ][ ][ ]

Date [ ][ ] / [ ][ ] / [ ][ ]

POD 3:

	True	False	Source P S C	Comments	Initials
Physical therapy twice a day	①	②	○ ○ ○		
Blood glucose levels < 200mg	①	②	○ ○ ○		
Patient had Diabetes Mellitus skills review	①	②	○ ○ ○		

Unit [ ][ ][ ][ ]

Date [ ][ ] / [ ][ ] / [ ][ ]

POD 4:

	True	False	Source P S C	Comments	Initials
Physical therapy twice a day	①	②	○ ○ ○		
Blood glucose levels < 200mg	①	②	○ ○ ○		
Patient educated re: hypoglycemic therapy	①	②	○ ○ ○		

Unit [ ][ ][ ][ ]

Date [ ][ ] / [ ][ ] / [ ][ ]

POD 5:

	True	False	Source P S C	Comments	Initials
Physical therapy twice a day	①	②	○ ○ ○		
Discharged to home	①	②	○ ○ ○		

B

Figure 57–3 *(cont.)*

TABLE 57–2 Critical Pathway Development and Implementation

1) Benchmark
2) Identify current process of delivering care
3) Identify variability in current process
4) Multidisciplinary collaboration to find solutions
5) Develop a tracking document
6) Implement critical pathway using standard orders and tracking document
7) Maintain critical pathway with variance and outcome reports
8) Modify critical pathway based on variances and outcomes

EFFECTS OF CRITICAL PATHWAYS

Most health-care institutions begin their orthopaedic experience with critical pathways by applying them to joint replacement surgery.

In total joint arthroplasty, the expense incurred arises from three dominant factors: length of hospitalization, time in the operating room, and cost of the implant. The critical pathway can address the former two factors by standardizing the care among the orthopaedic surgeons. The operating room staff will have less variability among surgeons, thus increasing the operating room staff's efficiency. The orthopaedic unit nurses will have a standard treatment plan focused on the patient and a postsurgical date that is independent of the operating surgeon.

When a critical pathway is properly applied to the delivery of care for a surgical procedure, the effect is abrupt. At Allegheny General Hospital, the Pittsburgh campus of Allegheny University for the Health Sciences, critical pathways were applied to THA in January, 1994 and to total knee arthroplasty (TKA) in May, 1994.

In Fig. 57–4, a comparison is made between the length of stay (LOS) during the 3 months prior to the initiation of the THA critical pathway and the first 3 months on the critical pathway. The mean LOS dropped from 9 days to 5.1 days, with the pathway goal set at 5 days. More significantly, the standard deviation dropped from 4.5 days down to 1.8 days, demonstrating the manner in which the pathway acts to decrease variability. The incidence of postoperative complications such as infection and deep venous thrombosis declined, demonstrating a positive patient outcome of the critical pathway. Hospital charges declined 28% through pathway controls.

Given this experience, a TKA critical pathway was started 5 months later. Figure 57–5 demonstrates, as was expected, a drop in the LOS from 7.2 days to 3.7, days with the pathway goal set at 3 days. Note that the standard deviation dropped from 3.4 days to 1.6 days. Once again, there was a positive effect on the complication rate to the patient's benefit and a 21% decline in hospital charges to the institution's benefit.

The experience at Allegheny General Hospital demonstrates the validity of the critical pathway concept as it is applied in the medical field. Similar gains are noted from pathways developed and implemented in the nonsurgical areas such as congestive heart failure, myocardial infarction, stroke, and diabetes.

A critical pathway cannot be a single-minded nor a mindless pursuit. Not every patient nor every disease state is a candidate for a pathway. A patient can leave the pathway at any point to be managed in the traditional fashion. Indeed, the patient may need to leave the pathway based on postsurgical complications such as infection. In general, it is a goal to develop critical pathways for approximately 60 to 80% of the patient population for a given institution.

PEARL

The critical pathway benefits occur abruptly, once the pathway is implemented.

PHYSICIAN CONCERNS

The initial reaction of many physicians to critical pathways is that of loss of control of the patient's care. One needs to understand that participation in the pathway is voluntary. The development team does not need to satisfy every surgeon's demands. If a physician cannot compromise and is skeptical of the pathway, then it should be initiated without his or her support. As data is collected from the pathway, the nonparticipating physician usually presents as an outlier in terms of the pathway goals. This information provides the outlier physician with the motivation for eventual participation in the critical pathway.

It is important to understand that a critical pathway is for process control not involuntary physician control. The physician, through consensus, does relinquish some control, but, as can be seen in the Allegheny General Hospital experience, this benefits not only the patient but the surgeon and the health-care institution as well.

With physician participation, the critical pathway serves as the vehicle that delivers the most current and proven treatments when the institution is benchmarked against national data. The local standard of care can be readily updated by revision to the tracking document. This provides continuing education for the individual physician with minimal effort.

Carried to its highest conceptual level, a critical pathway will not only control the parameters for which it is developed but also can serve as a research vehicle to pool patients with common diagnoses. By modifying the pathway to include study parameters, a controlled study can be readily performed on a large and accessible database of patients.

PEARL

The critical pathway is an ideal research vehicle.

The reporting of variances is at first met with the concern that an error has occurred and blame will be placed. The term variance has a dual meaning. Socially it denotes antagonism. Mathematically, it denotes a positive or negative difference

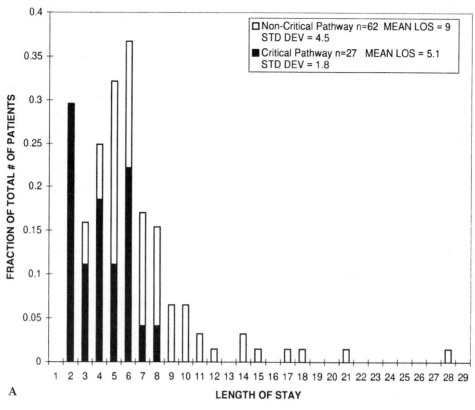

A

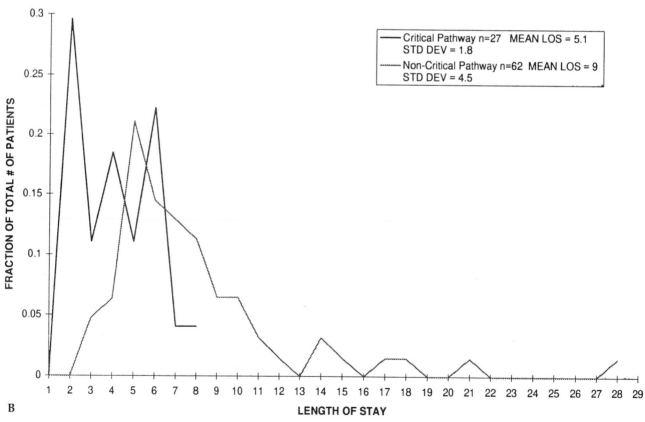

B

Figure 57–4 (A,B). Comparative analysis of using a critical pathway versus a noncritical pathway for total hip arthroplasty

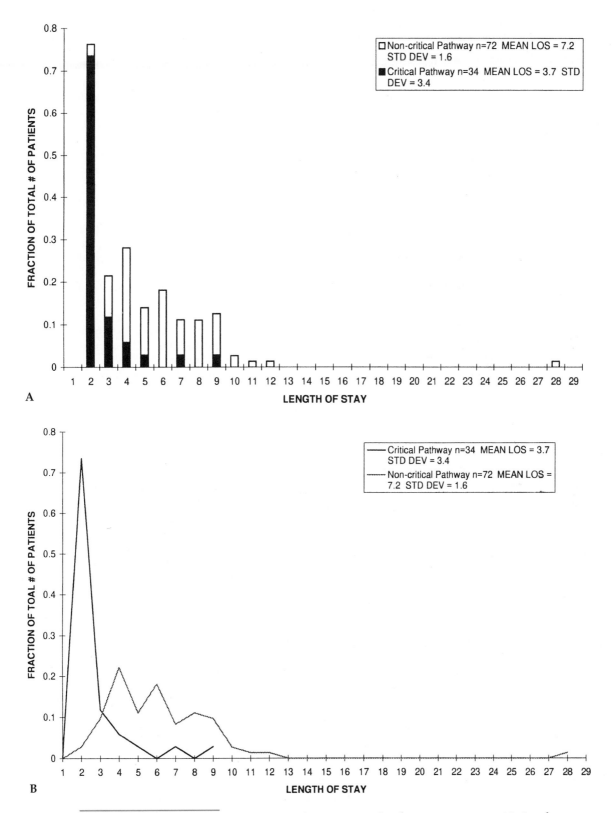

Figure 57–5   (A,B). Comparative analysis of using a critical pathway versus a noncritical pathway for total knee arthroplasty

between an expectation and an actual occurrence. It is the mathematical term that is used for critical pathway monitoring. Positive variances should be reinforced, and the source of negative variances located and modified. If variances are not recorded, there is no means to determine how well the pathway is performing. Variances, therefore, are a systems issue, not a personal issue.

The standard order set and the tracking document can be used to the benefit of the physician and nurse in decreasing the time spent on repetitious documentation. Very few if any orders need to be written if the patient is on a critical pathway. The tracking document at some institutions is used as the sole documentation of the patient's hospital stay and becomes part of the electronic medical record. Nurses typically spend one-third of their working hours documenting patient care. A tracking document allows the nursing staff to chart only the exceptions to the critical pathway care and allows increased time for patient contact.

One of the most important physician concerns is that of the relationship between medical liability and critical pathways. This concern centers on being held liable for an adverse patient outcome while following a pathway.

In addressing this fear, one first needs to consider that the onus of proving malpractice is upon the plaintiff and must satisfy the following four criteria:

1. The plaintiff was injured.
2. The defendant was negligent and did not meet the standard of care.
3. The negligence caused the injury.
4. There was a dutiful relationship between the patient and physician.

It is obvious that critical pathways, especially when benchmarked against nationwide care, can be construed as the standard of care. One of the primary goals of a critical pathway is to improve patient satisfaction and decrease the rates of medical injury. It can therefore become the standard of care in the local and national environments.

In the case of *Quigley v Jobe* in 1992 the plaintiff attempted to utilize insurance company risk-management guidelines in the construction of a claim. It was alleged that these guidelines were not followed by the defendant. The trial court held these guidelines to be inadmissible, as they did not necessarily reflect the standard of care within the industry.

In the case of *Roach v Springfield Clinic*, the court did admit guidelines from the American College of Obstetrics and Gynecology. The court specifically held that standards within a profession would be admissible in a negligence action. Of benefit for the physician is the fact that the court recognizes the expertise of the medical profession in the creation of guidelines rather than allowing case rulings to generate them.

In Maine, with the support of the Maine Medical Association, a 5-year project was initiated in 1992 to explore the relationship between practice guidelines and medical liability. Practice parameters, that is, practice guidelines, were passed into law thereby defining them as the standard of care. This provides the physician with some degree of liability protection if the patient is treated according to the guideline.

As experience with critical pathways evolves, it appears that deviation from a critical pathway in and of itself will not constitute negligence. However, when a critical pathway is deemed to be the standard for the industry, then such a possibility exists.

Given the rapidity with which critical pathways can affect positive change in the health-care industry, it appears that the risks of malpractice liability are outweighed by the benefits to patients in improvement in the standard of care, along with the benefits to physicians and hospitals, as shown in Tables 57–3 and 57–4. The final relationship between critical pathways and the judicial system will most likely take years to unfold and will occur on a case-by-case basis. The pressures of cost containment and the ability of critical pathways to accomplish this goal appear to have lent a degree of immunity to judicial interference in the propagation of critical pathways.

TABLE 57–3 The Benefits of Critical Pathways to Physicians

Ability to easily upgrade care through pathway modification
Benchmarking to the highest level of care
Improved clinical outcomes
Accurate and timely outcomes data
Increased patient satisfaction
Large accessible database for research
Possible reduction of malpractice liability

TABLE 57–4 The Benefits of Critical Pathways to Hospitals

Decreased health-care delivery costs
Decreased resource utilization
Improved clinical outcomes
Increased patient satisfaction
Enhanced ability to compete
Uniform delivery of care in a multicenter network

SELECTED BIBLIOGRAPHY

BADENHAUSEN WE. Improving patient outcomes following joint replacement surgery at Methodist Evangelical Hospital. *Quality Letter.* June 1993:11–13.

DEMOTT K. Critical pathways save $6.4 m, cut ALOS at the Christ Hospital. *Med Guidelines Outcomes Res.* 1994;5:1–3.

HADORN DC, BAKER D. Development of the AHCPR; sponsored heart failure guideline: methodologic and procedural issues. *J Quality Improvement.* 1994;20:539–554.

Institute Of Medicine; Bethesda, MD FIELDS MJ, ed. *Setting Priorities for Clinical Practice Guidelines.* National Academy Press; 1995.

MILLER FH. *Legal implications of practice guidelines:* Presented at Medical Outcomes Research Conference IV. Washington DC, May 12–13, 1994.

MUTSCHLER TA. Critical pathways development, implementation, and outcomes. Presented at Allegheny General Hospital, Pittsburgh, PA, March 3, 1994.

SMITH GH. A case study in progress: practice guidelines and the affirmative defense in Maine. *J Quality Improvement.* 1993;19:355–362.

WEST JC. The legal implications of medical practice guidelines. *J Health Hospital Law.* 1994;27:97–103.

SAMPLE QUESTIONS

1. Which care algorithm includes elements regardless of their effect on the clinical outcome:
   (a) clinical practice guideline
   (b) clinical pathway
   (c) critical pathway

2. Which care algorithm includes only the vital and proven elements of care that are delivered in a timely fashion:
   (a) clinical practice guideline
   (b) clinical pathway
   (c) critical pathway

3. A critical pathway:
   (a) is indigenous to the medical field
   (b) manages the process of care delivery
   (c) controls the physician involuntarily
   (d) is a static process without updating

4. Variance reporting:
   (a) is a systems issue
   (b) is a personal issue
   (c) monitors the pathway
   (d) always denotes negative events
   (e) a and c
   (f) b and d

5. Legally, critical pathways:
   (a) are viewed by the court as inadmissible
   (b) represent an industrial standard of care
   (c) limit malpractice liability in all states of the United States
   (d) if not followed constitute negligence
   (e) none of the above

GLOSSARY

Benchmarking   Comparison of the institution's local pathways and goals with the national experience

Clinical pathway   Algorithm or flowchart representation of a clinical practice guideline that includes all elements of care

Clinical practice guideline   Systemically developed statements to assist in the formulation of a treatment plan for a specific diagnostic group

Critical pathway   Treatment that includes only vital elements that are proven to positively affect the outcome and that are delivered in a timely fashion

Outcomes report   Periodic update of the ability to achieve the outcomes for which the pathway is constructed

Process management   Control of the process of the delivery of care to avoid costly variations

Tracking document   Process control document constructed on a per-day basis detailing the events that are to occur

Standard order set   Postoperative order set that encompasses the whole of the critical pathway

Variability   Unwanted differences in the delivery of care that do not positively affect the outcome and add unnecessarily to costs

Variance   The difference, positive or negative, between the expected and actual occurrence

Variance report   A periodic review of variances used to modify the pathway to reinforce the positive variances and obliterate the negative ones

Answers: 1) b; 2) c; 3) b; 4) e; 5) e

Chapter 58

Workers' Compensation Overview

Morton L. Kasdan, MD, FACS, Dean S. Louis, MD and Trevor Soergel, MD

Workers' compensation is an insurance program which provides economic security to workers who suffer injuries while on a reportable job. The employer is liable for an employee's injury. Under this no-fault system, the employee must prove causation but need not prove that the employer was culpable. The workers' compensation program, therefore, benefits both the employer and the employee. The employee relinquishes the right to sue the employer directly but is guaranteed coverage regardless of employer fault. Employers are guaranteed a monetary limit on their liability, allowing them to control the cost of workplace injuries without suffering the repercussions of unexpected and exorbitant lawsuits. This does not apply to the Federal Employees Liability Act, which includes railroads and waterways and is tried similar to tort litigation.

Causation is the essential element that the injured worker must prove in a workers' compensation claim. The worker has the burden of proving that the injury was caused by the work. In the early 1900s, workers' compensation laws regarded workplace injuries as those resulting from sudden traumatic events that immediately produced objective findings of an injury. These early laws, however, did not take into account an employee's long-term exposure to conditions at the workplace. Therefore, in the mid-1900s, many states expanded their workers' compensation laws to include recovery for occupational conditions that developed over time. These expanded workers' compensation laws initially focused on pulmonary diseases such as coal worker's pneumoconiosis, asbestosis, and silicoses. The employee was required to rule out other factors that might have caused the disease and to prove that the disease was caused by conditions peculiar to the occupation.

In the 1980s, an increasing number of workers began seeking recovery for a different type of "occupational disease." Workers claimed that regional musculoskeletal pain, classified under the broad terminology of so-called repetitive strain injuries (RSIs) or cumulative trauma disorders (CTDs), resulted from workplace conditions that required repetitive motion. This was seen in epidemic proportions at Telecom Australia, a government agency that provides telecommunications throughout Australia. Between 1981 and 1985, Hocking (1987) documented approximately 4000 reports of RSI at Telecom at a total cost of 15.5 million dollars and 293,600 lost work days, averaging approximately 74 lost days per case. The U.S. Department of Labor, Bureau of Labor Statistics reported that the number of CTDs in the United States

increased from 23,000 in 1981 to 223,600 in 1991. In 1981, CTDs represented only 18% of all occupational illnesses; whereas in 1991, they represented 61% of all reported occupational illnesses.

As a result of this epidemic, many states expanded workers' compensation laws to include recovery for injuries caused by conditions of employment in which "continual strain" disabled the employee. Unlike the previous occupational injuries covered by workers' compensation, no definite time and place of injury existed. The injured worker, therefore, had difficulty proving the element of causation necessary for monetary recovery. This difficulty resulted in increasing reliance on the expert testimony of physicians to prove the cause of the injury.

Physicians have problems in determining causation. The first difficulty physicians encounter is in reconstructing the worker's employment and medical history. Physicians tend to rely on the patient for this information. Patients' perceptions of their injuries, however, are likely to be influenced by the increasing media attention. If the worker is seeking compensation and perceives that the injury is work-related before the physician has even given a definite diagnosis, the patient is likely to give a history that reflects this perception. Patients' self-perceptions influence not only their subjective medical history, but also their recovery. A New York School of Medicine study (Jones, 1993) revealed that a patient's perception that a "CTD" is work-related or covered by workers' compensation can actually slow recovery and increase the period of time off work. Physicians, therefore, must look beyond the patients' subjective history to seek objective findings of causation. By examining the physical requirements of the job and the employee's activities outside of work, the physician should be able to construct a more accurate history.

Even if physicians are successful in obtaining an accurate medical history, the presence of confounding factors will hinder their ability to accurately determine causal inference. Symptoms occur gradually, rather than as a result of a single traumatic event. It is, therefore, difficult to determine when the injury began. Establishing the beginning of the onset of symptoms is important because it may or may not link the injury to the workplace. Numerous nonoccupational factors may also complicate the issue of causation. For example, medical conditions such as pregnancy, smoking, lack of fitness, or a family history of neurological and endocrine disorders can be risk factors for a peripheral neuropathy. In addition, psychosocial factors, such as job stress and job dis-

Orthopaedic Surgery: The Essentials. Edited by M.E. Baratz, A.D. Watson, and J.E. Imbriglia. Thieme Medical Publishers, Inc., New York © 1999

satisfaction, as well as iatrogenesis have been correlated to upper extremity pain. Finally, the employee's activities outside the workplace may also be a contributing cause.

Several studies have linked the patient's psychosocial work environment to upper extremity pain. Hocking (1987) observed that advanced technology in the workplace "has made work routine, which has led to decreased social contact and less job satisfaction, against a background of planned redundancy in a depressed economy." Linton and Kamwendo (1989) noted that high levels of work stress, increased isolation, monotony of tasks, and increased workload—characterize the modern psychosocial work environment. Linton and Kamwendo also found a correlation between psychosocial factors and reported neck and shoulder pain in secretaries. Although the increasing numbers of work-related neck and shoulder symptoms have been attributed to ergonomic factors such as repetitive work tasks and prolonged periods of a stationary posture (also vague terms), this study revealed that the cause may be psychosocial factors related to the organization of the workplace. Secretaries are often at the bottom of the work hierarchy. As a result, secretaries report feelings of helplessness because of unpredictable workplace demands. This same study concluded that these feelings, rather than the ergonomics of the workplace, caused the reports of pain.

The Telecom Australia study also noted a link between psychosocial factors and RSIs that was the result of the workers' low job satisfaction. Symptoms reported by part-time workers were as frequent and as severe as those of full-time workers. In addition, those with higher job satisfaction but a poor ergonomic environment reported fewer workplace injuries than those with lower job satisfaction and a better ergonomic environment. In fact, the worker's keystroke rate was inversely proportional to the number of reported RSIs. According to this study, new technology and poor ergonomics do not cause RSIs. Hocking concluded that "workers report more RSIs because of feelings of monotony and isolation associated with new technology."

Reports of upper extremity "injuries" may also be linked to the patient's increased awareness of symptoms. Patients have a heightened sensitivity to symptoms due to physicians' labeling of diagnoses and repeated exposure through the media and society. For example, patients become more aware of their own symptoms that fit the description of carpal tunnel syndrome (CTS). This concept is called *iatrogenesis* and can be divided into two categories: clinical iatrogenesis and social iatrogenesis.

Clinical iatrogenesis occurs when a physician's words or actions during an examination induce a patient to perceive the existence of an ailment. The physician's misuse of terminology can influence patients to perceive their symptoms as caused by work. For example, physicians use a multitude of terms to describe regional musculoskeletal pain, such as tendonitis or neuritis, without adequate objective findings. These terms also include: CTD, repetitive trauma disorder, occupational musculoskeletal disorders, overuse syndrome, repetitive motion disorder, and repetitive stress injury. Words such as "trauma" and "injury" imply that there is actual damage to underlying tissue. Furthermore, the adjectives physicians use to describe these conditions—cumulative, repetitive, and strain—imply that repetitive motions cause these disorders.

The physician's use of this terminology has adverse effects on the patient's perception of symptoms and causation. When physicians make diagnoses using terminology that implies a tissue injury secondary to work, (but the symptoms actually point only to musculoskeletal pain), patients assume that the symptoms arise from definite disease or injury caused by work. Furthermore, some physicians treat such musculoskeletal pain by having the patient avoid the use of the affected body part. This increased patient focus on use as the cause can exacerbate the patient's perception of symptoms and conditions and retard recovery.

Social iatrogenesis occurs when patients develop a heightened sensitivity to symptoms commonly associated with societal influences. Beginning in the 1980s, social programs and media messages were designed to increase public awareness of potential injuries in the workplace. This has oversensitized those people who perceive themselves to be at risk and has induced a heightened awareness of musculoskeletal pain.

The employee's activities outside the workplace result in another factor that confounds the correlation of "repetitive motion" at work. People use their hands for extracurricular activities as well as for the activities of daily living, not just in the workplace. Simple calculations show that if one considers a person who works a total of 47 years, beginning at age 18 and retiring at age 65, approximately 16% of that person's 65 years is spent at work. This takes into consideration that within the 365 days in a year there are a total of 246 working days(52 weekends, 10 vacation days, 5 holidays) at an average of 8 hours per day. Additionally, most people do not work the first 18 years. Therefore, in analyzing a 30-year-old patient with a claim of pain symptoms related to repetitive work, it can be logically inferred that if the patient had been working since age 18, 12 years were spent at that job. The total time spent at work over the span of 30 years accounts for less than 9% of the patient's total hours. It would, therefore, be difficult to hypothesize that only the patient's work activities caused the symptoms. This is especially difficult in cases in which there are no objective findings.

Workers' compensation was intended to protect both employees and employers in the event of unfortunate accidents in the workplace. The increasing incidence of work-related claims involving upper extremity pain, however, has overloaded this system. Employees have the burden of proving that the repetitive nature of their work is the cause of their symptoms. Causal inference is not easy to prove because of numerous confounding factors that have to be considered: the lack of objective findings to substantiate the subjective symptoms, numerous psychosocial issues, and clinical and social iatrogenesis. There is a definite lack of epidemiological evidence to support the theory that work causes the so-called cumulative trauma disorders.

Unfortunately, many of the misconceptions concerning cumulative trauma disorders are related to the failure to understand the literature. In the 1996 edition of *Accident Facts*, the National Safety Council compiled statistics on CTS. They reported that nearly 1.87 million workers *self-reported* CTS. In addition, 675,000 workers stated their CTS was identified by a medical person, and in half of these cases, the medical person *suggested* a work-related cause. The misconception of causation about CTDs results from studies like this in which statistical data is collected from self-reports and suggestions of cause and effect relationships without objective data and sound scientific method. It is assumed that CTS is a cumulative trauma disorder and that *self-reports* and *suggested* etiology are accurate. A diagnosis is assumed without confirmation, making the statistics invalid.

If workers' compensation is to benefit both employer and employee as was originally intended, then the evaluating and treating physician is encouraged to seek a more thorough understanding of the patient's upper-extremity activities before assuming that a "syndrome" is caused by work. It is equally important to distinguish between symptoms and a disease (or injury) before labeling with a diagnosis that has no foundation in *objective* findings. Finally, an attempt should be made to determine the incidence and prevalence of the diagnosis in a given workplace.

SELECTED BIBLIOGRAPHY

BERNARD B, SAUTER SL, FINE LJ et al. Psychosocial and work organization risk factors for cumulative trauma disorders in the hands and wrists of newspaper employees. *Scand J Work Environ Health*. 1992;18(suppl 2):119–120.

Brooks P. RSI—regional pain syndrome: the importance of nomenclature. *Br J Rheum*. 1988;28:180–181.

BROOKS P. Repetitive strain injury: does not exist as a separate medical condition. *Br Med J*. 1993;307:1298.

CLELAND LG. "RSI": a model of social iatrogenesis. *Med J Aust*. 1987;147:236–239.

HADLER NM. Occupational illness: the issue of causality. *J Occup Med*. 1984;26:587–593.

HADLER NM. Cumulative trauma disorders: an iatrogenic concept. *J Occup Med*. 1990;32:38–41.

HOCKING B. Epidemiological aspects of "repetitive strain injury" in Telecom Australia. *Med J Aust*. 1987;147:218–222.

JONES HD, JACKSON C. *Cumulative Trauma Disorders: A Repetitive Strain on the Workers' Compensation System*, 20 N Ky L Rev 765, 778–779 (1993).

JUGE DP, STOKES HM, PINE JC: *Cumulative Trauma Disorders—"The Disease of the '90s": An Interdisciplinary Analysis*, 55 La L Rev 895, 900–901 (1995).

KASDAN ML. Medical and surgical management of cumulative trauma disorders of the wrist and hand. In: *Trends in Ergonomics/Human Factors IV*. New York, NY: Elsevier; 1987;1029–1033.

KASDAN ML. Occupational cumulative trauma: a small fraction of life. *J Hand Surg*. 1994;19A:523.

KASDAN ML, MILLENDER LH. Occupational soft tissue and tendon disorders. *Orthop. Clin N Am*. 1996;27:795–803.

LINTON SJ, KAMWENDO K. Risk factors in the psychosocial work environment for neck and shoulder pain in secretaries. *J Occup Med*. 1989;31:609–613.

LOUIS DS. A question of causality. *AAOS Bulletin*. 1996;Jan.16.

National Safety Council. *Accident Facts*. 1996 Ed. Itasca, IL: National Safety Council; 1996.

SEMPLE JC. Tenosynovitis, repetitive strain injury, cumulative trauma disorder, and overuse syndrome, et cetera. *J Bone Jt Surg*. 1991;73B:536–538.

WEBSTER BS, SNOOK SH. The cost of compensable upper extremity cumulative trauma disorders. *J Occup Med*. 1994;36:713–717.

WRIGHT GD. The failure of the "RSI" concept. *Med J Aust* 1987;147:233–136.

Chapter 59

A Defense Attorney's Perspective: The Impact of Workers' Compensation on Disability

George N. Stewart, Esq.

Outline

Workers' compensation (WC) systems exist in all 50 states. These systems serve to compensate employees who have been injured in the scope of their employment or who suffer from work-related conditions or illnesses. Workers' compensation replaces the common-law remedies that would otherwise be available to such employees. Instead of determining the liability of the employer for each employee's injury, the employer bears the economic loss resulting from the work-related injury or condition, regardless of fault. The employee's financial recovery is determined by the WC system, not a jury.

The magnitude of the WC system and its costs should not be underestimated. A recent report noted that occupational injuries and illnesses in the United States contribute significantly to the total costs of health care (*Arch Intern Med*, 1997;). The cost to the nation of such job-related injuries and diseases are more than the costs associated with AIDS or Alzheimer's disease, as well as those associated with cancer or heart disease. Direct costs (i.e., medical and hospital bills) of occupational injuries and illnesses totaled $65 billion in 1992. Indirect costs, including lost wages, were $106 billion. (This yielded a combined daily total of $460 million.) Researchers determined that in 1992, approximately 6,500 Americans died and 13.2 million were injured as a result of work-related causes.

Workers' compensation has had unintended effects on the delivery of medical care to injured employees, as well as on the frequency, duration, severity, and permanency of disability sustained as a result of employment. This phenomenon has been termed *secondary gain*. Secondary gain usually refers to the monetary benefits that an employee receives as a result of an injury. The concept of secondary gain also encompasses such benefits as freedom from an unsatisfying job and receipt of sympathy and attention. Secondary gains experienced by employees have a significant impact on the claimants and employers within the WC system, as well as on the system itself. The effects of such secondary gains are discussed in detail below.

EFFECT OF WORKERS' COMPENSATION ON FREQUENCY OF CLAIMS

In recent years, the frequency with which WC claims are filed has increased dramatically. Evidence exists that the frequency of WC claims filed is tied to injury rate and the level of benefits available. (Note that an injured employee is not required to file a WC claim; filing a claim is voluntary.) Worrall and Appel (1987) analyzed data gathered by various researchers in the early and mid-1980s. As the amount of WC benefits increases, the frequency of claim filing increases. External economic factors such as the unemployment rate have been linked to filing frequency. Job dissatisfaction and depression have also been found to prompt injured employees to file claims (Hadler, 1993).

Another study reported that approximately 50% of the working population experiences work-related back pain each year. Fewer than 5% of those employees file WC claims (Skol Corp., 1994). Job-related stress that existed before the injury occurred has been identified as the most significant factor in determining whether an employee will file a WC claim (Skol Corp., 1994). This past decade has witnessed explosive growth in a particular area of concern—claims of repetitive-strain injuries (RSIs) and cumulative trauma disorders (CTDs).

The 1990s saw a massive rise in workers compensation and civil actions consisting of claims that RSI and CTD is work-related or proximately related to the tortious conduct of third parties including:

1. computer keyboard manufacturers

2. manufacturers of other industrial machinery

3. job configuration components (nonadjustable chairs, desk design, etc.)

Socioeconomic factors appear to have at least some impact on claims of RSI/carpal tunnel syndrome (CTS) and complaints of symptoms. In one analysis, Japanese workers were studied in an effort to compare them with American workers as to prevalence of nerve conduction abnormalities, median entrapment neuropathy, and reporting of symptoms. The Japanese workers exhibited similar findings as to nerve conduction abnormalities (prevalence magnitude, etc.). However, the Japanese workers exhibited a far different response with rare reports of symptoms. Decreased sensitivity was

915

speculated to stem in part from greater exercise and better general physical condition. The Japanese workforce exhibited more positive attitudes concerning their jobs and significantly longer employment, and they demonstrated less financial incentive to file a compensation claim for CTS. (Nathan et al, 1994).

In July 1997, the National Institute for Occupational Safety and Health (NIOSH) issued an update on musculoskeletal disorders and workplace factors, setting forth what it deemed "the most comprehensive compilation to date of the epidemiologic research on the relationship between selected musculoskeletal disorders and exposure to physical factors at work." The institute "concludes that a large body of credible epidemiologic research exists which shows a consistent relationship between musculoskeletal disorders and certain physical factors, especially at higher exposure levels." In its reviews of RSI and CTD conditions (in chapters focused on carpal tunnel syndrome, hand-arm vibration syndrome, epicondylitis, etc.), NIOSH discusses numerous Nathan (1988, 1992) studies and follow-up reports, as well as the Silverstein (1987) studies, which appear to be mutually critical of each other. The NIOSH commentators appeared to go to great lengths to embrace the Silverstein studies, which more aggressively enunciate causal relationship.

An entire continent was afflicted by massive numbers of repetitive-motion injury claims. In the late 1970s and early 1980s, Australia experienced voluminous increases in the reporting rates of repetitive-strain injuries, thought to be driven by the workers compensation delivery system. One-third of the work force was reported affected by repetitive-strain injuries, with as many as 76% of the claimants out of work for some period of time. Beginning in 1985, Australia undertook numerous new legislative promulgations with initiatives involving the form, adequacy, and duration of benefits. The number of reported RSI injuries rapidly declined from the 1983 and 1984 reporting highs. The benefit delivery system when paired with the third-party civil action tort mechanism creates at least the potential for impact on disability and the employee's desire to return to work. Under most private workers compensation systems, the provider of workers' compensation benefits has a subrogation right to any recovery made by the injured employee against any third party. In some instances, it may be the workers' compensation carrier, in pursuit of its subrogation interests, who initiates the claim against a third party perceived to be responsible for the work-related injury, such as a product manufacturer or driver of another motor vehicle. If the third party denies responsibility, the matter can be pushed to litigation. In this event, compensable damages are not limited to incurred medical bills. Lost wages (indemnity benefits) may include items of noneconomic detriment such as pain and suffering, loss of consortium or services, as well as claims for future damages. Once counseled by a lawyer, a claimant will learn that jurors tend to award more for the noneconomic items of damages such as pain and suffering. The entire process may be driven with a negative incentive to return to work and conclude treatment. This "caps" special damages until the matter is either heard by a jury or concludes in a settlement of the third-party claim.

The workers' compensation system has led to the development of ever-increasing tort litigation in emerging areas.

The mass toxic tort litigation had its genesis in workers' compensation-type systems. Originally focusing upon occupational illnesses such as black lung, silicosis, and asbestos-related illness, the WC system has exploded in the 1990s to far-reaching litigation including claims for: multiple chemical sensitivity (MCS), fibromyalgia; indoor air quality sick-building syndrome; latex sensitivity and allergy; and illness due to solvents, benzene, isocyanate, "toxic" carpeting, fiberglass insulation, pesticide/herbicides, and electromagnetic fields (EMFs).

Access to health coverage for a worker may depend entirely on whether the condition from which the worker suffers is deemed work-related. If the employee does not have his or her own private coverage, the delivery system may enhance the tendency for the treating physician to provide a causal nexus in a debatable area to increase the possibility of the patient having insurance coverage.

EFFECT OF WORKERS' COMPENSATION ON DURATION OF DISABILITY

The duration of disability has been linked to benefits. Worrall and Appel (1987) have reported that duration of disability lengthens as the amount of WC benefits increases. Wage replacement programs such as WC have been reported to have an inverse relationship to an injured employee's return to work (Martin et al, 1994). Researchers have found that workers who receive WC for work-related injuries remain disabled longer than people who have sustained injuries outside of work (Martin et al, 1994). Headley (1989) has also reported that external economic, psychological, and medical factors combine to influence the duration of disability. He cited a 1983 study by Svensson and Andersson, in which low, work satisfaction; an unpleasant or stressful position; and uncertainty of future employment provide a disincentive to return to work. This is especially true when the injured employee is receiving WC or is in the midst of litigation (Sullivan et al, 1991).

In 1991, Battie and Bigos reported on a study in which injured workers who received WC were compared with those who did not. Those authors found that job satisfaction and emotional distress correlated significantly with the onset of injury for workers who were receiving WC but not for those who were not (Battie and Bigos, 1991; Conte and Banerjee, 1993). After surgical intervention, fewer employees receiving WC returned to work than did employees who were not receiving WC (Battie and Bigos, 1991; Conte and Banerjee, 1993).

Researchers have also found that WC claimants are less likely to plan to return to work after an injury than are employees who are not receiving WC (Skol Corp., 1994). It is clear that nonmedical issues play a role in disability development and duration. Sensitive areas that have been examined in analyzing work injuries include the effects of higher benefits on claim frequency and duration, insurer adjustment activity, and the retention of legal counsel by the injured employee. (Thomason and Burton, 1993) Among the more emboldened conclusions of Thomason and Burton is that the retention of legal counsel increases the probability of settlement of a workers' compensation claim on a lump-sum basis.

This suggests that claimant attorneys are acting contrary to their clients' interests and inducing claimants to accept smaller settlements. Thomason and Burton concluded that a lump-sum settlement was less likely if benefits were provided by either self-insuring employers or the state insurance fund rather than by a private insurer. The statistics are troublesome in that they suggest that involvement of a lawyer for the claimant increases the likelihood of a lump-sum settlement and does not increase the benefits to nor advance the medical care of the injured employee. The method used to determine claimant attorneys fees through a contingency basis, which links the amount of the fee to the size of a lump-sum settlement, may be directly at odds with efforts to reemploy the worker or to provide the optimum environment for recovery.

SUGGESTIONS FOR THE FUTURE

One possible antidote to the low return-to-work rate among WC claimants is patient education. LaCroix and associates (1990) reported that 94% of WC claimants who were judged to have a good understanding of their injuries did return to work, whereas only 33% of those who had a poor understanding of their injuries returned to work. WC systems should acknowledge the role that job-related stress plays in the decisions of employees to file claims and in the duration of their disabilities. Rehabilitation programs should provide medical care and support directed at alleviating WC claimants' work-related stress (Skol Corp., 1994).

Although the WC system is aimed at providing compensation and rehabilitation while encouraging injured employees to return to work, the design of the WC system has been assailed for perpetuating disability. Because the claimant must prove persistent pain and disability to remain eligible for benefits, he or she does not focus on recovery but instead dwells on the injury (Hadler 1994). It seems clear that the WC system subverts its own goal of providing cost-effective remuneration to employees for a limited time. An employee who must concentrate on providing continued disability will not get well. Hadler (1990) calls this internal contradiction within the WC system "the vortex of disability determination."

Permitting companion third-party tort actions or vesting in a workers compensation insurer, a subrogation right may further perpetuate the need to remain "injured or disabled." WC systems must evaluate the effect that increases in benefits have in increasing injury rates. Society must be concerned about the possibility that higher, disability payment levels may remove the worker's economic incentive to prevent injuries. As such, although better patient education is stressed to aid return-to-work rates, changes in worker behavior prior to injury through increased education is necessary for improvements in occupational safety.

Safety legislation should be a primary component of any workers' compensation reform. Workers' compensation should be a vehicle for the promotion of increased safety to reduce the number of injuries.

The current level of workers' compensation costs appear to be sufficiently high to encourage prevention efforts by employers. Various states and federal agencies have discussed reforms with categories including premium discounts, safety and health training and consultation services, safety and health committees, as well as enforcement and penalty provisions. It is clear that workers' compensation benefits will not be the sole remedy available to an injured employee permitted to pursue a third-party tort action. The employer, if at fault (for example who removes safety devices from machinery to increase production), should be subject to third-party suits for contribution or indemnity or to direct action by the injured employee under some increased gross negligence threshold. Such limitations on WC immunity will further pre-injury safety initiatives.

Workers' compensation systems must remain dedicated to rehabilitation and remuneration. These systems must address the legal, social, economic, and psychological factors that combine with a claimant's medical condition to influence the rise in claims filed and the increase in disability duration.

Several states provide incentives to both employers and injured workers for speedy return to work, including higher permanent partial disability benefits for workers who are not rehired, penalties for employers who unreasonably refuse to rehire injured workers, as well as subsidies and special incentives to return to work quickly. A recent study by the Workers' Compensation Research Institute (1998) concluded that important factors shaping return to work are: returning to work for the pre-injury employer, worker and employer attitudes and motivations about returning to work, firm size, determining that employees at smaller firms are much less likely to return to the pre-injury employer (and thereby incur longer periods off work than those at larger firms), and economic incentives such as the ability to return to better-paying jobs. Improved claimant education appears to be a good starting point for increasing the return-to-work rate.

SELECTED BIBLIOGRAPHY

BIGOS SJ, BATTIE MC. Acute care to prevent back disability. *Clin Orthop.* 1987;221:121–130.

CONTE LE, BANERJEE T. The rehabilitation of persons with low back pain. *J Rehab.* 1993;59:18.

HADLER NM. *Occupational Musculoskeletal Disorders.* New York, NY: Raven Press; 1993:249–262.

HADLER NM. The injured worker and the internist. *Ann Intern Med.* 1994;120:163–164.

HADLER NM. From arm pain to cumulative trauma disorder: an untenable conceptual leap with injurious consequences!

In: Burton JF, ed. 1995 *Workers' Compensation Yearbook.* Horsham, PA: LRP Publications; 199A: I-38–I-43.

HEADLEY BJ. Delayed recovery: taking another look. *J Rehab.* 1989;55:61–66.

LACROIX JM, POWELL J, LLOYD GJ, DOXEY NC, MITSON GL, ALDAM CF. Low back pain: factors of value in predicting outcome. *Spine.* 1990;15:495–499.

MARTIN KJ, EISENBERG C, MCDONALD G, SHORTRIDGE LA. Application of the Menninger return-to-work scale among injured workers in a production plant. *J Rehab.* 1994;60:42.

Menninger Return-to-Work Center. Available online at: http://spiderman. menninger. edu/tmc_prv_rtn wrk.ntml

Nathan PA, Keniston RC, Meyers LTD, Meadows KD. Obesity as a risk factor for slowing a sensory conduction of the median nerve in industry: a cross-sectional and longitudial study involving 429 workers. *J Occup Med*. 1992;34: 379–383.

Nathan PA, Meadows KD, Doyle LS. Occupation as a risk factor for impaired sensory conduction of the median nerve at the carpal tunnel. *J Hand Surg*. 1988;13B:167–170.

Nathan PA, Takigawak, Keniston RC, LocKwood RS. Slowing of sensory conduction of the median nerve and carpal tunnel syndrome in Japanese and American industrial workers. *J Hand Surg Br*. 1994; Vol. 19 p9 30–34.

National Institute for Occupational Safety and Health. *Criteria for a Recommended Standard Occupational Exposure to Dioisocynates*. U.S. Department of Health, Education, and Welfare 1978; publication 73-11022.

Sandler HM. The pain of work: occupational injury. *Occup Hazards*. 1995;57:51.

Silverstein BA, Fine LJ, Armstrong TJ. Hand wrist cumulative trauma disorders in industry. *Br J Indust Med*. 1986;43:779–784.

Silverstein BA, Fine LJ, Armstrong TJ. Occupational factors and the carpal tunnel syndrome. *Am J Indust Med*. 1987;11:343–358.

Skol Corporation. Ignoring job dissatisfaction and stress can be a potent prescription for treatment failure: addressing workplace issues is vital to recovery. *The Back Letter*. 1994;9:121.

Sullivan MD, Turner JA, Romano J. Chronic pain in primary care: identification and management of psychosocial factors. *J Fam Pract*. 1991;32:193.

Svensson HO, Andersson GBJ. Low back pain in 40- to 47-year-old men: work history and environmental factors. *Spine*. 1993;18:272–276.

Thomason T, Burton JF, Jr. Economic effects of workers compensation in United States: private insurance and the administration of compensation claims. *J Labor Econom*. 1993;11(no 1, pt 2):S1–S37.

Workers' Compensation Research Institute. What are the most important factors shaping return to work? In: *Workers' Compensation Yearbook. Vol 1–4. Horsham, PA*: Workers' Compensation Research Institute; 1998.

Worrall JD, Appel D. The impact of workers' compensation benefits on low-back claims. In: Hadler NM, ed. *Clinical Concepts in Regional Musculoskeletal Illness*. Stratton, Orlando, FL:Grune & Stratton; 1987;281–297.

Hadler NM. The vortex of disability determination: The object lesson of impairment rating for axial pain. In: Hadler NM, Bunn WB, eds. *Occupational Problems in Medical Practice*, New York: Della Corte; 1990:261–266.

Chapter 60

The Independent Medical Examination: The Orthopaedic Surgeon as a Medical Expert

Jon B. Tucker, MD

Outline

In our society, many patients seek compensation for the pain, suffering, and impairment and/or disability they sustain as a result of trauma. Most orthopaedic surgeons are aware that patients respond differently to stresses in life; for some, redress through the legal system plays a large (sometimes overwhelming) role in their recovery.

Human nature combined with the fiduciary basis of the physician-patient relationship form the one-two punch that can knock an otherwise rational surgeon unconscious when it comes time to frame a patient's case in medicolegal terms. At such a time, an orthopaedic surgeon is susceptible to losing objectivity. In fact, the surgeon may unwittingly become an overzealous patient advocate, turning a blind eye to the factual basis on which medical opinions should reside. Because of the physician's desire to avoid conflict with the patient, a treating physician may render an opinion that casts the most favorable light on the compensability or causality of a patient's claim.

This sequence of events often leads to excessive and unnecessary medical care, poor outcomes, and protracted litigation. Because of this, most states have evolved a system whereby injured patients can be compelled to submit to an independent examination by a peer physician. Depending on the jurisdiction, the milieu (workers' compensation, auto, third-party liability), and the timing, the examiner may be called upon to perform an analysis of a case. This independent medical examination (IME) plays a pivotal role in a patient's journey through the medicolegal system.

The IME is an important tool that is difficult to do well. A surgeon's ability to perform a competent IME results from the synthesis of analytical skills, organized thinking, an eye for detail, and the ability to impartially render an opinion based on fact. Surgeons interested in pursuing this aspect of practice need to have a working knowledge of the regulations governing peoples' behaviors, including their own, during the course of an examination and its aftermath. The surgeon-evaluator should also know the range of medicolegal matters on which it is ethically appropriate to comment, and those on which it is not. Finally, good communication and writing skills are a must. None of these talents receive much attention during residency training!

This chapter will provide a template for a typical IME. Depending on circumstances unique to each case, a surgeon may find that certain areas require more detailed analysis. The hints provided in each section provide an idea of how to frame opinions logically, concisely, and definitively.

PRODUCING AN INDEPENDENT MEDICAL EXAMINATION: FOUR STEPS TO A QUALITY EVALUATION

Cover Letter and Review of Records

Review the cover letter carefully. Often, the consulting entity (third party administrator, insurer, attorney) will be clear as to the subject of the IME. In complex cases with multiple injuries, multiple injury dates, and pre-existing conditions, this step is absolutely necessary before proceeding. You should have a clear idea of the questions you will need to answer after you complete the IME. Caveat: do not be influenced by opinions in a cover letter. Your opinion as an expert is the valued work product!

Complete your detailed medical records review before meeting the examinee. This is likely to be the most time-consuming and ultimately crucial part of the IME. *Do Not* skimp on this part of the exam: make a note of any missing records and attempt to obtain them, take written notes if necessary, organize a chronology of events, highlight unusual or important facts, and disregard the opinions of treating physicians noted in the chart. Formulate your own opinion!

Direct History and Examination

Obtain a careful verbal history from the examinee. It is important to perform a detailed first-person interview. Take written notes, documenting or paraphrasing the examinee's recapit-

Orthopaedic Surgery: The Essentials. Edited by M.E. Baratz, A.D. Watson, and J.E. Imbriglia. Thieme Medical Publishers, Inc., New York © 1999

ulation of his or her history. This is an important legal step, which must be taken to avoid the trap of hearsay evidence. This demonstrates your interest in the case and what the examinee has to say about it. *Remember*—the examinee is usually compelled to submit to the exam and is not happy to be seeing you! Respect for, and interest in the patient's history will make the evaluation better for everyone.

The physical examination will probably be the shortest part of the IME. As a surgeon, this will be the most familiar role you will play. You must be complete and methodical when the complaints are diffuse. I discourage a "cookbook" physical exam because the important elements become lost in the minutiae. A concise, well-documented exam is very powerful if and when you are called to testify! Pay special attention to inconsistencies on exam with respect to history, paradoxical findings, sham tests, and so forth.

Written Report

Your written report is the entire work product of the IME. There is no follow-up care, no surgery, and usually no further contact with the examinee. Many people, including some that may be opposed to your opinion, will examine the report very carefully. You may be deposed to give testimony under oath regarding your examination and will be expected to explain and defend your findings and opinions. A well written, organized, and meticulous report is mandatory.

The best way to construct a report is to recapitulate the totality of the encounter with the examinee. This method is especially helpful in organizing complex cases, in which the chronology may stretch over a decade or longer. Below is a suggested outline:

1. State the purpose of the examination.
2. Transcribe the history and complaints according to the examinee's recollection using information obtained during the interview.
3. Transcribe a synopsis of the medical records review. Pay careful attention to dates, pivotal medical findings, tests, procedures, quality of documentation, missing or incomplete documents, and contradictory findings. Organize in chronological order.
4. Dictate a review of all imaging studies, including your interpretation, and indicate if you reviewed any films personally (preferred). Indicate any review of new studies, (e.g., x-rays which you obtained at the time of the IME).
5. Document the physical examination in detail. Record all pertinent positives, negatives, and paradoxical findings. If global phrases are used, be sure to place them in the appropriate context, with no allowance for multiple interpretations.
6. Record your impression, loud and clear, in its own paragraph. Keep it short.
7. Dictate a recommendations section. Explain the basis of your conclusions in clear and unambiguous terms. Answer all questions posed by the consulting party in the cover letter, and explain them based on the IME.
8. Complete any necessary forms (e.g., job capabilities, estimated impairments, AMA guides rating). Correlate these figures with the text of your IME.

Understanding Common Medicolegal Terms

Accuracy in your report is extremely important. One of the easiest ways to create trouble is to use terms or phrases that can be misinterpreted. Below are some hints that should serve as a guide when writing your report:

Causation: Legal Definition

Direct causal relationship
Indirect causal relationship
Aggravation of prior injury
Reoccurrence of prior injury

Causation: Medical Definition

Injury mechanism
Magnitude of injury
Symptom complex, chronology
Pre-existing condition (temporary exacerbation with resolution vs. aggravation with acceleration of disease)

Legal definitions have *significant* meaning to attorneys and judges. You may not understand the nuance of these terms and the implications of their use on the causality of the injury. Medical experts often confuse these terms and use them liberally and interchangeably, without regard to their legal meaning. Strive to limit your written comments to the medical definitions of causation. If the legal terms need to be used, seek guidance regarding exact definitions.

Symptom Magnification

Overblown subjective complaints
Inexplicable, nonanatomic, diffuse
No pain-free intervals
Intolerance of treatments

Pain Behavior

Objective finding!
Grunting, grimacing, posturing
Withdrawal, giveaway weakness
Nonanatomic or paradoxical findings

Any symptom magnification or pain behavior should be documented in the written report, as they speak to the credibility of the claimant *and* the examiner. Many experts tend to shy away from accurate reporting of these elements. In cases in which subjective complaints are predominant, you will enhance your credibility by documenting and explaining these findings.

Malingering

Malingering is volitional, active illness behavior in the absence of objective disease process. True malingering is quite rare. To meet this definition, one must find evidence of deception. A claimant may have had an injury in the past and still qualify as a malingerer. These claimants are often very interesting individuals who have developed complex mannerisms. They are relatively easy to identify because they derive emotional satisfaction from their attention-drawing tactics.

Residual Impairment and Maximum Improvement

There are commonly used yet poor definitions that reside in the "purgatory" of the medicolegal arena.

Subjective Residuals—Functional Capacity

A qualified expert's estimate of residual impairment is just as, or more accurate than a formal capacities evaluation performed by a multidisciplinary group. In cases where a "credible" 'expert witness' opinion is recognized, this estimate must be supported logically and methodically.

Objective Residuals—Loss of Use

The AMA guidelines regarding loss of use, required in many jurisdictions, function under the concept of loss of use (impairment). These guidelines, while objective, also have shortcomings. They are purely based upon diagnosis-related estimates or composite estimates calculated using tables.

Maximum Medical Improvement

Maximum medical improvement (MMI) is a reasoned medical opinion by an expert. This term is useful in defining an endpoint to a claimant's case. If residuals are present that prevent a claimant from returning to a pre-injury functional status *and* no further reasonable medical treatment will improve function, then the criteria for MMI are met.

THE DEPOSITION

The "final common pathway" of the medicolegal process is the testimony of the medical expert under oath and the chance for these opinions to be challenged by others in any legal proceedings affected by the expert's opinion. This is the essence of the deposition. Physicians and surgeons usually feel uncomfortable in the role of a witness. This emotion is especially strong when the physician is cross-examined by a "hostile" attorney. Scientific, medical, and logical conclusions are questioned as to their accuracy. The physician's credibility is attacked, and his or her prowess as a diagnostician is held suspect. Medical credentials, impeccable as they might be, are picked apart, ridiculed, and belittled. The physician may even be accused of selling an opinion to the requesting party!

A clear understanding of your role and the roles of the attorneys participating in the deposition helps to defuse tempers and allows for a balanced perspective on the process. The physician must understand that the deposition is under the control of the attorneys and the legal system. Unlike the collegial medical field, the legal system thrives on the adversarial process, with zealous attorneys representing each side of an argument. Their obligation is to present their case in the best possible light, as advocates for the interest of their respective clients. Their job is to do this irrespective of the merits of the case.

Remember that you are not in the operating room, and you are not in charge. You are a servant to this process. Remember your role as an expert witness. Never become an advocate for either side. Preserve your integrity and credibility! Never be quick to anger under cross-examination and try not to overpower or control the deposition process. Answer questions honestly, factually, and concisely. When you are asked to comment beyond factual conclusions, indicate you are stating your opinion; if asked to speculate, decline to do so. When you recognize that an attorney is asking you to stretch facts beyond reasonable limits, you should decline to go along. It is the job of the attorneys to take you as far as they can, but your obligation is to stop when you become uncomfortable. Remember that recanting any of your opinions during cross-examination will completely obliterate your credibility. You must be sure that all of your opinions are based on accepted medical knowledge and a coherent interpretation of the facts.

SUMMARY

This chapter is intended to give the reader a framework for producing a coherent independent medical evaluation. The making of a good expert witness, like the making of a good physician, is an amalgamation of experience, knowledge, and skill. Although some of the skills are acquired, the talent required to be a good expert witness/independent evaluator escapes many of the most intelligent physicians. The field is unnatural to the practice of medicine, with adversaries battling for their positions. By virtue of their training and collegial predilections, most physicians find this environment foreign. For this reason, there is a shortage of qualified professionals in this field.

The most elementary concepts have been reviewed. Surgeons interested in developing additional expertise are urged to attend the course offered by the American Academy of Orthopaedic Surgeons each year on disability and worker's compensation. The American Academy of Disability Evaluating Physicians (AADEP) and the American Academy of Occupational and Environmental Physicians (ACOEM) sponsor courses that teach the same fundamentals.

SELECTED BIBLIOGRAPHY

AMA Guides to Permanent Impairment. 4th Ed.

Chapter 61

Workers' Compensation Depositions—Attorney's Perspective

James D Strader, Esq.

In most workers' compensation proceedings, the physician's testimony is taken through the use of a deposition, as opposed to having the physician appear in person before the workers' compensation judge or hearing officer. A deposition is testimony of a witness under oath taken in question and answer form. Opportunity is given to the opposing side to be present and cross-examine the witness. The deposition is stenographically reported and then presented to the judge or hearing officer as evidence.

A physician can be expected to become involved in workers' compensation litigation through several different routes and may be called on to testify either for the injured worker, the employer, or the insurance carrier. Some physicians become involved in cases because they have been treating an individual. Their testimony concerning the history, diagnosis, treatment, and opinion concerning causal relationship is important to the case. Other physicians, because of the nature of their practices, are called on to examine an injured worker either by an attorney representing the injured worker or by an insurance carrier or employer who is liable for the payment of workers' compensation benefits. Regardless of how the physician becomes involved in a workers' compensation case, the guidelines and procedures followed concerning depositions are essentially the same.

The attorney who will be using the physician as an expert witness should plan for the deposition long before the actual date of the deposition. In fact, unless the physician is a treating physician, that planning should begin with selection of the physician who will be called on to be deposed. An important factor in determining which physician will perform the examination is the physician's effectiveness as a witness. The best examination and opinion are useless unless the physician can effectively relate his or her opinion to the adjudicator.

The physician will be asked to provide a report of the evaluation. Prior to the examination, it is the attorney's responsibility to provide the physician with as much information as possible. This includes records of treatment by other physicians, hospital admissions, emergency department records, results of all diagnostic tests performed, and copies of all imaging studies.

The physician should make the report as complete as possible, summarizing the available information on diagnosis and prior treatment. The physician should indicate an opinion concerning causal relationship between an alleged injury and the worker's disability. The physician may also be asked to comment on the extent to which the worker is disabled. If the physician is unsure as to what question or questions the attorney wishes to be answered in the report, the physician should clarify that prior to preparing the report. If the physician misunderstands or is not sure of the question to be addressed and prepares a report and mails it, it becomes difficult to change the contents of that report in a supplemental report or at the time of the deposition.

The attorney or a member of the attorney's staff will contact the physician to schedule a time and place for the deposition. Usually, the deposition takes place at the physician's office. Occasionally, the deposition is videotaped. The physician should make sure that the deposition is scheduled at a convenient time to leave ample time for testimony and cross examination.

Time needs to be set aside before the deposition for the physician to consult with the attorney concerning the subject matter of the deposition. This predeposition can take place just before the deposition or at a separate time. When the physician and attorney know one another and have previously consulted on similar issues, it is often possible to conduct this predeposition meeting immediately prior to the taking of the deposition. However, if the physician does not know the attorney well or if the case involves a unique or complex issue, the attorney and physician should meet at a separately scheduled time to discuss the case and the doctor's impending testimony. If a physician believes such a meeting is necessary and it is not requested by the attorney, the physician should make this view known so that such a meeting takes place.

At the predeposition meeting, the physician and attorney should make sure that the physician has seen all the information that is available. When a case involves a litigated workers' compensation matter, there may be records that have been generated since the time of the physician's examination, and there may have been depositions of other witnesses and other physicians taken in the case. All that information should be provided to the physician prior to the deposition and should be reviewed by the doctor prior to the predeposition meeting. This is particularly important if the opposing side's physician has testified. It will be helpful for the physician about to be deposed to know what the other side's physician has indicated in his or her testimony. Even if the other physicians in the case have not already testified by deposition, their records and reports may well have become available and they should be reviewed.

Orthopaedic Surgery: The Essentials. Edited by M.E. Baratz, A.D. Watson, and J.E. Imbriglia. Thieme Medical Publishers, Inc., New York © 1999

The attorney must make sure that the physician understands the issues in the case and how his or her testimony fits into the overall case. In other words, the physician must know what the attorney is trying to prove so that his or her testimony will assist in reaching that goal. This is not to say that the physician is expected to testify to anything but the truth. However, unless the physician knows where the attorney is trying to go, the physician will have a difficult time testifying in a manner that will be of assistance to the attorney.

There are some guidelines that the physician must remember when testifying. The physician must always remember that the testimony is being taken under oath. Regardless of personal feelings concerning the litigation, the physician must tell the truth. He or she must listen to the question that has been asked and then answer that question. The physician should not guess at what additional information the attorney is trying to seek. It is not acceptable to volunteer additional information. The attorney may not want that information in the record, and the information may be irrelevant to the issue at hand. The physician should keep in mind that if the attorney wants additional information, the attorney will, in all likelihood, ask additional questions.

When questioned, the physician should remember that the attorney cannot ask leading questions. Leading questions are generally defined as those types of questions that call for "yes" or "no" as an answer. The questions should, thus, be framed in such a manner as to allow the witness to give a narrative answer. That answer should be on point and should not be an exaggeration.

It is important for a physician testifying as a witness to remember that the judge or hearing officers reading the transcript of the deposition have different levels of sophistication regarding medical information. Both the attorney and the physician should strive to make sure the testimony is presented in language that is easily understood by the average person. Attorneys who are familiar with medical terminology often forget this point and mistakenly believe that the person adjudicating the claim will understand the medical terminology. Thus, it is important to explain medical terms, tests, and diagnoses to properly serve the client and patient.

The deposition will proceed according to a format that should be discussed between the attorney and physician at the predeposition meeting. The first thing that must be established after the physician is identified is the qualifications of the physician as an expert medical witness. This testimony is often shortened by reference to and admission of the physician's curriculum vitae into evidence. The attorney should make sure that the physician has an accurate and up-to-date curriculum vitae available for use in the deposition, and that an adequate number of copies are available at the time of the deposition.

The physician will then be asked a series of questions as to how the injured worker came to his or her attention, whether as a treating or examining physician, and the identity of the individual or party that referred the matter to the physician. The deposition will proceed with questions concerning the patient's presenting symptoms followed by a recitation of the history received directly from the injured worker. At this point, it is well to caution both attorneys and physicians that allowing the physician to merely read into the record what is contained in the physician's report is not only boring but

can be detrimental to the case. There are obviously things contained in the physician's report that are not relevant to the deposition; and as indicated above, there is terminology that may need to be explained. Therefore, if the physician is merely reciting the contents of the report, the attorney should interrupt the physician to request explanations or definitions of terminology and tests.

It cannot be stressed enough that a good deposition will read well and tell an accurate story to the judge or hearing officer. Questions and answers with explanations in understandable terms, flowing in a logical sequence is much better than a recitation of highly technical terms.

In addition to testifying about the history received directly from the patient, the physician should also be able to testify about the history received from the various records that were made available to the physician. There may be a conflict between the histories, and this should be commented upon if relevant to the case.

The results of the physical examination of the injured worker should also be presented. If a physical examination reveals no positive objective findings, that testimony can be presented by the attorney and physician either as a long recitation of normal findings or a simple statement that there were not positive findings on physical examination. Depending on the case, one or the other technique may be the most effective way to present that information.

The physician will then be asked to state a diagnosis and whether he or she has an opinion within a reasonable degree of medical certainty as to the cause of the diagnosis and whether it is any way related to the injury that is the subject of the litigation. The physician should then render an opinion and be prepared to support that opinion.

A word or two about the use of hypothetical questions in medical depositions. There are times when the physician may not have received a full history or where certain witnesses have not yet testified but an attorney is aware that they will testify and anticipates what they will say at the time of their testimony. This type of information may be put together in a hypothetical question to the physician and the physician may be asked to provide an opinion. The attorney, when asking such a question, must be extremely careful to only put into their hypothetical question facts that will be established in the course of testimony. The opposing attorney can and should object to each individual item in the hypothetical question that has either not yet been proven in the case or whose proof is questionable. If the opposing counsel does not object at the time the question is asked and before the answer given, the counsel may have waived the right to object. The testimony of the witness may be admissible even though the hypothetical facts are never proven in the course of the litigation.

After testifying on direct testimony, the physician is subject to cross-examination. The possible areas of cross-examination should be discussed at the predeposition meeting. An experienced attorney should be able to anticipate areas of cross-examination to help prepare the physician. In cross-examination, unlike direct examination, leading questions can be used by the attorney. The witness should remember to answer only the question asked and to make sure that he or she understands the question before answering. If the witness is asked a question that requires a simple "yes" or "no" answer but such an answer will, in the opinion of the witness, result in a misinterpretation, then it is clearly appropriate for the witness to testify "yes, but…" and provide some explanation for the "yes" or "no" answer.

One area in which witnesses and physicians may find themselves in difficulty is when they are asked to admit something as being a fact yet are unwilling to admit it even though they know that they should. In other words, they find themselves becoming too much of an advocate. They feel that if they agree with the opposing attorney's question, they are not furthering the cause of the party for whom they are testifying. In actuality, a medical witness who admits things that should be admitted is a more credible witness than the physician who takes the advocate's role and is unwilling to provide the opposing counsel with an admission on any point.

When discussing cross-examination, it is appropriate to note that there can be cross-examination concerning the doctor's qualifications and questions should be answered directly and truthfully as all testimony given by the physician. Some attorneys may ask the physician if he or she is being paid for the testimony; however, this is less common in workers' compensation proceedings than in jury trial. The physician obviously is being paid and should so state.

SELECTED BIBLIOGRAPHY

BOND TR, DUHL JZ. Understanding causation in workers' compensation cases. In: Goodmann HF, ed. *Orthopaedic Disability and Expert Testimony*. 4th ed. supl. New York: Wiley Law Publications; 1996:168–180.

CHURRIE JC, HODGE SD. Direct examination of an orthopaedic surgeon. In: Goodmann HF, ed. *Orthopaedic Disability and Expert Testimony*. 4th ed. New York: Wiley Law Publications; 1991:179–210.

FRIEDLAND S. The expert witness. In Goodmann HF, ed. *Orthopaedic Disability and Expert Testimony*. 4th ed. New York: Wiley Law Publications; 1991:123–147.

Chapter 62

Medical Malpractice: Perspective of the Physician's Team

Clayton A. Peimer, MD and Samuel Goldblatt, JD

Many perceive medical practice to be under assault, particularly from the legal profession. Medicolegal issues have insinuated themselves into medical practice and frequently influence medical decision making. Emphasizing legal aspects of medical practice has improved practice standards and peer review. Medical practice does not occur in a vacuum; therefore, clinicians, educators, and trainees must understand the legal, ethical, and medical implications of their actions.

LITIGATION PREVENTION

Patients often expect a perfect outcome when they allow physicians to assume the tremendous responsibility for their welfare when providing medical services. Physicians also expect the best outcomes possible from their intervention. However, medicine remains an imperfect science in an imperfect world, and suboptimal outcomes can and do occur.

Practices that can prevent litigation when undesirable outcomes occur include thoroughly discussing reasonable expectations of treatment with patients, diligent documentation, asking for help when needed, and ongoing self-evaluation as a medical practitioner.

Communication

Effective communication between a physician and patient requires a thorough, honest, easily understood description of the proposed treatment options, expected outcomes of each option, and potential complications and their treatment. The patient should be encouraged to ask questions. The physician should ask if the patient understands the discussion. It is unsafe and unfair to the patient to simply assume understanding. Full disclosure and honest interaction are essential moral imperatives.

Discussion is an essential element of medical care delivery and requires the same patience and attentiveness as the actual surgery. Assume that the patient wants to know what you would want to know if you were the patient.

Record Keeping

The fundamental purpose of written medical records is to document observations and treatments and to facilitate communication among the various providers of care such as nurses, therapists, and physicians. Medical records play an important role in medicolegal action because they document the patient's course and communication among the medical providers. Medical records alone can support or subvert allegations in a case.

All findings and events that affect the patient's well-being should be completely recorded as contemporaneously as possible. Documentation should include findings and events that influence the prognosis or outcome, either positively or adversely. The absence of relevant findings should be documented. Omission may suggest that the physician did not attempt to elucidate the relevant finding. It is not acceptable to state that because a finding is not documented, it was therefore negative. It is better to document at the time of evaluation that a finding was negative or absent.

PITFALL

In court, exclusion of a portion of the physical examination does not implicitly mean the examination was negative, only that it was not performed.

Once a written record is in the patient's chart, do not alter it at a later date. Noncontemporaneous "additions" for

Orthopaedic Surgery: The Essentials. Edited by M.E. Baratz, A.D. Watson, and J.E. Imbriglia. Thieme Medical Publishers, Inc., New York © 1999

PEARL

The physician should always ask him- or herself whether the patient's evaluation and treatment has been appropriately documented at the time of the visit to avoid retrospectively lamenting "if only I had written..." A few moments now may save years of misery later.

---

enhancement, clarification, or correction can be considered evidence tampering in the courtroom. Simply write a new note that enhances, clarifies, or corrects a previous note. The new note should be dated at the time it is written and not "predated" to act as an addendum. Later addendums better than nothing, and *much* better than altering a previous note.

Consultants

It is often useful to ask for help from an expert in another specialty or even one in the same specialty who has a different perspective to maximize the patient's potential outcome. A physician should be able to recognize when help is needed and should not be afraid to ask for it when the patient's condition, attitude, or treatment requires it. Patients generally prefer that their physicians involve the appropriate consultants in their care rather than attempting to "go it alone." However, it is not appropriate to request consultation simply to "cover oneself" in the event of possible or impending medicolegal action.

Care Monitoring

Quality assurance (QA) and total quality management (TQM) are methods that depend on peer review to evaluate and optimize medical care delivery. One element of evaluation that focuses on physicians is the "morbidity and mortality conference." The purpose is to determine at what point medical care with delivery failed so that appropriate measures can be taken to prevent similar suboptimal outcomes in the future.

Quality assurance can be expanded to evaluate the complete course of patient care by defining optimal outcomes for a given diagnosis and then trying to determine what led to those outcomes not being achieved. These methods help the medical care delivery team develop the ideal of "best case management" for a given diagnosis and assure that all participants share information that can impact medical care delivery and training.

The threat of potential litigation is minimized by quality assurance methods because the lessons from a single mistake are rapidly disseminated among the health care delivery team so that the mistake is not repeated by any other member of the team in the future. In effect, one's learning curve slopes upward more steeply when one can learn from another's mistake before making the same mistake.

THE TROUBLESOME PATIENT

Difficult patients and situations can make medical care delivery uncomfortable and can increase medicolegal risk. Anticipating problems and responding appropriately to difficult patients and situations minimizes clinical and medicolegal disruptions.

Office staff should be encouraged to alert the physician about an unreasonable patient, one who makes unreasonable demands on the staff with regard to appointment scheduling, therapy, and nurse callbacks. Potential problems in the office may be anticipated from the patient's behavior on the phone or in the waiting room. Difficult patients often "tone down" their behavior when the physician is present; therefore, do not minimize your office staff's observation of the patient's behavior. Expect courtesy for yourself, for your patients, and for those with whom you work.

Ask a difficult patient about his or her behavior. It is essential that this is done objectively and for the purposes of gathering medical information. The behavior should be thoroughly documented. Nurses, therapists, and other office staff should document difficult situations as well. Documentation should be very objective and nonjudgmental to avoid compromising medicolegal defense that may become necessary.

The difficult patient's behavior and its implications should be discussed with the patient. The patient may not be "reformed" by an honest nonemotional discussion with the physician about the offending or difficult behavior, but it is likely that the behavior will either be modified or that the patient will seek care elsewhere. Written "information brochures" can help patients develop reasonable expectations about their medical care, but personal communication has no equal.

Physicians and their staffs must be alert to sexually suggestive or dangerously noncompliant patients because the behavior of such patients can negatively influence outcomes or even be dangerous. The behavior must be documented; the patient must be informed of the problem and how it should be corrected. The physician should also document that the patient was confronted about the behavior and a solution discussed. Noncompliant patients should be followed closely with a deadline and parameters for appropriate behavior established.

In the few extreme cases wherein a patient's misconduct persists and compromises the quality of care, it may be appropriate and necessary to terminate the physician-patient relationship. This action is fraught with numerous logistic and medicolegal complications and requires judicious handling. Hospital administration and legal resources should be consulted because exact procedures vary by locale.

THE BAD RESULT

Untoward results can be either *acceptable* or *unacceptable* to the patient and the patient's family. Poor outcomes may result from bad luck, patient noncompliance, or mismanagement. The situation often engenders disappointment, frustration, and fear in the patients and physician.

Increasing the acceptableness of a potential untoward result begins with a thorough, comprehensible discussion of potential complications, their effects, and their treatments prior to onset of care. Patients must understand preoperatively that further care may become necessary if the outcome is suboptimal. Medically appropriate treatment options and the natural history and expectations of each option must be offered to the patient, and the patient must be allowed to choose. As a result, the patient shares responsibility for the medical decision making.

Most suboptimal results are not the impetus for litigation. By making the patient an integral member of his or her care team, the patient will recognize the physician's diligence and dedication and will be better able to accept any suboptimal or adverse outcomes.

Once the result has been deemed suboptimal, the physician and patient should discuss the short- and long-term implications of the result and whether or not improvement is possible and warranted. Both the physician and the patient must have reasonable expectations regarding the natural history, with and without further intervention. Unbridled optimism may lead to disappointment with an otherwise acceptable outcome, whereas excessive pessimism may result in lost opportunity for improvement.

GETTING SUED

Notification of impending legal action may begin by a seemingly simple request for medical records from an attorney who "represents the interests" of the patient, by formal notification that the case is being reviewed in consideration of a possible lawsuit, or by "serving papers" to the physician. The latter is generally done by an individual who appears at the reception desk explaining to the staff that he or she must see the doctor for a moment about a "legal matter" or to "serve papers." The staff and physician should respond calmly, considerately and professionally; accept the "papers" and return to patient care.

The physician should notify his or her professional liability insurance carrier as soon as feasible. No communication should be attempted or allowed with any attorney until after the professional liability insurance carrier has been notified, and only with the carrier's direct consent. The patient must *not* be contacted regarding the case. If the patient needs and wants continuing care after filing suit, professional, considerate, and empathic care should continue to be provided. The legal action should not be discussed.

The office chart and imaging records must be secured as soon as possible. They must not be altered in any way. Two copies of all office and imaging records should be made. The originals are then sent to a secure location off the office premises. One copy of the complete records is forwarded to the insurance carrier by certified mail, and the second copy becomes the working office chart and imaging records.

After initial review, a representative of the professional liability insurance carrier will interview the physician regarding the case. Counsel may be assigned at the time of the interview or shortly thereafter. The physician should inform the professional liability insurance carrier at the outset if he or she prefers specific defense attorneys in the community.

Preparation for malpractice defense consumes considerable effort, energy, and time. It is imperative that the physician is comfortable with the malpractice defense team.

DEFENDING YOURSELF

Interface with Counsel

The relationship between the physician and his/her lawyer must be open and honest. Discussion of the case requires complete candor. All communications between attorney and client, like those between doctor and patient, are privileged and not discoverable by third parties. No one may inquire into communications between the physician and the representing attorney unless the privilege is waived or certain conditions apply that are generally inapplicable in malpractice claims.

The physician should meet with the lawyer retained to defend the claim as soon as possible. Adequate time should be arranged to brief the attorney on the facts of the case and the pertinent medical records. The physician should be thoroughly familiar with the history of the case and records before meeting with the attorney. The records, imaging studies, pathology specimens, and medical devices should be brought to the meeting, and the physician should be prepared to review all aspects of the case.

The physician should determine early on his or her preferred level of involvement and communicate this decision to the attorney. Some physicians want only limited contact with their attorney, but an active role generally improves the defense. Regular contact with the defending attorney to review the timetable and the different phases of the proceedings will allay anxiety and maximize the effectiveness of the physician's involvement. It is helpful to routinely receive copies of important "pleadings" that describe the claims and defenses of the parties, the "theories of recovery" or the claim of wrongdoing, information about the identity of the witnesses including expert witnesses, and correspondence between counsel. Review of these materials will help the physician prepare for pretrial testimony (deposition) and trial.

Seek First to Understand then to be Understood

Understanding the opponents and their claims facilitates defense preparation; particularly in the early stages of litigation when the physician knows much more about the patient history than the opposition knows about the physician's position. Invest time thinking about the case from the patient's point of view. Disappointment with the outcome of a procedure or care is frequently at the root of malpractice claims.

The physician must challenge him- or herself to understand why the patient was disappointed. Was the outcome within the range of foreseeable possibilities? Were potential adverse outcomes explained in advance? Is the patient in denial or unreasonably refusing to accept the outcome of a known risk? The answers will help the attorney understand the basis for the patient's motivations. The physician should identify "fact witnesses" such as family members, caregivers, or other medical providers who can provide additional support for the defense. Defense experts should be identified who can explain the reasonableness of the outcome and define the local standard of care. Other important information to provide to the defense attorney includes texts, monographs, and important articles about the procedure, disease process, outcome, and device or pharmaceuticals at issue.

Carefully consider the patient's role in the outcome. In most states, patient conduct that causes or contributes to the outcome is a partial defense to the claim and may be persuasive to jurors who have to comparatively judge the conduct of all parties involved in the suit.

The physician should review a copy of the patient's answers to *interrogatories*, which are written questions submitted by each attorney to the other's client that must be answered under oath. This is an excellent opportunity to determine the specifics of the claims; interrogatories often provide insight into the basis for the lawsuit. It is helpful to suggest questions to include in the interrogatories.

Expert testimony is required in virtually all malpractice cases tried in the United States and is often a key factor in the jury's decision. The physician should review the expert witness disclosure statement or the reports of the adverse experts. The background, experience, credentials, and publications of the expert witness require careful study to understand the basis and biases for the expert witness's position and opinions. Previous cases in which the expert witness has testified may offer additional insight. Equally important is thoughtful selection of defense experts. Their background, experience, credentials, and publications should be scrutinized to mitigate against destructive cross-examination by the patient's attorney.

Background information about the opposing lawyers, their experience in medical litigation, the judge, and demographic information about the jurors is useful for preparing a defense. The physician should likewise evaluate the defense attorney's experience and *insist* on representation by counsel with substantive competence in professional negligence law.

Communicating Your Position

The suit begins with *preliminary pleading* wherein the patient's attorney formally presents the patient's claim to the court and the physician's attorney formally responds to the claim. *Paper discovery* then takes place as documents and records are exchanged between the attorneys and the court. The attorneys then question the parties under oath at a *deposition*. A stenographer records the questions and answers and produces a transcript of the proceeding. Depositions are often videotaped to provide a visual record. In most states, deposition testimony may be read or shown to the jury.

Depositions serve several practical and tactical purposes, but they are essentially intended to help the attorneys discover the facts and prevent surprise at trial. The physician must be thoroughly prepared at deposition because answers are given under oath and are recorded. It is very difficult to change testimony later. A witness who answers questions differently at trial will be confronted with their prior answers under oath, and will thereby be "impeached" with great fan-

fare and damage to credibility. The defense attorney usually spends several hours with the physician to prepare for the deposition.

In most states, any of the involved parties have the right to attend all depositions and court hearings. The physician will be better able to prepare a defense and give depositions if he or she attends the depositions of key witnesses including the patient and plaintiff's expert witnesses. The physician can often help the defense attorney formulate questions by integrating the depositions of others with his or her knowledge of the patient's history, medical care, and records.

PEARL

When testifying at the deposition or trial:

- **The physician must be persuasive, but never argumentative or hostile. It is appropriate to show compassion and caring for the patient. Expression of those feelings must not compromise the expression of the physician's belief in the correctness of his or her position. The physician must be confident and caring, but not arrogant.**

- **Thorough preparation and attention to details improves confidence. No questions should take the physician by surprise lest he or she appear indecisive or unfamiliar with the patient and the case.**

- **The patient should be referred to by name. The physician should know the names of other medical care providers involved with the case and important dates.**

- **The medical records should be available at trial or deposition, and the physician should freely refer to them instead of relying on "guesses" or recollections.**

- **Insist that a poorly worded, multiple part, convoluted question be clarified before answering it. It is imperative that an answer to a question have only one interpretation to avoid being "tripped up" by one's own testimony. This requires a focused question. The physician must fight for a good question without appearing uncooperative or defensive. A mock examination or observing a skilled witness may be useful to develop skilled witness techniques.**

- **The physician's presence in the court room *throughout* the trial helps demonstrate care, commitment, and concern for the patient.**

EXPERT REVIEWS

Review of medical malpractice cases can be an intellectually stimulating endeavor. It makes one more comfortable with legal procedures and protocol. The reviewer develops an understanding of alternative treatment methods and potential complications that may be applicable to his or her own practice. Legal case review improves one's own medical record-keeping, patient care, and malpractice prevention.

Expert reviewers undertake an important responsibility because they can prevent unnecessary lawsuits and ensure that wrongfully harmed individuals receive the support their problems merit. Expert reviewers should be willing to review both plaintiff's and defendant's cases to maintain objectivity. It is important not to be labeled as a physician who "only testifies for one side" because the jury may perceive a biased perspective regardless of the thickness of your curriculum vitae. Reviewing plaintiff's cases will afford the opportunity to learn how the opposition is thinking.

SUMMARY

Medicolegal issues can produce significant anxiety for physicians. Prevention can be the "best medicine." Effective communication with the patient; detailed, accurate, and thorough record-keeping; availing oneself of appropriate consultations; and comprehensive monitoring of quality of care are effective methods of litigation prevention. Calm, professional interaction with difficult patients and patients with suboptimal outcomes helps defuse potential litigation. A thorough understanding of and active involvement in the legal process improves one's own defense.

SELECTED BIBLIOGRAPHY

BRENNAN TA, SOX CM, BURSTIN HR. Negligent adverse events and the outcomes of medical-malpractice litigation: relation between negligent adverse events and the outcomes of medical-malpractice litigation. *N Eng J Med.* 1996;335: 1963–1967.

SAMPLE QUESTIONS

1. One of the first things a physician should do on learning a malpractice suit has been filed against him or her is to:
   (a) contact the patient to learn why suit has been filed
   (b) notify the professional liability insurance carrier
   (c) make corrections in the medical records
   (d) forward a copy of the patient's medical records to the patient's attorney
   (e) none of the above

2. Purpose(s) of quality assurance programs include(s):
   (a) Defining measures to prevent adverse outcomes
   (b) reprimanding physicians with adverse outcomes
   (c) identifying possible factors that lead to adverse outcome
   (d) a and c
   (e) a, b, and c

3. True or false: A physician who is a defendant in a malpractice suit is allowed to refer to the patient's medical record during testimony.
   (a) true
   (b) false

4. Which of the following is (are) true:
   (a) A physician may attend the deposition of the patient filing suit against him or her.
   (b) A plaintiff may review correspondence between a physician and his or her defense attorney.
   (c) Patient noncompliance is admissible in court and can lead to a defense verdict.
   (d) a and c
   (e) a, b, and c

5. Option(s) for dealing with a difficult patient whose behavior jeopardizes his or her medical care include:
   (a) telling the patient that he or she will no longer be seen in the office if the prescribed care is not accepted
   (b) informing the patient that his or her behavior could jeopardize the outcome and then proposing methods and deadlines for correcting the behavior
   (c) releasing the patient from care
   (d) a and c
   (e) none of the above

Answers: 1) b; 2) d; 3) a; 4) d; 5) b

Chapter 63

Medical Malpractice: The Attorney

Fredrick W. Bode III, Esq.

Professional negligence actions have become a reality in the practice of medicine. Most physicians see lawyers as the reason for the boom in these types of actions. In reality, lawyers are but one element in a group of factors that have coalesced to cause a tremendous increase in the number of lawsuits. Other factors include the litigious nature of society; the willingness of our judges and politicians to permit the redistribution of wealth from insurance carriers to injured patients (government to society in general); and doctors. If the last statement appears a bit incongruous, a closer analysis reveals that physicians are a crucial element in every malpractice case. Simply stated, there would be no malpractice cases if doctors would not testify against other doctors. Put another way, for a professional negligence action to lie, one physician must provide testimony that the care rendered by another physician was substandard and resulted in injury to the plaintiff. Without this testimony, there would be no professional negligence actions.

Although the pendulum has swung toward reform, professional negligence actions against physicians will not be eliminated by tort reform as long as society, the elected state and federal legislatures, the elected and/or appointed judiciary, and the media favor redistribution of wealth through these types of actions. On an almost monthly basis, one can view any of a number of television news magazine productions and see firsthand that medical negligence cases are alive and well.

Having said this, it is incumbent to have a basic understanding of how a professional negligence action arises, what efforts can be undertaken to limit claims, and what actions should be taken when suit is commenced.

In most states, a professional negligence action occurs when a physician or some medical provider under that physician's control renders *substandard* care that results in injury or damages to a patient. Some professional negligence cases can also stem from the failure to provide adequate information to the patient relative to the treatment being rendered. This hybrid claim is sometimes known as an informed consent action.

Although most professional negligence actions follow the common law of the state in which the treatment or care occurred, many states have enacted legislation that controls the breath and scope of professional negligence actions and informed consent claims. While these laws have the appearance of limiting exposure, largely they narrow the focus of the lawsuit and, in some instances, limit the extent of damages.

Whereas the American Medical Society and other groups have attempted to alter the landscape concerning these types of claims, the reality is that, for the foreseeable future, they are here to stay. As such, it is imperative that each physician understand how to limit exposure to these types of claims. It is also important to understand what should be accomplished when suit has been commenced.

Communication and expectations are behind most lawsuits. One can ensure that a malpractice suit will be filed by adhering to the following principles:

1. Display arrogance towards patient and family.
2. Have contempt for your patients and their "stupid" questions.
3. Do not return phone calls or, better yet, have phone calls returned by an inexperienced practitioner who is unable to communicate the requisite information.
4. Play God with your patients; do not explain care or treatment and, if the outcome is unfortunate, blame your colleagues or physicians from prior institutions.
5. Hire office personnel who parallel your self-importance and arrogance.

At first blush, the above elements may appear both silly and condescending. A careful analysis of most lawsuits will reveal that several of the elements are present. Most patients will weather a bad result if they are properly apprised of the risks and benefits of a procedure before it is commenced. Similarly, most patients will not be inclined to bring an action against a physician if the physician and his or her office staff (this is important) have a good rapport with the patient. Nothing destroys rapport with your patients faster than a lack of communication and/or availability, which will often be perceived as either arrogance and/or insensitivity. Moreover, no physician enhances his or her reputation by criticizing the care and/or treatment of a prior-treating physician.

Such conduct increases the possibility that the patient will consult counsel regarding care and treatment; ensures that if counsel is contacted the physician will be a witness in the lawsuit; and serves to diminish referrals and communications from one physician to another. Except in the most egregious of circumstances, this type conduct should never be condoned.

Obviously, although the above elements serve as the foundation for most professional negligence actions, avoidance of same through proper communication and retention of excel-

Orthopaedic Surgery: The Essentials. Edited by M.E. Baratz, A.D. Watson, and J.E. Imbriglia. Thieme Medical Publishers, Inc., New York © 1999

lent assistants (either in the operating room or in the office) will serve to radically diminish the potential for litigation.

A medical malpractice defense lawyer understands the physician's perspective and realizes that more is at stake than merely establishing the validity of the underlying case. Prevailing in a professional negligence action requires excellent communication between the physician and lawyer, preparation, and a thorough understanding of the arena in which the matter is to be decided. When a malpractice action is commenced, the defendant physician must adhere to the following rules:

1. Do not destroy and/or alter the medical chart in any manner.
2. Resolve that sufficient time will be set aside for thorough and complete meetings with your attorney.
3. Educate your attorney in the key medical issues involved in the lawsuit and provide your attorney with the appropriate journal articles that support your position.
4. Understand that a lawsuit is far different from a morbidity and mortality conference.

Each physician must realize that attorneys are lay people who have a modest understanding of medicine. One must never assume that counsel understands the medicine, and every effort must therefore be taken to apprise your lawyer of the central medical issues in the case. It is equally important that each defendant physician not underestimate plaintiff's counsel. If there are weaknesses in the care and treatment rendered to the patient (plaintiff), those weaknesses must be divulged to defense counsel so that proper representation can be accomplished. A rude awakening lies in wait for those who assume that a problem area will be missed. The rationale for this is simple: The plaintiff will retain a physician who will pour over the records and discern this weakness.

As such, to secure the best defense possible, full disclosure is not only important, it is mandatory to a successful outcome.

The attorney-client privilege protects such disclosure and prohibits the discovery of same by other parties to the lawsuit.

At the outset of this chapter, the role of the physician as witness against the defendant-physician was referenced. Professional negligence defense lawyers know that most malpractice cases ineluctably turn on a battle of the experts and on whom the lay people who constitute the jury believe. Factors that a physician must consider when selecting an expert include:

1. the ability of the expert to communicate and teach;
2. whether that physician will testify live before the jury (as opposed to on videotape);
3. the credentials of the expert; and
4. how that expert will relate to the jury

As in every other aspect of the defense of a medical malpractice case, it is imperative that adequate time and preparation be set aside for selection of an expert, conference with counsel, preparation for depositions, medical research, and preparation for and attendance at trial. Adoption of an ostrichlike approach will not cause the matter to disappear and will result in an outcome that is less than satisfactory in the circumstances.

From the defense lawyer's perspective, good communication and thorough, prompt preparation are crucial to the successful outcome of a professional negligence action. Whereas failure to adhere to the above rules might not immediately cripple the defense of a claim, it is a given that following the guidelines will enhance the defendant's chances of prevailing and will make the defense lawyer's role significantly easier.

SELECTED BIBLIOGRAPHY

American Academy of Orthopaedic Surgeons. *Medical Malpractice. A Primer for Orthopaedic Residents and Fellows.* Rosemont, IL: American Academy of Orthopaedic Surgeons; 1993.

American Academy of Orthopaedic Surgeons. *Managing Orthopaedic Malpractice Risk.* Rosemont IL: American Academy of Orthopaedic Surgeons; 1996.

Moore MN. Orthopaedic pitfalls in emergency medicine. *South Med J.* 1988;81:371–378.

Chapter 64

Telemedicine Technology

Jory D. Richman, MD and Ario B. Keyarash, MD

Telemedicine may be defined as the transfer of medical information between remote sites using telecommunications technology. Telemedicine, in its literal sense, has been with us since the advent of telephone. The new age of telemedicine, however, is only 3 decades old. The facsimile machine and clinical telemetry are two recent technologies that have supplemented and further defined our new idea of telemedicine. Telemedicine now encompasses an array of technologies not even imaginable a decade ago. The purpose of this chapter is to outline the telemedicine technologies available and to discuss orthopaedic applications, challenges, limitations and future capabilities. It is imperative that young orthopaedic surgeons become familiar and comfortable with the use of telemedicine so that they may communicate effectively among themselves and with their patients.

THE CURRENT STATE AND DRIVING FORCES OF TELEMEDICINE

Telemedicine has it roots in the 1960s when several federally funded programs were begun in United States and Canada to develop the technologies necessary for transmitting video and radiographic images between remote sites. Nearly all the programs started before 1986 are no longer in existence because these early endeavors were neither cost-effective nor self-sustaining. During the past decade telemedicine has enjoyed a period of rapid growth. The revitalization of telemedicine has come about for a variety of reasons. Telemedicine technology has improved in quality with a simultaneous decrease in cost. Recent developments in digitization and data compression technologies now allow for the transfer of large bundles of information required for successful transmission of video images. Telemedicine no longer

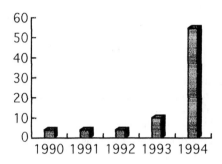

Figure 64–1 Total IATV consultation projects by year in early 1990s.

implies the need for supercomputers or federally funded projects costing hundreds of thousands of dollars. Consequently, the number of two-way interactive television systems (IATV) has increased exponentially in the United States over the past decade (Fig. 64–1).

The two most important factors driving the development of telemedicine are the reorganization of health-care delivery through managed care networks and the deregulation of the telecommunications industry. As the price of telecommunications link-ups becomes less expensive, many third-party payers are exploring the idea of using telemedicine to deliver health care services in rural area where managed care has traditionally not had much impact. Telemedicine has been increasingly viewed as a means of expanding the catchment area of a tertiary-care facility by linking rural or underserved populations in a single network. Several well-known institutions, such as the Mayo Clinic and the Massachusetts General Hospital, have formed for-profit telemedicine ventures that provide services well beyond their geographic catchment areas. Academic medical centers in the United States and Europe have also begun to compete for patients overseas using telecommunications technology.

Federal and state deregulation of the telecommunications industry has also served to increase the demand for telemedicine. Long distance phone carriers, regional telephone companies, satellite providers, cellular phone companies, cable television companies, and internet computer network providers are all competing for health-care dollars in this rapidly expanding market. In addition, manufacturers of computer, multimedia, and video conferencing equipment

935

have been attracted to the field of telemedicine communications. Until recently, transmission of full-motion video signals required satellite links costing several hundred dollars per hour. With recent developments in digitization technology, images can now be transmitted at greatly reduced bandwidth. Transmission of these digitized signals now costs only one tenth as much as satellite communication. The current cost of installing IATV telemedicine sites is between $70,000 and $100,000; however, full motion IATV may soon be available to medical clinics at a fraction of that cost.

Although telemedicine is often perceived as the ability to interact simultaneously between remote sites using video transmission, "store-and-forward" technologies are equally promising. These technologies involve the transmission of static images, such as radiographs, that are received and stored at a remote storage site for later retrieval for review and consultation by a physician. Such technologies have the advantage of not requiring the simultaneous availability of both consulting parties. They permit a practitioner at one site to digitally scan an image that can be sent to another physician for opinion or interpretation. These technologies require far less bandwidth for transmission of data or computer memory for data storage and are available at a fraction of the cost of IATV systems. With the installation of a simple and inexpensive software package, two physicians can relay images to each other using a laptop computer and a modem.

TELEMEDICINE AND ORTHOPAEDIC SURGERY

The field of orthopaedic surgery is well suited for the emerging capabilities of telemedicine. Orthopaedic surgeons have traditionally relied on the interpretation of radiographic images to guide clinical decisions. Using store-and-forward technology, a practitioner can instantaneously scan and transmit an x-ray image to an orthopaedic colleague for interpretation. The almost universal accessibility and low cost of this technology may one day replace the need for mailing x-rays between an outlying rural hospital and a tertiary, academic medical center. Store-and-forward image transmission can also give a young surgeon reassuring advice from a more experienced colleague thousands of miles away in a matter of minutes. In addition to radiographic images, clinical photographs are equally amenable to digitization and rapid transmission. The scanners used for digitizing x-rays are readily available at many hospitals already, and commercially available software for performance of this task may be purchased for less than $1000. The fields of radiology and pathology have already made extensive use of the above mentioned technology. The Internet is increasingly being used to transmit virtual images or short audiovisual clips and has enormous potential for further utilization.

> **PEARL**
>
> **Telemedicine has tremendous potential as a tool for consultation and education.**

The use of IATV technology has been employed by a number of orthopaedic surgery organizations, including the American Academy of Orthopaedic Surgery (AAOS). This technology allows for interactive surgical demonstrations from a central site, which may then be viewed by subscribing physicians across the world. Each year, the AAOS serves as telemedicine host to allow members to view the latest advances in surgical technique. Through video conferencing of orthopaedic grand rounds, many academic centers are beginning to conduct monthly programs on topics of general interest to participating orthopaedic surgeons in their respective communities This technology will enhance continuing medical education by allowing participation at national or regional meetings without the need for travel. The possible uses for telemedicine technologies cover a wide spectrum from simple radiographic consultation or tele-education to complex "virtual reality" tele-robotic surgery.

CHALLENGES AND LIMITATIONS

There are many challenges to the successful implementation of telemedicine technology. Despite all the recent advances in telecommunications, matching technology to clinical needs still remains a challenge. Although it is simple to diagnose a given fracture with the image resolution of most telemedicine software, many diagnoses remain in the realm of direct physician-patient interaction. Aside from this obvious limitation, economic and legal issues are the main barriers to successful implementation of a nationwide telemedicine network.

Economic Issues

Because of the cost involved in establishing a telemedicine network, telecommunications technologies are currently being funded largely by federal or state-subsidized grants or through venture capital programs. The central, unresolved issue that is limiting the widespread use of telemedicine technology concerns the issue of reimbursement. The Health Care Financing Administration (HCFA) has issued reimbursement guidelines for teleradiology interpretations only. Currently, teleradiology and telepathology are the only telemedicine-based services that receive full reimbursement. A number of unresolved issues stand as barriers to federal financing of telemedicine technology. It is not clearly established whether telemedicine is truly cost-effective as a diagnostic or therapeutic modality. Does the advantage of an immediate opinion merit the increased expense? It is difficult for the financing agency or insurance company to factor in the intangible qualities such as lowered travel costs or time off from work, costs generally incurred by the patients. By making subspecialty consultation easier, telemedicine may paradoxically increase the cost of health-care delivery. It is also unclear which types of telemedicine consultations are true patient examinations subject to reimbursement. Without the ability to generate a fee, most telemedicine projects will not be able to survive.

Because insurance companies and managed care networks do not reimburse for these technologies at this time, federal and state support will continue to be required for further development of telemedicine programs. The federal government is currently providing grants totaling more than 100 million dollars a year to fund telemedicine applications. Some states with large, underserved rural populations have also been investing in the telecommunications infrastructure for telemedicine. Georgia has allocated approximately 8 million dollars for a program that links multiple sites to the Medical College of Georgia. Texas and Pennsylvania are two other states that have explored the possibility of telemedicine consultations for the state prison population to avoid the unnecessary transfer of inmates to the medical facilities. Preliminary data from the Texas program suggests that more than 70% of such inmate transfers to community hospitals may not be necessary. This remains one of the few areas in which telemedicine is undeniably cost-effective. All branches of the armed forces, the National Health Service, and the Department of Veteran's Affairs have active telemedicine programs to facilitate home and international consultation.

Legal Issues

The application of telemedicine technology creates many legal challenges that have not been resolved. Telemedicine consultations frequently cross state and national boundaries that involve issues of cross-licensure and remote malpractice liability. Because each state maintains a separate licensing board responsible for registering and disciplining physicians, there are no universally accepted national practice guidelines. This patchwork of state regulations and accreditation is incompatible with the widespread use of electronic telemedicine programs. It remains uncertain whether a physician in one state can legally offer a medical opinion used to guide treatment to a patient or a physician residing in another state. If such opinion is offered, it is unclear which state guidelines apply to the consulting physician's telemedicine practice. Only the department of Veteran's Affairs and the Indian Health Service have established universal cross-state licensure. These issues have yet to be tested in state or federal courts.

PITFALL

The liability associated with offering a medical opinion based on information conveyed through telemedicine remains unresolved, particularly when transmitted from one state to another.

Several other legal issues in this arena have remained untested. It is not clear which community standards of practice will apply. Will the standards be rural or urban, subspecialist or general practitioner, when telemedicine consultations are used between two physicians? If a poor outcome results when telemedicine services are available but are not used, will these be viewed as a form of malpractice by the courts? Well-intentioned physicians who try to guide clinical decisions through electronic media may find themselves exposed to unanticipated liability.

THE FUTURE

The growth of telemedicine programs in the United States will hinge on a number of key issues in the coming decade. Clear goals and priorities must be defined when planning any local, regional, or national telemedicine project. Clinicians and hospital administrators must determine the needs of the communities that they are serving to assess whether electronic transmission of images and data will have a positive impact. They must determine if the most cost-effective solutions to their health-care delivery problems will come in the form of outreach clinics or telemedicine. Once the needs have been assessed, planners then may design the appropriate system with the modalities that fit those needs. The effects of telemedicine on conventional medical practices and its impact in different clinical situations remain unknown.

For telemedicine programs to grow, universal standards of communication must be established by regulatory bodies and medical societies. Licensure issues will need to be addressed on a national and perhaps even an international level to allow for effective use of electronic communication between practitioners. Our outdated system of medical societies is insufficient for development or governance of telemedicine technology. National and international medical societies, including the AAOS and subspecialty orthopaedic groups, must develop standards and guidelines for educational and clinical use of this technology. Although not intended to replace physical participation at regional and national meetings, telemedicine is an exceptional educational tool, which will not expand without the active encouragement of the various specialty boards. Reimbursement policies will need to be instituted by HCFA as well as third-party payers before telemedicine can become readily available. Physicians and administrators must decide whether the use of telemedicine can provide the desired clinical outcome at the most reasonable cost. Ultimately, the decision to implement telemedicine programs must be based on the services that can be provided, not the technology that is available.

In the future orthopaedic surgeons and other physicians will be able to consult on patients at remote sites using desktop computers in a wireless configuration. They will be able to choose between interactive video and store-and-forward technologies as required by task. Patients records will increasingly be stored in the form of digitized radiographic images, pathology slides, operative findings, pharmaceutical records, and electronic charts. Physicians will be able to benefit from instant, on-line access to medical bibliographies as well as interactive surgical demonstrations. Continuing medical education will be enhanced by the ability to participate in seminars and meetings electronically. Young orthopaedic surgeons should view this technology as both a means of communication with their colleagues and as a way to facilitate clinical decision making for unusual problems.

In the new millennium, the practice of medicine will be transformed by the information age and its by-products. Practitioners of the art of medicine, including orthopaedic surgeons, will ultimately find their practices altered to include telemedicine consultations. This will open new avenues of communication and foster a few new headaches. The challenge in this rapidly developing field will be to remove the economic, legal, and technological barriers to its advancement and implementation.

SELECTED BIBLIOGRAPHY

BASHUR RL. On the definition and evaluation of telemedicine. *Telemed J.* 1995;1:19–30.

DAKINS DR, JONES E. Cream of the crop: 10 outstanding telemedicine programs. *Telemed J.* 1996;2:24–41.

PEREDNIA DA, ALLEN A. Telemedicine technology and clinical applications. *JAMA.* 273:483–488.

JOHNSON E, DEBOLD VP et al. Telemedicine; an annotated bibliography: part I. *Telemed J.* 1995;1:155–165.

JOHNSON E, DEBOLD VP et al. Telemedicine; an annotated bibliography: part II. *Telemed J.* 1995;1:257–293.

INDEX